NOLTE'S *the* HUMAN BRAIN

An Introduction to its Functional Anatomy

TODD W. VANDERAH, PhD

Professor and Head
Department of Pharmacology
University of Arizona
Tucson, Arizona

DOUGLAS J. GOULD, PhD

Professor and Vice Chair
Department of Biomedical Sciences
Oakland University William Beaumont School
of Medicine
Rochester, Michigan

ELSEVIER

ELSEVIER

1600 John F. Kennedy Blvd.
Ste 1800
Philadelphia, PA 19103-2899

Library of Congress Cataloging-in-Publication Data

Vanderah, Todd W., author.
  Nolte's The human brain : an introduction to its functional anatomy / Todd W. Vanderah,
Douglas J. Gould.—Seventh edition.
    p. ; cm.
  Human brain : an introduction to its functional anatomy
  Preceded by: The human brain / John Nolte. 6th ed. c2009.
  Includes bibliographical references and index.
  ISBN 978-1-4557-2859-6 (pbk. : alk. paper)
  I. Gould, Douglas J., author. II. Nolte, John. Human brain. Preceded by
(work): III. Title. IV. Title: Human brain : an introduction to its functional anatomy.
  [DNLM: 1. Central Nervous System—anatomy & histology. 2. Brain—anatomy &
histology. 3. Nervous System Physiological Phenomena. WL 300]
  QM451
  611.8—dc23
                                                          2015008889

Content Strategist: Meghan Ziegler
Content Development Specialist: Marybeth Thiel
Publishing Services Manager: Catherine Jackson
Project Manager: Carol O'Connell
Design Direction: Amy Buxton

Printed in the United States of America

Last digit is the print number: 9 8 7 6 5 4 3 2 1

Preface

Over the past 5 to 6 years since the publication of the sixth edition, our understanding of the human brain has continued to rapidly grow with the human brain being the "unknown frontier" in understanding human behavior. Many new techniques are being developed to further measure and understand the functions of the human brain and its connections to the periphery. This new edition upholds the academic rigor and new technologies established by the previous editions written by Dr. Jack Nolte. The basic science of the nervous system continues to help in our clinical understanding of normal and abnormal behaviors, while emphasizing methods and treatments that are being used in practice today. Dr. Doug Gould and I have continued to stay true to the ideas on the inception of the book, keeping things simple to the facts and not trying to simply obfuscate. We have updated terminology that is slowly changing, such as the removal of names from when things were first discovered but no longer are correct. The new edition has made some changes in figures, tables, and illustrations to better understand and categorize important facts. The current edition continues to use the latest medical imaging, including diffuse tensor images to delineate neuronal pathways. Suggested readings have been emphasized and references listed for more detailed information in each area of the nervous system.

This edition continues to carry the tradition of cross-referencing from chapter to chapter in order that the reader understands how the nervous system all works together.

In addition to the many traditions held in this new edition, we have added multiple-choice questions to the end of each chapter on Student Consult that will allow for continued learning opportunities. In addition to these questions, other resources, including an electronic collection of images and videos, are also available. This includes the images from the book and a series of animations of three-dimensional brain reconstructions produced by Drs. John Sundsten and Kathleen Mulligan of the University of Washington. Our hope is that students, enthusiasts, and other faculty find these materials useful in their own learning and teaching.

Our challenge in writing an up-to-date text in a rapidly growing field is to have a textbook that remains updated while not including overwhelming information that may make the function of the human brain difficult to understand. There is hope that the updated version along with added questions to each chapter will continue to aid in students' ability to learn. We welcome comments and suggestions for future editions and for our own knowledge.

Todd W. Vanderah

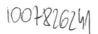

In Memoriam

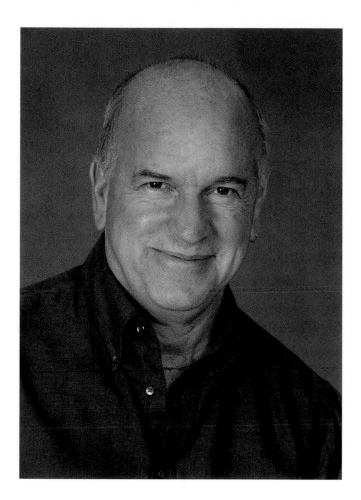

When it comes to learning the anatomy and basic functions of the human nervous system, John "Jack" Nolte has played a role as an author and/or a professor for hundreds of thousands of students, residents, and physicians. Jack viewed the human brain as an endlessly fascinating playground that is forever changing. His lifetime goal was not only to educate students but to educate future teachers as well. He continually scoured the primary literature and behaved with childhood excitement when discovering new explanations for human brain function. His own love and excitement for the nervous system would naturally bleed over to his students and colleagues, encouraging them to explore and question the human nervous system.

In working with Jack for over 15 years, my career and take on life changed from teaching as a "job" to teaching as an enjoyable hobby with benefits. His ability to make teaching fun, telling jokes and giving examples, led to an enriched student environment that resulted in students wanting more. Our meetings most often included discussions of how we could better educate students. Jack was on the cutting edge of designing "case-based" instruction, showing videos of patients for teaching purposes, having patients present in the classroom, and pushing ideas of working and taking exams as groups, using innovative technology, including the virtual brain and interconnected vocabulary terms across multiple fields of science. Jack's desire to create a textbook that was cutting edge yet to the point for learning purposes was his continual love. He shared with me chapters, images, and novel ideas while writing the next edition to continually produce a product that students would enjoy.

Our time together was not all work. Although most know him as a professor of the nervous system, Jack also enjoyed playing handball, woodworking, traveling, cooking, wonderful deep red wines, a martini with blue cheese olives, and the joy of eating oysters (things that often appeared in his textbook as examples of nervous system function). In closing, I dedicate this new edition to my teacher, colleague, and friend. I dearly miss Jack's enthusiasm for teaching, his humor, his friendship, and of course his infamous Birkenstocks.

Todd W. Vanderah

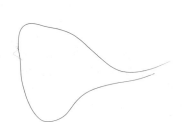

Contents

Video Contents

Introduction to the Nervous System

The aims of this book are to present and explain some basic anatomical facts about how the brain is put together and to discuss some aspects of how it works. This introductory chapter describes in a very general way the subdivisions of the nervous system, then focuses on the cellular elements found within it and the anatomical specializations that adapt these cellular elements to their respective functions.

The Nervous System Has Central and Peripheral Parts

The nervous system is broadly subdivided into the **peripheral nervous system** (PNS) and the **central nervous system** (CNS) (Fig. 1-1). The PNS is the collection of spinal and cranial nerves whose branches infiltrate virtually all parts of the body, conveying messages to and from the CNS. The CNS, ensconced in the skull and vertebral column, is composed of the **brain** and the **spinal cord** (Fig. 1-2). The brain itself has multiple subdivisions and is composed of the **forebrain,** the **cerebellum,** and the **brainstem.** The forebrain, in turn, is composed of the two massive **cerebral hemispheres** (separated from one another by the **longitudinal fissure**—a long cleft between the two hemispheres) and the **diencephalon**[a]; in an intact human brain most of the

---

[a]Much seemingly arcane neuroanatomical terminology has a Latin or Greek derivation that actually makes sense. In this case, *encephalon* is Greek for "in the head" (i.e., "brain"). *Diencephalon* means "in between brain," signifying that this part of the CNS is interposed between the cerebral hemispheres and the brainstem.

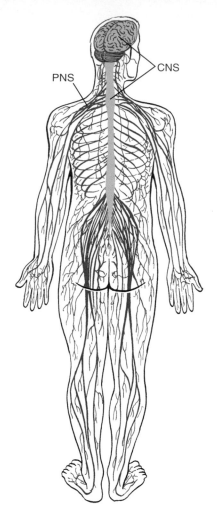

PNS

CNS

Figure 1-1 Central and peripheral nervous systems. The central nervous system (CNS) is encased in the skull and vertebral canal. The peripheral nervous system (PNS) is attached to the CNS, but its nerve fibers are distributed throughout the body. *(Redrawn from Krstić RV: General histology of the mammal, Berlin, 1985, Springer-Verlag.)*

diencephalon is hidden from view by the massive cerebral hemispheres. The brainstem is that part of the CNS, exclusive of the cerebellum, that lies between the forebrain and the spinal cord.

The Principal Cellular Elements of the Nervous System Are Neurons and Glial Cells

Despite the large size and widespread distribution of the nervous system, it contains only two principal categories of cells—**nerve cells,** or **neurons,** which are the information-processing and signaling elements, and **glial cells,** which play a variety of supporting roles. Both neurons and glial cells are present in enormous

numbers. There are around 100 billion[b] neurons in the human nervous system and a similar number of glial cells.

Neurons Come in a Variety of Sizes and Shapes, yet All Are Variations on the Same Theme

Neurons are in the business of conveying information. They do so by a combination of electrical and chemical signaling mechanisms: electrical signals are used to convey information rapidly from one part of a neuron to another, whereas chemical messengers are typically used to carry information between neurons. Hence there are anatomically specialized zones for collecting, integrating, conducting, and transmitting information (Fig. 1-3, Table 1-1). All neurons have a cell body (or **soma**[c]) that supports the metabolic and synthetic needs of the rest of the neuron. Most neurons have a series of branching, tapering processes called **dendrites** (Greek for "like a tree") that receive information from other neurons at junctions called **synapses**[d] and one long, cylindrical process called an **axon** that conducts information away from the cell body. The axon gives rise to a series of terminal branches that form synapses on other neurons. Hence neurons are anatomically and functionally polarized, with electrical signals traveling most often in only one direction under ordinary physiological circumstances. (The molecular underpinnings of this anatomical and functional polarization are discussed in Chapters 7 to 9.)

Despite the basic similarity of neurons to one another, there is wide variability in the details of their shapes and sizes (Fig. 1-4). Certain aspects of somatic, dendritic, and axonal morphology give rise to a descriptive terminology for neurons. The vast majority of vertebrate neurons are **multipolar,** meaning that there are multiple dendritic projections from the cell body and almost always an axon as well (see Fig. 1-4A to E); in many cases the pattern of the dendritic processes is characteristic of that type of neuron. Some neurons are **bipolar** (see Fig.

---

[b]It is hard to get a sense of how big numbers like this really are, so analogies sometimes help. If you could count one neuron per second, and took no breaks for anything else, it would take you more than 3000 years to count 100 billion neurons!

[c]Sometimes also referred to as the **perikaryon.** *Karyon* is Greek for "nucleus," and, strictly speaking, the perikaryon is the cytoplasm surrounding the nucleus of a neuron. However, the term is commonly used to refer to the entire cell body.

[d]"Synapse" is derived from two Greek words meaning "to fasten together."

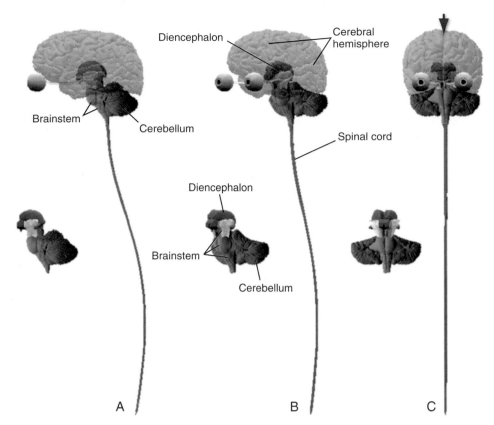

Figure 1-2 Three-dimensional reconstruction of the entire CNS, seen from the left side **(A)**, from directly in front **(C)**, and from halfway between **(B)**. The eyes are included with the reconstruction because, as described in Chapter 2, the retina develops as an outgrowth from the same neural tube that becomes the CNS. The *arrow* in **C** indicates the longitudinal fissure that separates the two cerebral hemispheres. (See Video 1-1.) *(Courtesy Dr. John W. Sundsten, Department of Biological Structure, University of Washington School of Medicine.)*

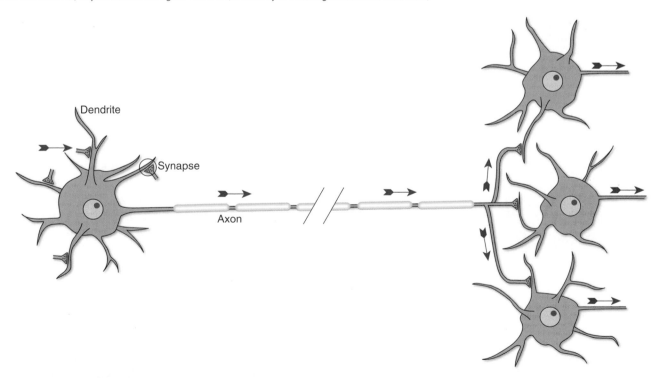

Figure 1-3 Schematic view of a typical neuron, indicating synaptic inputs to its dendrites (although other sites are possible) and the flow of electrical information down its axon, reaching synaptic endings on other neurons. Electrical information flow is unidirectional due to molecular specializations of various parts of neurons, as described in Chapters 7 and 8. The pink segments covering the axon represent the myelin sheath that coats many axons (see Figs. 1-27 and 1-33), and the gap in the axon represents a missing extent that might be as long as a meter in the longest axons.

| Table 1-1 | Parts of a Typical Neuron | | |

Table 1-1 Parts of a Typical Neuron

Part	Description	Major Organelles	Primary Functions
Dendrites	Tapered extensions of cell body	Cytoskeleton, mitochondria	Collect information from other neurons
Soma (cell body)	May have one, two, or many processes; typically one axon, many dendrites	Nucleus, Golgi apparatus, Nissl substance, cytoskeleton, mitochondria	Synthesize macromolecules, integrate electrical signals*
Axon	Single, cylindrical; may be many centimeters long; may be myelinated or unmyelinated	Cytoskeleton, mitochondria, transport vesicles	Conduct information to other neurons
Axon terminals (synaptic endings)	Vesicle-filled apposition to part of another neuron; most are axodendritic or axosomatic, but other configurations occur	Synaptic vesicles, mitochondria	Transmit information to other neurons

*As discussed in Chapter 7, the final integration of electrical signals (i.e., conversion of synaptic potentials to trains of action potentials) typically occurs at the beginning of the axon.

1-4F) or **unipolar**[e] (see Fig. 1-4G), having two processes or only one, respectively. There is a broad spectrum not only of neuronal shapes but also of neuronal sizes. Cell bodies range from about 5 to 100 μm in diameter. Many axons are short, only a millimeter or so in length; but some, like those that extend from the cerebral cortex to the sacral spinal cord, measure a meter or more.[f] For many years, the major technique available for studying the shapes and sizes of neurons was Golgi staining, a method that infiltrates all the processes of a small

percentage of neurons with heavy metals, causing them to stand out from an unstained or counterstained background (see Figs. 1-4 and 1-16A). More recently, however, a variety of methods relying on microinjection, immunocytochemical, or other techniques have become available (Box 1-1). These now make it possible to correlate the structure of an individual neuron with aspects of its function.

Neurons can also be classified according to their connections. **Sensory neurons** either are directly sensitive to various stimuli (e.g., touch or temperature changes) or they receive direct connections from nonneuronal **receptor cells. Motor neurons** end directly on muscles, glands, or other neurons in PNS ganglia. Most sensory and motor neurons live partly in the PNS and partly in the CNS (see Fig. 1-10), whereas almost all other neurons reside entirely in the CNS and interconnect other neurons. Some are local **interneurons** and have all their processes confined to a single small area of the CNS. Others are **projection neurons,** with long axons connecting different areas, as in a neuron in the cerebral cortex whose axon reaches the spinal cord. In a strict sense, the human nervous system is composed almost entirely of interneurons and projection neurons: there are at most 20 million sensory fibers in all of the spinal and cranial nerves combined and no more than a few million motor neurons. Even taking into account the autonomic neurons that innervate muscles and glands (see Chapter 10), more than 99% of our neurons are interneurons or projection neurons. However, the words "sensory" and "motor" are often used in a much broader sense to refer to cells and axons that carry information related to sensory stimuli and to the generation of responses, respectively.

---

[e]Although true unipolar neurons are common in invertebrate nervous systems, vertebrate neurons with a unipolar appearance are actually **pseudounipolar.** They start out as bipolar neurons, but during development the cell body expands asymmetrically (below), leaving behind a stalk from which both processes emerge.

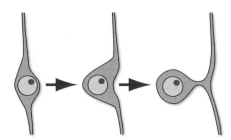

[f]Diagrams and drawings such as those in Figures 1-3 and 1-4 do not convey a sense of the relative sizes of neurons and their parts. If you envision the cell body of the spinal motor neuron shown in Figure 1-4D as being the size of a tennis ball, then its dendrites would spread out through a room-size volume and its axon would correspond to a garden hose half a mile or so in length. Using the same scale, the small interneuron shown in Figure 1-4B would be a few pinheads in diameter; its axon would be a hair-thin process only 1 or 2 feet long.

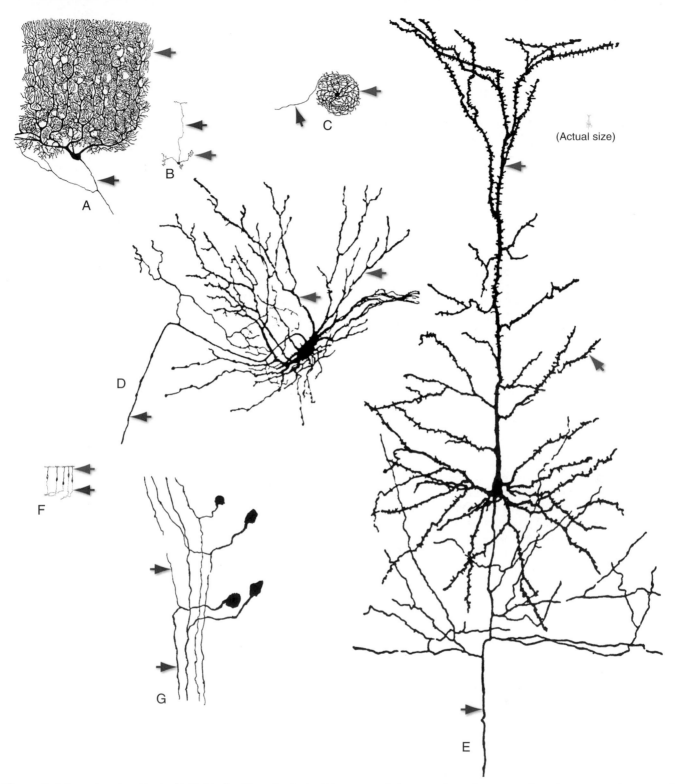

(Actual size)

Figure 1-4 Examples of multipolar **(A-E),** bipolar **(F),** and unipolar **(G)** neurons, all drawn to about the same scale to demonstrate the range of neuronal sizes and shapes. All were stained by the Golgi method (see Fig. 1-16A); dendrites are indicated by *green arrows,* axons by *blue arrows.* **A,** Purkinje cell from the cerebellar cortex; **B,** granule cell from the cerebellar cortex; **C,** projection neuron from the inferior olivary nucleus; **D,** spinal cord motor neuron; **E,** large pyramidal neuron from the cerebral cortex; **F,** olfactory receptor neurons; **G,** dorsal root ganglion cells (whose processes have axonal properties along almost their entire course). The tiny inset at the upper right shows the actual size of the pyramidal neuron in **E.** *(Modified from Ramón y Cajal S: Histologie du système nerveux de l'homme et des vertébrés, Paris, 1909, 1911, Maloine.)*

Making the Morphology of Individual Neurons Visible

One drawback of Golgi staining is that it stains a subset of neurons indiscriminately (see Fig. 1-16A), revealing relatively little about the function of an individual cell.

The last few decades have seen the development of increasingly sophisticated techniques for demonstrating the morphology of functionally identified neurons.

A mainstay in the study of the electrophysiological properties of individual neurons has been the use of micropipette electrodes that either impale single neurons or attach to their surfaces (see Chapter 7). The same electrodes can be used as tiny hypodermic needles to inject a dye or marker substance, allowing study of the anatomy of the same neuron (Fig. 1-5). Such injections can reveal morphological detail comparable to that shown by Golgi staining (Figs. 1-5 and 1-6).

Different classes of neurons also have chemically different interiors, and it is possible to make labeled antibodies that demonstrate some of these differences (see Fig. 1-6D). Correlations of neuronal morphology and location with neurotransmitter content have been particularly instructive. For example, neurons that use norepinephrine as the chemical transmitter at their synapses contain this substance throughout their axons and cell bodies. Appropriate fixation and processing causes these neurons to be fluorescent. Alternatively, it is possible to make a labeled antibody to an enzyme involved in the formation of a neurotransmitter or a labeled antibody to a receptor for a given transmitter. Such methods have made it possible to map out "chemically coded" neural pathways (see Chapter 11). Methods for studying neurotransmitter content and electrophysiological properties can be combined to produce particularly elegant structure-function correlations (see Fig. 1-6).

Genetic techniques have assumed a progressively more prominent role in mapping the structure and connections of neuronal populations. An early method involved engineering neurons and other cells to express green fluorescent protein (Fig. 1-7), a small protein originally isolated from the jellyfish *Aequorea victoria*. Mutated versions of this protein fluoresce in colors other than green, and animals can be genetically manipulated in such a way that different neurons express distinctive mixtures of multiple fluorescent proteins (Fig. 1-8). The effect is almost one of having multiple distinguishable populations of Golgi-stained neurons, so that the interconnections of networks of neurons can be traced.

Neuronal Cell Bodies and Axons Are Largely Segregated Within the Nervous System

For the most part, the CNS is easily divisible into **gray matter** and **white matter** (Fig. 1-9). *Gray matter* refers to areas where there is a preponderance of cell bodies and dendrites. (In life, however, gray matter is actually a pinkish-gray color because of its abundant blood supply.) *White matter* refers to areas where there is a preponderance of axons; many axons have a **myelin** sheath (described later in this chapter) that is mostly lipid and therefore has a fatty, white appearance.

Specific areas of gray matter are often called **nuclei,**[g] particularly if the contained cell bodies are functionally related to one another. An area where gray matter forms a layered surface that covers some part of the CNS is referred to as a **cortex.** The cerebral and cerebellar cortices are the two most prominent examples. Occasionally, descriptive names are used for particular areas of gray matter (e.g., the putamen, a nucleus in each cerebral hemisphere named for its shape and location), but these are relatively infrequent.

In contrast, subdivisions of white matter (i.e., collections of axons) go by a bewildering variety of names,[h] such as **fasciculus, funiculus, lemniscus, peduncle,** and, most commonly, **tract.** Many tracts have two-part names that provide some free information about the nature of the tract: The first part of the name refers to the location of the neuronal cell bodies from which these axons originate, and the second part refers to the site where they terminate. Thus a *spinocerebellar tract* is a collection of axons with cell bodies in the spinal cord and synaptic endings in the cerebellum.

The spinal cord provides a reasonably clear example of the separation of neural tissue into gray matter and white matter (Fig. 1-10). Sensory axons, whose pseudounipolar cell bodies are located in the dorsal root ganglia of spinal nerves, enter the spinal cord and divide into a large number of branches, most of which terminate on neuronal processes in the spinal gray matter. Motor axons emerge from multipolar cell bodies located in the spinal gray matter, leave the spinal cord, and travel with spinal nerves and innervate skeletal muscle. The white matter contains **long descending tracts** (from the brainstem and forebrain), **long ascending tracts** (to

---

[g]Thus the term *nucleus* has two meanings in the CNS—it can mean either the nucleus of an individual cell or a collection of neuronal cell bodies.

[h]These are mostly descriptive terms that also make sense, carried forward from the days when the appearances of these structures were better known than their functions. *Fasciculus* and *funiculus* mean "little bundle" and "string," respectively. *Lemniscus* means "ribbon" and is used for tracts that are flattened out in cross section. *Peduncle* means "little foot," and is used for a site where axons funnel down into a compact bundle.

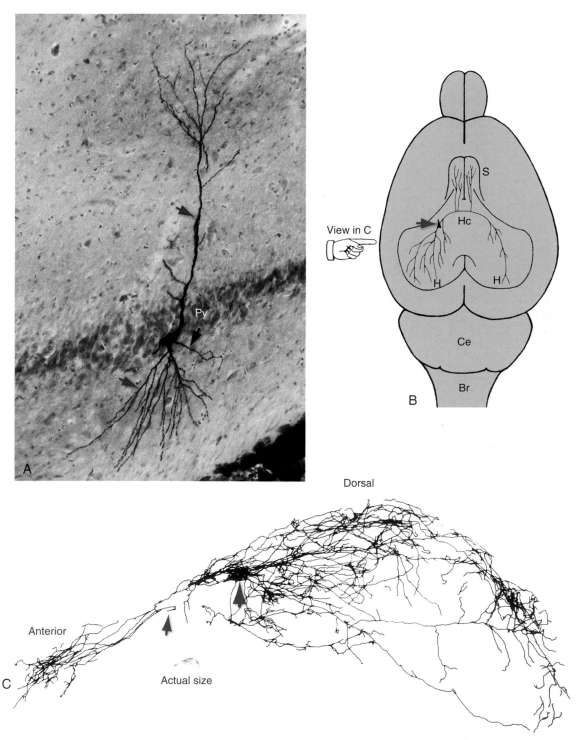

Dorsal

Anterior

Actual size

Figure 1-5 Morphology of an individual neuron revealed by injection of a marker substance from an intracellular recording electrode. This study not only shows the striking degree of anatomical detail that can be demonstrated using this technique but also shows that, although we tend to draw neurons as fairly simple cells with a single axon going from one place to another, they are in reality far more complicated. **A,** A pyramidal neuron from the hippocampus of a rat, injected with horseradish peroxidase. The marker was subsequently visualized using an immunocytochemical technique, and the cell body *(blue arrow)* of the injected neuron stands out from the neighboring neurons in the pyramidal cell layer (Py); dendrites *(red arrows)* and a single axon *(black arrow)* emerge from the cell body. Examining stained processes of this neuron in many adjacent sections led to the conclusion that the axon had a long, complex set of branches, shown schematically in **B.** This is a view of the dorsal surface of a rat's brain. The hippocampus (H) is a specialized area of cerebral cortex buried within each cerebral hemisphere (see Chapter 24). The labeled hippocampal pyramidal neuron *(blue arrow)* sent axonal branches to the septal nuclei (S) bilaterally, to the hippocampus in which the neuron resided, and to the opposite hippocampus by way of the hippocampal commissure (Hc). Br, brainstem; Ce, cerebellum. **C,** Drawing of a reconstruction of the neuron and its branches in the injected hemisphere, compiled from numerous adjacent parasagittal sections. The view is from the side, as indicated by the pointing finger in **B.** At this magnification the cell body is a small structure *(large blue arrow)* surrounded by dendrites. The axon branches extensively and sends projections both anteriorly and posteriorly. In this reconstruction, it ends at the point *(small blue arrow)* where one of its branches prepares to cross the midline and project to the contralateral hemisphere. *(Modified from Tamamaki N, Watanabe K, Nojyo Y: Brain Res 307:336, 1984.)*

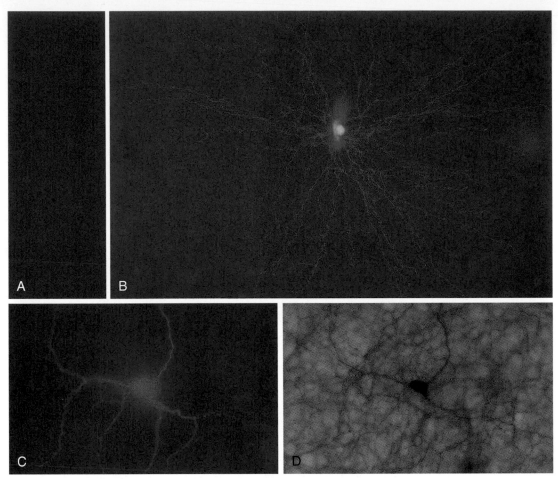

Figure 1-6 Combined use of neurotransmitter identification techniques and intracellular injection of dye. A subset of retinal amacrine cells (see Chapter 17) uses serotonin as a neurotransmitter. These neurons accumulate serotonin from the surrounding medium and accumulate certain analogs of serotonin. **A,** A fluorescent analog (5,7-dihydroxytryptamine) was applied to a living, flat-mounted rabbit retina, which was then viewed using ultraviolet illumination. Serotonin-accumulating amacrine cells fluoresce blue under these conditions, allowing chemically identified neurons to be impaled by dye-filled micropipette electrodes. **B,** A serotonin-containing amacrine cell injected with a fluorescent dye (Lucifer yellow). Details of the long, mostly unbranched dendrites of this neuron are readily apparent. **C** and **D,** An additional example of combined use of a neurotransmitter identification technique and intracellular injection of dye. Another subset of retinal amacrine cells uses dopamine as a neurotransmitter. One such amacrine cell was first injected with a fluorescent dye (Lucifer yellow, **C**). The same area of retina was then stained with an antibody to tyrosine hydroxylase (an enzyme involved in the synthesis of dopamine) as shown in **D.** The obvious correspondence between the two images indicates that the injected amacrine cell manufactures dopamine. (*A and B courtesy Dr. David I. Vaney, National Vision Research Institute of Australia. **C** and **D** courtesy Dr. Dennis M. Dacey, University of Washington School of Medicine.*)

the brainstem, cerebellum, and forebrain), and local axons interconnecting different spinal levels. The gray matter, on the other hand, contains motor neuron cell bodies, the endings of incoming sensory axons, the second order sensory cell bodies (whose axons enter long ascending tracts of white matter to relay sensory information to the brainstem and forebrain), and endings of long descending tracts and local interneurons. This division into white and gray matter is rarely absolute; for example, axons in long descending tracts obviously must pass through some gray matter before reaching their targets (see Chapter 10).

Peripheral nerves are, for most of their courses, collections of axons on their way to or from places such as skin, muscle, or internal organs, accompanied by glial and connective tissue sheaths (see Fig. 9-19). Many of these axons have cell bodies that also reside in the PNS, and these somata are typically clustered in **ganglia** (Greek for "swellings") at predictable sites along the nerve (see Fig. 1-10).

Neuronal Organelles Are Distributed in a Pattern That Supports Neuronal Function

Neurons need mechanisms to deal not only with their electrical and chemical signaling functions but also with other consequences of their extended anatomy. A large neuron with a long axon (e.g., one of the neurons shown in Fig. 1-4D and E) may have 99% of its cytoplasm in the axon, much of it many centimeters away from the

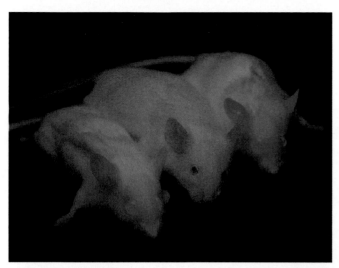

Figure 1-7 Three mice illuminated by ultraviolet light. The mice to the left and right had been bred to express the gene for green fluorescent protein. *(From Moen I, Jevne C, Wang J, et al: BMC Cancer 12:21, 2012.)*

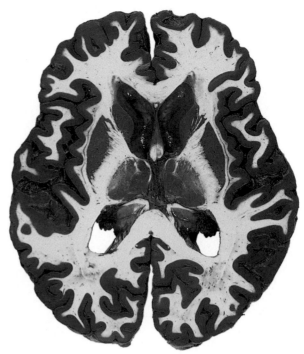

Figure 1-9 Axial (horizontal) slice of a whole human forebrain, approximately 6 mm thick, stained by a method that differentiates between gray and white matter. Pretreatment with phenol makes the white matter resistant to the blue copper sulfate stain, so white matter appears white and gray matter appears bright blue. *(Prepared by Pamela Eller and Jack Nolte, University of Colorado Health Sciences Center.)*

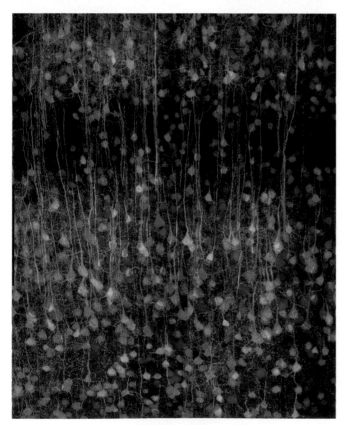

Figure 1-8 Layers of neurons in the cerebral cortex of a mouse from a line (dubbed Brainbow mice) in which the neurons were engineered to express distinctive mixtures of different fluorescent proteins. Notice the uniform color of each neuronal cell body and its processes. *(Courtesy Dr. Jeff W. Lichtman, Harvard University.)*

cell body; hence its single nucleus and associated synthetic apparatus must have efficient mechanisms for communicating with distant parts of its appendages. In addition, brains have no bones, but neurons have long, delicate processes, so there is a need for mechanical sta-

bilization that can be met only partially by the external suspension mechanisms described in Chapters 4 and 5. To address these issues, neurons, like other cells, contain a nucleus and an assortment of organelles—mitochondria, endoplasmic reticulum, Golgi apparatus, and cytoskeletal elements—but the abundance and configuration of these organelles in different parts of a neuron reflect the function of each of these parts.

Neuronal Cell Bodies Synthesize Macromolecules

The neuronal cell body is the site of synthesis of most of the neuron's enzymes, structural proteins, membrane components, and organelles, as well as some of its chemical messengers. Its structure (Fig. 1-11) reflects this function. The nucleus is large and pale when stained for neurofibril, with most of its chromatin dispersed and available for transcription; it contains one or more prominent nucleoli, which are actively involved in the transcription of ribosomal RNA. The cytoplasm contains abundant rough endoplasmic reticulum and free ribosomes for protein synthesis, together with stacks of Golgi cisternae for further processing and packaging of synthesized proteins. Many mitochondria are also present, to meet the energy requirements of continuous, very active protein synthesis.

Ribosomes, whether studding the surface of the rough endoplasmic reticulum or free in the cytoplasm between

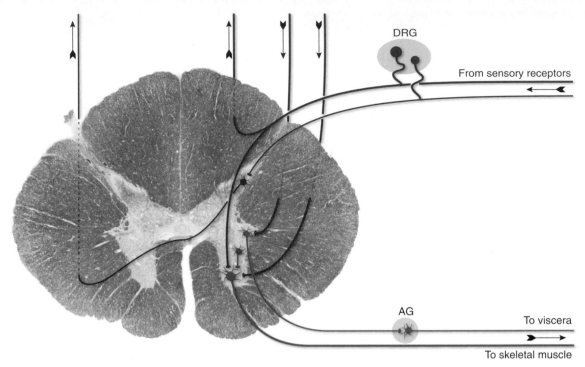

DRG

From sensory receptors

AG

To viscera

To skeletal muscle

Figure 1-10 Division of the CNS into gray matter and white matter, as typified by the thoracic spinal cord in cross section; in this case, white matter was stained blue. The core of gray matter contains interneurons, projection neurons, motor neurons, and endings of sensory fibers and fibers arriving from other parts of the CNS. The surrounding white matter contains ascending and descending pathways. Neurons in the peripheral nervous system are clustered in ganglia, some containing sensory neurons (DRG, dorsal root ganglion) and some containing autonomic neurons (AG, autonomic ganglion).

the cisternae, are stained intensely by basic dyes, appearing light microscopically as clumps called **Nissl bodies** or **Nissl substance** (Fig. 1-12). Nissl bodies are particularly prominent in large neurons, a consequence of the large total volume of cytoplasm contained in their processes, and appear in characteristic configurations in different neuronal types.

The organelles just described are embedded in a network of three kinds of filamentous protein polymers that extend throughout the neuron and its processes, collectively comprising the neuronal **cytoskeleton**. **Microtubules** are cylindrical assemblies, about 25 nm in diameter, of 13 strands (protofilaments) of protein arranged around a hollow core. Each protofilament is a polymer of the protein **tubulin;** an assortment of additional proteins associated with the microtubules links them to each other, to other cytoskeletal elements, and to various organelles as they travel toward or away from the cell body. **Neurofilaments,** the neuron's version of the intermediate filaments found in most cells, are multiply twisted, ropelike assemblies of strands that are polymers involving at least three different proteins from the cytokeratin family. Neurofilaments are about 10 nm in diameter, much too small to be seen under the light microscope, but they aggregate in response to certain chemical fixatives. When silver stains are applied, such aggregates can be visualized as **neurofibrils** (Fig. 1-13). Finally, **microfilaments,** the thinnest cytoskeletal element (7 nm), are twisted pairs of actin filaments. All three kinds of cytoskeletal elements contribute to maintaining the shape of the neuron. Microtubules also serve as the substrate along which organelles are transported through neuronal processes (as described in more detail later in the chapter). Microfilaments are important for anchoring membrane molecules in place (e.g., receptor molecules at synapses), for shuttling things to and from the cell membrane, and for movement of the advancing tip of growing axons.

Dendrites Receive Synaptic Inputs

Dendrites are tapering extensions of the neuronal cell body that collectively provide a great increase in the surface area available for synaptic inputs; the total dendritic surface area of a typical spinal cord motor neuron, for example, may be 30 or more times that of the cell body. Although the total array of dendrites—a neuron's **dendritic tree**—can have an elaborate structure (see Fig. 1-4), each individual dendrite has a cytoplasmic construction similar to that of the cell body. Hence microtubules, neurofilaments, and microfilaments

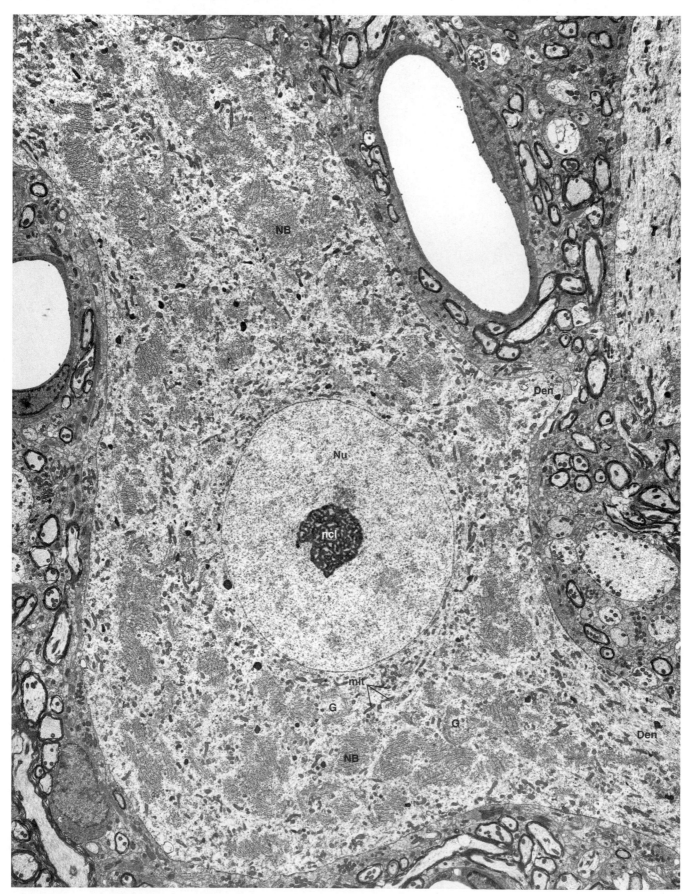

Figure 1-11 Cell body and some of the proximal dendrites (Den) of a spinal cord motor neuron. The nucleus (Nu) and prominent nucleolus (ncl) are apparent, as are other organelles typical of neuronal cell bodies—Nissl bodies (NB), Golgi cisternae (G), and mitochondria (mit). Cytoskeletal elements, although present, are difficult to resolve at this low magnification. The actual size of the area shown in this micrograph is about 55 µm × 70 µm. *(From Peters A, Palay SL, Webster H deF: The fine structure of the nervous system: neurons and their supporting cells, ed 3, New York, 1991, Oxford University Press.)*

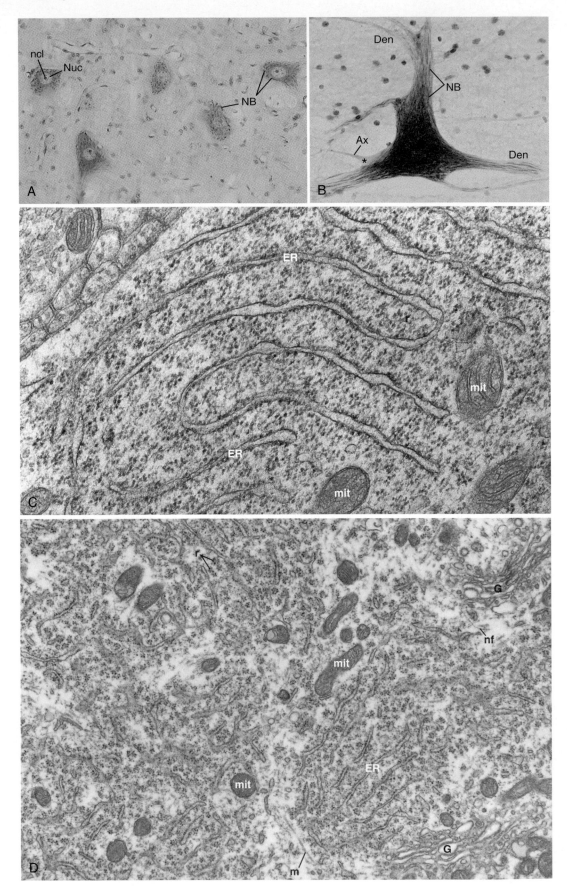

Figure 1-12 Nissl bodies in spinal cord motor neurons. At the light microscopic level (**A** and **B**), Nissl bodies (NB) appear as clumps of basophilic material distributed throughout the cell body and extending into dendrites (Den) but not axons (Ax) or their point of origin (the axon hillock, [*]). Electron microscopy (**C** and **D**) reveals that Nissl bodies are stacks of rough endoplasmic reticulum (ER) with interspersed clusters of free ribosomes (r), embedded in neuronal cytoplasm containing Golgi cisternae (G), mitochondria (mit), microtubules (m), and neurofilaments (nf). The actual size of the Nissl body in **C** is about 3 μm × 2 μm. Ncl, nucleolus; Nuc, nucleus. (*A courtesy Dr. Nathaniel T. McMullen, University of Arizona College of Medicine. B courtesy Dr. Allen L. Bell, University of New England College of Osteopathic Medicine. C from Pannese E: Neurocytology: fine structure of neurons, nerve processes, and neuroglial cells, New York, 1994, Thieme Medical Publishers, Inc. D from Peters A, Palay SL, Webster H deF: The fine structure of the nervous system: neurons and their supporting cells, ed 3, New York, 1991, Oxford University Press.*)

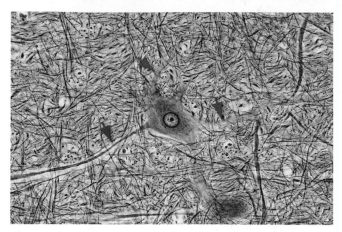

Figure 1-13 Neurofibril stain (Bodian method) applied to an area of spinal cord gray matter reveals a dense thicket of neuronal processes surrounding a motor neuron. The neurofibrils extend into virtually all parts of the neuron, including its axon *(blue arrow)* and dendrites *(green arrows)*. *(Courtesy Dr. Nathaniel T. McMullen, University of Arizona College of Medicine.)*

extend into the dendrites (Figs. 1-14 and 1-15). Nissl bodies may extend into the proximal parts of dendrites (see Fig. 1-12), as may parts of the Golgi apparatus. Mitochondria are abundant, particularly near synaptic endings where they meet the energy requirements of the synaptic signaling processes described in Chapter 8. As the principal input structures of neurons, dendrites are surrounded by a dense meshwork of synaptic terminals and processes of glial cells (see Figs. 1-14 and 1-23). The dendrites of many neurons are studded with small protuberances called dendritic **spines** (Fig. 1-16), which are the preferred sites for some kinds of synapses. Although dendrites are the principal input structures of neurons, recent findings support the notion of minor communication from dendrites to the axon endings in order to give feedback resulting in either the strengthening or weakening in synapses (see Chapter 24).

Axons Convey Electrical Signals Over Long Distances

The single axon of each neuron looks different from the dendrites. Rather than being a tapered extension of the neuronal cell body, the axon is a cylindrical process that arises abruptly from an **axon hillock** on one side of the neuronal cell body or one of its proximal dendrites. Bundles of microtubules, accompanied by neurofilaments and mitochondria, funnel through the axon hillock into the **initial segment** of the axon (Fig. 1-17). Some RNA makes it into the axon, but Nissl substance stays behind (see Fig. 1-12B); despite some local axonal protein synthesis, the relatively vast volume of axonal cytoplasm depends on the soma for most of the macromolecules needed by it and its synaptic terminals. The initial segment is typically the most electrically excitable part of the neuron; as described in Chapters 7 and 8, all the synaptic inputs to the dendrites, cell body, and initial segment itself are summed up here to determine the electrical response that will be propagated along the axon.

Beyond the initial segment, many axons are encased in a spiral wrapping of glial membranes called **myelin** (Fig. 1-18). As discussed in Chapter 7, myelin is a mammalian invention that greatly increases the speed of propagation of electrical signals along axons.

Organelles and Macromolecules Are Transported in Both Directions Along Axons

Axons are much too long to depend on diffusion for the delivery of macromolecules and organelles synthesized in the soma; it would take weeks for something to diffuse down the axon of a small interneuron, and decades to diffuse down a long PNS axon. For this reason, neurons depend on an active process of **axonal transport** for normal function. Similarly, a variety of substances ranging from "used" organelles to intracellular chemical messengers need to be transported from synaptic endings back to the soma. Transport away from the soma is termed **anterograde,** and transport toward the soma is termed **retrograde.** There are two general categories of axonal transport in terms of speed, appropriately enough called **slow** and **fast.** Slow axonal transport moves soluble proteins—such as cytoskeletal proteins and cytoplasmic enzymes—in the anterograde direction at rates of a few millimeters a day; the mechanism of this movement is still not understood.[i] Fast axonal transport moves membrane-associated substances—mitochondria, lysosomes, vesicles of neurotransmitter precursors, and membrane components—at rates up to 400 mm a day. Microtubules serve as the "railroad tracks" for fast transport. Some things move preferentially in the anterograde direction, others in the retrograde direction. This is made possible by the longitudinal polarity of microtubules: tubulin is a structurally polarized molecule and can only be added in one orientation to one end (called the *plus end*) of an existing microtubule. Axonal microtubules are oriented with their plus ends pointing away from the soma. Two ATPases associated with microtubules serve as the motors for fast transport. **Kinesin** bridges between microtubules and some membrane-associated cell components and moves them toward

Text continued on p. 18

---

[i]At a transport rate of a few millimeters a day, it would take substances a year or so to reach the terminals of a long axon. Proteins typically have a lifetime of only weeks before being replaced, and it is slowly becoming clear that ribosomes sparsely distributed along axons are actually responsible for the synthesis of many cytoskeletal proteins and cytoplasmic enzymes.

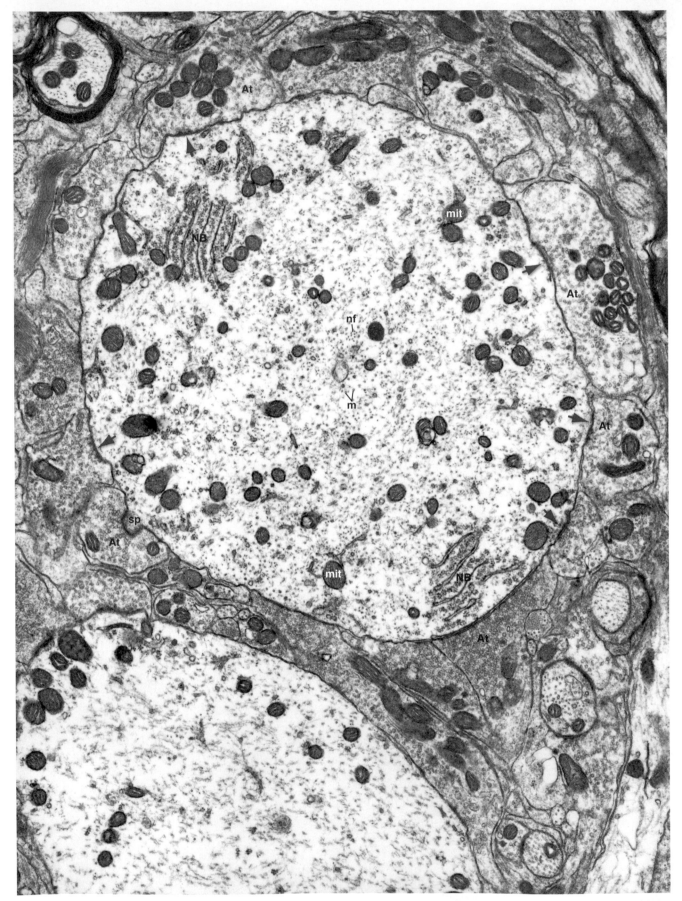

Figure 1-14 Cytoskeletal elements and other organelles of dendrites, seen in a transverse section of a spinal cord motor neuron dendrite. Microtubules (m) and neurofilaments (nf) extend longitudinally through the dendrites, accompanied by mitochondria (mit) and, because this section is close to the soma, Nissl bodies (NB). As the principal input site of neurons, dendrites are typically surrounded by axon terminals (At), forming synaptic endings either directly on the shaft of the dendrite *(arrows)* or on small spines (sp) protruding from the dendrite. The actual diameter of this dendrite is about 7 μm. *(From Peters A, Palay SL, Webster H deF: The fine structure of the nervous system: neurons and their supporting cells, ed 3, New York, 1991, Oxford University Press.)*

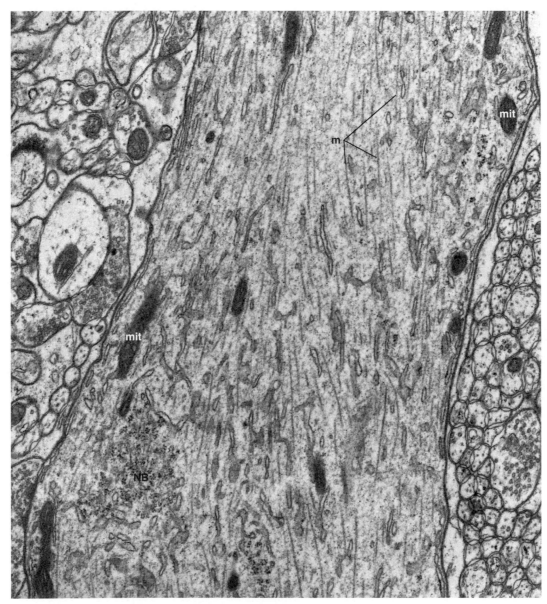

Figure 1-15 Cytoskeletal elements and other organelles of dendrites, seen in a longitudinal section of a cerebellar Purkinje cell dendrite. Microtubules (m) extend longitudinally through the dendrites, accompanied by mitochondria (mit) and, in parts close to the soma, Nissl bodies (NB). The actual diameter of this dendrite is about 4 μm. *(From Pannese E: Neurocytology: fine structure of neurons, nerve processes, and neuroglial cells, New York, 1994, Thieme Medical Publishers.)*

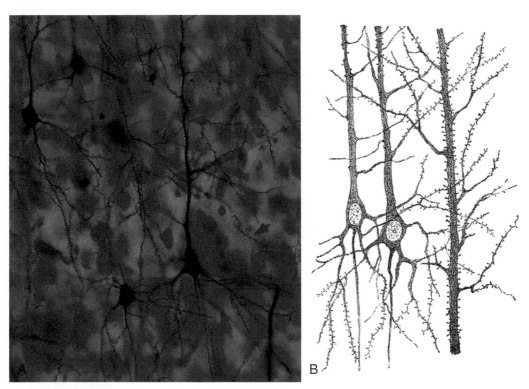

Figure 1-16 Dendritic spines on pyramidal neurons of the cerebral cortex, visible as tiny protuberances *(arrows)* from the dendrites of neurons stained by a Golgi/Nissl method **(A)** or with methylene blue **(B).** (*A courtesy Dr. Nathaniel T. McMullen, University of Arizona College of Medicine. B from Ramón y Cajal S: Histologie du système nerveux de l'homme et des vertébrés, Paris, 1909, 1911, Maloine.)*

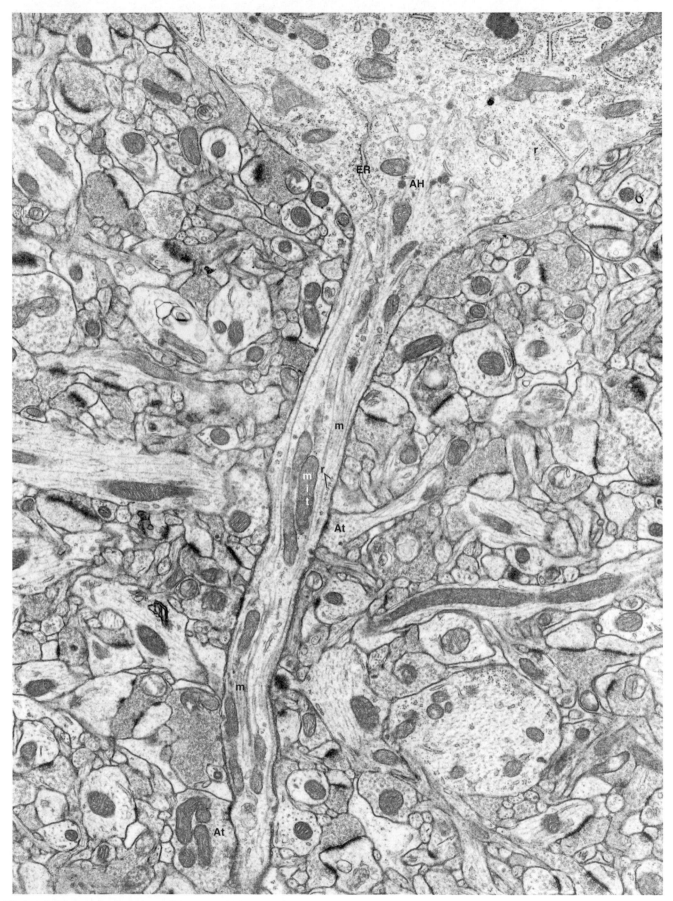

Figure 1-17 The initial segment of the axon of a pyramidal neuron in the cerebral cortex. Many microtubules (m) funnel into the axon from the axon hillock (AH). The axon also contains mitochondria (mit), clusters of ribosomes (r), and scattered bits of endoplasmic reticulum (ER), but no Nissl bodies. Axon terminals (At) also reach the initial segment, but not more distal portions of the axon (except for the axon terminals, which can receive synaptic inputs). The actual diameter of this axon is about 1 μm. *(From Peters A, Palay SL, Webster H deF: The fine structure of the nervous system: neurons and their supporting cells, ed 3, New York, 1991, Oxford University Press.)*

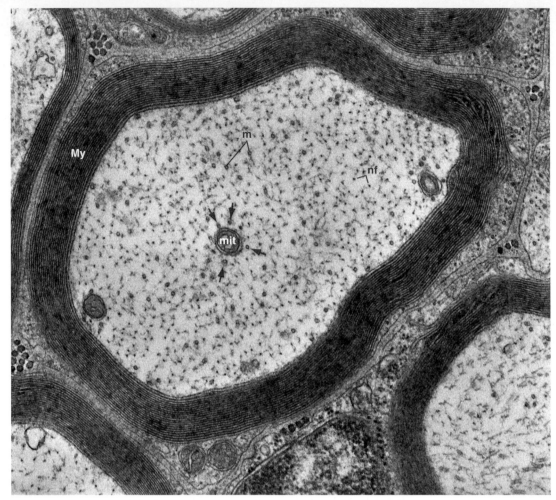

Figure 1-18 Cross section of a myelinated axon in the peripheral nervous system. Beyond the initial segment, many axons of the CNS and PNS acquire a myelin sheath (My) provided by glial cells (see Figs. 1-26 and 1-32) in addition to the usual complement of mitochondria (mit), microtubules (m), and neurofilaments (nf). Microtubules are involved in the transport of organelles along axons (see Figs. 1-15 and 1-19) and are often found closely associated with mitochondria *(arrows)*. The actual diameter of this axon is about 1.5 μm, and the thickness of the myelin sheath is about 0.25 μm. *(From Pannese E: Neurocytology: fine structure of neurons, nerve processes, and neuroglial cells, New York, 1994, Thieme Medical Publishers.)*

the plus end of the microtubule (i.e., in the anterograde direction). **Dynein** moves some components in the retrograde direction (Fig. 1-19).

Modern neuroanatomical techniques take advantage of axonal transport to map out the connections between neurons (Box 1-2 and Fig. 1-20). Appropriate tracer substances injected into or near known neuronal cell bodies are transported anterogradely, revealing the locations of the neurons' synaptic terminals. Conversely, tracers injected near synaptic endings are taken up by the endings and transported retrogradely to the cell bodies (a method used covertly by some viruses [e.g., herpes] to gain access to the nervous system, and now overtly to trace connections).

Synapses Mediate Information Transfer Between Neurons

Information is collected and integrated by a neuron's dendrites and cell body, transmitted along its axon, and finally conveyed to other neurons at synapses (see Fig. 1-3). The vast majority of vertebrate synapses are variations on a common theme. An enlargement (the **presynaptic** element) of a distal axonal branch abuts part of another neuron (the **postsynaptic** element), separated from it by a **synaptic cleft** 10 to 20 nm across. The presynaptic ending contains membrane-bound packets **(synaptic vesicles)** of neurotransmitter molecules (Fig. 1-21); some vesicles release their contents into the synaptic cleft in response to electrical activity. The neurotransmitter diffuses across the synaptic cleft, binds to receptor molecules in the postsynaptic membrane, and causes an electrical signal in the postsynaptic neuron. At first telling, this seems like an inordinately labor-intensive way to transfer a message from one neuron to another. However, there are major computational advantages to this strategy, as discussed further in Chapter 8.

Most synapses have an axonal ending as the presynaptic element and part of a dendrite as the postsynaptic

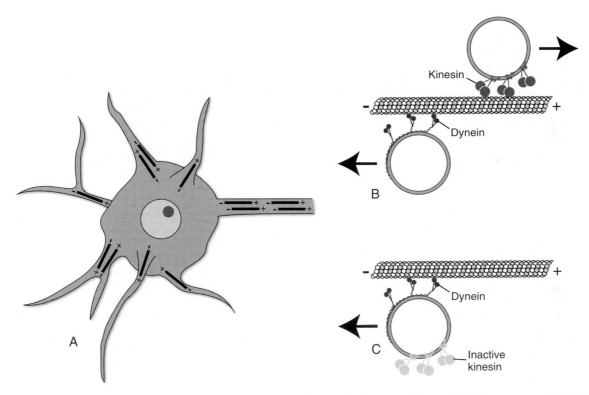

Figure 1-19 Mechanism of fast axonal transport. **A,** Schematic neuron with microtubules arranged longitudinally in its axon and dendrites. Axonal microtubules are arranged with plus ends directed away from the cell body and toward the axon's terminals. In contrast, dendritic microtubules can be oriented in either direction. Part of a single microtubule is shown enlarged in **B** and **C,** with tubulin molecules shown as small spheres. The two slightly different forms of tubulin (shaded and white in the figure) are arranged in strands, like beads on a string, with 13 longitudinally oriented strands forming the walls of each microtubule. Tubulin "beads" can only be added at the plus end. Kinesin and dynein bind to membranous organelles (e.g., mitochondria, vesicles) and form temporary cross-bridges with microtubules, allowing the organelles to "walk" along the microtubule toward its plus (kinesin) or minus (dynein) end. Because all the plus ends of axonal microtubules point in the same direction, kinesin mediates anterograde transport and dynein mediates retrograde transport. Some types of organelles may bind just one of these motor molecules preferentially **(B).** Alternatively, organelles may bind both but only have one of the two in an active state at any given time **(C).** (*A based on an illustration in Pannese, E: Neurocytology: fine structure of neurons, nerve processes, and neuroglial cells, New York, 1994, Thieme Medical Publishers. B and C, redrawn from Vallee RB, Bloom GS: Annu Rev Neurosci 14:59, 1991.*)

BOX 1-2

Using Axonal Transport to Study Neuronal Connections

Neurons are embedded in a seemingly impenetrable thicket of processes of other neurons (see Figs. 1-13 and 1-17), but are nevertheless interconnected in systematic ways. Mapping these interconnections has been a formidable challenge. Degeneration techniques were introduced in the 19th century and are based on the reactions of neurons to injury (see Chapter 24). If an axon is severed, its formerly attached cell body undergoes a characteristic series of cytological changes (chromatolysis). Therefore examining brain sections for chromatolytic cells can reveal the locations of the cell bodies of origin of the severed axons. While the cell body undergoes chromatolysis, the portion of the axon distal to the cut degenerates (wallerian degeneration). The same distal changes occur if the damage is inflicted at the ultimate proximal location (that is, if the cell body is destroyed). Special staining methods can be used to selectively stain degenerating axons or their synaptic terminals. Therefore if a particular nucleus or cortical area is destroyed, the path of axons originating there and the sites of their termination can be determined.

Although a great deal of information was gained over the years with the aid of degeneration techniques, their use is not without pitfalls. It is technically difficult, and sometimes impossible, to completely destroy a particular structure without also damaging nearby structures. In addition, because the segregation of gray and white matter is not absolute, axons passing through a given nucleus can be destroyed along with the cell bodies forming the nucleus. For these and other reasons, techniques that take advantage of axonal transport proved to be a great advance. Early methods of this type used

radioactive substances (usually tritiated amino acids) that were introduced into an area of gray matter, taken up by the resident neurons, incorporated into macromolecules, and transported down the axons of these neurons. Eventually, the synaptic terminals of these axons become radioactive. Subsequent methods have used the introduction of a marker substance (often a protein) into selected areas of gray matter, where it encounters synaptic terminals. The terminals take up the protein and transport it back to the parent neurons. A protein commonly used in such experiments is an enzyme called horseradish peroxidase, which can be detected with great sensitivity and resolution by appropriate histochemical procedures (see Fig. 1-5). Although this technique is typically used for retrograde transport studies, it can be used simultaneously for anterograde transport studies, labeling not only the neurons that project to a given area of gray matter but also the targets of axons that leave it (see Fig. 1-20). Certain fluorescent dyes can also be used in retrograde transport studies. By injecting two different dyes at two different sites in the nervous system, it is possible to determine whether any neurons have branching axons that project to both sites.

One disadvantage of these tract-tracing markers is that they become greatly diluted each time a synapse is crossed. More recently, techniques have been devised to use the transport of viruses, sometimes genetically modified in various ways, to map connections. The viruses replicate each time they enter a new neuron, solving the dilution problem, and the number of synapses they cross can be controlled.

---

element, but in fact any part of a neuron can be presynaptic to any part of another neuron (or sometimes even to itself). This gives rise to names for categories of synapses based on the identities of the presynaptic and postsynaptic elements (Fig. 1-22).

The total number of synapses in a human CNS is almost unimaginably huge (Fig. 1-23) and ultimately makes possible our complex mental abilities. The number of synapses on a given neuron is roughly related to the extent of its dendrites and ranges from a few dozen on a small neuron such as a cerebellar granule cell (see Fig. 1-4B) to hundreds of thousands on the elaborate dendritic tree of a cerebellar Purkinje cell (see Fig. 1-4A).

Schwann Cells Are Glial Cells of the PNS

Neurons in the PNS (Table 1-2) and their parts, with few exceptions, are almost completely enveloped by processes of glial cells. The general roles of these glial

processes are to provide metabolic support and electrical insulation; PNS neurons and processes, unlike those in the CNS, are mechanically supported by connective tissue sheaths (see Chapter 9). All PNS glial cells are variants of one cell type, the **Schwann cell.** Some Schwann cells are flattened out as **satellite cells** that surround the neuronal cell bodies in PNS ganglia (Fig. 1-24). Most, however, envelop axons as they travel through peripheral nerves.

PNS Axons Can Be Myelinated or Unmyelinated

Many peripheral nerve fibers are **myelinated,** vaguely resembling a string of sausages. Each link of sausage corresponds to a length of axon wrapped in myelin, with adjacent links separated by a gap in the myelin. The gaps are **nodes of Ranvier** (Fig. 1-25), sites about 1 μm long where the axon exposed to extracellular space, partly separated from it only by fingerlike projections from Schwann cells. The myelin between two nodes is an **internode** and is formed by a single Schwann cell

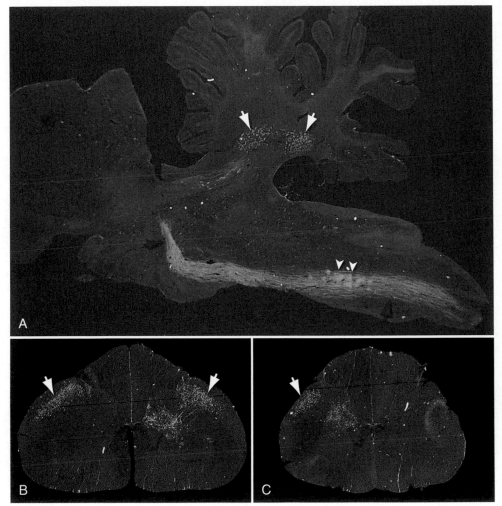

Figure 1-20 Use of bidirectional transport to demonstrate projections to and from the red nucleus, an area of gray matter in the rostral brainstem. Inputs to the red nucleus include projections from the cerebellum; outputs include projections to the spinal cord. Both inputs and outputs are organized topographically so that a given part of the red nucleus receives inputs from a specific part of the contralateral half of the cerebellum and sends outputs to specific parts of the contralateral half of the brainstem and spinal cord. These connections were traced in the CNS of a cat by injecting a marker substance (horseradish peroxidase conjugated with wheat germ agglutinin [WGA-HRP] for increased sensitivity and specificity), localizing it histochemically, and viewing labeled CNS sections with polarized darkfield microscopy. **A,** Parasagittal section through one side of a cat's brainstem after injection of WGA-HRP into the contralateral red nucleus; rostral is to the left. The red nucleus itself cannot be seen in this plane of section, but retrogradely labeled neurons can be seen in two deep cerebellar nuclei (anterior and posterior interposed nuclei; *white arrows*), and anterogradely labeled fibers of the rubrospinal tract *(red arrows)* can be seen traversing the brainstem. Along the course of the rubrospinal tract, some fibers terminate in the lateral reticular nucleus of the brainstem *(arrowheads)*. **B,** Section through the cervical spinal cord of a cat after injection of WGA-HRP into the forelimb area of the left red nucleus and the hindlimb area of the right red nucleus. Because both red nuclei were injected, both rubrospinal tracts are labeled *(white arrows),* but only fibers contralateral to the forelimb area injection terminate in the spinal gray matter at this level *(red arrow)*. **C,** Section through the lumbar spinal cord of the same cat as in **B**. No labeled rubrospinal fibers remain on the right side, contralateral to the forelimb area injection, because they all terminated rostral to this level. However, labeled fibers can be seen in the left rubrospinal tract *(white arrow)* and ending in the spinal gray matter on the left side *(red arrow)*, contralateral to the hindlimb area injection. *(From Robinson FR, Houk JC, Gibson AR: J Comp Neurol 257:553, 1987.)*

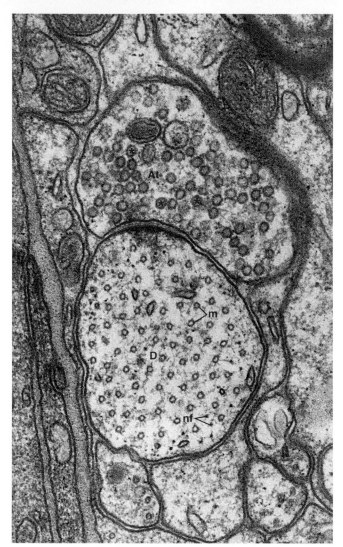

Figure 1-21 A synapse in the gray matter of a rat's spinal cord. The presynaptic element is an axon terminal (At), filled with synaptic vesicles (*) and abutting the postsynaptic element, which is a dendrite (D) of another neuron. The two elements are separated by a synaptic cleft, and the postsynaptic membrane is thickened, an indication of the presence of specialized molecules in and near the membrane at this site. The dendrite is cut transversely in this image, and microtubules (m) and neurofilaments (nf) can be seen cut in cross section. The actual diameter of the postsynaptic dendrite is about 0.75 μm. *(From Pannese E: Neurocytology: fine structure of neurons, nerve processes, and neuroglial cells, New York, 1994, Thieme Medical Publishers.)*

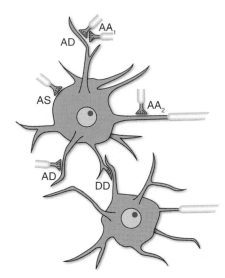

Figure 1-22 Potential sites of synaptic contacts. Most synapses consist of an axon terminal contacting a dendrite, and so are called *axodendritic synapses* (AD). However, all other possible combinations occur at least occasionally, giving rise to two-part names for the synapse type, with the first part indicating the presynaptic element and the second part indicating the postsynaptic element. These include axosomatic (AS) and dendrodendritic (DD) synapses and axoaxonic synapses with the postsynaptic element being another axon terminal (AA$_1$) or the initial segment of an axon (AA$_2$). *(Based on an Illustration in Pannese E: Neurocytology: fine structure of neurons, nerve processes, and neuroglial cells, New York, 1994, Thieme Medical Publishers.)*

individual Schwann cells (Fig. 1-28). This lack of myelin, together with their small diameter, leads to relatively slow conduction of electrical signals by unmyelinated axons (see Chapter 7).

Although the enhancing of axonal conduction velocity by myelin is their best-understood function, Schwann cells have been implicated in several other functions, including facilitating the regrowth of axons after peripheral nerve injury, helping to regulate extracellular ionic concentrations around neurons and their processes, and collaborating with neurons in some developmental and metabolic processes. Some Schwann cells located next to the cell bodies in the DRG called satellite cells may not necessarily completely myelinate a segment of the axon but may play a role in supporting the neuron.

CNS Glial Cells Include Oligodendrocytes, Astrocytes, Ependymal Cells, and Microglial Cells

Glia is Greek for "glue." Historically, glia were so named because they fill up most of the spaces between neurons and appear to hold them in place. Although some glial cells do provide structural support, it is now clear that CNS glial cells, like Schwann cells, play a wide variety of additional roles. In contrast to the PNS, there are multiple kinds of glial cells in the CNS (Fig. 1-29, Table 1-3).

(Fig. 1-26); adjacent internodes form the projections that partly cover the node between them (Fig. 1-27). Internodes range in length from about 0.2 to 2 mm, with larger diameter axons having longer internodes and thicker myelin sheaths. As explained in Chapter 7, this arrangement is part of what allows larger axons to conduct electrical signals more rapidly.

Most of the smaller axons in peripheral nerves do not acquire myelin sheaths. Rather groups of up to a dozen or so **unmyelinated** axons are simply embedded in

Text continued on p. 29

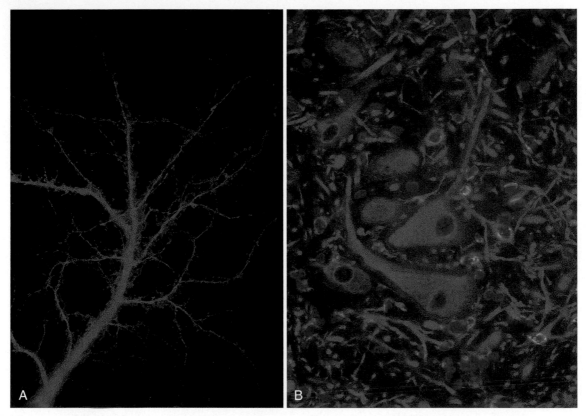

Figure 1-23 Synapses densely distributed over the surface of CNS neurons. **A,** Double immunofluorescence micrograph of a dendrite of a hippocampal neuron developing in tissue culture. The cell body (not seen in this field of view) and dendrites were stained with a fluorescent antibody directed against MAP2, a microtubule-associated protein restricted to the soma-dendritic region of neurons *(green fluorescence)*. Axon terminals originating from other neurons not visible in this field form a dense network of synaptic contact sites and were stained with a fluorescent antibody directed against synaptotagmin, an integral membrane protein of synaptic vesicles. (Overlapping red and green fluorescence, from sites where an axon terminal is superimposed on part of the dendrite, appears yellow.) **B,** Triple fluorescence micrograph of CNS gray matter (deep cerebellar nuclei of a rat). MAP2 was stained as in **A,** showing neuronal cell bodies and dendrites *(green fluorescence)*. Axon terminals, which almost completely cover the cell bodies and dendrites, were stained with a fluorescent antibody directed against synaptojanin, another protein concentrated in presynaptic terminals *(red fluorescence)*. A third dye (DAPI) was used to stain the nuclei of neurons and glial cells *(blue fluorescence)*. *(**A** courtesy Drs. Olaf Mundigl and Pietro De Camilli, Yale University School of Medicine. **B** from the cover photograph accompanying McPherson PS, Garcia EP, Slepnev VI, et al: Nature 379:353, 1996.)*

Table 1-2	Components of the Peripheral Nervous System	
Cells/Parts of Cells	**Types**	**Locations/Forms**
Neuronal cell bodies	Sensory neurons	Spinal and cranial nerve ganglia, some sensory epithelia
	Autonomic ganglion cells	Sympathetic, parasympathetic, enteric ganglia
Parts of neurons	Axons of motor neurons, axons of autonomic neurons, peripheral processes of sensory neurons	Spinal and cranial nerves
Glial cells	Schwann cells	Myelin sheaths, sheaths of unmyelinated axons, satellite cells

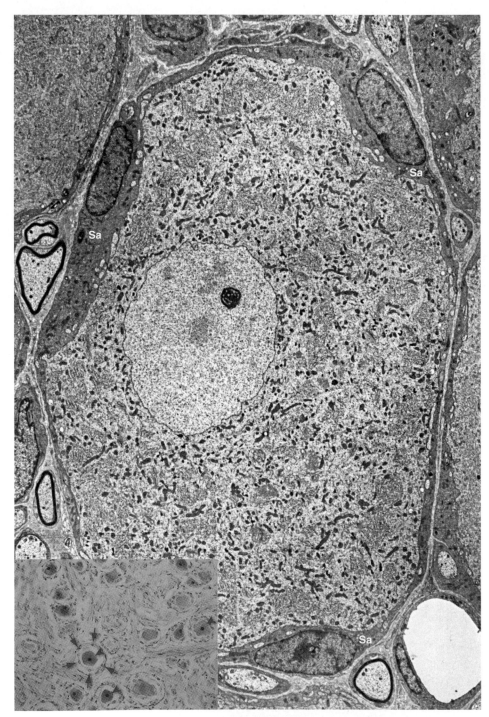

Figure 1-24 Schwann cells flattened out as satellite cells (Sa) surrounding a single dorsal root ganglion cell from a rat. The actual size of the cell is about 20 μm × 30 μm. The inset at the lower left is a light micrograph of part of a dorsal root ganglion, in which the nuclei *(arrows)* can be seen in flattened satellite cells surrounding individual, much larger, dorsal root ganglion cells *(arrowheads). (Electron micrograph from Pannese E: Neurocytology: fine structure of neurons, nerve processes, and neuroglial cells, New York, 1994, Thieme Medical Publishers. Inset courtesy Dr. Nathaniel T. McMullen, University of Arizona College of Medicine.)*

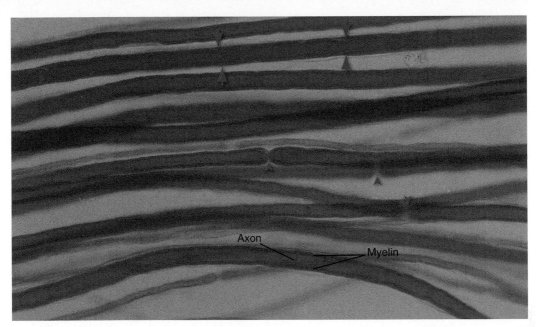

Figure 1-25 Myelin sheaths and nodes of Ranvier in peripheral nerve fibers. A fixed peripheral nerve was teased apart into individual nerve fibers and stained with osmium (a lipophilic stain for membranes). The axon is the central pale area in each fiber, and the myelin sheath stands out on both sides of each axon as a more densely stained area; a few nodes of Ranvier *(arrowheads)* are visible. The occasional diagonal clefts *(arrows)* that appear to cross the myelin sheaths are known as *Schmidt-Lanterman incisures;* they correspond to thin extensions of Schwann cell cytoplasm that spiral around with the myelinating membranes (see Fig. 1-27). *(Courtesy Dr. Nathaniel T. McMullen, University of Arizona College of Medicine.)*

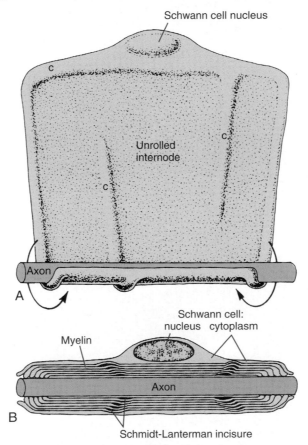

Figure 1-26 Schematic diagram of the formation of myelin in the PNS. **A,** The single Schwann cell that forms an internode, unrolled from the axon it would normally be wrapped around. The cell is flattened into a two-membrane-thick sheet, with cytoplasm (c) remaining only as a thin rim around the periphery and as a few thin fingers extending between the membranes. **B,** A longitudinal section through the internode resulting from the Schwann cell in **A** spiraling around the axon. Most of the internode consists simply of tightly wrapped Schwann cell membranes. Some cytoplasm remains on the surface of the internode near the nucleus, as small pockets near the node, and as Schmidt-Lanterman incisures. *(Redrawn from Krstić RV: Illustrated encyclopedia of human histology, Berlin, 1984, Springer-Verlag.)*

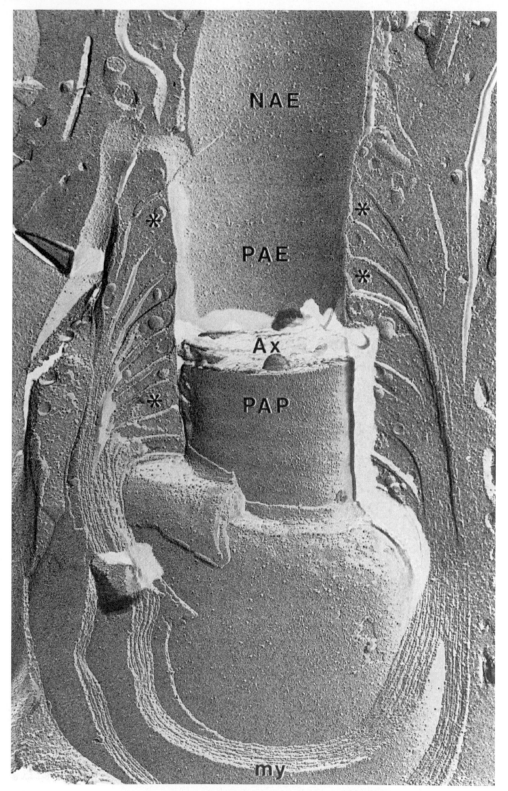

Figure 1-27 Freeze-fracture preparation of a node of Ranvier from a cat peripheral nerve. This technique involves freezing and splitting a tissue sample, then coating the exposed surfaces with a heavy metal, such as gold or platinum, and examining them with a scanning electron microscope. Sometimes the fracture cuts across cell membranes, but it often splits membranes in two, revealing their interiors. In the latter case, the part of the membrane whose other side faces the extracellular space is called the *E* (for external) *face* and the part whose other side faces the cell's interior is called the *P* (for protoplasmic) *face*. (Imagine a cell membrane as a peanut butter and jelly sandwich oriented so that the peanut butter is closer to the cell interior, then freeze-fracturing would involve prying the sandwich apart; the *P* face would correspond to the peanut butter, and the *E* face would correspond to the jelly.) In part of the picture, the fracture cuts through the myelin (my) near the node, through pockets of Schwann cell cytoplasm (*) adjacent to the node, or through the axon itself (Ax) near the node. On either side of the transection of the axon, its membrane is split, revealing the P face (PAP) and the E face (PAE) of the paranodal axonal membrane. The split through the membrane continues into the node, revealing the E face of the axonal membrane there (NAE). The numerous particles exposed on the E face of the nodal membrane correspond to the voltage-gated Na⁺ ion channels that are concentrated in this region (see Chapter 7). *(From Pannese E: Neurocytology: fine structure of neurons, nerve processes, and neuroglial cells, New York, 1994, Thieme Medical Publishers.)*

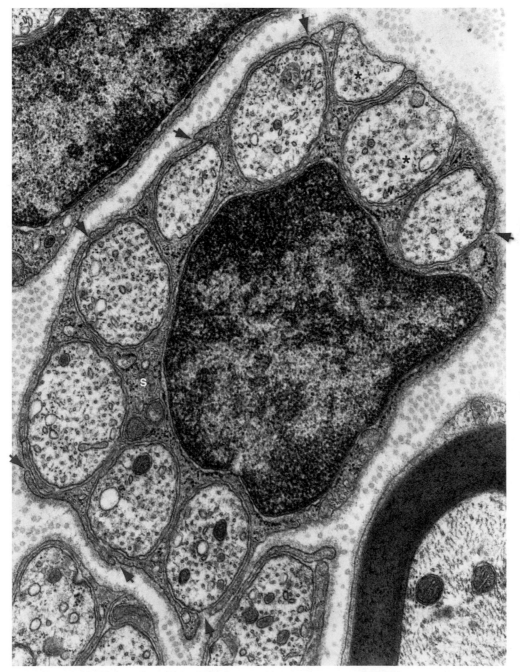

Figure 1-28 Unmyelinated nerve fibers in a dorsal root of a rat. Nine axons, each with the usual complement of microtubules, neurofilaments, and mitochondria, are embedded in a single Schwann cell (S). Even though no myelin is present, seven of the axons are almost completely ensheathed, communicating with the adjacent extracellular spaces only through small clefts *(arrows)* in the Schwann cell wrapping. The other two axons *(*)* are partially exposed at the surface of the Schwann cell. *(From Pannese E: Neurocytology: fine structure of neurons, nerve processes, and neuroglial cells, New York, 1994, Thieme Medical Publishers.)*

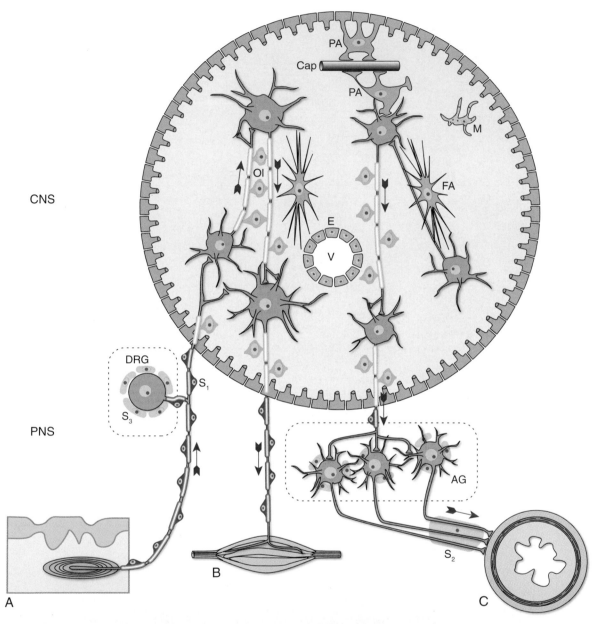

Figure 1-29 Summary diagram of cell types in the nervous system, showing the distribution of glial cell types in the CNS and PNS. A layer of end-feet of protoplasmic astrocytes (PA) forms a leaky membrane that covers the surface of the CNS, separating it from the PNS. Other end-feet of protoplasmic astrocytes are distributed in the gray matter, abutting either neurons or capillaries (Cap). Fibrous astrocytes (FA) are interspersed among nerve fibers in the white matter, many of which are myelinated by oligodendrocytes (Ol). Small microglial cells (M) act as scavengers in response to injury, and ependymal cells (E) line the ventricular cavities (V) of the CNS. Schwann cells and their variants are the principal glial cells of the PNS, forming the myelin of peripheral nerve fibers (S_1), enveloping unmyelinated axons (S_2), and forming satellite cells (S_3) surrounding sensory neurons in peripheral ganglia such as dorsal root and autonomic ganglia (DRG, AG). The direction of information flow in various neurons is indicated by *arrows*. Processes of sensory neurons convey information to the CNS (**A,** in this case from skin). Information leaves the CNS to reach skeletal muscle directly **(B)** or to reach smooth muscle and glands **(C)** after a synapse in an autonomic ganglion (AG). *(Based on a drawing in Krstić RV: General biology of the mammal, Berlin, 1985, Springer-Verlag.)*

Table 1-3	Cell Types in the Central Nervous System	
Cells/Parts of Cells	**Principal Locations**	**Principal Functions**
Neurons, dendrites, synapses	Gray matter	Collect, integrate, transmit information; synthesize macromolecules
Axons	White matter	Conduct information
Oligodendrocytes	White (and gray) matter	CNS myelin sheaths
Protoplasmic astrocytes	Gray matter	Mechanical and metabolic support, response to injury
Fibrous astrocytes	White matter	Mechanical and metabolic support, response to injury
Microglia	Gray (and white) matter	Phagocytosis, response to injury
Ependymal cells	Walls of ventricles	Line ventricles and choroid plexus, secrete cerebrospinal fluid

Some CNS Axons Are Myelinated by Oligodendrocytes, but Others Are Unmyelinated

Many CNS axons are wrapped in myelin sheaths (Figs. 1-30 and 1-31) that are fundamentally similar to those of PNS axons, except that in the CNS the sheaths are formed by a different population of glial cells called **oligodendrocytes.** As in the periphery, larger axons have thicker myelin and longer internodes. However, as the name implies (*oligodendro-* is Greek for "tree with a few branches"), individual oligodendrocytes produce internodes on multiple axons (compare Figs. 1-26 and 1-32). A single oligodendrocyte may have dozens of branches, each ending as an internode (Figs. 1-33 and 1-34; see Fig. 1-37C). Unlike Schwann cells, oligodendrocyte processes do not envelop unmyelinated CNS axons, which can be directly exposed to the extracellular environment (Fig. 1-35). Given their role as myelin-producing cells, oligodendrocytes are most prominent in white matter, but they are also found in gray matter. Here they provide myelin sheaths for axons traversing the gray matter and also participate (along with other glial cell types) in surrounding neurons and their processes in a manner analogous to satellite cells in the PNS.

Astrocytes Provide Structural and Metabolic Support to Neurons

Astrocytes, named for their typical star shapes, form the second major category of CNS glial cells. Most adult astrocytes fall into two broad classes—a heterogeneous population of **protoplasmic** astrocytes (Figs. 1-36 and 1-37A), found in gray matter, and **fibrous** astrocytes (see Fig. 1-37B), found in white matter. (Astrocytes of a third category, called **radial glia,** are present during development and form a scaffolding that helps guide growing axons.) Despite their somewhat different appearances, protoplasmic and fibrous astrocytes have basically similar characteristics. Astrocytes have a well-developed cytoskeleton (Fig. 1-38) that is dominated by intermedi-

ate filaments but also includes microtubules and actin filaments, consistent with a role as structural support elements in the CNS. In addition, some astrocyte processes have enlarged end-feet that are applied either to the surface of CNS capillaries or to the surface of the CNS itself (see Fig. 1-36); other processes abut neurons, dendrites, synaptic endings, and nodes of Ranvier. This carpeting of otherwise exposed surfaces with astrocyte processes underlies many of the diverse functions of these cells: their roles in the regulation of extracellular ionic concentrations, in transferring metabolites to and from neurons and controlling CNS blood flow (see Chapter 6), and in modulating synaptic function (see Chapter 8). Finally, astrocytes are a major part of the limited armamentarium available to the CNS in responding to injury; they multiply, increase their production of intermediate filaments, and form dense, gliotic scars.

Ependymal Cells Line the Ventricles

The CNS, as described in Chapter 2, develops embryologically from a neuroepithelial tube. The cavity of the tube persists in the adult CNS as a system of ventricles (see Chapter 5) with an epithelial lining of **ependymal cells.** In some locations the ependymal cells are specialized as a secretory epithelium that produces the cerebrospinal fluid (CSF) that fills the ventricles and bathes the CNS (see Fig. 5-6).

Microglial Cells Respond to CNS Injury

Microglial cells (see Fig. 1-37A and D), as their name implies, are smaller than oligodendrocytes and astrocytes (which together are sometimes called **macroglia**). Microglia seem not to be involved in the minute-to-minute metabolism and electrical signaling of the nervous system. Instead, they play the other major role in the nervous system's response to injury. In the normal, healthy nervous system they use their numerous

Text continued on p. 38

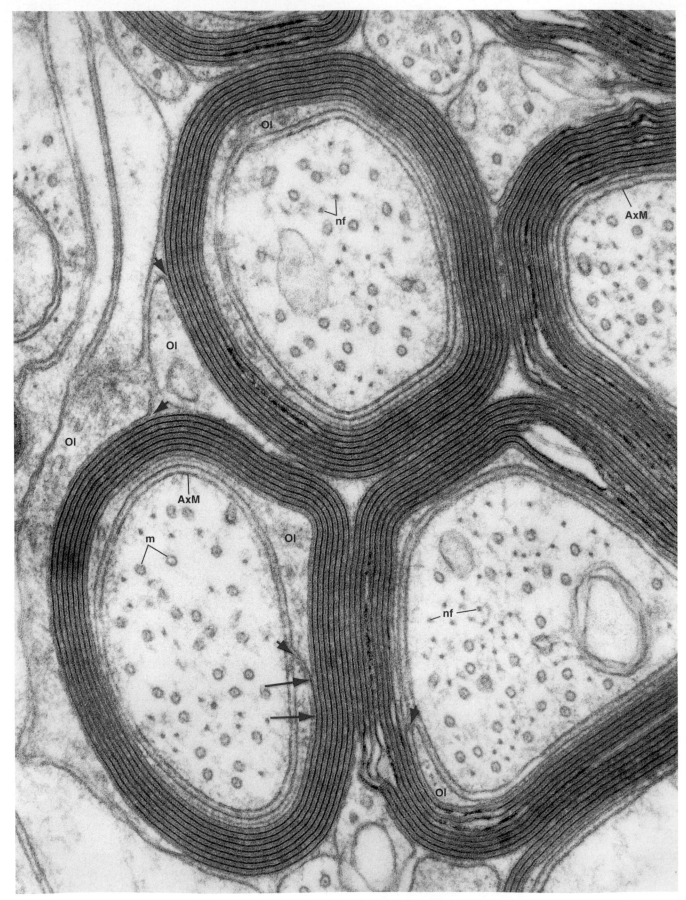

Figure 1-30 CNS myelin sheaths, here in a transverse section of a rat's optic nerve. Each axon contains microtubules (m) and neurofilaments (nf) and is bounded by a cell membrane (AxM). Processes of oligodendrocytes (Ol) wrap around each axon to form its myelin sheath. Tongues of oligodendrocyte cytoplasm at the inside and outside of the myelin sheath narrow until the inner surfaces of their membranes fuse, forming the dense line that spirals through the myelin *(long arrows)*. The clefts between adjoining oligodendrocyte processes *(short arrows)* lead to the fainter zones between the dense lines. The actual diameter of each axon is about 0.5 μm. *(From Peters A, Palay SL, Webster H deF: The fine structure of the nervous system: neurons and their supporting cells, ed 3, New York, 1991, Oxford University Press.)*

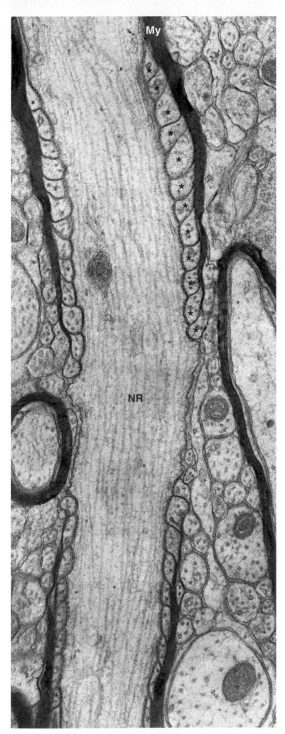

Figure 1-31 Longitudinal section of a myelinated axon and node of Ranvier in a rat spinal cord. Numerous microtubules run longitudinally through the axon. At the node (NR) the myelin (My) ends as a series of pockets of oligodendrocyte cytoplasm (*), leaving the axon bare. The actual diameter of this axon is about 1 μm. *(From Pannese E: Neurocytology: fine structure of neurons, nerve processes, and neuroglial cells, New York, 1994, Thieme Medical Publishers.)*

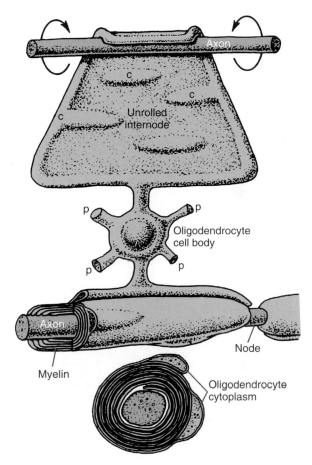

Figure 1-32 Schematic diagram of the formation of myelin in the CNS. A series of processes (p) emanate from an oligodendrocyte, each one giving rise to a flattened expansion that wraps around an axon to form an internode. As in the case of PNS myelin (see Fig. 1-26), most of the internode consists of tightly wrapped membranes, but small rims and fingers of oligodendrocyte cytoplasm (c) are also carried along. *(Redrawn from Krstić RV: Illustrated encyclopedia of human histology, Berlin, 1984, Springer-Verlag.)*

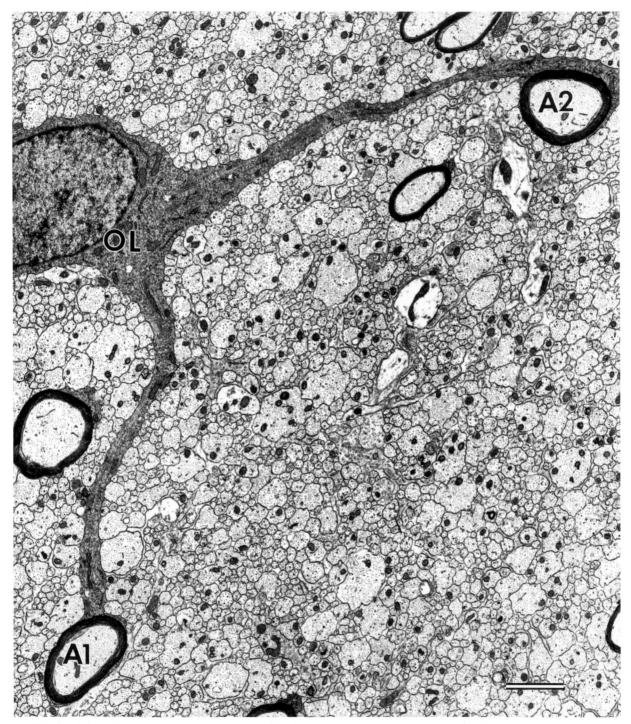

Figure 1-33 A single oligodendrocyte (OL) in the spinal cord white matter of a young rat, myelinating two different axons (A1, A2). This cell and its processes stand out because in young rats, like many other young mammals, myelin has not yet developed around many axons. Note that the oligodendrocyte is connected to its myelin sheaths via thin processes; this tenuous connection has been cited as a possible reason for the paucity of remyelination after injury to myelin sheaths in the brain and spinal cord. Scale mark equals 2 μm. *(From Waxman SG, Sims TJ: Brain Res 292:179, 1984.)*

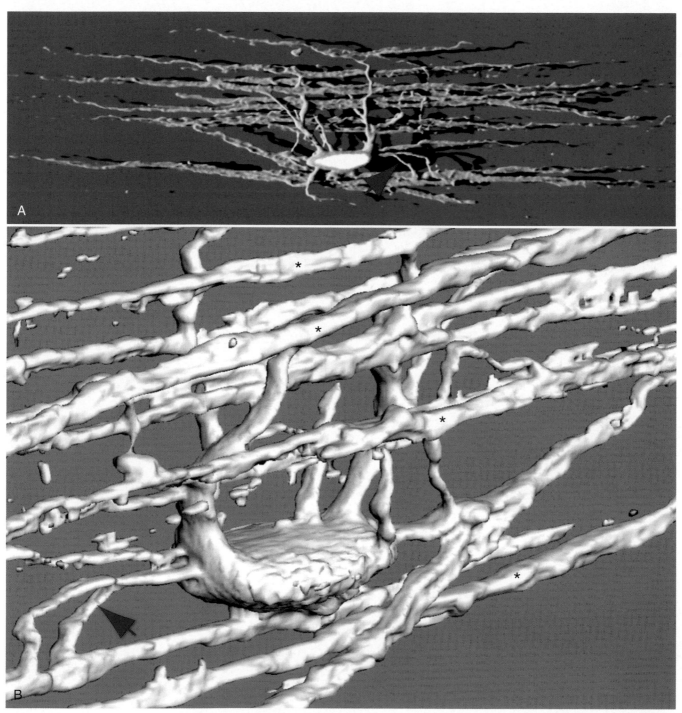

Figure 1-34 Two views of a single oligodendrocyte from the cerebellar white matter of a rat. Individual cells in fixed brain tissue were injected with Lucifer yellow using a dye-filled micropipette and reconstructed with a confocal laser scanning microscope. Digital processing yielded the three-dimensional reconstruction seen in **A** and, at higher magnification and from a different viewpoint, in **B**. Numerous processes emerge from the cell body (the same one is indicated by an arrow in both parts of the figure). Each process ends as an internode (*). The actual size of the area shown in **A** is about 330 μm × 100 μm, and the actual longest diameter of the oligodendrocyte's cell body is about 25 μm. *(Courtesy Dr. Peter S. Eggli, Institute of Anatomy, University of Bern.)*

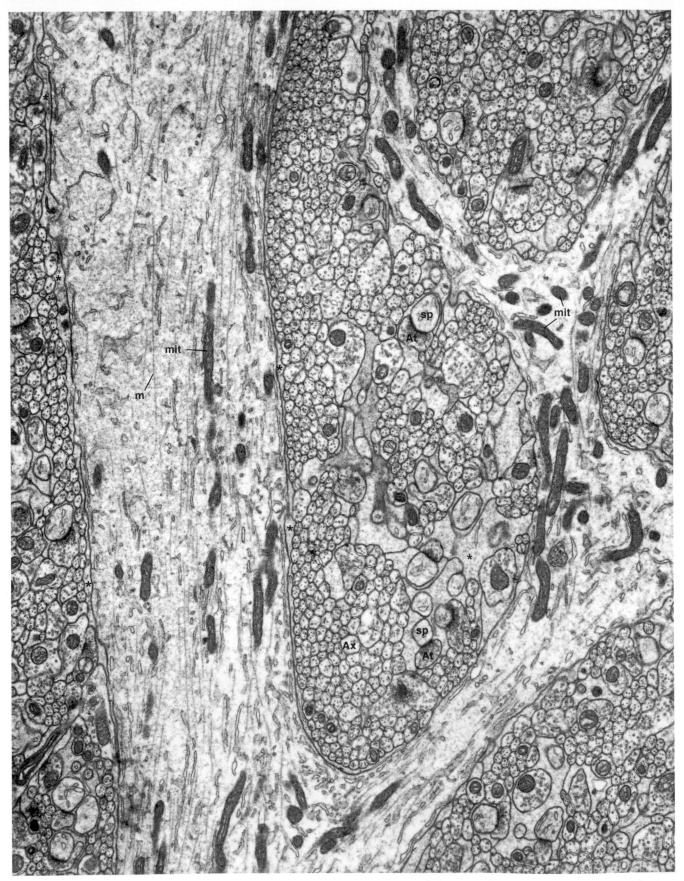

Figure 1-35 Unmyelinated axons in the CNS. Hundreds of tiny axons (Ax, actual diameter about 0.25 μm) are cut transversely as they pass between large branches of a Purkinje cell dendrite in the cerebellar cortex. The dendrite contains longitudinally oriented microtubules (m) and mitochondria (mit) and is almost completely covered by thin processes of astrocytes (*), except where dendritic spines (sp) are contacted by the terminals of the unmyelinated axons (At). In contrast to the glial covering of unmyelinated PNS axons, unmyelinated axons in the CNS are typically bare. *(From Peters A, Palay SL, Webster H deF: The fine structure of the nervous system: neurons and their supporting cells, ed 3, New York, 1991, Oxford University Press.)*

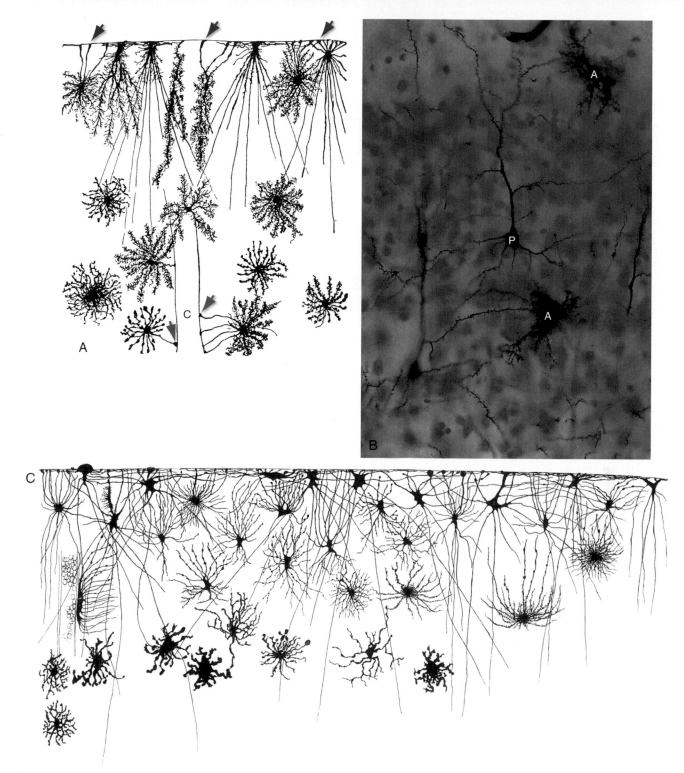

Figure 1-36 Protoplasmic astrocytes in the cerebral cortex, stained by the Golgi method. **A,** Astrocytes have enlarged end-feet, covering the surface of the CNS *(blue arrows)*, contacting capillaries (C, *green arrows)* and contacting neurons (not shown). **B,** Golgi-stained astrocytes (A) and pyramidal neurons (P). **C,** Golgi-stained astrocytes from the frontal cortex of a 42-year-old woman, demonstrating their morphological diversity. (*A from Ramón y Cajal S: Histologie du système nerveux de l'homme et des vertébrés, Paris, 1909, 1911, Maloine. **B** courtesy Dr. Nathaniel T. McMullen, University of Arizona College of Medicine. **C** from Retzius, G., 1894. Biologische Untersuchungen. Die Neuroglia des Gehirns beim Menschen und bei Saeugethieren, Vol. 6. Verlag von Gustav Fischer, Jena.)*

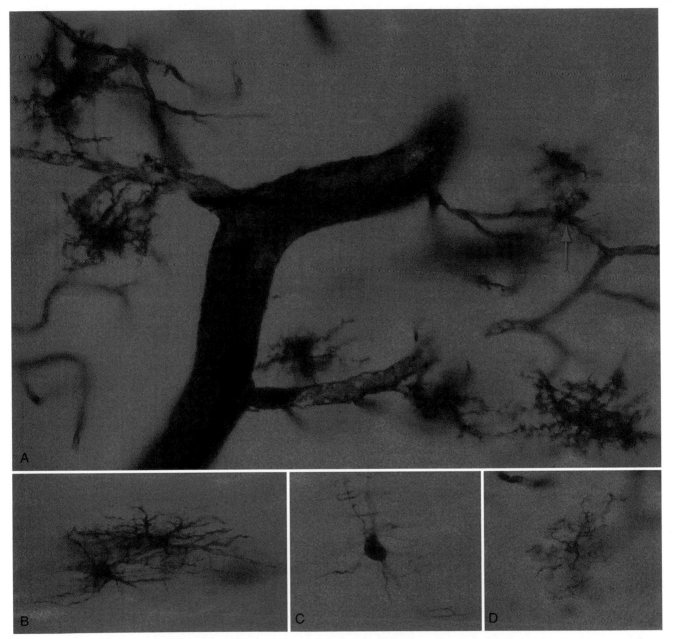

Figure 1-37 Glial cells from rabbit CNS, stained by the Golgi method (del Rio Hortega modification) and all shown at the same magnification. **A,** Protoplasmic astrocytes and one microglial cell *(arrow)* associated with thalamic capillaries. **B,** Two fibrous astrocytes in subcortical white matter. **C,** An oligodendrocyte in subcortical white matter. **D,** A microglial cell in the thalamus. *(Courtesy Dr. Nathaniel T. McMullen, University of Arizona College of Medicine.)*

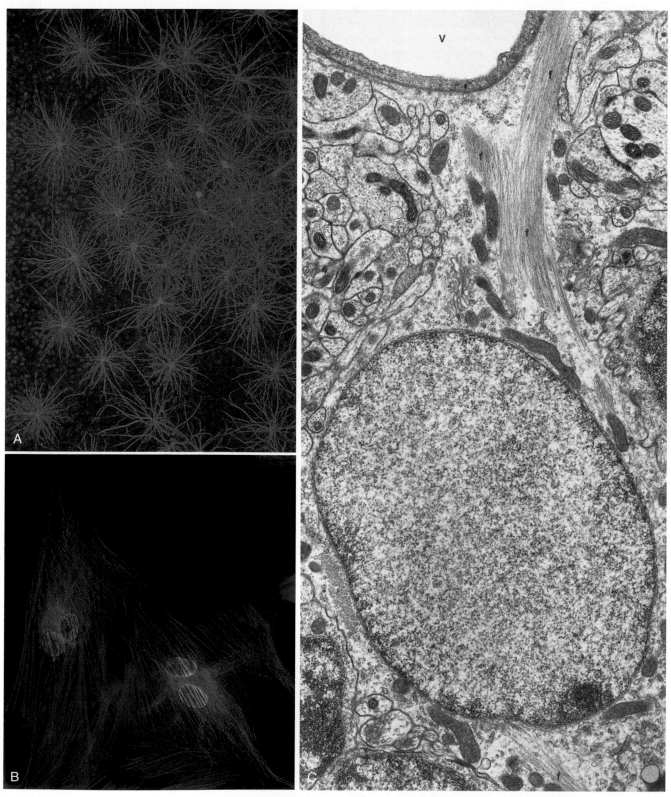

Figure 1-38 Cytoskeletal elements of astrocytes. **A,** Retinal astrocytes stained with a fluorescent antibody directed against a specific protein in astrocyte intermediate filaments (glial fibrillary acidic protein, or GFAP). This spectacular image illustrates why astrocytes (Greek for "star cell") got their name. **B,** Triple fluorescence micrograph of astrocytes isolated from rat cerebral cortex and developing in tissue culture. Actin filaments were stained with fluorescent phalloidin *(red fluorescence)*, microtubules with a fluorescent antibody directed against tubulin *(green fluorescence)*, and cell nuclei with DAPI *(blue fluorescence)*. **C,** Electron micrograph of a fibrous astrocyte in the cerebellum of a rat. Prominent bundles of intermediate filaments (f) are apparent, one of them leading into an expanded end-foot that partly surrounds a blood vessel (V). (*A courtesy Dr. Andreas Karschin, Max-Planck-Institut für Biophysikalische Chemie. B courtesy Drs. Olaf Mundigl and Pietro De Camilli, Yale University School of Medicine. C from Pannese E: Neurocytology: fine structure of neurons, nerve processes, and neuroglial cells, New York, 1994, Thieme Medical Publishers.*)

processes (see Fig. 1-37D) to sweep through extracellular spaces looking for damage or disease. When they find some, they proliferate, migrate to the affected site, transform into macrophages,[j] and devour pathogens and neuronal debris.

---

[j]The origin of microglia has long been controversial. Their resemblance to white blood cells after neuronal injury is consistent with the conventional view that many or most of them are derived from primitive macrophages that invade the nervous system early in embryogenesis.

SUGGESTED READINGS

Angevine JB: The nervous tissue. In Fawcett DW, editor: Bloom and Fawcett: a textbook of histology, ed 12, New York, 1994, Chapman and Hall.

Azevedo FAC, et al: Equal numbers of neuronal and nonneuronal cells make the human brain an isometrically scaled-up primate brain. J Comp Neurol 513:532, 2009.
  For a long time it was conventional wisdom that glial cells are 10-fold more numerous than neurons. Newer counting methods indicate this is probably not correct.

Baumann N, Pham-Dinh D: Biology of oligodendrocyte and myelin in the mammalian central nervous system. Physiol Rev 81:871, 2001.

Brown A: Axonal transport of membranous and nonmembranous cargoes: a unified perspective. J Cell Biol 160:817, 2003.

Davalos D, et al: ATP mediates rapid microglial response to local brain injury in vivo. Nature Neurosci 8:752, 2005.
  Microglia were once thought to sit there quietly in healthy CNS, but time-lapse studies like this show otherwise.

DeFelipe J: Cajal's butterflies of the soul: science and art, New York, 2010, Oxford University Press.
  A strikingly beautiful collection of illustrations of neural tissue made by a variety of investigators in the 19th and early 20th centuries.

Fawcett JW, Asher RA: The glial scar and central nervous system repair. Brain Res Bull 49:377, 1999.

Ginger M, et al: Revealing the secrets of neuronal circuits with recombinant rabies virus technology. Front Neural Circuits 7:2, 2013.

Ginhoux F, et al: Fate mapping analysis reveals that adult microglia derive from primitive macrophages. Science 330:841, 2010.

Goldstein LSB, Yang Z: Microtubule-based transport systems in neurons: the roles of kinesins and dyneins. Annu Rev Neurosci 23:39, 2000.

Haydon PG, Carmignoto G: Astrocyte control of synaptic transmission and neurovascular coupling. Physiol Rev 86:1009, 2006.

Ibrahim M, Butt AM, Berry M: Relationship between myelin sheath diameter and internodal length in axons of the anterior medullary velum of the adult rat. J Neurol Sci 133:119, 1995.

Jung H, Yoon BC, Holt CE: Axonal mRNA localization and local protein synthesis in nervous system assembly, maintenance and repair. Nature Rev Neurosci 13:308, 2012.

Kasischke KA, et al: Neural activity triggers neuronal oxidative metabolism followed by astrocytic glycolysis. Science 305:99, 2004.

Kettenmann H, et al: Physiology of microglia. Physiol Rev 91:461, 2011.

Lee MK, Cleveland DW: Neuronal intermediate filaments. Annu Rev Neurosci 19:187, 1996.

Lichtman JW, Denk W: The big and the small: challenges of imaging the brain's circuits. Science 334:618, 2011.
  A nice overview of the difficulties inherent in studying the structural biology of the brain in detail and of some recent technological advances that help.

Lichtman JW, Livet J, Sanes JR: A technicolour approach to the connectome. Nature Rev Neurosci 9:417, 2008.

Mai JK, Paxinos G, editors: The human nervous system, ed 3, San Diego, 2012, Elsevier Academic Press.
  A detailed, extensive review of human neuroanatomy.

Matyash V, Kettenmann H: Heterogeneity in astrocyte morphology and physiology. Brain Res Rev 63:2, 2010.

Palay SL, et al: The axon hillock and initial segment. J Cell Biol 38:193, 1968.

Pannese E: The histogenesis of the spinal ganglia. Adv Anat Embryol Cell Biol 47(5):1974.

Pannese E: Neurocytology: fine structure of neurons, nerve processes, and neuroglial cells, New York, 1994, Thieme Medical Publishers.
  A succinct yet thorough review, and the source of a number of beautiful micrographs in this book.

Peters A, Palay SL, Webster H deF: The fine structure of the nervous system: the neurons and their supporting cells, ed 3, New York, 1991, Oxford University Press.
  A classic reference work on electron microscopy of neural tissues and also the source of a number of beautiful micrographs in this book.

Ramón y Cajal S: Histology of the nervous system of man and vertebrates, Swanson N, Swanson LW, trans, New York, 1995, Oxford University Press.
  An English translation of the monumental 1909 treatise.

Stuart G, Spruston N, Häusser M, editors: Dendrites, New York, 1999, Oxford University Press.
  Dendrites increase the surface area available for synaptic inputs, but they contribute much more than this to the computational capabilities of neurons.

Trivedi N, Jung P, Brown A: Neurofilaments switch between distinct mobile and stationary states during their transport along axons. J Neurosci 27:507, 2007.
  Some parts of what seems to be slow axonal transport may be an illusion created by brief periods of fast transport interspersed with longer periods of nonmovement.

Ulfhake B, Kellerth J-O: A quantitative light microscopic study of the dendrites of cat spinal α-motoneurons after intracellular staining with horseradish peroxidase. J Comp Neurol 202:571, 1981.

Vallee RB, Bloom GS: Mechanisms of fast and slow axonal transport. Annu Rev Neurosci 14:59, 1991.

Volterra A, Meldolesi J: Astrocytes, from brain glue to communication elements: the revolution continues. Nature Rev Neurosci 6:626, 2005.

Waxman SG, Kocsis JD, Stys PK, editors: The axon: structure, function, and pathophysiology, New York, 1995, Oxford University Press.
  A terrific compendium of work on all aspects of axonal structure and function—central and peripheral, myelinated and unmyelinated.

Weruaga-Prieto E, Eggli P, Celio MR: Topographic variations in rat brain oligodendrocyte morphology elucidated by injection of Lucifer yellow in fixed tissue slices. J Neurocytol 25:19, 1996.

Winckler B, Forscher P, Mellman I: A diffusion barrier maintains distribution of membrane proteins in polarized neurons. Nature 397:698, 1999.
  Elegant experiments providing hints about how different regions of neurons stay specialized at a molecular level.

Yamazaki Y, et al: Oligodendrocytes: facilitating axonal conduction by more than myelination. Neuroscientist 16:11, 2010.

Zaborszky L, Wouterlood FG, Lanciego JL: Neuroanatomical tract-tracing 3: molecules, neurons, and systems, ed 3, New York, 2006, Springer.
  It's come a long way since the first edition in 1981.

Zhang Y, Barres BA: Astrocyte heterogeneity: an underappreciated topic in neurobiology. Curr Opin Neurobiol 20:588, 2010.

Development of the Nervous System

As complex as the human nervous system is, it starts out embryonically as a simple, tubular, ectodermal structure. An understanding of the development of the nervous system helps make sense of its adult configuration and organization. Similarly, congenital malformations of the central nervous system (CNS) are more easily understood in light of its embryological development; such malformations provide clues that aid in the understanding of normal development.

The focus in this chapter is on the events that lead to the formation of the CNS and the configuration of its major components. There is clearly much more to building a nervous system than this—neurons must proliferate in enormous numbers, migrate from their places of birth to their final destinations, and establish appropriate connections with other neurons. Some of these aspects are touched on in Chapter 24.

The Neural Tube Gives Rise to the Central Nervous System

During the third week of embryonic development, in response to chemical signals released by the underlying midline mesoderm, a longitudinal band of ectoderm thickens to form the **neural plate.** Shortly thereafter, the neural plate begins to fold inward, forming a longitudinal **neural groove** in the midline flanked by a parallel **neural fold** on each side (Figs. 2-1 and 2-2). The neural groove deepens, and the neural folds approach each other in the dorsal midline. At the beginning of the fourth week, the two folds begin to fuse midway along the neural groove at a level corresponding to the future cervical spinal cord, starting the formation of the **neural tube** (Fig. 2-3), the open ends of which are the cranial

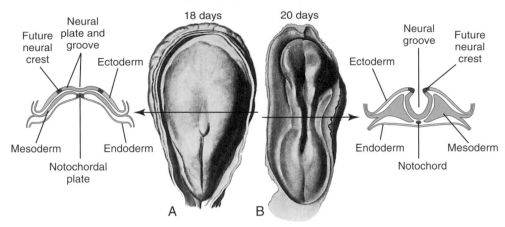

Figure 2-1 The neural plate and beginning neural groove at about 18 days of development **(A)**, and the neural groove 2 days later **(B)**, shortly before the neural tube begins to close. The schematic cross sections to the left and right are at the levels indicated by *arrows* in **A** and **B**, respectively. *(A and B from Arey LB: Developmental anatomy, ed 4, Philadelphia, 1941, WB Saunders.)*

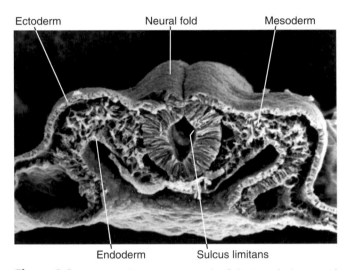

Figure 2-2 Scanning electron micrograph of the just-closing neural tube of a chick embryo, fractured at about the level of the future mid-brain. *(From the cover photograph accompanying Schoenwolf GC, Smith JL: Development 109:243, 1990.)*

and caudal neuropores. Fusion proceeds cranially and caudally, and the entire neural tube is closed by the end of the fourth week. This process is referred to as **primary neurulation.** As the neural tube closes, it progressively separates from the ectodermal (i.e., skin) surface, leaving behind groups of cells from the crest of each neural fold (Fig. 2-4). These **neural crest cells** develop into a variety of cell types (see Fig. 2-19), including the peripheral nervous system (PNS). The neural tube, on the other hand, develops into virtually the entire CNS; its cavity becomes the ventricular system of the brain and the central canal of the spinal cord.

The sacral spinal cord forms by a slightly different mechanism. After the neural tube closes, a secondary cavity extends into the solid mass of cells at its caudal end during the fifth and sixth weeks, in a process of **secondary neurulation.**

The Sulcus Limitans Separates Sensory and Motor Areas of the Spinal Cord and Brainstem

A recurring theme in neural development is the creation of concentration gradients of various signaling molecules, which in turn guide the development of different cell types or the growth of neuronal processes; one prominent example is dorsal-ventral patterning in the spinal cord and brainstem. The ectoderm near what will become the dorsal surface of the neural tube and the mesodermal **notochord** near the ventral surface produce different signaling molecules early in development. The opposing concentration gradients of these signaling molecules induce distinctive patterns of subsequent development in these two regions of the neural tube (Fig. 2-5). This becomes morphologically apparent during the fourth week, when a longitudinal groove (the **sulcus limitans**) appears in the lateral wall of the neural tube, separating it into a dorsal half and a ventral half throughout the future spinal cord and brainstem. The gray matter of the dorsal half forms an **alar plate** and that of the ventral half a **basal plate** (Fig. 2-6; see also Fig. 2-2). This is a distinction of great functional importance because alar plate derivatives are primarily concerned with sensory processing, whereas motor neurons are located in basal plate derivatives. In the adult spinal cord, even though the sulcus limitans is no longer apparent, the central gray matter can be divided into a **posterior (dorsal) horn** and an **anterior (ventral) horn** on each side (see Fig. 2-6C). The central processes of sensory neurons (derived from neural crest cells) end mainly in the posterior horn, which contains cells whose axons form ascending sensory pathways. In contrast, the anterior horn contains the cell bodies of somatic and autonomic motor neurons, whose axons leave the spinal cord and innervate skeletal muscles and autonomic ganglia. The same distinction between sensory alar plate derivatives and motor basal plate derivatives holds true in the

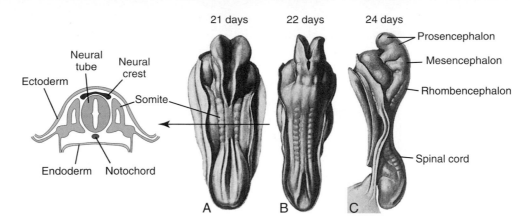

Figure 2-3 Neural tube closure during the fourth week. **A,** Neural folds begin to fuse at the cervical level of the future spinal cord at about day 21. The total length of the neural tube at this time is about 2.5 mm. **B,** This and additional areas of fusion expand rapidly in both rostral and caudal directions. **C,** By about day 24, the rostral end of the neural tube has closed; the caudal end will close 2 to 3 days later. Even before the neural tube has finished closing, local enlargements (the primary vesicles) and bends begin to appear **(C).** The notochord is the forerunner of the skeletal axis, helping to form the vertebral column. The mesodermally derived somites, adjacent to the neural tube, go on to form most of the vertebral column, as well as segmental structures such as skeletal muscle and dermis corresponding to spinal cord segments (see Chapter 10). **(A-C** from Arey LB: Developmental anatomy, ed 4, Philadelphia, 1941, WB Saunders.)

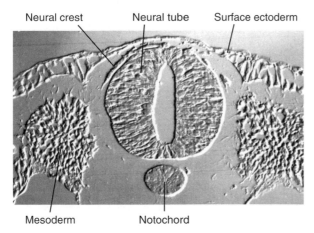

Figure 2-4 Section through the just-closed neural tube of a chick embryo at the level of the future spinal cord. Neural crest cells have been pinched off as the neural tube closed. (From Schoenwolf GC, Smith JL: Development 109:243, 1990.)

brainstem, as discussed briefly in this chapter and in more detail in Chapter 12. (The sulcus limitans probably does not extend beyond the brainstem in any meaningful way, although concentration gradients of various signaling molecules induce other distinctive dorsal/ventral patterns of development in the forebrain. Hence the alar/basal plate distinction is not useful for forebrain structures, even though some deal primarily with sensory processes and others with motor processes.)

The Neural Tube Has a Series of Bulges and Flexures

Similar strategies, involving concentration gradients of signaling molecules, come into play in specifying the

longitudinal development of the neural tube. The neural tube is never a simple, straight cylinder. Even before it has completely closed, bulges begin to appear in the rostral end of the neural tube in the region of the future brain, and bends begin to appear as well (see Fig. 2-3C).

There Are Three Primary Vesicles

During the fourth week, three bulges, or vesicles, are apparent and are referred to as the **primary vesicles** (Fig. 2-7). From rostral to caudal, these are the **prosencephalon** (Greek for "front brain," or forebrain), the **mesencephalon** (Greek for "midbrain"), and the **rhombencephalon** (named for its rhomboidal shape—see Figs. 2-7B and 2-8B), which merges smoothly with the caudal (spinal) portion of the neural tube. The prosencephalon develops into the forebrain. The mesencephalon becomes the midbrain of the adult brainstem, and the rhombencephalon (sometimes referred to as the **hindbrain**) becomes the rest of the brainstem and the cerebellum (Table 2-1).

The three primary vesicles are not arranged in a straight line, but rather are associated with two bends or flexures in the neural tube (see Fig. 2-7A). One of these, the **cervical flexure,** occurs between the rhombencephalon and the spinal cord but straightens out later in development, thus rendering it of little significance in the adult. The second, the **cephalic** (or **mesencephalic**) **flexure,** occurs at the level of the future midbrain and persists in the adult as an 80- to 90-degree bend between the axes of the brainstem and the forebrain (see Fig. 3-1). This is the bend that is not present in animals that walk on four legs but exists in humans and other animals that walk on two legs.

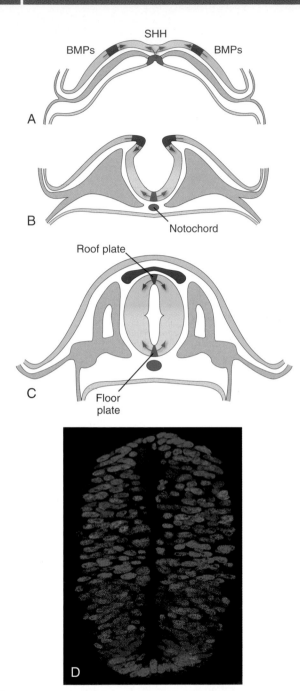

Figure 2-5 Two of the best known signaling proteins involved in the induction of dorsal-ventral patterns of differentiation in the spinal cord by concentration gradients. **A,** At the neural plate stage, midline mesoderm and later the notochord produce a signaling protein called *sonic hedgehog* (SHH; so named because the gene that specifies it is similar to a gene called *Hedgehog* that serves a similar purpose in invertebrates). Simultaneously, ectoderm adjacent to the neural plate produces another set of signaling proteins from a group called *bone morphogenetic proteins* (BMPs). **B,** Under the continued influence of the notochord, cells near the ventral midline of the neural groove (the **floor plate**) begin to express sonic hedgehog themselves. Ectoderm near the crests of the neural folds continues to produce BMPs. **C,** After the neural tube closes, cells near the dorsal midline (the **roof plate**) produce BMPs, continuing the opposing SHH/BMP concentration gradients. **D,** Staining a developing chick spinal cord with fluorescent antibodies to various proteins shows how SHH-BMP (and other) concentration gradients result in discrete populations of different cell types. (*A-C based on a drawing in Tanabe Y, Jessell TM: Science 274:1115, 1996. D from Le Dréau G, Martí E: Devel Neurobiol 72:1471, 2012.*)

There Are Five Secondary Vesicles

As the brain continues to develop, two of the primary vesicles become subdivided. During the fifth week, five **secondary vesicles** can be distinguished (see Fig. 2-8). The prosencephalon gives rise to the **telencephalon** (Greek for "end-brain") and the **diencephalon** (Greek for "in-between-brain"); the mesencephalon remains undivided; the rhombencephalon gives rise to the **metencephalon** and the **myelencephalon.** The telencephalon becomes the cerebral hemispheres of the adult brain. The diencephalon gives rise to the **thalamus** (a large mass of gray matter interposed between the cerebral cortex and other structures), the **hypothalamus** (an autonomic control center), the retina, and several other small structures.

The mesencephalon develops into the midbrain, while the metencephalon becomes the **pons** and the **cerebellum.** The myelencephalon becomes the **medulla** (the part of the brainstem that merges with the spinal cord).

In addition, a **pontine flexure** appears in the dorsal surface of the brainstem between the metencephalon and the myelencephalon (see Fig. 2-8A). This flexure does not persist as a bend in the axis of the brainstem, but it does have important consequences for the configuration of the caudal brainstem. As the flexure develops, the walls of the neural tube spread apart to form a diamond-shaped cavity (hence the name *rhombencephalon*) so that only a thin membranous roof remains over what will become the **fourth ventricle** (Fig. 2-9). Thus the alar and basal plates, still separated by the sulcus limitans, come to lie in the floor of the fourth ventricle. The result is that in the corresponding part of the adult brainstem (rostral medulla and caudal pons), sensory nuclei are located lateral, rather than posterior, to motor nuclei. As discussed further in Chapter 12, this is of some utility in making sense of the arrangement of cranial nerve nuclei.

Lateral portions of the alar plate in the rostral metencephalon thicken considerably and form the **rhombic lips.** Parts of the rhombic lips migrate into the brainstem to form cerebellum-related nuclei; remaining parts continue to enlarge, finally fusing in the midline to form a transverse ridge that will eventually become the cerebellum[a] (Fig. 2-10).

Growth of the Telencephalon Overshadows Other Parts of the Nervous System

Subsequent events are dominated by the tremendous growth of the telencephalon. This portion of the neural

---

[a]Although the cerebellum develops from the alar plate, it is involved in motor functions in the sense that cerebellar lesions cause impairments of posture and movement but not of sensation (see Chapter 20).

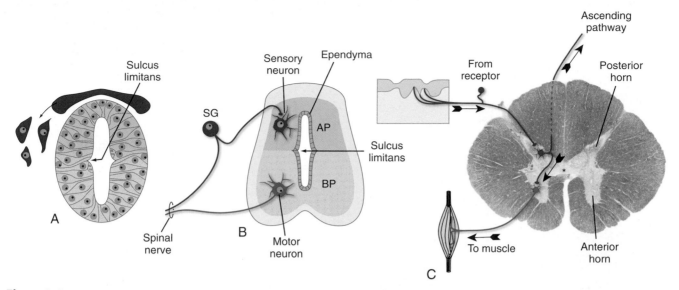

Figure 2-6 Sulcus limitans and alar and basal plates. **A,** Neural tube during the fourth week. **B,** Embryonic spinal cord during the sixth week; spinal ganglion (SG) cells, derived from the neural crest, send their central processes into the spinal cord to terminate mainly on alar plate (AP) cells; many basal plate (BP) cells become motor neurons, whose axons exit in the anterior roots. **C,** Adult spinal cord. *Asterisk* indicates the location of the central canal.

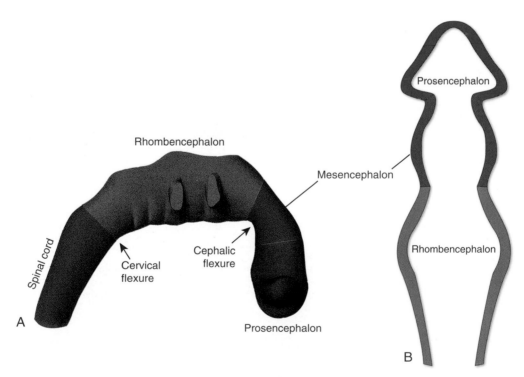

Figure 2-7 Primary vesicles at the end of the fourth week. **A,** Lateral view of the neural tube, showing vesicles and flexures. **B,** Schematic longitudinal section, as though the flexures are straightened out. (***A*** *modified from Hochstetter F: Beiträge zur Entwicklungsgeschichte des menschlichen Gehirns. I. Teil, Vienna, 1919, Franz Deuticke.*)

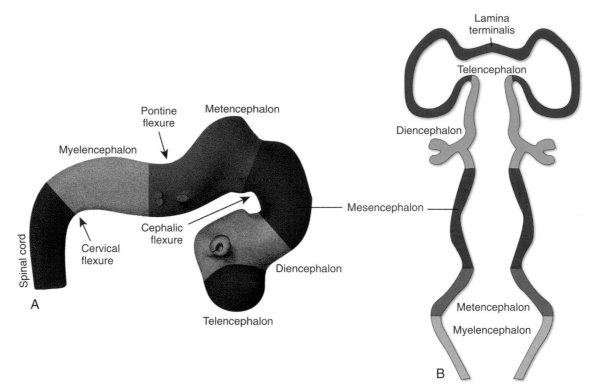

Figure 2-8 Secondary vesicles during the sixth week. **A,** Lateral view of the neural tube, showing vesicles and flexures. **B,** Schematic longitudinal section, as though the flexures are straightened out. (**A** modified from Hochstetter F: Beiträge zur Entwicklungsgeschichte des menschlichen Gehirns. I. Teil, Vienna, 1919, Franz Deuticke.)

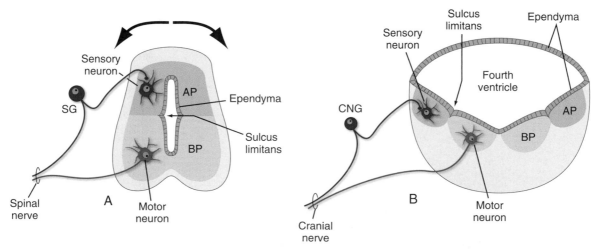

Figure 2-9 Formation of the floor of the fourth ventricle. The walls of the neural tube are spread apart by the pontine flexure so that they and the sulcus limitans become the floor of the ventricle and the roof stretches out into a thin membrane. The dorsal-ventral arrangement of sensory and motor areas in the spinal cord (**A**) becomes a lateral-medial arrangement in the brainstem (**B**). AP, alar plate; BP, basal plate; CNG, cranial nerve ganglion cell; SG, spinal ganglia.

Table 2-1	Derivatives of Vesicles of the Neural Tube		
Primary Vesicle	**Secondary Vesicle**	**Neural Derivatives**	**Cavity**
Prosencephalon (forebrain)	Telencephalon	Cerebral hemispheres	Lateral ventricles
	Diencephalon	Thalamus, hypothalamus, retina, other structures	Third ventricle
Mesencephalon	Mesencephalon	Midbrain	Cerebral aqueduct
Rhombencephalon (hindbrain)	Metencephalon	Pons, cerebellum	Part of fourth ventricle
	Myelencephalon	Medulla	Part of fourth ventricle, part of central canal

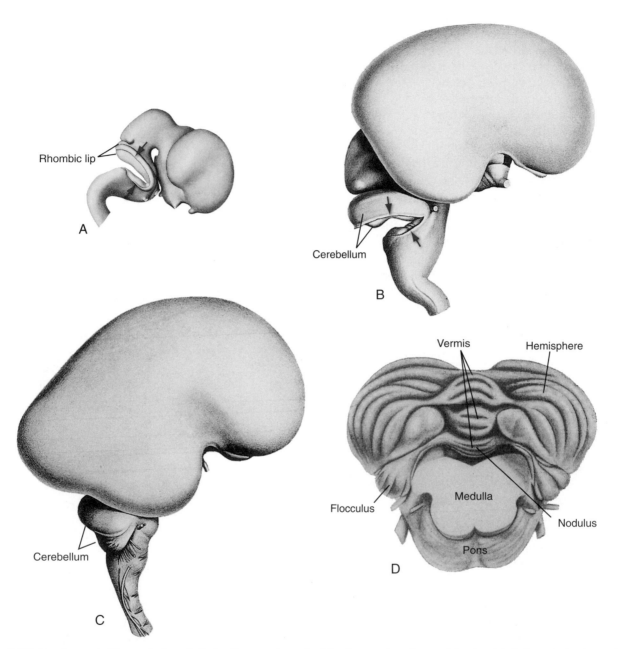

Figure 2-10 Development of the cerebellum. **A,** During the second month of development lateral parts of the alar plate in the rostral metencephalon thicken to form rhombic lips. These continue to enlarge during the third and fourth month (**B** and **C**), forming the cerebellum. **D,** By about 5 months, a series of deep fissures develops in the cerebellar surface, and both midline (vermis) and lateral (hemisphere) zones are apparent. (The nodulus is a special part of the vermis, continuous laterally with the flocculus; see Chapter 20 for additional details.) *Arrows* in **A** and **B** indicate the cut edge of the thin roof of the fourth ventricle, which becomes overgrown and mostly hidden from view as the cerebellum develops. (*A-C from Hochstetter F: Beiträge zur Entwicklungsgeschichte des menschlichen Gehirns. I. Teil, Vienna, 1919, Franz Deuticke. **D** from Hochstetter F: Beiträge zur Entwicklungsgeschichte des menschlichen Gehirns. II. Teil, Vienna, 1929, Franz Deuticke.*)

tube begins as two swellings connected across the midline by a thin membrane, the **lamina terminalis**[b] (see Fig. 2-8B). The basal part of the wall of the telencephalon, adjacent to the diencephalon, thickens to form the primordia of gray masses called the **basal ganglia** or **basal nuclei.** At the same time, the walls of the diencephalon thicken to form the thalamus and hypothalamus, separated by the **hypothalamic sulcus.** With continued growth, the telencephalon folds down alongside the diencephalon until eventually the two fuse (Fig. 2-11). The telencephalic surface overlying the area of fusion develops into a portion of the cerebral cortex called the **insula.** The cortex adjoining the insula expands greatly during the ensuing months (Fig. 2-12) until the insula itself is completely hidden from view (see Fig. 2-11C). Each cerebral hemisphere ultimately assumes the shape of a great arc encircling the insular cortex, and parts of the hemisphere that started out dorsal to the insula get pushed around into the temporal lobe (see Fig. 2-12). As discussed and demonstrated in the next chapter, knowledge of this growth of each cerebral hemisphere in a great C shape is of considerable importance for understanding the anatomical organization of the forebrain (see Fig. 3-18).

The expansion of cortical area that begins as an evagination of two telencephalic vesicles, and continues as the growth of each hemisphere into a C shape, concludes with development of extensive folds in the surface of the hemisphere. Thus each cerebral hemisphere starts out with a smooth surface (Fig. 2-13) and becomes progressively more convoluted (Figs. 2-14 and 2-15). A critical part of this growth of the cerebral cortex (and of the cerebellum [see Fig. 2-10] and other parts of the CNS) is massive proliferation and migration of neurons and glial cells. Most neuronal production and migration occurs during the third through fifth months of development, but the formation of neuronal connections continues well after birth; production of myelin sheaths mainly occurs postnatally (Fig. 2-16).

The Cavity of the Neural Tube Persists as a System of Ventricles

The cavity of the neural tube persists as the ventricular system of the adult brain and the central canal of the spinal cord (Fig. 2-17; see also Figs. 5-1 and 5-2). The cavity of the pons and rostral medulla is the fourth ventricle; that of the diencephalon is the **third ventricle.** A

---

[b]The lamina terminalis thus starts out as a bridge between the two cerebral hemispheres and as such is the site where bundles of fibers interconnecting the hemispheres begin to grow. In the adult brain, the two most prominent of these commissures, or crossing bundles—the anterior commissure and the corpus callosum—are still attached to the thin lamina terminalis (see Figs. 3-2 and 3-15).

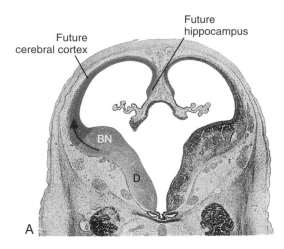

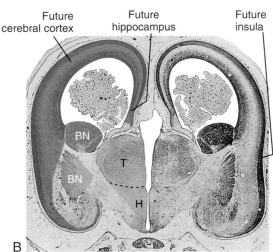

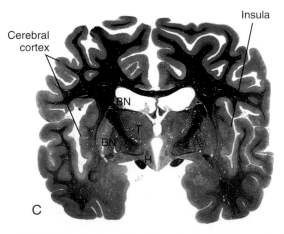

Figure 2-11 Fusion between the diencephalon and telencephalon as the cerebral hemispheres enlarge. **A,** During the second month, the telencephalic vesicles, including zones that will become the cerebral cortex and basal nuclei (BN), are separate from but continuous with the diencephalon and its cavity. As a result of subsequent rapid telencephalic growth, the basal nuclei portion folds down toward the diencephalon. At the end of the third month **(B)** the telencephalon and diencephalon have fused. After further rapid growth, the insula, overlying the point of fusion, becomes overgrown by other cerebral cortex in the adult brain **(C).** H, hypothalamus; T, thalamus. *(A and B from Hochstetter F: Beiträge zur Entwicklungsgeschichte des menschlichen Gehirns. I. Teil, Vienna, 1919, Franz Deuticke.)*

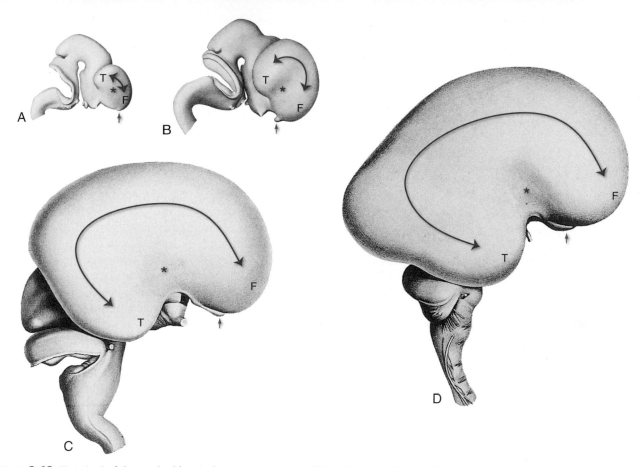

Figure 2-12 "Rotation" of the cerebral hemispheres into a C shape. Although commonly described as a rotation, the change in shape is actually caused by disproportionate growth of cortex (neocortex, described in Chapter 22) above the location of the future insula (*). The frontal (F) and temporal (T) poles actually move little, but expansion of the cortex between them causes development of the C shape during the second (**A** and **B**), third (**C**), and fourth **(D)** months. The olfactory bulb is indicated by *green arrows. (From Hochstetter F: Beiträge zur Entwicklungsgeschichte des menschlichen Gehirns. I. Teil, Vienna, 1919, Franz Deuticke.)*

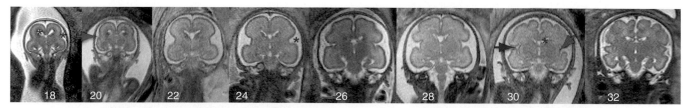

Figure 2-13 Coronal magnetic resonance images of 18- to 32-week-old (gestational age) fetuses in utero. Fluid-filled spaces are bright in these T2-weighted images (see Chapter 5), and the lateral ventricles (*blue asterisks*) and the abundant subarachnoid space *(red asterisks)* surrounding the brain can be seen. The surface of the cerebral hemispheres starts out smooth. A depression *(green arrows)* at the site of the insula is apparent in the second trimester, and during the third trimester the cortical surface becomes progressively more convoluted and the insula winds up hidden from view in the depths of the lateral sulcus *(red arrow). (Adapted from Dittrich E et al: Top Magn Res Imaging 22:107, 2011.)*

large C-shaped **lateral ventricle** occupies each cerebral hemisphere. Each lateral ventricle communicates with the third ventricle through an **interventricular foramen** (Fig. 2-18), and the third ventricle communicates with the fourth ventricle through the **cerebral aqueduct** of the midbrain.

Where the walls of the rhombencephalon spread apart to form the fourth ventricle, the roof of the

ventricle becomes extremely thin (see Fig. 2-9). An area covering the roof of the third ventricle and extending onto the surface of the telencephalon becomes similarly thin (see Fig. 2-18). At each of these locations, tufts of small blood vessels invaginate the ventricular roof to form the **choroid plexus,** which is responsible for the production of most of the **cerebrospinal fluid (CSF)** that fills the ventricles (see Fig. 5-6). As each cerebral

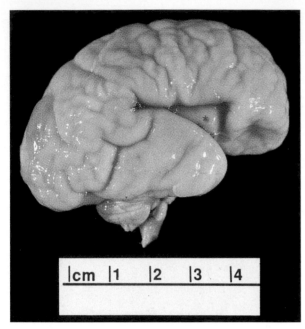

Figure 2-14 The brain of a 26-week-old who died shortly after birth as the result of an intraventricular hemorrhage. Sulci are still few and shallow, and the insula (*) is still exposed. *(Courtesy Dr. Naomi Rance, University of Arizona College of Medicine.)*

hemisphere grows around in a C shape, so too does the choroid plexus that protrudes into its lateral ventricle (see Fig. 5-7).

The Neural Crest and Cranial Placodes Give Rise to the Peripheral Nervous System

The neural crest pinches off as continuous bilateral strands of cells as the neural tube closes, extending as far as the future diencephalon. These cells go on to form essentially the entire PNS of the trunk and limbs, including sensory and autonomic ganglion cells and Schwann cells, as well as cutaneous pigment cells and secretory cells of the adrenal medulla (Fig. 2-19). They also move into the head and from there contribute to a surprising array of structures—bones of the skull and face, smooth muscles, connective tissues, more pigment cells, glomus cells that monitor blood-oxygen levels, even arteries leaving the heart.

A strip of ectoderm adjacent to the brainstem neural crest, continuing around the rostral end of the neural plate (see Fig. 2-19A), thickens in places to form a series of **cranial placodes** (see Fig. 2-19B). These placodes, in collaboration with parts of the neural crest, form sensory components of the PNS of the head. The

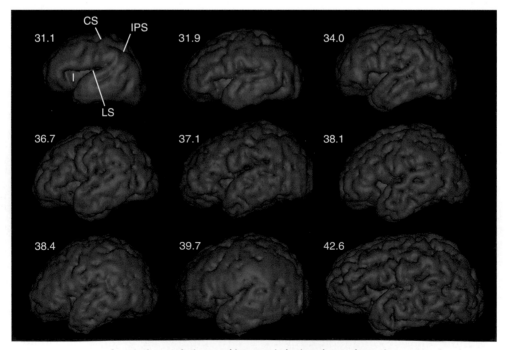

Figure 2-15 Progressive development of cortical convolutions and increase in brain volume, shown in a series of neonatal brains reconstructed in three dimensions from magnetic resonance images. The gestational age of each infant (in weeks) is indicated. The central (CS), intraparietal (IPS), and lateral (LS) sulci are apparent early on; in succeeding weeks more sulci and gyri appear, and the two banks of the lateral sulcus grow closer together, covering up the insula (I). Some of the older brains (especially 39.7 weeks) appear smoother than they actually were, because the sulci were so narrow they could not be reconstructed accurately. *(From Nishida M et al: Neuroimage 32:1041, 2006.)*

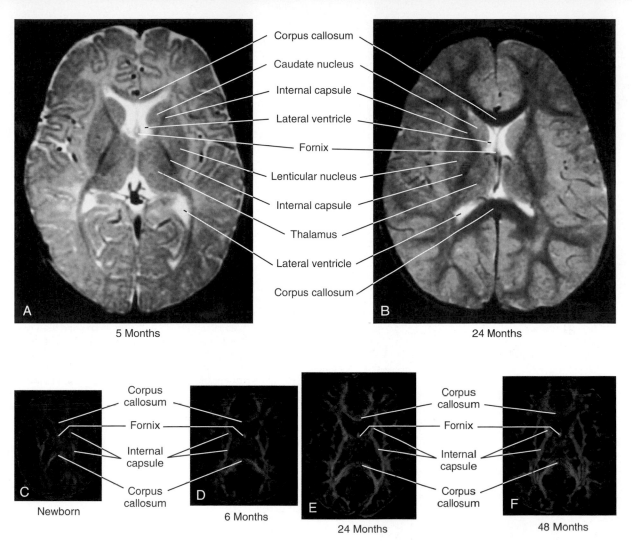

Figure 2-16 Postnatal production of myelin. In T2-weighted magnetic resonance images (see Chapter 5) from a 5-month-old **(A)** and a 2-year-old **(B)** child, fluid-filled spaces are bright and areas with a lot of myelin are dark. (Both brains are shown the same size, although a 2-year-old brain is typically about 50% larger than a 5-month-old brain.) Relatively little myelin has developed yet in the 5-month-old in areas that will contain many myelinated fibers at 2 years of age (e.g., internal capsule, corpus callosum, and especially deep cerebral white matter). **C** to **F,** Diffusion tensor images (see Box 5-1) demonstrate the orientation of axons and show that axons, even though unmyelinated, are present in their normal orientations at birth. In these color maps, red indicates areas where axons are mostly oriented transversely (e.g., corpus callosum), green indicates areas where axons are mostly oriented in an anterior-posterior direction (e.g., fibers moving toward or away from the frontal and occipital lobes), and blue indicates areas where axons are mostly oriented perpendicular to the page (e.g., fornix, parts of the internal capsule). (**A** and **B** courtesy Dr. Roger Bird, St. Joseph's Hospital and Medical Center, Phoenix, Arizona. **C** to **F** from Hermoye L et al: Neuroimage 29:493, 2006.)

unpaired **adenohypophyseal placode** forms the anterior pituitary (see Fig. 23-9). The **lens placode** on each side goes on to form the lens of the eye (see Fig. 17-1). Migrating neural crest cells go on to form most or all of the glia in cranial ganglia and sensory organs,[c] and team up with placodes in varying proportions to yield the olfactory epithelium and nerve, the trigeminal ganglion, the inner ear, and the sensory ganglia of cranial nerves VII, IX, and X.

---

[c]Except for those of the retina, which forms from an outgrowth of the neural tube (see Fig. 17-1).

Adverse Events During Development Can Cause Congenital Malformations of the Nervous System

A large number of intricate events need to happen in a precisely coordinated fashion for the nervous system to develop properly. Sometimes a flaw in the process causes a congenital malformation of the nervous system, and the characteristics of the malformation frequently provide clues about the timing of the defect (Table 2-2). Although the nature of the insults and events responsible for many malformations are still unknown, in many

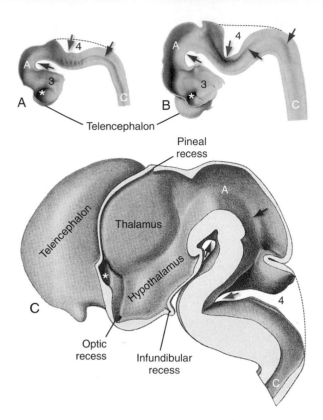

Figure 2-17 Development of the ventricular system at 37 days **(A)**, 41 days **(B)**, and 50 days **(C)**. By 50 days the thalamus and hypothalamus form the walls of the slit-shaped midline third ventricle (3); several small recesses (see Fig. 5-4) protrude from this ventricle. As each cerebral hemisphere grows around in a C shape (see Fig. 2-12), so too does its lateral ventricle; the adult configuration is shown in Figures 5-1 and 5-2. The location of the thin, membranous roof of the fourth ventricle (4) is indicated by *dotted lines. Blue arrows,* cephalic flexure; *green arrows,* pontine flexure; *red arrows,* sulcus limitans; *,* interventricular foramen; *A,* cerebral aqueduct; *C,* central canal of the spinal cord and caudal medulla. (*A and B from Hines M: J Comp Neurol 34:73, 1922.* **C** *from Hochstetter F: Beiträge zur Entwicklungsgeschichte des menschlichen Gehirns. II. Teil, Vienna, 1929, Franz Deuticke.*)

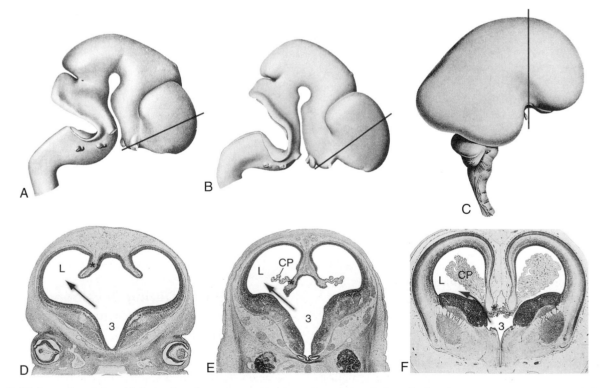

Figure 2-18 Formation of choroid plexus. **A** to **C** are nervous systems at about 6, 7, and 15 weeks; **D** to **F** are sections in the indicated planes. At 6 weeks (**A** and **D**) the third (3) and lateral (L) ventricles are in open continuity through the interventricular foramen *(arrow);* the thinned-out roof of the neural tube begins to invaginate into the lateral ventricle at the choroid fissure (*). At 7 weeks (**B** and **E**), fronds of choroid plexus (CP) begin to form at the site of invagination. By 15 weeks (**C** and **F**), the choroid plexus is a vascular, convoluted mass occupying much of the lateral ventricle; both the choroid fissure and choroid plexus curve around in a C shape with the cerebral hemisphere. Similar but less extensive choroid plexus forms in the roof of the third ventricle **(F)** and in the roof of the fourth ventricle (not shown). (*From Hochstetter F: Beiträge zur Entwicklungsgeschichte des menschlichen Gehirns. I. Teil, Vienna, 1919, Franz Deuticke.*)

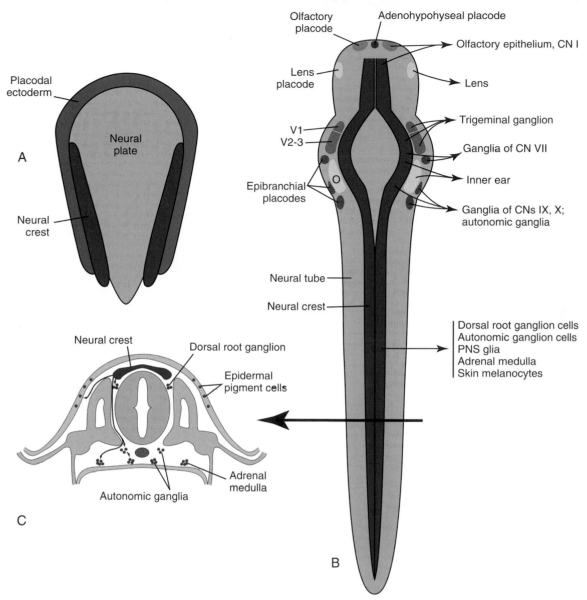

Figure 2-19 Formation of the PNS by neural crest and cranial placodes. **A,** Schematic view of the neural plate during the third week of development, flanked by strands of neural crest. The neural crest is flanked in turn by a strip of ectoderm that continues over the rostral end of the neural crest and will soon form cranial placodes. **B,** Migratory paths and some fates of neural crest and cranial placode cells. Neural crest cells give rise to an extraordinary variety of tissues and structures, only some of which are indicated here. The adenohypophyseal and lens placodes give rise to the anterior pituitary and the lens of the eye, respectively. The remaining placodes, in collaboration with cranial neural crest cells, develop into various sensory structures of the head. The **olfactory placode** develops into the sensory neurons of the olfactory epithelium and their axons (cranial nerve I). The trigeminal ganglion starts out as two placodes, the **ophthalmic** (V1) and **maxillomandibular** (V2-3) **placodes**, which subsequently fuse. The **otic placode** goes on to form the inner ear. Three **epibranchial placodes** on each side, so called because each arises at the top of a branchial arch (see Chapter 12), go on to form sensory ganglia of cranial nerves VII, IX, and X. **C,** Cross section of the developing neural tube and, neural crest cells which give rise to the dorsal root ganglia (also known as spinal ganglia), autonomic ganglia, the adrenal medulla, and epidermal pigment cells. *(Based in part on Grocott T, Tambalo M, Streit A: Dev Biol 370:3, 2012.)*

cases their genetic, environmental, and molecular bases are becoming clear.

The discussion that follows focuses on CNS malformations. However, accurate PNS construction also depends on genetic programs and signaling molecules (often genes and molecules similar or identical to those involved in CNS development), and there is likewise a spectrum of PNS malformations. For example, particular mutations affecting differentiation or migration of neural crest cells can cause congenital deafness and autonomic, pigmentary, and cardiac abnormalities.

Defective Closure of the Neural Tube Can Cause Spina Bifida or Anencephaly

Defective closure of the neural tube is a frequent cause of congenital malformations of the nervous system—about 1 per 1000 live births. Complete failure of the

Table 2-2 Timing of Developmental Events

Week	Major Developments	Appearance*	Malformations
3	Neural groove and folds Three primary vesicles visible Cervical and cephalic flexures Motor neurons appear		Neural tube defects
4	Neural tube starts to close (day 22) Rostral end of neural tube closes (day 24) Caudal end of neural tube closes (day 26) Neural crest cells begin to migrate Secondary neurulation starts Motor nerves emerge		Neural tube defects, holoprosencephaly
5	Optic vesicle, pontine flexure Five secondary vesicles visible Sulcus limitans, sensory ganglia Sensory nerves grow into CNS Rhombic lips Basal nuclei begin Thalamus, hypothalamus begin Autonomic ganglia, lens, cochlea start		Holoprosencephaly, sacral cord abnormalities
6-7	Telencephalon enlarged Basal nuclei prominent Secondary neurulation complete Cerebellum and optic nerve begin Choroid plexus Insula		
8-12	Neuronal proliferation Cerebral and cerebellar cortex begin Anterior commissure, optic chiasm Internal capsule Reflexes appear		Migration/proliferation problems (e.g., abnormal cortex or gyri)
12-16	Neuronal proliferation and migration Glial differentiation Corpus callosum		Migration/proliferation problems (e.g., abnormal cortex or gyri)
16-40	Neuronal migration Cortical sulci Glial proliferation Some myelination (mostly postnatal) Synapse formation		Hemorrhage, other destructive events

*Top two illustrations from Arey LB: Developmental anatomy, ed 4, Philadelphia, 1941, WB Saunders. Bottom illustration courtesy Dr. Naomi Rance, University of Arizona College of Medicine; all others from Hochstetter F: Beiträge zur Entwicklungsgeschichte des menschlichen Gehirns. I. Teil, Vienna, 1919, Franz Deuticke.

neural tube to close results in a fatal deformity called **craniorachischisis** (from Greek words meaning "cleft skull and spine"), in which the CNS appears as an open furrow on the dorsal surface of the head and body. Failure of the caudal end of the tube to close can result in a severe form of **spina bifida** called **myelomeningocele** (from Greek words meaning "herniated spinal cord and meninges"). In myelomeningocele, the alar and basal plates of the two sides are visible as four distinct bands on the exposed neural plate. The sulcus limitans on each side and the midline ventral groove between the basal plates also are visible on the body surface. Vertebrae fail to form over the defect, the caudal walls of the neural tube are still continuous with the skin of the back, and the cord and meninges are displaced into a saclike cavity on the back. Myelomeningocele is accompanied by a **Chiari type II malformation** in which the cerebellum and caudal brainstem are elongated and pushed down into the foramen magnum. Frequently there is obstruction to the flow of CSF and hydrocephalus results. The reason these two deformities accompany one another is not known with certainty, but it has been proposed that the decreased pressure inside the developing neural tube caused by the open neural tube results in abnormal development of the cerebellum and rhombencephalon. Prenatal surgical techniques are now available that improve the outcome in many cases of caudal neural tube closure defect.

If the rostral end of the neural tube fails to close, **anencephaly,** in which much of each cerebral hemisphere is absent, can result. As in spina bifida, the walls of the neural tube then may be continuous with the skin of the head, and the central cavity of the neural tube may be open to the outside.

Neural tube defects can be detected by clinical imaging studies or indicated by elevated levels of **alpha-fetoprotein.** This protein is a major component of fetal serum, and an open neural tube allows some to leak out into amniotic fluid (and ultimately to reach the maternal circulation, another place where it can be detected). Although the causes of many cases of neural tube defect remain unknown, the majority can be prevented if the maternal diet contains sufficient levels of **folic acid** at the time of neural tube closure. Because closure occurs at the end of the first month of gestation, when a woman may be unaware of the pregnancy, routine folic acid supplementation has been recommended for potentially childbearing women, and folic acid is now added to fortified grain products in the United States.

Defective Secondary Neurulation Can Cause a Distinctive Set of Abnormalities

The cell mass at the caudal end of the neural tube gives rise not only to the sacral spinal cord but also to some adjacent tissues. Hence defective secondary neurulation can be associated with a unique spectrum of abnormalities, including traction injuries to the spinal cord as a result of tethering of its caudal end, and a variety of cysts and tumors. Dimpling, hairiness, or discoloration of the overlying skin may provide an indication of an otherwise hidden defect.

The Forebrain Can Develop Abnormally Even If Neural Tube Closure Is Complete

The complex changes and subdivisions in the forebrain develop under the influence of multiple signaling molecules and differentially expressed genes. Disruption of the production or action of even one of these signaling molecules can cause profound defects in the formation of the forebrain. A spectrum of malformations known as **holoprosencephaly** (from Greek words meaning "affecting the entire forebrain") results from partial or complete failure of the prosencephalon to separate into the diencephalon and the paired telencephalic vesicles (Fig. 2-20), a process normally initiated during the fourth week of development and completed during the second month. Holoprosencephaly is also common and is usually fatal, affecting about 1 in 250 embryos, but only a few percent of these survive. Because of overlap in the processes that induce formation of the forebrain and the face, holoprosencephaly is typically associated with marked facial abnormalities as well; in extreme cases, there may be a single midline eye with a rudimentary nose above it. A variety of other influences during early

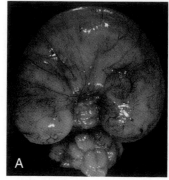
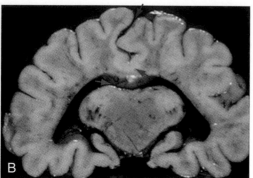

Figure 2-20 A, Anterior view of the brain of 20-week fetus with a severe form of holoprosencephaly in which the fissure normally present between the hemispheres is completely missing. **B,** A newborn with a slightly less severe form of holoprosencephaly. Part of the longitudinal fissure is present *(red arrow),* but cortex continues across the midline *(blue arrow),* the corpus callosum is missing, a single lateral ventricle spans the midline *(green arrow),* and the diencephalon is fused into a single structure. *(Courtesy Dr. Jeffrey A. Golden, University of Pennsylvania School of Medicine.)*

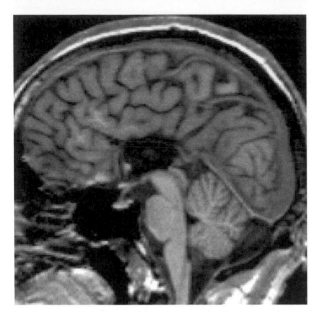

Figure 2-21 Another malformation not related to defective neural tube closure. This magnetic resonance image of a 26-year-old man with fetal alcohol syndrome, a common cause of congenital malformations of the face and CNS, shows complete absence of the corpus callosum (compare to Figs. 3-2 and 5-18). This individual also had mild facial abnormalities and an IQ of 77. *(From Swayze VW et al: Pediatrics 99:232, 1997.)*

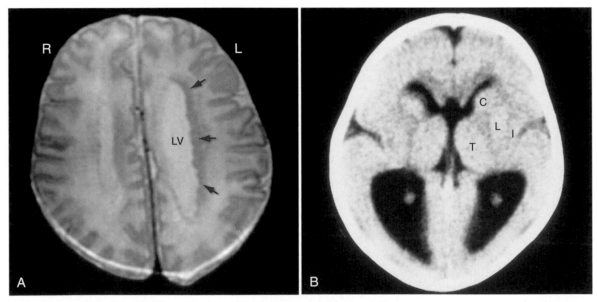

Figure 2-22 Malformations caused by defective proliferation or migration of neurons. **A,** Magnetic resonance image of a 2-week-old female infant with a somewhat enlarged left lateral ventricle (LV) and a layer of gray matter *(arrows)* in its wall, caused by failure of these neurons to migrate to the cerebral cortex. Displaced areas of gray matter such as this, called *heterotopias* (Greek for "in a different place"), can occur in the ventricular wall or as bands or nodules in the white matter and are commonly a source of seizure activity. **B,** Computed tomography image of a 5-month-old male infant with a seizure disorder and developmental delay. Although all of the major elements of the CNS appear to be present, including the thalamus (T), caudate nucleus (C), lenticular nucleus (L) and insula (I), cortical folding is almost completely absent. This condition, called lissencephaly (Greek for "smooth brain"), is thought to be due to defective migration of neurons during the third and fourth month of development. *(Courtesy Dr. Raymond F. Carmody, University of Arizona College of Medicine.)*

development, such as environmental insults, can cause less profound structural abnormalities that may still have major neurological consequences (Fig. 2-21).

Disruptions occurring later in development may affect neuronal proliferation or migration. This can lead to abnormal gyral patterns or ectopic areas of gray matter, even though all of the basic elements of the CNS may be present (Fig. 2-22).

SUGGESTED READINGS

Adzick NS, et al: A randomized trial of prenatal versus postnatal repair of myelomeningocele. New Engl J Med 364:993, 2011.

Barkovich AJ: Current concepts of polymicrogyria. Neuroradiology 52:479, 2010.

Barraud P, et al: Neural crest origin of olfactory ensheathing glia. Proc Natl Acad Sci U S A 107:21040, 2010.

"…overturns the existing dogma on the developmental origin of OECs."

Blom HJ, et al: Neural tube defects and folate: case far from closed. Nature Rev Neurosci 7:724, 2006.

Bronner ME, LeDouarin NM: Development and evolution of the neural crest: an overview. Dev Biol 366:2, 2012.
The introductory paper to a special issue on neural crest.

Clouchoux C, et al: Quantitative in vivo MRI measurement of cortical development in the fetus. Brain Struct Funct 217:127, 2012.
Careful measurements of the pattern of sulcal development from 25 to 35 weeks of gestation.

Copp AJ, Greene NDE: Neural tube defects—disorders of neurulation and related embryonic processes. Wiley Interdiscip Ref Dev Biol 2:213, 2013.

Crelin ES: Development of the nervous system. CIBA Clin Symp 26(2):1974.

ten Donkelaar HJ, Lammens M, Hori A: Clinical neuroembryology: development and developmental disorders of the human central nervous system, New York, 2006, Springer.

Drews U: Color atlas of embryology, Stuttgart, 1995, Georg Thieme Verlag.
A compact, well-illustrated review.

Francis F: Human disorders of cortical development: from past to present. Eur J Neurosci 23:877, 2006.

Freyer L, Aggarwal V, Morrow BE: Dual embryonic origin of the mammalian otic vesicle forming the inner ear. Development 138:5403, 2011.
Indications that cranial sensory structures long considered to be placodal derivatives are actually derived in part from neural crest.

Garel C, et al: Fetal cerebral cortex: normal gestational landmarks identified using prenatal MR imaging. Am J Neuroradiol 22:184, 2001.

Golden JA: Towards a greater understanding of the pathogenesis of holoprosencephaly. Brain Dev 21:513, 1999.

de Graaf-Peters VB, Hadders-Algra M: Ontogeny of the human central nervous system: what is happening when? Early Hum Devel 82:257, 2006.

Grocott T, Tambalo M, Streit A: The peripheral sensory nervous system in the vertebrate head: a gene regulatory perspective. Dev Biol 370:12, 2012.

Hayhurst M, McConnell SK: Mouse models of holoprosencephaly. Curr Opin Neurol 16:135, 2003.

Haynes RL, et al: Axonal development in the cerebral white matter of the human fetus and infant. J Comp Neurol 484:156, 2004.
The relative timing of axonal growth, functionality, and myelination.

Hermoye L, et al: Pediatric diffusion tensor imaging: normal database and observation of the white matter maturation in early childhood. Neuroimage 29:493, 2006.

Hong SE, et al: Autosomal recessive lissencephaly with cerebellar hypoplasia is associated with human RELN mutations. Nat Genet 26:93, 2000.

Huang X, Saint-Jeannet J-P: Induction of the neural crest and the opportunities of life on the edge. Dev Biol 275:1, 2004.

Huttenlocher PR: Morphometric study of human cerebral cortex development. Neuropsychologia 28:517, 1990.
A look at developmental changes in numbers of neurons and numbers of synapses, with some consideration of how these might relate to the development of cognitive abilities.

Jennings MT, et al: Neuroanatomic examination of spina bifida aperta and the Arnold-Chiari malformation in a 130-day human fetus. J Neurol Sci 54:325, 1982.

Kiecker C, Lumsden A: The role of organizers in patterning the nervous system. Annu Rev Neurosci 35:347, 2012.
A recent, concise review of the multiple concentration gradients underlying regional development of the CNS.

Kier EL, Fulbright RK, Bronen RA: Limbic lobe embryology and anatomy: dissection and MR of the medial surface of the fetal cerebral hemisphere. Am J Neuroradiol 16:1847, 1995.

Lim Y, Golden JA: Patterning the developing diencephalon. Brain Res Rev 53:17, 2007.

Marcorelles P, Laquerriere A: Neuropathology of holoprosencephaly. Am J Med Genet Part C Semin Med Genet 154C:109, 2010.

Marti E, Bovolenta P: Sonic hedgehog in CNS development: one signal, multiple outputs. Trends Neurosci 25:89, 2002.
Sonic hedgehog is a signaling molecule critically involved in inducing formation of ventral midline parts of most of the CNS.

Moore KL, Persaud TVN, Torchia MG: The developing human: clinically oriented embryology, ed 9, Philadelphia, 2011, WB Saunders.

Nakatsu T, Uwabe C, Shiota K: Neural tube closure in humans initiates at multiple sites: evidence from human embryos and implications for the pathogenesis of neural tube defects. Anat Embryol 201:455, 2000.
Although the primary site of neural tube closure described in this chapter is the longitudinally most extensive closure, there are probably at least two other sites that start shortly thereafter; failure of any one of these closures can cause a neural tube defect in a distinctive pattern.

Nishida M, et al: Detailed semiautomated MRI based morphometry of the neonatal brain: Preliminary results. Neuroimage 32:1041, 2006.

O'Rahilly R, Müller F: The embryonic human brain: an atlas of developmental stages, ed 3, New York, 2006, Wiley-Liss.

Paus T, et al: Maturation of white matter in the human brain: a review of magnetic resonance studies. Brain Res Bull 54:255, 2001.

Raybaud C: The corpus callosum, the other great forebrain commissures, and the septum pellucidum: anatomy, development, and malformation. Neuroradiology 52:447, 2010.

Richardson WD, Kessaris N, Pringle N: Oligodendrocyte wars. Nat Rev Neurosci 7:11, 2006.
They originate from multiple sites in the neural tube and compete with each other to stay around.

Sanes DH, Reh TA, Harris WA: Development of the nervous system, ed 3, San Diego, 2012, Academic Press.

Schlosser G: Making senses: development of vertebrate cranial placodes. Int Rev Cell Mol Biol 283:129, 2010.

Smith JL, Schoenwolf GC: Neurulation: coming to closure. Trends Neurosci 20:510, 1997.
A review of the sources of the forces that cause the neural plate to indent and form the neural groove and tube.

Suzuki K: Neuropathology of developmental abnormalities. Brain Dev 29:129, 2007.
A recent review of the distinctive kinds of abnormalities associated with different stages of development.

Swayze VW, et al: Magnetic resonance imaging of brain anomalies in fetal alcohol syndrome. Pediatrics 99:232, 1997.

Tanabe Y, Jessell TM: Diversity and pattern in the developing spinal cord. Science 274:1115, 1996.
How concentration gradients of signaling molecules lead to differentiation of the spinal cord gray matter.

Tortoni-Donati P, Rossi A, Cama A: Spinal dysraphism: a review of neuroradiological features with embryological correlations and proposal for a new classification. Neuroradiology 42:471, 2000.
The spectrum of neural tube defects affecting the spinal cord.

Volpe JJ: Neurology of the newborn, ed 5, Philadelphia, 2008, WB Saunders.

Wallingford JB, et al: The continuing challenge of understanding, preventing, and treating neural tube defects. Science 339:1047, 2013.

Wilson L, Maden M: The mechanisms of dorsoventral patterning in the vertebrate neural tube. Dev Biol 282:1, 2005.

Wilson YM, et al: Neural crest cell lineage segregation in the mouse neural tube. Development 131:6153, 2004.

Gross Anatomy and General Organization of the Central Nervous System

3

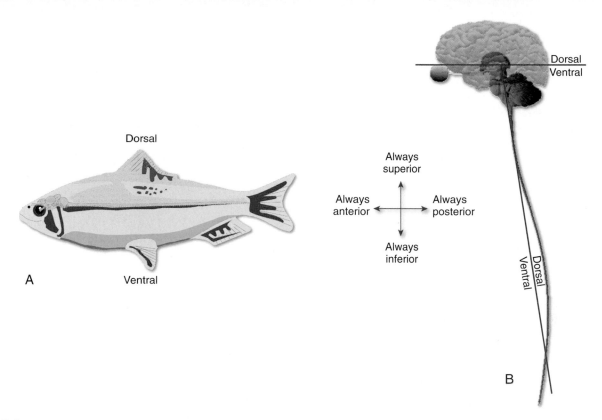

Figure 3-1 Various directional terms used when referring to different parts of the CNS. For animals that move through the world horizontally **(A),** dorsal and ventral are always equivalent to superior and inferior. Because humans stand upright posture and because of the cephalic flexure **(B),** dorsal-ventral is equivalent to superior-inferior in the forebrain and to posterior-anterior in the spinal cord and brainstem. *(Courtesy Dr. John W. Sundsten, University of Washington School of Medicine.)*

The human central nervous system (CNS) is composed of the brain and spinal cord. This chapter briefly discusses the major surface and internal structures of the brain (summarized in Fig. 3-26) and, together with the following six chapters, lays the groundwork for the more detailed discussions of the functional anatomy of the CNS in ensuing chapters.

The Long Axis of the CNS Bends at the Cephalic Flexure

Before considering the parts of the brain in more detail, it is helpful to discuss some terms used for planes and directions in the nervous system. The **sagittal** plane goes through the midline and divides the brain into two symmetrical halves. **Parasagittal** planes are those parallel to the sagittal plane. **Coronal** planes (also called **frontal** planes) are parallel to the long axis of the body and perpendicular to the sagittal plane (e.g., a vertical plane passing through both of your ears). **Axial** planes (also called **transverse** or **horizontal** planes) are perpendicular to the long axis of the body. These terms are fairly straightforward and have the same meaning with respect to any part of the nervous system. However,

directional terms such as **anterior, dorsal,** and **rostral** change their meanings relative to each other in different parts of the nervous system. The reason for this, as indicated in Figure 3-1, is that walking upright necessitates a bend of about 80 degrees in going from the long axis of the spinal cord and brainstem to the long axis of the forebrain. This bend is a consequence of the **cephalic flexure,** which appears early in the embryological development of the nervous system (see Fig. 2-7) and persists in the mature brain. Dorsal-ventral terminology ignores this bend, as though we had a linear CNS and walked around on all fours like most other vertebrates, so that the directional meaning of "dorsal" changes by 80 degrees at the midbrain-diencephalon junction. The terms *anterior* and *superior,* in contrast, retain a constant meaning relative to the normal upright orientation of the body as a whole. This means, for example, that the ventral surface of the spinal cord is also its *anterior* surface, but the ventral surface of the forebrain is its *inferior* surface. Rostral-caudal terminology may cause additional confusion. Anatomically, *rostral* means "toward the nose." However, it also has a functional connotation for many (implying "toward the telencephalon"), so that the posterior end of the cerebral hemispheres could be

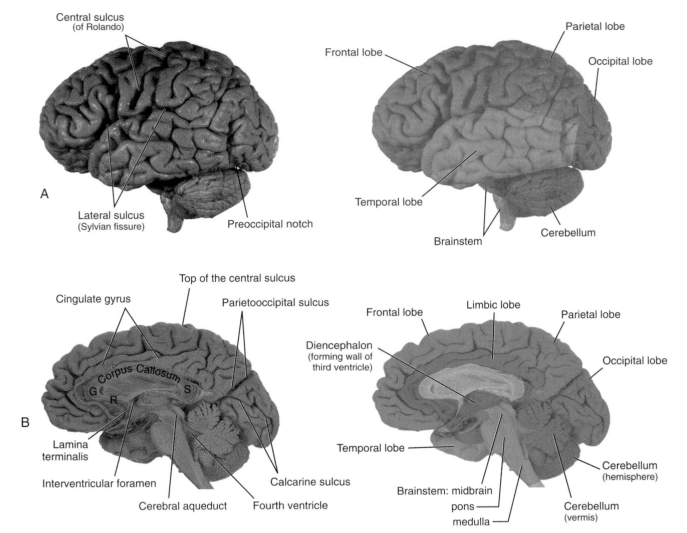

Figure 3-2 Major regions of the adult brain as seen in a lateral view **(A)** and in a medial view of a hemisected brain **(B)**. G, genu; R, rostrum; S, splenium of the corpus callosum. *(Dissection courtesy of Grant Dahmer, Department of Cell Biology and Anatomy, University of Arizona College of Medicine.)*

considered rostral to all parts of the diencephalon. Use of anterior-posterior and superior-inferior terminology in reference to the cerebrum avoids any ambiguity.

Hemisecting a Brain Reveals Parts of the Diencephalon, Brainstem, and Ventricular System

Hemisection of the brain reveals many parts of the diencephalon, brainstem, and cerebellum, and additional features of the cerebral hemispheres (Fig. 3-2B). The cephalic flexure is visible at the junction between the brainstem and the diencephalon. The brainstem itself is subdivided into the **midbrain,** which is continuous with the diencephalon, the **pons,** and the **medulla,** which is continuous with the spinal cord. The two cerebral hemispheres are joined by a huge fiber bundle, the **corpus callosum,** which has an enlarged and rounded posterior

splenium, a **body,** and an anterior, curved **genu,** which tapers gently into a ventrally directed **rostrum** that merges into the lamina terminalis—the site of closure of the rostral neuropore.

The nervous system develops embryologically from a neuroectodermal tube; the cavity of the tube persists in adults as a system of ventricles (see Fig. 5-1), part of which is apparent in the sagittal plane (see Fig. 3-2B). Portions of the medial surfaces of the diencephalon form the walls of the narrow, slitlike **third ventricle,** which opens into the large **lateral ventricle** of each cerebral hemisphere through an **interventricular foramen (foramen of Monro).** Posteriorly, the third ventricle is continuous with a narrow channel through the midbrain, the **cerebral aqueduct (aqueduct of Sylvius).** The aqueduct in turn is continuous with the **fourth ventricle** of the pons and medulla, and the fourth ventricle is continuous with the microscopically tiny **central canal** of the caudal medulla and the spinal cord.

Humans, Relative to Other Animals, Have Large Brains and Many Neurons

One impressive feature of the human brain is its size, to which distinctively human mental capacities are commonly attributed. An average human brain weighs about 400 g at birth; this weight triples during the first 3 years of life (resulting from addition of myelin and growth of neuronal processes, rather than the addition of more neurons). The rate of growth then slows, and the maximum brain weight of around 1400 g (Table 3-1) is reached at about age 11 years. This weight holds steady until about the age of 50 years, when a slow decline sets in (Fig. 3-3). The weight of 1400 g is only an average figure; brain weights for normal individuals range from 1100 g (or less) to around 1700 g. This large range of sizes is surprising, and its significance is not well understood; there is only a modest correlation between brain size and mental ability.

Part of the large brain size is simply a reflection of body size: big animals tend to have big brains (Fig. 3-4).

Elephants, for example, have 5000-g brains. Similarly, the size difference between the bodies of human males and females explains, at least in part, why male brains are slightly larger than female brains (see Fig. 3-3). However, many animals that are larger than humans nevertheless have smaller brains (Fig. 3-5). In different kinds of animals, brain size increases at different rates with increasing body size; primates have relatively large brains for their body size.[a] A rodent with a brain the same size as a human's, for example, would be predicted to have a body dozens of times larger than a typical human. Humans have the largest brains among primates and it is tempting to attribute human mental abilities to these relatively large brains, but this is an oversimplification. Not only is the size of the brain scaled to the size of the body in different ways in different kinds of animals, but also different numbers of neurons grow in given volumes of these brains. In primates, many neurons are packed into the gray matter; the same hypothetical rodent with a human-size brain would contain fewer than 15% as many neurons. The net result is that humans have relatively large brains with perhaps more neurons than any other species, mostly located in the cerebral and cerebellar cortices (Fig. 3-6).

Table 3-1	Approximate Average Volumes of Intracranial Contents	
		Volume (cm³)
Brain		1365
Gray matter		695
White matter		670
Cerebrospinal fluid		180
Forebrain		1200
Basal nuclei*		8
Cerebellum		135
Brainstem		30

*Caudate nucleus, putamen, and globus pallidus.
Based on Anastasi et al (2006), Kruggel (2006), and Makris et al (2003).

Named Sulci and Gyri Cover the Cerebral Surface

A striking aspect of human cerebral hemispheres is the degree to which their surface is folded and convoluted.

[a]There are exceptions to the various brain-scaling rules found in various animal groups. In the case of primates, for example, great apes have smaller brains than would be expected for their body sizes, perhaps because they evolved to eat a diet inadequate to support the energy requirements of larger brains. Nevertheless, these smaller-than-expected brains have the neuronal packing densities and ratios of neurons to nonneuronal cells expected for primate brains.

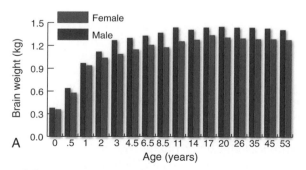

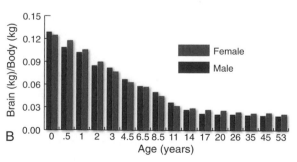

Figure 3-3 A, Average brain weights of human males and females at different ages. Notice how the brain grows rapidly after birth, doubling in the first year of life, before reaching its full size at about the age of 11 years. At all ages, male brains have a greater average weight than female brains. However, as indicated in **B,** adult female brains account for a greater percentage of body weight than do adult male brains. After the rapid brain growth in the first 1 to 3 years of life, body growth takes over and the brain weight/body weight ratio declines progressively until about age 17 years. *(Plotted from the data in Dekaban AS, Sadowsky D: Ann Neurol 4:345, 1978.)*

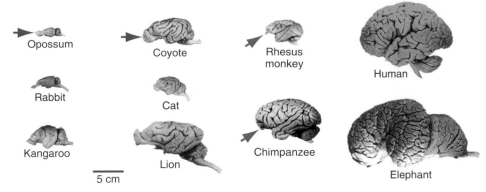

Figure 3-4 Brains of a series of representative mammals, all reproduced at the same scale. Brain size is partly related to body size (e.g., cat vs. lion, human vs. elephant) and partly related to mental abilities (e.g., lion vs. human). Not all parts of the brain change size in proportion to each other. For example, the olfactory bulbs of opossums and coyotes *(blue arrows)* are relatively large, those of monkeys and chimpanzees *(green arrows)* are proportionally much smaller, and those of humans are barely discernible at this magnification. *(From www.brainmuseum.org, courtesy Dr. Wally Welker; supported by NSF grant 0131028.)*

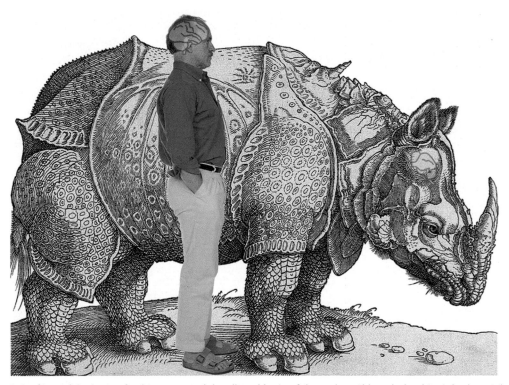

Figure 3-5 The relative sizes of the brain of a rhinoceros and the alleged brain of the author. Although the rhino's body weight is about 30 times greater, its brain weight is likely to be only half as great. *(Drawing of rhino produced by Albrecht Dürer; author produced by Mr. and Mrs. Nolte; suggested by an illustration in Cobb S: Arch Neurol 12:555, 1965.)*

Each ridge is called a **gyrus,** and each groove between ridges is called a **sulcus;** particularly deep sulci are often called **fissures.** This folding into gyri and sulci is a mechanism for increasing the total cortical area (and the total number of cortical neurons). Each of us has enough cortex to command a surface area of about 2.5 ft^2 (about 2300 cm^2), two thirds of which is hidden from view in the walls of sulci. The appearance of various gyri and sulci varies considerably from one brain to another (Fig. 3-7), to the point that they may not even be continuous structures (e.g., a particular gyrus may be transected by one or more sulci). Major features, however, are reasonably constant.

In the discussion that follows, the principal surface features of the hemispheres are described, with some broad generalizations regarding the function of various cortical areas. These functional descriptions are highly oversimplified and are offered primarily for purposes of initial orientation. Cortical function is discussed in more detail in Chapter 22.

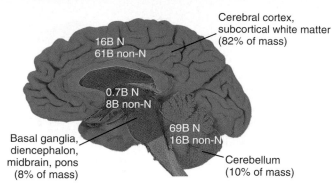

Figure 3-6 Numbers of neurons (N) and numbers of nonneuronal cells (non-N) in different parts of the brain. Nonneuronal cells are mostly glia, but also include other cell types such as the ependymal cells lining the ventricles and the endothelial cells of blood vessels. *(Based on Azevedo FAC et al: J Comp Neurol 513:532, 2009.)*

Each Cerebral Hemisphere Includes a Frontal, Parietal, Occipital, Temporal, and Limbic Lobe

Four prominent sulci—the **central sulcus,** the **lateral sulcus** (fissure), the **parietooccipital sulcus,** and the **cingulate sulcus**—together with the **preoccipital notch** and parts of a few other sulci are used to divide each cerebral hemisphere into five lobes (Fig. 3-8, Video 3-1):

1. The **frontal lobe** extends from the anterior tip of the brain (the **frontal pole**) to the central sulcus (**sulcus of Rolando**). On the lateral surface of the hemisphere, the lateral sulcus (**Sylvian fissure**) separates it from the temporal lobe. On the medial surface of the brain, it extends to the cingulate sulcus and posteriorly to an imaginary line from the top of the central sulcus to the cingulate sulcus. Inferiorly it continues as the **orbital** part of the frontal lobe (named for its location above the orbit).

2. The **parietal lobe** extends from the central sulcus to an imaginary line connecting the top of the parietooccipital sulcus and the preoccipital notch. Inferiorly it is bounded by the lateral sulcus and the imaginary continuation of this sulcus to the posterior boundary of the parietal lobe. On the medial surface of the brain, it is bounded inferiorly by the **subparietal** and **calcarine sulci,** anteriorly by the frontal lobe, and posteriorly by the parietooccipital sulcus.

3. The **temporal lobe** extends superiorly to the lateral sulcus and the line forming the inferior boundary of the parietal lobe; posteriorly it extends to the line connecting the top of the parietooccipital sulcus and the preoccipital notch. On the medial surface, its posterior boundary is an imaginary line extending from the preoccipital notch toward the splenium of the corpus callosum, and part of its superior boundary is the **collateral sulcus.**

4. The **occipital lobe** is bounded anteriorly by the parietal and temporal lobes on both the lateral and medial surfaces of the hemisphere.

5. The **limbic lobe** is a strip of cortex that appears to more or less encircle the telencephalon-diencephalon junction. It is interposed between the corpus callosum and the frontal, parietal, and occipital lobes, and curves around to occupy part of the medial surface of what would otherwise be called the temporal lobe.

These separations correspond only approximately to functional subdivisions, but they do provide a meaningful basis for discussion and reference.

An additional area of cerebral cortex not usually included in any of the five lobes discussed lies buried in the depths of the lateral sulcus, concealed from view by portions of the frontal, parietal, and temporal lobes. This cortex, called the **insula,** overlies the site where the telencephalon and diencephalon fuse during embryological development (see Chapter 2). It can be revealed by prying open the lateral sulcus or by removing the overlying portions of other lobes (Fig. 3-9). The portion of a given lobe overlying the insula is called an **operculum** (Latin for "lid"); there are frontal, parietal, and temporal opercula. The **circular sulcus** outlines the insula and marks its borders with the opercular areas of cortex.

The Frontal Lobe Contains Motor Areas

Four gyri make up the lateral surface of the frontal lobe (Fig. 3-10). The **precentral gyrus** is anterior to the central sulcus and parallel to it, extending to the **precentral sulcus.** The **superior, middle,** and **inferior frontal gyri** are oriented parallel to one another and roughly perpendicular to the precentral gyrus. The superior frontal gyrus continues onto the medial surface of the hemisphere as far as the cingulate sulcus. The inferior frontal gyrus is visibly divided into three parts: (1) the **orbital part,** which is most anterior and is continuous with the inferior (orbital) surface of the frontal lobe; (2) the **opercular part,** which is most posterior and forms a portion of the frontal operculum; and (3) the wedge-shaped **triangular part,** which lies between the other two. The inferior, or orbital, surface of the frontal lobe is mostly occupied by a group of gyri of somewhat variable appearance that usually are collectively referred to simply as **orbital gyri** or **orbitofrontal cortex.** The only consistently named gyrus on this surface is **gyrus rectus** (Greek for "straight gyrus"), which is most medial and extends onto the medial surface of the hemisphere. Between gyrus rectus and the orbital gyri is the **olfactory sulcus,** which contains the olfactory bulb and tract. The medial surface of the lobe contains extensions of the superior frontal gyrus, precentral gyrus, and gyrus rectus; certain small cortical areas near the rostrum of the corpus callosum are part of the limbic lobe.

The frontal lobe contains four general functional areas:

1. Much of the precentral gyrus is the **primary motor cortex,** which contains many of the cells of origin of

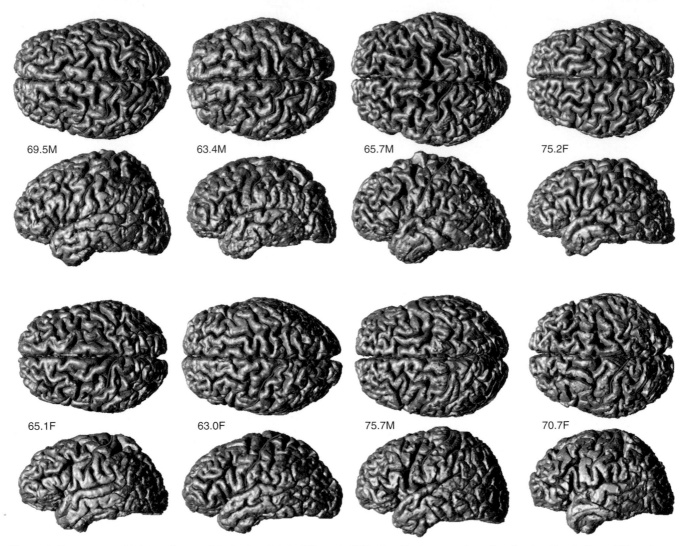

69.5M

63.4M

65.7M

75.2F

65.1F

63.0F

75.7M

70.7F

Figure 3-7 Superior and left lateral views of the brains of eight different individuals, with the age and gender of each subject indicated. These images were reconstructed from magnetic resonance imaging scans and show the range of sizes and shapes of normal brains. The left lateral sulcus *(green lines)* is in about the same place in each brain, has roughly the same configuration, but differs in its details from one brain to another. Other features (e.g., the folding pattern of the superior frontal gyrus, the configuration of the superior temporal sulcus) vary more substantially. *(Method from Tosun D et al: Neuroimage 23:108, 2004. Courtesy Dr. Jerry Prince, MR data of Baltimore Longitudinal Study of Aging; participants provided by the Intramural Research Program of the National Institute on Aging.)*

descending motor pathways and is involved in the initiation of voluntary movements.

2. The **premotor** and **supplementary motor areas** occupy the remainder of the precentral gyrus together with the posterior portions of the superior and middle frontal gyri; they are functionally related to the planning and initiation of voluntary movements.

3. **Broca's area,** the opercular and triangular parts of the inferior frontal gyrus of one hemisphere (usually the left), is important in the production (motor aspects) of written and spoken language.

4. The **prefrontal cortex,** a very large and somewhat confusingly named area (because it sounds like it is in front of the frontal lobe), occupies the remainder of the frontal lobe. Prefrontal cortex is involved with

what are often referred to as **executive functions**— what may very generally be described as personality, insight, and foresight.

The Parietal Lobe Contains Somatosensory Areas

The lateral surface of the parietal lobe is divided into three areas: the **postcentral gyrus** and the **superior** and **inferior parietal lobules** (Fig. 3-11). The postcentral gyrus is posterior to the central sulcus and parallel to it, extending to the **postcentral sulcus.** The **intraparietal sulcus** runs posteriorly from the postcentral sulcus toward the occipital lobe, separating the superior and inferior parietal lobules. The inferior parietal lobule in turn is composed of the **supramarginal gyrus,** which caps the upturned end of the lateral sulcus, and

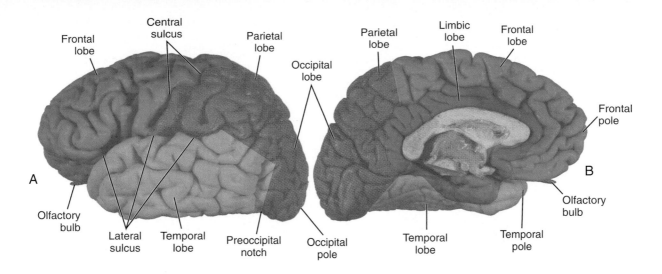

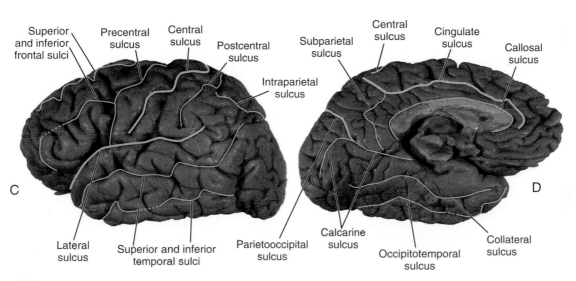

Figure 3-8 Lobes and sulci of the cerebral hemisphere. **A,** The boundaries of the frontal, parietal, occipital, and temporal lobes on the lateral surface of the hemisphere. **B,** The boundaries of the frontal, parietal, occipital, temporal, and limbic lobes on the medial surface of the hemisphere. **C,** Major sulci on the lateral surface of the hemisphere. **D,** Major sulci on the medial and inferior surfaces of the hemisphere. The subparietal sulcus of this hemisphere looks like a continuation of the cingulate sulcus, but in two thirds of brains they are separate sulci. (See Video 3-1.) *(Dissection courtesy of Grant Dahmer, Department of Cell Biology and Anatomy, University of Arizona College of Medicine.)*

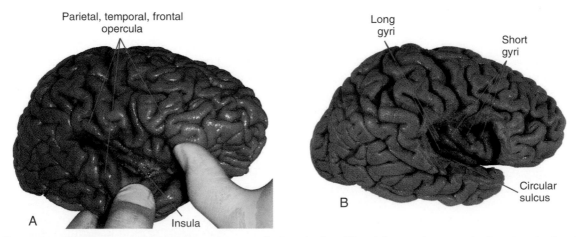

Figure 3-9 Location of the insula, demonstrated by prying open the lateral sulcus **(A)** and then cutting away the frontal, parietal, and temporal opercula **(B).** The surface of the insula is convoluted like other cortical areas, typically into about three short gyri and two long gyri. *(Dissection courtesy of Grant Dahmer, Department of Cell Biology and Anatomy, University of Arizona College of Medicine.)*

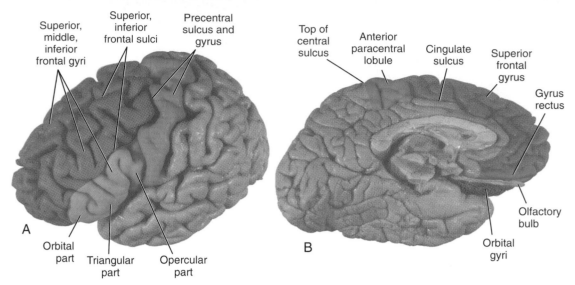

Figure 3-10 Lateral, medial, and inferior surfaces of the frontal lobe, seen from above and in front **(A)** and from medially and below **(B).** (The medial extensions of the precentral and postcentral gyri surround the end of the central sulcus, and for this reason are sometimes referred to as the *paracentral lobule.* Using this terminology, the medial extension of the postcentral gyrus is also called the *anterior paracentral lobule.*) *(Dissection courtesy of Grant Dahmer, Department of Cell Biology and Anatomy, University of Arizona College of Medicine.)*

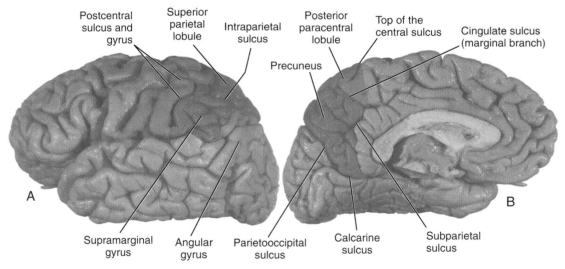

Figure 3-11 Lateral **(A)** and medial **(B)** surfaces of the parietal lobe. *(Dissection courtesy of Grant Dahmer, Department of Cell Biology and Anatomy, University of Arizona College of Medicine.)*

the **angular gyrus,** which similarly caps the **superior temporal sulcus.** The angular gyrus is typically broken up by small sulci and may overlap the supramarginal gyrus. The medial surface of the parietal lobe contains the medial extension of the postcentral gyrus (i.e., the **posterior paracentral lobule**) and is completed by an area called the **precuneus,** which is bounded by the subparietal and parietooccipital sulci, the **marginal branch** of the cingulate sulcus, and part of the calcarine sulcus.

The parietal lobe is associated, in a very general sense, with three functions:

1. The postcentral gyrus corresponds to **primary somatosensory cortex;** it is concerned with the initial

cortical processing of tactile and proprioceptive (sense of position) information; more specifically, it deals with sensory localization.

2. Much of the inferior parietal lobule of one hemisphere (usually the left), together with portions of the temporal lobe, is involved in the comprehension of language.

3. The remainder of the parietal cortex subserves complex aspects of spatial orientation and directing attention.

The Temporal Lobe Contains Auditory Areas

The lateral surface of the temporal lobe is composed of the **superior, middle,** and **inferior temporal gyri**

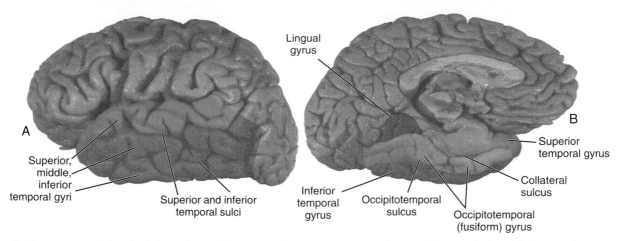

Figure 3-12 Lateral, medial, and inferior surfaces of the temporal lobe, seen from the side **(A)** and from medially and below **(B).** The superior and inferior temporal gyri meet at the temporal pole. *(Dissection courtesy of Grant Dahmer, Department of Cell Biology and Anatomy, University of Arizona College of Medicine.)*

(Fig. 3-12). The superior surface of the temporal lobe extends into the lateral sulcus, where it continues into the temporal operculum. The inferior temporal gyrus continues onto the inferior surface of the lobe. The rest of the inferior surface is made up of the broad **occipito-temporal (fusiform) gyrus**, which is separated from the limbic lobe by the collateral sulcus. The occipitotemporal gyrus, as its name implies, is partly in the occipital lobe and partly in the temporal lobe.

The temporal lobe is associated in a general way with four functions:

1. Part of the superior surface of the temporal lobe, continuing as a small area of the superior temporal gyrus, is the **primary auditory cortex.**
2. **Wernicke's area,** the posterior portion of the superior temporal gyrus of one hemisphere (usually the left), is important in the comprehension of language.
3. Much of the temporal lobe, particularly the inferior surface, is involved in higher order processing of visual information.
4. The most medial part of the temporal lobe[b] is involved in complex aspects of learning and memory.

The Occipital Lobe Contains Visual Areas

The lateral surface of the occipital lobe is of variable configuration, and its gyri are usually referred to simply as **lateral occipital gyri.** On the medial surface, the wedge-shaped area between the parietooccipital and calcarine sulci is called the **cuneus** (Latin for "wedge")

---

[b]The structures important in learning and memory (discussed in Chapter 23) are actually parts of the limbic lobe and underlying limbic-related structures and are not part of the temporal lobe as defined in this chapter. However, because of their gross anatomical location, these structures critical for memory are commonly referred to as *medial temporal.*

(Fig. 3-13). The gyrus inferior to the calcarine sulcus is the **lingual gyrus.** The lingual gyrus is adjacent to the posterior portion of the occipitotemporal gyrus, separated from it by the collateral sulcus, and usually continuous anteriorly with the **parahippocampal gyrus.** The transition from lingual to parahippocampal gyrus occurs at the **isthmus** of the cingulate gyrus (Fig. 3-14).

The occipital lobe is more or less exclusively concerned with visual functions. **Primary visual cortex** is contained in the walls of the calcarine sulcus and a bit of the surrounding cortex. The remainder of the lobe is referred to as **visual association cortex** and is involved in higher order processing of visual information; visual association cortex extends into the temporal lobe as well, reflecting the importance of vision in primates.

The Limbic Lobe Is Interconnected with Other Limbic Structures, Some Buried in the Temporal Lobe

The **limbic lobe** (see Fig. 3-14) is mostly composed of the **cingulate** and **parahippocampal gyri.** The cingulate gyrus, immediately superior to the corpus callosum, can be followed posteriorly to the splenium of the corpus callosum, where it turns inferiorly as the narrow isthmus of the cingulate gyrus and continues as the parahippocampal gyrus. These two gyri give the appearance of encircling the diencephalon and they, together with some small cortical areas near the lamina terminalis (paraterminal gyrus) and inferior to the genu of the corpus callosum (subcallosal area), make up the limbic lobe (from the Latin word *limbus,* meaning "border"). The anterior end of the parahippocampal gyrus hooks backward on itself, forming a medially directed bump called the **uncus.** The superior border of the parahippocampal gyrus is the **hippocampal sulcus** (see Fig. 3-24). Folded into the temporal lobe at the hippocampal sulcus is a differently structured area of cortex called the

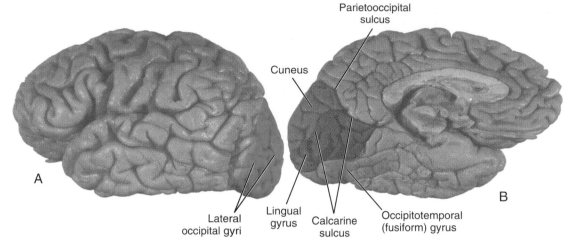

Figure 3-13 Lateral, medial, and inferior surfaces of the occipital lobe, seen from the side **(A)** and from medially and below **(B)**. *(Dissection courtesy of Grant Dahmer, Department of Cell Biology and Anatomy, University of Arizona College of Medicine.)*

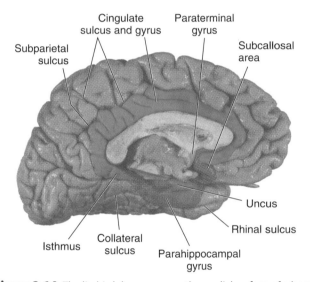

Figure 3-14 The limbic lobe as seen on the medial surface of a hemisected brain from which the brainstem and cerebellum were removed. The cingulate sulcus in most brains is separate from the subparietal sulcus, turning superiorly into a marginal branch and ending just behind the top of the central sulcus. About a third of the time (as in the brain in this figure), however, it gives off the marginal branch, then continues into the subparietal sulcus. *(Dissection courtesy of Grant Dahmer, Department of Cell Biology and Anatomy, University of Arizona College of Medicine.)*

hippocampus (Fig. 3-15). The limbic lobe is the cortical component of the **limbic system,** which is important in emotional responses, drive-related behavior, and memory.

The Diencephalon Includes the Thalamus and Hypothalamus

The diencephalon accounts for less than 2% of the weight of the brain, but nevertheless is extremely important. It has four divisions: **thalamus, hypothalamus, epithalamus,** and **subthalamus** (*thalamus* is Latin for "inner chamber"). Portions of three of these divisions can be seen on a hemisected brain (Fig. 3-16); the subthalamus is an internal structure that can be seen only in sections through the brain. The epithalamus comprises the midline **pineal gland** and several small nearby neural structures visible in sections.

The Thalamus Conveys Information to the Cerebral Cortex

The thalamus is an ovoid nuclear mass, part of which borders on the third ventricle. The line of attachment of the roof of this ventricle is marked by a horizontally oriented ridge, the **stria medullaris** ("white stripe") **of the thalamus.** Parts of the medial surfaces of the two thalami fuse in most younger brains in an area called the **interthalamic adhesion** or **massa intermedia.** (Because the massa intermedia is absent in many normal older brains, it apparently performs no unique function.) Posteriorly, the thalamus protrudes over the most superior portion of the brainstem. Anteriorly, it abuts the interventricular foramen.

The thalamus is a nuclear mass of major importance in most functional systems: Nearly every pathway carrying specific information bound for the cerebral cortex from a subcortical site includes a stop in the thalamus. No sensory information, with the exception of olfactory information, reaches the cerebral cortex without a synaptic stop in some part of the thalamus (see Fig. 3-28). In addition, the anatomical loops characteristic of motor systems, which involve pathways between the cerebellum and cerebral cortex and between basal nuclei and cerebral cortex, typically involve thalamic nuclei as well (see Figs. 3-34 and 3-35). Finally, limbic

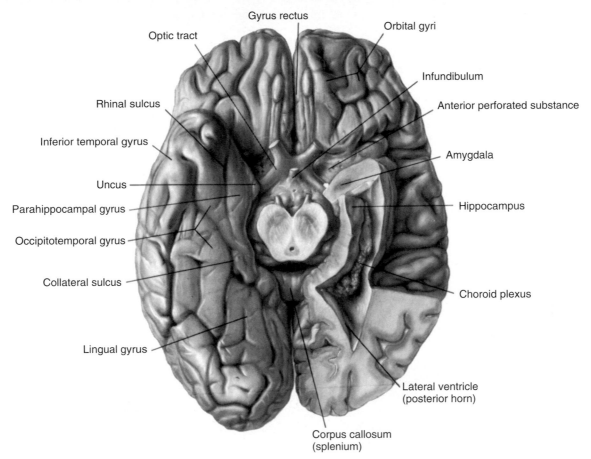

Figure 3-15 Dissection of the temporal lobe to demonstrate the hippocampus. The hippocampus is a specialized cortical area that has folded into the inferior horn of the lateral ventricle in the medial temporal (limbic) lobe. The anterior perforated area is an area of the base of the brain where many small blood vessels enter the forebrain. The rhinal sulcus often looks like an anterior continuation of the collateral sulcus (as in Fig. 3-8), but is actually a separate landmark. *(From Mettler FA: Neuroanatomy, ed 2, St. Louis, 1948, Mosby.)*

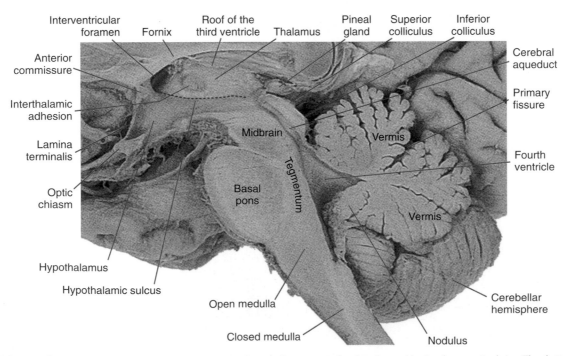

Figure 3-16 Major features of the diencephalon, brainstem, and cerebellum as seen in a hemisected brain, shown actual size. The dotted line in the wall of the third ventricle indicates the location of the hypothalamic sulcus.

projections to the cerebral cortex also traverse the thalamus.

The Hypothalamus Controls the Autonomic Nervous System

The hypothalamus is inferior and anterior (or rostral) to the thalamus, separated from it by the shallow **hypothalamic sulcus** in the wall of the third ventricle. It also forms the floor of this ventricle, and its inferior surface is one of the few parts of the diencephalon visible on an intact brain. This inferior surface (Figs. 3-17 and 3-18) includes the **infundibular stalk** (the connection between the hypothalamus and the pituitary gland) and two rounded protuberances called the **mammillary bodies.**

The hypothalamus is the major autonomic control center of the brain that is involved in a number of functions including regulating visceral responses, temperature, and even some limbic system functions.

Most Cranial Nerves Are Attached to the Brainstem

The brainstem plays major roles in cranial nerve functions, in conveying information to and from the forebrain, and in some special functions of its own. It is divided into the midbrain, the pons, and the medulla (see Fig. 3-2B). The **tectum** (Latin for "roof") of the midbrain, the portion posterior to the cerebral aqueduct,

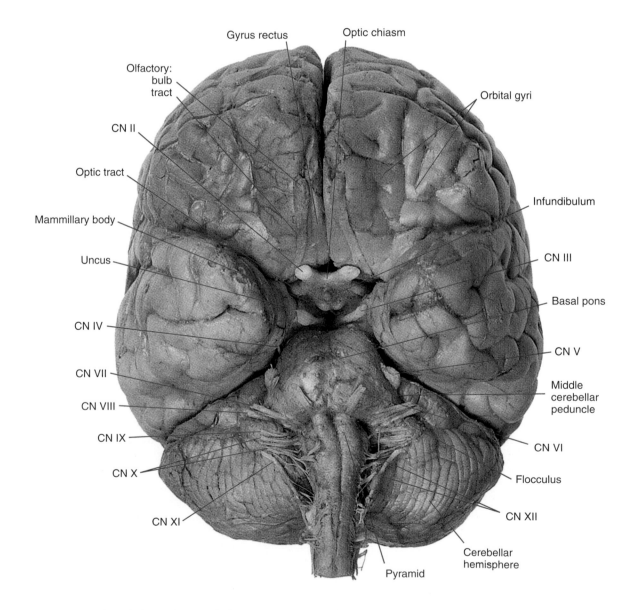

Figure 3-17 Inferior surface of a brain, showing the locations of cranial nerves II through XII. *(Dissection by Dr. Norman Koelling, University of Arizona College of Medicine.)*

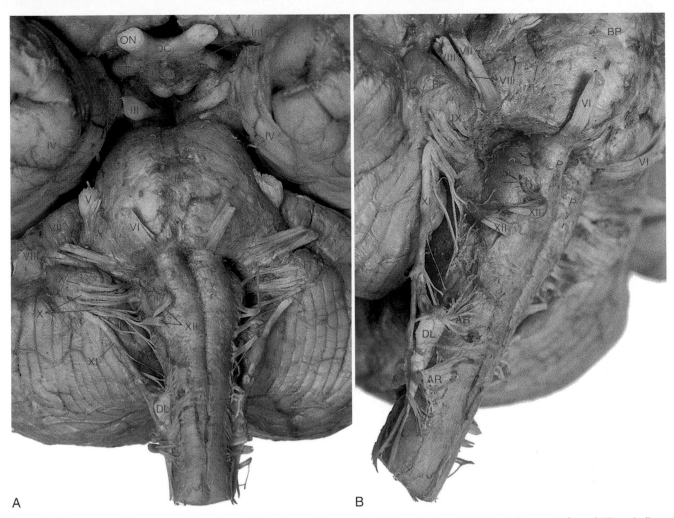

A   B

Figure 3-18 Closeups of the anterior **(A)** and lateral **(B)** surfaces of the same brain shown in Figure 3-17. Cranial nerves III through XII are indicated by Roman numerals. AR, cervical anterior root; BP, basal pons; CP, cerebral peduncle; DL, dentate ligament (suspensory ligament of the spinal cord); FI, flocculus; Inf, infundibulum (former attachment of the pituitary gland); MB, mammillary body; MCP, middle cerebellar peduncle; OC, optic chiasm; OI, olive; ON, optic nerve (cranial nerve II); OT, optic tract; Pyr, pyramid; U, uncus; VIIi, intermediate nerve (part of the facial nerve). *(Dissection by Dr. Norman Koelling, University of Arizona College of Medicine.)*

consists of paired bumps called the **superior** and **inferior colliculi** (Latin for "little hills"). The paired **cerebral peduncles** make up most of the remainder of the midbrain (see Figs. 3-23 and 3-24). The pons consists of a protruding **basal pons,** oval in sagittal section, and the overlying **pontine tegmentum,** which forms part of the floor of the fourth ventricle. The medulla consists of a rostral **open** portion, containing part of the fourth ventricle, and a caudal **closed** portion, continuous with the spinal cord (see Fig. 3-16).

The points of attachment of most cranial nerves, as well as additional brainstem structures, can be seen in an inferior view of the brain (see Figs. 3-17 and 3-18). The **olfactory tract** is located in the olfactory sulcus, lateral to gyrus rectus, and is attached directly to the cerebral hemisphere. **Cranial nerve I (olfactory)** is actually a collection of bundles of very fine axons called **olfactory fila** (Latin for "olfactory threads") that termi-

nate in the **olfactory bulb** at the anterior end of the tract. Slightly posterior to the attachment points of the olfactory tracts, the **optic nerves (cranial nerve II)** join to form the **optic chiasm,** in which half the fibers of each nerve cross to the opposite side (see Fig. 17-26). The **optic tract** proceeds from the optic chiasm to the thalamus. Embryologically, the optic nerves are outgrowths of the diencephalon (see Chapter 2) and properly are tracts of the CNS, but they are treated as cranial nerves because of their course outside the rest of the brain. Considered in this way, cranial nerve II is the only one that projects directly to the diencephalon.

Located farther posteriorly are the cerebral peduncles of the midbrain, each of which contains a massive fiber bundle that carries a great deal of the descending projection from the cerebral cortex to the brainstem and spinal cord. **Cranial nerve III (oculomotor)** emerges into the **interpeduncular fossa** between the cerebral peduncles. **Cranial nerve IV (trochlear)** emerges from the posterior surface of the brainstem just caudal to the inferior colliculi, then proceeds anteriorly through the space between the brainstem and the cerebral hemisphere.

Caudally, the cerebral peduncles disappear into the transversely oriented basal pons. Posterolaterally, the basal pons narrows into a large fiber bundle that enters the cerebellum. This is the **middle cerebellar peduncle (brachium pontis,** or "arm of the pons"), which carries the major input from the opposite cerebral hemisphere to the cerebellum by way of relays in the pontine nuclei (see Fig. 3-34). **Cranial nerve V (trigeminal)** emerges from the lateral aspect of the basal pons. **Cranial nerve VI (abducens)** emerges near the midline at the caudal edge of the pons. **Cranial nerves VII (facial)** and **VIII (vestibulocochlear)** emerge more laterally near the cerebellum, at the caudal edge of the pons. The area of attachment of cranial nerves VII and VIII is called the **cerebellopontine angle** and is a common site of development of tumors, particularly tumors of the Schwann cells of cranial nerve VIII.

Caudal to the pons are two thick fiber bundles that resemble the cerebral peduncles but are considerably smaller. These are the **pyramids** of the medulla, which carry those fibers of the cerebral peduncles destined for the spinal cord. The two pyramids decussatee[c] in the area of transition from brainstem to spinal cord. Posterolateral to each pyramid is an ovoid protuberance called the **olive. Cranial nerve XII (hypoglossal)** emerges from the sulcus between the pyramid and the olive. The more or less continuous series of filaments that will form **cranial nerves IX (glossopharyngeal)** and **X (vagus)** emerge from the sulcus posterior to the olive. **Cranial nerve XI (accessory)** emerges from the upper cervical spinal cord and ascends into the skull through the foramen magnum before reversing course and heading back into the neck.

The Cerebellum Includes a Vermis and Two Hemispheres

The cerebellum can be subdivided in several different ways (see Chapter 20), two of which are briefly considered here. In one sense the cerebellum comprises a midline **vermis,** which is hemisected in a hemisected brain (see Fig. 3-16), and a much larger, lateral

---

[c]A *decussation* is a site where nerve fibers joining unlike areas of the CNS cross, such as where fibers cross on their way from one side of the forebrain to the opposite side of the spinal cord. In contrast, a *commissure* is a crossing site for fibers connecting similar areas, such as the corpus callosum, a massive commissure that interconnects cortical areas.

hemisphere on each side (see Fig. 3-16). Using any other method of subdividing the cerebellum, a given division has both a vermal and a hemispheral component.

Lobes of the cerebellum, which roughly correspond to separate functional areas, are also recognized. The **anterior lobe** is that portion anterior to the **primary fissure** (see Fig. 3-16). This lobe receives a large proportion of its afferent inputs from the spinal cord and plays a prominent role in coordinating trunk and limb movements. The **flocculonodular lobe** consists of three small components: the **nodulus,** which is the vermal portion of the lobe (see Fig. 3-16), and a small **flocculus** on each side near the vestibulocochlear nerve (see Fig. 3-17). The nodulus is actually continuous with the flocculus of each side, but this continuity is difficult to see without dissecting the cerebellum. The flocculonodular lobe receives afferent inputs from the vestibular system and is involved in controlling eye movements and postural adjustments to gravity. All of the cerebellum posterior to the primary fissure, exclusive of the flocculonodular lobe, constitutes the **posterior lobe,** which is the largest of the three lobes. The posterior lobe receives the majority of the afferent input from the cerebral cortex by way of relays in **pontine nuclei** and transmission through the middle cerebellar peduncle. This lobe also plays a prominent role in the coordination of voluntary movements. (In reality, cerebellar function is not quite so neatly parceled out among these anatomical subdivisions, as discussed in more detail in Chapter 20.)

Sections of the Forebrain Reveal the Basal Nuclei and Limbic Structures

Many Parts of Each Cerebral Hemisphere Are Arranged in a C Shape

Before consideration of the internal structures of the brain, it is useful to discuss one of the major consequences of the shape of the cerebral hemispheres. As a result of the embryological development of the hemispheres (see Fig. 2-12), the cortical lobes are arranged in a C shape from the frontal lobe, through the parietal and occipital lobes, and into the temporal lobe. A number of other structures, such as the lateral ventricles (Fig. 3-19A), are similarly C-shaped, with the result that sections through the brain may cut these structures in two different places. The hippocampus, together with its efferent fiber bundle (the **fornix**), is another example (see Fig. 3-19B). The hippocampus is folded into the temporal lobe, forming part of the wall of the lateral ventricle there (see Fig. 3-15). It becomes smaller as the temporal lobe curves into the parietal lobe, and it ends near the splenium of the corpus callosum. The fornix continues this curved course, arching anteriorly under the corpus callosum, then turning inferiorly and

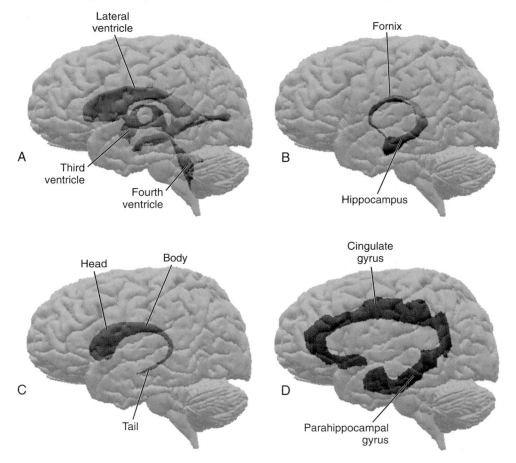

Figure 3-19 Four examples of C-shaped telencephalic structures: the lateral ventricle **(A)**, hippocampus/fornix system **(B)**, caudate nucleus **(C)**, and limbic lobe **(D)**. *(Courtesy Dr. John W. Sundsten, University of Washington School of Medicine.)*

posteriorly toward the hypothalamus, where many of its fibers end in the mammillary bodies.

The Caudate Nucleus, Putamen, and Globus Pallidus Are Major Components of the Basal Nuclei

The basal nuclei (ganglia) are a group of nuclei that lie deep to the cerebral cortex in each hemisphere. The major basal nuclei are the **caudate** and **lenticular nuclei** (together with some brainstem structures with which they are interconnected). The caudate nucleus, another example of a C-shaped structure, has an enlarged **head** deep in the frontal lobe, and its increasingly attenuated **body** and **tail** follow the lateral ventricle around into the temporal lobe (see Fig. 3-19C). The lenticular nucleus, which is subdivided into the **putamen** and the **globus pallidus,** lies lateral and partially anterior to the thalamus. It is separated from the thalamus and from much of the head of the caudate nucleus by a thick sheet of fibers called the **internal capsule.** The internal capsule contains most of the fibers interconnecting the cerebral cortex and deep structures such as the thalamus, basal nuclei, and brainstem.

The Amygdala and Hippocampus Are Major Limbic Structures

The **amygdala,** another nucleus contained within each cerebral hemisphere, together with the hippocampus are major components of the limbic system. The amygdala lies beneath the uncus of the temporal lobe (see Fig. 3-22). The hippocampus extends posteriorly from the level of the amygdala, underlying the medial temporal lobe.

Cerebral Structures Are Arranged Systematically

Figs. 3-20 to 3-25 are intended as an introduction to the configuration of internal structures of the brain. Each section is in a coronal plane and has been stained for myelin, thus differentiating gray matter from white matter. Only major structures are labeled, but the same sections are presented in more detail elsewhere in this book and in a companion atlas, *The Human Brain in*

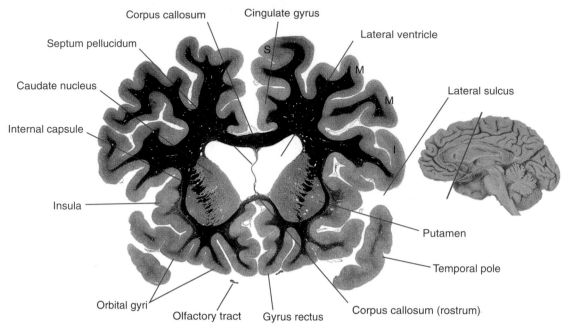

Corpus callosum   Cingulate gyrus
Septum pellucidum   Lateral ventricle
Caudate nucleus
                                          Lateral sulcus
Internal capsule
Insula
                                          Putamen
                                          Temporal pole
Orbital gyri   Corpus callosum (rostrum)
        Olfactory tract   Gyrus rectus

Figure 3-20 Sections through the frontal lobes. Inferior to the body of the corpus callosum is the septum pellucidum, a thin, bilaminar membrane that intervenes between the corpus callosum and the fornix and separates portions of the two lateral ventricles. At this level, which is anterior to the diencephalon, the basal nuclei are represented by the putamen and the head of the caudate nucleus, with part of the internal capsule between them. Inferiorly, note the continuity between these nuclei. I, Inferior frontal gyrus; M, middle frontal gyrus; S, superior frontal gyrus.

Photographs and Diagrams, ed 4. Figure 3-26 diagrams the interrelationships (and some of the functions) of the major structures that make up the CNS.

Parts of the Nervous System Are Interconnected in Systematic Ways (Generalizations)

The functional subdivisions of the CNS discussed thus far (see Fig. 3-26) interact with one another as the substrate for perception, motivation, and behavior. Despite the seemingly impenetrable thicket of interconnections among neurons in the nervous system (see Fig. 1-17), there are in fact some "wiring principles" that govern many of these interconnections. This section is an overview of such principles, primarily using somatic sensation and body movement as examples. None of these wiring principles is an absolute rule; rather, much like the "rules" of English grammar and spelling, they are guidelines rife with exceptions. Nevertheless, such general guidelines may be helpful in navigating subsequent chapters.

Axons of Primary Afferents and Lower Motor Neurons Convey Information to and From the CNS

Peripheral nerves, including the cranial nerves, are the electrical "cables" through which the CNS communicates with the body. Some peripheral nerve axons are those of **primary afferents,**[d] fibers that convey information into the CNS from the periphery. Others are axons of **lower motor neurons,** fibers that convey messages to skeletal muscles directing them to contract. (Peripheral nerves also contain autonomic fibers, contacting visceral structures. These are not included in this discussion but, as described in Chapters 10 and 23, similar wiring principles apply to them.)

Axons of Primary Afferents Enter the CNS Without Crossing the Midline

The only way the CNS can receive information about things touching the skin, or about the position of limbs, is as information conveyed by axons in peripheral nerves. Each primary afferent neuron involved has its cell body in a sensory ganglion, a peripherally directed process ending in skin, a muscle, or a joint, and a central process ending in the CNS (Fig. 3-27). Primary afferents terminate in the CNS on second-order neurons, which in turn project to third-order neurons. With few exceptions, the receptive ending, cell body, and central terminals of a primary afferent are all on the same side. That is, the central process ends on the side **ipsilateral**[e] (Latin for "same side") to the cell body.

---

[d]*Afferent* and *efferent* refer to the direction of information flow in an axon, relative to some structure. Hence axons that convey information from structure A to structure B are both efferent from structure A and afferent to structure B.

[e]*Ipsilateral* and *contralateral* are relative terms, just like *afferent* and *efferent*. Any site in the nervous system is ipsilateral to some structures and contralateral to others.

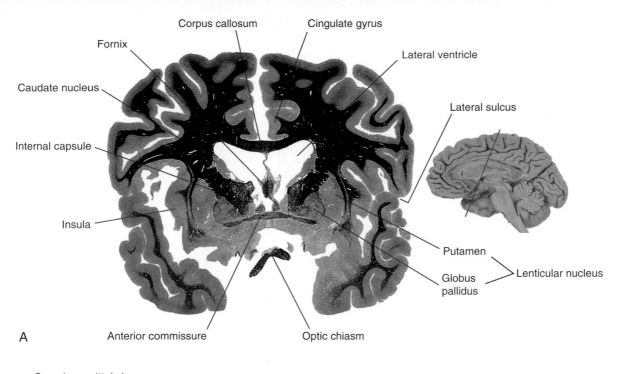

A

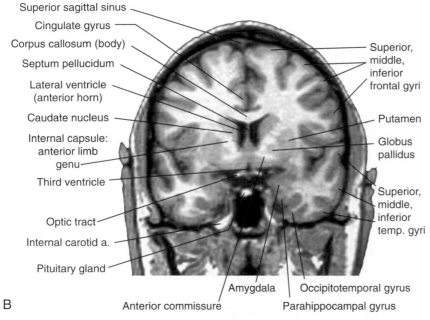

B

Figure 3-21 Sections through the anterior commissure, which interconnects portions of the temporal lobes, as well as certain olfactory structures. At this level both parts of the lenticular nucleus (the putamen and the globus pallidus) are present. **A,** The section is at the anterior end of both the interventricular foramen and the thalamus and cuts through the fornix tangentially as it curves down toward the hypothalamus. **B,** Magnetic resonance image. (**B** *from Nolte J, Angevine JB Jr: The human brain in photographs and diagrams, ed 4, Philadelphia, 2013, Elsevier Saunders. Courtesy Dr. Elena M. Plante.*)

Axons of Lower Motor Neurons Leave the CNS Without Crossing the Midline

Similarly, the only way the CNS can induce muscles to contract is by way of messages conveyed by axons of lower motor neurons. Lower motor neurons have their cell bodies within the CNS and axons that travel through peripheral nerves to end (again, with few exceptions) on ipsilateral muscle fibers (see Fig. 3-27).

Somatosensory Inputs Participate in Reflexes, Pathways to the Cerebellum, and Pathways to the Cerebral Cortex

Most types of sensory information do at least three different things. They feed into local functions such as reflexes, and they distribute to both the cerebral cortex (via the thalamus) and the cerebellum. An individual

Text continued on p. 78

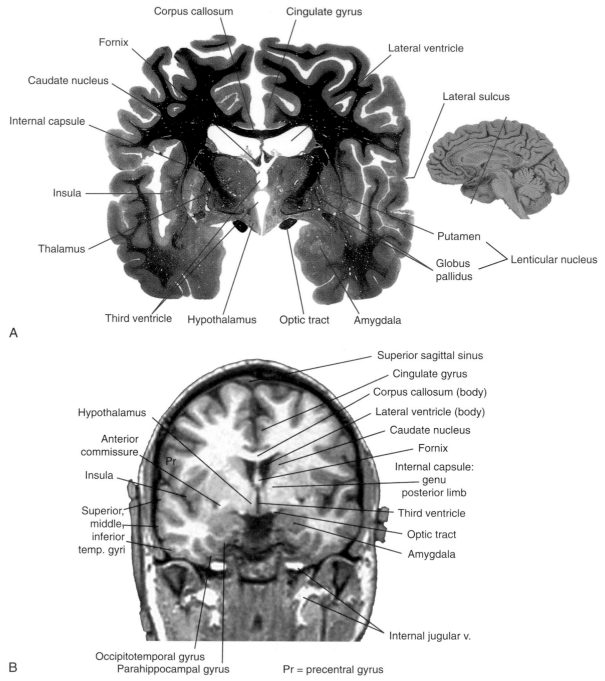

Figure 3-22 Section through the anterior part of the diencephalon. Parts of both the thalamus and the hypothalamus can be seen. At this level and at more posterior levels, the internal capsule is found between the lenticular nucleus and the thalamus. The third ventricle can be seen in the midline, above and below the interthalamic adhesion. **A,** The section passes through the anterior part of the uncus, revealing the amygdala. **B,** Magnetic resonance image. (*B from Nolte J, Angevine JB Jr: The human brain in photographs and diagrams, ed 4, Philadelphia, 2013, Elsevier Saunders. Courtesy Dr. Elena M. Plante.*)

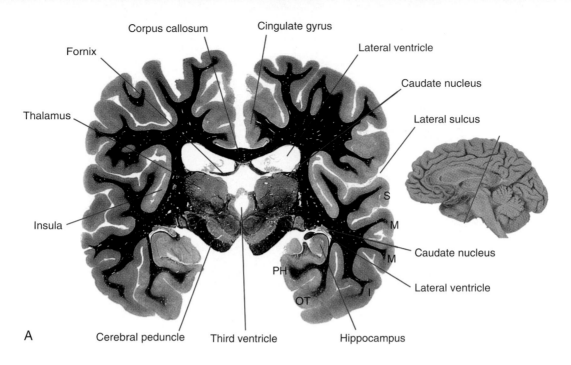

A

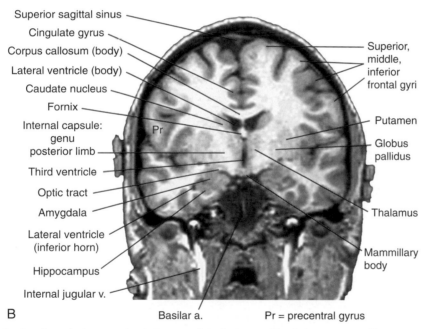

B

Pr = precentral gyrus

Figure 3-23 Section through the posterior thalamus and the brainstem. The thalamus is partially posterior to the lenticular nucleus, accounting for the presence of one but not the other at this level. The section is also posterior to the uncus, and the amygdala has been replaced by the hippocampus. **A,** The caudate nucleus and lateral ventricle can now be seen in two places; because of their C shapes, they were transected twice in this and the next section. **B,** Magnetic resonance image. I, inferior temporal gyrus; M, middle temporal gyrus; OT, occipitotemporal gyrus; PH, parahippocampal gyrus; S, superior temporal gyrus. (*B from Nolte J, Angevine JB Jr: The human brain in photographs and diagrams, ed 4, Philadelphia, 2013, Elsevier Saunders. Courtesy Dr. Elena M. Plante.*)

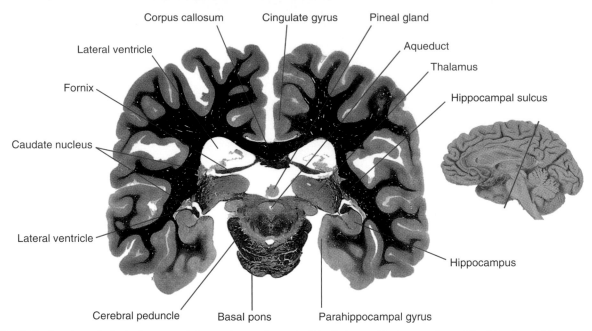

Figure 3-24 Section through the brainstem and the most posterior part of the thalamus. The two portions of the lateral ventricle on each side are closer together than in previous sections because the posterior edge of their C shape is being approached. The thalamus protrudes posteriorly and is superior and lateral to part of the midbrain.

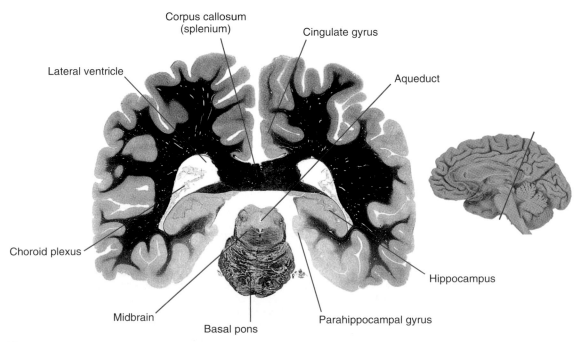

Figure 3-25 Section through the splenium of the corpus callosum. The lateral ventricle is no longer cut in two places because this section is tangential to the posterior edge of its C shape. The final portion of the hippocampus can be seen as it ends near the splenium.

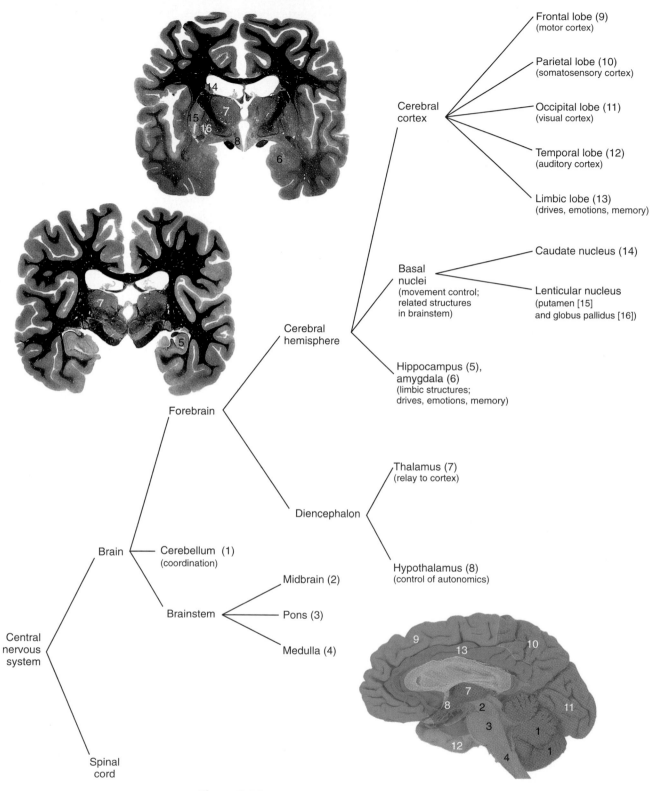

Figure 3-26 Overview of the subdivisions of the CNS.

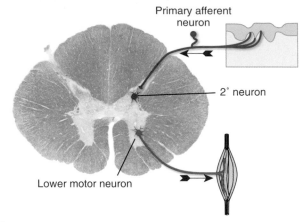

Figure 3-27 Wiring pattern of primary afferents and lower motor neurons.

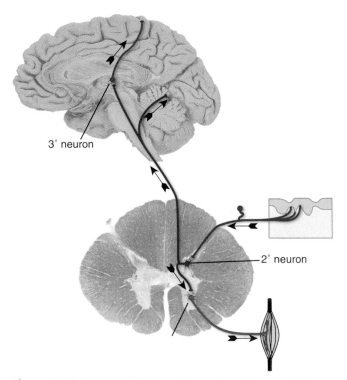

Figure 3-28 Typical distribution pattern of somatosensory information (and other types of sensory information) to reflex arcs, the cerebellum, and the cerebral cortex (via the thalamus). This is a schematic depiction of this distribution. In reality, single second-order neurons do not typically project in these three different ways. Instead, primary afferents distribute multiple branches to an assortment of interneurons and projection neurons.

primary afferent, together with the interneurons with which it is connected, commonly does all three (Fig. 3-28); that is, we have just one set of primary afferents, and these provide inputs to multiple CNS circuits. For simplicity, primary afferents are often drawn as though each has but a single central process, whereas in reality they typically have hundreds of branches.

The somatosensory system provides a nice example of this distribution in three different spheres. *Somato-*

sensory literally means "body sense," and encompasses several different types of sensation, including pain, temperature, simple touch, proprioception (perception of position), kinesthesia (perception of movement), and stereognosis (perception of the size and shape of objects by touch). In addition to sending their information to the thalamus and cerebellum, somatosensory afferents feed into things like stretch reflexes (e.g., the familiar knee-jerk reflex) and withdrawal reflexes (e.g., pulling away from something painful, blinking in response to something touching a cornea).

Somatosensory Pathways to the Cerebral Cortex Cross the Midline and Pass Through the Thalamus

Somatosensory *pathways* on their way to the cerebral cortex (not necessarily individual *fibers*) typically cross the midline someplace between their origin and their destination so that, for example, information about one hand reaches the **contralateral** (Latin for "opposite side") postcentral gyrus. This crossing of sensory pathways is a curious and unexplained fact of vertebrate evolution.[f] It applies not only to those pathways representing spinal nerves but often to those representing cranial nerves as well (except for taste and olfaction; see Chapter 13). A number of hypotheses have been advanced to explain this phenomenon, including the notion that it is an early evolutionary mistake still awaiting correction (Sasha N. Zill: Personal communication, 1977). Whatever its explanation, it would be even more peculiar if information from the *right* hand reached the left cerebral hemisphere, which in turn controlled the *left* hand. This is not the case, however, because descending pathways also cross the midline at some point between their origins and their terminations (see Fig. 3-33).

The thalamus and cerebral cortex of each side reside in the same half of the forebrain, and thalamocortical fibers are uncrossed. Because primary afferents are also uncrossed, this implies that the shortest path to the cerebral cortex is three neurons long: a primary afferent, a neuron that crosses the midline, and a thalamic neuron (Fig. 3-29). The location in the CNS where the midline crossing takes place is different for different pathways, and knowledge of these crossover points can be crucial in deciding where a lesion is. In the case of the somatosensory system, for example, the pain and temperature pathway crosses at a different level than the main pathway for touch (Fig. 3-30). Note that one-sided damage affecting these two pathways at level A would have the curious result of diminution of touch on the

---

[f]Not only is it curious, it may not even be necessary for proper functioning of the CNS. Rare cases have been reported of humans born without such crossing, or even with some pathways crossed and others uncrossed, but with normal sensation and dexterity.

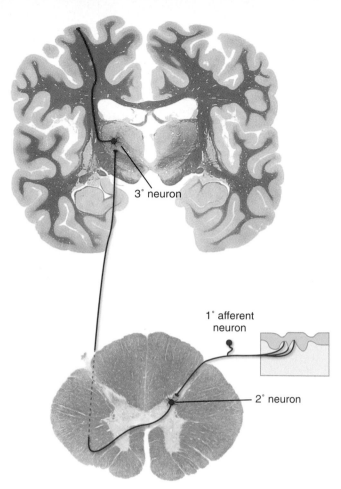

Figure 3-29 The shortest sensory pathway from the periphery to the cerebral cortex.

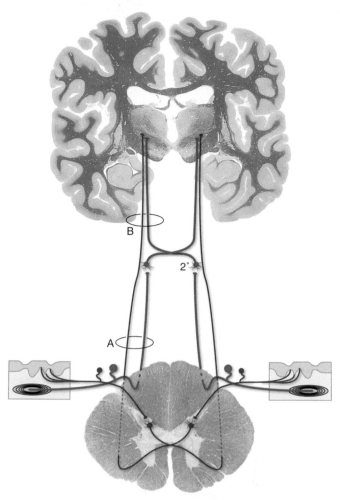

Figure 3-30 Implications of different sensory pathways crossing the midline at different CNS levels. In the somatosensory system, the second-order neurons for the principal pain/temperature pathway (the spinotha-lamic tract; *blue*) are located in the spinal cord and cross there. In contrast, the second-order neurons for the principal touch/position pathway (the posterior column–medial lemniscus pathway; *green*) are located in the medulla. Hence damage to one side of the spinal cord *(A)* would cause diminution of touch on the side ipsilateral to the lesion and diminution of pain on the side contralateral to the lesion. Damage rostral to the medulla *(B)*, on the other hand, would cause diminution of both touch and pain on the side contralateral to the lesion.

side ipsilateral to the lesion and diminution of pain on the side contralateral to the lesion. Reflexes would be unaffected because they are mediated by local connections near the level of entry of the primary afferents.

Somatosensory Cortex Contains a Distorted Map of the Body

Somatosensory information from different parts of the body enters the spinal cord at different levels (see Figs. 10-4 and 10-19). Representations of different parts within a pathway thereafter remain contiguous but separate (e.g., Fig. 10-22). The end result is that the contralateral half of the body is mapped out systematically in each postcentral gyrus in a little humanoid **somatotopic** map called a **homunculus** (Latin for "little human"). The map is spatially distorted, however, emphasizing areas such as the fingertips and lips, for which somatosensory acuity is most important (Fig. 3-31A). Systematic, distorted maps are a repeated theme in the CNS; many cases in which they have not been found are probably simply reflections of our not knowing which parameter to map.

Each Side of the Cerebellum Receives Information About the Ipsilateral Side of the Body

The cerebellum receives large amounts of sensory information and uses it not in perceptual processes but rather in helping with the design and coordination of movements; somatosensory information is particularly germane. The cerebellum is also a major exception to the generalization about pathways crossing the midline: a given side of the cerebellum is related to the ipsilateral side of the body. One of the anatomical bases for this uncrossed relationship is that somatosensory pathways from the periphery to the cerebellum are typically uncrossed. Somatosensory pathways

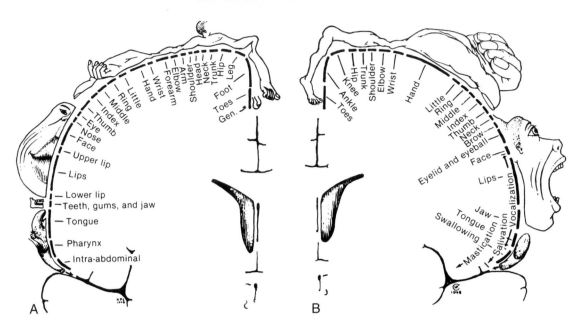

Figure 3-31 Somatotopic mapping in human somatosensory **(A)** and motor **(B)** cortex obtained by electrical stimulation of the surface of the brains of conscious patients during neurosurgery. The size of a given part of the homunculus is roughly proportional to the size of the cortical area devoted to that body part. *(From Penfield W, Rasmussen T: The cerebral cortex of man. © 1950 Macmillan Publishing Co., Inc., renewed 1978 by T. Rasmussen.)*

from the periphery to the cerebellum do not pass through the thalamus and can involve as few as two neurons (Fig. 3-32).

Other Sensory Systems Are Similar to the Somatosensory System

The somatosensory system is one of the better understood sensory systems, but others are organized according to similar anatomical principles—primary afferents that terminate without crossing, participation in reflexes, pathways to the cerebral cortex that involve at least three neurons and a relay in the thalamus, distorted maps, and projections to the cerebellum. One area of variability is the pattern of crossing the midline. Some systems project bilaterally to the thalamus. For example, the inputs from both ears need to be compared to localize sound; this comparison begins to take place in the brainstem, and each ear is represented bilaterally in the brainstem, thalamus, and cerebral cortex. The olfactory,[g] taste, and some visceral pathways are uncrossed, for reasons as unclear as those for the crossing of other pathways. Most or all kinds of sensory information reach the cerebellum, but many of the connections involved are not as well understood as the somatosensory connections.

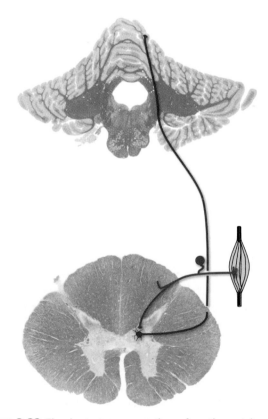

Figure 3-32 The shortest sensory pathway from the periphery to the cerebellum.

[g]The olfactory pathway is also unusual in bypassing the thalamus, at least initially. The olfactory bulb is an outgrowth of the telencephalon, and the olfactory nerve projects directly to it, and from there to certain cortical areas.

Higher Levels of the CNS Influence the Activity of Lower Motor Neurons

Lower motor neurons are subject to a variety of influences, such as reflex circuitry and descending impulses from the brainstem (e.g., the automatic posture adjustment signals from the vestibular nuclei). Most important in terms of voluntary movement is the **corticospinal tract,** a collection of fibers that, as the name implies, descend from cell bodies in motor areas of the cerebral cortex and terminate in the spinal cord. These are often referred to clinically as **upper motor neurons.**[h] Systematic maps are found in motor cortex just as in somatosensory cortex, and the cell bodies of corticospinal neurons are distributed in the precentral gyrus in a pattern parallel to the somatosensory homunculus (see Fig. 3-31B). Damage to the corticospinal tract causes weakness of half of the body, even though reflexes may still be functional (or even exaggerated).

The cerebellum and basal nuclei also influence movement but have few or no outputs of their own that reach the spinal cord. Rather, they act indirectly by affecting the activity of motor areas of the cerebral cortex. Damage to the cerebellum or basal nuclei leaves motor cortex and lower motor neurons intact, so movements are defective—they may, for example, be slow or uncoordinated—but weakness is not prominent.

Corticospinal Axons Cross the Midline

Just as somatosensory pathways cross the midline between the periphery and the cerebral cortex, so too does the corticospinal tract (Fig. 3-33). Hence damage to one cerebral hemisphere can result in both somatosensory deficits and weakness in the contralateral arm and leg. A relay in the thalamus is not required for outputs from the cortex, so single neurons with very long axons project all the way from motor cortex to the contralateral half of the spinal cord.

Each Side of the Cerebellum Indirectly Affects Movements of the Ipsilateral Side of the Body

The cerebellum (discussed further in Chapter 20), in a very general sense, helps to plan the details of movements and to correct them while they are still in progress. For example, to lift a glass to your lips you need to contract your biceps and relax your triceps, both by just the right amount at just the right time; as the glass approaches your lips, you need to make fine adjustments in its trajectory. The cerebellum plays a role in both processes. To do so, it needs to know not only what you intend to do (i.e., input from the cerebral cortex),

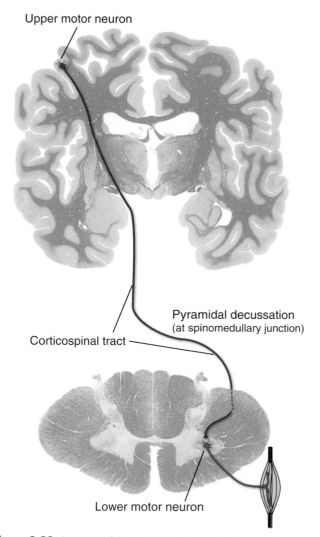

Figure 3-33 Overview of the corticospinal tract. Corticospinal neurons project directly to the spinal cord, bypassing the thalamus.

but also the moment-to-moment position of your arm (i.e., somatosensory inputs). Cerebellar outputs return to motor cortex, affecting corticospinal activity; this requires a stop in the thalamus. The final element in the general pattern of cerebellar connectivity is dictated by the fact that one side of the cerebellum is related to the ipsilateral side of the body. Because one side of the forebrain is related to the contralateral side of the body, this means that pathways interconnecting the cerebellum and forebrain must cross the midline (Fig. 3-34). Because cerebellar outputs are directed toward motor cortex (via the thalamus), cerebellar damage causes problems with movement but not with sensation.

The Basal Nuclei of One Side Indirectly Affect Movements of the Contralateral Side of the Body

The basal nuclei also participate in the planning of movements, although in a somewhat different way than the cerebellum does (see Chapter 19). Like the cerebellum, the basal nuclei receive input from the cerebral

---

[h]For the purposes of this discussion, *corticospinal neurons* are synonymous with *upper motor neurons.* As will be discussed further in subsequent chapters, however, the two terms are often used variably and inconsistently.

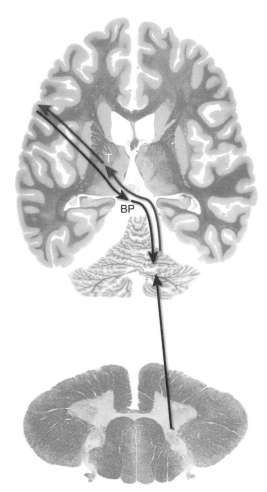

Figure 3-34 Overview of cerebellar connections, explained in more detail in Chapter 20. (The spinal cord section is inverted relative to its appearance in most other sections in this book, so that anterior is up in both parts of the figure.) BP, basal pons; T, thalamus.

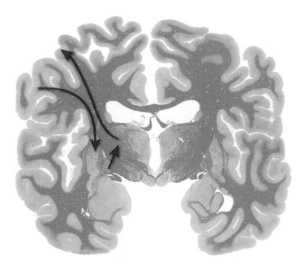

Figure 3-35 Overview of the major circuit involved in basal nuclei functions, explained in more detail in Chapter 19. Because the basal nuclei of one hemisphere influence motor cortex of the ipsilateral hemisphere, damage to the basal nuclei on one side can cause a contralateral movement disorder.

cortex and then influence movement by affecting the output of motor cortex (Fig. 3-35). One set of this cortex–basal nuclei–thalamus circuitry resides in each half of the forebrain, so damage to the basal nuclei on one side causes problems with movement on the contralateral side. The basal nuclei are not prominently involved in adjusting ongoing movements, so they do not receive sensory information as directly as the cerebellum does (compare Figs. 3-34 and 3-35).

SUGGESTED READINGS

Amoiridis G, et al: Patients with horizontal gaze palsy and progressive scoliosis due to ROBO3 E319K mutation have both uncrossed and crossed central nervous system pathways and perform normally on neuropsychological testing. J Neurol Neurosurg Psychiatry 77:1047, 2006.
  A remarkable report of two brothers with crossed spinothalamic tracts, uncrossed dorsal column-medial lemniscus and corticospinal pathways, and normal sensation and dexterity.

Anastasi G, et al: In vivo basal ganglia volumetry through application of NURBS models to MR images. Neuroradiology 48:338, 2006.

Armstrong E: Brains, bodies and metabolism. Brain Behav Evol 36:166, 1990.

Blinkov SM, Glezer II: The human brain in figures and tables, New York, 1968, Plenum Press and Basic Books.

Chiavaras MM, Petrides M: Orbitofrontal sulci of the human and macaque monkey brain. J Comp Neurol 422:35, 2000.

DeArmond SJ, Fusco MM, Dewey MM: Structure of the human brain: a photographic atlas, ed 3, New York, 1989, Oxford University Press.

Dekaban AS, Sadowsky D: Changes in brain weights during the span of human life: relation of brain weights to body heights and body weights. Ann Neurol 4:345, 1978.

Duvernoy HM: The human brain: surface, three-dimensional sectional anatomy and MRI, ed 2, Vienna, 1999, Springer-Verlag.

Gluhbegovic N, Williams TH: The human brain: a photographic guide, New York, 1980, Harper and Row.
  Includes a series of beautiful dissections.

Herculano-Houzel S: The human brain in numbers: a linearly scaled-up primate brain. Front Hum Neurosci 3:31, 2009.

Herculano-Houzel S: The remarkable, yet not extraordinary, human brain as a scaled-up primate brain and its associated cost. PNAS 109(Suppl 1):10661, 2012.

Igarashi S, Kamiya T: Atlas of the vertebrate brain: morphological evolution from cyclostomes to mammals, Baltimore, 1972, University Park Press.
  Ever wonder what an anteater's brain looks like?

Kruggel F: MRI-based volumetry of head compartments: normative values of healthy adults. Neuroimage 30:1, 2006.

Ludwig E, Klingler J: Atlas cerebri humani, Boston, 1956, Little, Brown.
  A series of technically spectacular dissections of human brains.

Mai JK, Assheuer J, Paxinos G: Atlas of the human brain, ed 2, San Diego, 2004, Academic Press.

Makris N, et al: Human cerebellum: surface-assisted cortical parcellation and volumetry with magnetic resonance imaging. J Cog Neurosci 15:584, 2003.

Nieuwenhuys R, Voogd J, van Hurjzen C: The human central nervous system: a synopsis and atlas, ed 4, New York, 2007, Springer.
  Includes many beautiful drawings of the brain and various subsystems of the CNS.

Nolte J, Angevine JB, Jr: The human brain in photographs and diagrams, ed 4, Philadelphia, 2013, Elsevier Saunders.

Ono M, Kubik S, Abernathey CD: Atlas of the cerebral sulci, New York, 1990, Thieme Medical Publishers.
A good place to get a sense of the variability of the cortical surface from one brain to another.

Schnitzlein HN, Murtagh FR: Imaging anatomy of the head and spine: a photographic color atlas of MRI, CT, gross, and microscopic anatomy in axial, coronal, and sagittal planes, ed 2, Baltimore, 1990, Urban and Schwarzenberg.

Toro R, et al: Brain size and folding of the human cerebral cortex. Cereb Cortex 18:2352, 2008.

Türe U, et al: Topographic anatomy of the insular region. J Neurosurg 90:720, 1999.

Vulliemoz S, Raineteau S, Jabaudon D: Reaching beyond the midline: why are human brains cross wired? Lancet Neurol 4:87, 2005.

Woolsey TA, Hanaway J, Gado MH: The brain atlas: a visual guide to the human central nervous system, ed 3, Hoboken, 2007, Wiley.

Meningeal Coverings of the Brain and Spinal Cord

Living brain is on the soft and mushy side, despite the network of cytoskeletal proteins contained in neurons and glial cells. Without support of some kind, the central nervous system (CNS) would be unable to maintain its shape, particularly as we walk and run around and occasionally bump our heads. The brain and spinal cord are protected from outside forces by their encasement in the skull and vertebral column, respectively. In addition, the CNS is suspended within a series of three membranous coverings, the **meninges** (from the Greek word *meninx,* meaning "membrane"), that stabilize the shape and position of the CNS in two different ways during head and body movements. First, the brain is mechanically suspended within the meninges, which in turn are anchored to the skull, so that the brain is constrained to move with the head. Second, there is a layer of **cerebrospinal fluid** (CSF) within the meninges; the buoyant effect of this fluid environment greatly decreases the tendency of various forces (e.g., gravity) to distort the brain. Thus a brain that weighs 1500 g in air effectively weighs less than 50 g in its normal CSF environment, where it is easily able to maintain its shape. In contrast, an isolated fresh brain, unsupported by its usual surroundings, becomes seriously distorted and may even tear under the influence of gravity (Fig. 4-1).

There Are Three Meningeal Layers: The Dura Mater, Arachnoid, and Pia Mater

The three meninges, from the outermost layer inward, are the **dura mater,** the **arachnoid mater,** and the **pia mater** (Fig. 4-2). In common usage, the "mater" is often

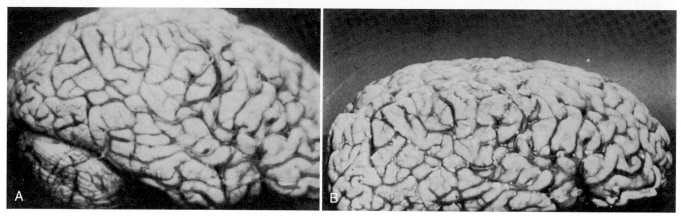

Figure 4-1 Effects of gravity and of partial flotation on brain. **A,** An unfixed human brain in a vat of isotonic saline; normal shape is maintained. **B,** The same brain in air, obviously distorted by its own weight. *(From Oldendorf W: The quest for an image of brain, New York, 1980, Raven Press.)*

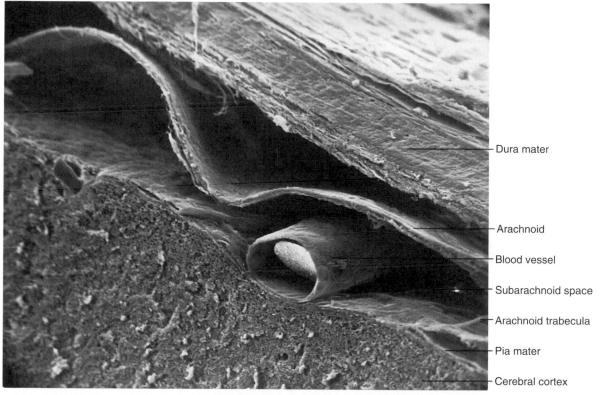

Dura mater

Arachnoid

Blood vessel

Subarachnoid space

Arachnoid trabecula

Pia mater

Cerebral cortex

Figure 4-2 Scanning electron micrograph of the cranial meninges of a young dog. The apparent space between the dura mater and the arachnoid is an artifact of processing and would not normally be present. *(Courtesy Dr. Delmas J. Allen, Medical College of Ohio.)*

dropped and the three are referred to simply as the *dura, arachnoid,* and *pia.* The dura mater is by far the most substantial of the meninges, and for this reason is also called the **pachymeninx** (from the Greek word *pachy* meaning "thick," as in thick-skinned pachyderms). The arachnoid and pia mater, in contrast, are thin and delicate. They are continuous with each other, often regarded as two parts of a single layer, and so are sometimes referred to together as the *pia-arachnoid* or the **lepto-meninges** (from the Greek word *lepto,* meaning "thin" or

"fine"). The dura mater is attached to the inner surface of the skull, and the arachnoid is adherent to the inner surface of the dura mater by dural border cells and pressure from the CSF. The pia mater is attached to the brain, following all its contours, and the space between the arachnoid and pia mater is filled with CSF.

The same three meningeal layers continue around the spinal cord but have a slightly different arrangement there, so spinal meninges are described separately toward the end of this chapter.

Table 4-1	Spaces in the Cranial Meninges

Space	Location
Epidural	Potential space between dura and calvaria
Subdural	Potential space in the innermost dural layer, near the dura-arachnoid interface
Subarachnoid	Normally present, CSF-filled space; enlarged in cisterns

The Dura Mater Provides Mechanical Strength

The cranial dura is a thick, tough, collagenous membrane that adheres firmly to the inner surface of the skull (*dura* is the Latin word for "hard," as in durable). It is often described as consisting of two layers: an outer layer that serves as the periosteum of the inner surface of the skull and an inner layer, the meningeal dura. Because these two layers are tightly fused, with no sharp histological boundary between them, the entire complex is ordinarily referred to as *dura mater*.

With few exceptions, no space exists on either side of the cranial dura under normal circumstances because one side is attached to the skull and the other side adheres to the arachnoid.[a] However, two **potential spaces,** the **epidural** and **subdural** spaces, are associated with the dura (Table 4-1; see Fig. 4-14). Epidural (or **extradural**) space refers to the potential space between the cranium and the periosteal layer. Subdural space is commonly described as potential space between dura and arachnoid and is sometimes said to contain a thin film of fluid. However, electron microscopic evidence indicates that the dura and arachnoid are normally attached to each other, and when they appear to separate the splitting actually occurs within the innermost cellular layers of the dura. Parts of these potential spaces can become actual fluid-filled cavities in certain pathological conditions, most often as a result of hemorrhage (see Fig. 4-14).

Dural Folds Partially Separate Different Intracranial Compartments

There are several places where the inner dural layer separates from its external counterpart and protrudes into

the cranial cavity. Such extensions of dura reflect back on themselves to form double-layered dural folds (dural reflections or dural septa). The principal dural folds are the **falx cerebri**[b] between the two cerebral hemispheres, and the **tentorium cerebelli** between the cerebral hemispheres and the cerebellum (Fig. 4-3). The **falx cerebelli** is a small reflection that partially separates the two cerebellar hemispheres. The **diaphragma sellae,** another small reflection, covers the pituitary fossa, admitting the infundibulum through a small perforation.

The falx cerebri is a long, arched, vertical dural fold (see Fig. 4-3; Fig. 4-4A) that occupies the longitudinal fissure and separates the two cerebral hemispheres. Anteriorly it is attached to the crista galli of the ethmoid bone. The falx curves posteriorly and fuses with the middle of the tentorium cerebelli, ending posteriorly at the internal occipital protuberance. The tentorium cerebelli separates the superior surface of the cerebellum from the occipital and temporal lobes, defining **supratentorial** and **infratentorial** compartments within the cranial vault. The supratentorial compartment contains the forebrain, and the infratentorial compartment (or **posterior fossa**) contains the brainstem and cerebellum. Because the cleft between the cerebral hemispheres and the cerebellum is not horizontal or flat, neither is the tentorium. Rather, it is roughly the shape of a bird with its wings extended in front of it; the bird's body would correspond to the midline region where the falx cerebri joins the tentorium, and its wings would correspond to the rest of the tentorium, which extends anteriorly (see Fig. 4-3). Posteriorly the tentorium is attached mainly to the occipital bone. This line of attachment continues anteriorly and inferiorly along the petrous part of the temporal bone. The free edge of the tentorium also curves anteriorly on each side, almost encircling the midbrain (see Figs. 4-3 and 4-4). This space in the tentorium, through which the brainstem passes, is called the **tentorial notch** (or **tentorial incisure**). It is of great clinical significance, as discussed later in this chapter.

The Dura Mater Contains Venous Sinuses That Drain the Brain

As noted previously, the two layers of the cranial dura are tightly fused, and there are no pathological conditions in which an intradural space (i.e., a space between the two layers) develops. However, at the attached edges of dural folds, the two layers are normally separated to form venous channels, called **dural venous sinuses,** into which the cerebral veins empty. These sinuses are roughly triangular in cross section and are lined with endothelium (Fig. 4-5). The locations of the major sinuses can be inferred by considering the lines of

---

[a]There are a few places near the inferior surface of the brain where a real intracranial epidural space between the inner layer of the dura and the intracranial periosteum exists. For example, the epidural venous plexus surrounding the dural sac of the spinal cord (described later in this chapter) continues through a similarly situated basilar venous plexus anterior to the brainstem and inferior to the diencephalon; this plexus in turn communicates with the cavernous sinus.

[b]Named for its shape—*falx* is Latin for "sickle."

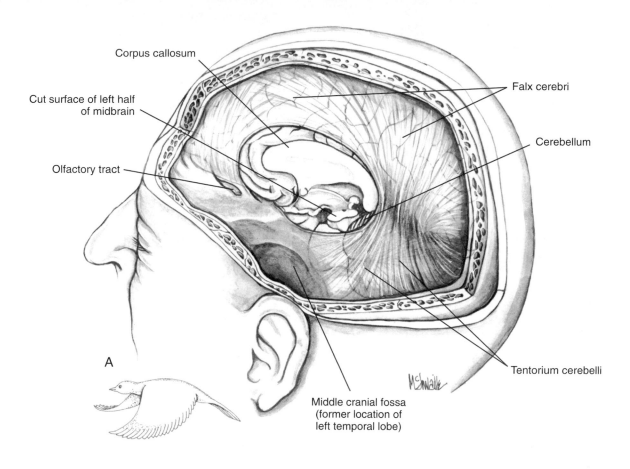

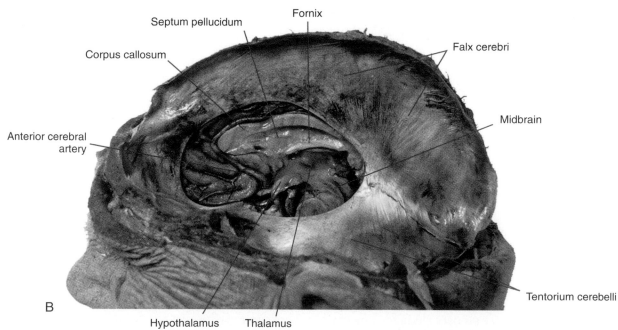

Figure 4-3 Shape and spatial relationships of the major dural folds. **A,** The cerebellum and the right cerebral hemisphere are drawn in on the other side of the tentorium cerebelli and falx cerebri. The small bird in the lower left corner reminds certain individuals of the shape of the tentorium cerebelli. **B,** A prosection similar to the drawing in **A,** showing the midbrain passing through the tentorial notch. (*A drawn from a dissection by Gary Jenison, University of Colorado Health Sciences Center. B courtesy Dr. John W. Sundsten, University of Washington School of Medicine.*)

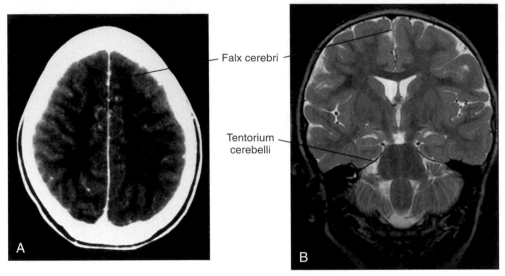

Figure 4-4 Major dural folds as seen in clinical images. **A,** A contrast-enhanced computed tomography scan (see Chapter 6) showing the falx cerebri between the two cerebral hemispheres. **B,** A coronal magnetic resonance image (see Chapter 5) showing the falx cerebri and tentorium cerebelli. *(Courtesy Drs. Raymond F. Carmody (**A**) and Joachim F. Seeger (**B**), University of Arizona College of Medicine.)*

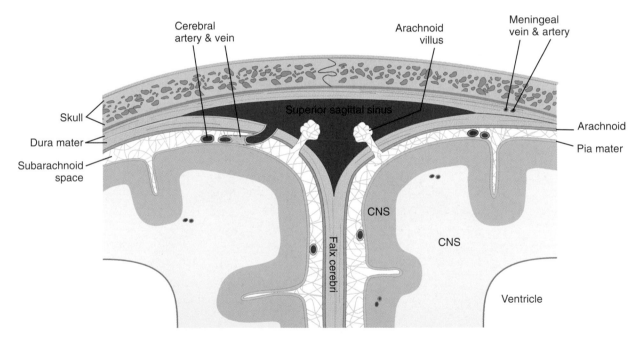

Figure 4-5 Coronal section through one of the major dural venous sinuses (the superior sagittal sinus). The movement of CSF from subarachnoid space, through the arachnoid villi, and into the sinus is described a little later in this chapter. *(Modified from Nolte J: Elsevier's Integrated Neuroscience, Philadelphia, 2007, Mosby/Elsevier.)*

attachment of the dural folds. The **superior sagittal sinus** is found along the attached edge of the falx cerebri, the left and right **transverse sinuses** along the posterior line of attachment of the tentorium cerebelli, and the **straight sinus** along the line of attachment of the cerebral falx and tentorium cerebelli to each other (Figs. 4-6 and 4-7). All four of these sinuses meet in the **confluence of the sinuses** (also called the **torcular,** or **torcular Herophili**—"the winepress of Herophilus") near the internal occipital protuberance. Venous blood flows posteriorly

in the superior sagittal and straight sinuses into the confluence, and from there through the transverse sinuses. Each transverse sinus continues, as the **sigmoid sinus,** which proceeds anteriorly and inferiorly through an S-shaped course and empties into the internal jugular vein (see Figs. 4-6 and 4-7; see also Fig. 6-32).

The confluence of the sinuses is generally not a symmetrical structure. Usually most of the blood from the superior sagittal sinus flows into the right transverse sinus, whereas blood from the straight sinus flows into

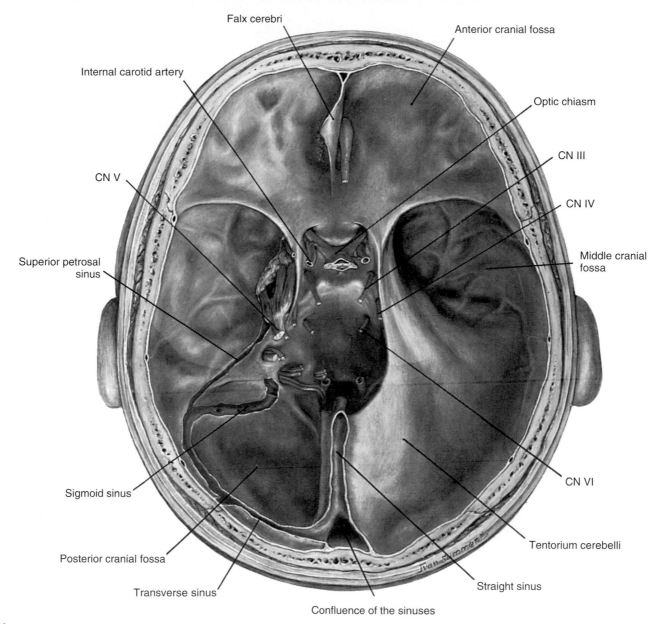

Figure 4-6 Dural lining of the base of the skull. The falx cerebri has been removed except for a small anterior portion. The left half of the tentorium has also been removed, exposing the posterior fossa (where the cerebellum was). *(From Mettler FA: Neuroanatomy, ed 2, St. Louis, 1948, Mosby.)*

the left transverse sinus (see Figs. 4-6 and 4-7; see also Fig. 6-31). Occasionally, the two transverse sinuses are not interconnected at all.

In addition to receiving cerebral veins, the major dural sinuses are connected with several smaller sinuses (see Fig. 6-31). The **inferior sagittal sinus,** in the free edge of the falx cerebri, empties into the straight sinus. The small **occipital sinus,** in the attached edge of the falx cerebelli, empties into the confluence of the sinuses (see Fig. 4-7). The **superior petrosal sinus,** in the edge of the tentorium attached to the petrous part of the temporal bone, carries blood from the cavernous sinus to the transverse sinus at the point where the latter leaves the tentorium to become the sigmoid sinus (see Fig. 4-6).

The **inferior petrosal sinus** follows a groove between the temporal and occipital bones, carrying blood from the cavernous sinus to the internal jugular vein.

The Dura Mater Has Its Own Blood Supply

The arterial supply of the dura comes from a collection of meningeal arteries. These are somewhat misnamed because they travel in the periosteal layer of the dura and function mainly in supplying the bones of the skull; however, many small arterial branches penetrate the dura itself. The largest of the meningeal arteries is the **middle meningeal artery,** a branch of the maxillary artery, which ramifies over most of the lateral surface of

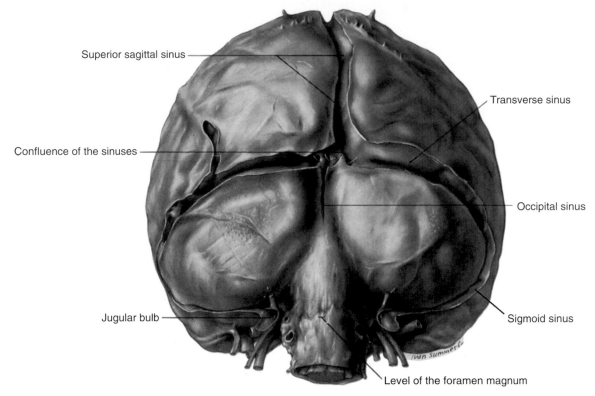

Superior sagittal sinus

Transverse sinus

Confluence of the sinuses

Occipital sinus

Jugular bulb

Sigmoid sinus

Level of the foramen magnum

Figure 4-7 The brain, still encased in dura, viewed from behind. Note the asymmetry of the confluence of the sinuses. Note also the jagged line at the foramen magnum level corresponding to the cut edge of the periosteal layer of the cranial dura. Below this line, a single-layered dural sheath continues around the spinal cord. *(From Mettler FA: Neuroanatomy, ed 2, St. Louis, 1948, Mosby.)*

the cerebral dura. Anteriorly the dura is supplied by branches of the ophthalmic artery, and posteriorly it is supplied by branches of the occipital and vertebral arteries. Meningeal veins, also located in the periosteal layer, generally parallel the arteries.

The Dura Mater Is Pain Sensitive

Remarkably, the brain itself, as well as the arachnoid and pia mater, is not sensitive to pain (in the sense that physical stimulation of these structures is not painful). As a consequence, some neurosurgical procedures can be carried out without general anesthesia. The principal pain-sensitive intracranial structures are the dura mater and proximal portions of blood vessels at the base of the brain.

Most of the cranial dura, except for that of the posterior fossa, receives sensory innervation from the trigeminal nerve. Dural nerves follow the meningeal arteries and end near either the arteries or the dural sinuses. Except in the floor of the anterior cranial fossa, areas of dura between branches of meningeal arteries are innervated sparsely, if at all. Deformation of these dural endings is painful and is the cause of certain types of headache (Fig. 4-8). Interestingly, the way the pain is perceived depends on whether endings near meningeal arteries or endings near dural sinuses are stimulated. In

the former case, the pain is fairly accurately localized to the area of stimulation. In the latter case the pain is referred to portions of the peripheral distribution of the trigeminal nerve, such as the eye, temple, or forehead.

The dura of the posterior fossa is supplied primarily by fibers of the vagus nerve and the second and third cervical nerves.[c] As in the case of supratentorial dural innervation, the pain-sensitive endings in the posterior fossa are mostly located near dural arteries and venous sinuses. Deformation in these areas causes pain referred to the area behind the ear or the back of the neck.

The Arachnoid Mater

The arachnoid is a thin, avascular membrane composed of a few layers of cells interspersed with bundles of collagen. It is semitransparent and resembles a substantial cobweb, for which it is named (the Greek word *arachne* means "spider's web"). The outer portion of the arachnoid consists of several layers of flattened cells adhering to the innermost cellular layer of the dura mater—the dural border cells. This interface region of cell layers,

[c]The sensory component of the first cervical nerve typically is minor and does not contribute substantially to this innervation.

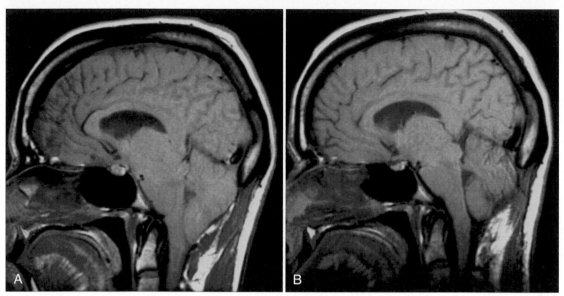

Figure 4-8 Headache caused by mechanical deformation of the meninges. This 41-year-old man had a 9-year history of debilitating headaches that were relieved by lying down. He was found to have a meningeal diverticulum at the level of the second lumbar vertebra, through which CSF presumably drained. This interfered with the normal flotation effect of the CSF, causing "sagging" of the brain **(A)** and consequent traction on the meninges. After ligation of the diverticulum, the brain assumed a nearly normal shape **(B)** and the headaches resolved. *(From Schievink WI et al: J Neurosurg 84:598, 1996.)*

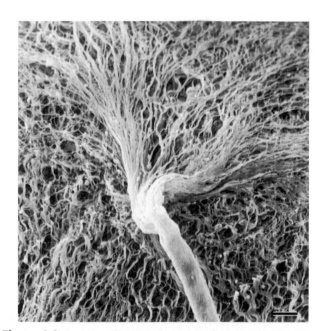

Figure 4-9 Scanning electron micrograph of a human arachnoid trabecula. The view is as though you were standing in the lateral sulcus looking out at the overlying arachnoid and dura mater. Collagen bundles spread out from the trabecula and merge with the arachnoid lining of the dura mater. Scale mark = 3 μm. *(From Alcolado R et al: Neuropath Applied Neurobiol 14:1, 1988.)*

partially dura and partially arachnoid, contains no collagen and is only about 100 μm thick. Small strands of collagenous connective tissue called **arachnoid trabeculae** (Fig. 4-9), covered with fibroblast-like arachnoid cells, extend to the pia, with which they merge. Arachnoid trabeculae help keep the brain suspended

within the meninges, much the way the Lilliputians stabilized Gulliver's position.[d] Dural septa extend this suspension system inward, preventing the cerebral hemispheres from bumping up against each other or the cerebellum.

The Arachnoid Bridges Over CNS Surface Irregularities, Forming Cisterns

Because the arachnoid is adherent to the inner surface of the dura mater, it (like the dura) conforms to the general shape of the brain but does not dip into sulci or follow the more intricate contours of the surface of the brain. Therefore there is a **subarachnoid space,** filled with CSF, between the arachnoid and the pia mater, because the pia closely covers all of the external surfaces of the CNS. This is the only substantial fluid-filled space normally found around the outside of the brain. The subarachnoid space is very narrow over the surfaces of gyri, relatively small where the arachnoid bridges over small sulci, and much larger in certain locations where it bridges over large surface irregularities (Fig. 4-10). An example of such a location is the space between the inferior surface of the cerebellum and the posterior surface of the medulla. Regions such as this, which contain a considerable volume of CSF, are called **subarachnoid cisterns.** This particular example is called the **cerebellomedullary cistern** on anatomical grounds, and because it is the largest cranial cistern it is also

---

[d]Thanks to Dr. Theodore J. Tarby for the analogy.

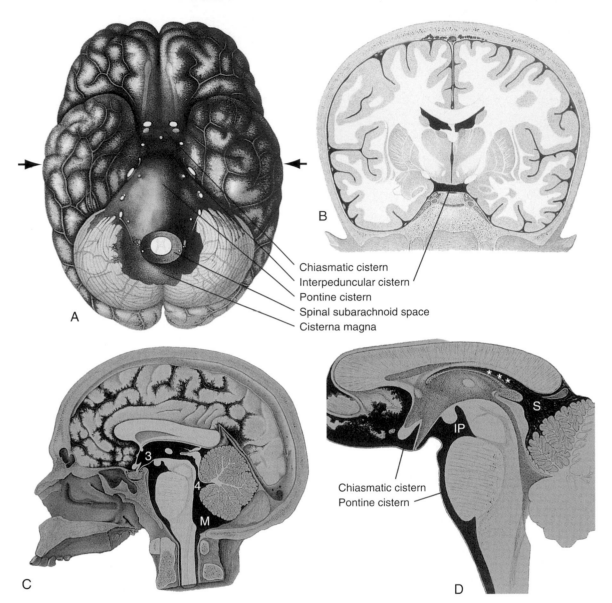

Chiasmatic cistern
Interpeduncular cistern
Pontine cistern
Spinal subarachnoid space
Cisterna magna

Chiasmatic cistern
Pontine cistern

Figure 4-10 Subarachnoid cisterns. **A,** Cisterns at the base of the brain, demonstrated by filling subarachnoid space with dyed gelatin. The dye fills prominent cisterns, as well as cerebral sulci, but is mostly excluded from the surface of gyri, where there is little subarachnoid space. **B,** A coronal section of a similar specimen, in the plane indicated by the arrows in **A.** Dye fills the ventricles and subarachnoid space, including the interpeduncular cistern. Low **(C)** and high **(D)** magnification views of the cisterns and ventricles near the midline, demonstrated by filling subarachnoid space (and in **C,** the ventricles as well) with dyed gelatin. As in **A** and **B,** the dye fills prominent cisterns, as well as cerebral sulci, but is mostly excluded from the surface of gyri. *, transverse cerebral fissure; 3, third ventricle; 4, fourth ventricle; IP, interpeduncular cistern; M, cisterna magna (cerebellomedullary cistern); S, superior (quadrigeminal) cistern. *(From Key A, Retzius G: Studien in der anatomie des nervensystems und des bindegewebes, Vol. 1, Stockholm, 1875, Norstad.)*

referred to as **cisterna magna** (literally, "great cistern"). Other prominent cisterns are shown in Figure 4-10 and include (1) the **pontine cistern,** which is located around the anterior surface of the pons and medulla and is continuous posteriorly with the cerebellomedullary cistern; (2) the **interpeduncular cistern,** which is located between the cerebral peduncles and contains the posterior part of the cerebral arterial circle (of Willis) (see Fig. 6-3); and (3) the **superior cistern** (also referred to as the **quadrigeminal cistern** and the **cistern of the great cerebral vein**), a radiological landmark above the midbrain

(see Fig. 5-15C). The superior cistern is continuous laterally with a thin, curved layer of subarachnoid space on each side that partially encircles the midbrain before opening into the interpeduncular cistern. The combination of the superior cistern and these sheetlike extensions is referred to as the **ambient cistern.**[e] The **transverse cerebral fissure,** a fingerlike extension of subarachnoid space between the fornix and the roof of

---

[e]Many use the term *ambient cistern* to refer to the sheetlike extensions alone.

the third ventricle, continues anteriorly from the superior cistern; it became trapped in this location as the cerebral hemispheres grew backward over the diencephalon during development (see Figs. 5-5 and 5-8).

Arachnoid trabeculae are particularly prominent in subarachnoid cisterns, sometimes coalescing into delicate membranes that partially occlude the subarachnoid space and separate cisterns from each other.

CSF Enters the Venous Circulation Through Arachnoid Villi

The CSF contained in the subarachnoid space generally is separated from the venous blood in dural sinuses by a layer of arachnoid, a thick layer of dura, and the endothelial lining of the sinus. However, at many locations along dural sinuses, particularly along the superior sagittal sinus, small evaginations of the arachnoid, called **arachnoid villi,** herniate through the wall of the sinus. At these sites the connective tissue of the dura is mostly missing, and only a loose layer of arachnoid cells and a layer of endothelium intervene between subarachnoid space and venous blood (see Fig. 4-5). Large clusters of arachnoid villi are called **arachnoid granulations,** and those that become calcified with age are referred to as **pacchionian bodies.** The villi are especially numerous in laterally directed dilations of the superior sagittal sinus, called **venous lacunae** or **lateral lacunae** (Fig. 4-11).

The arachnoid villi are the major sites of reabsorption of CSF into the venous system. Functionally, they behave like one-way valves, allowing flow from subarachnoid space into venous blood but not in the reverse direction. Because CSF pressure is ordinarily greater than venous pressure, the villi normally allow continuous movement of CSF, more or less as though by bulk flow, into the sinuses; however, even if the pressure gradient reverses, the flow does not. The exact mechanism of this flow has been the subject of debate for many years. Some authors have described open channels, micrometers in diameter, through the walls of the arachnoid villi, but others deny their existence. Others have suggested that giant vacuoles originate on the side of the endothelial cells facing subarachnoid space, travel across to the venous side, and sometimes are transiently open to both sides simultaneously (Fig. 4-12).

The Arachnoid Has a Barrier Function

The CNS is isolated in some respects from the rest of the body and lives in a tightly controlled environment (discussed in more detail in Chapters 5 and 6). This control is achieved partly by a system of diffusion barriers between the extracellular spaces in and around the nervous system and extracellular spaces elsewhere. One such barrier is between the CSF in the subarachnoid space and the extracellular fluids of the dura. Marker

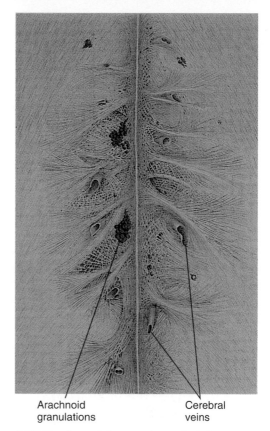

Arachnoid
granulations

Cerebral
veins

Figure 4-11 The floor of the superior sagittal sinus, penetrated by both arachnoid granulations and cerebral veins. *(From Key A, Retzius G: Studien in der anatomie des nervensystems und des bindegewebes, Vol. 1, Stockholm, 1875, Norstad.)*

substances injected into the middle meningeal artery spread throughout the dura but do not enter the subarachnoid space. The barrier resides in those cellular layers of the arachnoid in the interface region with the dura, where the cells are connected to each other by a series of tight junctions that occlude extracellular space (see Fig. 4-14).

Pia Mater Covers the Surface of the CNS

The pia mater (from the Latin word *pia,* meaning "tender") is a delicate membrane that, unlike the arachnoid, closely invests all external surfaces of the CNS. Pia follows all of the contours of the brainstem and all of the folds of the cerebral and cerebellar cortices, abutting the layer of astrocyte end-feet at the surface of the CNS. Arachnoid trabeculae span the subarachnoid space and merge with the pia mater so subtly that it is difficult to decide where the arachnoid ends and the pia begins. For this reason, some speak of the entire leptomeningeal complex as one entity—the pia-arachnoid.

Cerebral arteries and veins travel in subarachnoid space, invested by pia. As each small vessel enters or leaves the brain, it carries with it a sleeve of **perivascular**

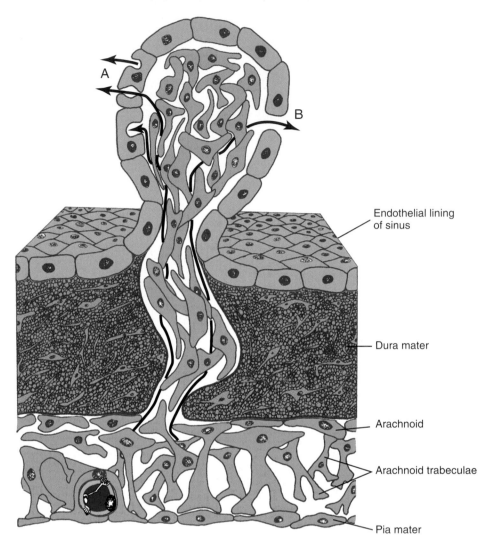

Figure 4-12 An arachnoid villus, showing the passage of CSF from subarachnoid space into a dural venous sinus. **A,** Cerebrospinal fluid movement through large vacuoles in endothelial cells, as described by some workers. **B,** Movement through channels between cells, as described by other authors. *(Modified from Shabo AL, Maxwell DS: J Neurosurg 29:451, 1968.)*

space (or **Virchow-Robin space**)—an extension of subarachnoid space. This space extends inward, filled with connective tissue and extracellular fluid, to the level at which the vessel becomes a capillary. The actual nature and extent of this microscopic space and the question of whether it provides a functional pathway of communication between the extracellular space around neurons and the subarachnoid space have been matters of controversy for decades. The traditional view holds that the connective tissue elements of the perivascular space arise as an inwardly directed cuff of pia that accompanies each vessel, but there are indications that in fact the pia may be left behind on the surface of the CNS. Similarly, some claim that perivascular space is small and restricted, although there are indications that it may provide an important route for movement of extracellular fluid that may even be continuous with the cervical lymphatics through the adventitia of larger vessels.

The Vertebral Canal Contains a Spinal Epidural Space

The meningeal coverings of the spinal cord are fundamentally similar to those of the brain, but there are some important differences (Table 4-2).

The spinal dura mater has no periosteal component. Instead, the cranial dura splits at the foramen magnum (Fig. 4-13): The periosteal layer continues around onto the outside of the skull, and the meningeal layer continues as the single-layered dura of the spinal cord. The spinal dura mater is separated from the vertebral periosteum by an epidural space. Thus there are two basic differences between cranial and spinal epidural spaces:

1. Cranial epidural space is a potential space in almost all parts of the skull, whereas spinal epidural space is an actual space.

Table 4-2	Differences Between Cranial and Spinal Meninges	
	Cranial	**Spinal**
Dura mater	Double layered, attached to inner calvarial surface	Single layered, suspended in vertebral canal
Epidural space	Potential space between periosteum and calvaria	Real space between dura and vertebral periosteum
Arachnoid	Attached to inner surface of dura	Attached to inner surface of dura
Pia mater	Attached to CNS surface	Attached to CNS surface, expanded as denticulate ligaments

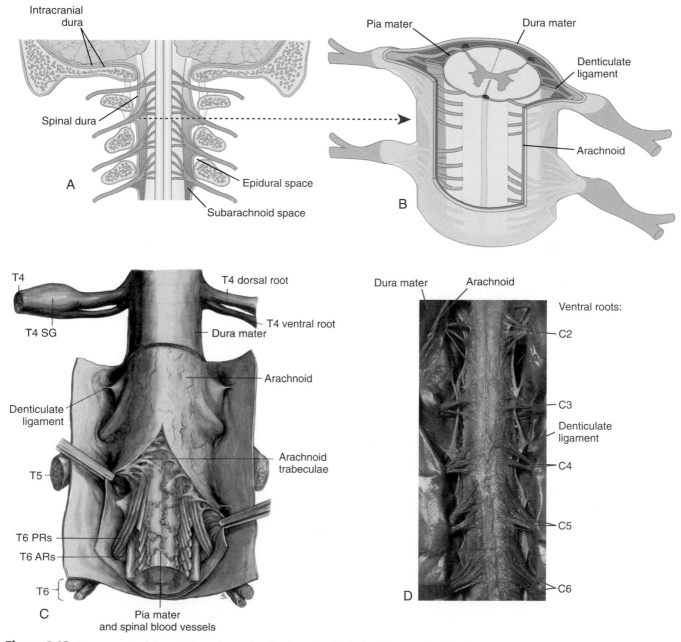

Figure 4-13 Arrangement of the spinal meninges showing how the denticulate ligaments anchor the spinal cord to its dural sheath through the arachnoid. **A** and **B** show how the double-layered cranial dura mater is continuous with the single-layered dural sheath of the spinal cord. **C,** A drawing of a posterior view. **D,** Anterior view of a dissection in which the dural sheath was cut open longitudinally. ARs, anterior rootlets; PRs, posterior rootlets; SG, spinal ganglion. (*A and B modified from Nolte J: Elsevier's Integrated Neuroscience, Philadelphia, 2007, Mosby/Elsevier. C from Mettler FA: Neuroanatomy, ed 2, St. Louis, 1948, Mosby. D courtesy Dr. Normal Koelling, University of Arizona College of Medicine.*)

2. Cranial epidural space, when present in pathological conditions, is located between periosteal dura and cranium. Spinal epidural space is located between periosteum and dura. This spinal epidural space is filled with fatty connective tissue and the external vertebral venous plexus.

The spinal arachnoid mater, like its cranial counterpart, is closely applied to the inner surface of the dura mater, leaving a CSF-filled subarachnoid space between itself and the pia mater that invests the spinal cord surface (see Fig. 4-13). The spinal dura and its arachnoid lining end at about the second sacral vertebra, whereas the spinal cord itself ends at about the level of the disk between the first and second lumbar vertebrae (see Fig. 10-2). There is, therefore, a large subarachnoid cistern, the **lumbar cistern,** between these two points. This is the favored site for sampling CSF, because a needle can be inserted here with relatively little risk of damaging neural structures.

The pial covering of the spinal cord is relatively thick and gives rise to a pair of longitudinal projections on each side called **denticulate (dentate) ligaments.** Each denticulate ligament exhibits 21 toothlike extensions that anchor the spinal cord to the arachnoid and through it to the dura mater. In addition, another pial projection, the **filum terminale** internus (the "terminal thread"), anchors the caudal end of the spinal cord (the **conus medullaris**) to the caudal end of the spinal dural sheath (see Fig. 10-3). The caudal end of the dural sheath, in turn, is anchored to the caudal end of the vertebral canal by the filum terminale externus.

Bleeding Can Open Up Potential Meningeal Spaces

As discussed previously, the three meningeal coverings of the brain have various real or potential spaces associated with them (Fig. 4-14). There is no significant space between the pia and the brain, but there is a subarachnoid space between the pia and the arachnoid, along with potential subdural and epidural spaces. Both of these potential spaces can become actual fluid-filled spaces under certain conditions (Table 4-3).

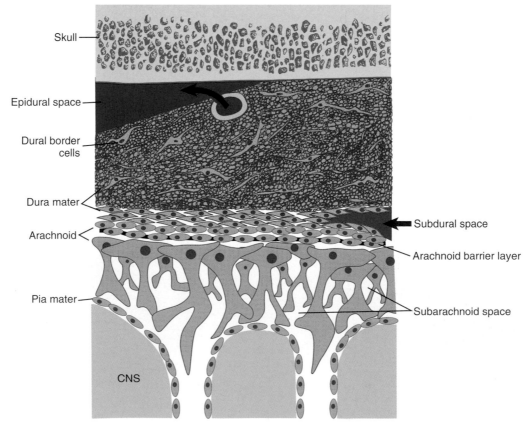

Figure 4-14 Actual spaces and potential spaces in and around the cranial meninges. Epidural space (not normally present) between dura and skull may be opened up by blood from a ruptured meningeal artery or, less commonly, a torn dural venous sinus. Subdural space (not normally present), typically within the dura near the latter's junction with the arachnoid, may be opened up by blood from a vein that tears as it crosses the arachnoid to enter a dural sinus. Dark bars joining superficial arachnoid cells represent the tight junctions that are the basis of the barrier properties of this portion of the arachnoid.

Tearing of Meningeal Arteries Can Cause an Epidural Hematoma

The meningeal arteries run in the periosteal layer of the dura. If one of these arteries is torn (typically as a result of traumatic skull injury), bleeding occurs between the periosteum and the skull, opening up the potential epidural space and causing an **epidural** (or **extradural**) **hematoma.** As the hematoma expands, it compresses and distorts the underlying brain (Fig. 4-15) and is likely to be fatal unless promptly treated surgically. Less commonly, tearing of a dural venous sinus can cause an epidural hematoma (Fig. 4-16).

Table 4-3	Locations of Hematomas	
Source of Blood	**Nature of Bleeding or Hematoma**
Meningeal artery	Epidural hematoma
Dural venous sinus	Subdural or epidural hematoma
Vein at attachment to sinus	Subdural hematoma
Cerebral artery or vein	Subarachnoid hemorrhage
	Intraparenchymal hemorrhage
	Intraventricular hemorrhage

Tearing of Veins Where They Enter Venous Sinuses Can Cause a Subdural Hematoma

Bleeding can also occur into the potential subdural space, resulting in a **subdural hematoma.** The most common cause of subdural hematomas is tearing of a cerebral vein as it penetrates the arachnoid and enters a dural sinus. This can result from rapid accelerations or decelerations of the head (Fig. 4-17): the venous sinuses are attached to the skull and move with it, but the brain can lag behind, so a vein extending from the brain to a sinus can tear at the point where it penetrates the arachnoid. Some subdural hematomas are acute and produce symptoms much like those of an epidural hematoma, whereas others may progress very slowly and become surprisingly large before producing symptoms.

Parts of the CNS Can Herniate from One Intracranial Compartment Into Another

Dural reflections such as the falx cerebri and the tentorium cerebelli are firmly attached to the cranium. These reflections are taut, which allows them to perform their mechanical support function, but this very tautness can result in additional problems in cases

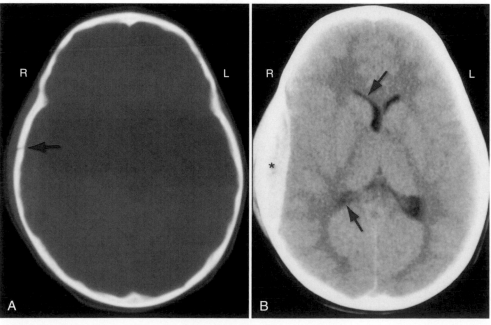

Figure 4-15 Epidural hematoma in a 3-year-old girl who hit her head in an automobile accident. About 2 hours after the accident she complained of a severe headache and nausea and became lethargic. Computed tomography (CT) set to show bony details **(A)** revealed a fracture of the right temporal bone *(arrow)*. CT set to reveal soft tissue details **(B)** revealed a lens-shaped epidural hematoma (*) and compression of the right lateral ventricle *(arrows)*. After rapid neurosurgical treatment she made a full recovery. L, left side; R, right side. *(Courtesy Dr. Raymond F. Carmody, University of Arizona College of Medicine.)*

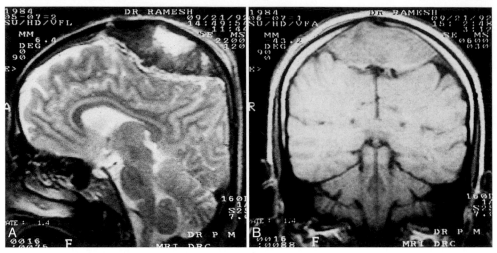

Figure 4-16 Epidural hematoma, seen in sagittal (**A**) and coronal (**B**) magnetic resonance images, resulting from laceration of the superior sagittal sinus several days previously. This very large hematoma has the characteristic lens shape of epidural hematomas and crosses the midline (**B**). R, right side. (Subdural hematomas typically are crescent shaped [see Figs. 4-17 and 4-18] and do not cross the midline because they cannot get past the falx cerebri.) In this case, a 43-year-old medical practitioner presented with severe generalized headache of 4 days' duration. Four days earlier, he had fallen from a scooter while trying to avoid a collision with a cyclist. He had transient loss of consciousness lasting a few minutes, following which he was hospitalized elsewhere for a day and discharged. The patient was treated surgically and recovered. *(From Ramesh VG, Sivakumar S: Surg Neurol 43:138, 1995.)*

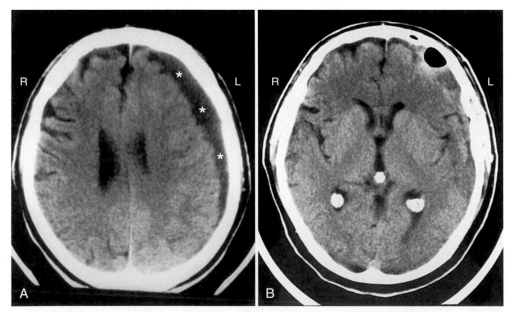

Figure 4-17 A, Crescent-shaped subdural hematoma (*) over the surface of the left cerebral hemisphere, compressing its subarachnoid spaces and lateral ventricle and shifting midline structures to the right. L, left side; R, right side. Although subdural hematomas are commonly caused by a blow to the head, they can also be caused by other mechanical disturbances (as in the shaken-baby syndrome). This is the case of a 64-year-old man whose headaches developed gradually after he began riding a roller coaster at an amusement park. The roller coaster, he reported, "swings people upside down as many as six times." He rode the roller coaster on 11 different occasions until his headaches became so severe that he was unable to continue. After surgical removal of the hematoma (**B**), subarachnoid spaces and ventricular symmetry returned and the patient recovered uneventfully. (*A from Bo-Abbas Y, Bolton CF: N Engl J Med 332:1585, 1995. Copyright © 1995 Massachusetts Medical Society. All rights reserved. B courtesy Dr. Y. Bo-Abbas, Victoria Hospital, London, Ontario, Canada.*)

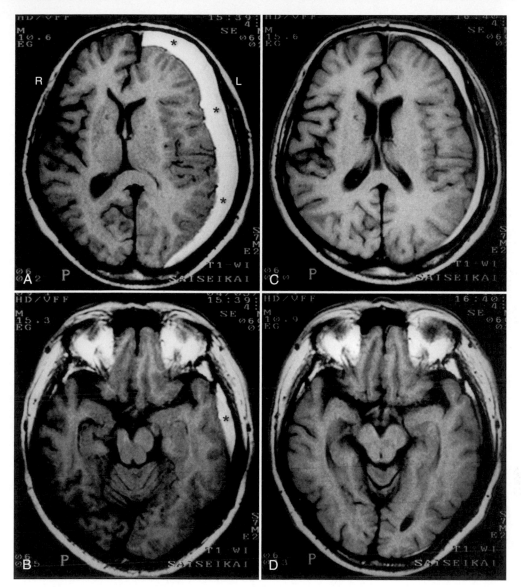

Figure 4-18 Chronic subdural hematoma (*) over the surface of the left cerebral hemisphere, compressing its subarachnoid spaces and lateral ventricle **(A),** shifting midline structures to the right and deforming the right cerebral peduncle *(arrow,* **B)** by pressing it against the edge of the tentorium cerebelli. L, left side; R, right side. This deformation of the cerebral peduncle caused left-sided weakness, which improved when surgical removal of the hematoma resolved the compression (**C** and **D**). *(From Itoyama Y, Fukioka S, Ushio Y: J Neurosurg 82:645, 1995.)*

of increasing intracranial pressure (for example, a subdural hematoma or an expanding tumor). The midbrain may be pushed against the edge of the tentorium while passing through the tentorial notch (Fig. 4-18), causing damage to a cerebral peduncle and one or more cranial nerves (typically the oculomotor nerve). Also, depending on where the expanding mass causing the increased pressure is located, certain portions of the brain may herniate from one side of a dural reflection to another (Figs. 4-19 and 4-20). For example, increased pressure on the lateral surface of one cerebral hemisphere can cause the hemisphere to be displaced inferiorly and medially, in turn causing the uncus and adjacent portions of the temporal lobe to herniate through the tentorial notch and compress the midbrain. Such pressure could also cause one cingulate

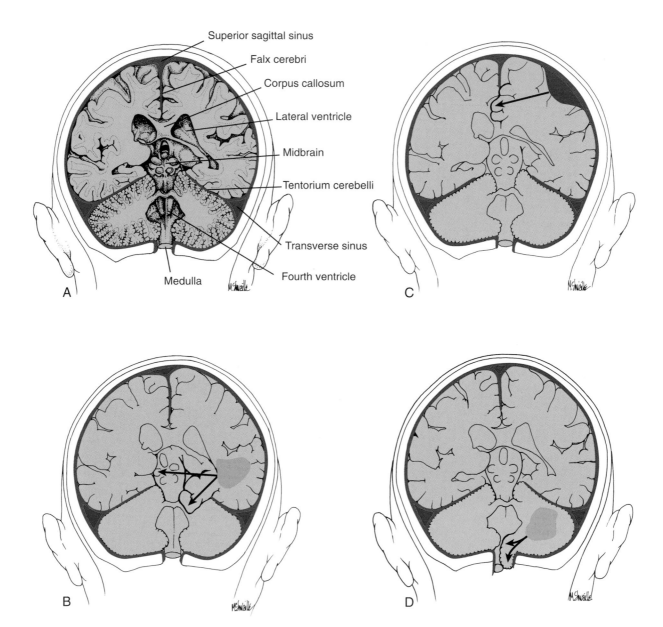

Superior sagittal sinus
Falx cerebri
Corpus callosum
Lateral ventricle
Midbrain
Tentorium cerebelli
Transverse sinus
Fourth ventricle
Medulla

Figure 4-19 The three most common ways in which portions of the brain herniate from one compartment into another. **A,** The normal configuration in a plane approximately parallel to the long axis of the brainstem. **B,** As a result of pressure from a subdural hematoma, one cingulate gyrus can slip under the falx cerebri and press on the opposite cingulate gyrus; this can happen with no serious neurological consequences. **C,** As a result of pressure from an expanding mass in one temporal lobe, part of the medial temporal lobe can herniate through the tentorial notch and press the midbrain against the free edge of the tentorium. The midbrain contains structures essential for consciousness, and this type of herniation typically produces coma, often followed by death. **D,** As a result of pressure from an expanding cerebellar mass, one tonsil of the cerebellum can herniate through the foramen magnum, compressing the medulla against the margin of the foramen. The medulla contains respiratory and cardiovascular centers, and pressure on it is usually rapidly fatal.

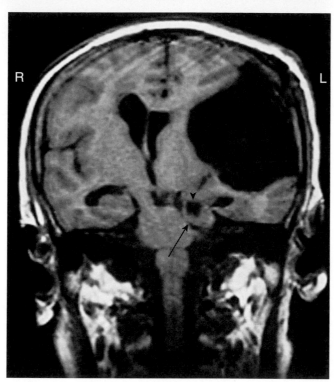

Figure 4-20 Magnetic resonance image of uncal herniation. L, left side; R, right side. A 62-year-old woman experienced slowly progressive weakness over a period of 2 years. She was found to have a large cyst that distended the left lateral sulcus. This pushed the left uncus, adjacent portions of the parahippocampal gyrus, and part of the inferior horn of the lateral ventricle *(arrowhead)* through the tentorial notch. Note how the herniated temporal lobe distorts the midbrain and rostral pons *(arrow)*, and how the large cyst pushed the bodies of both lateral ventricles to the right. Uncal herniation is usually a neurosurgical emergency, and images like this are rarely obtained. *(From Iwama T et al: Neuroradiol 33:346, 1991.)*

gyrus to herniate under the falx. Similarly, downward pressure can cause portions of the cerebellum to herniate into the foramen magnum and compress the medulla. Herniations that compress the brainstem are likely to have grave consequences.

SUGGESTED READINGS

Alcolado R, et al: The cranial arachnoid and pia mater in man: anatomical and ultrastructural observations. Neuropathol Applied Neurobiol 14:1, 1988.
Argues that cerebral vessels enter the brain beneath the pia, rather than through subarachnoid space.

Bo-Abbas Y, Bolton CF: Roller-coaster headache. New Engl J Med 332:1585, 1995.
One way that rapid accelerations and decelerations can cause subdural hematoma.

Boon JM, et al: Lumbar puncture: anatomical review of a clinical skill. Clin Anat 17:544, 2004.

Davson H, Hollingsworth G, Segal MB: The mechanism of drainage of the cerebrospinal fluid. Brain 93:665, 1970.
Physiological experiments supporting the concept of bulk flow of CSF through arachnoid villi.

Esiri MM, Gay D: Immunological and neuropathological significance of the Virchow-Robin space. J Neurol Sci 100:3, 1990.
Reviews the evidence for a connection between Virchow-Robin spaces and the lymphatic system and the idea that this connection can be significant in CNS diseases involving the immune system.

Fox RJ, et al: Anatomic details of intradural channels in the parasagittal dura: a possible pathway for flow of cerebrospinal fluid. Neurosurg 39:84, 1996.

Froelich SC, et al: Microsurgical and endoscopic anatomy of Liliequist's membrane: a complex and variable structure of the basal cisterns. Neurosurg 63(Suppl 1):ONS1, 2008.

Groeschel S, et al: Virchow-Robin spaces on magnetic resonance images: normative data, their dilatation, and a review of the literature. Neuroradiology 48:745, 2006.

Inoue K, et al: Microsurgical and endoscopic anatomy of the supratentorial arachnoidal membranes and cisterns. Neurosurg 65:644, 2009.
Beautifully illustrated.

Itoyama Y, Fujioka S, Ushio Y: Kernohan's notch in chronic subdural hematoma: findings on magnetic resonance imaging. J Neurosurg 82:645, 1995.
Kernohan's notch is the impression made in the midbrain in situations where it is pressed against the free edge of the tentorium by an expanding mass.

Keller JT, et al: Innervation of the posterior fossa dura of the cat. Brain Res Bull 14:97, 1985.

Kobayashi K, et al: Anatomical study of the confluence of the sinuses with contrast-enhanced magnetic resonance venography. Neuroradiology 48:307, 2006.

Krahn V: The pia mater at the site of the entry of blood vessels into the central nervous system. Anat Embryol 164:257, 1982.

Laine FJ, et al: Acquired intracranial herniations: MR imaging findings. Am J Roentgenol 165:967, 1995.
A nice pictorial review of conditions causing herniation under the falx, through the tentorial notch, or through the foramen magnum.

Liang L, et al: Normal structures in the intracranial dural sinuses: delineation with 3D contrast-enhanced magnetization prepared rapid acquisition gradient-echo imaging sequence. Am J Neuroradiol 23:1739, 2002.
Magnetic resonance imaging demonstration of the distribution of arachnoid villi in the superior sagittal, straight, and transverse sinuses.

Liliequist B: The subarachnoid cisterns: an anatomic and roentgenologic study. Acta Radiol Suppl 185, 1959.

Livingston RB: Mechanics of cerebrospinal fluid. In Ruch TC, Patton HD, editors: Physiology and biophysics, ed 19, Philadelphia, 1965, WB Saunders.
Explains why a brain suspended in CSF has an effective weight of only 50 g.

Matsuno H, Rhoton AL, Jr, Peace D: Microsurgical anatomy of the posterior fossa cisterns. Neurosurg 23:58, 1988.

May PRA, et al: Woodpecker drilling behavior: an endorsement of the rotational theory of impact brain injury. Arch Neurol 36:370, 1979.
Not closely related to the meninges, but an interesting discussion of suspension of the brain within the cranium and protection of the brain from injury. Imagine what would happen if you banged your beak on a tree as often and as hard as a woodpecker does.

Messlinger K, Strassman AM, Burstein R: Anatomy and physiology of pain-sensitive cranial structures. In Silberstein SD, Lipton RB, Dodick DW, editors: Wolff's headache and other head pain, ed 8, New York, 2007, Oxford University Press.
A lucid review of sometimes conflicting reports.

Meyer A: Herniation of the brain. Arch Neurol Psychiatr 4:387, 1940.

Millen JW, Woollam DHM: On the nature of the pia mater. Brain 84:514, 1961.
A lucid discussion of the appearance of the pia at the light microscopic level.

Nabeshima S, et al: Junctions in the meninges and marginal glia. J Comp Neurol 164:127, 1975.
    Ultrastructural appearance of the meninges, the arachnoid barrier layer, and subdural space.

Parkinson D: Extradural neural axis compartment. J Neurosurg 92:585, 2000.
    A brief description of the continuation of spinal epidural space along the base of the skull, past the cavernous sinus, and into the orbits.

Pease DC, Schultz RL: Electron microscopy of rat cranial meninges. Am J Anat 102:301, 1958.

Penfield W, McNaughton F: Dural headache and innervation of the dura mater. Arch Neurol Psychiatr 44:43, 1940.
    A long but interesting account of the gross anatomy of dural innervation, headaches resulting from dural distortion, and surgical methods for providing relief from such headaches.

Ramesh VG, Sivakumar S: Extradural hematoma at the vertex: a case report. Surg Neurol 43:138, 1995.
    An example of epidural hematoma caused by laceration of a venous sinus.

Ray BS, Wolff HG: Experimental studies on headache: pain-sensitive structures of the head and their significance in headache. Arch Surg 41:813, 1940.

Schachenmayr W, Friede RL: The origin of subdural neomembranes. I. Fine structure of the dura-arachnoid interface in man. Am J Pathol 92:53, 1978.

Schievink WI: Spontaneous spinal cerebrospinal fluid leaks and intracranial hypotension. J Am Med Assoc 295:2286, 2006.

Schievink WI, et al: Spontaneous spinal cerebrospinal fluid leaks and intracranial hypotension. J Neurosurg 84:598, 1996.
    An illustration of the painful consequences of partial loss of the buoyant effect of CSF.

Shabo AL, Maxwell DS: The morphology of the arachnoid villi: a light and electron microscopic study in the monkey. J Neurosurg 29:451, 1968.

Tripathi BJ, Tripathi RC: Vacuolar transcellular channels as a drainage pathway for cerebrospinal fluid. J Physiol 239:195, 1974.

Upton ML, Weller RO: The morphology of cerebrospinal fluid drainage pathways in human arachnoid granulations. J Neurosurg 63:867, 1985.

Vandenabeele F, Creemers J, Lambrichts I: Ultrastructure of the human spinal arachnoid mater and dura mater. J Anat 189:417, 1996.

Waggener JD, Beggs J: The membranous coverings of neural tissues: an electron microscopy study. J Neuropathol Exp Neurol 26:417, 1967.

Yaşargil MG, et al: Anatomical observations of the subarachnoid cisterns of the brain during surgery. J Neurosurg 44:298, 1976.

Zhang ET, Inman CBE, Weller RO: Interrelationships of the pia mater and the perivascular (Virchow-Robin) spaces in the human cerebrum. J Anat 170:111, 1990.

Zouaoui A, Hidden G: Cerebral venous sinuses: anatomical variants or thrombosis? Acta Anat 133:318, 1988.

Ventricles and Cerebrospinal Fluid

5

The cavity of the embryonic neural tube develops into a continuous, fluid-filled system of ventricles lined with **ependymal cells** in adults; each division of the central nervous system (CNS) contains a portion of this ventricular system. Cerebrospinal fluid (CSF) is formed within the ventricles, fills them, and emerges from apertures in the fourth ventricle to fill the subarachnoid space. CSF is responsible for suspension of the brain through its partial flotation, as discussed in Chapter 4, but it does much more—it is an important component of the system that regulates the composition of the fluid bathing the neurons and glial cells of the CNS and provides a route through which certain chemical messengers can be widely distributed in the nervous system.

The Brain Contains Four Ventricles

Within each cerebral hemisphere is a relatively large **lateral ventricle.** The paired lateral ventricles communicate with the **third ventricle** of the diencephalon through the **interventricular foramina (of Monro).** The third ventricle in turn communicates with the **fourth ventricle** of the pons and medulla through the narrow **cerebral aqueduct (of Sylvius)** of the midbrain. The fourth

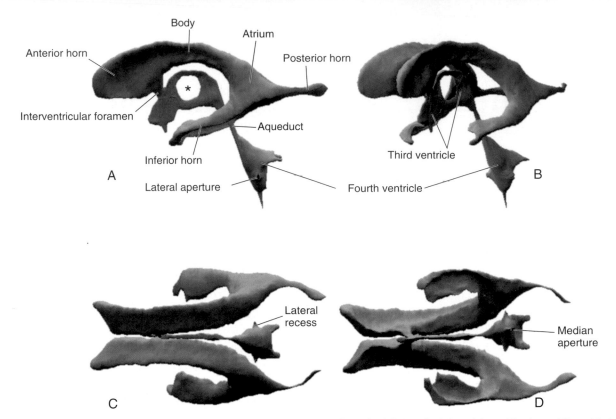

Figure 5-1 Three-dimensional reconstruction of the ventricular system, seen from the left **(A)**, the left and front **(B)**, above **(C)**, and below **(D)**. The location of the interthalamic adhesion is indicated by an asterisk. (See Video 5-1.)

ventricle continues caudally as the central canal of the caudal medulla and spinal cord; this canal is usually not patent over much of its extent.

A Lateral Ventricle Curves Through Each Cerebral Hemisphere

Each lateral ventricle follows a long C-shaped course through all the lobes of the cerebral hemisphere in which it resides. It is customarily divided into five parts (Figs. 5-1 and 5-2): (1) an **anterior** (or **frontal**) **horn** in the frontal lobe, anterior to the interventricular foramen; (2) a **body** in the frontal and parietal lobes, extending posteriorly to the region of the splenium of the corpus callosum; (3) a **posterior** (or **occipital**) **horn** projecting posteriorly into the occipital lobe; (4) an **inferior** (or **temporal**) **horn** curving inferiorly and anteriorly into the temporal lobe; and (5) an **atrium,** or **trigone,** the region near the splenium where the body and the posterior and inferior horns meet. The body, atrium, and inferior horn of each lateral ventricle represent the original C-shaped development of the ventricle; the anterior and posterior horns are extensions from this basic shape.

Various structures form the borders of the lateral ventricle in its course through the cerebral hemisphere; many of them can be seen easily in coronal sections (see

Figs. 3-20 to 3-24) or in brains dissected from above (Fig. 5-3). The similarly C-shaped caudate nucleus (see Fig. 3-19) is a constant feature in sections through the ventricle. Its enlarged head forms the lateral wall of the anterior horn (see Fig. 3-20), its somewhat smaller body forms most of the lateral wall of the body of the ventricle (see Fig. 3-22), and its attenuated tail lies in the roof of the inferior horn (see Figs. 3-23 and 5-8C). Proceeding posteriorly, as the caudate nucleus becomes smaller, the thalamus becomes larger and forms the floor of the body of the ventricle (compare Figs. 3-21, 3-22, and 3-23). The corpus callosum and **septum pellucidum** give a good indication of the size and location of the anterior horn and body of the ventricle. The body of the corpus callosum forms the roof of these parts of the ventricle, and the genu of the corpus callosum curves inferiorly to form the anterior wall of the anterior horn. The septum pellucidum forms the medial wall of the body and anterior horn, and its termination near the splenium marks the site where the bodies of the ventricles diverge from the midline and begin to curve around into the inferior horns (compare Figs. 3-22 and 3-24).

The posterior horn is phylogenetically the most recently developed part of the lateral ventricle and is also the most variable in size, sometimes being rudimentary. There are a number of slight asymmetries

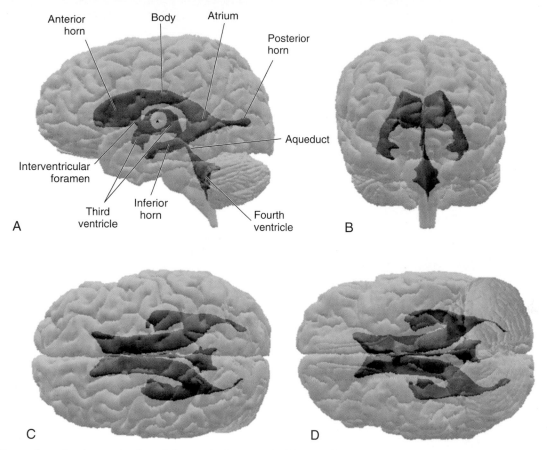

Figure 5-2 Three-dimensional reconstruction of the ventricular system inside a translucent brain, seen from the left **(A)**, front **(B)**, above **(C)**, and below **(D)**. The location of the interthalamic adhesion is indicated by an asterisk. (See Video 5-2.)

between the cerebral hemispheres of the human brain, and the left posterior horn tends to be longer than the right, particularly in right-handed individuals. The two lateral ventricles are otherwise quite symmetrical.

The hippocampus forms most of the floor and medial wall of the inferior horn (see Fig. 5-8C), which ends anteriorly at about the level of the uncus.

The Third Ventricle Is a Midline Cavity in the Diencephalon

The narrow, slit-shaped third ventricle occupies most of the midline region of the diencephalon (see Figs. 5-1 and 5-2), so its entire outline can be seen in a hemisected brain (see Fig. 3-16). It often looks like a misshapen doughnut in casts or reconstructions of the ventricular system (see Fig. 5-1). The hole in the doughnut corresponds to the **interthalamic adhesion,** which joins the thalami and crosses the ventricle in most human brains.

Anteriorly the third ventricle ends at the **lamina terminalis,** the remnant of the rostral neuropore. Much of the medial surface of the thalamus and hypothalamus forms the wall of the third ventricle, and part of the

hypothalamus forms its floor. It has a thin, membranous roof containing choroid plexus (discussed in the next section). At the posterior end of the mammillary bodies, the third ventricle narrows fairly abruptly to become the cerebral aqueduct (of Sylvius), which traverses the midbrain. The interventricular foramen, in the anterior part of each wall of the third ventricle, is an important radiological landmark because its location can be visualized by several different methods and it bears a known anatomical relationship to a number of deep structures (e.g., it is at the anterior end of the thalamus). Blockage of one of the interventricular foramen is a common cause of obstructive or noncommunicating hydrocephalus (discussed later).

An outline of the third ventricle reveals four protrusions, called **recesses** (Fig. 5-4), corresponding to structures that have evaginated from the diencephalon. Inferiorly the **optic recess** lies anterior to the optic chiasm at the base of the lamina terminalis; the **infundibular recess** lies immediately posterior to the chiasm. Superiorly the **pineal recess** invades the stalk of the pineal gland, and the **suprapineal recess** lies just anterior to this stalk.

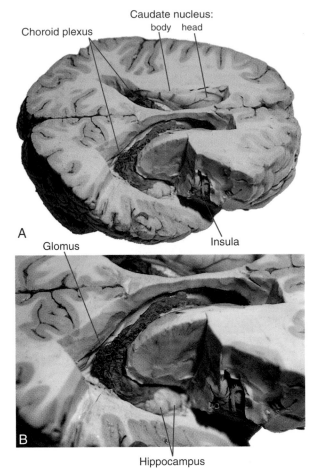

A

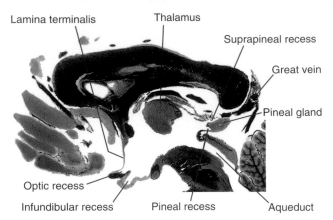

Figure 5-4 Recesses of the third ventricle, as seen in a sagittal section near the midline. *(Adapted from Nolte J, Angevine JB Jr: The human brain in photographs and diagrams, ed 3, St. Louis, 2007, Mosby.)*

Figure 5-3 Dissection demonstrating the lateral ventricles, viewed from above and to the right. **A,** A horizontal cut was made to expose the ventricles, and most of the corpus callosum was removed. Some white matter was removed on both sides to expose the posterior horns. The superior portions of the right temporal lobe and most of the insula were also removed so that the inferior horn could be seen on that side. **B,** Continuous choroid plexus follows a C-shaped course from the inferior horn through the atrium, through the body of the lateral ventricle, and into the interventricular foramen (not visible from this angle). There is no choroid plexus in the anterior or posterior horn.

The Fourth Ventricle Communicates with Subarachnoid Cisterns

The fourth ventricle is sandwiched between the cerebellum posteriorly and the pons and rostral medulla anteriorly (see Fig. 5-2). The floor is relatively flat, and because it narrows rostrally into the cerebral aqueduct and caudally into the central canal of the spinal cord, it is somewhat diamond shaped (see Fig. 11-3A). For this reason, the floor is sometimes referred to as the **rhomboid fossa.** At the location where the lateral point of the diamond would be expected, the entire ventricle becomes a narrow tube that proceeds anteriorly and curves around the brainstem, ending adjacent to the flocculus of the cerebellum. This tubular prolongation is the **lateral recess** of the fourth ventricle (see Fig. 5-1).

The rostral portion of the roof is the **superior medullary velum,** and the caudal portion is the **inferior medullary velum.** The superior medullary velum is a thin layer of white matter related to the cerebellum, whereas the inferior medullary velum is a membrane containing choroid plexus, similar to the roof of the third ventricle.

The lateral and third ventricles are nearly closed cavities, communicating only with other parts of the ventricular system. In contrast, there are three apertures in the fourth ventricle through which the ventricular system communicates freely with subarachnoid space. These are the unpaired **median aperture** (or **foramen of Magendie**) and the two **lateral apertures** (or **foramina of Luschka**) of the fourth ventricle (see Fig. 5-10). The median aperture is simply a hole in the inferior medullary velum (Fig. 5-5); it is as though the caudal end of the membrane, where it should have closed off the ventricle at its junction with the central canal, was instead lifted up and attached to the inferior surface of the cerebellar vermis. The result is a funnel-shaped opening from the subarachnoid space (the cerebellomedullary cistern, or cisterna magna) into the ventricle. The inferior medullary velum also covers the lateral recess, and at the end of each recess is another opening in the velum, the lateral aperture.

The Ventricles Contain Only a Fraction of the CSF

The ventricles are both smaller and more variable in size than one might expect. Although there is an average total of approximately 200 mL of CSF within and around the brain and spinal cord, only about 25 mL of this fluid is contained within the ventricles. The rest occupies subarachnoid space. The third and fourth ventricles together have a volume of only about 2 mL, and the volumes of the aqueduct and central canal are negligible, so the lateral ventricles contain nearly all the ventricular CSF. The total volume of 25 mL is only an average figure, and

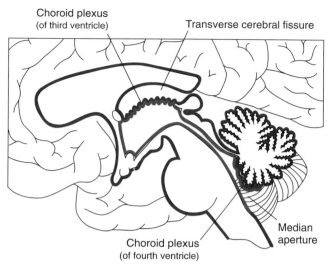

Choroid plexus
(of third ventricle)

Transverse cerebral fissure

Choroid plexus
(of fourth ventricle)

Median
aperture

Figure 5-5 Disposition of the pia mater and ependyma in and around the third and fourth ventricles. Colored lines indicate the edges of the pia mater (blue) and ependymal lining (green) that would have been cut during hemisection. Areas where pia and ependyma are directly applied to each other form part of the choroid plexus.

the ventricles of some apparently normal brains have been found to have total volumes of less than 10 mL or more than 30 mL (however, volumes greater than 30 mL are usually considered suspicious).

Choroid Plexus Is the Source of Most CSF

All four ventricles contain strands of highly convoluted and vascular membranous material called **choroid plexus** that secretes most of the CSF. The composition of choroid plexus can be appreciated by first considering, for example, the anatomy of the roof of the third ventricle (see Figs. 2-19 and 5-5). This roof is simply a layer of ependymal cells overlain by a layer of pia. As in all other locations, the pial layer also faces subarachnoid space. At certain locations this pia-ependyma complex invaginates into the ventricle with a collection of capillaries (Fig. 5-6). Here the ependymal layer is specialized as a cuboidal, secretory epithelium, the **choroid epithelium;** the whole ependyma-pia-capillary complex is the choroid plexus. There is a long, continuous band of choroid plexus reflecting the original C-shaped course of each lateral ventricle, extending from near the tip of the inferior horn, through the body of the ventricle, and reaching the interventricular foramen (Fig. 5-7 and see Fig. 5-3). There is no choroid plexus in the anterior or posterior horn. The plexus is enlarged in the region of the atrium, and here it is called the **glomus** (Latin for "ball of thread"). Choroid plexus becomes calcified with age, and the glomus can often be seen in x-ray studies (see Fig. 5-15D). The choroid plexus of each lateral ventricle grows through the interventricular foramen, forming part of its posterior wall, and becomes one of

the two narrow strands of choroid plexus in the roof of the third ventricle (see Fig. 5-7). It does not continue through the cerebral aqueduct, which is lined with ependyma and completely surrounded by neural tissue.

The choroid plexus of the fourth ventricle is formed from a similar invagination of the inferior medullary velum into the caudal half of the ventricle. It is T shaped, with the vertical part of the T consisting of two adjacent longitudinal strands of plexus. These frequently extend as far as the median aperture, where they are directly exposed to subarachnoid space (see Fig. 5-5). The transverse portion of the T consists of one strand of plexus, which extends into each lateral recess. Each end reaches a lateral aperture, where a small tuft of choroid plexus generally protrudes through the aperture and is exposed directly to subarachnoid space.

Because one side of pia mater always faces subarachnoid space, choroid plexus must always be adjacent to subarachnoid space on its pial side and to intraventricular space on its choroid epithelial side. Although this may seem contrary to the plexus's apparent location deep within each cerebral hemisphere (see Fig. 5-3), it can be easily demonstrated in coronal sections (Fig. 5-8). The location of the invagination of choroid plexus into the lateral ventricle is called the **choroid fissure.** The choroid fissure is a C-shaped slit of subarachnoid space that accompanies the fornix from the inferior horn to the interventricular foramen. By the same reasoning, the space above the roof of the third ventricle, which continues laterally into the choroid fissure, is also subarachnoid space (see Figs. 5-5 and 5-8). This is the **transverse cerebral fissure,** a long finger of subarachnoid space trapped in the middle of the cerebrum by growth of the cerebral hemispheres posteriorly over the diencephalon and brainstem. The transverse cerebral fissure continues posteriorly into the superior cistern.

The Ependymal Lining of Choroid Plexus Is Specialized as a Secretory Epithelium

Choroid plexus is functionally a three-layered membrane between blood and CSF (Fig. 5-9). The first layer is the endothelial wall of each choroidal capillary. This wall is fenestrated, allowing easy movement of substances out of the capillary (in contrast to capillary walls elsewhere in the brain, which, as discussed in Chapter 6, are tightly sealed). The second layer, consisting of scattered pial cells and some collagen, is fragmentary. The third layer, derived from the same layer of cells that forms the ependymal lining of the ventricles, is the choroid epithelium. The choroid epithelial cells look as though they are specialized for secretion because they have many basal infoldings, numerous microvilli on the side facing the CSF, and abundant mitochondria. In addition, adjacent cells are connected to one another by arrays of tight junctions that occlude the extracellular

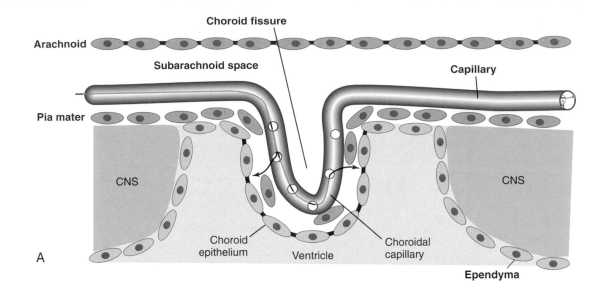

A

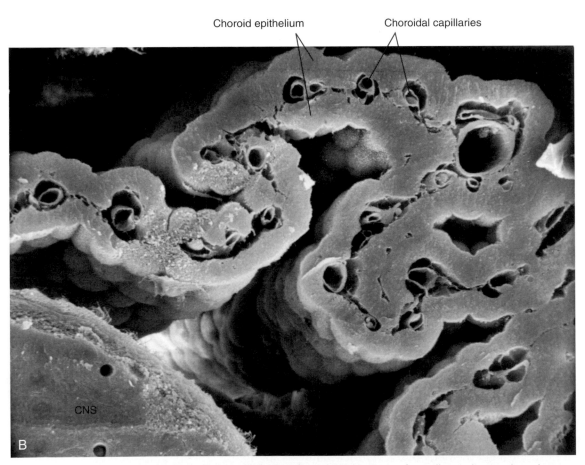

B

Figure 5-6 **A,** Composition of choroid plexus. Fenestrations are shown in the choroidal segment of a capillary, indicating that substances can escape from blood into the choroid plexus. However, they are stopped by arrays of tight junctions (represented here as dark bars) between choroid epithelial cells. **B,** Scanning electron micrograph of a freeze-fractured preparation of choroid plexus. Note that choroid epithelium almost completely surrounds the choroidal capillaries, being separated from the capillaries only by attenuated pial elements. *(B, from Kessel RG, Kardon RH: Tissues and organs: a text-atlas of scanning electron microscopy, New York, 1979, WH Freeman.)*

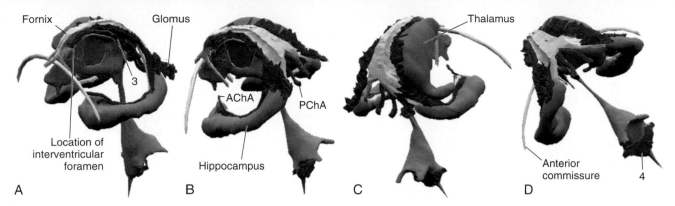

Figure 5-7 Three-dimensional reconstruction showing the location of choroid plexus, seen from the left and front **(A)**, left and rear **(B)**, right and rear **(C)**, and obliquely above and behind **(D)**. The cerebral hemispheres, lateral ventricles, and left thalamus were removed for clarity. A C-shaped strand of choroid plexus curves around with the medial wall of the inferior horn and body of each lateral ventricle, forms part of the wall of the interventricular foramen, and continues into the roof of the third ventricle (3). Separate strands of choroid plexus invaginate the roof of the fourth ventricle (4). (See Video 5-3.)

space between them. As in the case of the arachnoid barrier layer discussed in Chapter 4, these junctions help limit the movement of substances across the choroid epithelium; some ions are able to diffuse across these tight junctions, but peptides and other larger molecules are blocked.

The surface area of the choroid plexus is increased not only by the folding of individual cell membranes into microvilli but also by the macroscopic folding of the choroid plexus itself into numerous fronds and villi (see Fig. 5-8). This folding is so extensive that the total surface area of the human choroid plexus, neglecting the contribution of the microvilli, is more than 200 cm^2 or about two thirds of the total ventricular surface area.

CSF Is a Secretion of the Choroid Plexus

CSF is a clear, colorless liquid, low in cells and proteins but generally similar to plasma in its ionic composition. For this reason, it was considered for some time to be an ultrafiltrate of blood. However, careful analysis of the composition of CSF reveals that its content of various ions differs from that of plasma in a way that is not consistent with its being an ultrafiltrate. For example, compared with plasma, CSF contains a higher concentration of magnesium and chloride ions and a lower concentration of potassium and calcium ions. Furthermore, these concentrations are maintained at very stable levels in the face of changes in plasma concentrations—a constancy that would not be expected if CSF were an ultrafiltrate.[a] Finally, the formation of new CSF is

---

[a]Because the composition of CSF is so constant in health, changes in its composition can be very helpful in diagnosing neurological disease. For example, meningitis can be either viral or bacterial in origin. In the latter case, the glucose concentration in the CSF is markedly reduced (the bacteria eat the glucose), and the protein concentration is elevated. In viral meningitis, glucose is normal and protein is slightly elevated or normal.

depressed by certain metabolic inhibitors, as would be expected if it was formed by an active, energy-requiring process. From these and other observations, it is clear that CSF is an actively secreted product whose composition is dictated by specific transport mechanisms.

Most of the CSF is produced within the ventricles by their choroid plexuses. Production of fluid by the choroid plexus was demonstrated directly by a neurosurgeon, Harvey Cushing, early in the 20th century. During procedures in which it was necessary to open and drain a lateral ventricle, he noted that fluid could be seen accumulating on the surface of the choroid plexus; if he put a small silver clip on the artery supplying the choroid plexus, the fluid stopped appearing. A basically similar procedure has been used since then to study the composition of newly formed CSF: a micropipette in contact with oil-covered choroid plexus can collect the fluid as it is formed. Chemical analysis has shown that it is identical in composition to bulk CSF in normal ventricles.

CSF is formed by filtration of blood through the fenestrations of the choroidal capillaries, followed by the active transport of substances (particularly sodium ions) across the choroid epithelium into the ventricle. Water then flows passively across the epithelium to maintain osmotic balance. The barrier properties of the choroid epithelium prevent substances from diffusing across it in an uncontrolled manner. The total process is actually more complicated than this and involves a balance between active transport and some passive diffusion of ions and other substances either through or between the choroid epithelial cells. It is also known that some substances are transported in the reverse direction (i.e., from CSF to blood) and that there are specific transporters for certain nutrients, vitamins, and other substances.

Although CSF is secreted primarily by choroid plexus, lesser amounts are also secreted by the arachnoid, ependymal, and perivascular spaces of the brain. At any given

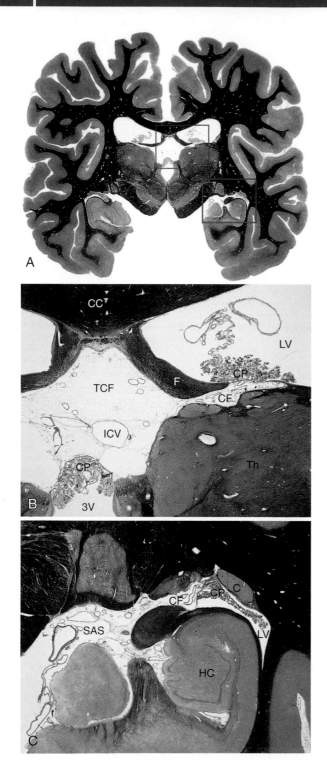

A

B

C

Figure 5-8 Coronal sections at different magnifications demonstrating how choroid plexus faces subarachnoid space on one side and ventricular space on the other. The areas outlined in **A** are enlarged in **B** and **C.** In **B,** choroid plexus (CP) separates the subarachnoid space of the transverse cerebral fissure (TCF) from the intraventricular spaces of the lateral ventricle (LV) and third ventricle (3V). Similarly, in **C,** choroid plexus (CP) separates subarachnoid space (SAS) of the ambient cistern from the intraventricular space of the inferior horn of the lateral ventricle (LV). The site of invagination of the choroid plexus in the medial wall of the lateral ventricle is the choroid fissure (CF). C, tail of the caudate nucleus; CC, corpus callosum; F, fornix; HC, hippocampus; ICV, internal cerebral vein (a major tributary of the great vein; see Chapter 6); Th, thalamus. (**A,** from Nolte J, Angevine JB Jr: The human brain in photographs and diagrams, ed 3, St. Louis, 2007, Mosby.)

time, there is approximately 150 mL of CSF circulating in the ventricles and subarachnoid space. The production of about 500 mL/day means that CSF is completely turned over three to four times per day. The rate of formation of new CSF is relatively constant and little affected by systemic blood pressure or intraventricular pressure.

One way this rate of formation can be modified is by the autonomic nervous system. Both sympathetic and parasympathetic fibers end not only on choroidal blood vessels but also near the bases of the choroid epithelial cells. Stimulating the sympathetic fibers, for example, causes a reduction of about 30% in the rate of CSF production. Little is known, however, about the significance of this autonomic innervation under ordinary circumstances.

CSF Circulates Through and Around the CNS, Eventually Reaching the Venous System

If the CSF is turned over several times per day, it must circulate from its site of formation to a site of removal. We have already discussed all the elements of the system involved (Fig. 5-10): CSF formed in the lateral ventricles passes through the interventricular foramina into the third ventricle, from there through the cerebral aqueduct into the fourth ventricle, and then through the median and lateral apertures into the cisterna magna and the pontine cistern. From these basal cisterns, the fluid slowly moves through the tentorial notch, up and over the cerebral hemispheres, through the arachnoid villi, and into the superior sagittal sinus. The movement should not be thought of as a slow and steady circulation, because arterial pulsations, respiratory movements, and vasomotor activity cause a constant ebb and flow, with a small net movement toward the superior sagittal sinus with each heartbeat.

In addition to this basic pattern of circulation, some CSF moves from the cisterns around the fourth ventricle into the subarachnoid space around the spinal cord. As might be expected from the effect of gravity, CSF in the lumbar cistern (inferior to the spinal cord) tends to be more static, the effects of which remain unclear. Eventually, most of this fluid is returned to the venous system through arachnoid villi that penetrate the dural sleeves accompanying spinal nerve roots.

CSF Has Multiple Functions

The CSF in the subarachnoid space plays a mechanically supportive role because of the buoyant effect discussed previously. In addition, CSF serves as part of a spatial buffering system necessitated by the fact that the brain lives inside a rigid skull: something inside the skull can enlarge only if something else leaves. For example, the heart pumps arterial blood into the brain with each beat.

Space is made for this arterial blood partly by venous blood leaving and partly by CSF leaving, either through the arachnoid villi or into spinal subarachnoid space. Hence a small volume of CSF sloshes back and forth through the foramen magnum with each heartbeat (Fig. 5-11). Similarly, but over a longer time, an expanding mass such as a tumor can be accommodated to some extent by decreased CSF volume (see Figs. 4-17A and 4-18A).

It seems apparent, however, that an actively secreted, constantly renewed fluid with a closely regulated composition must have other functions as well. Most of the functions that have been suggested involve regulation of the extracellular environment of neurons. This can happen in one or both of two ways. First, the CSF is in free communication with the extracellular fluid of the brain, so secretion of controlled CSF by the choroid plexus secondarily controls, to some extent, the composition of this extracellular fluid. Second, the CSF system probably exerts a reverse sort of control by acting as a "sink" for substances produced by the brain, which are then selectively absorbed from CSF by the choroid plexus or nonselectively removed by flow through arachnoid villi. It is also likely that the CSF is a route for the spread of neuroactive hormones through the nervous system.

Imaging Techniques Allow Noninvasive Visualization of the CNS

The neurological examination of a patient can often reveal a great deal about any underlying pathology, particularly its probable anatomical location. However, much additional information, sometimes critically important, can be provided in images of the CNS or its surroundings. Until fairly recently, the CNS of live, unopened people could not be imaged at all, and it was

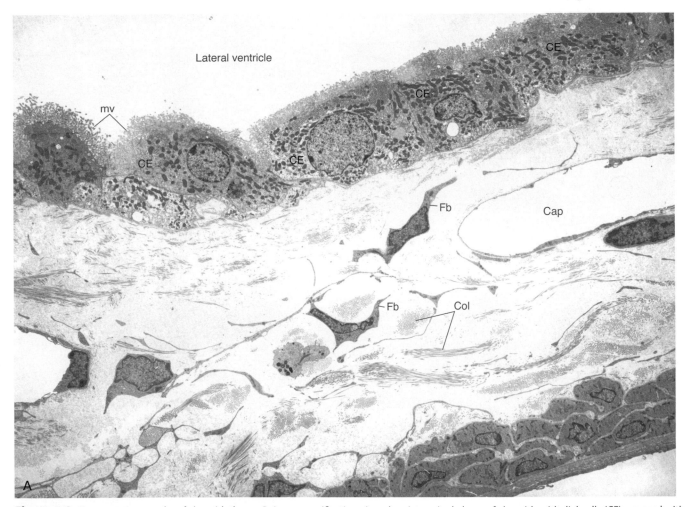

Figure 5-9 Electron micrographs of choroid plexus. **A,** Low-magnification view showing a single layer of choroid epithelial cells (CE), covered with microvilli (mv) that protrude into the ventricle. Near the basal surfaces of the choroid epithelial cells are thin-walled, fenestrated capillaries (Cap) embedded in a loose connective tissue matrix (Col, collagen; Fb, fibroblast) derived from the pia.

Continued

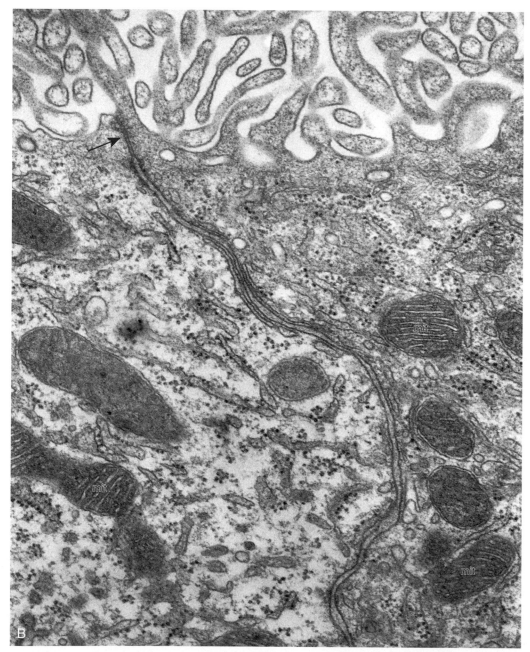

Figure 5-9, cont'd **B,** Higher-magnification view of two adjacent choroid epithelial cells, joined near their ventricular surfaces by a tight junction *(arrow)*. Abundant mitochondria (mit) subserve the energy requirements of CSF secretion. *(**A,** from Peters A, Palay SL, Webster H de F: The fine structure of the nervous system: neurons and their supporting cells, ed 3, New York, 1991, Oxford University Press. **B,** from Pannese E: Neurocytology: fine structure of neurons, nerve processes, and neuroglial cells, New York, 1994, Thieme Medical Publishers.)*

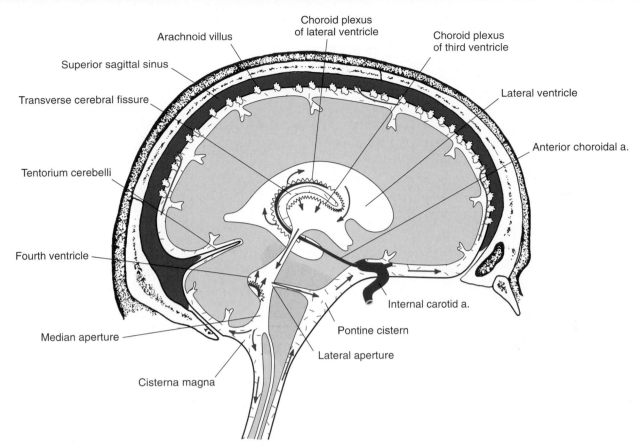

Figure 5-10 Path of CSF circulation from its formation in the ventricles to its absorption into the superior sagittal sinus. *(Redrawn from Hamilton WJ, editor: Textbook of human anatomy, ed 2, St. Louis, 1976, Mosby.)*

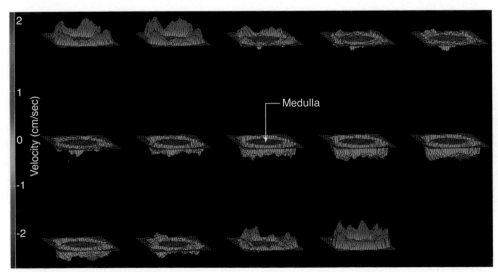

Figure 5-11 Magnetic resonance imaging is usually used to map out the concentration of water in different parts of the head and body (discussed later in this chapter). However, its parameters can also be adjusted to measure the velocity of water movement in some direction. This series of contour plots shows the velocity of CSF movement up and down through the foramen magnum in the subarachnoid space surrounding the medulla. The data were acquired in synchrony with a volunteer's electrocardiogram, and the time from the first image to the last corresponds to a single heartbeat. CSF moves upward (positive velocity) in phase with diastole, slows to zero, then moves downward in phase with systole. *(From Quigley MF et al: Radiology 232:229, 2004.)*

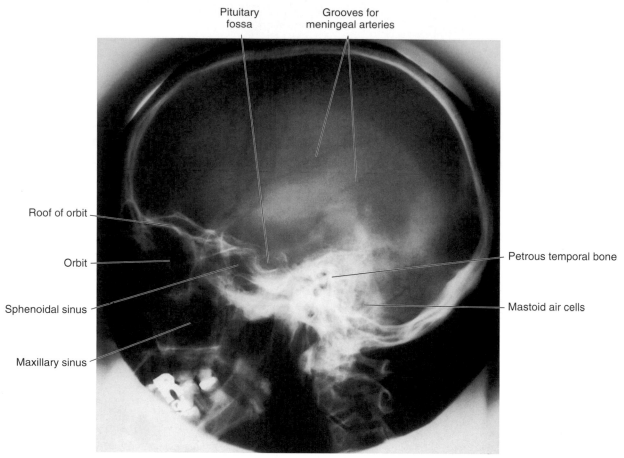

Pituitary
fossa

Grooves for
meningeal arteries

Roof of orbit

Orbit

Sphenoidal sinus

Maxillary sinus

Petrous temporal bone

Mastoid air cells

Figure 5-12 Normal skull x-ray image of a 67-year-old man. The CNS cannot be distinguished, and the x-ray densities of multiple spatially separated structures (e.g., sella turcica, both temporal bones) are collapsed onto one plane. *(Courtesy Dr. Raymond F. Carmody, University of Arizona College of Medicine.)*

necessary to make images of things within or around the brain and infer the shape of the brain from these images.

Conventional skull x-ray studies, the first clinical imaging modality used to provide indirect information about the brain, work by directing x-rays through a patient's head and using photographic film to record what comes out the other side; areas that are particularly x-ray dense (e.g., temporal bones) block transmission and are recorded as light areas on the film. This procedure has two major disadvantages: (1) it can record differences only between things that vary substantially in x-ray density (e.g., bone vs. brain vs. air), so different parts of the brain cannot be distinguished from one another; and (2) all the x-ray density between the source and the film gets "collapsed" into a single plane (Fig. 5-12). Both these problems have been overcome by the tomographic techniques described later.

One of the few ways to get hints about the shape of the brain using skull x-rays is to introduce air into the subarachnoid space or ventricles. (Another is to record the configuration of intracranial arteries and veins, as described in Chapter 6.) Air is much less x-ray dense than CSF, so the shape of air-filled ventricles can be recorded by x-ray photography in a procedure called **pneumoencephalography** (Fig. 5-13). The shape of the ventricles can yield information not only about the ventricles themselves (e.g., the presence and location of hydrocephalus, as discussed later) but also about masses pushing against the brain and distorting the ventricles. Pneumoencephalography is painful and dangerous, and fortunately, it has been replaced by other imaging techniques.

Tomography Produces Images of Two-Dimensional "Slices"

The Greek word *tomos* means "slice" (as in a microtome used to cut brain sections), and **tomography** means "constructing pictures of slices." Some photographic tricks can be used to get one plane of the skull in better focus than the rest of the skull—this is what tomography originally referred to—but the use of computers to

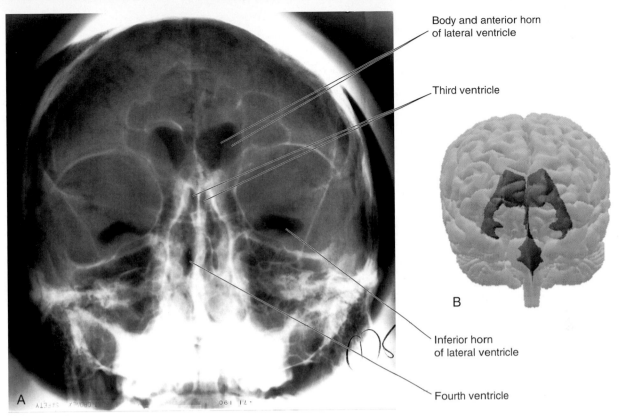

Body and anterior horn
of lateral ventricle

Third ventricle

Inferior horn
of lateral ventricle

Fourth ventricle

Figure 5-13 A, Normal pneumoencephalogram, anteroposterior view (as though looking into the patient's face). The body and inferior horn of each lateral ventricle are particularly dark because they are viewed approximately end-on, so that the x-rays traverse a relatively long path through air. **B,** Three-dimensional reconstruction of the ventricular system inside a translucent brain, seen in a similar orientation. **(A,** *courtesy Dr. John Stears, University of Colorado Health Sciences Center.)*

reconstruct slices using signals coming from or through the brain has revolutionized neuroradiology. Computed tomography (CT) can be based on any measurable parameter that varies in different parts of the brain.

The essence of the method of computation can be appreciated using the following example: If an x-ray source and an x-ray detector were coupled together and rotated around a person's head at ear level, the x-ray beam would be attenuated by varying amounts as the source-detector pair rotated. For example, the beam would be attenuated a lot when it passed through the petrous temporal bones, less so when it was oriented at other angles. The only x-ray density that would be present at every angle would be the density of the spot inside the head where all the beams intersected (Fig. 5-14); this would be a constant, to which a varying density that depended on the x-ray angle would be added. By repeating this procedure with many different centers of rotation and, in essence, subtracting the variable density each time, it is possible to compute the density at each point in the plane of rotation.

There are multiple techniques that produce reconstructed "slices" using some variant of this calculation.

The parameter mapped, as described further in this and the next chapter, can be x-ray density or the concentration of water or a variety of other substances.

CT Produces Maps of X-Ray Density

X-ray **computed tomography** (usually referred to simply as **CT**) is based on variations in x-ray density at different points in the head or body, as in the example just described. CT was the first of the new wave of techniques that have overcome the limitations referred to earlier: it can produce a picture of the brain itself, and it can do so in slices (rather than collapsing the whole brain into a single plane). CSF, gray matter, white matter, and bone can all be distinguished (Fig. 5-15). Because CT provides images based on x-ray density, structures such as bone that attenuate x-rays appear light; structures such as air and CSF that do not attenuate x-rays as much appear darker; blood (Fig. 5-16) and brain are intermediate. The spatial resolution of CT is not quite as good as that of skull x-rays, but for most purposes, its advantages far outweigh this limitation.

The range of x-ray densities in someone's head is much greater than can be displayed in a single gray-scale

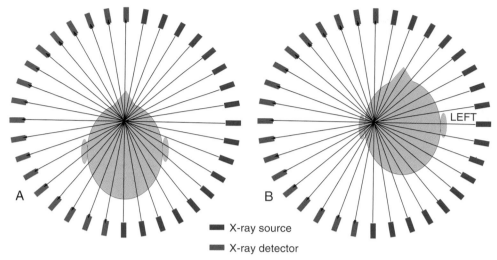

LEFT

■ X-ray source
■ X-ray detector

Figure 5-14 Principle of CT. **A,** The only x-ray density encountered by all the beams is that at their point of intersection. **B,** Moving the sources and detectors results in a change in the common density encountered by all beams. (By convention, images are constructed as though looking from below the patient's head, so the patient's left side is on the right side of the image.)

image,[b] so if the contrast "window" of the CT apparatus is set to display CSF–gray matter–white matter differences, bone will be solid white with little detail visible. The window can be reset to emphasize bone detail, turning soft tissue a more or less uniform dark gray (Fig. 5-17; see also Fig. 4-15A). Because x-ray CT produces maps of x-ray density, radiopaque dyes (called *contrast agents*) can be injected intravenously, and the portions of blood vessels in any given slice can be visualized (see Fig. 6-16).

MRI Produces Maps of Water Concentration

Because CT reconstructs images based on spatial variations in x-ray density, the relatively small density differences between gray and white matter limit its ability to differentiate between different areas of the brain. In addition, the much greater x-ray density of bone can overwhelm these small gray-white differences and cause

artifacts in bony areas such as the posterior fossa (see Fig. 5-15B).

Magnetic resonance imaging (MRI) overcomes these problems by being exquisitely sensitive to spatial variations in the concentration and physicochemical situation of particular atomic nuclei (almost always hydrogen nuclei). Nuclei with an odd number of protons or neutrons, such as hydrogen nuclei, behave like tiny magnets. Imposing a powerful magnetic field on something containing these nuclei (e.g., the head) causes a net tendency for the nuclei to align with the external field. Once so aligned, the nuclei preferentially absorb and then emit electromagnetic energy at a particular frequency (the resonant frequency for that nucleus in that situation). Hence applying radiofrequency pulses to a subject in a strong, static magnetic field, and then measuring the spatial distributions of various time constants with which the absorbed energy is reemitted, can provide data for the construction of extraordinarily detailed images (Fig. 5-18) based on different tissue properties. In addition, images can be reconstructed not only in approximately horizontal planes similar to those used for CT but also in coronal and parasagittal planes (Fig. 5-19).

Two time constants—T1 and T2—are important in clinical MRI (Fig. 5-20). T1 is the time constant with which nuclei return to alignment with the static field. T2 is the time constant with which nuclei, all perturbed at the same time by radiofrequency pulses, lose alignment with one another. T1- and T2-weighted images emphasize different tissue parameters in different ways. For example, CSF is dark in T1 images and light in T2 images; white matter is light in T1, dark in T2. Both types of images can be used to demonstrate various kinds of

[b]Our visual system can distinguish only a few hundred levels of gray between the parts of an image that are completely black and those that are completely white. The gray scale in printed images, for example, uses 256 levels of gray, so two things that differ in brightness by less than about 0.4% will look the same. The difference in x-ray density between gray matter and white matter accounts for less than 0.2% of the range between air and dense bone; even the difference between brain and CSF accounts for less than 1%. Hence CT images are constructed so that the available levels of gray are devoted to a restricted range of the x-ray densities present. In typical images, gray matter, white matter, and CSF are the center of attention; CSF and everything significantly less dense (e.g., fat, air) appears black, and everything significantly more dense than blood (e.g., all kinds of bone) appears white.

Text continued on p. 121

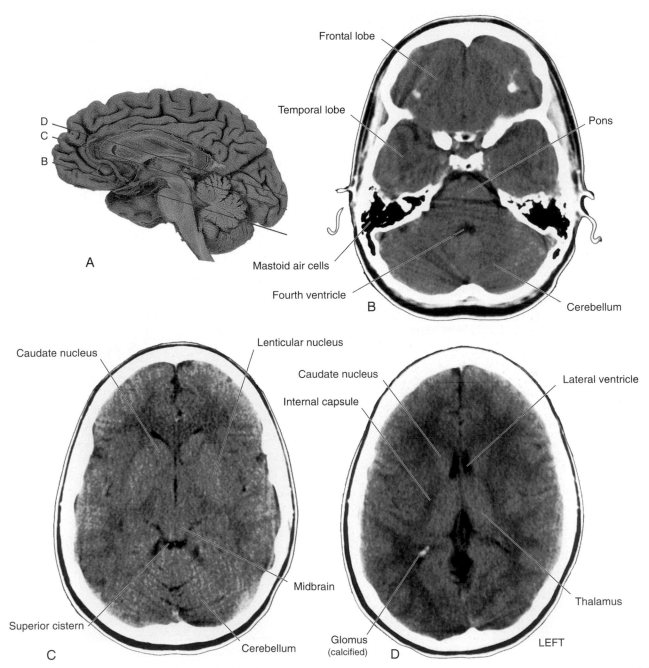

Figure 5-15 Examples of CT scans. CSF is dark in these scans and fills the ventricular system, subarachnoid cisterns, and cerebral sulci around the edge of the brain. Bone is white, air is black, and gray matter is slightly lighter than white matter. **A,** Planes of section produced by the computer and displayed as **B, C,** and **D.** The streaks cutting across the brainstem and cerebellum in **B** are artifacts reflecting the dense bone surrounding these regions. *(Courtesy Dr. Raymond F. Carmody, University of Arizona College of Medicine.)*

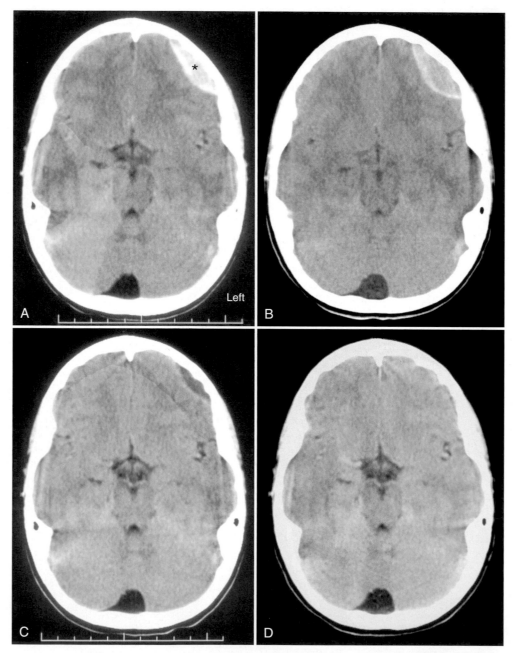

Figure 5-16 Progressive changes in the appearance of blood as demonstrated by CT. A 13-year-old boy fell from his bicycle, struck his head, and incurred an epidural hematoma overlying his left frontal lobe. He did not lose consciousness, and surgery was thought to be unnecessary; instead, he was followed clinically, and sequential CT scans were obtained. A day after the accident **(A),** the high hemoglobin concentration in the clot (*) makes it more x-ray dense than brain. The hemoglobin slowly breaks down, and at 8 days **(B),** the hematoma is about the same density as brain; at 23 days **(C),** it is smaller and less dense; and by 38 days **(D),** it is almost completely resorbed. *(Courtesy Dr. Raymond F. Carmody, University of Arizona College of Medicine.)*

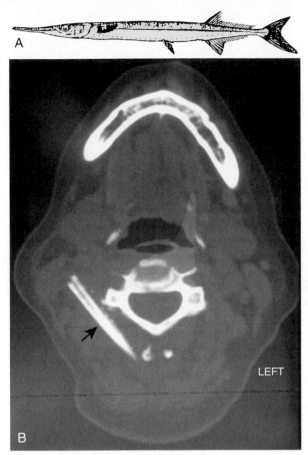

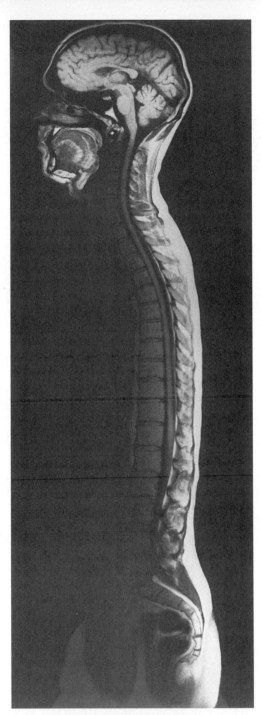

Figure 5-17 Imaging of calcified objects using CT. A 53-year-old woman was swimming in the Red Sea when a needlefish (*Tylosorus crocodilus,* **A**) leaped from the water about 20 m away, flew through the air, and struck her on the neck. At the time, an x-ray of her neck revealed nothing abnormal, so her wound was dressed and she was released. She had neck pain of increasing intensity, and a bone-window CT scan **(B)** a month later revealed the calcified beak of the needlefish *(arrow)* adjacent to the transverse process of the C4 vertebra. The beak was removed successfully. *(From Bendet E et al: Ann Otol Rhinol Laryngol 104:248, 1995.)*

Figure 5-18 Midsagittal magnetic resonance image, demonstrating the extraordinary anatomical detail possible with this technique. *(Courtesy Philips Medical Systems.)*

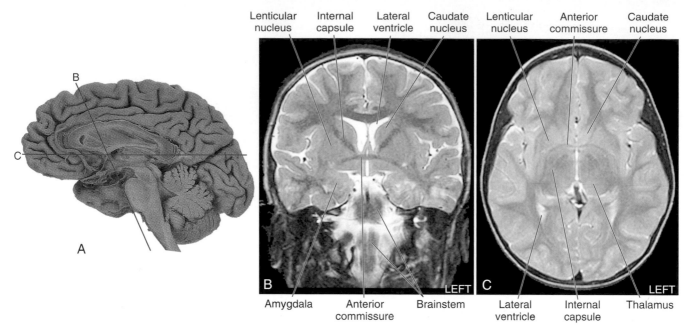

Figure 5-19 Examples of magnetic resonance images (T2-weighted). **A,** Planes of section produced by the computer and displayed as **B** and **C.** Magnetic resonance images can be produced not only in axial planes but also in coronal and parasagittal planes. By convention, coronal images are constructed as though looking at the patient's face, so the patient's left side is on the right side of the image. *(Courtesy Dr. Joachim F. Seeger, University of Arizona College of Medicine.)*

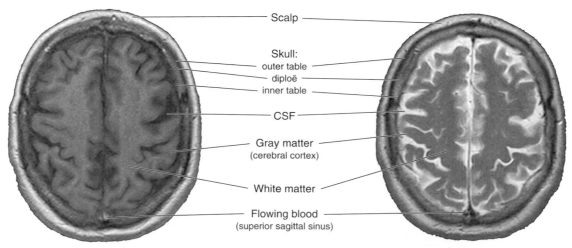

Figure 5-20 T1-weighted (left) and T2-weighted (right) magnetic resonance images. In T1-weighted images, white matter is lighter than gray matter, and CSF is dark. Conversely, in T2-weighted images, white matter is darker than gray matter, and CSF is bright and prominent. In both, air and dense bone, which contain relatively few hydrogen nuclei, are dark. (The spongy, marrow-containing diploic layer of the skull, in contrast, can be seen.) The appearance of flowing blood depends on a number of technical parameters, but in many instances, such as the T2-weighted image on the right, perturbed nuclei have left the area before the imaging measurement is made, so the blood vessel appears dark, as though no hydrogen nuclei were present. *(Courtesy Dr. Raymond F. Carmody, University of Arizona College of Medicine.)*

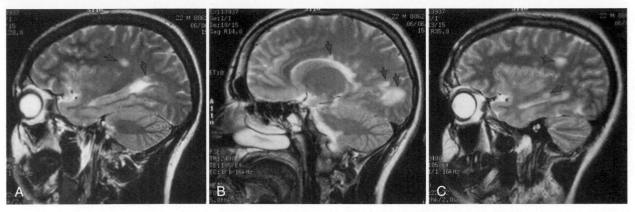

Figure 5-21 Multiple sclerosis demonstrated by MRI. The hallmark of multiple sclerosis is multiple areas of demyelination, separated in space and typically in time. The demyelinated plaques appear as areas of increased signal intensity *(arrows)* in T2-weighted magnetic resonance images in the left hemisphere **(A)**, near the midline **(B)**, and in the right hemisphere **(C)** of this 22-year-old man. *(Courtesy Dr. Raymond F. Carmody, University of Arizona College of Medicine.)*

BOX 5-1

Diffusion Tensor Imaging: *Using Magnetic Resonance Imaging to Visualize Tracts in the White Matter*

Contrasts in T1- and T2-weighted MRI reflect the concentration and physical environment of water, which is relatively constant throughout areas of gray matter; it is also relatively constant throughout areas of white matter (although slightly different than in gray matter). The result is that gray and white matter can be differentiated from each other (see Fig. 5-19), but each looks relatively uniform. Despite its uniformity in these images, white matter contains multiple tracts that interdigitate with one another in complex patterns. Until recently, it was possible to study these tracts only using experimental techniques in animals or following damage in humans (see Box 1-2). Diffusion tensor imaging (DTI) now allows tracts in normal human white matter to be visualized noninvasively.

DTI is based on MRI techniques that measure how easily water is able to diffuse in a given direction in any small volume of the nervous system. Water is able to diffuse equally easily in any direction in bulk CSF; this is referred to as *isotropic diffusion.* Similarly, water diffuses isotropically in gray matter because neuronal cell bodies and dendrites and the clefts between them are not oriented in any systematic way. In white matter, however, it is easier for water to diffuse longitudinally along bundles of axons than transversely: longitudinal travel is unobstructed, but the transverse route requires circuitous travel around axons. This *anisotropic diffusion* can be demonstrated with MRI (Fig. 5-23). The degree of anisotropy in any small volume can be quantified as a *diffusion tensor* (hence the name), which specifies the direction of the anisotropy and its magnitude, and the diffusion tensors in an MRI slice can be converted into a color-coded map (Fig. 5-24). By connecting related diffusion tensors in successive MRI slices, remarkable three-dimensional images of white matter tracts can be reconstructed (Fig. 5-25).

Thanks to Dr. Susumu Mori for help with the preparation of this box.

---

intracranial pathology, often in ways that cannot be accomplished with CT (Figs. 5-21 and 5-22).

More recent MRI techniques allow the mapping of local changes in blood flow during brain activity (see Fig. 6-21) and the reconstruction of tracts in white matter (Box 5-1).

Disruption of CSF Circulation Can Cause Hydrocephalus

Because the rate of production of CSF is relatively independent of blood pressure and intraventricular pressure, fluid continues to be produced even if the path of its circulation is blocked or is otherwise abnormal. When this happens, CSF pressure rises, and ultimately the ventricles expand at the expense of surrounding brain tissue, creating a condition known as **hydrocephalus** (Fig. 5-26). In principle, hydrocephalus can result from excess production of CSF, blockage of CSF circulation, or a deficiency in CSF reabsorption. All three types occur, but that caused by a blockage of circulation is by far the most common.

Tumors of the choroid plexus, called *papillomas*, are sometimes associated with hydrocephalus. In some of these cases, a much greater than normal production of

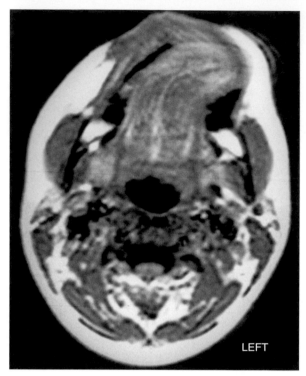

Figure 5-22 An unusual case of linguobuccal dislocation demonstrated by MRI. In this case, "a 48-year-old, 160-pound white man was admitted to our hospital for evaluation of a distended left cheek and pain in his neck. The man reported that while dining, his head became entangled in the purse strap of a female diner walking behind his chair. The force of the strap pulled his head backward, overturning the chair, and forcing his head against the bowling bag belonging to another diner. He was dragged a distance of 14 ft before the woman realized she had snared him. In the emergency room, a protrusion of the left cheek was noted and evaluated with a 0.5-T magnetic resonance (MR) scanner … [which] revealed the patient's tongue in his cheek." *(From IM Fasesjas, Jess Kidden. Am J Neuroradiol 16:777, 1995.)*

CSF has been shown directly and is believed to be the cause of the hydrocephalus.

Circulation of CSF can be obstructed at any point in the pathway, although one of the bottlenecks is the most likely site. A tumor can occlude one interventricular foramen (or both of them), in which case the lateral ventricle involved becomes hydrocephalic and the remainder of the ventricular system remains normal. Tumors of the pineal gland sometimes push down on the midbrain, squeeze the aqueduct shut, and cause hydrocephalus of the third ventricle and both lateral ventricles. In some congenital abnormalities, all three apertures of the fourth ventricle may either fail to develop or be occluded, resulting in hydrocephalus of the entire ventricular system. Finally, circulation may be obstructed outside the ventricular system in the subarachnoid space. For example, a relatively common cause of hydrocephalus in adults is subarachnoid bleeding, which can result in clogging of arachnoid villi by erythrocytes. As another example, meningitis is sometimes followed by meningeal adhesions around the base of the brain that block the flow of CSF through the tentorial notch. (CSF passes from the fourth ventricle into the posterior fossa, so it must ordinarily pass through the tentorial notch before reaching the arachnoid villi of the superior sagittal sinus.) Both of these conditions cause hydrocephalus of the entire ventricular system.

Persistent defects in the reabsorption of CSF are not common, but rare cases have been reported in which an apparent congenital absence of arachnoid villi was associated with hydrocephalus. Also, there are occasional reports of obstruction of the superior sagittal sinus

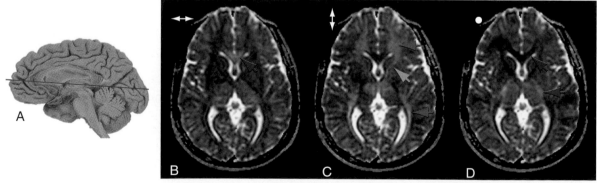

Figure 5-23 Anisotropic diffusion measured with MRI. **A,** The plane of section shown in **B** to **D.** The ease of left-right **(B)**, anteroposterior **(C)**, and up-down **(D)** diffusion is indicated by the lightness of a given area. The appearance of ventricular CSF and of gray matter does not vary, because diffusion is isotropic in these areas. In contrast, the appearance of the genu of the corpus callosum *(red arrows)* does change, from light in **B** (indicating many fibers traveling in a left-right direction) to dark in **C** and **D** (indicating few fibers traveling in any other direction). Similarly, the appearance of frontal and parietal-occipital white matter *(green arrows)* and of the anterior limb of the internal capsule *(light green arrow)* in **C** indicates the presence of many fibers traveling in an anterior-posterior direction. Finally, the appearance of the posterior limb of the internal capsule *(blue arrow)* in **D** indicates the presence of vertically oriented fibers. *(B to D, from Mori S et al: MRI atlas of human white matter, Amsterdam, 2005, Elsevier.)*

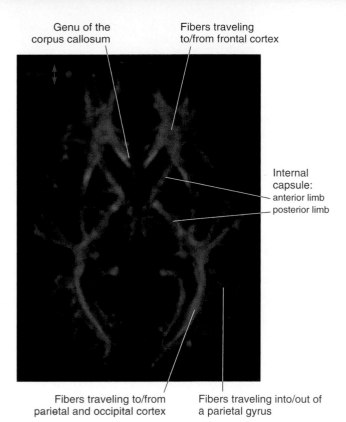

Genu of the corpus callosum

Fibers traveling to/from frontal cortex

Internal capsule:
anterior limb
posterior limb

Fibers traveling to/from parietal and occipital cortex

Fibers traveling into/out of a parietal gyrus

Figure 5-24 Conversion of a series of diffusion measurements (such as those in Fig. 5-23) into a color-coded diffusion tensor map. Red, green, and blue indicate the direction of anisotropy: left-right, anterorposterior, and up-down, respectively. Anisotropy along oblique angles is some mixture of the three primary colors. The brightness of each area indicates the degree of anisotropy there. Isotropic areas (e.g., cortex, CSF) are dark. *(Courtesy Dr. Susumu Mori, Johns Hopkins University School of Medicine.)*

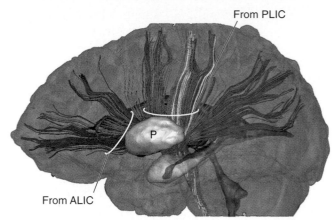

From PLIC

From ALIC

Figure 5-25 Three-dimensional reconstruction of fibers entering and leaving the internal capsule, based on a series of color maps such as that in Figure 5-24. Fibers in the anterior limb of the internal capsule (ALIC) travel mostly in an anteroposterior direction, whereas those in the posterior limb of the internal capsule (PLIC) travel mostly in a vertical direction, many of them continuing down into the brainstem or spinal cord (see Chapter 16 for more details on the internal capsule). P, putamen. *(From Mori S et al: MRI atlas of human white matter, Amsterdam, 2005, Elsevier.)*

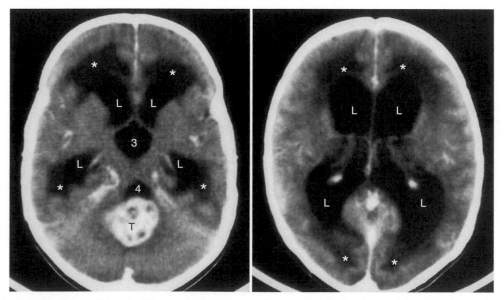

Figure 5-26 Hydrocephalus demonstrated by CT. A tumor (T)—an ependymoma—in the fourth ventricle of this 2-year-old girl obstructed CSF outflow pathways and caused noncommunicating hydrocephalus involving the third (3), fourth (4), and lateral (L) ventricles. The increased intraventricular pressure also caused areas of edema (*) adjacent to the lateral ventricles. *(Courtesy Dr. Raymond F. Carmody, University of Arizona College of Medicine.)*

causing hydrocephalus, presumably because venous pressure becomes high enough to prevent CSF movement through the arachnoid villi.[c]

Clinically, hydrocephalus caused by blockage of CSF circulation is divided into **communicating** and **noncommunicating** types. Communicating (nonobstructive) hydrocephalus occurs in the absence of a blockage of CSF flow, resulting from a failure of resorption, while noncommunicating (obstructive) hydrocephalus results from a blockage of flow through the system. Once diagnosed, many cases of hydrocephalus can be treated surgically by implanting a shunt that extends from the locus of increased pressure to sites such as the peritoneal cavity. The implanted catheter must contain a valve to prevent reverse flow. A more recent alternative is the creation of a hole in the floor of the third ventricle, through which CSF can escape into basal cisterns such as the interpeduncular cistern. There were many early attempts to treat hydrocephalus by removing the choroid plexus, but they were generally unsuccessful, probably because of the continued extrachoroidal production of CSF.

---

[c]Hydrocephalus has been taken as evidence that the arachnoid villi are not the sole route by which CSF can leave the subarachnoid space. Possible alternative routes include movement along the adventitia of blood vessels and the sheaths of cranial and spinal nerves.

SUGGESTED READINGS

Arriada N, Sotelo J: Review: treatment of hydrocephalus in adults. Surg Neurol 58:377, 2002.

Atlas SW, editor: Magnetic resonance imaging of the brain and spine, ed 3, Philadelphia, 2001, Lippincott-Raven.

Beaulieu C: The basis of anisotropic water diffusion in the nervous system: a technical review. NMR Biomed 15:435, 2002.

Brightman MW, Reese TS: Junctions between intimately apposed cell membranes in the vertebrate brain. J Cell Biol 40:648, 1969.
  An important paper that discusses, among other things, the barrier properties of the choroid epithelium.

Brown PD, et al: Molecular mechanisms of cerebrospinal fluid production. Neuroscience 129:955, 2004.

Bruni JE, DelBigio MR, Clattenburg RE: Ependyma: normal and pathological—a review of the literature. Brain Res Rev 9:1, 1985.

Bull JWD: The volume of the cerebral ventricles. Neurology 11:1, 1961.

Cushing H: Studies in intracranial physiology and surgery, London, 1926, Oxford University Press.
  Contains the classic account of the direct observation of CSF forming on the surface of human choroid plexus.

Cutler RWP, et al: Formation and absorption of cerebrospinal fluid in man. Brain 91:707, 1968.
  Direct measurement of the rate of formation of CSF in humans.

Dandy WE: Experimental hydrocephalus. Ann Surg 70:129, 1919.
  The classic description of the production of hydrocephalus by obstruction of an interventricular foramen, cerebral aqueduct, or subarachnoid space around the base of the brain. It appears that, in the light of subsequent work, some of the experiments were technically flawed, but the conclusions are basically sound.

Davson H, Segal MB: Physiology of the CSF and blood-brain barriers, Boca Raton, Fla, 1996, CRC Press.

De Rougemont J, et al: Fluid formed by choroid plexus. J Neurophysiol 23:485, 1960.
  Experiments in which droplets of CSF were collected, under oil, from the surface of the choroid plexus and their composition analyzed.

DiChiro G: Observations on the circulation of the cerebrospinal fluid. Acta Radiol (Diagn) 5:988, 1966.
  Description of the time course and pattern of movement of tracer substances through subarachnoid space on their way toward the venous system.

Dohrmann GJ, Bucy PC: Human choroid plexus: a light and electron microscopic study. J Neurosurg 33:506, 1970.

Duyn JH, et al: High-field MRI of brain cortical substructure based on signal phase. Proc Natl Acad Sci U S A 104:11796, 2007.

Eisenberg HM, McComb JG, Lorenzo AV: Cerebrospinal fluid overproduction and hydrocephalus associated with choroid plexus papilloma. J Neurosurg 40:381, 1974.

Gudeman SK, et al: Surgical removal of bilateral papillomas of the choroid plexus of the lateral ventricles with resolution of hydrocephalus. J Neurosurg 50:677, 1979.

Gutierrez Y, Friede RL, Kaliney WJ: Agenesis of arachnoid granulations and its relationship to communicating hydrocephalus. J Neurosurg 43:553, 1975.

Haaxma-Reiche H, Piers DO, Beekhuis H: Normal cerebrospinal fluid dynamics: a study with intraventricular injection of 111In-DTPA in leukemia and lymphoma without meningeal involvement. Arch Neurol 46:997, 1989.
  A discussion of the time course of tracer movement out of the ventricles and through subarachnoid space.

Hewitt W: The median aperture of the fourth ventricle. J Anat 94:549, 1960.

Kier EL: The cerebral ventricles: a phylogenetic and ontogenetic study. In Newton TH, Potts DG, editors: Radiology of the skull and brain, vol 3, Anatomy and pathology, St Louis, 1977, Mosby.
  A long but fascinating and beautifully illustrated account.

Kruggel F: MRI-based volumetry of head compartments: normative values of healthy adults. Neuroimage 30:1, 2006.

Lindvall M, Owman C: Autonomic nerves in the mammalian choroid plexus and their influence on the formation of cerebrospinal fluid. J Cereb Blood Flow Metab 1:245, 1981.

Lowhagen P, Johansson BB, Nordborg C: The nasal route of cerebrospinal fluid drainage in man: a light-microscope study. Neuropathol Appl Neurobiol 20:543, 1994.

Matsumae M, et al: Age-related changes in intracranial compartment volumes in normal adults assessed by magnetic resonance imaging. J Neurosurg 84:982, 1996.
  Measurements of age-related and gender-related differences in brain volume, ventricular volume, and total CSF volume.

Matsushima T, Rhoton AL, Jr, Lenkey C: Microsurgery of the fourth ventricle. Part 1. Microsurgical anatomy. Neurosurgery 11:631, 1982.
  Finely detailed and beautifully illustrated.

McConnell H, Bianchine J, editors: Cerebrospinal fluid in neurology and psychiatry, London, 1994, Chapman & Hall.

McRae DL, Branch CL, Milner B: The occipital horns and cerebral dominance. Neurology 18:95, 1968.

Milhorat TH: Choroid plexus and cerebrospinal fluid production. Science 166:1514, 1969.
  An account of the continued production of CSF in the lateral ventricles of monkeys after removal of the choroid plexus.

Mori S, et al: MRI atlas of human white matter, Amsterdam, 2005, Elsevier.
  A stunningly beautiful book of diffusion tensor images.

Mori S, Zhang J: Principles of diffusion tensor imaging and its applications to basic neuroscience research. Neuron 51:527, 2006.

Nagata S, Rhoton AL, Jr, Barry M: Microsurgical anatomy of the choroidal fissure. Surg Neurol 30:3, 1988.

Naidich TP, Valvanis AG, Kubik S: Anatomic relationships along the low-middle convexity. Part I. Normal specimens and magnetic resonance imaging. Neurosurgery 36:517, 1995.

A beautifully illustrated paper showing techniques for identifying gyri and sulci in parasagittal magnetic resonance images.

Nicholson C: Signals that go with the flow. Trends Neurosci 22:143, 1999.

A summary of a 1998 workshop on chemical communication via CSF pathways.

Nilsson C, Lindvall-Axelsson M, Owman C: Neuroendocrine regulatory mechanisms in the choroid plexus–cerebrospinal fluid system. Brain Res Rev 17:109, 1992.

Choroid epithelial cells have receptors for a host of hormones and neurotransmitters, the function of which is just beginning to be understood.

Oka K, et al: An observation of the third ventricle under flexible fiberoptic ventriculoscope: normal structure. Surg Neurol 40:273, 1993.

Peering into the ventricles during neurosurgery.

Oldendorf WH: The quest for an image of brain, New York, 1980, Raven Press.

A thoroughly delightful, nontechnical book by one of the founders of CT, tracing the history of various imaging techniques.

Pollay M, Curl F: Secretion of cerebrospinal fluid by the ventricular ependyma of the rabbit. Am J Physiol 213:1031, 1967.

Technically admirable experiments demonstrating the production of CSF within the aqueduct and rostral fourth ventricle.

Quigley MF, et al: Cerebrospinal fluid flow in foramen magnum: temporal and spatial patterns at MR imaging in volunteers and in patients with Chiari I malformation. Radiology 232:229, 2004.

Spector R, Johanson CE: The mammalian choroid plexus. Sci Am 261:68, 1989.

Strazielle N, Ghersi-Egea J-F: Choroid plexus in the central nervous system: biology and physiopathology. J Neuropathol Exp Neurol 59:561, 2000.

Timurkaynak E, Rhoton AL, Jr, Barry M: Microsurgical anatomy and operative approaches to the lateral ventricle. Neurosurgery 19:685, 1986.

Finely detailed and beautifully illustrated.

Torzewski M, et al: Integrated cytology of cerebrospinal fluid, New York, 2008, Springer.

Voetmann E: On the structure and surface area of the human choroid plexus. Acta Anat(Suppl 10):1949.

Welch K, Pollay M: The spinal arachnoid villi of the monkeys Cercopithecus aethiops sabaeus and Macaca irus. Anat Rec 145:43, 1963.

Yamamoto I, Rhoton AL, Jr, Peace DA: Microsurgery of the third ventricle. Part 1. Microsurgical anatomy. Neurosurgery 8:334, 1981.

Finely detailed and beautifully illustrated.

Blood Supply of the Brain

Turtles can walk around for hours with no oxygen supply to their brains. In contrast, our brains are absolutely dependent on a continuous supply of well-oxygenated blood. After just 10 seconds of brain ischemia, we lose consciousness. After 20 seconds, electrical activity ceases, and after just a few minutes, irreversible damage usually begins. Corresponding to this metabolic dependence, blood vessels in the central nervous system (CNS), particularly in gray matter, are arranged in a dense meshwork (Fig. 6-1). An understanding of the brain's blood supply is essential to an understanding of its normal function and of the consequences of cerebrovascular disease. This chapter provides a general overview of the circulatory system of the CNS. Subsequent chapters include a more detailed discussion of the arterial supply of individual portions of the CNS.

The Internal Carotid Arteries and Vertebral Arteries Supply the Brain

The arterial supply of the brain and much of the spinal cord is derived from two pairs of vessels, the **internal carotid arteries** and the **vertebral arteries** (Fig. 6-2). The internal carotid arteries provide about 80%, supplying most of the telencephalon and much of the diencephalon. The vertebral system provides the remaining 20%, supplying the brainstem and cerebellum, as well as parts

Arteries

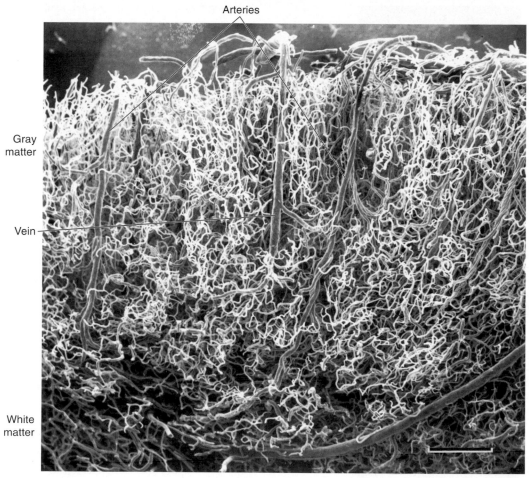

Gray matter

Vein

White matter

Figure 6-1 Arrangement of blood vessels in the cerebral cortex of the temporal pole of a 66-year-old man. The blood vessels were injected with plastic, the surrounding tissues were dissolved away, and an image of the resulting cast was made with a scanning electron microscope (the scale mark corresponds to 500 μm). Notice that the meshwork of vessels is more dense in gray matter than in white matter, corresponding to the greater metabolic needs of neuronal cell bodies. In gray matter, the vessels are so tightly packed that no neuron is more than 100 μm or so from a capillary. *(From Duvernoy HM, Delon S, Vannson JL: Brain Res Bull 7:519, 1981.)*

of the diencephalon, spinal cord, and occipital and temporal lobes (Table 6-1).

The Internal Carotid Arteries Supply Most of the Cerebrum

An internal carotid artery ascends through each side of the neck, traverses the petrous temporal bone, passes through the cavernous sinus, and finally reaches the subarachnoid space at the base of the brain (see Fig. 6-15). Just as it leaves the cavernous sinus, it gives rise to the **ophthalmic artery,** which travels along the optic nerve to the orbit, where it supplies the eye, other orbital contents, and some nearby structures.[a] The internal carotid artery then proceeds superiorly alongside the

optic chiasm (Fig. 6-3) and bifurcates into the **middle** and **anterior cerebral arteries.** Before bifurcating, it gives rise to two smaller branches, the **anterior choroidal artery** and the **posterior communicating artery.** The anterior choroidal artery is a long, thin artery that can be significant clinically in that it supplies a number of different structures and is frequently involved in cerebrovascular accidents. Along its course (see Fig. 6-6) it supplies the optic tract; the choroid plexus of the inferior horn of the lateral ventricle; and some deep brain structures such as portions of the internal capsule, thalamus, and hippocampus (see Fig. 6-22). The posterior communicating artery passes posteriorly, inferior to the optic tract and toward the cerebral peduncle, and joins the **posterior cerebral artery** (part of the vertebral artery system).

The anterior cerebral artery runs medially, superior to the optic nerve, and enters the longitudinal fissure (see Fig. 6-3). The two anterior cerebral arteries, near their entrance into the longitudinal fissure, are connected by the **anterior communicating artery** (see Figs. 6-6 and

[a]The ophthalmic artery, being one of the first divisions of the internal carotid arteries, is vulnerable to atherosclerotic plaques causing a transient ischemic attack referred to as amaurosis fugax (see later).

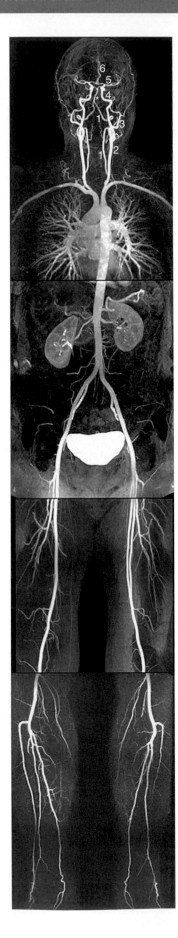

Figure 6-2 Origins of the arterial supply of the brain, seen in a remarkable contrast-enhanced whole-body magnetic resonance angiogram (see Box 6-1) of a healthy 56-year-old man. The vertebral (1) and common carotid (2) arteries can be seen ascending through the neck. The two vertebral arteries fuse to form the basilar artery (*), and each common carotid bifurcates into an external (3) and internal (4) carotid artery. Each internal carotid then ends at the base of the brain by dividing into a middle (5) and anterior (6) cerebral artery. *(From Nael K et al: Radiology 242:865, 2007.)*

6-11). The anterior cerebral arteries then arch posteriorly, following the corpus callosum, to supply medial parts of the frontal and parietal lobes (Fig. 6-4A). Some of the smaller branches extend onto the posterolateral surface of the hemisphere (see Fig. 6-4B). Distal to the anterior communicating artery, the anterior cerebral artery continues as the **pericallosal artery,** which stays immediately adjacent to the corpus callosum. Near the genu of the corpus callosum, the **callosomarginal artery** typically branches off from the pericallosal artery and follows the cingulate sulcus (see Fig. 6-4A). Parts of the precentral and postcentral gyri extend superiorly onto the medial surface of the frontal and parietal lobes, so occlusion of an anterior cerebral artery causes restricted contralateral motor and somatosensory deficits (affecting the leg more than other parts of the body, because of the somatotopic arrangement shown in Fig. 3-30).

The large middle cerebral artery proceeds laterally into the lateral sulcus (see Fig. 6-3). It divides into a number of branches that supply the insula, emerge from the lateral sulcus, and spread out to supply most of the lateral surface of the cerebral hemisphere (Fig. 6-5 and see Fig. 6-4B). Most of the precentral and postcentral gyri are within this area of supply, so occlusion of a middle cerebral artery causes major motor and somatosensory deficits. In addition, if the left hemisphere is the one involved, language deficits are almost invariably found.

Small Perforating Arteries Supply Deep Cerebral Structures

Along its course toward the lateral sulcus, the middle cerebral artery gives rise to as many as a dozen very small branches that penetrate the brain near their origin and supply deep structures of the diencephalon and telencephalon (Figs. 6-6 to 6-8). These particular arteries are called the **lenticulostriate arteries,** but similar small branches, referred to collectively as **perforating** (or **ganglionic) arteries,** arise from all the arteries around the base of the brain. Perforating arteries are particularly numerous in the area adjacent to the optic chiasm and in the area between the cerebral peduncles; for this reason they are called the **anterior** and **posterior perforated substances,** respectively. The narrow, thin-walled

Table 6-1	Arterial Supply of the Central Nervous System*

Anatomical Area	Artery
Cerebral Hemisphere	
Cortical Areas	
Frontal lobe	
Lateral surface	MCA
Medial surface	ACA
Inferior surface	ACA, MCA
Parietal lobe	
Lateral surface	MCA
Medial surface	ACA
Occipital lobe	
Lateral surface	MCA[†]
Medial, inferior surfaces	PCA
Temporal lobe	
Lateral surface	MCA
Medial, inferior surfaces	PCA
Temporal pole	MCA
Limbic lobe	
Cingulate gyrus	ACA
Parahippocampal gyrus	PCA
Insula	MCA
Basal Ganglia	
Caudate nucleus (head)	ACA*p*, MCA*p*
Putamen	MCA*p*, ACA*p*
Globus pallidus	AChA, MCA*p*
Limbic Structures	
Amygdala	AchA
Hippocampus	PCA, AchA
Internal Capsule	MCA*p*, AChA, ACA*p*, ICA*p*
Corpus Callosum	
Genu, body	ACA
Splenium	ACA, PCA
Diencephalon	
Thalamus	PCA*p*, PCom*p*, AChA
Hypothalamus	PCom*p*, ICA*p*, ACom*p*
Cerebellum	
Superior surface	SCA
Inferior, anterior surfaces	PICA, AICA
Brainstem	
Midbrain	PCA, SCA, BA
Pons	BA, AICA
Medulla	VA, PICA
Spinal Cord	
Anterior two thirds	ASpA
Posterior third	PSpA

*Includes major arteries only; does not include areas of overlap such as ACA-MCA overlap on the lateral surface near the longitudinal fissure. For a pictorial representation, see Figure 6-22. More details on particular areas of supply are included in subsequent chapters.
†Middle cerebral and posterior cerebral territories overlap at the occipital pole. This has important implications for the kinds of visual deficits that follow strokes involving a posterior cerebral artery (see Fig. 17-33).
ACA, anterior cerebral artery; AChA, anterior choroidal artery; ACom, anterior communicating artery; AICA, anterior inferior cerebellar artery; ASpA, anterior spinal artery; BA, basilar artery; ICA, internal carotid artery; MCA, middle cerebral artery; *p*, perforating branches of the artery; PCA, posterior cerebral artery; PCom, posterior communicating artery; PICA, posterior inferior cerebellar artery; PSpA, posterior spinal artery; SCA, superior cerebellar artery; VA, vertebral artery.

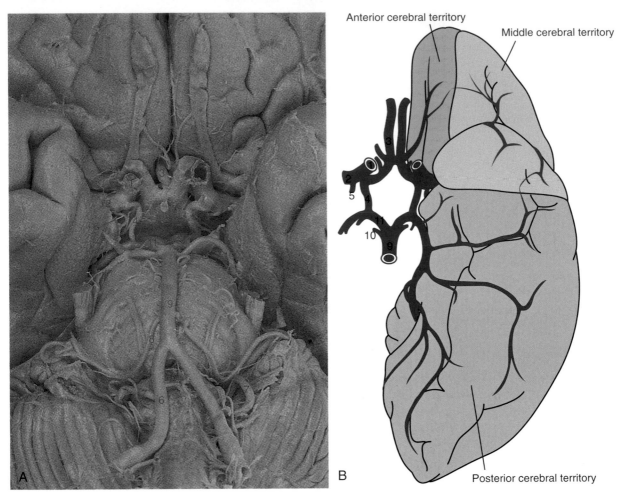

Figure 6-3 Arteries on the inferior surface of the brain **(A)** and sources of arterial supply to cortical areas **(B).** The internal carotid artery (1) divides into the middle (2) and anterior (3) cerebral arteries after giving rise to the posterior communicating (4) and anterior choroidal (5) arteries. Collectively, these vessels supply anterior and lateral parts of the cerebrum. The vertebral arteries (6) join to form the basilar artery (9) after giving rise to the posterior inferior cerebellar artery (7). The basilar artery in turn gives rise to the anterior inferior (8) and superior (10) cerebellar arteries before bifurcating into the posterior cerebral arteries (11). Collectively, the vertebral-basilar system supplies the brainstem, much of the diencephalon, and inferior and posterior parts of the cerebral hemispheres. The apparently very large left posterior communicating artery in this specimen is actually a relatively common variant in which the posterior cerebral artery on one side originates from the internal carotid artery instead of the basilar artery (see Fig. 6-12). (*A, from Nolte J, Angevine JB Jr: The human brain in photographs and diagrams, ed 3, St. Louis, 2007, Mosby; dissection courtesy Grant Dahmer, University of Arizona College of Medicine. **B,** modified from Mettler FA: Neuroanatomy, ed 2, St. Louis, 1948, Mosby.*)

vessels of the anterior perforated substance are involved frequently in strokes (Fig. 6-9). The deep cerebral structures they supply are such that damage to these small vessels can cause neurological deficits out of proportion to their size. For example, the somatosensory projection from the thalamus to the postcentral gyrus must pass through the internal capsule; damage to a small part of the internal capsule from rupture or occlusion of a perforating artery can cause deficits similar to those resulting from damage to a large expanse of cortex.

The Vertebral-Basilar System Supplies the Brainstem and Parts of the Cerebrum and Spinal Cord

The two vertebral arteries run rostrally alongside the medulla and fuse at the junction between the medulla

and pons to form the midline **basilar artery,** which proceeds rostrally along the anterior surface of the pons (see Fig. 6-3).

Before joining the basilar artery, each vertebral artery gives rise to three branches: the **posterior spinal artery, anterior spinal artery,** and **posterior inferior cerebellar artery.** The posterior spinal artery runs caudally along the posterolateral aspect of the spinal cord and supplies the posterior third of the cord. The anterior spinal arteries join together forming a single anterior spinal artery that runs caudally along the anterior midline of the spinal cord, supplying the anterior two thirds of the cord (see Figs. 10-29 and 10-30). These small spinal arteries cannot carry enough blood from the vertebral arteries to supply more than the cervical segments of the spinal cord and must be refilled at various points caudal to this (discussed in Chapter 10). The posterior inferior

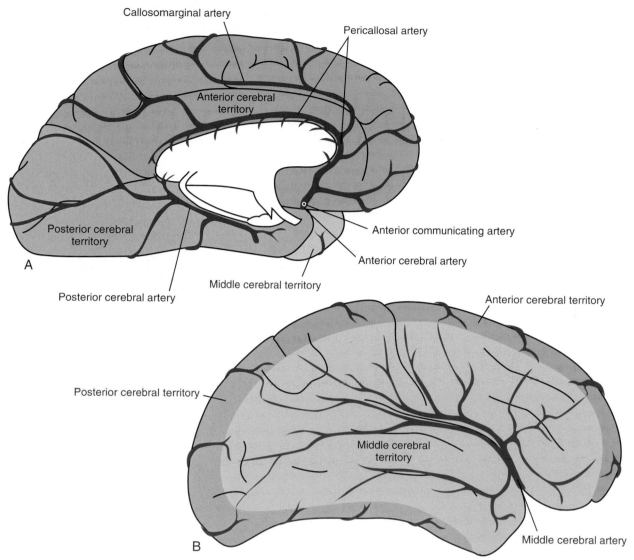

Figure 6-4 Arteries on the medial **(A)** and lateral **(B)** surfaces of the brain, with their areas of supply indicated. *(Modified from Mettler FA: Neuroanatomy, ed 2, St. Louis, 1948, Mosby.)*

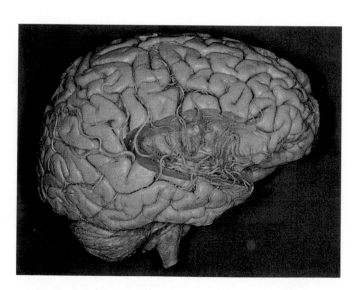

Figure 6-5 Branches of the right middle cerebral artery on the surface of the insula, revealed by removing the opercula of the right hemisphere. *(From Yaşargil MG: Microneurosurgery, vol 4A, CNS tumors: surgical anatomy, neuropathology, neuroradiology, neurophysiology, clinical considerations, operability, treatment options, New York, 1994, Thieme Medical Publishers.)*

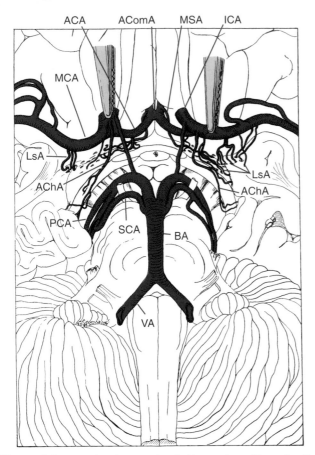

Figure 6-6 Lenticulostriate arteries (LsA), together with perforating branches of the anterior cerebral artery (ACA) and anterior choroidal artery (AChA), entering the anterior perforated substance. Similar perforating branches arise from other arteries of the cerebral arterial circle and from the basilar artery (BA), but these are not included in this drawing. The medial striate artery (MSA), also called the recurrent artery (of Heubner) because of the way it runs back along the anterior cerebral artery, is a major perforating branch important for the supply of the basal ganglia (see Fig. 6-8 and Video 6-1). AComA, anterior communicating artery; ICA, internal carotid artery; MCA, middle cerebral artery; PCA, posterior cerebral artery; SCA, superior cerebellar artery; VA, vertebral artery. *(From Alexander L: Res Pub Assoc Res Nerv Ment Dis 21:77, 1942.)*

cerebellar artery (often referred to by the acronym **PICA**), as its name implies, supplies much of the inferior surface of the cerebellar hemisphere (Fig. 6-10); however, it sends branches to other structures on its way to the cerebellum. As it curves around the brainstem, the PICA supplies much of the lateral medulla, as well as the choroid plexus of the fourth ventricle. This is a uniform occurrence in the large named branches of the vertebral-basilar system, directly comparable to the perforating branches from vessels such as the middle cerebral artery: on their way to their major area of supply, arteries in the vertebral-basilar system send branches to brainstem structures. By knowing the brainstem level at which these large named branches emerge, one can make reasonably accurate inferences about the blood supply of any given region of the brainstem (see Figs. 11-29 and 11-30). The basilar artery proceeds rostrally and, at the level of the midbrain, bifurcates into the two **posterior cerebral arteries.** Before this bifurcation, it gives rise to numerous unnamed branches and two named branches, the **anterior inferior cerebellar artery** and the **superior cerebellar artery.**

The anterior inferior cerebellar artery (or **AICA**) arises just rostral to the origin of the basilar artery and supplies the more anterior portions of the inferior surface of the cerebellum (e.g., the flocculus), as well as parts of the caudal pons. The superior cerebellar artery arises just caudal to the bifurcation of the basilar artery and supplies the superior surface of the cerebellum and much of the caudal midbrain and rostral pons. The many smaller branches of the basilar artery, collectively called **pontine arteries,** supply the remainder of the pons. One of these, the **internal auditory** or **labyrinthine artery** (which is often a branch of the AICA), although hard to distinguish from the others by appearance, is functionally important because it also supplies the inner ear. Its occlusion can lead to vertigo and ipsilateral deafness.

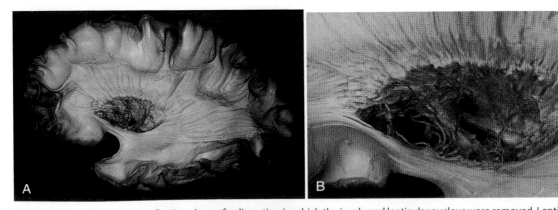

Figure 6-7 Low **(A)** and high **(B)** magnification views of a dissection in which the insula and lenticular nucleus were removed. Lenticulostriate arteries remain, crossing the space formerly occupied by the lenticular nucleus and entering the internal capsule. *(From Yaşargil MG: Microneurosurgery, vol 4A, CNS tumors: surgical anatomy, neuropathology, neuroradiology, neurophysiology, clinical considerations, operability, treatment options, New York, 1994, Thieme Medical Publishers.)*

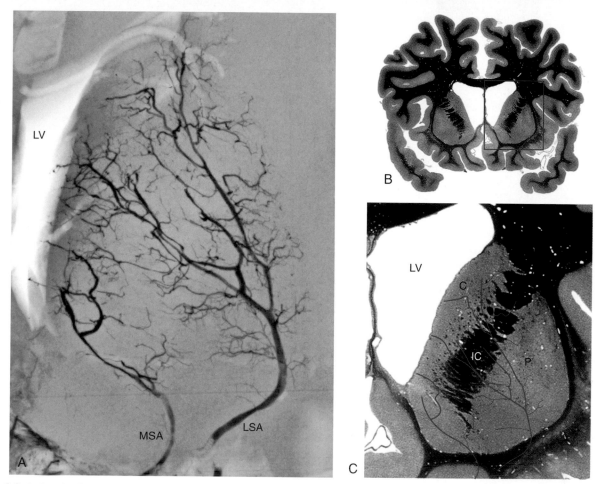

Figure 6-8 A, Supply of parts of the basal ganglia by perforating branches of the anterior and middle cerebral arteries, shown in an x-ray photograph of a brain slice after injection with barium sulfate. The medial striate artery (MSA) is a branch of the anterior cerebral artery, and the lenticulostriate arteries, one of which is seen here (LSA), are branches of the middle cerebral artery. **B,** Brain section in about the same plane shown in **A,** with the area enlarged in **C** indicated. C, caudate nucleus; IC, internal capsule; LV, lateral ventricle; P, putamen. (**A,** *from Feekes JA et al: Ann Neurol 58:18, 2005.*)

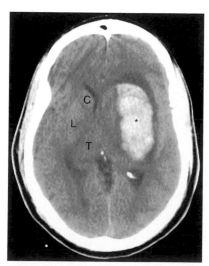

Figure 6-9 Computed tomography scan of a 39-year-old hypertensive man in whom one of the lenticulostriate arteries has ruptured, causing an intracerebral hemorrhage (*) mostly in the basal ganglia. C, caudate nucleus; L, lenticular nucleus; T, thalamus. (*Courtesy Dr. Raymond F. Carmody, University of Arizona College of Medicine.*)

The posterior cerebral artery curves around the midbrain and passes through the superior cistern; its branches spread out to supply the medial and inferior surfaces of the occipital and temporal lobes (see Figs. 6-3, 6-4A, and 6-10). Along the way, it sends branches to the rostral midbrain and posterior parts of the diencephalon including the thalamus. It also gives rise to several **posterior choroidal arteries,** which supply the choroid plexus of the third ventricle and the body of the lateral ventricle. The anterior and posterior choroidal arteries form anastomoses[b] in the vicinity of the glomus. The primary visual cortex is located in the occipital lobe, so occlusion of a posterior cerebral artery at its origin leads to visual field losses in addition to other deficits referable to the midbrain and diencephalon.

[b]Anastomosis comes from the Greek meaning to provide with an outlet or to connect—described as the reconnection of two streams that previously branched out.

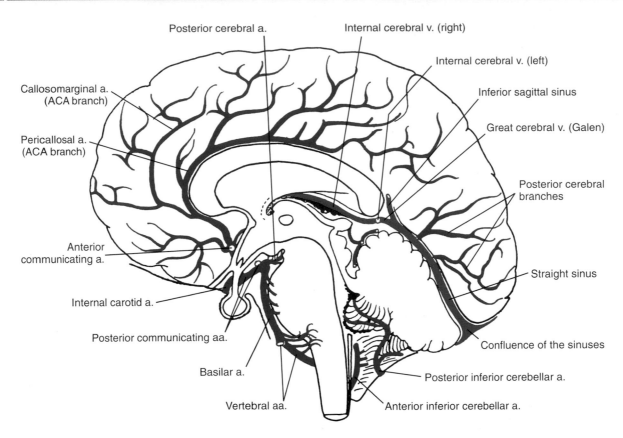

Figure 6-10 Hemisected brain, showing the arterial supply to its medial surface (and part of the venous return as well). ACA, anterior cerebral artery. *(Modified from Mettler FA: Neuroanatomy, ed 2, St. Louis, 1948, Mosby.)*

The Cerebral Arterial Circle (Circle of Willis) Interconnects the Internal Carotid and Vertebral-Basilar Systems

The posterior cerebral artery is connected to the internal carotid artery by the posterior communicating artery. This completes an arterial polygon called the **cerebral arterial circle** (circle of Willis) (Fig. 6-11 and see Fig. 6-3), through which the anterior cerebral, internal carotid, and posterior cerebral arteries of both sides are interconnected. Normally, due to pressure differentials very little blood flows around this circle: the arterial pressure in the internal carotid arteries is about the same as that in the posterior cerebral arteries, so little blood flows through the posterior communicating arteries. However, if one major vessel becomes occluded, either within the cerebral arterial circle or proximal to it, the communicating arteries may allow critically important anastomotic flow and prevent neurological damage. By such a mechanism it would be theoretically possible (though highly unlikely) for the entire brain to be perfused by just one of the four major arteries that normally supply it. The anterior and posterior communicating arteries are quite variable in size (see later), so the establishment of effective anastomotic flow in the event of an arterial occlusion may also depend on the time course of the

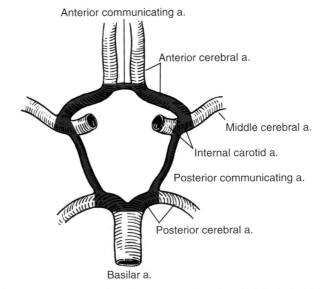

Figure 6-11 The normal cerebral arterial circle, which includes the anterior cerebral artery, the anterior and posterior communicating arteries, and short segments of the internal carotid and posterior cerebral arteries. The middle cerebral artery, the major source of supply to lateral parts of the cerebral hemispheres, is outside the circle. *(Modified from Hodes PJ et al: AJR Am J Roentgenol 70:61, 1953.)*

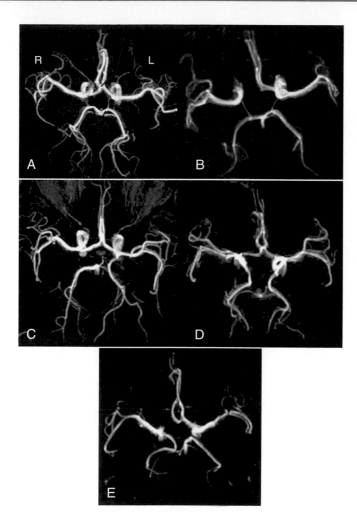

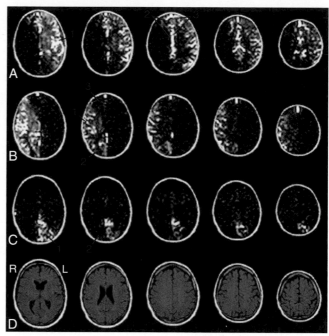

Figure 6-13 Magnetic resonance imaging maps of the areas perfused by different arteries in a brain with the cerebral arterial circle variant shown in Figure 6-12E. **A,** The left internal carotid supplies the territory of the left middle cerebral artery (1) and both the right (2) and left (3) anterior cerebral arteries. **B,** The right internal carotid supplies the territory of the right middle (1) and posterior (2) cerebral arteries, but not the right anterior cerebral artery (3). **C,** The vertebral-basilar system supplies the territory of the left (1) but not the right (2) posterior cerebral artery. **D,** The brain sections mapped. *(From van Laar PJ et al: Neuroimage 29:136, 2006.)*

Figure 6-12 Variants of the cerebral arterial circle, demonstrated by magnetic resonance angiography (see Box 6-1). **A,** Normal circle: 1, anterior cerebral artery; 2, anterior communicating artery; 3, internal carotid artery; 4, posterior communicating artery; 5, posterior cerebral artery. **B,** Circle with a hypoplastic initial segment of the right anterior cerebral artery; both anterior cerebral arteries *(red arrows)* arise from the left internal carotid. This occurs in 5% to 10% of the general population. **C,** The left posterior cerebral artery *(red arrows)* arises from the internal carotid, and the posterior communicating artery *(green arrow)* connects it to the basilar artery and the other posterior cerebral artery. This occurs in about 20% of the population. **D,** Both posterior cerebral arteries *(red arrows)* arise from the internal carotids. This variation is found about 5% of the time. **E,** Both anterior cerebral arteries *(green arrows)* arise from the left internal carotid, and the right posterior cerebral artery *(red arrows)* arises from the right internal carotid. *(A to D, from Hendrikse J et al: Radiology 235:184, 2005. E, from van Laar PJ et al: Neuroimage 29:136, 2006.)*

occlusion. A small communicating artery can enlarge slowly to compensate for a slowly developing occlusion, but in such a case an abrupt blockage might cause serious damage.

Designating the cerebral arterial circle shown in Figure 6-11 as "normal" is largely a nod to an aesthetic need, because fewer than half the circles have this appearance. Some frequently seen "abnormalities" are indicated in Figure 6-12. Asymmetries are common (as in the brain shown in Fig. 6-3A): one or more of the communicating arteries may be very small (hypoplastic) or absent[c]; one anterior cerebral artery may be much smaller at its origin than the other; one posterior cerebral artery may retain its embryological origin from the internal carotid and be connected to the basilar artery through a posterior communicating artery. These asymmetries in the cerebral arterial circle lead to corresponding asymmetries in the way the brain is supplied (Fig. 6-13).

Other routes of collateral circulation are available, although the cerebral arterial circle is likely to be the most important. There are anastomoses at the arteriolar and capillary levels between terminal branches of the cerebral arteries. These are usually inadequate in adults for maintaining the entire territory of a major cerebral artery if it becomes occluded, but occasionally they may be sufficient for maintaining a large part of this territory. In addition, well-defined arterial anastomoses may enlarge to a remarkable degree to compensate for slowly developing occlusions. For example, there have been documented cases in which the territory of one

---

[c]Although parts of the circle are seldom missing entirely, vessels smaller than 0.5 to 1 mm in diameter carry so little blood that they are functionally ineffective and are considered "missing."

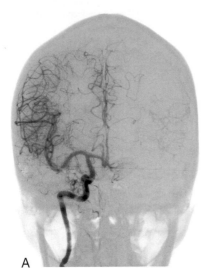 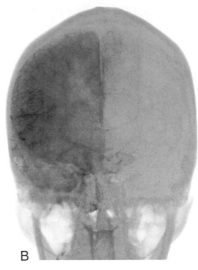 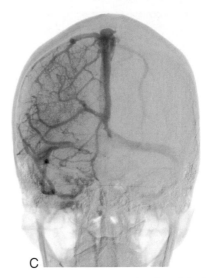

A   B   C

Figure 6-14 Movement of contrast material through the intracranial vasculature, as seen in a series of anteroposterior views (as though looking diagonally downward at the patient's forehead) after injection of the right internal carotid artery. **A,** About 2 seconds after injection, the arteries are filled. **B,** About 5 seconds after injection, the contrast agent has moved out of the arteries and into the capillary beds, resulting in a diffuse image. **C,** About 7 seconds after injection, the contrast agent has moved into veins and venous sinuses. *(Courtesy Dr. Joachim F. Seeger, University of Arizona College of Medicine.)*

posterior cerebral artery was supplied by the internal carotid artery on that side by means of flow through the anterior choroidal artery and, from there, through a posterior choroidal artery and into the posterior cerebral artery.

Finally, there are a limited number of intracranial-extracranial anastomoses that can enlarge to a functional degree. The most important are anastomoses in the orbit between the ophthalmic artery and branches of the external carotid artery. If an internal carotid artery becomes occluded, it is possible for blood from the external carotid artery to flow backward through the ophthalmic artery to reach internal carotid territory.

Imaging Techniques Allow Arteries and Veins to Be Visualized[d]

Blood vessels can be visualized with most imaging techniques by finding a way to make the blood contained within them differ in some way from surrounding structures. Cerebral **angiography** utilizes the intravenous injection of iodinated dyes to make blood much more opaque than brain to x-rays. A cerebral angiogram is typically produced by introducing a catheter into the femoral artery, threading it (under fluoroscopic guidance) up the aorta and into the aortic arch, then steering the catheter tip into the artery of interest. In this way, the contrast material can be introduced into a single vertebral or internal carotid artery. Once the dye

has been introduced, a rapid series of x-ray pictures can follow it as it flows through the artery, into capillaries, and then into veins (Fig. 6-14). Finally, photographic[e] (as in Fig. 6-14) or digital techniques can be used to remove bone images and reveal blood vessels in relative isolation.

Angiography was the first technique developed for making images of normal and diseased vessels, and for decades it was also a major tool for inferring changes in the brain that caused distortion of the vasculature. It still produces the most detailed images of cerebral vasculature (Fig. 6-15). Computed tomography (CT) and magnetic resonance imaging (MRI), however, are less invasive and can simultaneously show the CNS itself. Hence they have become widely used for imaging studies of blood vessels (Box 6-1).

Blood Flow to the CNS Is Closely Controlled

The brain is very active metabolically but has no effective way to store oxygen or glucose. A stable and copious blood supply is therefore required, and the brain, which represents only 2% of the total body weight, uses about 15% of the normal cardiac output and accounts for nearly 25% of the body's oxygen consumption. The

---

[d]Parts of this discussion were adapted from Nolte J, Angevine JB Jr: The human brain in photographs and diagrams, ed 3, St. Louis, 2007, Mosby.

[e]An x-ray image is made before injection of the iodinated dye, and its contrast is reversed (i.e., a positive image is made so that bone is dark). The reverse-contrast image is stacked on top of the image made after dye injection, and a print is made of both together. The reciprocally contrasting portions of the two images thus provide a relatively uniform background from which the blood vessels stand out.

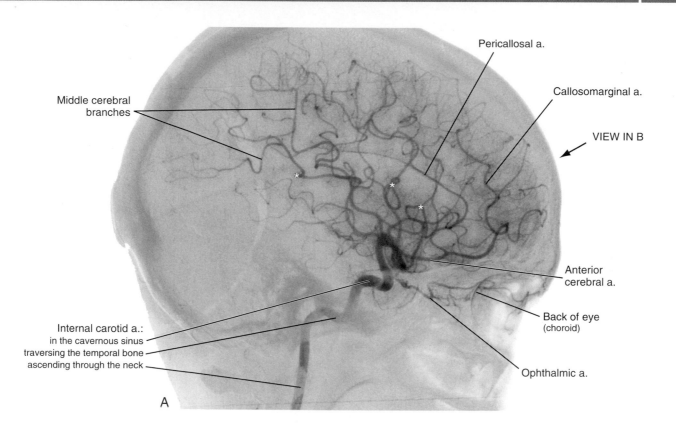

Pericallosal a.

Callosomarginal a.

VIEW IN B

Middle cerebral branches

Anterior cerebral a.

Internal carotid a.:
in the cavernous sinus
traversing the temporal bone
ascending through the neck

Back of eye
(choroid)

Ophthalmic a.

A

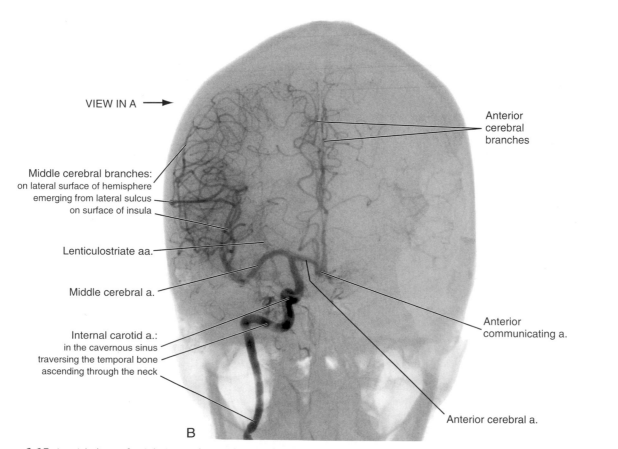

VIEW IN A

Anterior cerebral branches

Middle cerebral branches:
on lateral surface of hemisphere
emerging from lateral sulcus
on surface of insula

Lenticulostriate aa.

Middle cerebral a.

Anterior communicating a.

Internal carotid a.:
in the cavernous sinus
traversing the temporal bone
ascending through the neck

Anterior cerebral a.

B

Figure 6-15 Arterial phase of a right internal carotid angiogram. **A,** Lateral view; anterior is to the right. The *asterisks* indicate sites where middle cerebral branches turn superiorly or inferiorly as they emerge from the lateral sulcus. **B,** Anteroposterior view—as though looking at the patient's forehead. *(Courtesy Dr. Joachim F. Seeger, University of Arizona College of Medicine.)*

Imaging Blood Vessels with Computed Tomography and Magnetic Resonance Imaging

Computed tomography (CT) and magnetic resonance imaging (MRI) techniques can be used to produce not only images of CNS planes but also images of the cerebral vasculature. The x-ray density of blood is not different enough from that of CNS to allow the imaging of blood vessels in ordinary CT scans. However, prior intravenous injection of an x-ray–dense contrast agent such as those used in angiography allows images of both CNS and blood vessels to be created (Fig. 6-16). The spatial resolution of contrast-enhanced CT scans is not as good as that of angiography, but the need to thread catheters into places such as the aortic arch is avoided. In addition, computer processing can remove the CNS from the images and allow three-dimensional reconstructions of arteries or veins (see Figs. 6-23 and 6-32). Various MRI parameters can be adjusted to emphasize the intrinsic properties of flowing blood, making vessels visible even without the use of an intravenous contrast agent (Fig. 6-17). As in the case of contrast-enhanced CT scans, three-dimensional reconstructions—magnetic resonance angiograms—can be produced (see Fig. 6-12).

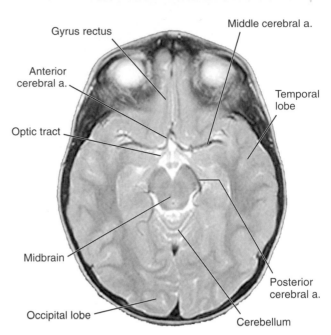

Figure 6-17 T2-weighted magnetic resonance image in which the major arteries of the cerebral arterial circle can be seen, even without injection of a contrast agent. *(Courtesy Dr. Joachim F. Seeger, University of Arizona College of Medicine.)*

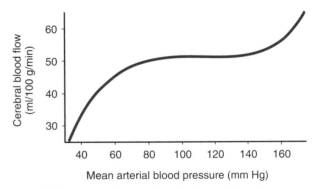

Figure 6-18 Autoregulation of cerebral blood flow. Over a broad range of blood pressures, cerebral vessels dilate as pressure decreases, keeping flow constant. Outside the range in which autoregulation functions, increases or decreases in pressure cause increases or decreases in flow.

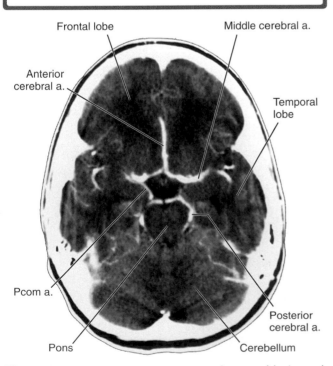

Figure 6-16 Computed tomography scan of a normal brain, made after the injection of an iodinated contrast agent. Pcom a., posterior communicating artery. *(Courtesy Dr. Raymond F. Carmody, University of Arizona College of Medicine.)*

overall flow rate is normally maintained at a very constant level, but this rate may increase or decrease in particular regions of the brain, in a pattern correlated with neural activity.

The Overall Flow Rate Is Constant, but There Are Regional Changes in Blood Flow

Three major kinds of mechanisms are known to be involved in the control of cerebral blood flow. The first is a process termed **autoregulation** (Fig. 6-18), by which cerebral blood vessels themselves act to maintain constant flow. Arterial and arteriolar smooth muscle cells are directly stretch sensitive, so the vessels constrict (thus increasing their resistance) in response to increased blood pressure, and they relax in response to decreased pressure.

The second factor is a collaborative local response of neurons, astrocytes, and cerebral vessels to increased neural activity. Multiple mechanisms are involved, but one of the best studied relies on the astrocytic end-feet applied to neurons and to CNS arterioles and capillaries (see Fig. 1-36C). A large majority of CNS synapses use glutamate as a neurotransmitter (see Chapter 8), so increased synaptic activity causes increased release of glutamate. Some of this spills out of the synaptic cleft and reaches nearby astrocytic end-feet, which also contain glutamate receptors. Binding of glutamate to these receptors causes the increase of intracellular calcium within the astrocyte resulting in the release of vasodilating factors (prostaglandins and others) from end-feet applied to nearby blood vessels, thereby causing a local increase in blood flow. Measuring these regional changes in blood flow in active areas of the brain during various mental activities is, in a very real sense, watching the mind at work. A number of methods for doing this are now available (Box 6-2). The same methods can be

---

BOX 6-2

Watching Changes in Blood Flow: *Images of the Brain at Work*

The electrical signals generated by neurons as they communicate with one another are difficult to localize from outside the head. Hence there has been great interest in indirect measures of neuronal activity, such as increases in blood flow to active areas of the brain. Methods are now available for measuring the regional blood flow in normal human cerebral hemispheres and, by inference, measuring the varying levels of metabolic activity of different areas of the brain during different types of mental activity. An early, conceptually straightforward technique involves the injection of a small amount of an inert, radioactive gas (such as ^{133}Xe, a gamma-emitting isotope of xenon) into the cerebral circulation. After the injection, a bank of gamma-ray cameras records the inflow and washout of the gas while the patient performs various tasks. The spatial resolution of this method is not very good, and it suffers from one of the same drawbacks as plain skull x-rays: the signals from all parts of the three-dimensional brain are collapsed onto one plane. The latter difficulty can be addressed by using intravenously injected gamma-emitting isotopes, a ring of gamma-ray detectors, and tomographic calculations similar to those used in x-ray computed tomography. Because the signal used to construct the tomographic images consists of gamma-ray photons, the process is referred to as single photon emission computed tomography (SPECT). Although technical limitations of SPECT imaging result in a spatial resolution of only 10 mm or so, it is nevertheless a useful clinical method for demonstrating regional changes in brain blood flow.

Positron emission tomography (or PET scanning) is related to SPECT but has twice the spatial resolution. PET scanning relies on the fact that certain isotopes decay by emitting a positron. The emitted positron quickly combines with a nearby electron, and the two particles annihilate each other, producing two gamma rays that travel in opposite directions. By surrounding a patient's head with a ring of gamma-ray detectors, it is possible to localize the positron-emitting isotope within the brain. One way to utilize this phenomenon is to label deoxyglucose with the positron emitter ^{18}F and inject the resulting compound. Active neurons take up deoxyglucose as readily as glucose but metabolize it much more slowly. Therefore the ^{18}F remains in the active neurons long enough for computer-generated tomographic images to be formed (Fig. 6-19). More commonly, a positron emitting isotope of oxygen (^{15}O) is incorporated into water as $H_2{}^{15}O$, which is used to track changes in blood flow. Although expensive and technologically complex, PET scanning has resulted in striking images depicting brain function. Many different compounds can be labeled with positron-emitting isotopes, making it possible to map out not only glucose metabolism and blood flow but also oxygen consumption and the locations of receptors for neurotransmitters and hormones. It is even possible to combine PET and MRI data from single individuals to produce remarkable images of brain activity (Fig. 6-20).

More recently, MRI protocols that emphasize changes in blood flow have been devised. The most common method takes advantage of the differences between the paramagnetic properties of hemoglobin and deoxyhemoglobin. Active areas of brain receive an even greater increase in blood flow than they need, so blood leaving active areas actually has a higher concentration of oxygen than blood leaving inactive areas. Hence MRI signals that reflect hemoglobin-deoxyhemoglobin ratios can provide a measure of regional changes in blood flow. Because these magnetic resonance images (Fig. 6-21) demonstrate areas of brain activity, the process is referred to as functional magnetic resonance imaging (fMRI). Although fMRI is the newest of the activity-imaging techniques, it has rapidly become the most widely used because it uses readily available equipment and, like MRI in general, has the major advantage of being completely noninvasive.

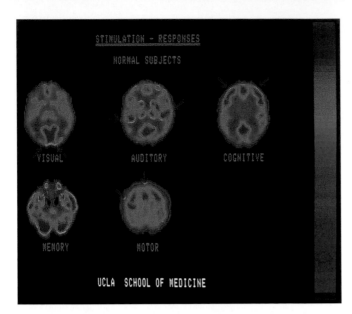

Figure 6-19 Use of positron emission tomography scanning and ^{18}F-fluorodeoxyglucose to map increased glucose consumption in distinctive areas of the brain during different kinds of tasks. All images are in computed tomography planes, with anterior at the top. Yellow and orange areas correspond to areas of increased glucose consumption. A checkerboard visual stimulus activates the medial parts of the occipital lobes. An auditory stimulus causes increased glucose consumption in the superior parts of the temporal lobes; the areas of increase have different shapes in the two hemispheres, reflecting the anatomical asymmetry of the surface of the superior temporal gyrus (see Chapter 22). When an individual is involved in an active, cognitive task rather than the passive perception of stimuli, glucose consumption increases in the frontal lobes. Subjects trying to remember information from a verbal stimulus (a story) show increased glucose consumption in the medial parts of the temporal lobes, consistent with increased metabolism in the hippocampus and amygdala (see Chapters 23 and 24). Sequential movements of the fingers of the right hand activate motor cortex on the left, as well as the supplementary motor area *(vertical arrow)*. *(Courtesy Drs. Michael E. Phelps and John C. Mazziotta, UCLA School of Medicine.)*

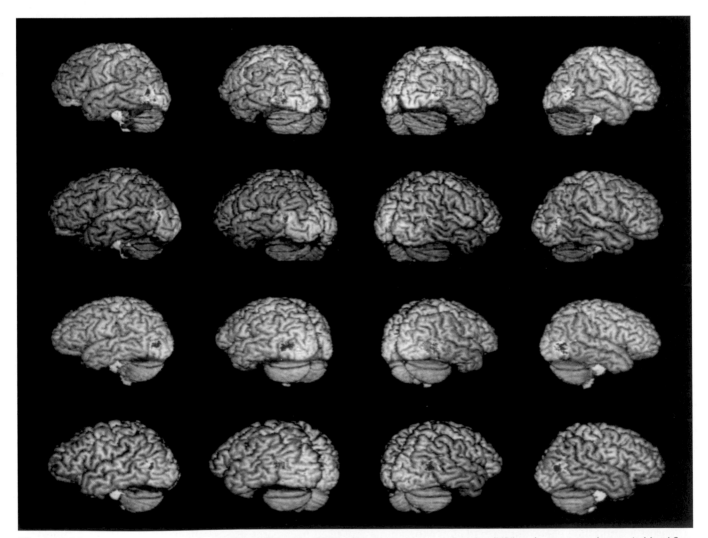

Figure 6-20 Combined use of positron emission tomography (PET) and magnetic resonance imaging (MRI) to demonstrate changes in blood flow as subjects watch moving visual stimuli (versus stationary stimuli); each row of four images is from a different subject. Blood flow was mapped using PET scanning after intravenous injection of $H_2^{15}O$, an image of the surface of each subject's brain was reconstructed from T1-weighted MRI scans, and the two sets of data were co-registered. Moving visual stimuli activate an area on the lateral surface of each occipital lobe, near its junction with the temporal lobe (see Chapter 17). *(From Watson JDG et al: Cereb Cortex 3:79, 1993.)*

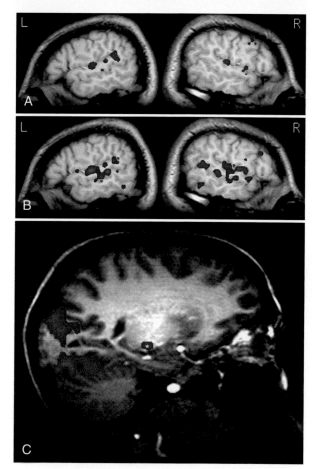

Figure 6-21 Use of functional magnetic resonance imaging (fMRI) to demonstrate human auditory and visual cortex. fMRI data from a 30-year-old man listening to white noise **(A)** and to spoken words **(B)** were superimposed on T1-weighted parasagittal slices of his left (L) and right (R) hemispheres. Yellow and orange areas correspond to areas of increased blood flow. Both stimuli activate the superior temporal gyrus, but spoken words activate a more extensive area of this gyrus. **C,** fMRI data from another subject watching a red and black checkerboard in which the squares reversed color 8 to 10 times per second, again superimposed on a T1-weighted parasagittal slice. The stimulus activates not only occipital cortex above and below the calcarine sulcus but also the principal thalamic nucleus relaying visual information (the lateral geniculate nucleus, *; see Chapter 16). (*A and B,* from Binder JR et al: Ann Neurol 35:662, 1994. *C,* from Chen W et al: Magn Reson Med 39:89, 1998.)

used to study regional metabolic or vascular abnormalities, in some cases when CT and MRI studies appear normal.

Finally, cerebral vessels are innervated both by sympathetic autonomic fibers and by fibers from several locations within the brain. The evidence concerning the role of this innervation is incomplete and somewhat conflicting, but the current consensus is that neural control is of relatively minor importance. It may play a part in adapting to stress of various sorts and in sustaining the extremes of the autoregulation range, but under ordinary circumstances, local control and direct autoregulatory mechanisms seem to predominate.

Strokes Result From Disruption of the Vascular Supply

Cerebrovascular disease and accidents are the most common causes of neurological deficits. Normally, about 55 mL of blood flows through each 100 g of CNS per minute. This is a little more than the CNS needs to survive, but any significant reduction of this perfusion rate rapidly causes malfunction or even death of neurons. Reduction of the flow rate to about 20 mL/100 g/min causes neurons to stop generating electrical signals. Neurons can survive in this condition for a while, and timely restoration of normal flow can restore their function. Reduction to about 10 mL/100 g/min for more than a few minutes initiates processes that result in necrosis of the involved brain tissue. A necrotic region of tissue is called an **infarct.** An abrupt incident of vascular insufficiency is called a **stroke**; bleeding into or immediately adjacent to the brain can also have stroke-like consequences called a hemorrhagic stroke.

Ischemic strokes (those caused by sudden blockage of blood flow to some part of the CNS) are most commonly caused by a **thrombus** (a blood clot formed within a vessel) or an **embolus** (a bit of foreign matter, such as part of a blood clot or an atherosclerotic plaque, carried along in the bloodstream). Either can cause occlusion of an artery supplying the brain, and both are highly correlated with atherosclerosis (although this is by no means the only cause). If the occlusion occurs within or proximal to the cerebral arterial circle, there is a possibility of adequate collateral circulation, particularly if the involved artery slowly became occluded before the stroke. In contrast, anastomoses between arteries distal to the cerebral arterial circle are variable, and collateral circulation is less likely to be adequate, so occlusion of one of these vessels typically results in an infarct in a predictable territory (Fig. 6-22). The size of the infarct is obviously related to the size of the occluded vessel, ranging from tiny lesions (called **lacunes**) caused by occlusion of a small perforating artery to infarcts that affect large expanses of a cerebral hemisphere. However, as pointed out earlier in this chapter, the magnitude of a neurological deficit is not necessarily related to the size of the infarct causing it. A very small lesion in the brainstem or internal capsule can have a much more devastating neurological effect than damage to certain relatively large areas of the cerebellum or cerebral hemispheres. The size and distribution of the infarct are also related to the location of the occlusion along the course of an artery. For example, occlusion of a middle cerebral artery in the lateral sulcus causes a large cortical infarct; occlusion of the same artery as it leaves the cerebral arterial circle also blocks flow into the lenticulostriate arteries on that side, damaging deep structures as well.

Damage to an ischemic area of brain is not all or nothing; rather, it involves multiple processes with

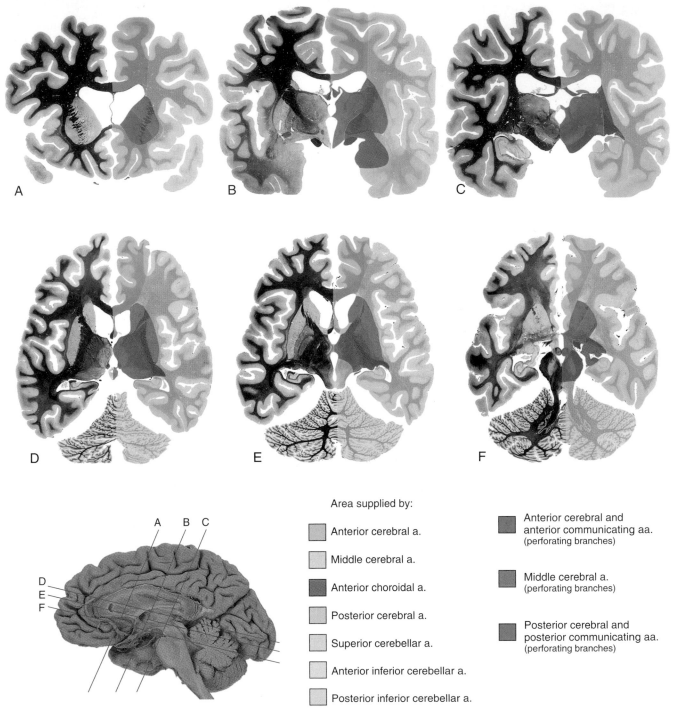

Area supplied by:

Anterior cerebral a.

Middle cerebral a.

Anterior choroidal a.

Posterior cerebral a.

Superior cerebellar a.

Anterior inferior cerebellar a.

Posterior inferior cerebellar a.

Anterior cerebral and anterior communicating aa. (perforating branches)

Middle cerebral a. (perforating branches)

Posterior cerebral and posterior communicating aa. (perforating branches)

Figure 6-22 Areas of the cerebrum and cerebellum supplied by major arteries and their perforating branches shown in coronal (**A** to **C**) and axial (**D** to **F**) sections. Details of the spinal cord and brainstem supply are provided in Chapters 10 and 11.

varying time courses. Profound ischemia rapidly depletes the energy stores of neurons and glial cells, the energy-requiring processes that maintain membrane potentials (see Chapter 7) fail, and the cells depolarize. This in turn causes excessive release of excitatory neurotransmitters, further depolarization, and the initiation of multiple destructive cascades of events that result in relatively rapid death of the cells involved. Simultaneously, slower

destructive processes (e.g., inflammatory responses) that act over a period of days are set in motion; these become apparent only in partially ischemic areas, where blood flow is sufficient to keep cells alive that long. Occlusion of a cerebral artery typically results in a CNS area (the "core") so severely ischemic that it is irreversibly damaged within minutes or hours, surrounded by a less ischemic **penumbra** of neural tissue that may be temporarily inactivated but able to survive for days. Current therapies for stroke are designed to restore blood flow to the ischemic area and to protect neurons from the destructive processes triggered by the ischemia. These therapies include drugs that can break up the clot (i.e., tissue plasminogen activator, tPA), allowing blood to reflow into the ischemic area; however, if there are any damaged blood vessels, tPA may cause excessive bleeding within the brain, causing more damage, and therefore must be used with caution. The core zone can be treated effectively for only a few hours (at most) after the occlusion, but the realization that neurons in the penumbra can still be saved for days afterward has spurred intense research efforts in this area. Therapies after an ischemic stroke include drugs that prevent further emboli and blood clotting including antiplatelets such as aspirin and clopidogrel.

Another vascular event with symptoms somewhat similar to an ischemic stroke is a **transient ischemic attack (TIA).** The crucial difference between a TIA and an ischemic stroke is that the deficits associated with a transient ischemic attack (as the name implies) persist for only a few minutes to a few hours and are followed by an essentially complete recovery. TIAs are usually caused by minute emboli that originate from atherosclerotic plaques or thrombi, partially occlude brain arteries, and are then broken down by normal body mechanisms. A classic example of a TIA syndrome is **transient monocular blindness** or **amaurosis fugax** (Greek for "fleeting darkness"), typically caused by emboli that detach from a plaque in the internal carotid artery, enter the ophthalmic artery, and render the retina temporarily ischemic.

Intracerebral or **intraparenchymal hemorrhage** (see Fig. 6-9) is often considered a type of stroke, although the pathophysiology is different from that of ischemic stroke. Such hemorrhages most commonly result from the rupture of small perforating arteries, such as the lenticulostriate arteries. These are particularly thin-walled vessels, and the likelihood of their spontaneous rupture is increased greatly in individuals suffering from hypertension. The lenticulostriate arteries supply some important deep cerebral structures, and hemorrhage there can be rapidly fatal. Hemorrhage can also occur secondary to an infarct in which tissue and blood vessels begin to die resulting in blood leaking into the infarcted area.

Aneurysms (Greek for "dilation") are balloon-like swellings of arterial walls. They occur most frequently at or near arterial branch points. Those close to the brain usually occur in or near the anterior half of the cerebral arterial circle (Fig. 6-23A), although they are also found at other locations (see Fig. 6-23B). An aneurysm can cause neurological deficits in two ways. As it grows (some can become huge), it may push against and compress brain structures, much as a growing tumor would.

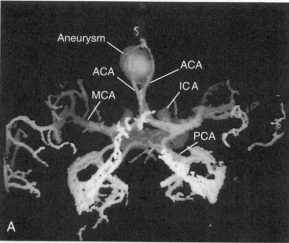

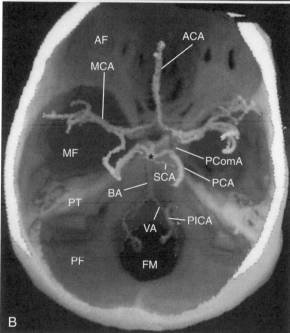

Figure 6-23 Intracranial aneurysms. **A,** Aneurysm near the anterior half of the cerebral arterial circle. The patient was a 58-year-old woman who presented with headache and altered mental status. Computed tomography (CT) studies without contrast revealed subarachnoid hemorrhage, and a three-dimensional rendering of the cerebral arterial circle reconstructed from contrast-enhanced CT scans demonstrated an aneurysm of the left anterior cerebral artery. ACA, anterior cerebral artery; ICA, internal carotid artery; MCA, middle cerebral artery; PCA, posterior cerebral artery. **B,** Aneurysm in a less typical location—the posterior half of the cerebral arterial circle. The patient was a 46-year-old woman being evaluated for what she described as the worst headache of her life. A three-dimensional rendering reconstructed from contrast-enhanced CT scans demonstrated a small aneurysm (*) at the rostral end of the basilar artery. Most of the arteries at the base of the brain can be seen clearly in this reconstruction, including the anterior cerebral (ACA), basilar (BA), middle cerebral (MCA), posterior cerebral (PCA), posterior communicating (PComA), posterior inferior cerebellar (PICA), superior cerebellar (SCA), and vertebral (VA) arteries. Features of the base of the skull are also apparent, including the anterior, middle, and posterior fossae (AF, MF, PF, respectively); foramen magnum (FM); and petrous temporal bone (PT). *(Courtesy Dr. Sean O. Casey, University of Minnesota Medical School.)*

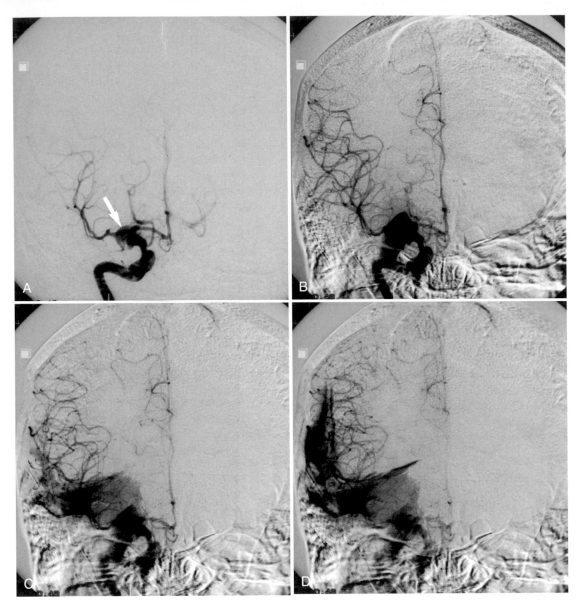

Figure 6-24 Four consecutive images obtained at 0.5-second intervals, showing subarachnoid bleeding from an aneurysm. Angiography of the right internal carotid artery of a 48-year-old woman being evaluated for the sudden onset of severe headache revealed an aneurysm of the internal carotid artery (*arrow* in **A**). As the angiographic procedure began, blood and contrast agent escaped from the aneurysm and spread through the subarachnoid space (**B** to **D**). *(From Franke CL, Engelshove H: J Neurol Neurosurg Psychiatry 60:140, 1996.)*

It also can rupture (Fig. 6-24) and cause a **subarachnoid hemorrhage** (Fig. 6-25) that, depending on its size and location, can have disastrous consequences. Many aneurysms, particularly if they are detected before they become too large, can be corrected surgically.

Another type of vascular problem is an **arteriovenous malformation (AVM).** This is a congenital malformation in which large anastomoses exist between arteries and veins in a relatively circumscribed area circumventing the capillary system (Fig. 6-26). These malformations may become larger with age and can cause neurological problems, either by "stealing" blood from adjacent normal brain tissue as a result of their low resistance or by hemorrhaging.

A System of Barriers Partially Separates the Nervous System From the Rest of the Body

The concept of a **blood-brain barrier** arose from the early observation that many substances, when injected into the bloodstream, do not gain access to the brain. Such a barrier must consist of more than just an impediment at the junction between blood vessels and brain, because this alone would not prevent substances in tissues around the brain from diffusing into it. The term *blood-brain barrier* therefore is commonly used in a more general sense to refer to the anatomical and physiological complex that controls the movement of substances from the general extracellular fluid of the body to the extracellular fluid of the brain. Using the term in this way, the barrier includes three regions of the CNS: (1) the arachnoid barrier layer, (2) the blood–cerebrospinal fluid (CSF) barrier (Fig. 6-27) and what is often referred to as the true blood-brain barrier, and (3) rows of tight junctions between adjacent endothelial cells of CNS capillaries together with a lack of pinocytotic vesicles in these endothelial cells (Fig. 6-28). As in the case of the blood-CSF barrier, this barrier is selective. Lipid-soluble substances can diffuse across it, and glucose can cross it by a process of facilitated diffusion,

but other molecules of similar size and solubility cannot. In addition, various substances can be actively transported in both directions across this endothelial wall. The permeability and transport properties of the barrier are under a degree of neural control and may be influenced in pathological and injured states. Astrocytes are believed to play an important role in relaying chemical messages to endothelial cells within the CNS parenchyma to form tight junctions.

This complex barrier system can be a mixed blessing. For example, it is efficient at keeping microorganisms out of the brain, but it is equally efficient at keeping many drugs such as antibiotics out. An intracranial infection therefore can be difficult to treat. The development of techniques for reversibly opening the blood-brain barrier and the synthesis of therapeutic agents that can cross an intact blood-brain barrier are both active areas of research.

As discussed in Chapter 5, the capillaries of the choroid plexus are fenestrated, and substances can leave them only to be stopped by the arrays of tight junctions between adjacent choroid epithelial cells. There are several other locations where the cerebral capillaries are fenestrated and allow free communication between the blood and the brain's extracellular fluid. These additional sites are in contact with the walls of the third and fourth ventricles and collectively are termed the **circumventricular organs** (Fig. 6-29). They include the pineal gland, the median eminence of the hypothalamus (Fig. 6-30), the posterior lobe of the pituitary gland, and a few other structures. Some circumventricular organs have a sensory function: they contain cell bodies of sensory neurons that monitor the composition of the general extracellular fluid and project their axons to other parts of the CNS. Others are sites where hormones are released

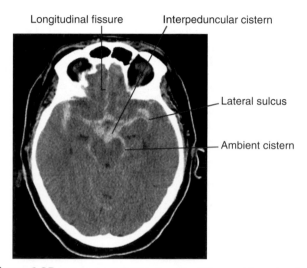

Figure 6-25 Subarachnoid hemorrhage in a 51-year-old man involved in a motor vehicle accident. In contrast to lens-shaped epidural hematomas (see Fig. 4-15) and crescent-shaped subdural hematomas (see Fig. 4-17), subarachnoid hemorrhages spread through the cisterns and fissures surrounding the brain. *(Courtesy Dr. Raymond F. Carmody, University of Arizona College of Medicine.)*

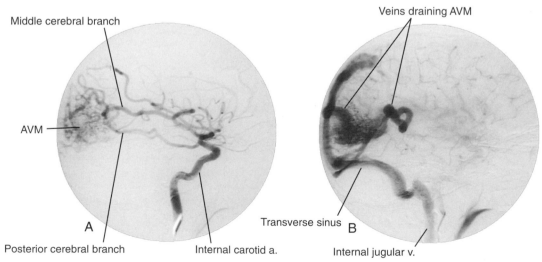

Figure 6-26 Occipital lobe arteriovenous malformation (AVM)—lateral view, with anterior to the right. The AVM is supplied **(A)** by enlarged branches of the middle and posterior cerebral arteries and drains **(B)** through distended venous channels into the straight and superior sagittal sinuses. *(Courtesy Dr. Raymond F. Carmody, University of Arizona College of Medicine.)*

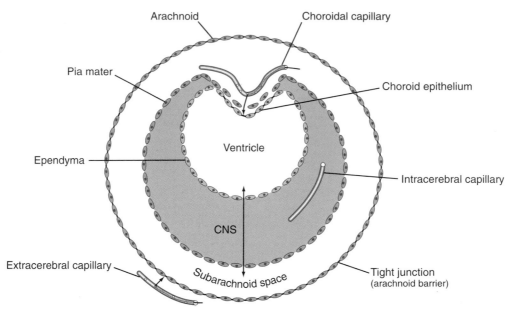

Figure 6-27 Barrier systems in and around the brain. Substances can leave extracerebral capillaries but are then blocked by the arachnoid barrier. They can also leave choroidal capillaries but are then blocked by the choroid epithelium. They cannot leave any other capillaries that are inside the arachnoid barrier (except for those in the circumventricular organs). The ventricular and subarachnoid spaces are in free communication with each other, and both communicate with the extracellular spaces of the brain.

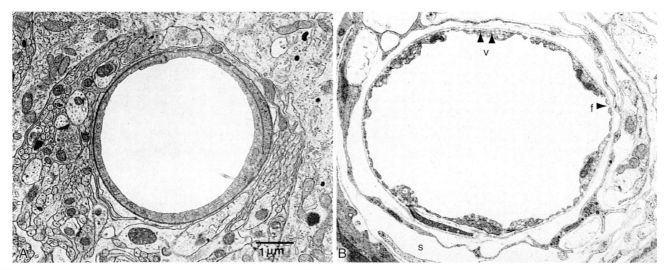

Figure 6-28 CNS capillaries with and without barrier properties. **A,** Capillary in a hypothalamic nucleus (supraoptic nucleus) of a rat. The continuous endothelial wall and the lack of pinocytotic vesicles are apparent; tight junctions are also present between endothelial cells but cannot be seen at this magnification. **B,** Capillary in the subfornical organ, which is a circumventricular organ near the roof of the third ventricle adjacent to the interventricular foramen. The walls of this capillary are quite permeable and are characterized by fenestrations (f), pinocytotic vesicles (v), and substantial spaces (s) around the capillary. *(From Gross PM: Brain Res Bull 15:65, 1985.)*

from neuronal endings for blood-borne distribution. In both varieties, free access to the bloodstream is essential for efficient operation. Specialized ependymal cells called **tanycytes** (specialized ependymal cells) that overlie each circumventricular organ form a barrier between the organ and the ventricular CSF. Tanycyte processes interconnected by tight junctions also form a barrier between the median eminence and adjacent

parts of the hypothalamus, and other circumventricular organs may have a similar barrier.

Superficial and Deep Veins Drain the Brain

The principal route of venous drainage of the brain is through a system of cerebral veins that empty into the

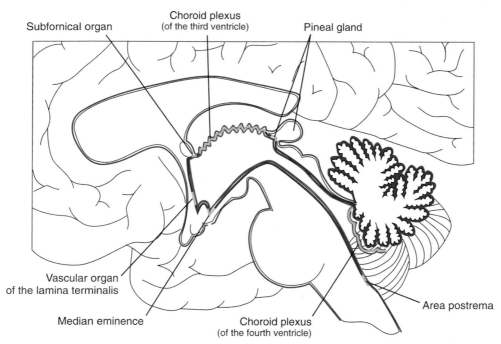

Figure 6-29 Sites in the walls of the third and fourth ventricles where a blood-brain barrier is lacking. Blue and green represent pia mater and ependyma, respectively, as in Figure 5-5. Red represents areas where capillaries in the ventricular wall are part of the blood-brain barrier, and pink represents areas where the capillaries are leaky. The **subfornical organ** is a small nodule in the anterior, superior corner of the third ventricle, adjacent to the interventricular foramina; it has been implicated in the control of fluid balance and drinking behavior (see Chapter 23). The **vascular organ of the lamina terminalis,** as its name implies, is embedded in the lamina terminalis; it participates in the control of fluid balance and may be involved in neuroendocrine functions as well. The **median eminence** and the **posterior lobe of the pituitary** (not shown) are major elements of the neuroendocrine system and are discussed further in Chapter 23. The **pineal gland** secretes melatonin, which participates in the control of seasonal reproductive cycles in many animals; in humans, melatonin plays a role in regulating circadian rhythms (see Chapter 23). The **area postrema,** located in the walls of the caudal end of the fourth ventricle, monitors blood for the presence of toxins and triggers vomiting when appropriate. Some authors also include the choroid plexuses of the lateral, third, and fourth ventricles in the list of circumventricular organs because they lack a blood-brain barrier and are located in ventricular walls.

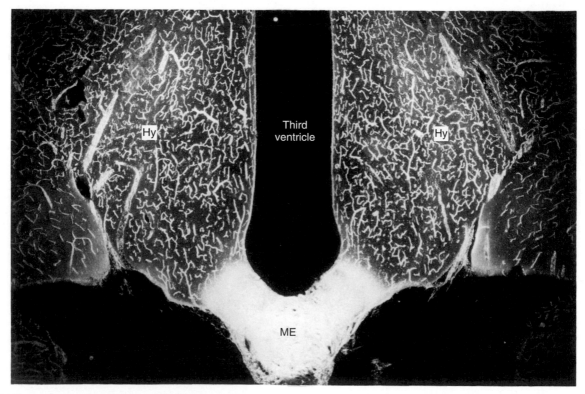

Figure 6-30 Macroscopic demonstration of capillaries inside and outside the blood-brain barrier. Horseradish peroxidase was administered intravenously to a monkey, demonstrated histochemically, and viewed in coronal sections using darkfield microscopy. Reaction product fills the median eminence (ME), an area of the hypothalamus that has no blood-brain barrier and is one of the circumventricular organs. However, no reaction product is seen around the numerous capillaries in the remainder of the hypothalamus (Hy). *(From Broadwell RD et al: J Comp Neurol 260:47, 1987.)*

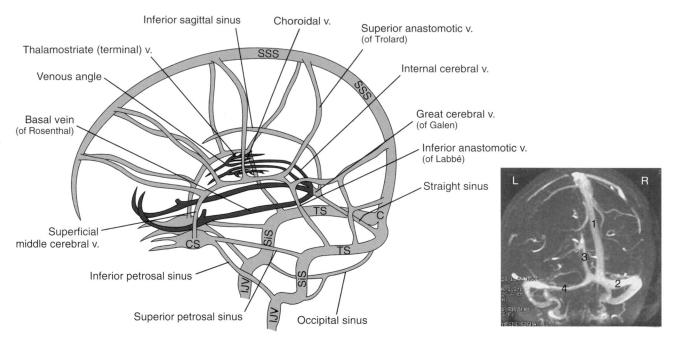

Figure 6-31 Overview of the venous system of the brain. Dural sinuses and superficial veins are light blue; deep veins are bright blue. The inset is a contrast-enhanced magnetic resonance venogram showing a common variant of the confluence of the sinuses, with blood from the superior sagittal sinus (1) flowing mostly into the right transverse sinus (2), and blood from the straight sinus (3) flowing mostly into the left transverse sinus (4). C, confluence of the sinuses; CS, cavernous sinus; IJV, internal jugular vein; SIS, sigmoid sinus; SSS, superior sagittal sinus; TS, transverse sinus. *(Modified from Warwick R, Williams PL, editors: Gray's anatomy, ed 35 Br, Philadelphia, 1973, WB Saunders. Inset, courtesy Dr. Keiko Kobayashi, Kanazawa University School of Medicine.)*

dural venous sinuses and ultimately into the **internal jugular veins** (Fig. 6-31). The internal jugular veins drain into the **basilar venous plexus** around the base of the brain that communicates with the **epidural venous plexus** of the spinal cord.[f] These veins, like cerebral arteries, can be visualized by angiographic (see Fig. 6-14C) or digital (Fig. 6-32) techniques. There is also a collection of **emissary veins** connecting extracranial veins with dural sinuses. These play a relatively minor role in the normal circulatory pattern of the brain but can be important clinically as a path for the spread of infection into the cranial cavity.

Cerebral veins are conventionally divided into **superficial** and **deep** groups. In general, the superficial veins lie on the surface of the cerebral hemispheres, and most empty into the superior sagittal sinus, whereas the deep veins drain internal structures and eventually empty into the straight sinus. The **basal vein (of Rosenthal),** described later in this section, drains some cortical areas but is nevertheless considered a deep vein because it

also drains some deep structures and eventually empties into the straight sinus.

Cerebral veins are valveless and, in contrast to cerebral arteries, are interconnected by numerous functional anastomoses, both within a group and between superficial and deep groups.

Most Superficial Veins Empty Into the Superior Sagittal Sinus

The superficial veins are quite variable and consist of a superior group that empties into the superior and inferior sagittal sinuses and an inferior group that empties into the transverse and cavernous sinuses (Fig. 6-33). Only three of these veins are reasonably constant from one brain to another: (1) the **superficial middle cerebral vein,** which runs anteriorly and inferiorly along the lateral sulcus, draining most of the temporal lobe into the cavernous sinus or into the nearby sphenoparietal sinus; (2) the **superior anastomotic vein** (or **vein of Trolard**), which typically travels across the parietal lobe and connects the superficial middle cerebral vein with the superior sagittal sinus; and (3) the **inferior anastomotic vein** (or **vein of Labbé**), which travels posteriorly and inferiorly across the temporal lobe and connects the superficial middle cerebral vein with the transverse sinus.

---

[f]The internal jugular veins are often considered the only significant routes through which venous blood can leave the head. This is true, however, only when in a supine position. When we sit up or walk around upright, the internal jugulars collapse, and blood leaves through the vertebral venous plexus instead.

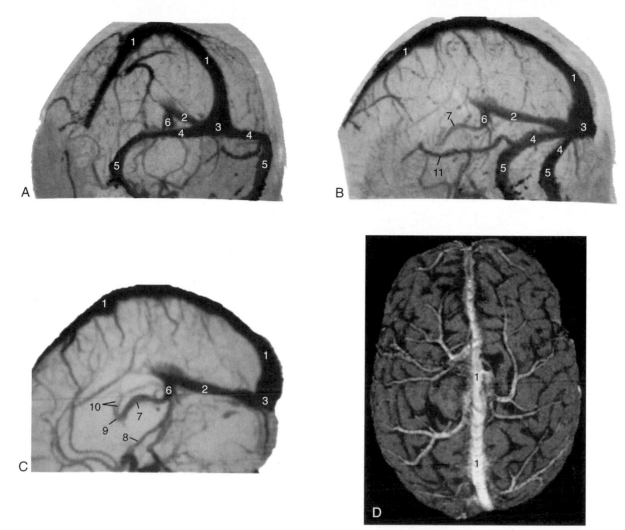

Figure 6-32 Cerebral veins reconstructed from contrast-enhanced computed tomography scans **(A** to **C)** or magnetic resonance images **(D)** and viewed from the left and behind **(A** and **B),** from the left **(C),** and from above **(D).** Blood in the superior sagittal (1) and straight (2) sinuses reaches the confluence of the sinuses (3) and flows from there into the transverse (4) and sigmoid (5) sinuses. Most superficial cortical veins empty into the superior sagittal sinus **(D),** although some empty into other sinuses, such as the vein of Labbé (11) joining the transverse sinus. Deep cerebral veins empty into the great vein (6), which in turn joins the straight sinus. The internal cerebral (7) and basal (8) veins are major tributaries of the great vein. The choroidal, thalamostriate (10), and other veins join at the interventricular foramen and turn posteriorly in the venous angle (9) to form the internal cerebral vein of each side. **(A** and **D,** courtesy Dr. Sean O. Casey, University of Minnesota Medical School. **B** and **C,** from Casey SO et al: Radiology 198:163, 1996.)

Deep Veins Ultimately Empty Into the Straight Sinus

The deep veins are more constant in configuration than are the superficial veins. Because they are found deep in the brain in locations where arteries are small, the deep veins form clinically useful radiological landmarks.

The major deep vein is the **internal cerebral vein** (Fig. 6-34), which is formed at the interventricular foramen by the confluence of two smaller veins: the **septal vein** (so named because it runs posteriorly across the septum pellucidum) and the **thalamostriate** (or **terminal) vein,** which travels in the groove between the thalamus and the caudate nucleus (Fig. 6-35), draining much of both these structures. Near the interventricular foramen, the

thalamostriate vein is joined by the **choroidal vein,** a tortuous vessel that drains the choroid plexus of the body of the lateral ventricle.

Immediately after forming, the internal cerebral vein bends sharply in a posterior direction. This bend is called the **venous angle** and is used in imaging studies as an indication of the location of the interventricular foramen (see Fig. 6-32). The paired internal cerebral veins proceed posteriorly through the transverse cerebral fissure and fuse in the superior cistern to form the unpaired **great cerebral vein** (or **vein of Galen).** The great vein turns superiorly and joins the inferior sagittal sinus to form the straight sinus.

Along its short course, the great vein is joined by the basal veins. On each side the basal vein is formed near

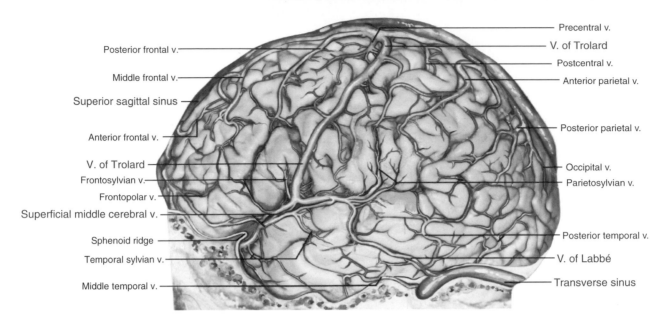

Figure 6-33 Superficial veins of the lateral surface of the brain. Anterior is to the left, and the names of the major veins mentioned in the text are shown in blue. *(From Oka K et al: Neurosurgery 17:711, 1985.)*

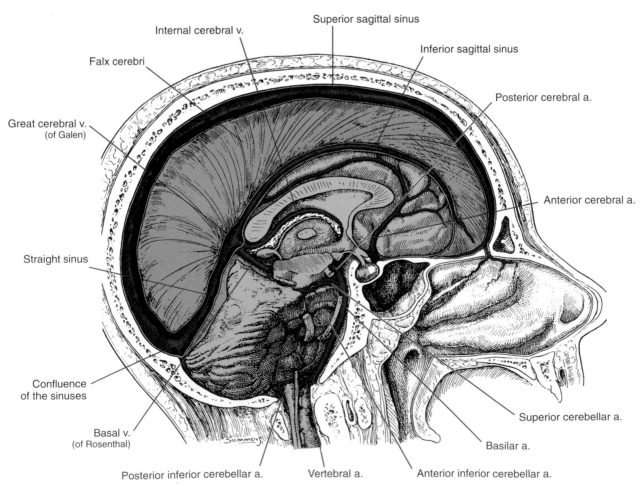

Figure 6-34 Major tributaries of the straight sinus. *(Modified from Mettler FA: Neuroanatomy, ed 2, St. Louis, 1948, Mosby.)*

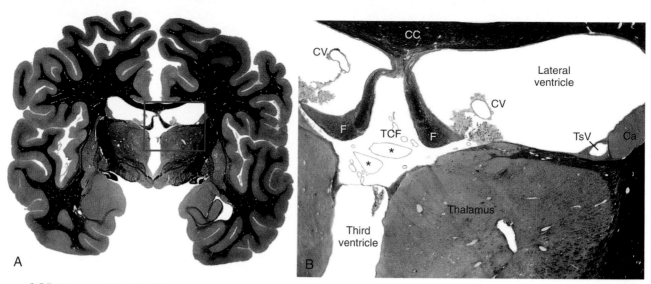

Figure 6-35 Deep cerebral veins. The area outlined in the coronal section in **A** is enlarged in **B**. The thalamostriate vein (TsV) of each hemisphere, in the groove between the thalamus and the caudate nucleus (Ca), joins the choroidal vein (CV) and other deep veins at the interventricular foramen to form the internal cerebral vein. The paired internal cerebral veins (*) turn posteriorly, forming the venous angle, and travel through the transverse cerebral fissure (TCF) before joining to form the great vein. CC, corpus callosum; F, fornix.

the optic chiasm by the **deep middle cerebral vein,** which drains the insula, and several other tributaries that drain inferior portions of the basal ganglia and the orbital surface of the frontal lobe. It then proceeds along the medial surface of the temporal lobe, curves around the cerebral peduncle, and enters the great vein.

In addition to the superficial and deep veins already described, there is a separate, complex collection of veins that serves the cerebellum and brainstem. These drain into the great vein and into the straight, transverse, and petrosal sinuses.

The venous system of the spinal cord includes interior small veins draining into either the posterior spinal vein or the anterior spinal vein eventually drains into the azygos system, a vein running up the right side of the thoracic vertebral column.

Vascular problems involving the venous system are not seen nearly as often as those involving the arterial supply. This is partly because occlusions and hemorrhages occur less often in the venous system and partly because of the large number of functional anastomoses. Thus a slowly developing occlusion of the anterior portion of the superior sagittal sinus probably would be asymptomatic. Even if such an occlusion developed rapidly, the symptoms might be no more than a transient headache. However, if the occlusion were in a more critical location, such as the posterior portion of the superior sagittal sinus, the consequences would be much more serious and might include headache (due to increased intracranial pressure), seizures, and motor problems. Occlusion of the great vein, although unusual, is particularly serious and can result in coma and death.

SUGGESTED READINGS

Alpers BJ, Berry RG, Paddison RM: Anatomical studies of the circle of Willis in normal brain. Arch Neurol Psychiatry 81:409, 1959.

Attwell D, Laughlin SB: An energy budget for signaling in the grey matter of the brain. J Cereb Blood Flow Metab 21:1133, 2001.

Banerjee S, Bhat MA: Neuron-glial interactions in blood-brain barrier formation. Annu Rev Neurosci 30:235, 2007.

Bogousslavsky J, Caplan L, editors: Stroke syndromes, ed 2, New York, 2001, Cambridge University Press.

Bousser M-G, Ferro JM: Cerebral venous thrombosis: an update. Lancet Neurol 6:162, 2007.

Brightman MW, Reese TS: Junctions between intimately apposed cell membranes in the vertebrate brain. J Cell Biol 40:648, 1969.
A classic paper describing the ultrastructural basis of the blood-brain barrier and blood-CSF barrier.

Brisman JL, Song JK, Newell DW: Cerebral aneurysms. N Engl J Med 355:928, 2006.

Casey SO, et al: Cerebral CT venography. Radiology 198:163, 1996.

Chaynes P: Microsurgical anatomy of the great cerebral vein of Galen and its tributaries. J Neurosurg 99:1028, 2003.

Choi JH, Mohr JP: Brain arteriovenous malformations in adults. Lancet Neurol 4:299, 2005.

Chorobski J, Penfield W: Cerebral vasodilator nerves and their pathway from the medulla oblongata: with observations on the pial and intracerebral vascular plexus. Arch Neurol Psychiatry 28:1257, 1932.

Cobb S, Finesinger JE: Cerebral circulation. XIX. The vagal pathway of the vasodilator impulses. Arch Neurol Psychiatry 28:1243, 1932.
Although not all subsequent investigators agree with the findings, this paper provides a straightforward and convincing demonstration of a pathway through the vagus nerve into the brainstem and out through the facial nerve, causing dilation of cortical vessels.

Duvernoy HM: Human brainstem vessels, ed 2, Heidelberg, 2003, Springer-Verlag.
A painstakingly detailed and magnificently illustrated book.

Duvernoy HM, Risold P-Y: The circumventricular organs: An atlas of comparative anatomy and vascularization. Brain Res Rev 56:119, 2007.
Beautifully illustrated.

Feekes JA, et al: Tertiary microvascular territories define lacunar infarcts in the basal ganglia. Ann Neurol 58:18, 2005.
Beautiful pictures of some of the perforating arteries.

Fisher CM: Lacunes: small, deep cerebral infarcts. Neurology 15:774, 1965.

Frackowiak RSJ, et al: Human brain function, ed 2, San Diego, 2004, Academic Press.
An extensive review of functional imaging studies.

Fry M, Ferguson AV: The sensory circumventricular organs: brain targets for circulating signals controlling ingestive behavior. Physiol Behav 91:413, 2007.

Galatius-Jensen F, Ringberg V: Anastomosis between the anterior choroidal artery and the posterior cerebral artery demonstrated by angiography. Radiology 81:942, 1963.

Grand W, Hopkins LN: Vasculature of the brain and cranial base: variations in clinical anatomy, New York, 1999, Thieme Medical Publishers.

Harik SI: Blood-brain barrier sodium/potassium pump: modulation by central noradrenergic innervation. Proc Natl Acad Sci U S A 83:4067, 1986.

Hendrikse J, et al: Distribution of cerebral blood flow in the circle of Willis. Radiology 235:184, 2005.

Howarth C: The contribution of astrocytes to the regulation of cerebral blood flow. Front Neurosci 8:103, 2014.

Huettel SA, Song AW, McCarthy G: Functional magnetic resonance imaging, Sunderland, Mass, 2004, Sinauer.

Hupperts RMM, et al: Infarcts in the anterior choroidal artery territory: anatomical distribution, clinical syndromes, presumed pathogenesis and early outcome. Brain 117:825, 1994.

Iadecola C, Nedergaard M: Glial regulation of the cerebral microvasculature. Nat Neurosci 10:1369, 2007.

Kakou M, Destrieux C, Velu S: Microanatomy of the pericallosal arterial complex. J Neurosurg 93:667, 2000.

Kapp JP, Schmidek HH: The cerebral venous system and its disorders, Orlando, Fla, 1984, Grune & Stratton.

Kidwell CS, Wintermark M: Imaging of intracranial haemorrhage. Lancet Neurol 7:256, 2008.

Kobayashi K, et al: Anatomical study of the confluence of the sinuses with contrast-enhanced magnetic resonance venography. Neuroradiology 48:307, 2006.

Lassen NA, Ingvar DH, Skinhøj E: Brain function and blood flow. Sci Am 239:62, 1978.
One of the original techniques for studying the activity of different areas of the brain by measuring, with an external gamma-ray camera, the amounts of radioactive isotope delivered to different areas through the arterial circulation.

Lipton P: Ischemic cell death in brain neurons. Physiol Rev 79:1432, 1999.

Long JB, Holaday JW: Blood-brain barrier: endogenous modulation by adrenal-cortical function. Science 277:1580, 1980.

McCulloch J: Perivascular nerve fibers and the cerebral circulation. Trends Neurosci 7:135, 1984.

McKinley MJ, Oldfield BJ: Circumventricular organs. In Paxinos G, editor: The human nervous system, ed 2, San Diego, 2003, Academic Press.

Millen JW, Woollam DHM: Vascular patterns in the choroid plexus. J Anat 87:114, 1953.

Muir KW, et al: Imaging of acute stroke. Lancet Neurol 5:755, 2006.

O'Connell JEA: Some observations on the cerebral veins. Brain 57:484, 1934.
A lucid description of the developmental patterns of the superficial cerebral veins and their relationship to the superior sagittal sinus.

Oka K, et al: Microsurgical anatomy of the superficial veins of the cerebrum. Neurosurgery 17:711, 1985.

Oktar SO, et al: Blood-flow volume quantification in internal carotid and vertebral arteries: comparison of 3 different ultrasound techniques with phase-contrast MR imaging. AJNR Am J Neuroradiol 27:363, 2006.

Ono M, et al: Microsurgical anatomy of the deep venous system of the brain. Neurosurgery 15:621, 1984.

Peruzzo B, et al: A second look at the barriers of the medial basal hypothalamus. Exp Brain Res 132:10, 2000.
Demonstration of the walling off of the median eminence by junctions between tanycytes.

Raichle ME, Mintun MA: Brain work and brain imaging. Annu Rev Neurosci 29:449, 2006.
Sorting out the functions that functional imaging images.

Rhoton AL, Jr: The posterior cranial fossa: microsurgical anatomy and surgical approaches. Neurosurgery 47(Suppl), 2000.
An exhaustive and beautifully illustrated description.

Rhoton AL, Jr, Fujii K, Fradd B: Microsurgical anatomy of the anterior choroidal artery. Surg Neurol 12:171, 1979.
Finely detailed and beautifully illustrated.

Robin ED: The evolutionary advantages of being stupid. Perspect Biol Med 16:369, 1972-1973.
Turtles may not be very smart, but they do not need much oxygen and have been around for a long, long time.

Rothwell PM, Buchan A, Johnston SC: Recent advances in management of transient ischaemic attacks and minor ischaemic strokes. Lancet Neurol 5:323, 2006.

Smith PM, Beninger RJ, Ferguson AV: Subfornical organ stimulation elicits drinking. Brain Res Bull 38:209, 1995.

Stephens RB, Stilwell DL: Arteries and veins of the human brain, Springfield, Ill, 1969, Charles C Thomas.
A well-photographed series of dissections of brains in which the arteries or veins were injected.

Suzuki Y, et al: Variations of the basal vein: identification using three-dimensional CT angiography. AJNR Am J Neuroradiol 22:670, 2001.

Takano T, et al: Astrocyte-mediated control of cerebral blood flow. Nat Neurosci 9:260, 2006.
Elegant experiments showing a direct connection among glutamate, astrocytes, and local changes in blood flow.

Tatu L, et al: Arterial territories of human brain: brainstem and cerebellum. Neurology 47:1125, 1996.

Tatu L, et al: Arterial territories of human brain: cerebral hemispheres. Neurology 50:1699, 1998.

Toole JF: Cerebrovascular disorders, ed 5, Philadelphia, 1999, Lippincott Williams & Wilkins.

Tsukada H, et al: Regulation of cerebral blood flow response to somatosensory stimulation through the cholinergic system: a positron emission tomography study in unanesthetized monkeys. Brain Res 749:10, 1997.

Valdueza JM, et al: Postural dependency of the cerebral venous outflow. Lancet 355:200, 2000.

Van Gijn J, Kerr RS, Rinkel GJE: Subarachnoid haemorrhage. Lancet 369:306, 2007.

Van Laar PJ, et al: In vivo flow territory mapping of major brain feeding arteries. Neuroimage 29:136, 2006.
Using MRI to map out the territories supplied by major vessels of the circle of Willis.

Vander Eecken HM, Adams RD: The anatomy and functional significance of the meningeal arterial anastomoses of the human brain. J Neuropathol Exp Neurol 12:132, 1953.
Injection studies of the end-to-end anastomoses between intracranial arteries.

Wackenheim A, Braun JP: The veins of the posterior fossa, New York, 1978, Springer-Verlag.

Weinberger JM: Evolving therapeutic approaches to treating acute ischemic stroke. J Neurol Sci 249:101, 2006.

A recent discussion of the state of the art in using thrombolytics to restore blood flow and in identifying and protecting the penumbra.

Welch K, et al: The collateral circulation following middle cerebral branch occlusion. J Neurosurg 12:361, 1955.

Discussion of two cases in which much of the middle cerebral artery filled through the anterior cerebral artery.

Yaşargil MG: Microneurosurgery, vol 3A, AVM of the brain, history, embryology, pathological considerations, hemodynamics, diagnostic studies, microsurgical anatomy, vol 4A, CNS tumors: surgical anatomy, neuropathology, neuroradiology, neurophysiology, clinical considerations, operability, treatment options, Stuttgart, 1987, 1994, Georg Thieme Verlag.

Beautifully illustrated books with extensive discussions of cerebrovascular anatomy.

Electrical Signaling by Neurons

We depend on our brains to process and convey huge quantities of information rapidly and reliably. As a biological system, the brain must do this using neurons and their axons and synapses rather than wires and transistors. This makes the task more difficult, because it is substantially harder to move electrical signals around in the aqueous medium inside and surrounding neurons than in more conventional electronic devices.[a] The solution used by neurons allows current to be carried not by electrons but rather by the movement of ions, driven by the energy stored in ionic

---

[a]For example, Hodgkin (1964) pointed out that an axon 1 µm in diameter and 1 m long has the same electrical resistance as 10^{10} miles of 22-gauge copper wire—a length of wire 10 times the distance from here to Saturn.

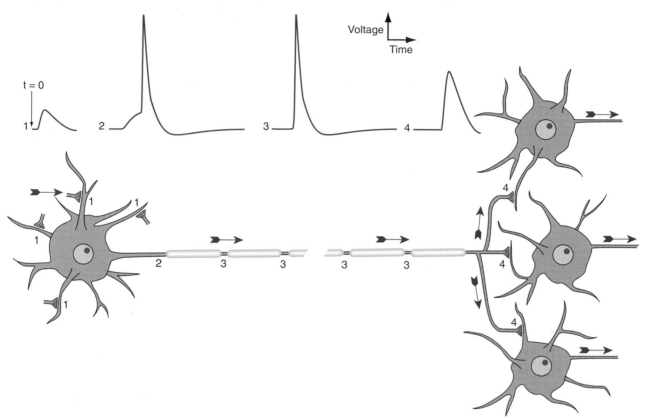

Figure 7-1 General scheme of distribution of electrical signals in the nervous system, with the direction of information flow indicated by arrows. Release of neurotransmitter by synaptic terminals causes slow postsynaptic potentials, as discussed further in Chapter 8. Some are positive-going, or excitatory (1); some are negative-going, or inhibitory (not indicated). Synaptic potentials spread passively to a trigger zone where, if threshold is reached, action potentials are initiated (2). The synaptic potentials die out near the neuronal cell body, but action potentials are propagated actively and without decrement along the axon (3). Action potentials then spread passively into axon terminals (4) and cause the release of neurotransmitter onto other neurons.

concentration gradients and controlled by molecular switches.

Neurons, as described in Chapter 1, have a complement of organelles comparable to that of other cells, but arrayed in a fashion supporting their signaling functions and their unusual shapes. Like other cells, neurons are also bounded by a semipermeable membrane that is electrically polarized, in this case to a **resting membrane potential** of about −65 mV. (By convention, the extracellular fluid is considered to be at 0 mV, so a resting potential of −65 mV means that the inside of the cell is 65 mV negative to the outside.) Neurons, however, are masters of moment-to-moment modulation of this membrane potential and use the changes as a signaling mechanism. They use a combination of (1) graded, local potential changes that typically develop and decay relatively slowly and can be compared and summed (e.g., **synaptic potentials, receptor potentials**) and (2) brief, actively propagated potentials (**action potentials**) for conveying information over long distances (Fig. 7-1). This chapter describes the biophysical bases for the resting potential, the spread of slow potentials, and the generation and propagation of action potentials. Synaptic potentials are

discussed in Chapter 8, and the potentials produced by sensory receptors are addressed in Chapter 9.

A Lipid-Protein Membrane Separates Intracellular and Extracellular Fluids

The electrical signaling capabilities of neurons are based on ionic concentration gradients between the intracellular and extracellular compartments (Table 7-1). The cell membrane, a complex of a bilayer of lipid molecules with an assortment of protein molecules embedded in it (Fig. 7-2), separates these two compartments. Concentration gradients are maintained by a combination of selective permeability characteristics and active pumping mechanisms.

The Lipid Component of the Membrane Is a Diffusion Barrier

The lipid component of the membrane is a double sheet of phospholipids, elongated molecules with polar groups at one end and fatty acid chains at the other (see

Table 7-1	Extracellular and Intracellular Ionic Concentrations of Typical Mammalian Neurons		
Ion	Extracellular Concentration (mM)	Intracellular Concentration (mM)	Equilibrium Potential* (37°C)
Na+	140	15	+60 mV
K+	4	130	−94 mV
Ca2+	2.5	0.0001†	+136 mV
Cl−	120	5	−86 mV

*The potential at which there is no net tendency for a particular ionic species to move in either direction across the membrane, that is, the electrical gradient balances the concentration gradient. See Calculating the Membrane Potential for details.
†The total intracellular Ca^{2+} concentration is 1 to 2 mM, but almost all of it is bound or sequestered. The free cytoplasmic Ca^{2+} concentration is $\leq 10^{-7}$ M.

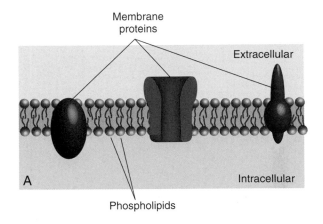

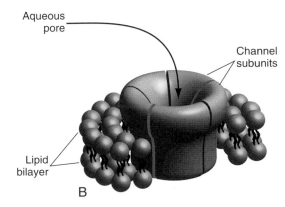

Figure 7-2 A, Schematic view of part of a neuronal cell membrane, with membrane proteins embedded in a phospholipid bilayer. **B,** An ion channel consisting of multiple subunits, embedded in the lipid bilayer.

Fig. 7-2). This structure leads to differential activities of the two parts of the molecule when exposed to water (itself a polar molecule): the polar groups are **hydrophilic,** interacting with water, and the fatty acid tails are **hydrophobic,** interacting with each other. The consequence is a lipid arrangement in which the fatty acid tails face each other in the center of the membrane and the polar groups face the aqueous solutions inside and outside the neuron. Development of the lipid bilayer was a pivotal event in the evolution of life, because the

hydrophobic core prevents diffusion of water-soluble substances and allows the maintenance of concentration gradients across the membrane. The ions that carry the currents used for neuronal signaling are among these water-soluble substances, so the lipid bilayer is also an insulator, the barrier across which membrane potentials develop (see Fig. 7-25). In biophysical terms, the lipid bilayer is not **permeable** to ions. In electrical terms, it functions as a **capacitor,** able to store charges of opposite sign that are attracted to each other but unable to cross the membrane, creating an "excitable" cell (see Resistors, Capacitors, and Neuronal Membranes).

Membrane Proteins Regulate the Movement of Solutes Across the Membrane

Embedded in the lipid bilayer is a large assortment of proteins, some exposed mainly on the outer or inner surface, but many completely spanning the membrane (see Fig. 7-2). Different categories of these proteins have distinctive functions. Some serve as anchor points for cytoskeletal elements; some are surface recognition molecules, participating in physical interactions between neurons and their neighbors or other elements of their extracellular surroundings; some facilitate the movement of lipid-insoluble nutrients such as glucose into neurons. Most important for the purposes of this chapter are proteins that regulate the passage of ions into or out of the cell. Because a lipid bilayer by itself does not allow ions to cross, it cannot be the entire basis for electrical signaling. Certain membrane-spanning proteins confer this ability, either by allowing selected ions to flow down electrical or concentration gradients or by pumping them across.

Ions Diffuse Across the Membrane Through Ion Channels—Protein Molecules With Pores

Some membrane-spanning proteins consist of several subunits surrounding a central aqueous pore (see Fig. 7-2B). Ions whose size and charge "fit" the pore can diffuse through it, allowing these proteins to serve as **ion channels.** Hence unlike the lipid bilayer, ion channels

BOX 7-1

Methods of Measuring Voltages and Currents Across Neuronal Membranes

Knowledge of the mechanism of electrical signaling by neurons grew during the 20th century and continues to expand with the development of more sophisticated techniques. Very early work depended on indirect methods, such as measuring currents and voltages in extracellular spaces outside neurons. In the 1930s, Hodgkin, Huxley, Katz, Cole, and others began to take advantage of the huge axons that certain invertebrates have developed as a means of increasing conduction velocity (see Fig. 7-22). Methods were devised to thread wires longitudinally through these axons and record currents and voltages directly across the axon membrane.

At about the same time, other workers found that controlled heating and stretching of capillary tubing until it snaps can produce micropipettes with tip diameters smaller than 1 μm. Filled with a salt solution, these micropipettes can be used as electrodes for recording

voltages and currents across neuronal membranes; the tip diameter is small enough to puncture many kinds of relatively large neurons without damaging them too much (Fig. 7-3A).

Micropipette electrodes were a mainstay of neurophysiologists for decades, but they always had shortcomings. They damaged small cells and processes, and even when the method was successful, it was possible to record events only across relatively large expanses of membranes. A technique that opened up new horizons appeared in the late 1970s, when Neher and Sakmann developed patch clamping (see Fig. 7-3B). Patch clamping makes it possible to record events across the membranes of small cells and processes; even more remarkably, it allows the recording of the activity of individual ion channels in patches of membrane (see Fig. 7-17).

have an appreciable permeability (or **conductance**[b]) to some ions. In electrical terms, they function as **resistors,**[c] allowing a predictable amount of current flow in response to a voltage across them (see Resistors, Capacitors, and Neuronal Membranes). Although hundreds of different ion channels have been described, they have some characteristics in common:

Multiple states. Most or all ion channels can exist in two or more different, stable conformations. The different conformations fall into two general categories: open, in which the pore is available for ions to traverse, and closed, in which the pore is occluded enough to prevent ion flow. Open channels have high conductance, and closed channels have low conductance, so ion channels are variable resistors; this is the key to their role in membrane potential changes. Remarkably, the transitions between these different conductance states can be observed directly using **patch-clamp** techniques (Box 7-1; see Fig. 7-17). Most channels in resting neuronal membranes are closed and respond to particular stimuli by opening, although the opposite is also found.

Gating. The opening and closing of an individual ion channel is a probabilistic event, and the channel can flip between these states nearly instantaneously. Most channels are tuned to certain factors that affect their

probability of being open or closed.[d] Some channels open in response to changes in membrane potential and are referred to as **voltage-gated** channels (Fig. 7-4A and B). The best understood of these is the voltage-gated sodium channel that underlies action potentials (see Fig. 7-10), but there are also voltage-gated potassium, calcium, and chloride channels. Other channels open or close in response to the binding of signaling molecules (see Fig. 7-4C and D). The bound molecule is called a **ligand** (from the Latin *ligare*, "to bind"), so these are **ligand-gated** channels. The best known of these are postsynaptic receptors that bind specific neurotransmitters and change their permeability in response (see Chapter 8), but other channels bind intracellular ligands released in response to various stimuli. Some channels are **thermally gated,** allowing the neurons that contain them to function as miniature thermometers or as thermal injury detectors (see Chapters 9 and 23). Finally, some channels are **mechanically gated.** A prominent example is the receptor cells of the inner ear (see Fig. 14-7), but others are known (e.g., see Fig. 23-7).

Selectivity. The central pores of ion channels are not wide enough to let any and all ions traverse them. Rather, the size of the pore and the nature of the

[b]*Conductance* and *permeability* technically have slightly different meanings but are commonly used interchangeably. A membrane permeable to a given ion easily conducts currents carried by that kind of ion.

[c]Resistance is simply the inverse of conductance. A channel with high conductance has little resistance to current flow, and vice versa.

[d]Discussions in this and other chapters may seem to imply that populations of channels as a whole open or close (slowly or suddenly) in response to some stimulus. The individual channels in such populations, however, exist in an equilibrium state, flipping back and forth between different states; the only thing that changes is the probability of being in one or another state. A population of channels, each with a slowly increasing probability of being open, would seem macroscopically like a population of channels all opening slowly at the same time.

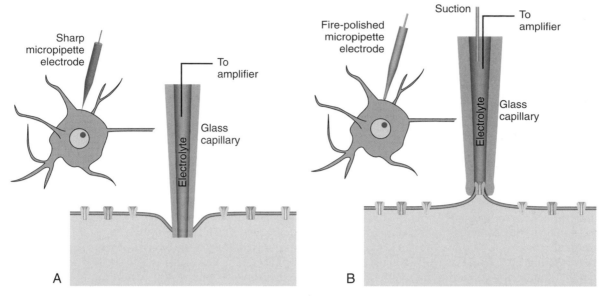

A

B

Figure 7-3 Recording electrical activity across neuronal membranes using sharp microelectrodes **(A)** and patch-clamp electrodes **(B)**. If the tip of a sharp micropipette electrode is small enough, it can be used to impale relatively large neurons with minimal injury. The punctured cell membrane seals around the electrode, and resting transmembrane potentials and potential changes such as those shown in Figure 7-1 can be recorded. Patch-clamp electrodes are generally larger and are prepared with smooth, fire-polished tips. Contact with the surface of a neuron, combined with gentle suction, causes the neuronal membrane to seal onto the pipette tip. Once the seal is established, a series of additional maneuvers allows various recording arrangements: current passing through the attached area of membrane can be measured (see Fig. 7-17); the attached area of membrane can be perforated, creating electrical continuity between the pipette and the cell's interior and allowing measurement of voltage changes across the cell membrane (referred to as *whole-cell recordings;* see Fig. 7-13); or the attached membrane patch can be torn away from the cell and exposed to controlled solutions of various sorts while measuring current flows.

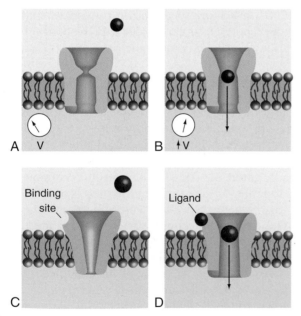

A V

B ↑V

C

D

Figure 7-4 Gating properties of ion channels. Voltage-gated channels respond to appropriate voltage changes (in this example, to decreased negativity inside the cell, as in the case of voltage-gated sodium channels) by switching from a closed **(A)** to an open **(B)** state. Ligand-gated channels bind specific ligands when available and, in this example, switch from a closed **(C)** to an open **(D)** state.

amino acid residues lining it are such that some ions can diffuse through more easily than others. Some channels are minimally selective and may simply distinguish between small anions and small cations. Others are highly selective and may be, for example, hundreds of times more permeable to sodium ions than to potassium ions.

The many different types of ion channels generally are not distributed uniformly in neuronal membranes. Rather, neurons somehow manage to place them preferentially in sites that make functional sense. For example, although the channels that determine the resting membrane potential are widely distributed, voltage-gated sodium channels are grouped so that only certain regions of a neuron can generate action potentials. Similarly, appropriate ligand-gated channels are located in postsynaptic membranes across from presynaptic terminals and not in other locations. This selective regional distribution of channels and other membrane proteins forms much of the basis for the functional specialization of different parts of each neuron.

Small differences in amino acid sequences are sufficient to change the selectivity of a channel, and many channel types are closely related to each other. All the voltage-gated cation channels are the products of one closely related family of genes; some ligand-gated postsynaptic receptors are related to the voltage-gated

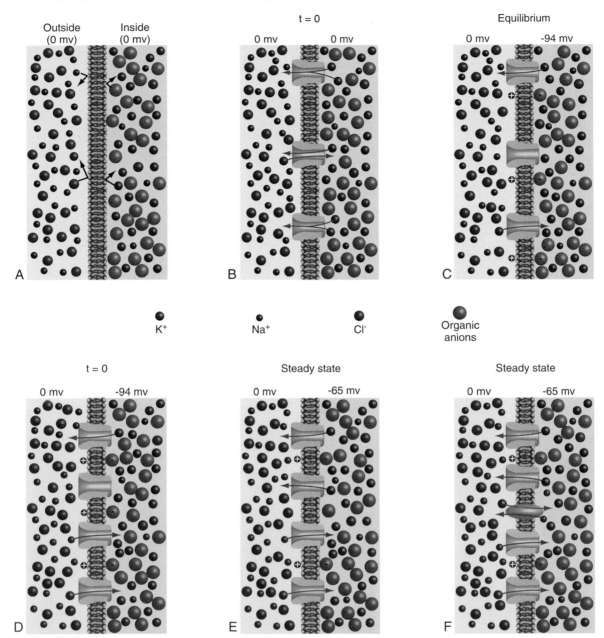

Figure 7-5 Development and maintenance of a resting membrane potential. **A,** A lipid bilayer by itself is impermeable, allowing no charge separation to develop. **B,** Adding K⁺ channels initially results in net movement of K⁺ ions out of the cell (K⁺ ions are free to move in either direction, but because there are more inside the cell, more move from inside to outside than in the opposite direction). **C,** At equilibrium, a vanishingly small number of excess extracellular K⁺ ions results in cations (mostly Na⁺ ions) lining up on the outside of the membrane, counterbalanced by anions on the inner surface of the membrane. This accounts for the resting membrane potential, which develops abruptly across the membrane. K⁺ ions still flow through their channels, but now equal numbers move out (down the concentration gradient) and in (down the voltage gradient). **D,** Addition of a small number of Na⁺ channels causes a small inward movement of Na⁺ ions, driven not just by the Na⁺ concentration gradient but also by the intracellular negativity. **E,** A steady state is reached in which equal numbers of cations move inward and outward across the membrane. However, there is a net inward movement of Na⁺ and outward movement of K⁺. **F,** The Na⁺/K⁺ ATPase is an exchange pump that compensates for the net Na⁺ and K⁺ fluxes in **E.**

channels, and others evolved independently. Although the chemical differences between channel types are often subtle, they are nevertheless sufficient to allow pharmacological manipulation of particular channels. This is commonly exploited in the treatment of disease states. Conversely, some diseases are themselves the result of abnormal functioning of particular channel types (see Box 7-2).

The Number and Selectivity of Ion Channels Determine the Membrane Potential

The importance of ion channels in the development of the resting membrane potential is indicated in Figure 7-5. A lipid bilayer separating intracellular and extracellular fluids with the ionic concentrations shown in Table 7-1 would not develop a membrane potential.

Even though all the ion species involved (including Ca^{2+}, which is not indicated in Fig. 7-5, to keep things a little simpler) are unequally distributed, the impermeability of the membrane would prevent them from moving down their concentration gradients (see Fig. 7-5A). The number of positive charges and negative charges on each side of the membrane would be identical.

Consider what would happen if ion channels selectively permeable only to K^+ were added to such a membrane (Fig. 7-5B). K^+ ions would be equally free to diffuse into or out of the cell through these channels. However, simply because there are so many more K^+ ions inside the cell than outside, more K^+ ions would move out than in (i.e., K^+ ions would flow out of the cell down the K^+ concentration gradient). This would leave behind a number of intracellular negative charges. Because opposite charges attract each other, the excess intracellular negative charges would attract K^+ ions back into the cell. At a time determined by the number of channels available for K^+ ion movement, the concentration gradient driving K^+ out of the cell would be exactly counterbalanced by the intracellular negativity; the K^+ current moving out of the cell would be equal and opposite to the K^+ current moving into the cell (see Fig. 7-5C). The system at this point is in **equilibrium:** no energy is required to maintain it in this state. The membrane potential at which this equilibrium is reached is the **potassium equilibrium potential (V_K);** its value can be calculated using a logarithmic relationship called the **Nernst equation,** knowing only the intracellular and extracellular K^+ concentrations, the temperature, and some physical constants (see Calculating the Membrane Potential). Each ion species that is unequally distributed across the membrane has an equilibrium potential that can be calculated in the same way (see Table 7-1), indicating the membrane potential that would develop if the membrane were permeable solely to this type of ion (and the potential at which there would be no net movement of that ion in either direction).

The initial net outward movement of K^+ ions required to establish this membrane potential is actually extremely small, just enough to charge up the membrane capacitance—and no significant change in intracellular or extracellular K^+ concentration results. For example, the net outward movement of only about 175 million K^+ ions is enough to establish the predicted membrane potential of -94 mV across the membrane of a spherical cell 100 μm in diameter. Although this sounds like a lot of ions, a cell this size with an intracellular K^+ concentration of 130 mM contains about 4×10^{13} K^+ ions, so the net loss of K^+ ions required to establish this membrane potential is less than 0.001% of the starting number. This is a common theme in electrical signaling by neurons: substantial electrical signals can be generated by moving relatively minuscule numbers of ions, so that intracellular and extracellular ionic concentrations

change little over brief periods of time. (As seen later in this chapter, however, active pumping mechanisms are required to maintain ionic concentration gradients over long periods.) Knowing the equilibrium potential of the different ions aids in understanding how the movement of ions across the membrane for normal function, disease states, and under conditions of treatment relate to the function of neurons. For example, if a treatment is given allowing potassium to freely move into the neuron while all other ions are held constant (not allowed to move), the resting membrane becomes more negative (close to -94 mV, the equilibrium potential for K^+) and the cell is less likely to become excited. Therefore, drugs that may enhance the opening of potassium channels are more likely to slow neuronal function.

The Resting Membrane Potential of Typical Neurons Is Heavily Influenced, but Not Completely Determined, by the Potassium Concentration Gradient

The scenario just developed is actually close to the situation in typical neurons, whose membrane at rest is dominated by a steady potassium conductance. Hence the resting membrane potential of typical neurons is near the potassium equilibrium potential. Increases in extracellular potassium concentration cause the membrane potential to become less negative, by almost the amount predicted by the Nernst equation (Fig. 7-6). However, the membrane is never quite as negative as the

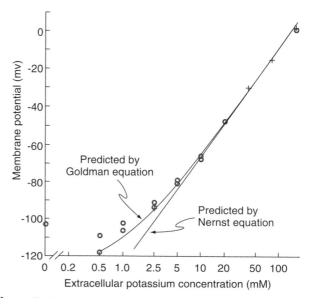

Figure 7-6 The membrane potential of frog muscle fibers at different K^+ concentrations in the bathing solution. (The membranes of skeletal muscle fibers have properties similar to those of neurons.) Crosses indicate measurements made after the muscle fiber had equilibrated with a new K^+ concentration for 10 to 60 minutes, blue circles 20 to 60 seconds after an abrupt increase in K^+ concentration, and green circles 20 to 60 seconds after an abrupt decrease. The curves fitted to the data are provided by equations described in Calculating the Membrane Potential. *(Redrawn from Hodgkin AL, Horowicz P: J Physiol 148:127, 1959.)*

potassium equilibrium potential, and the deviation becomes greater the lower the extracellular potassium concentration becomes. Clinically relevant is when a person becomes hypokalemic (low potassium), excitable cells like neurons can become even more excitable in that the resting membrane potential becomes less negative or, in other words, the cell becomes more excitable.

The basis for this deviation from the membrane potential predicted by the Nernst equation is the additional presence of a relatively small resting permeability to Na$^+$ ions, as indicated in Figure 7-5D and E. If one imagines this permeability being added to the K$^+$-permeable membrane of Figure 7-5C, an inward flow of Na$^+$ ions results, driven not only by the interior negativity of the cell but also by the Na$^+$ concentration gradient (Fig. 7-5D). The inward Na$^+$ current would be small because the Na$^+$ conductance is small, but it would nevertheless move positive charges into the cell, making its interior less negative. This in turn would cause the membrane potential to move slightly away from V_K, creating a small voltage gradient that drives K$^+$ ions out of the cell. Assuming that concentrations remain constant, a **steady state** is reached in which the small inward Na$^+$ current (small because the Na$^+$ conductance is small) is exactly counterbalanced by a small outward K$^+$ current (small because the conductance is relatively large but the voltage gradient is small). The exact membrane potential at this steady state is somewhere between V_K and V_{Na}, dictated by the relative magnitudes of the K$^+$ and Na$^+$ permeabilities (see Calculating the Membrane Potential). Typical neurons have resting Na$^+$ permeabilities that are 1% to 10% as great as the resting K$^+$ permeability, so the resting membrane potential is a weighted average of V_K and V_{Na}, or around –65 mV (closer to V_K than to V_{Na} because of the greater K$^+$ permeability).

Concentration Gradients Are Maintained by Membrane Proteins That Pump Ions

There is a major difference between the equilibrium condition that exists when the membrane is permeable to only one ion (see Fig. 7-5C) and the steady state that is achieved when the membrane is permeable to more than one ion (see Fig. 7-5E). In the equilibrium condition the equal and opposite current flows involve the same ion (e.g., K$^+$), so no concentration changes ensue and no energy is required to maintain the condition. In the steady-state condition, the equal and opposite current flows involve different ions and eventually result in concentration changes. In the typical neuronal situation, the small but constant inward Na$^+$ and outward K$^+$ currents, if uncompensated, would slowly dissipate the Na$^+$ and K$^+$ concentration gradients across the membrane. The equilibrium potential for ions with no concentration gradient is 0 mV, so the membrane potential would slowly fade away. Another class of membrane proteins

called **ion pumps** allows this dilemma to be circumvented by neurons and, indeed, by all cells. The best studied of these is a membrane-spanning **Na$^+$/K$^+$ ATPase,** so called because it uses the energy released by hydrolysis of adenosine triphosphate (ATP) to move Na$^+$ ions out of the cell and K$^+$ into the cell (Fig. 7-5F). These Na$^+$/K$^+$ pumps move three Na$^+$ ions out of the cell and two K$^+$ ions into the cell per hydrolysis of an ATP. The inhibition of these pumps results in the loss of the cells' excitability characteristics and their ability to function. In addition, Ca^{2+} ions and Cl$^+$ ions can also move into cells in response to certain kinds of stimuli, and specific membrane pumps are available to redistribute them as well. All of them pump at concentration-sensitive rates, so they speed up when there are more ions to be extruded or recaptured.

Inputs to Neurons Cause Slow, Local Potential Changes

We think of conventional electronic devices as designed not to distort but rather to transmit signals over long distances unchanged, accurately amplifying them as necessary. Neurons do not seem to be very well designed for transmitting information over long distances. Axons, relative to metal wires, are poor conductors; their insulation (except where myelin is present) is not very good, and the input signals to neurons become smeared out over space and time because of membrane resistance and capacitance. As is discussed in this chapter and the next, however, these apparent shortcomings are precisely what allow neurons to compare and summate numerous inputs and make determinations about appropriate outputs.

Changes in the relative permeability of the membrane to ions such as K$^+$ and Na$^+$ (and Ca^{2+} and Cl$^+$) are the basis for electrical signaling by neurons. Increasing the Na$^+$ permeability, for example, would cause an increased inward Na$^+$ current and **depolarization**[e] of the membrane (i.e., decreased internal negativity; opening Na$^+$ channels drives the resting membrane potential toward the Na$^+$ equilibrium potential of +60 mV; see Table 7-1). Increasing the K$^+$ permeability would **hyperpolarize** the membrane (i.e., make the inside more negative by moving its potential even closer to V_K). Such permeability changes may be caused by the action of ligand-gated channels at postsynaptic sites (Chapter 8) or by the action of stimulus-gated channels in the membranes of

---

[e]Strictly speaking, *depolarization* ("removing the polarization") should mean a movement of the membrane potential toward 0 mV. As the terms are commonly used, however, *depolarization* and *hyperpolarization* mean changes of the membrane potential in a positive or negative direction from some starting point.

sensory receptors (Chapter 9). In either case, the net effect is a change in current flow through the affected channels for as long as the probability of their being open remains altered. The consequences of local current flow such as this are dictated largely by the passive electrical properties of adjacent areas of neuronal membrane—their resistance and capacitance. These passive electrical properties are referred to as the **cable properties** of neurons.

Membrane Capacitance and Resistance Determine the Speed and Extent of the Response to a Current Pulse

Abruptly increasing the membrane conductance to some kind of ion causes an abrupt change in the rate at which it crosses the membrane (i.e., it causes a rapid change in current flow either into or out of the neuron's cytoplasm). The time course and spatial distribution of the voltage changes caused by this current flow depend on the properties of both the cytoplasm and the membrane of the neuron, with major implications for the way signals spread along neuronal membranes. The following discussion of applicable principles is based on inward current flow (e.g., of Na⁺ ions), but the same considerations apply for outward current flow.

Membranes Have a Time Constant, Allowing Temporal Summation

In the simple (albeit unlikely) case of uniform conductance changes over the entire surface of a spherical cell, the current flow and voltage changes across all parts of the membrane are identical. A step increase in conductance, producing a step increase in current flow, causes an exponential decrease in membrane voltage because of the parallel resistance and capacitance of the membrane (Fig. 7-7). The final value of the voltage change is determined by the product of the current and the membrane resistance ($V = IR$), whereas the **time constant** for reaching this final voltage—the time required to get 63% ($1 - 1/e$) of the way there—is determined by the product of the membrane resistance and capacitance ($\tau = RC$; see Resistors, Capacitors, and Neuronal Membranes). Hence membranes with many open channels (high conductance, low resistance) have relatively short time constants, and membranes with few open channels have longer time constants. A typical neuronal time constant is 10 msec, although shorter and longer values are common.

The membrane capacitance similarly slows the decay of voltage at the end of a conductance change, with a similar time constant. A brief conductance change may

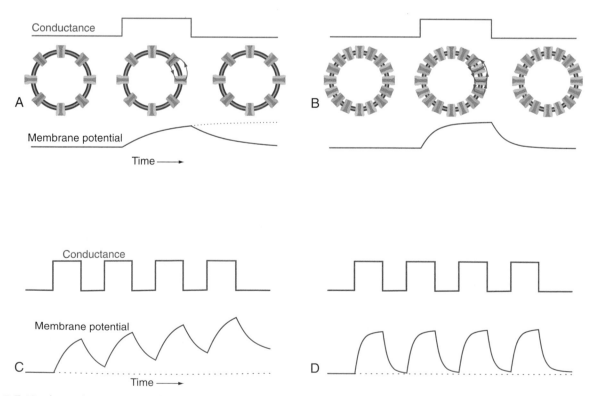

Figure 7-7 Membrane time constants and temporal summation. **A,** High membrane resistance results in a long time constant; the membrane capacitance may not be completely charged *(dashed line)* at the end of a relatively brief conductance change. **B,** Low membrane resistance results in a short time constant. Neurons or neuronal processes with long time constants **(C)** display more temporal summation than neurons with short time constants **(D).**

cause only partial charging of the membrane capacitance (Fig. 7-7C). This seemingly disadvantageous slowing of electrical signals actually has an important function. Because signals are spread out over time, multiple inputs that occur at not quite the same time can partially reinforce each other. This phenomenon is called **temporal summation,** and its limits are dictated largely by the membrane time constant.

Larger-Diameter Neuronal Processes Have Longer Length Constants

Conductance changes in real neurons are usually localized (e.g., to a postsynaptic site on a dendrite), so the effects of distance from the conductance change must also be considered in determining the resulting potential changes. The effects of just the resistive elements are indicated in Figure 7-8A. Current entering a dendrite (or any other part of a neuron) begins to leak out immediately and cause a voltage change across the membrane, so less is present a few micrometers from the site of entry. At this point a few micrometers away, some percentage of the remaining current leaks out (causing a

smaller voltage change), so even less remains. The amount of current remaining at any given point declines exponentially with distance from the site of entry, until eventually all the current leaks out. The distance required for the current (and for the voltage change) to decline to 1/e (37%) of the value at the site of entry is called the **length constant.** Typical length constants for neuronal processes are a few hundred micrometers, and constants of more than a millimeter or two are unusual. Hence the passive spread of signals in neurons (called **electrotonic spread** or **electrotonic conduction**) is said to be **decremental,** indicating that the signal becomes smaller with distance.

The factors influencing the length constant of a neuronal process can be appreciated by considering the locations of conductance in the path of current flow (Fig. 7-8B). At any given point along the interior of the process, current has two alternative paths: either it can cross the membrane and leave, or it can continue along longitudinally through the process. The higher the membrane conductance, the more likely the current is to leave; the higher the longitudinal conductance of the process, the

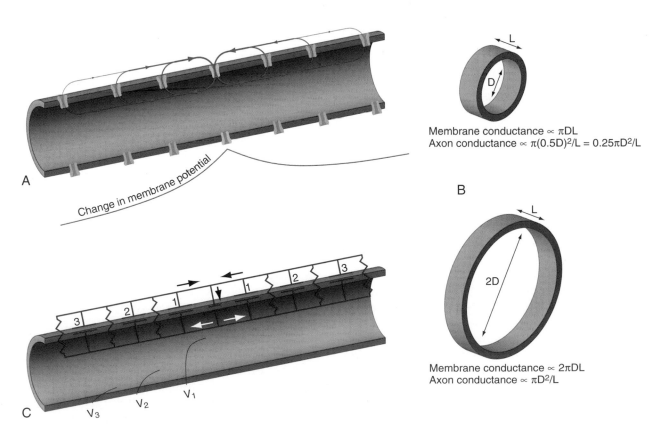

Figure 7-8 Passive spread of voltage changes in neuronal processes. **A,** Progressively less of a steady current entering a neuronal process at one location remains as the distance from the point of entry increases. Hence the voltage change declines exponentially with distance from the point of entry. **B,** Influence of the diameter of a neuronal process on its length constant. Membrane area (and conductance) increases directly with the diameter, whereas cross-sectional area (and conductance) increases with its square. Hence doubling the diameter doubles the membrane conductance but quadruples the longitudinal conductance. **C,** Effects of membrane capacitance on the longitudinal spread of voltage changes. The final value of the voltage change at any given point is dictated by membrane and longitudinal (not indicated) resistances. However, the rate of reaching this final value becomes progressively slower with distance, as more and more capacitance is added.

more likely the current is to continue flowing longitudinally. For a given length of neuronal process, the conductance of the membrane is determined by the number of available ion channels, which in turn is proportional to the area of membrane covering the process. The membrane area, and therefore its conductance, is proportional to the *diameter* of the process. In contrast, each little cross-sectional bit of cytoplasm represents a longitudinal path for current flow, so the longitudinal conductance increases with the cross-sectional area of the process and is proportional to the *square of the diameter.* Hence as dendrites and axons get larger, the longitudinal conductance increases more than the membrane conductance does, so the length constant increases. (Alternatively, keeping the diameter of the process constant and decreasing the number of ion channels would also increase the length constant.[f])

Membrane capacitance, as in the case of uniform current flow, does not affect the final value of the voltage change at any point along the dendrite. It does, however, cause the rate at which the voltage changes to diminish progressively with distance, because the total capacitance increases with distance (Fig. 7-8C).

Just as multiple inputs that are temporally close to one another can summate, inputs that are physically close to one another can exhibit **spatial summation** (Fig. 7-9).

Action Potentials Convey Information Over Long Distances

Spatial summation has computational advantages for neurons because the degree of interaction between signals can be influenced by their relative locations. But it comes at a price. The decremental conduction of slow potentials, such as synaptic potentials, means that they will die out completely within a few millimeters of the site where they are generated. Some neurons are small and only need to convey information over distances that are short relative to their length constants, so they can rely on electrotonic conduction. Most neurons, however, must convey signals over distances equal to hundreds or even thousands of length constants. **Action potentials** (commonly referred to as **spikes** or **nerve impulses** because of their shape in time), actively propagated over long distances and mediated by special voltage-gated ion channels, take care of this part of the signaling process (see Fig. 7-1).

[f]Continuing with the water-flow analogy used in Resistors, Capacitors, and Neuronal Membranes, a dendrite with a very short length constant is like a garden hose with many gaping holes in its walls; a dendrite with a very long length constant is like a fire hose with a few pinholes.

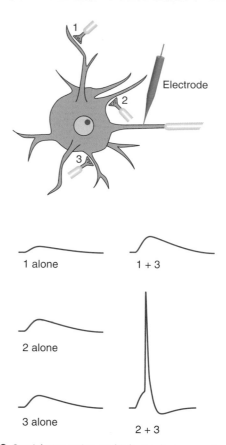

Figure 7-9 Spatial summation. Multiple simultaneous voltage changes (in this example, synaptic potentials) add to one another, to a degree determined by their relative proximity to one another and by various space constants. Summation may be sufficient to bring the neuron's trigger zone to threshold.

Opening and Closing of Voltage-Gated Sodium and Potassium Channels Underlie the Action Potential

We are accustomed to thinking about voltages much larger than membrane potentials, such as the 110-volt circuits that run U.S. household appliances and the 1.5- to 9-volt batteries that power portable electronic devices. By comparison, a membrane potential of –65 mV seems puny. However, the membrane potential is developed across a membrane only 5 to 10 nm thick, resulting in a very large electric field across the membrane (130,000 V/cm across a 5-nm membrane). Neuronal membranes contain an assortment of ion channels whose conformations change in response to fluctuations in this electric field, changing their probability of being open or closed. Two of these in particular, a voltage-gated Na^+ channel and a voltage-gated K^+ channel, are centrally involved in the generation of typical action potentials. (Neurons also contain several varieties of voltage-gated Ca^{2+} channels, but these are usually not major factors in carrying the current for electrical signaling. Instead, they often admit sufficient Ca^{2+} to trigger other intracellular processes, described more in Chapter 8.)

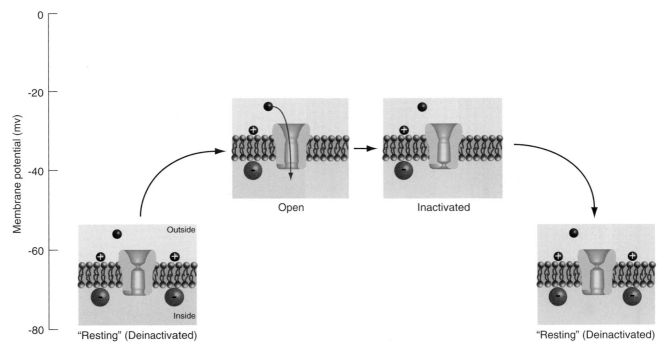

Figure 7-10 The Na$^+$ channel cycle. At the normal resting membrane potential, most voltage-gated Na$^+$ channels are closed. Depolarization increases the probability of opening. Once open, the channels enter a closed, inactivated state until the membrane is repolarized.

The voltage-gated Na$^+$ channels have three states (Fig. 7-10). In their "resting" state at the normal neuronal resting potential, the probability of being open is very low. Membrane depolarization rapidly increases their probability of being open. After a millisecond or so in this mostly open state, the channels spontaneously move into an **inactivated** state in which they are closed and will not reopen in response to further depolarization. Repolarizing the membrane toward resting potential moves the channels from this inactivated state back to the original resting state (also called the **deinactivated** state). Voltage-gated K$^+$ channels also open in response to depolarization, but more slowly. Once open, however, they do not inactivate; their probability of being open remains high as long as the membrane is depolarized.

Membranes with sufficient densities of these channels have the special property of **electrical excitability** (Fig. 7-11). In response to hyperpolarizing current, they show normal charging curves, but depolarization is different. In a membrane without voltage-gated Na$^+$ channels, depolarization draws K$^+$ ions out of the cell, at a rate determined by the resting K$^+$ conductance and the magnitude of the depolarization. In an excitable membrane, depolarization begins to cause the voltage-gated Na$^+$ channels to open, and a small inward Na$^+$ current develops. For small depolarizations, the expected outward K$^+$ current is equal and opposite and balances the Na$^+$ influx. At some level of depolarization, the inward Na$^+$ current exceeds the driving force for the compensating

K$^+$ current and adds a little extra depolarization of its own. Reaching this **threshold** causes more voltage-gated Na$^+$ channels to open and more depolarization, initiating an explosive increase in Na$^+$ conductance. In less than a millisecond, most available Na$^+$ channels enter the mostly open state, Na$^+$ conductance reaches a level as much as 50 times greater than the K$^+$ conductance, and the membrane potential moves past 0 mV and almost reaches V$_{Na}$ (Fig. 7-12). As the membrane potential moves toward V$_{Na}$, two things happen to terminate the action potential: the voltage-gated Na$^+$ channels inactivate and close due to the fact that they are unstable in the open state and stoichiometrically will only stay open for a very short time, and the voltage-gated K$^+$ channels open. The K$^+$ channels stay open for a few milliseconds, causing a brief **afterhyperpolarization,** during which the membrane potential moves even closer to V$_K$ than it is in the resting state. This repolarization allows the voltage-gated Na$^+$ channels to return to the resting state, ready for the initiation of another action potential.

Action potentials are stereotyped, **all-or-none** events—if the threshold is reached they occur, if not they do not. The generation of action potentials requires the opening of many voltage-gated sodium channels to occur at the same time. Action potentials are always depolarizing events, and for a given neuronal type, they are all the same size and duration. In these and several other ways they are fundamentally different from the

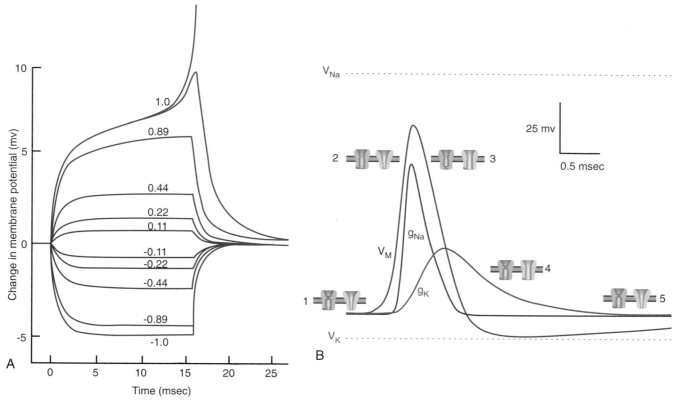

Figure 7-11 Generation of action potentials. **A,** Small hyperpolarizing current pulses (negative numbers) delivered to an unmyelinated axon (from a crab) result in smooth charging curves. Depolarizing current pulses result in almost mirror-image charging curves until a critical level of depolarization is reached (current magnitude = 1.0). At this threshold level, half the current pulses are followed by a return to baseline, and half induce an action potential that drives the membrane potential off scale. The magnitude of each current pulse is indicated as a fraction of the threshold value. **B,** Changes in Na$^+$ and K$^+$ conductance (g_{Na}, g_K) and in channel states underlying action potentials. At rest (1) most voltage-gated Na$^+$ channels and many voltage-gated K$^+$ channels are closed; many more K$^+$ channels than Na$^+$ channels are open, however, so the membrane potential (V_M) is near the K$^+$ equilibrium potential (V_K). Suprathreshold depolarization causes most voltage-gated Na$^+$ channels to open (2), and the membrane potential moves toward the sodium equilibrium potential (V_{Na}). Thereafter (3) the Na$^+$ channels inactivate, and voltage-gated K$^+$ channels begin to open. The resulting decrease in Na$^+$ conductance and increase in K$^+$ conductance repolarize the membrane, and the voltage-gated Na$^+$ channels revert to their resting state (4); extra K$^+$ channels that remain open during this period cause an afterhyperpolarization until the baseline state is reached again (5). (**A,** redrawn from Hodgkin AL, Rushton WAH: Proc Royal Soc B133:444, 1946. Voltage and conductance records in **B,** redrawn from Hodgkin AL, Huxley AF: J Physiol 117:500, 1952.)

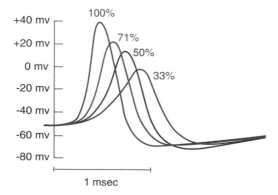

Figure 7-12 Dependence of the peak voltage reached during action potentials on the extracellular Na$^+$ concentration. The number accompanying each record is the percentage of seawater in a seawater–isotonic dextrose solution bathing a squid axon. (Redrawn from Hodgkin AL, Katz B: J Physiol 108:37, 1949.)

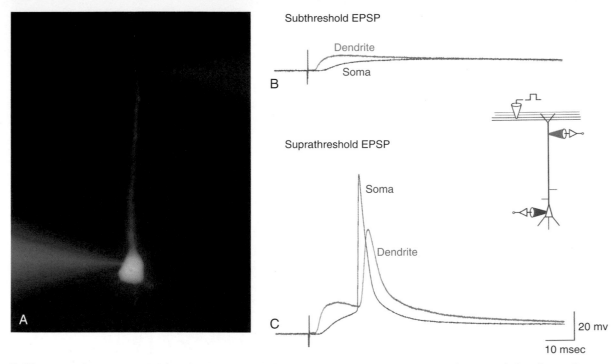

Figure 7-13 Spread of synaptic potentials and action potentials through the dendrites and soma. **A,** Simultaneous whole-cell recordings were made from the soma and apical dendrite of a pyramidal neuron in rat cerebral cortex, using patch-clamp electrodes filled with two different fluorescent dyes. **B,** Weak stimulation of the superficial layer of cortex (arrangement shown in inset) caused a depolarizing synaptic potential (EPSP) in the dendrite, which spread passively into the soma and arrived there later, slower, and smaller. **C,** Stronger stimulation of the superficial layer of cortex caused a large depolarizing synaptic potential in the dendrite, in this case large enough by the time it reached the action potential trigger zone (in the axon) to trigger an action potential that could be recorded in the soma. The action potential in turn spread back into the dendrite, arriving there later, slower, and smaller. (The dendritic action potential is actually larger than would be expected based on passive electrical properties because the dendrites of these neurons contain some voltage-gated Na^+ channels. However, there are not enough to initiate action potentials, just enough to "boost" signals that would otherwise spread passively.) *(From Sakmann B, Neher E: Single-channel recording, ed 2, New York, 1995, Plenum Press.)*

Table 7-2	Contrasting Properties of Slow Potentials and Action Potentials	
Property	**Slow Potentials**	**Action Potentials**
Amplitude	Graded, typically a few millivolts	All or none, typically about 100 mV
Duration	Graded according to stimulus	1-2 msec
Polarity	+ or −	Always +
Threshold	None (graded)	10-20 mV above resting potential
Summation	Temporal and spatial	None
Conduction	Decremental, passive	Nondecremental, active
Direction of propagation	All directions from stimulus	Unidirectional

a low threshold for generating action potentials (Fig. 7-13). The low-threshold zone (thought in most instances to be the initial segment of the axon) is a kind of analog-to-digital converter, the site where slowly fluctuating membrane potential changes are converted into a series of brief action potentials separated by varying intervals.[g] These areas of the axon segments contain large quantities of the voltage-gated sodium channels required to generate an action potential.

Mammalian Neurons Contain Multiple Types of Voltage-Gated Na^+ and K^+ Channels

The mechanism of action potential generation described in the preceding section was first unraveled in experiments on squid giant axons (see Fig. 7-22). The same basic mechanism applies in our axons, but in some places there are subtle differences. Mammals make several kinds of voltage-gated Na^+ channels, all very

slow potentials discussed earlier in this chapter (Table 7-2). Neurons use both kinds of potential changes to perform their information-processing roles. They receive a variety of inputs that spread electrotonically, summing spatially and temporally, eventually reaching a zone with

---

[g]A more apt analogy would be to say that the electrical coding strategy changes at the low-threshold zone from amplitude modulation (like AM radio) to frequency modulation (like FM radio).

similar to one another but can be found in differing quantities depending on the type of neurons (i.e., neurons of the heart will have one variety of voltage-gated Na⁺ channels while neurons of the cerebellum will have a different variety). Mammals also make a wide variety of voltage-gated K⁺ channels that differ from one another in such properties as the rate at which they respond to voltage changes and whether they inactivate after opening. Different neurons, and even different parts of individual neurons, contain distinctive mixtures of these channel types. This is part of the reason why toxins, medications, and disease processes can affect distinctive subsets of neurons.

Action Potentials Are Followed by Brief Refractory Periods

The two-part repolarization process used by neurons to terminate an action potential has consequences for the production of subsequent action potentials. For a brief period after the peak of an action potential, so many Na⁺ channels are inactivated that another impulse cannot be generated, no matter how much the membrane is depolarized. This is the **absolute refractory period** (Fig. 7-14A). This grades into a **relative refractory period** during which some but not all Na⁺ channels have returned to the resting state. A larger percentage of this reduced population of Na⁺ channels must be activated to initiate an impulse, and this in turn requires more depolarization than after full recovery. In addition, the voltage-gated K⁺ channels are still open. This shortens the time constant and the length constant, making it more difficult to depolarize the membrane to threshold. Both refractory periods together last only a few milliseconds, but they have important implications for the production and propagation of action potentials—they set limits on the frequency with which neurons can produce action potentials and on the directions in which they can propagate.

Refractory Periods Limit the Repetition Rate of Action Potentials

Continuous depolarization of a neuron, by current injection through an electrode (Fig. 7-15) or through a post-synaptic ion channel, causes the production of repetitive action potentials. The greater the depolarization, the more frequent the action potentials. The details of the train of action potentials are determined by the mix of ion channels contained in the membrane of a given neuron: at low frequencies, the firing rates of some neurons are remarkably linear functions of the depolarizing stimulus (Fig. 7-16A), whereas others fire in bursts or have other nonlinear characteristics (Fig. 7-16B and C); some can even switch between different functional states (e.g., see Fig. 16-15). The refractory periods, however, set upper limits on firing frequency (see Fig.

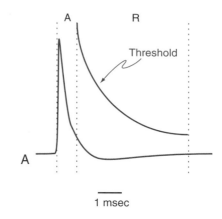

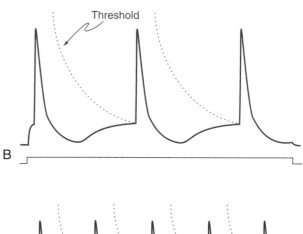

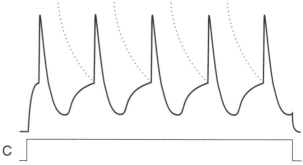

Figure 7-14 Refractory periods and their effects on neuronal firing rates. **A,** Threshold during the absolute refractory period (A, infinite) and the relative refractory period (R). **B** and **C,** Idealized neurons fire repetitively in response to a sustained depolarization, at a rate determined by the time it takes for the membrane potential to reach the declining threshold during the relative refractory period.

7-14B and C). A second impulse cannot be generated during the rising phase of an action potential (because all the voltage-gated Na⁺ channels are already in the process of opening) or during most of the falling phase (the absolute refractory period). Because these two phases together typically last 1 to 2 msec, the absolute upper limit on action potential frequency is about 1 kHz. In addition, the relative refractory period makes it difficult to reach this upper limit, and most neurons have maximum firing frequencies considerably lower than 1 kHz. In patients with epilepsy, seizures are due to the

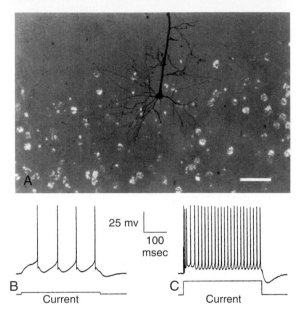

Figure 7-15 Repetitive action potentials recorded from a corticospinal neuron. **A,** The cell bodies of corticospinal neurons were labeled by retrograde transport of a fluorescent marker injected into the spinal cord. One of the resulting fluorescent neurons was impaled with a dye-filled micropipette and stained. **B,** A small amount of depolarizing current injected into the neuron in **A** caused repetitive firing at a slow, regular rate. **C,** A larger current injected into the same neuron caused a brief burst of action potentials, followed by repetitive firing at a regular rate faster than that in **B.** *(From Tseng G-F, Parada I, Prince DA: J Neurosci Methods 37:121, 1991.)*

frequent and uncontrollable rapid succession of action potentials. Medications used for seizures include drugs that will prolong the refractory states of the voltage-gated sodium channels, hence slowing or even stopping the action potentials.

Pathological Processes and Toxins Can Selectively Affect Voltage-Gated Channels

The dependence of neuronal electrical processes on particular ion channels makes them vulnerable to genetic mutation, disease processes, and toxins. For example, certain genetic diseases of neurons, muscle (which has an action potential mechanism similar to that of neurons), and other tissues are caused by mutations that affect various kinds of ion channels, resulting in disorders that are now known as **channelopathies.** In some instances the relationship between the channel defect and clinical symptoms is reasonably well understood (Box 7-2). There are also dozens of other neurological and neuromuscular disorders that are known to be associated with particular ion channel defects—some familial seizure disorders, episodic ataxias, and headache syndromes, among others—but in most cases the relationship between the defect and the symptoms has not yet been clarified.

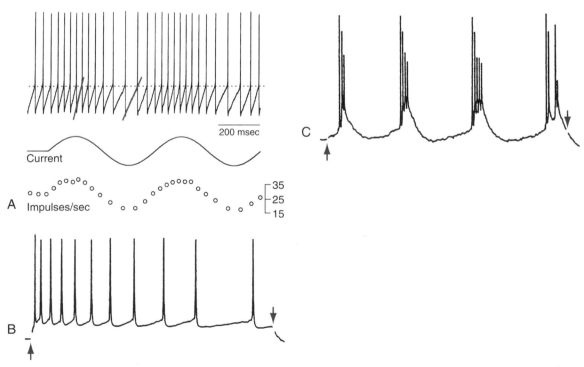

Figure 7-16 Varying patterns of repetitive firing in different types of neurons. **A,** A neuron in one of the vestibular nuclei whose firing rate varied linearly with the amount of depolarizing current injected into it. The action potentials were all of uniform size, and threshold *(dashed line)* remained constant, but the rate *(green lines)* at which the membrane potential reached threshold varied with the amount of current injected. **B** and **C,** Some cortical neurons respond to steady depolarization (beginning and end indicated by arrows) with a declining frequency **(B)** or a series of bursts **(C).** *(A, from du Lac S, Lisberger SG: J Neurosci 15:8000, 1995. B and C, from Agmon A, Connors BW: J Neurosci 12:319, 1992.)*

BOX 7-2

Channelopathies: *Diseases Caused by Defective Ion Channels*

Two hereditary muscle diseases with contrasting symptoms provide instructive examples of channelopathies. Patients with periodic paralysis, as the name of the syndrome suggests, have episodes of weakness. Patients with myotonia ("muscle tone") have difficulty getting muscles to relax once they have contracted.

Individuals with hyperkalemic periodic paralysis (one of several types of periodic paralysis) have episodes of weakness and decreased muscle tone that may follow exercise or the consumption of potassium-rich foods, such as fruit juice or bananas. During the attacks, the involved muscle fibers are depolarized by 30 to 40 mV and are unable to fire action potentials. The disorder is caused by a mutation of muscle voltage-gated Na^+ channels that prevents some percentage of them from inactivating completely after depolarization (Fig. 7-17). This results in a small but constant inward Na^+ current that depolarizes the fibers, inactivates normal channels, and renders the muscle inexcitable for a period of minutes to hours.

Thomsen's disease and Becker's disease are two similar forms of myotonia, inherited in an autosomal dominant and recessive fashion, respectively. The muscles of affected individuals relax unusually slowly following a sudden contraction. It may take several seconds, for example, to unclench a fist, to open a hand after a handshake, or to open the eyes after squinting during a sneeze or during exposure to bright sunlight. Abrupt attempts to run or jump may cause leg muscles

to stiffen, resulting in a fall. The mechanism of this form of myotonia was first unraveled by studying the muscle fibers of a strain of goats afflicted by basically the same disease. Myotonic goats, known since the 1880s as "nervous" or "fainting" goats, stiffen up and may fall over when startled.* Normal skeletal muscle fibers, unlike neurons, have a relatively high Cl^- permeability, so their resting membrane potential is determined largely by the Cl^- concentration gradient. This form of myotonia, in goats as in humans, is caused by a mutation of the Cl^- channels that account for most of this resting membrane conductance. The resulting increase in resistance not only makes the membrane time constant longer, so that muscle fibers take longer to repolarize after an action potential, but also reduces the amount of depolarizing current required to reach threshold (Fig. 7-18A and B). In addition, the muscle membrane potential now becomes dominated by the K^+ concentration, so that small increases in the extracellular K^+ concentration cause more depolarization than normal. The net result is that a depolarizing stimulus that would cause a single action potential in a normal muscle fiber causes a train of action potentials in a myotonic fiber, in turn causing contraction that is maintained for several seconds. One indication that reduced Cl^- conductance is responsible for these properties is the observation that replacing the Cl^- in the fluid bathing a normal fiber with an impermeant anion has the same effect (see Fig. 7-18C).

*"If these goats are suddenly surprised or frightened they become perfectly rigid. While in this condition they can be pushed or turned over as if they were carved out of a single piece of wood. This spell or 'fit' usually lasts only a short time—about ten to twenty seconds … if two or three men, who had crept up close without being observed, would suddenly rush toward the flock yelling and waving coats in the air a considerable number of the goats would be sure to fall to the ground and most of the rest would become rigid in the upright position for several seconds." (From Lush JL: *J Hered* 21:243, 1930.)

Toxins that affect voltage-gated channels would obviously be powerful weapons for animals that could dispense them. They are also powerful tools for studying neuronal physiology and for developing pharmacological agents useful for treating neurological problems. One of the best known neurotoxins is **tetrodotoxin,** which is concentrated in the liver and ovaries of some species of puffer fish and found in a few other animal species as well. Tetrodotoxin binds tightly to the extracellular part of voltage-gated Na^+ channels, preventing Na^+ ions from entering. As might be expected, this makes tetrodotoxin a potent poison (Box 7-3), but it has also proved invaluable in experimental studies. For example, tritium-labeled tetrodotoxin has been used to map out the locations of Na^+ channels in neuronal membranes. Plants and animals have developed a host of other toxins that affect various aspects of Na^+ channels and other channels.

Action Potentials Are Propagated Without Decrement Along Axons

The series of channel openings and closings just described not only generates an all-or-none action potential but also triggers the propagation of the action potential along adjacent areas of membrane that contain similar voltage-gated channels—primarily down the axon to ultimately cause the release of neurotransmitter from its synaptic terminals.

Propagation Is Continuous and Relatively Slow in Unmyelinated Axons

Propagation of action potentials along unmyelinated axons is straightforward though relatively slow. The inward current flowing through voltage-gated Na^+ channels during an action potential spreads longitudinally in both directions from the trigger zone, depolarizing

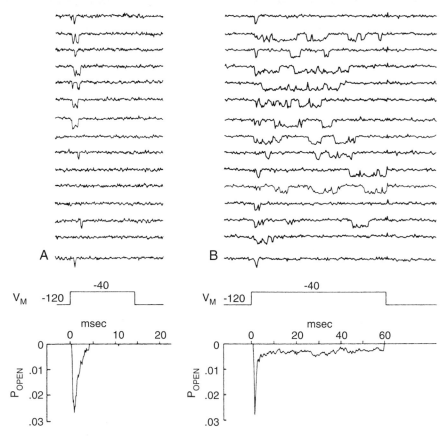

Figure 7-17 Abnormal voltage-gated Na⁺ channels in a patient with periodic paralysis. Repeated patch-clamp recordings of the current flowing through single channels of normal muscle membranes **(A)** and those of the patient **(B)** during depolarization from 120 to 40 mV indicate that the patient's channels do not inactivate rapidly. Averages of many such records were used to calculate the probability of channels being open (P$_{OPEN}$) over time. The continued, albeit reduced, probability of the patient's channels being open corresponds to a small but constant inward Na⁺ current that depolarizes the fiber. *(From Cannon SC: Trends Neurosci 19:3, 1996.)*

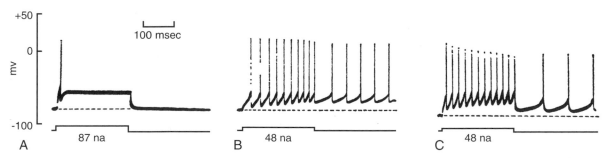

Figure 7-18 Effects of decreased Cl⁻ conductance on goat muscle fibers. **A,** Injection (through a microelectrode) of 87 nanoamperes of current into an intercostal muscle fiber from a normal goat elicits a single action potential. At the termination of the current pulse the membrane potential decays quickly to the original resting potential. **B,** Injection of little more than half as much current into a muscle fiber from a myotonic goat elicits a train of action potentials. At the termination of the current pulse the membrane stays somewhat depolarized (due to extracellular K⁺ accumulation), and action potentials continue at a slower rate. **C,** Replacing the Cl⁻ in the solution bathing a normal goat muscle fiber with an impermeant cation (sulfate) causes it to behave like a myotonic fiber. *(From Adrian RH, Bryant SH: J Physiol 240:505, 1974.)*

BOX 7-3

Puffer Fish and Sodium Channels

Puffer fish (Fig. 7-19) are scaleless, spiny fish that live mostly in warm tropical seas. They get their name from a striking ability to inflate themselves when provoked by sucking large amounts of water or air into a sac connected to the stomach. Some species of puffer fish in Asia have been known for thousands of years to be poisonous. In fact, one Chinese proverb says, "To throw away life, eat puffer fish." Despite this warning, puffer fish are also considered a culinary delicacy, particularly in Japan, where they are called *fugu*. Because tetrodotoxin, the active ingredient in puffer fish poison, is concentrated in internal organs such as the liver and gonads and is not destroyed by cooking, puffer fish is served publicly in Japan only by specially trained fugu chefs who are skilled at avoiding contamination of the meal.

Europeans were unaware of the poisonous nature of puffer fish until the 18th century. One of the first recorded European victims of tetrodotoxin poisoning was Captain James Cook, more widely known for naval explorations of the Pacific Ocean. On September 7, 1774, during his second voyage to the Pacific, a crew member traded some cloth for a puffer fish offered by the inhabitants of New Caledonia. Two naturalists on board tried to convince Cook not to eat it, but he insisted that he had eaten such fish before and that they should all have some. All three had a taste—fortunately, a small taste—of the liver and roe the next evening. Captain Cook, in his journal, described what happened next:

> About three o'clock in the morning we found ourselves seized with an extraordinary weakness and numbness all over our limbs. I had almost lost the sense of feeling; nor could I distinguish between light and heavy bodies of such as I had strength to move, a quart pot full of water and a feather being the same in my hand.*

Late in the 19th century it was demonstrated that crude extracts containing puffer fish poison block the responses of frog motor nerves to stimulation. In the 1960s intracellular recordings during the application of purified tetrodotoxin demonstrated that it selectively blocks current flow through voltage-gated Na^+ channels. Blocking the Na^+ channels of the peripheral nerves of victims explains tetrodotoxin's effects; larger doses than those consumed by Captain Cook can cause respiratory paralysis and death in minutes. Tetrodotoxin was the first studied of a long line of naturally occurring toxins that selectively affect various aspects of electrical signaling by neurons. Collectively they have been extremely helpful in unraveling the multiple processes involved in bioelectric phenomena (e.g., see Fig. 8-7).

*From Cook J: A voyage towards the South Pole and around the world, vol 2, London, 1777, Straham & Cadell; quoted in Kao CY: Pharmacol Rev 18:997, 1966.

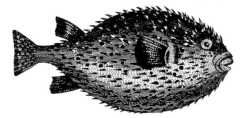

Figure 7-19 A puffer fish. *(From Heck JG: Heck's pictorial archive of nature and science, New York, 1851, Rudolph Garrigue.)*

adjacent areas of membrane (Fig. 7-20A). What happens next depends on the density of voltage-gated Na^+ channels in these adjacent regions. If the density is high enough to sustain an action potential, the electrotonically conducted depolarization will reach threshold and trigger one; if it is not, the depolarization will diminish with distance according to the space constant of the neuronal process. Most neuronal cell bodies and dendrites are thought not to be electrically excitable (although some contain enough Na^+ channels to propagate impulses under some circumstances). Axons, however, contain such channels in relative abundance, either distributed uniformly along unmyelinated axons or concentrated at the nodes of Ranvier along myelin-

ated axons. Hence the initial action potential will propagate along the axon toward its distal terminals, each segment of axonal membrane depolarizing the next segment to threshold (see Fig. 7-20B). Unlike electrotonically conducted slow potentials, action potentials move down the axon in a **nondecremental** fashion.

The rate at which an action potential propagates down an axon—the **conduction velocity**—is directly related to the length constant of the axon: the longer the length constant, the farther down the axon the depolarization reaches and the sooner the next segment of membrane will reach threshold (see Fig. 7-20C and D). Because larger-diameter axons have longer length constants, they also have faster conduction velocities. The thinnest unmyelinated axons in our peripheral nerves are 0.2 μm in diameter[h] and conduct at 0.5 m/sec; the largest are 1.5 μm and conduct at 2.5 m/sec. Some invertebrates have taken the strategy of speeding conduction velocity by increasing axonal diameter to extremes, typi-

[h]This is about as thin as axons can be and still be useful for conveying information accurately. Beginning at about 0.1 μm, the random opening of a single voltage-gated Na^+ channel would let in enough current to set off an action potential, making axons susceptible to thermal noise.

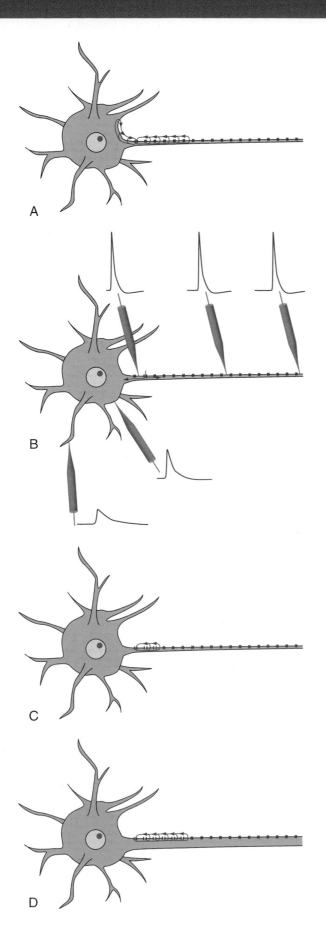

Figure 7-20 Propagation of action potentials along unmyelinated axons. **A,** Initiation of an action potential in the axonal trigger zone close to the cell body causes the spread of depolarizing current in both directions—into the electrically inexcitable cell body and into adjacent, electrically excitable parts of the axon. **B,** The action potential waveform spreads passively into the cell body and dendrites, becoming progressively later, slower, and smaller. In contrast, each successive part of the axon reaches threshold and generates its own action potential, so the spike becomes progressively later but not slower or smaller. **C,** Thin axons have relatively short space constants, so a shorter length of axon is depolarized to threshold at any given time (i.e., conduction velocity is relatively slow). **D,** Thick axons have relatively long space constants, so a greater length of axon is depolarized to threshold at any given time (i.e., conduction velocity is relatively rapid).

cally in axons that mediate rapid escape responses. The most celebrated example is the giant axons that innervate the mantle muscle of squid. They may be up to 500 μm in diameter, allowing them to conduct at 25 m/sec (see Fig. 7-22).

Refractory Periods Ensure That Action Potentials Are Propagated in Only One Direction

Action potentials can propagate from their point of initiation into any nearby excitable membrane. Experimental initiation of an action potential midway along an axon, for example, would cause impulses to propagate not only **orthodromically** toward the distal terminals of the axon but also **antidromically** toward the cell body (Fig. 7-21A). Under normal physiological conditions, however, impulses travel only orthodromically.[i] This is the second major consequence of the refractory periods that follow production of an action potential. Action potentials typically are initiated at a trigger zone in the axon near the cell body and then spread antidromically and passively into the inexcitable cell body and propagate orthodromically down the axon. As an impulse travels down an axon, inward Na+ current travels both orthodromically and antidromically. However, the part of the axon most recently traversed by the impulse is refractory, and an antidromic impulse cannot be initiated (see Fig. 7-21B).

Action Potentials "Jump" Rapidly from Node to Node in Myelinated Axons

Although the giant axons of invertebrates are effective at propagating impulses rapidly, this speed has a cost: they take up a lot of space (Fig. 7-22). (If the million axons in a human optic nerve were all 500 μm in diameter, the nerve would need to be larger than a typical human

---

[i]The exception is sensory axons with branches in the periphery. Action potentials that reach a branch point on their way to the CNS can propagate in both directions from that point—both toward the CNS and back toward the periphery over other branches (see Fig. 9-13).

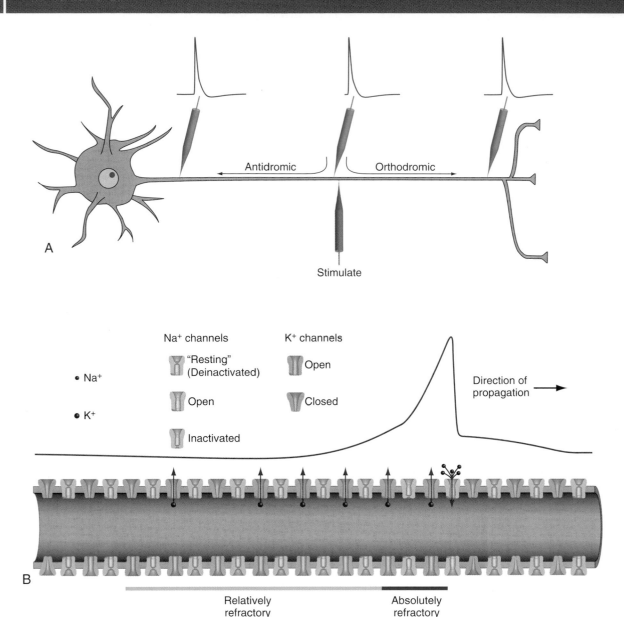

Figure 7-21 Normally unidirectional propagation of action potentials. **A,** An action potential artificially induced partway along an axon would encounter excitable membrane in both directions and so would propagate both orthodromically and antidromically. Because the typical zone where action potentials begin under normal physiological conditions is flanked on one side by inexcitable membrane (the cell body) and on the other side by excitable membrane (the rest of the axon), propagation normally proceeds only in the orthodromic direction. **B,** An action potential "frozen" in one instant of time as it propagates orthodromically. A relatively small number of Na⁺ ions rush in at the site of action potential generation and depolarize membrane segments in both directions. However, the trailing zones of absolutely and relatively refractory membrane ensure that the action potential continues to propagate only orthodromically. Notice that current enters the axon in the form of Na⁺ ions but leaves in the form of K⁺ ions. Although it is tempting to think of current flowing in loops through axonal membranes as being carried by the same ions, in fact, ions that enter at one site repel ions of like charge, which repel other ions of like charge in succession, until finally ions at some distance away leave the axon almost instantaneously. This is a lot like water emerging promptly when a faucet is turned on, even though the water may be entering the system far away. (This drawing is a schematic representation and is not to scale. In the case of an unmyelinated axon with a typical conduction velocity of 1 m/sec and an action potential and afterhyperpolarization of 3-msec total duration, the action potential and its afterhyperpolarization would be spread out along 3 mm of axon [1 m/sec × 3 × 10⁻³ sec]. Because a typical unmyelinated axon might be 1 μm in diameter, on the scale of this figure the action potential should be spread out over 60 m.)

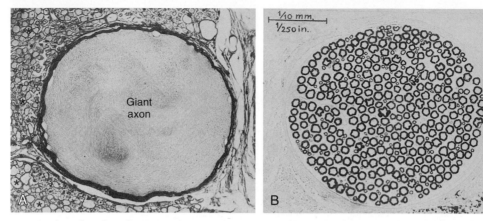

Figure 7-22 Space-saving benefits of myelin. **A,** Squid giant axon, surrounded by axons of more typical size (*). The giant axon, because of its size, conducts at 20 to 25 m/sec and is used by the squid to make its mantle muscle contract quickly when trying to escape. Also because of their size, squid giant axons were the subject of most early experiments on the mechanism of action potential generation and conduction. They were, for example, the source of the data in Figure 7-11B. **B,** The motor nerve to a rabbit's gastrocnemius, at the same magnification as the squid nerve in **A.** About 400 myelinated fibers fit into the space occupied by a single giant axon and, because of their myelin, are able to conduct at speeds up to 90 m/sec. *(From Young JZ: Doubt and certainty in science, New York, 1960, Oxford University Press.)*

neck). Vertebrates take the alternative approach to increasing conduction velocity: rather than simply increasing the diameter of the axon, they increase the length constant by adding myelin, which prevents longitudinal current from leaking out.[j] The result is a major saving of space, because a myelinated axon with a conduction velocity of 25 m/sec needs to be only 4 to 5 μm in diameter (including the myelin). Our largest myelinated fibers are about 20 μm in diameter and conduct at about 100 m/sec.

Even though the addition of myelin greatly increases the length constant of the axon, some current still leaves, and an action potential initiated only at a trigger zone such as the axon's initial segment would die out after a few millimeters. This is prevented by the presence of nodes of Ranvier (see Figs. 1-23, 1-25, and 1-29) every millimeter or so. The nodal membrane contains a very high concentration of voltage-gated Na[+] channels[k] (Fig. 7-23A and B; see also Fig. 1-25). Action potentials spread electrotonically along internodal parts of the axon, depolarize one node after another to threshold, and are regenerated at each node sequentially (see Fig. 7-23C). The electrotonic spread is very rapid, but the regeneration at each node takes a little time, so the action potential appears to skip from one node to the next (see Fig. 7-23C). Hence this is called **saltatory conduction** (from a Latin word meaning "to leap" or "to dance"). The larger the diameter of a myelinated axon, the more rapidly it conducts (Fig. 7-24), in part because of lower longitudinal resistance and because of the more widely spaced nodes of Ranvier.

Demyelinating Diseases Can Slow or Block Conduction of Action Potentials

Some disease processes selectively affect myelin in either the peripheral or central nervous system. Nodal membrane contains 1000 to 2000 voltage-gated Na[+] channels/μm²; internodal axonal membrane contains fewer than 25/μm². The membranes of unmyelinated axons contain from 100 to 200 channels/μm², so loss of myelin slows conduction drastically and may even cause failure of propagation. The two following examples in which the patient's own immune system attacks and destroys myelin are illustrative.

Guillain-Barré syndrome is an inflammatory process that typically begins a week or two after a viral infection, which is thought to trigger an immune response. In the most common form, infiltrating macrophages selectively attack and damage PNS myelin, mainly but not exclusively that of motor nerves. Over a period of a week or so patients become progressively weaker, often in an ascending pattern, and may become almost completely paralyzed and require ventilatory assistance. Conduction in proximal parts of motor nerves is slowed and may

[j]The successive layers of membranes in the myelin sheath act like a succession of resistors and capacitors wired in series, so electrically the sheath has high resistance and low capacitance (see Resistors, Capacitors, and Neuronal Membranes). Little current leaves through the myelin resistance, and little is needed to charge the myelin capacitance.

[k]Only voltage-gated Na[+] channels are concentrated in mammalian nodal membranes, and nodal action potentials are apparently terminated primarily by inactivation of these channels. Several kinds of K[+] channels are concentrated in paranodal and internodal axonal membranes (see Fig. 7-23B), where they maintain the axonal membrane potential and participate in axonal physiology in other less well understood ways. This is in contrast to unmyelinated fibers, in which Na[+] and K[+] channels are interspersed and the opening of voltage-gated K[+] channels plays an important role in terminating action potentials.

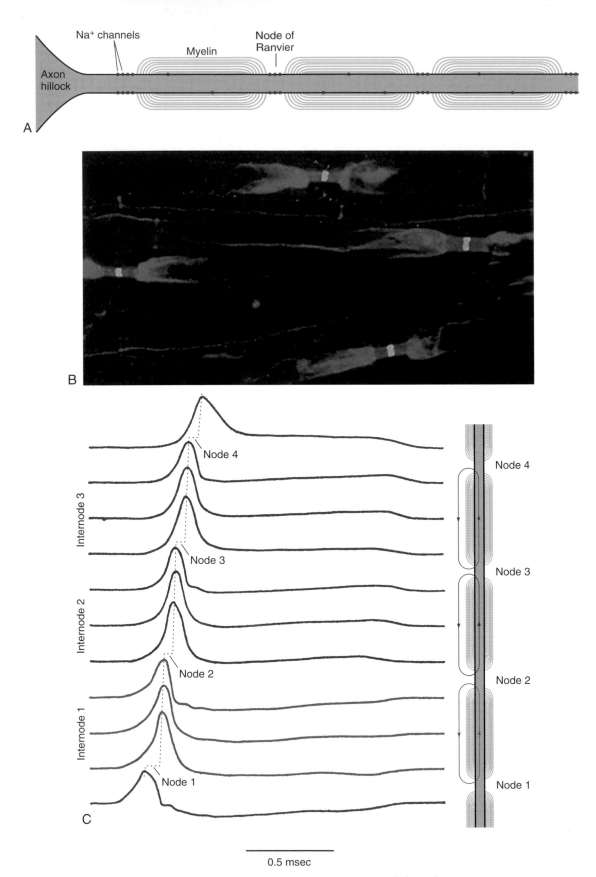

Figure 7-23 Propagation of action potentials along myelinated axons. **A,** Voltage-gated Na⁺ channels are concentrated in areas of the axon near the cell body and at nodes of Ranvier. **B,** Myelinated axons teased from the sciatic nerve of a mouse and stained with three different fluorescent antibodies to demonstrate some aspects of the molecular organization of nodes of Ranvier. Green fluorescence indicates voltage-gated Na⁺ channels, which are selectively concentrated in the nodes. Blue fluorescence indicates a protein called NCP1, which is part of the circumferential junctions between paranodal axonal membranes and the membranes of adjoining pockets of Schwann cell or oligodendrocyte cytoplasm (see Figs. 1-25 and 1-29). Not all the functions of NCP1 are known, but one of them may be to separate nodal membranes rich in voltage-gated Na⁺ channels from nearby membranes rich in voltage-gated K⁺ channels (red fluorescence). **C,** Measurements of extracellular current flow as an action potential propagates along a myelinated axon from a frog. Little current leaks across myelin, and current flows almost instantaneously along each internode. A little time is required at each internode for the voltage-gated Na⁺ channels to open and regenerate the action potential, which therefore appears to "skip" from node to node. (**B,** courtesy Dr. Manzoor A. Bhat, Mount Sinai School of Medicine. **C,** modified from Huxley AF, Stämpfli R: J Physiol 108:315, 1949.)

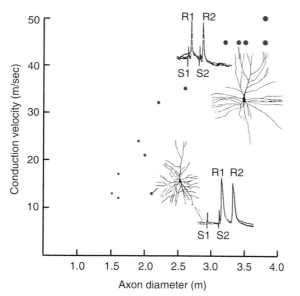

Figure 7-24 Conduction velocity of myelinated corticospinal axons as a function of axon diameter. Measurements were made of dye-injected neurons and axons and do not include myelin. Reconstructions of two of the corticospinal neurons are shown; larger-diameter axons generally arise from larger cell bodies. The electrical records accompanying the reconstruction of each neuron show pairs of antidromically conducted action potentials (R) recorded in the neuronal cell body in response to pairs of brief shocks (S) delivered to the corticospinal tract. The time between a stimulus and a response (e.g., from S1 to R1) provides a measure of conduction velocity. *(Modified from Sakai H, Woody CD: Brain Res 460:1, 1988.)*

be blocked. Fortunately, most patients recover over a period of weeks to months, although residual disabilities are common.

Multiple sclerosis is named for the multiple **plaques** of demyelinated CNS white matter (see Fig. 5-21) that often wax and wane over time. The plaques are the result of an autoimmune attack on focal areas of CNS myelin. The demyelination can occur at any CNS site, but some locations are more common than others: the optic nerve, the deep cerebral white matter (especially around the ventricles), the cerebellar peduncles, and particular parts of the brainstem and spinal cord. A genetic predisposition, together with unknown environmental exposures, is thought to trigger the immune response. Multiple sclerosis is relatively common, particularly in young adults, and can be a seriously debilitating chronic disorder. A variety of immunosuppression strategies are currently used as treatment approaches.

Resistors, Capacitors, and Neuronal Membranes

Most of the voltage and current changes that develop across biological membranes can be understood and described in terms of simple electrical circuits made up of batteries, switches, resistors, and capacitors. These electrical circuits themselves are a lot like networks of fluid-filled pipes, in which water pressure is equivalent to voltage, water flow to current, switches to valves, and resistors to constrictions in pipes (the analogy becomes a little strained in the case of capacitors).

Just as water pressure drives water flow through pipes, voltage drives electrical current through wires or across biological membranes. (In the latter case, the voltage source is the energy stored in the form of concentration gradients across the membrane.) For a pipe of a given size or a membrane of a given resistance, flow (current) increases linearly with pressure (voltage). This is Ohm's law:

$$V = IR \qquad [7\text{-}1]$$

or

$$V = \frac{I}{G} \qquad [7\text{-}2]$$

where V = voltage, I = current, R = resistance, and G = conductance (1/R).

Current always flows in complete circuits (so does water, although sometimes all the parts of the circuit may not be obvious), and all the voltage is dissipated in moving current through the resistances of the circuit (Fig. 7-25). Two resistors strung end to end (in series) present more of an impediment to current flow than does a single resistor, so resistors in series add:

$$R_{series} = R_1 + R_2 + R_3, etc. \qquad [7\text{-}3]$$

In contrast, two resistors connected side by side (in parallel) offer two paths through which current can flow simultaneously, so the total resistance diminishes. In other words, *conductances* (reciprocals of resistance) in parallel add:

$$G_{parallel} = G_1 + G_2 + G_3, etc. \qquad [7\text{-}4]$$

or

$$\frac{1}{R_{parallel}} = \frac{1}{R_1} + \frac{1}{R_2} + \frac{1}{R_3}, etc. \qquad [7\text{-}5]$$

Voltage changes in response to current flows in purely resistive networks happen almost instantaneously. Capacitors add a dimension of time. As an electrical device, a capacitor is simply two plates of conducting material separated by an insulating layer—for instance, two sheets of aluminum foil separated by a sheet of plastic film. If the two conducting sheets are connected to a circuit in which current is flowing, positive charges collect on one sheet and repel positive charges on the other. Therefore current, at least initially, continues to flow in the circuit, even though none actually crosses the insulating layer of the capacitor (Fig. 7-26). The separation of charges across the plates of the capacitor

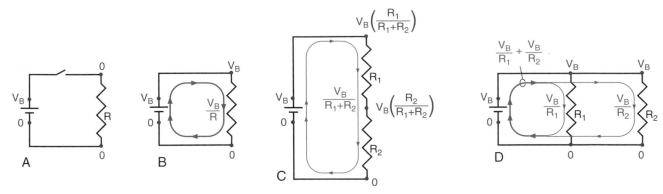

Figure 7-25 Voltages and current flows in purely resistive circuits. **A,** With a switch open, the battery voltage (V_B) drives no current flow around the circuit, and there is no voltage across the resistor (R). **B,** Closing the switch allows current flow according to Ohm's law, and the entire battery voltage is seen across the resistor. **C,** Resistors in series add, and the total current flow through both is predicted by Ohm's law. The battery voltage is divided between the resistors, in a proportion again predicted by Ohm's law. **D,** Resistors in parallel add as reciprocals. In this case the voltage across both resistors is the same, but the current is divided between them, as predicted by Ohm's law.

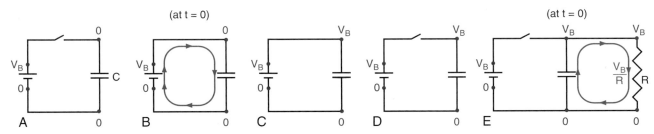

Figure 7-26 Storage of charge by capacitors. **A,** With a switch open, the battery voltage (V_B) drives no current flow around the circuit, and there is no voltage across the capacitor (C). Closing the switch allows rapid current flow **(B)** until the capacitor is charged to the battery voltage **(C).** The charge remains stored on the capacitor even if the switch is reopened **(D).** **E,** Addition of a leakage path (resistor R) allows charge to leave the capacitor, initially at a rate (i.e., current flow) predicted by Ohm's law. As charge progressively leaves the capacitor, its voltage declines (see Equation 7-7), so the current through and the voltage across the resistor decline exponentially.

constitutes a voltage across the capacitor, which continues to increase as long as current continues to flow (in real-life situations, until the voltage across the capacitor is equal to the battery voltage). Once accumulated on the plates of the capacitor, charge stays there until it is given a path through which to leak away (see Fig. 7-26). Hence capacitors store charge and build up voltage in response to current flow:

$$V = \frac{Q}{C} \qquad [7\text{-}6]$$

and

$$\Delta V / \Delta t = \frac{\Delta Q / \Delta t}{C} = \frac{I}{C} \qquad [7\text{-}7]$$

where V = voltage, Q = charge, C = capacitance, ΔV = change in voltage, and $\Delta Q/\Delta t$ = change in charge over time (i.e., $\Delta Q/\Delta t$ = current = I).

Capacitors act like a very low resistance when a voltage change is first applied, allowing current to flow easily in the circuit, and they behave like an open switch once they are charged up. Connecting two capacitors side by side is like having one capacitor with larger plates, so capacitors in parallel add:

$$C_{parallel} = C_1 + C_2 + C_3, etc. \qquad [7\text{-}8]$$

Conversely, capacitors in series add reciprocally, and the total capacitance diminishes:

$$\frac{1}{C_{series}} = \frac{1}{C_1} + \frac{1}{C_2} + \frac{1}{C_3}, etc. \qquad [7\text{-}9]$$

Biological membranes, like real electrical circuits, include combinations of resistances and capacitances. In the case of a patch of membrane, the lipid bilayer acts like the insulating layer in a capacitor, and the ion channels act like resistors in parallel with this capacitor (Fig. 7-27). Parallel resistor-capacitor combinations change the time course of signals. An injection of constant current, for example, initially flows easily through the capacitor, causing a change in voltage dictated by I/C (see Equation 7-7). As soon as voltage begins to develop across the capacitor, the same voltage is present across the resistor. Some of the current then begins flowing through the resistor, slowing the rate at which the capacitor charges. Eventually the capacitor is

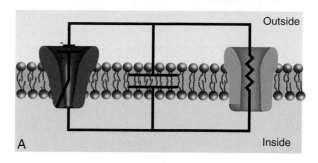

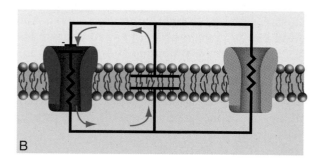

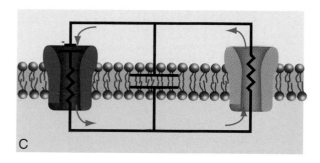

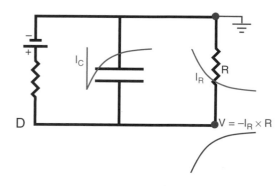

Figure 7-27 Neuronal membranes as parallel circuits of resistors and capacitors. **A,** The lipid bilayer, together with the conductive solutes on either side of it, is electrically equivalent to a series of capacitors in parallel; ion channels are electrically equivalent to variable resistors. Considering only the voltages and currents attributable to the channel on the left, when the channel is closed, no current flows through the membrane resistance or capacitance. **B** and **C,** Opening this channel initiates current flow through the membrane resistance and capacitance, dictated by a voltage corresponding to the gradient for the ion passing through this channel. Current flows initially through the membrane capacitance (**B**), then switches to open ion channels as the capacitance charges up (**C**). **D,** An electrical equivalent circuit (neglecting extracellular and cytoplasmic resistances). At time = 0 the capacitance acts like a very small resistance, so initial current flow is through the membrane capacitance (I_C), no current flows through the membrane resistance (I_R), and no change in membrane potential develops. At steady state, the capacitance is fully charged, and an amount of current predicted by Ohm's law flows through the membrane resistance. The time course of the voltage change (V) between time = 0 and steady state is an exponential curve whose duration depends on both membrane resistance and capacitance.

not respond instantaneously to changes in current flow. Instead they have exponential charging curves with a **time constant:**

$$\tau = RC \qquad [7\text{-}10]$$

where τ is the time constant, the time required for the voltage to reach 63% $(1 - 1/e)$ of its final value.

Calculating the Membrane Potential[i]

Walther Nernst in 1888 studied quantitatively the equilibrium condition for membranes permeable to only one ion, deriving an equation that still bears his name. The conceptual basis for the Nernst equation is simply that at equilibrium the work required to move a given ion across the electrical potential gradient is equal and opposite to the work required to move it against its concentration gradient. The work (W_e) required to move a mole of an ion across voltage V is:

$$W_e = zFV \qquad [7\text{-}11]$$

where z is the valence of the ion and F is Faraday's constant (the charge in 1 mole of monovalent ions). Hence it takes work to move positive ions to a more positive potential, whereas moving them to a less positive potential can be a source of work.

The work (W_c) required to change the concentration of a mole of the same ion (X) from $[X]_1$ to $[X]_2$ is:

$$W_c = RT \ln \frac{[X]_2}{[X]_1} \qquad [7\text{-}12]$$

charged and all the current flows through the resistor. The voltage across both at this point is dictated by IR (see Equation 7-1). The rate at which the current flow moves from the capacitor to the resistor is influenced by their size. The larger the capacitance, the longer the duration of current flow required to charge it. The larger the resistance, the less current flows through it at a given capacitor voltage, so the longer it takes for all the current flow to move to the resistor (i.e., if the resistance is large, the final voltage change will also be large, but it will take a long time to get there). Thus membranes do

[i]This account draws on the excellent discussion by Katz B: Nerve, muscle and synapse, New York, 1966, McGraw-Hill.

where R is the gas constant and T is the temperature in °K. Hence it takes work to concentrate the ion ($[X]_2 > [X]_1$), whereas diluting a solution can be a source of work ($[X]_2 < [X]_1$).

At equilibrium $W_e + W_c = 0$, so

$$zFV_X = -RT\ln\frac{[X]_2}{[X]_1} = RT\ln\frac{[X]_1}{[X]_2} \qquad [7\text{-}13]$$

Rearranging terms yields the Nernst equation:

$$V_X = \frac{RT}{zF}\ln\frac{[X]_1}{[X]_2} \qquad [7\text{-}14]$$

Combining all the constants (at $T = 37°C = 310°K$) and converting natural logs to $\log_{10}$ yields

$$V_X = 62\log_{10}\frac{[X]_1}{[X]_2} \qquad [7\text{-}15]$$

for monovalent cations such as Na^+ and K^+. For Cl^- the lumped constant would be −62 (because of the negative valence), and for Ca^{2+} it would be 31.

If we consider the example of a membrane permeable only to K^+, make $[K^+]_1$ and $[K^+]_2$ the extracellular and intracellular K^+ concentrations ($[K^+]_o$ and $[K^+]_i$, respectively, and use the values in Table 7-1, then

$$V_K = 62\log_{10}\frac{[K^+]_o}{[K^+]_i} = 62\log_{10}\frac{4}{130} = -94mv \qquad [7\text{-}16]$$

Once it became apparent that real membranes are permeable not just to K^+ but also, to some extent, to Na^+ and Cl^-, Goldman, and at about the same time Hodgkin and Katz, developed an equation describing the predicted membrane potential (V_m):

$$V_m = 62\log_{10}\frac{P_K[K^+]_o + P_{Na}[Na^+]_o + P_{Cl}[Cl^-]_i}{P_K[K^+]_i + P_{Na}[Na^+]_i + P_{Cl}[Cl^-]_o} \qquad [7\text{-}17]$$

where P_K, P_{Na}, and P_{Cl} are the permeabilities of the membrane to K^+, Na^+, and Cl^-, respectively.

Although this equation initially looks terrifying, it simply describes a weighted average of V_K, V_{Na}, and V_{Cl}, with permeability as the weighting factor. As the permeability to a particular ion increases, the membrane potential moves closer to the equilibrium potential for that ion. This is shown most dramatically during an action potential, when a large but transient increase in Na^+ permeability causes the membrane potential transiently to approach V_{Na} (see Fig. 7-11B). For situations in which the membrane is permeable to only one ion, the Goldman-Hodgkin-Katz equation reduces directly to the Nernst equation. Hence the equation indicates limiting conditions for the membrane potential: no combination of permeability changes to Na^+, K^+, or Cl^- can make the membrane potential more negative than V_K or more positive than V_{Na}.

The ratio of $P_K:P_{Na}:P_{Cl}$ in a typical resting neuronal membrane might be $1:0.1:0.25$, although there is considerable variation among different types of neurons. P_K is always substantially greater than P_{Na}, however, so the resting membrane potential is closer to V_K than to V_{Na} and is determined by the Na^+ and K^+ concentration gradients maintained by Na^+/K^+ ATPase. In some neurons, Cl^- is passively distributed across the membrane, adjusting its concentration gradient to counterbalance the membrane potential. Others, however, contain a Cl^- pump that pumps Cl^- out of the cell (or, in rare instances, *into* the cell). In neurons such as these, the resulting Cl^- concentration gradient contributes to the resting membrane potential, and alterations in Cl^- conductance can cause changes in the membrane potential. Some neurotransmitters, for example, cause an increase in the Cl^- conductance of the postsynaptic membrane and consequent inward Cl^- movement and hyperpolarization.

SUGGESTED READINGS

Adams ME, Swanson G: Neurotoxins, ed 2. Trends Neurosci 19(Suppl), 1996.
  An extensive listing of toxins that affect a variety of ion channels.
Bernard G, Shevell MI: Channelopathies: a review. Ped Neurol 38:73, 2008.
Bhat MA, et al: Axon-glia interactions and the domain organization of myelinated axons requires Neurexin IV/Caspr/Paranodin. Neuron 30:369, 2001.
  Elegant work on the molecular organization of nodes of Ranvier.
Black JA, Kocsis JD, Waxman SG: Ion channel organization of the myelinated fiber. Trends Neurosci 13:48, 1990.
Cannon SC: Pathomechanisms in channelopathies of skeletal muscle and brain. Annu Rev Neurosci 29:387, 2006.
Catterall WA: From ionic currents to molecular mechanisms: the structure and function of voltage-gated sodium channels. Neuron 26:13, 2000.
Colbert CM, Johnston D: Axonal action-potential initiation and Na^+ channel densities in the soma and axon initial segment of subicular pyramidal neurons. J Neurosci 16:6676, 1996.
  Standard teaching for a long time has been that the trigger zone for action potential initiation is in the axon initial segment. This paper provides evidence that it is actually more distal in at least some neurons—at the beginning of the myelin sheath or at the first node of Ranvier.
Faisal AA, White JA, Laughlin SB: Ion-channel noise places limits on the miniaturization of the brain's wiring. Curr Biol 15:1143, 2005.
Forsythe ID, Redman SJ: The dependence of motoneuron membrane potential on extracellular ion concentrations studied in isolated rat spinal cord. J Physiol 404:83, 1988.
Gouaux E, MacKinnon R: Principles of selective ion transport in channels and pumps. Science 310:1461, 2005.
Hartline DK, Colman DR: Rapid conduction and the evolution of giant axons and myelinated fibers. Curr Biol 17:R29, 2007.
  A scattering of invertebrate species also develop myelin-like sheaths on some of their axons, although it is not exactly clear why an earthworm needs the increased conduction velocity more than a lobster does.
Hauser SL, Oksenberg JR: The neurobiology of multiple sclerosis: genes, inflammation, and neurodegeneration. Neuron 52:61, 2006.
Hille B: Ionic channels of excitable membranes, ed 3, Sunderland, Mass, 2001, Sinauer.

Hodgkin AL: The conduction of the nervous impulse, Liverpool, 1964, Liverpool University Press.

Hodgkin AL, Huxley AF: A quantitative description of membrane current and its application to conduction and excitation in nerve. J Physiol 117:500, 1952.

The Nobel Prize–winning work that first established the ionic basis of the action potential, taking advantage of the large size of squid giant axons.

Hughes RAC, Cornblath DR: Guillain-Barré syndrome. Lancet 366:1653, 2005.

Isbister GK, Kiernan MC: Neurotoxic marine poisoning. Lancet Neurol 4:219, 2005.

Kandel ER, Schwartz JH, Jessell TM: Principles of neural science, ed 4, New York, 2000, McGraw-Hill.

Kao CY: Tetrodotoxin, saxitoxin and their significance in the study of excitation phenomena. Pharmacol Rev 18:997, 1966.

Katz B: Nerve, muscle and synapse, New York, 1966, McGraw-Hill.

A lucid introduction to neurophysiology by a Nobel laureate who did much of the early work on action potentials and on neuromuscular transmission.

Lai HC, Jan LY: The distribution and targeting of voltage-gated ion channels. Nat Rev Neurosci 7:548, 2006.

How do neurons get particular kinds of channels where they need to go, and then keep them there?

London M, Häusser M: Dendritic computation. Annu Rev Neurosci 28:503, 2005.

Dendrites actually do much more than serve as passive conduits for electrical signals.

Neher E, Sakmann B: Single-channel currents recorded from membrane of denervated frog muscle fibres. Nature 260:799, 1976.

The introduction of the patch-clamp technique.

Nicholls JG, et al: From neuron to brain, ed 4, Sunderland, Mass, 2001, Sinauer.

Sakai H, Woody CD: Relationships between axonal diameter, soma size, and axonal conduction velocity of HRP-filled, pyramidal tract cells of awake cats. Brain Res 460:1, 1988.

Salzer JL: Polarized domains of myelinated axons. Neuron 40:297, 2003.

Nodes of Ranvier look so simple on first inspection, but they are actually flanked by elaborately organized molecular zones that support their function.

Terlau H, Olivera BM: Conus venoms: a rich source of novel ion channel-targeted peptides. Physiol Rev 84:41, 2004.

A fascinating review of a family of predatory snails with beautiful shells; they produce an astonishing array of peptides that selectively target a wide range of ion channels.

Verkhratsky A, Krishtal OA, Petersen OH: From Galvani to patch clamp: the development of electrophysiology. Pflugers Arch 453:233, 2006.

Waxman SG, Kocsis JD, Stys PK, editors: The axon: structure, function, and pathophysiology, New York, 1995, Oxford University Press.

Synaptic Transmission Between Neurons

Early in the last century, Ramón y Cajal and others used the Golgi stain to demonstrate that the nervous system is a collection of individual neurons (e.g., see Fig. 1-14A) rather than a vast syncytial network, as some had alleged. An obvious corollary of this demonstration is that neurons must have mechanisms by which they communicate with one another. Although there are some instances in which neurons are directly coupled, allowing ionic currents to flow from one into another (discussed at the end of this chapter), in most cases neurons communicate with one another by releasing neuroactive chemical transmitters, typically at specialized sites called **synapses.**[a]

---

[a]The term *synapse* started out as a noun, derived from two Greek words meaning "to fasten together." It is now also used commonly as a verb, referring to one neuron making a synaptic contact with another.

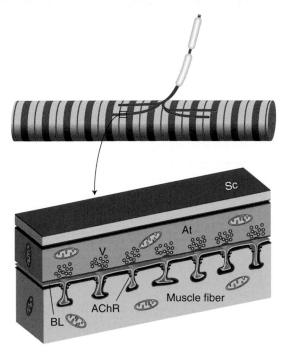

Figure 8-1 General arrangement of a neuromuscular junction (see Fig. 8-11 for a scanning electron micrograph of a real junction). A motor axon loses its myelin sheath and divides into several terminal branches (At) covered by processes of Schwann cells (Sc; not indicated in the upper drawing). Each terminal contains a series of clusters of vesicles (V) filled with acetylcholine. Invasion of a terminal by an action potential causes some of the vesicles to merge with the terminal membrane and dump their contents into the cleft between the terminal and the muscle fiber. The liberated acetylcholine diffuses across the cleft and through the basal lamina (BL) and reaches acetylcholine receptor molecules (AChR) at the entrance to troughs in the muscle surface across from each vesicle cluster. These acetylcholine receptors are ligand-gated cation channels, and binding acetylcholine causes depolarization of the muscle fiber (see Fig. 8-10). The action of acetylcholine is temporally limited by the enzyme acetylcholinesterase, associated with the basal lamina, which competes for and hydrolyzes acetylcholine.

The first insights into how synapses between neurons might work came from studies of the **neuromuscular junction.** There the endings of motor neurons release a small-molecule transmitter (**acetylcholine**), which diffuses across the cleft between neuronal ending and muscle fiber, attaches to receptor molecules in the muscle fiber membrane, and initiates permeability changes and consequent rapid depolarization (Fig. 8-1; see also Figs. 8-10 and 8-11). The depolarization is short-lived because an enzyme (acetylcholinesterase) simultaneously competes for acetylcholine and hydrolyzes it, making acetylcholine inactive. It is now apparent that the neuromuscular junction is representative of only one type of synaptic interaction. Several dozen **neurotransmitters** have been described to date. Some are small molecules such as acetylcholine (see Figs. 8-18, 8-19, and 8-21 to 8-23), whereas others are larger peptide molecules or diffusible gases; some produce brief depolarizing or hyperpolarizing changes in membrane potential, whereas others produce prolonged potential

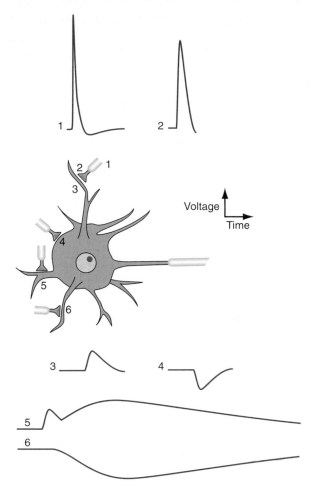

Figure 8-2 Schematic overview of the electrical events at typical chemical synapses. Action potentials (1) spread electrotonically into axon terminals (2) and cause the release of neurotransmitter molecules. Neurotransmitter then diffuses to postsynaptic membranes and elicits electrical responses determined by postsynaptic receptors; these include brief depolarizing (3) and hyperpolarizing (4) responses as well as slower responses, either preceded by a brief response (5) or not (6). The release and diffusion of neurotransmitter take hundreds of microseconds or longer, and as a result, postsynaptic signals are delayed slightly.

changes (Fig. 8-2) or changes in membrane properties that last for days or longer.[b]

There Are Five Steps in Conventional Chemical Synaptic Transmission

Chemical synapses come in a variety of shapes and sizes, but they all include as their essential components a

---

[b]Alternative terms such as *neuromodulator* or *neurohormone* are used by many authors to refer to neuroactive substances that have long-lasting effects or that diffuse from sites that are not typical synapses. However, there is not yet general agreement on how these terms should be defined, and a number of intermediate cases are known. Hence for the sake of simplicity, all such molecules are referred to as *neurotransmitters* in this chapter.

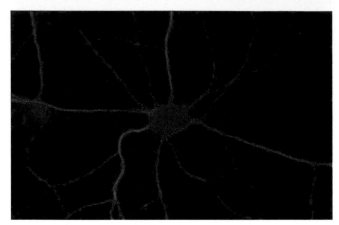

Figure 8-3 Synapses densely distributed over the surface of hippocampal neurons developing in tissue culture. The cell bodies and dendrites were stained with a fluorescent antibody directed against MAP2, a microtubule-associated protein restricted to the perikaryal-dendritic region of neurons (green fluorescence). Axon terminal projections originating from other neurons not visible in this field form a dense network of synaptic contact sites and were stained with a fluorescent antibody directed against synaptotagmin (red fluorescence), an integral membrane protein of synaptic vesicles. Overlapping red and green fluorescence, from sites where an axon terminal is superimposed on part of a dendrite, appears yellow. *(Courtesy Drs. Olaf Mundigl and Pietro De Camilli, Yale University School of Medicine.)*

presynaptic ending and a **postsynaptic** element, separated by a 10- to 20-nm **synaptic cleft** (see Fig. 1-19). The presynaptic elements are usually either terminal expansions of axons (see Fig. 8-2) or expansions of axons as they pass by other neuronal elements (referred to as **boutons terminaux** and **boutons en passage,** respectively—French for "terminal buttons" and "buttons along the way"). In some instances, however, dendrites or even parts of neuronal cell bodies can be presynaptic elements. Similarly, the postsynaptic element is usually part of the surface of a dendrite, but alternatively, it can be located on a cell body, axon initial segment, or another synaptic terminal (Fig. 8-3; see also Fig. 1-22). All these locations have functional implications, as described later in this chapter.

The presynaptic and postsynaptic elements are the principal sites involved in the five essential components of conventional chemical synaptic transmission:
1. Synthesis of neurotransmitter
2. Concentration and packaging of neurotransmitter in the presynaptic element in preparation for its release
3. Release of neurotransmitter from the presynaptic element into the synaptic cleft
4. Binding of neurotransmitter to receptor molecules embedded in postsynaptic membranes
5. Termination of neurotransmitter action

Although portions of the membranes of both presynaptic and postsynaptic elements appear thickened called the active zone (as **presynaptic** and **postsynaptic densi-** ties that contain parts of the release mechanism and most of the receptors, respectively), the presynaptic element is distinguished by the presence of a swarm of neurotransmitter-filled **synaptic vesicles.** This anatomical asymmetry corresponds to the functional unidirectionality of synaptic transmission: in response to depolarization, the presynaptic ending releases the neurotransmitter contents of one or more vesicles, the transmitter diffuses across the synaptic cleft and binds to receptor molecules embedded in the postsynaptic membrane, and the postsynaptic neuron responds in some way. Although, as described later in this chapter, chemical messages can also move in a retrograde direction across synapses.

Neurotransmitters Are Synthesized in Presynaptic Endings and in Neuronal Cell Bodies

Nearly all known or suspected neurotransmitters fall into one of two general categories: some are small molecules such as amines or amino acids, and the others are larger peptides (**neuropeptides**) or modified lipids. Small-molecule transmitters are synthesized in presynaptic cytoplasm, using locally available substrates (e.g., acetate and choline) and soluble enzymes that arrive by slow axonal transport (Fig. 8-4A). Making peptide transmitters, in contrast, requires the protein synthesis machinery that resides in the neuronal cell body. Neuropeptides start out there as larger precursor proteins that are packed into vesicles and dispatched by fast axonal transport to synaptic endings. Along the way, the precursors are cleaved and processed into the final, biologically active neuropeptides (see Fig. 8-4B).

Neurotransmitters Are Packaged Into Synaptic Vesicles Before Release

Synaptic vesicles are the units of currency at chemical synapses, the sites where neurotransmitters are packaged, concentrated, and protected from catabolism while awaiting release. All presynaptic endings contain small vesicles (about 40 nm), and many also contain less numerous but larger vesicles (≥100 nm). Depending on the preparation conditions used for electron microscopy, some of the small vesicles may appear dark, and others may look clear and either round or flattened; each large vesicle contains a dark core (Fig. 8-5). These differences in appearance correspond to differences in neurotransmitter content. For example, endings with clear, flattened vesicles usually contain neurotransmitter that more likely will result in inhibitory effects on the postsynaptic cell.

Small synaptic vesicles contain small-molecule transmitters, concentrated to levels far beyond that found in the cytoplasm by specific transporters in the vesicle walls. Large dense-core vesicles contain neuropeptides

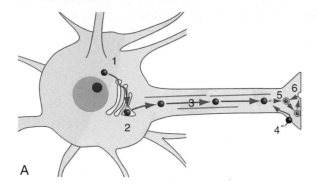

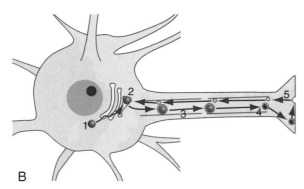

Figure 8-4 Life cycles of small-molecule neurotransmitters **(A)** and neuropeptides **(B)**. **A,** Enzymes required for the synthesis and packaging of small-molecule neurotransmitters are themselves synthesized in the cell body (1), released from the Golgi apparatus (2), and conveyed to presynaptic terminals by slow axonal transport (3). The neurotransmitters are then synthesized from substrates transported into the terminals (4) and concentrated in vesicles (5) that were either recycled from the presynaptic membrane (6) or assembled from components transported from the cell body. **B,** Precursors of neuropeptides are synthesized in the cell body (1) and packaged in the Golgi apparatus into vesicles (2), which are conveyed to presynaptic terminals by fast axonal transport along microtubules (3). Either in the cell body or during the journey down the axon, the precursor proteins are modified and become neuropeptides (4). After exocytosis, the membranes of large, dense-core vesicles are returned to the cell body for recycling (5).

at lower concentrations and may contain one or more small-molecule transmitters as well. The two kinds of vesicle, like the different neurotransmitters, are manufactured and recycled differently (see Fig. 8-4). Small-molecule transmitters are synthesized by cytoplasmic enzymes and can therefore be manufactured and packaged for release in individual synaptic endings. Small synaptic vesicles can therefore be recycled entirely within a presynaptic ending, whereas large dense-core vesicles must be created anew in the cell body. Modified lipid neurotransmitters do not use vesicles but are stored and released directly from the lipid membrane upon activation of enzymes.

Presynaptic Endings Release Neurotransmitters Into the Synaptic Cleft

Release of vesicle containing neurotransmitter is a Ca^{2+}-mediated secretory process. Each presynaptic density, or **active zone,** contains an abundance of voltage-gated Ca^{2+} channels, together with anchoring sites for a cluster of small vesicles that are held there ("docked") by a Ca^{2+}-sensitive system of proteins. Depolarization of the presynaptic terminal, such as by propagation of an action potential down the axon and subsequent electrotonic spread into the terminal, causes opening of the voltage-gated Ca^{2+} channels. Because the free intracellular Ca^{2+} concentration is only about 10^{-7} M, Ca^{2+} ions flow in through these channels and momentarily elevate the Ca^{2+} concentration near the active zone by as much as 1000-fold. During the brief period before the excess Ca^{2+} diffuses away or is sequestered, a vesicle docked nearby may fuse with the presynaptic membrane and discharge its contents into the synaptic cleft in a process called **exocytosis** (Fig. 8-6A). The whole process, from the arrival of an action potential to the release of a small vesicle's contents, can take less than 100 μsec. Because the large, dense-cored vesicles are not located adjacent to active zones, repetitive action potentials, additional Ca^{2+} entry, and more time (tens of milliseconds) are typically required for their exocytosis (see Fig. 8-6B). This exocytotic addition of membrane clearly cannot continue for very long, or else presynaptic endings would expand continuously. In fact, vesicle membranes are taken back up (by **endocytosis**), and those used for small-molecule transmitters can be recycled in less than a minute (see Fig. 8-4A).

Because neurotransmitter release is dependent on the entry of Ca^{2+}, the modulation of the voltage-gated calcium channels can have a large physiological response. Several toxins as well as several drugs have been known to modulate these channels in order to inhibit or increase neuronal activity. In addition, there are known toxins, such as botulinum toxin, that interfere with the ability of the acetylcholine-containing vesicles, inhibiting their release, and resulting in the relaxation of skeletal muscles (see Box 8-1).

Neurotransmitters Diffuse Across the Synaptic Cleft and Bind to Postsynaptic Receptors

Neurotransmitters released from small vesicles find postsynaptic receptor molecules waiting for them directly across the synaptic cleft (Fig. 8-7). For this reason, it takes the contents of such vesicles very little time to exert their effects. The total synaptic delay from presynaptic action potential to postsynaptic effect can be less than 200 μsec. The contents of large vesicles, in contrast, take longer to be released and often diffuse to receptors relatively far away (see Fig. 8-9), so their effects

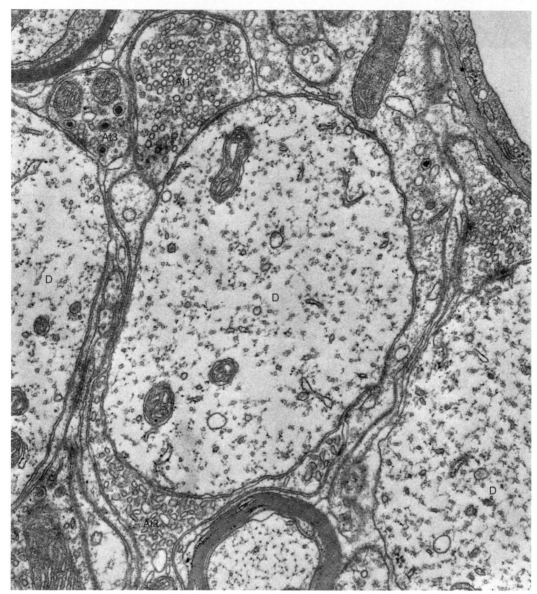

Figure 8-5 Types of synaptic vesicles in axon terminals (At) making synaptic contact with transversely sectioned dendrites (D) in the anterior horn of rat spinal cord. Two of the terminals (At1) contain clear, round vesicles; one (At2) contains clear, flattened vesicles; and one (At3) contains a mixture of small, round vesicles and large, dense-cored vesicles. The actual size of the dendrite in the center of the micrograph is about 2.5 × 1.5 μm. *(From Pannese E: Neurocytology: fine structure of neurons, nerve processes, and neuroglial cells, New York, 1994, Thieme Medical Publishers.)*

develop more slowly. As a self-regulation of transmitter release, at times the presynaptic neuron will also contain receptors (**autoreceptors**) that often result in the slowing of neurotransmitter release.

Neurotransmitter Action Is Terminated by Uptake, Degradation, or Diffusion

Neurotransmitter molecules need to be removed quickly once they have had a chance to bind to receptors, so that the postsynaptic membrane will be prepared for subsequent releases of transmitter. This is accomplished by virtually every means imaginable (Fig. 8-8). Binding of neurotransmitter and receptor is a reversible event, so

receptors and removal mechanisms compete for transmitter. Some transmitter simply diffuses away, but this is too slow a process to be the principal mechanism. In most synapses, transmitter is reabsorbed into the presynaptic ending or taken up by neighboring glial cells or even by the postsynaptic process. In others, enzymes in the synaptic cleft degrade free transmitter. Reabsorbed transmitters or their metabolic products, like vesicle membranes, are often recycled for use in a subsequent synaptic event.

Different kinds of neurotransmitters have different preferred mechanisms of removal. For example, serotonin, norepinephrine, and dopamine are transported rapidly back into the presynaptic ending through large

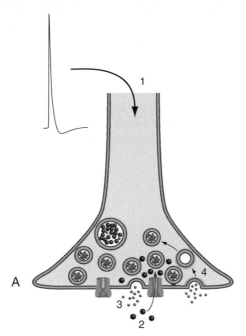

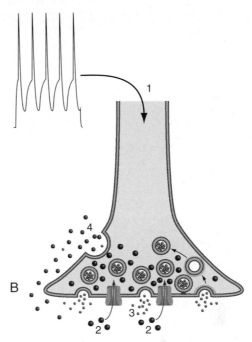

Figure 8-6 Ca²⁺-triggered release of neurotransmitter. **A,** Invasion of a presynaptic terminal by a single action potential (1) causes brief opening of voltage-gated Ca²⁺ channels (2) and a local increase in Ca²⁺ concentration. One or more nearby small vesicles may fuse with the presynaptic membrane (3) and discharge their contents into the synaptic cleft; they are then recycled (4) in the synaptic terminal. **B,** Repetitive action potentials (1) cause opening of more voltage-gated Ca²⁺ channels for longer periods (2) and a correspondingly more widespread increase in Ca²⁺ concentration. This causes fusion not only of small vesicles docked at active zones (3) but also of larger vesicles away from active zones (4).

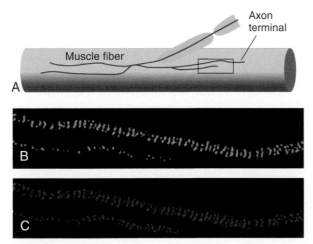

Figure 8-7 Juxtaposition of presynaptic voltage-gated Ca²⁺ channels and postsynaptic neurotransmitter receptors, shown at a neuromuscular junction by using toxins coupled to fluorescent dyes. The area of a frog neuromuscular junction outlined in **A** is enlarged in **B** and **C. B,** A marine snail toxin (ω-conotoxin) that binds selectively to voltage-gated Ca²⁺ channels demonstrates these channels' locations in the presynaptic terminal. **C,** Staining the same area with a snake toxin (α-bungarotoxin) that binds to nicotinic acetylcholine receptors (the type found at neuromuscular junctions) demonstrates that these receptors have an almost exactly parallel distribution in the postjunctional muscle membrane. *(From Robitaille R, Adler EM, Charlton MP: Neuron 5:773, 1990.)*

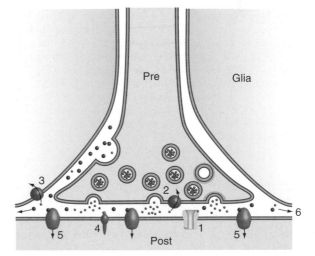

Figure 8-8 Neurotransmitter binds to postsynaptic receptors (1) while other mechanisms compete for the transmitter, trying to remove it from the synaptic cleft. Although it is unlikely that all these mechanisms would be used at a single synapse, different synapses use various combinations of reuptake of neurotransmitter by the presynaptic terminal (2) or nearby glial cells (3), enzymatic inactivation of neurotransmitter (4), and uptake by the postsynaptic terminal (5). Finally, some neurotransmitter simply diffuses out of the synaptic cleft (6).

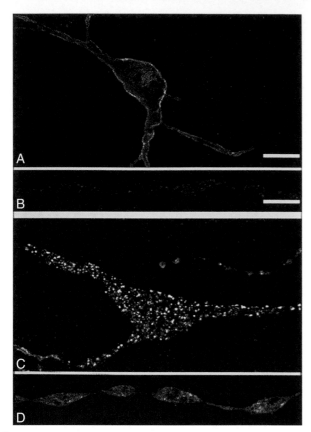

Figure 8-9 Endocytotic removal of a neuropeptide (substance P) and its receptor by postsynaptic neurons, demonstrated by staining substance P receptors using a fluorescent antibody technique. In the absence of stimulation, substance P receptors coat the somatic and dendritic membranes of pain-sensitive second-order neurons in the spinal cord posterior horn (**A,** red and yellow fluorescence), and the distal dendrites of these cells have a uniform diameter (**B**). Five minutes after a painful stimulus on the ipsilateral side, most of the substance P receptor has left the surface membranes and is found intracellularly (**C**), and distal dendrites have a beaded appearance, with varicosities filled with endosomes containing substance P receptor (**D**). Over about the next hour, the internalized substance P receptor molecules are recycled to the cell surface. The scale mark in **A** (also applies to **C**) is 20 µm. The scale mark in **B** (also applies to **D**) is 10 µm. *(From Mantyh PW et al: Science 268:1629, 1995.)*

protein transporters for repackaging into synaptic vesicles. Acetylcholine, in contrast, is split into acetate and choline by acetylcholinesterase in the synaptic cleft; the choline is then transported back into the presynaptic ending and used for the synthesis of more acetylcholine. Neuropeptides are either degraded by extracellular peptidases or swallowed up by the postsynaptic cell while still attached to their receptors (Fig. 8-9).

Synaptic Transmission Can Be Rapid and Point-to-Point, or Slow and Often Diffuse

Postsynaptic events in response to transmitter-receptor binding fall into two general categories—fast and slow. Some postsynaptic responses involve electrically silent metabolic or membrane changes, but most involve depolarizing or hyperpolarizing potential changes across the postsynaptic membrane. A depolarizing response brings the postsynaptic element closer to its threshold for firing an action potential and so is referred to as an **excitatory postsynaptic potential** (or **EPSP**). Conversely, a hyperpolarizing response moves the membrane away from the threshold and so is referred to as an **inhibitory postsynaptic potential** (or **IPSP**). Hence there are fast and slow EPSPs, and fast and slow IPSPs.

Fast synaptic potentials are used for point-to-point transfer of specific bits of information—for example, by motor neurons projecting to particular muscle fibers or by tract cells projecting to particular parts of the thalamus (e.g., see Fig. 10-19). Slow synaptic potentials are sometimes used in this way too, but many are generated by diffusely projecting neurons with hundreds of branches that regulate the overall activity level of broad expanses of the nervous system (e.g., see Figs. 11-24 and 11-26 to 11-28).

Rapid Synaptic Transmission Involves Transmitter-Gated Ion Channels

Early studies of synaptic transmission demonstrated that a single action potential in the motor nerve ending at a neuromuscular junction causes a large but brief EPSP,[c] sufficient to cause an action potential and contraction in the muscle fiber (Fig. 8-10B). Closer analysis revealed small, brief depolarizing events in the postjunctional muscle membrane during the periods between action potentials (see Fig. 8-10A), each corresponding to a brief period of channel opening and depolarizing current flow. We now know that each of these small depolarizing events is the response of the postsynaptic membrane to the spontaneous release of one synaptic vesicle. Each vesicle contains about 10,000 acetylcholine molecules, which diffuse across the synaptic cleft and bind briefly to acetylcholine receptors, which themselves are ligand-gated ion channels permeable to both Na^+ and K^+ ions. Acetylcholinesterase competes with the receptors for the released acetylcholine, so the channels stay open for only a millisecond or two. During this time, they allow a current flow that tries to move the membrane potential to a value around 0 mV (between the Na^+ and K^+ equilibrium potentials; see Chapter 7, Calculating the Membrane Potential, Equation 7-17). Because 2 msec is considerably less than the time constant of the muscle membrane, the membrane potential never reaches 0 mV. Instead, it rises rapidly at the beginning of the postsynaptic current flow and then decays slowly at the end of the current flow (see Fig. 8-10A). Entry of depolarizing current is localized to the site of the

---

[c]Often referred to as an **end-plate potential** because **motor end plate** is another term for neuromuscular junction.

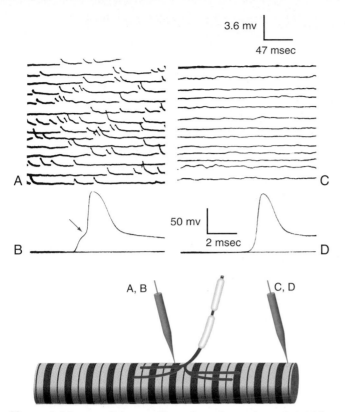

Figure 8-10 Intracellular recordings of muscle membrane potential at the motor end plate of a frog muscle fiber (**A** and **B**) and about 2 mm away from the end plate (**C** and **D**), demonstrating the localization of postjunctional potentials to the region of the neuromuscular junction. At rest, small depolarizing events (referred to as miniature end-plate potentials), each corresponding to the release of a single acetylcholine-filled vesicle, can be recorded at the end plate (**A**). At a point 2 mm away, they have almost completely died out because of electrotonic spread (**C**). An action potential in the motor axon elicits a large postjunctional potential at the end plate (**B;** note the different time and voltage scale), rapidly reaching threshold *(arrow)* and triggering a muscle action potential. At 2 mm away (**D**), only the propagated action potential remains. *(Electrical recordings, from Fatt P, Katz B: J Physiol 117:109, 1952.)*

receptors, so the postsynaptic potential decays electrotonically (see Fig. 8-10C and D). However, the presynaptic ending at each neuromuscular junction contains upwards of 1000 active zones (Fig. 8-11 and see Fig. 8-7), so a single action potential in the motor axon causes the nearly simultaneous release of hundreds of vesicles full of acetylcholine at closely spaced sites, which in turn causes the large EPSP normally seen (see Fig. 8-9B).

The basic elements of neuromuscular transmission have proved to be generally true of fast synaptic transmission throughout the nervous system (Fig. 8-12A). Depolarization-induced Ca^{2+} entry causes the release of one or more packets of neurotransmitter, called **quanta,** each of which is generally assumed to be the contents of a single vesicle docked at an active zone. The neurotransmitter then diffuses across the synaptic cleft and binds transiently to a **transmitter-gated** (i.e., ligand-gated) **ion channel.** The selectivity of the channel determines the postsynaptic effect. Opening channels selective for

monovalent cations, as in the example of the neuromuscular junction, causes an EPSP. Opening channels selective for Cl^-, in contrast, moves the membrane potential toward the Cl^- equilibrium potential; this is the most common basis of fast IPSPs in the central nervous system (CNS). The selective concentration of receptors on the postsynaptic membrane ensures that fast postsynaptic potentials are localized spatially. Transmitter-gated ion channels are also referred to as **ionotropic receptors** (from the same Greek word that gave rise to *tropism,* a movement toward or away from a stimulus, as in the heliotropic growth of plants in the direction of sunlight).

Slow Synaptic Transmission Usually Involves Postsynaptic Receptors Linked to Intracellular Proteins

Slow synaptic potentials are also caused by changes in current flow through membrane ion channels, but in this case a multistep process is involved in which binding of neurotransmitter leads to altered concentrations of **second messengers,** which in turn can modulate a number of other proteins including enzymes, channel conductance, and gene transcription. Because of the intermediate metabolic events, the receptors are referred to as **metabotropic receptors.** Many metabotropic receptors are membrane-spanning proteins linked to adjacent guanine nucleotide-binding proteins (**G proteins**). Transmitter binding by a **G protein–coupled receptor** causes dissociation of subunits of the G protein, which are then able to move laterally in the postsynaptic membrane and exert a cascade of effects (see Fig. 8-12B).

In the simplest scenario, a G protein subunit directly influences the state of ion channels, for example, causing K^+ or Ca^{2+} channels to open; in this instance, the G protein subunit itself is the second messenger. In most cases, however, the G protein subunit increases or decreases the activity of an enzyme, which in turn causes changes in the concentration of something else.

Multistep pathways such as this are slow and seem unwieldy, but they actually have considerable advantages. Synaptic inputs can be amplified, because a single receptor can cause the dissociation of multiple G proteins, and changing the activity of an enzyme can cause the synthesis or degradation of thousands of second messenger molecules. In addition, because there are many types of G protein–coupled receptors and many types of G proteins, a wide array of postsynaptic effects can result. Some, as indicated previously, are as simple as opening or closing an ion channel. Others may actually be electrically silent, causing things such as changes in sensitivity to other transmitters or changes in gene transcription. This kind of strategy is so versatile that it is not restricted to synapses. G proteins and second messengers are the basis for the receptor potentials

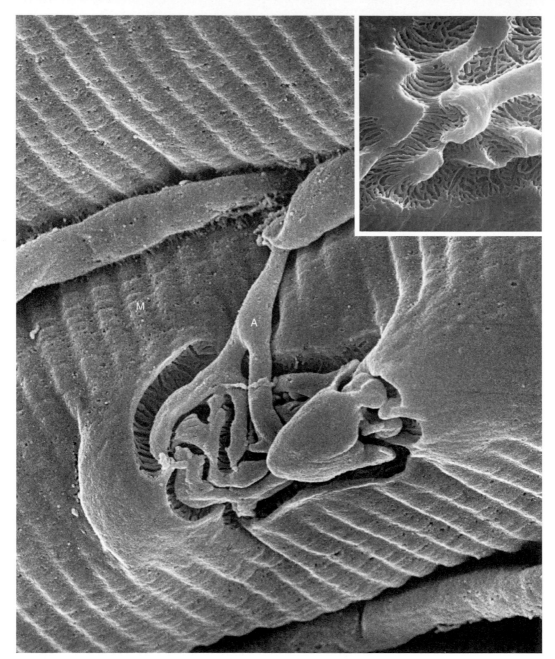

Figure 8-11 Three-dimensional structure of a neuromuscular junction. This scanning electron micrograph shows a motor axon (A) approaching a muscle fiber (M) in a calf muscle (peroneus longus) of a hamster. The axon divides into a series of terminal branches that occupy grooves in the surface of the muscle fiber. Removing these branches from a similar neuromuscular junction reveals a series of troughs traversing the grooves, each corresponding to one of the troughs in Figure 8-1 and containing acetylcholine receptors. The actual size of the end plate is about 7×12 μm. *(From Pannese E: Neurocytology: fine structure of neurons, nerve processes, and neuroglial cells, New York, 1994, Thieme Medical Publishers.)*

generated by retinal rods and cones, olfactory sensory neurons, and some other receptor cells (see Chapter 9).

The Postsynaptic Receptor Determines the Effect of a Neurotransmitter

There is nothing intrinsically "excitatory" or "inhibitory" about any neurotransmitter. The effect of a transmitter at any given synapse is instead determined by the nature of the receptor to which it binds. Because there are mul-

tiple types of receptors for most or all neurotransmitters, most transmitters can have more than one effect. This is well illustrated by acetylcholine, which causes fast excitatory events at some synapses and slow excitatory or inhibitory events at others. The reason for these differences is the fact that there are two categories of acetylcholine receptors. **Nicotinic** acetylcholine receptors (so called because they bind nicotine as well as acetylcholine), the kind found at neuromuscular junctions, are ionotropic receptors. **Muscarinic** acetylcholine

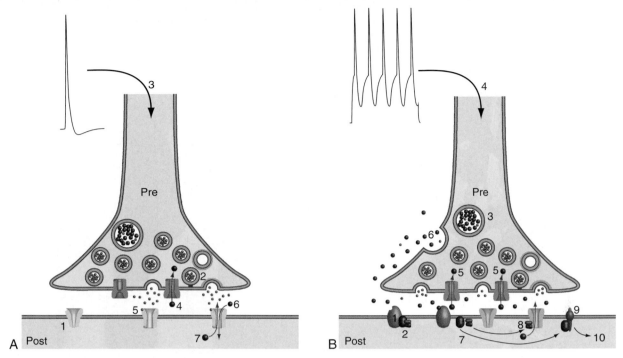

Figure 8-12 Basic events in typical fast **(A)** and slow **(B)** synaptic transmission. **A,** At rest, ligand-gated ion channels (ionotropic receptors) in the postsynaptic membrane are closed (1), and vesicles are docked in the presynaptic terminal (2) awaiting release. Depolarization of the terminal (3) causes Ca^{2+} influx (4), transmitter exocytosis, binding of transmitter to postsynaptic ligand-gated ion channels (5), and opening of the channels. In this example, open channels allow Na^+ influx (6) and K^+ efflux (7), depolarizing the postsynaptic membrane. **B,** Most slow synaptic responses involve metabotropic receptors (1) coupled at rest to a three-subunit G protein (2), as well as transmitters in large, dense-core vesicles (3) or in certain small vesicles. Prolonged or repetitive depolarization (4) of the presynaptic terminal causes widespread Ca^{2+} influx (5), exocytosis of transmitter from large, dense-core vesicles (6), and binding to G protein–coupled receptors (some of which may be located some distance from the presynaptic terminal; see Fig. 8-9). This binding causes dissociation of the G protein into subunits (7), which can have a variety of effects. They may bind to ion channels and alter their conductance (8); activate an enzyme (9), which in turn alters the concentration of a second messenger (e.g., cyclic adenosine monophosphate, inositol triphosphate, arachidonic acid metabolites); or have even more complex effects (10), such as altering gene expression.

receptors (which bind muscarine, a substance derived from the mushroom *Amanita muscaria*), found on smooth and cardiac muscle fibers and on many neurons, are G protein–coupled receptors. Acetylcholine applied to cardiac muscle, for example, causes increased opening of K^+ channels, allowing K^+ to flow out of the cell, resulting in a slow IPSP.

In addition to the two categories of acetylcholine receptors, there are multiple subtypes in each category—many different nicotinic receptors and at least five different muscarinic receptors—with different distributions. For example, the nicotinic receptor of skeletal muscle fibers is different from that of parasympathetic ganglion cells. This multiplicity of subtypes, which is true of neurotransmitter receptors in general, has made it possible to design drugs that target very specific neuronal subsystems[d] (see Fig. 8-26). The location of the receptors is important to the overall physiological process. The dif-

ferent flavors of receptors are expressed in different parts of the nervous system.

The Size and Location of a Synaptic Ending Influence the Magnitude of Its Effects

Neurons usually receive hundreds or even thousands of synaptic inputs from other neurons (see Fig. 8-3), combining their effects at the trigger zone to determine whether and how often to fire an action potential. This ability of neurons to compare and combine many different inputs is in great part responsible for the computational power of the nervous system. The net impact of any individual synapse obviously depends on the amount of transmitter released there and the number of postsynaptic receptors present, as well as on the distance from there to the trigger zone. In addition, the strength of a synapse can be influenced, sometimes profoundly and for long periods, by the history of activity at that synapse.

Synapses With Many Active Zones Have a Greater Effect

Muscle fibers do not need to do much computing—it makes functional sense for every action potential in the

---

[d]Nature, of course, has a head start on pharmacologists in this regard. A wide variety of toxins and other naturally occurring substances—nicotine and muscarine, for example—interact with specific receptor types or even subtypes.

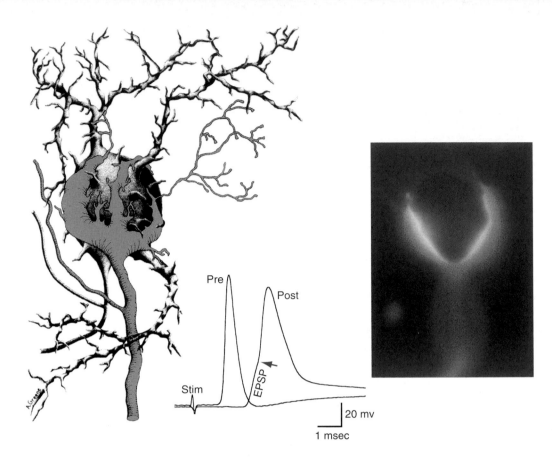

Figure 8-13 Simultaneous recordings from the presynaptic and postsynaptic elements at a CNS synapse with many active zones. Certain afferents to a brainstem nucleus in the auditory pathway form large, cuplike presynaptic endings (called *calyces of Held*) that partially envelop the neurons on which they synapse, as indicated in the drawing on the left. Two patch-clamp electrodes filled with different fluorescent dyes were used to record from and stain both elements. This yielded the electrical records in the center and the photograph on the right, in which the presynaptic ending is yellow and the postsynaptic neuron is blue. After stimulation of the afferent axon (Stim), it takes about 1 msec for an action potential to be conducted to the presynaptic ending and spread into it (Pre). After about another millisecond for Ca²⁺ influx and transmitter exocytosis and diffusion, a rapidly rising EPSP is recorded in the postsynaptic neuron (Post), quickly bringing it to threshold *(arrow)*. This type of CNS synapse is unusual in terms of the magnitude of the postsynaptic potential elicited—a reflection of the hundreds of active zones in the presynaptic terminal. *(Drawing, from Morest DK et al: Stimulus coding at caudal levels of the cat's auditory nervous system. II. Patterns of synaptic organization. In Møller AR, editor: Basic mechanisms in hearing, New York, 1973, Academic Press. Electrical records and photograph, from Borst JGG, Helmchen F, Sakmann B: J Physiol 489:825, 1995.)*

motor axon to trigger a twitch of the muscle fiber. Release of a single quantum of neurotransmitter has only a small effect (see Fig. 8-10A), so neuromuscular transmission calls for a very large presynaptic ending with many active zones at the neuromuscular junction (see Figs. 8-7 and 8-11). There are a few other instances in the peripheral nervous system (PNS) or the CNS where one input is of overwhelming functional importance and the presynaptic ending is very large (Fig. 8-13). Most synapses, however, are minute—less than 1 μm in diameter (see Figs. 1-21 and 8-5)—and individually release just one or a few quanta and produce very small postsynaptic potentials, usually less than a millivolt. Hence concerted activity at many synapses, and spatial and temporal summation of their effects, is likely to be required to substantially alter the firing frequency of most neurons.

Synapses Closer to the Action Potential Trigger Zone Have a Greater Effect

Synaptic potentials are generated focally at sites where neurotransmitter receptors are located, and they spread electrotonically from their point of origin. Hence things such as time constants and space constants become critical determinants of the effects that synaptic potentials cause in other parts of the postsynaptic neuron. A synapse on an axon's initial segment (see Fig. 1-15), close to the trigger zone, has a relatively powerful effect. In contrast, a postsynaptic potential of the same size generated far out on a distal dendrite would be expected to decay during electrotonic spread toward the trigger zone. (In fact, some dendritic membranes have a sprinkling of voltage-gated channels—usually not enough to generate action potentials on their own, but enough to give postsynaptic potentials a little boost along the way.)

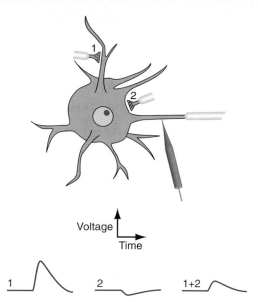

Figure 8-14 Interactions of a dendritic excitatory synapse (1) and a somatic inhibitory synapse (2), as recorded at the initial segment. The inhibitory synapse by itself produces a small IPSP, typically the result of increased conductance to K^+ or Cl^-, ions whose equilibrium potential is close to the resting membrane potential. However, simultaneous activation of both synapses causes a marked diminution of the EPSP because much of the current flowing in at the excitatory synapse flows out at the inhibitory synapse and never reaches the initial segment.

Synapses on neuronal cell bodies and initial segments are often inhibitory, making them particularly influential for two reasons. Besides being close to the trigger zone in an electrotonic sense, they are also in a position to diminish the effects of EPSPs generated more distally (Fig. 8-14) by, in effect, shortening the length constant of the neuron. In contrast, synapses on dendrites are often excitatory.

Presynaptic Endings Can Themselves Be Postsynaptic

Presynaptic terminals themselves contain the same kinds of receptors found in postsynaptic membranes. These receptors are involved in two different kinds of processes that control the amount of transmitter released by the terminal.

Some presynaptic terminals receive axoaxonic synaptic inputs that oppose the entry of Ca^{2+} into the presynaptic terminal. Because Ca^{2+} entry is the critical element in vesicle exocytosis, this decreases the amount of transmitter released in response to an action potential arriving at the terminal. This in turn decreases the likelihood of depolarizing the postsynaptic neuron to threshold, almost as though it had received an inhibitory input. The critical difference is that there is no IPSP in the postsynaptic neuron and no effect on its other inputs. In addition, only the terminal receiving the axoaxonic synapse has its transmitter release affected. Thus **presynaptic inhibition** (Fig. 8-15) is a clever mechanism for affecting only selected branches of an axon and for selectively suppressing only certain inputs to a postsynaptic

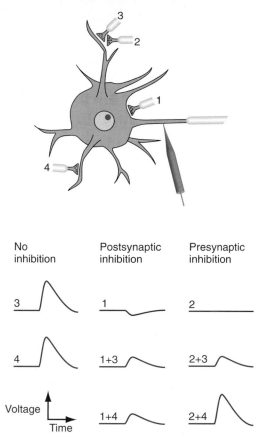

Figure 8-15 Presynaptic and postsynaptic inhibition. Standard inhibitory synapses (1), as indicated in Figure 8-14, generate an IPSP in the postsynaptic neuron and diminish the effect of all excitatory synapses on the same neuron (1 + 3, 1 + 4). Presynaptic inhibition, in contrast, results in no IPSP (2), except perhaps in the inhibited terminal, and diminishes the effect of only a subset of excitatory synapses (2 + 3 vs. 2 + 4).

neuron. Other axoaxonic synapses enhance the entry of Ca^{2+} into presynaptic terminals, mediating an analogous process of **presynaptic facilitation.**

Many presynaptic terminal membranes also contain receptors for their own transmitters, called **autoreceptors.** Some fraction of the transmitter released into the synaptic cleft binds to these autoreceptors. The most common effect is inhibition of further transmitter release.

Synaptic Strength Can Be Facilitated or Depressed

An action potential arriving at a presynaptic terminal does not necessarily always produce the same postsynaptic response. Presynaptic inhibition or facilitation can meet specific functional needs by temporarily altering the effectiveness of a terminal, but in addition, the properties of both a terminal and its postsynaptic process can vary depending on the history of activity at that synapse.

Given the molecular workings of synapses, it is easy to imagine that a brief, high-frequency burst of action potentials arriving at a synaptic terminal could cause the entry of too much Ca^{2+} to diffuse away or to be sequestered for a few seconds or, alternatively, that a longer high-frequency burst could deplete the terminal's supply of available vesicles. An elevated Ca^{2+} concentration increases the odds of vesicle exocytosis the next time an action potential arrives at the terminal, and a depleted vesicle pool decreases the odds. Both of these phenomena, called **potentiation** and **depression,** respectively, occur to varying degrees at many synapses, depending on the pattern of stimulation and the characteristics of a particular synapse. These effects usually last no more than seconds.

Learning and memory (see Chapter 24) involve long-term, even permanent, changes in the way neurons respond to particular stimuli. Short-lived changes such as brief periods of synaptic potentiation and depression are clearly inadequate for this kind of role. Other, much longer-lasting changes in synaptic efficacy are thought to be critical for this function. **Long-term potentiation,**

lasting for days, weeks, or even longer after a tetanic input delivered to some synaptic terminals, has taken center stage as a model for learning and memory. Long-term potentiation depends on activation of a particular receptor for the neurotransmitter **glutamate** (described later in this chapter) and may involve long-term increases in transmitter release, postsynaptic sensitivity, or both. Synaptic spines (see Fig. 1-14) have long been considered candidate sites for the synaptic changes of learning and memory, in part because of the cells on which they occur (e.g., cortical neurons) and in part because of their geometry (Fig. 8-16). Spines are connected to the main shaft of the dendrite by a narrow neck, and small changes in something such as the diameter of the neck could produce large changes in a spine's electrical properties or its ability to maintain altered concentrations of second messengers. Supporting spines' role in long-term changes in the CNS are observations that they are favored sites for the development of long-term potentiation (or the complementary phenomenon of **long-term**

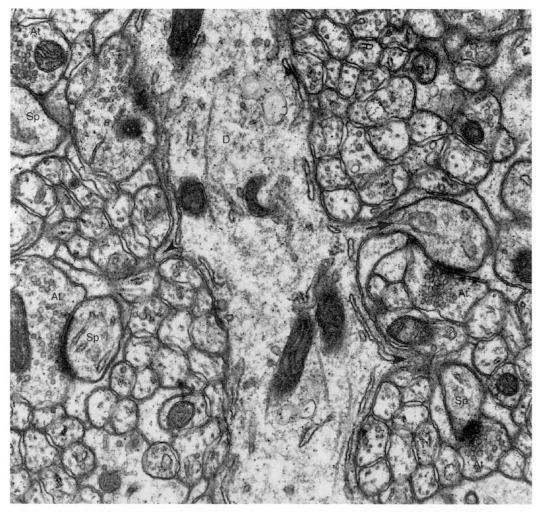

Figure 8-16 Synapses on spines of cerebellar Purkinje cells. A Purkinje cell dendrite (D) runs vertically through the micrograph, and the narrow neck *(arrow)* of one spine leads to an enlargement on which an axon terminal (At) ends. The necks of two other spines *(arrowheads)* can also be seen, as can sections through parts of other spines (Sp) contacted by axon terminals. The actual diameter of this dendrite is about 1 μm. *(From Pannese E: Neurocytology: fine structure of neurons, nerve processes, and neuroglia cells, New York, 1994, Thieme Medical Publishers.)*

depression) and that their shapes and numbers can change when learning occurs.

Messages Also Travel Across Synapses in a Retrograde Direction

The preceding account makes it sound as though all information flow at chemical synapses is unidirectional. However, postsynaptic elements have several electrically silent, nonvesicular mechanisms at their disposal to influence the properties of presynaptic terminals and neurons. For example, **growth factors** released by postsynaptic cells and transported back to the cell bodies of presynaptic neurons are important for the development and maintenance of synaptic connections (see Chapter 24). Several other mechanisms play important roles in regulating the release of transmitter by presynaptic endings on a shorter-term basis. One such mechanism, only recently clarified, is that which underlies the effects of marijuana. Humans have used extracts of *Cannabis sativa* both recreationally and medicinally for thousands of years, producing a variety of CNS effects that include mild euphoria, tranquility, appetite enhancement, impaired attention and memory, and alterations in sensory perception and coordination. These widespread effects reflect the binding of Δ^9-tetrahydrocannabinol (Δ^9-THC, the principal active ingredient of marijuana) to CB1 receptors (CB for cannabinoid), the most abundant G protein–coupled receptors in the nervous system.[e] Most CB1 receptors are located on presynaptic terminals, and their role in the normal functioning of the nervous system is mediated by the binding of **endocannabinoids** (endogenous cannabinoids) that are released by postsynaptic neurons. The first of these to be discovered was **anandamide** (arachidonylethanolamide), named from a Sanskrit word meaning "inner bliss," although 2-arachidonoylglycerol is a much more abundant endocannabinoid. Endocannabinoids, unlike conventional neurotransmitters, are not stored in vesicles. Instead, they are synthesized from membrane phospholipids at a rate determined by postsynaptic Ca^{2+} concentration, which increases in response to depolarization (either by entry through postsynaptic NMDA channels or voltage-gated Ca^{2+} channels or by release from internal stores). They then leave the postsynaptic membrane and diffuse to presynaptic CB1 receptors. G protein subunits dissociate from the receptors and temporarily decrease subsequent transmitter release, in part by blocking presynaptic voltage-gated Ca^{2+} channels (Fig. 8-17). Endocannabinoid signaling is now thought to be critically involved in the experience-dependent changes

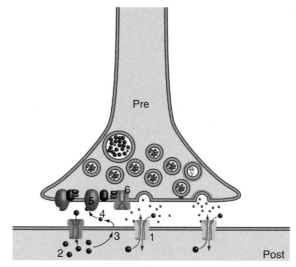

Figure 8-17 Retrograde signaling by endocannabinoids. Postsynaptic depolarization (1) causes an increase in Ca^{2+} concentration (2), in turn activating enzymes that synthesize endocannabinoids from membrane phospholipids (3). Endocannabinoids then diffuse across the synaptic cleft (4) and bind to presynaptic G protein–coupled (CB1) receptors (5). G protein subunits then suppress transmitter release, partly by blocking voltage-gated Ca^{2+} channels (6) and partly by causing presynaptic K^+ channels to open (thus hyperpolarizing the ending and reducing the effect of presynaptic action potentials).

in synaptic strength that normally occur throughout life (see Chapter 24).

A second form of retrograde signaling is mediated by **adenosine,** a breakdown product of extracellular adenosine triphosphate (ATP). Adenosine binds to another set of G protein–coupled receptors (P1 receptors) that are located mostly on presynaptic endings, suppressing transmitter release.

Finally, increased postsynaptic Ca^{2+} concentration also activates enzymes that produce **nitric oxide** (NO) or **carbon monoxide** (CO). These are small, mobile gases that can diffuse easily through neuronal membranes without even binding to a receptor, reaching parts of other cells 10s of micrometers away. Even though they have a short lifetime, they can enter nearby presynaptic terminals, where they activate guanylate cyclase and increase the presynaptic cyclic guanosine monophosphate (GMP) concentration. This in turn can modulate subsequent transmitter release for many minutes.[f]

---

[e]A second cannabinoid receptor type, CB2, is distributed outside the nervous system, primarily on cells of the immune system. These receptors account for the additional medicinal effects of marijuana.

[f]NO signaling is not restricted to the nervous system, but is widespread in other tissues. Its mode of action was first unraveled in the circulatory system, where smooth muscle cells in vascular walls relax in response to the increased cyclic GMP caused by NO released from nearby endothelial cells. This is exploited clinically by the use of nitroglycerin, a source of NO, to increase cardiac blood flow. It is also indirectly the basis for the use of sildenafil (Viagra), which inhibits phosphodiesterase V. This is the enzyme that breaks down cyclic GMP in selected smooth muscles, including those of the corpus cavernosum, so inhibiting it results in increased cyclic GMP levels and relaxation of these muscles.

Table 8-1	Major Neurotransmitters
Type	**Major Transmitters**
Amines	Acetylcholine
	Catecholamines
	Dopamine
	Norepinephrine
	Serotonin
	Histamine
Amino acids	Glutamate
	GABA (γ-aminobutyric acid)
	Glycine
Other small molecules	Adenosine triphosphate (ATP)
Neuropeptides	Angiotensin II
	β-endorphin
	Cholecystokinin
	Corticotropin-releasing factor (CRF)
	Enkephalin
	Neuropeptide Y
	Orexin
	Somatostatin
	Substance P
	Many others

Table 8-2	Typical Effects of Major Transmitters*
Effect	**Major Transmitters**
Fast excitatory	PNS: acetylcholine (nicotinic receptors)
	CNS: glutamate
	ATP (P2X receptors)
Fast inhibitory	GABA (GABA$_A$ receptors, mostly in the brain)
	Glycine (mostly in the spinal cord)
Second-messenger effects	Catecholamines
	Serotonin
	Acetylcholine (muscarinic receptors)
	Glutamate (metabotropic receptors)
	GABA (GABA$_B$ receptors)
	ATP (P2Y receptors)
	Neuropeptides

*These are typical but not exclusive effects. For example, one type of serotonin receptor is ionotropic.

Most Neurotransmitters Are Small Amine Molecules, Amino Acids, or Neuropeptides

There are only about a dozen known small-molecule transmitters (of which nine are particularly prominent [Table 8-1]), whereas there are more than 100 neuroactive peptides. Each kind of transmitter has a characteristic major role (Table 8-2).

Acetylcholine Mediates Rapid, Point-to-Point Transmission in the PNS

Acetylcholine (Fig. 8-18) was the first neurotransmitter to be discovered. It plays an especially prominent role in the PNS as the transmitter released by motor neurons at neuromuscular junctions and by many neurons of the autonomic nervous system (Table 8-3). Its distribution in the CNS is more restricted, and its role is quite different. Other than motor neurons, the **cholinergic** neurons of the CNS (see Fig. 11-28) are concentrated in parts of the brainstem, the base of the forebrain, and the basal ganglia (see Table 8-3). The cholinergic neurons in the brainstem and basal forebrain have extensively branching axons that innervate wide areas of the CNS, a pattern not suited for the point-to-point transfer of information. They are thought instead to play a role in regulating the general level of activity of CNS neurons, especially

Table 8-3	Locations of Cholinergic Neurons and Synapses	
Location of Neurons	**Location of Terminals**	**Principal Receptor**
Motor neurons	Skeletal muscle	Nicotinic
Preganglionic autonomics*	Autonomic ganglia	Nicotinic, muscarinic
Parasympathetic ganglia*	Smooth and cardiac muscle, glands	Muscarinic
Reticular formation†	Thalamus	Muscarinic
Basal nucleus†‡	Cerebral cortex, amygdala	Muscarinic
Septal nuclei†‡	Hippocampus	Muscarinic
Caudate nucleus, putamen	Local connections	Muscarinic

*Chapter 10.
†Chapter 11.
‡Chapter 22.

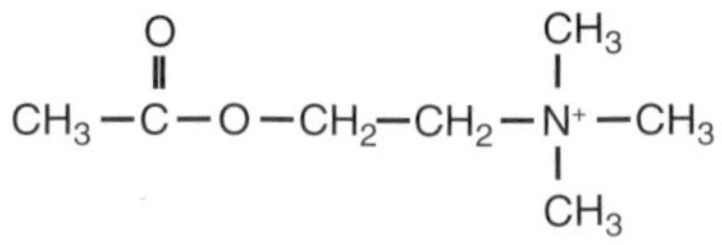

$$CH_3-\overset{\overset{\displaystyle O}{\|}}{C}-O-CH_2-CH_2-\overset{\overset{\displaystyle CH_3}{|}}{\underset{\underset{\displaystyle CH_3}{|}}{N^+}}-CH_3$$

Figure 8-18 Acetylcholine, which is manufactured by the acetylation of choline, a reaction catalyzed by the enzyme choline acetyltransferase.

during different phases of the sleep-wake cycle and during learning.

The physiological action of acetylcholine is different at central and peripheral endings. As noted earlier, there are nicotinic and muscarinic acetylcholine receptors. Nicotinic receptors are ionotropic receptors, transmitter-gated ion channels that mediate fast EPSPs. Muscarinic receptors are metabotropic receptors, G protein–coupled receptors that mediate a variety of second-messenger effects. Nicotinic receptors are more common in the PNS and muscarinic receptors in the CNS, although there is overlap. For example, single autonomic ganglion cells may possess both nicotinic and muscarinic receptors, and acetylcholine produces both fast and slow postsynaptic potentials in these cells.

Amino Acids Mediate Rapid, Point-to-Point Transmission in the CNS

Certain amino acids serve double duty, involved not only in intermediary metabolism and protein synthesis but also as neurotransmitters. The most important of these are **glutamate** and its derivative **γ-aminobutyric acid,** which is commonly referred to by its acronym **GABA** (Fig. 8-19). Glutamate is the major transmitter for brief, point-to-point, excitatory synaptic events in the CNS, playing a role analogous to that of acetylcholine in the periphery. Conversely, GABA and **glycine** are the major transmitters for brief, point-to-point, inhibitory synaptic events in the CNS. The distributions of GABA and glycine synapses overlap, but glycine is particularly prominent in the spinal cord and GABA everyplace else.

As might be expected from these roles, neurons containing glutamate or GABA are very widespread in the nervous system (Tables 8-4 and 8-5). For example, the endings of primary afferents in the spinal cord, the endings of ascending pathways in the thalamus, and the myriad outputs from the cerebral cortex all use glutamate as an excitatory neurotransmitter. In fact, it is estimated that glutamate is one of the transmitters at upwards of 90% of CNS synapses. Inhibitory connections using GABA are also abundant, as noted in a number of subsequent chapters.

Although there are several subtypes of metabotropic glutamate receptors, most are ionotropic. One of the latter, called the **NMDA receptor** because it also binds the compound *N*-methyl-D-aspartate, has both transmitter-gated and voltage-gated properties (Fig. 8-20) and is the channel responsible for some forms of long-term potentiation. NMDA receptors are found side by side on postsynaptic membranes with the more conventional glutamate-gated cation channels responsible for fast EPSPs. At the normal resting potential, a Mg^{2+} ion occupies the NMDA receptor channel and prevents current flow, even in the presence of glutamate. Depolarizing the postsynaptic membrane—for example, as a result of repetitive presynaptic activity and release of neuropeptides as well as substantial glutamate—expels the Mg^{2+} ion and allows the NMDA channel to open. This means that NMDA receptors can operate as molecular

Table 8-4	Major Locations of Neurons and Synapses That Use Glutamate
Location of Neurons	**Location of Terminals**
Interneurons in many CNS sites	Local connections
Projection neurons	CNS destinations of long tracts
Primary sensory neurons	Second-order neurons in the CNS
Pyramidal cells of cerebral cortex*	Basal ganglia, thalamus, spinal cord, other cortical areas

*Chapter 22.

Table 8-5	Major Locations of Neurons and Synapses That Use GABA (or Glycine)
Location of Neurons	**Location of Terminals**
Interneurons in many CNS sites	Local connections
Cerebellar cortex (Purkinje cells*)	Deep cerebellar nuclei*
Caudate nucleus, putamen	Globus pallidus, substantia nigra
Globus pallidus, substantia nigra	Thalamus, subthalamic nucleus[†]
Thalamic reticular nucleus[‡]	Other thalamic nuclei

*Chapter 20.
[†]Chapter 19.
[‡]Chapter 16.

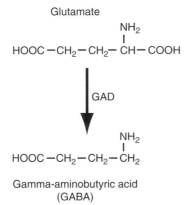

Glutamate

$$HOOC-CH_2-CH_2-\underset{\underset{NH_2}{|}}{CH}-COOH$$

GAD

$$HOOC-CH_2-CH_2-\underset{\underset{NH_2}{|}}{CH_2}$$

Gamma-aminobutyric acid
(GABA)

Figure 8-19 The two most prominent amino acid neurotransmitters, glutamate and γ-aminobutyric acid (GABA). GABA is synthesized from glutamate via a decarboxylation catalyzed by glutamic acid decarboxylase (GAD).

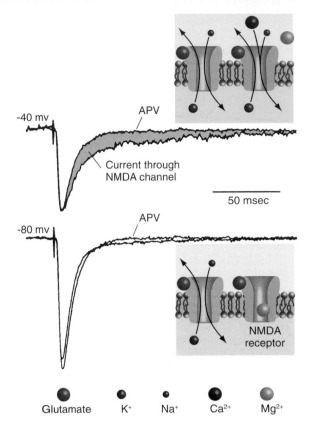

-40 mv

APV

Current through
NMDA channel

50 msec

APV

-80 mv

NMDA
receptor

Glutamate   K⁺   Na⁺   Ca²⁺   Mg²⁺

Figure 8-20 Properties of NMDA receptors, shown in patch-clamp recordings of postsynaptic currents in hippocampal pyramidal neurons. Near the normal resting membrane potential (−80 mVfv), most of the postsynaptic current in response to electrical stimulation of presynaptic fibers flows through non-NMDA channels, because the NMDA channels are blocked by Mg^{2+}. Hence application of the NMDA receptor antagonist 2-amino-5-phosphonovalerate (APV) causes no change in the postsynaptic current. Depolarization to −40 mV removes the Mg^{2+} block, and the same stimulus allows an additional, slower Na^+-K^+-Ca^{2+} current, blocked by APV, to flow through the NMDA channels. *(Electrical recordings, from Hestrin S et al: J Physiol 422:203, 1990.)*

computing elements, opening only if glutamate is present *and* there is preexisting depolarization. Open NMDA receptor channels are also unusual in that they permit the passage of not only Na^+ and K^+ ions but also large numbers of Ca^{2+} ions. The resulting postsynaptic increase in Ca^{2+} concentration activates second-messenger cascades, which in turn augment transmission at the synapse. NMDA receptors are found in other locations as well, such as the presynaptic terminals of some sensory neurons, and they may be widely involved in adjusting the strength of synapses.

As in the case of acetylcholine, there are both ionotropic and metabotropic GABA receptors. **GABA$_A$** receptors (as well as glycine receptors) are transmitter-gated ion channels, structurally similar to nicotinic receptors except for the fact that when open they are permeable to Cl^- ions. The less numerous **GABA$_B$** receptors are G protein–coupled receptors that cause slow IPSPs by opening K^+ channels.

Excessive Levels of Glutamate Are Toxic

Most neurons have receptors for glutamate, the principal excitatory neurotransmitter in the CNS, and this amino acid is available in high concentrations in excitatory synaptic terminals. Ordinarily, glutamate released at synapses is rapidly taken back up into the presynaptic terminal or surrounding glial cells, so that postsynaptic membranes are exposed to this amino acid only briefly. This is important, because more than a brief dose is toxic—prolonged exposure to glutamate triggers a sequence of events that can injure or even kill neurons, a phenomenon called **excitotoxicity.** Excessive Ca^{2+} entry through NMDA receptor channels is thought to initiate many aspects of the toxicity. Overexposure to glutamate can arise from either excessive release or deficient reuptake, and both mechanisms may play a role in some forms of neuropathology. Part of the mechanism of brain damage in stroke may involve the release of toxic amounts of glutamate in response to anoxia, and some degenerative diseases of the nervous system may result from localized defects in glutamate reuptake.

ATP Is Not Just an Energy Source but Also a Neurotransmitter

ATP is widely known as the dispenser of chemical energy in cells, but like glutamate, it serves double duty by also being a generally excitatory neurotransmitter contingent on the type of receptor it interacts with. Depending on the particular type of synapse, ATP may be stored in and released from the same vesicles as another transmitter (e.g., acetylcholine) or stored in separate vesicles; in a few instances, it is apparently the sole excitatory transmitter. Also as in the case of glutamate, there are both ionotropic and metabotropic ATP receptors (P2X and P2Y receptors, respectively, named for the purine ring in adenosine). Although far less prominent than glutamate receptors, ATP receptors are particularly important for transmission in some sensory systems and in the autonomic nervous system.

Amines and Neuropeptides Mediate Slow, Diffuse Transmission

The other amine transmitters, called **biogenic amines** (or **monoamines,** because each has a single amine group), are derived fairly directly from amino acids. Two of the four most prominent of these molecules, **norepinephrine** and **dopamine** (Fig. 8-21), are derived from tyrosine. (They are also referred to as **catecholamines** because of the catechol nucleus that forms part of each.) The third major biogenic amine transmitter, **serotonin** (Fig. 8-22), is derived from tryptophan, and the fourth, **histamine** (Fig. 8-23), from histidine. Nearly all biogenic amine receptors are G protein–coupled receptors. The

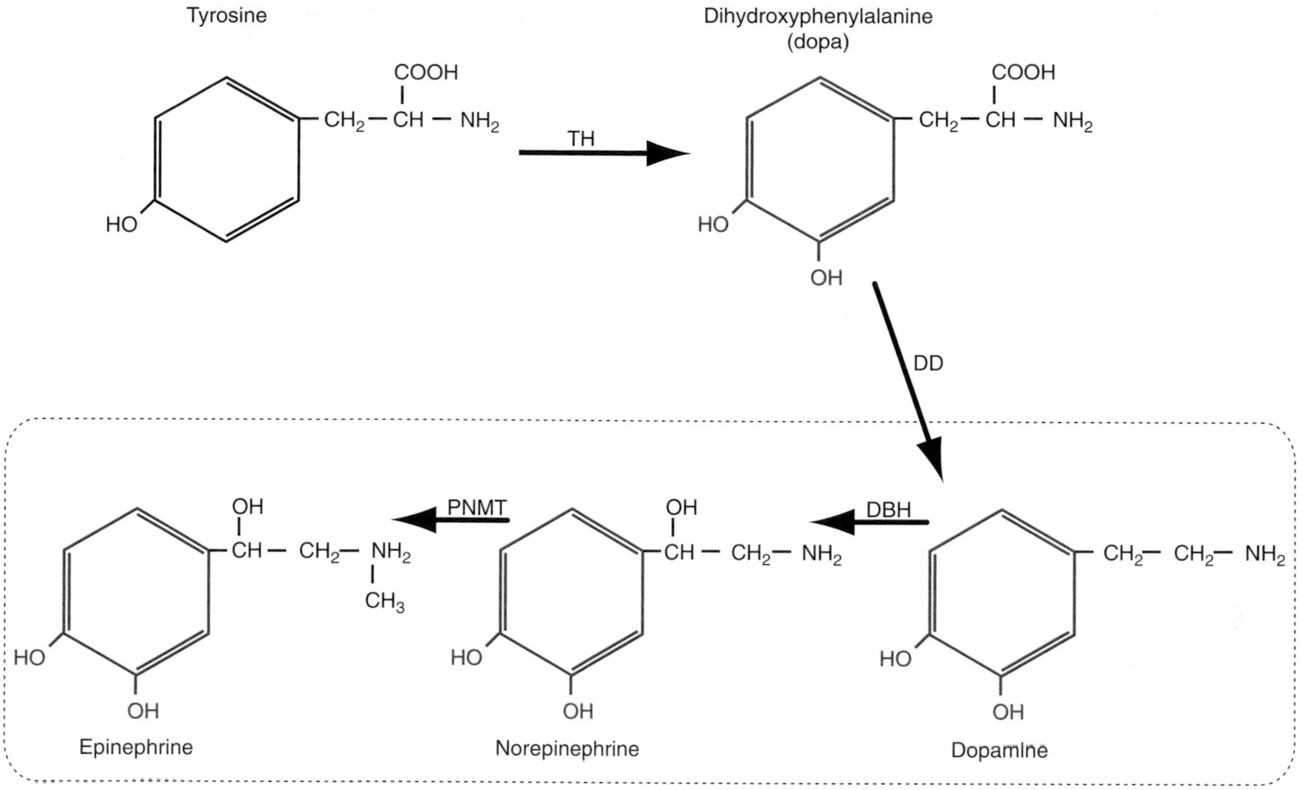

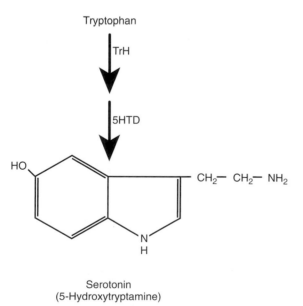

Figure 8-21 The catecholamine neurotransmitters (enclosed in the *dashed box*), so named because each includes a catechol group, which is the substituted benzene ring shown in color. These neurotransmitters are synthesized in a series of reactions that start with the amino acid tyrosine. Epinephrine plays a relatively minor role as a neurotransmitter in the human CNS, but dopamine and norepinephrine are widely distributed. DBH, dopamine β-hydroxylase; DD, dopa decarboxylase; PNMT, phenylethanolamine-N-methyltransferase; TH, tyrosine hydroxylase (the rate-limiting enzyme for the whole pathway).

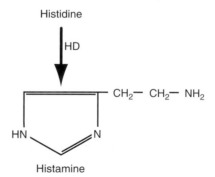

Figure 8-23 Structure and synthesis of histamine, which is synthesized in one step by decarboxylation of histidine. HD, histidine decarboxylase.

Figure 8-22 Structure and synthesis of serotonin. The pathway begins with the amino acid tryptophan, which is hydroxylated in a rate-limiting step catalyzed by tryptophan hydroxylase (TrH). The resulting 5-hydroxytryptophan is decarboxylated in a reaction catalyzed by 5-hydroxytryptophan decarboxylase (5HTD), resulting in serotonin.

only exception is one type of serotonin receptor, which is ionotropic.

Biogenic amine-containing CNS neurons are concentrated in the brainstem and hypothalamus (Table 8-6). Despite this restricted distribution, these neurons, like those of some central cholinergic nuclei, have far-flung connections (see Figs. 11-24, 11-26, 11-27, and 22-31), suggesting that they too are involved in regulating or tuning the activity of large portions of the CNS. Nevertheless, there are characteristic differences among the

Table 8-6	Major Locations of Neurons and Synapses That Use Biogenic Amines	
Transmitter	**Location of Neurons**	**Location of Terminals**
Norepinephrine	Sympathetic ganglia* Locus ceruleus,[†] reticular formation[†]	Smooth and cardiac muscle, glands Widespread CNS areas
Dopamine	Substantia nigra[††] (compact part) Ventral tegmental area[†§] Hypothalamus[§] Retina (some amacrine cells)[¶]	Caudate nucleus, putamen Limbic structures, cerebral cortex Infundibulum[§] Local connections
Serotonin	Raphe nuclei[†]	Widespread CNS areas
Histamine	Hypothalamus[§]	Widespread CNS areas

*Chapter 10.
[†]Chapter 11.
[‡]Chapter 19.
[§]Chapter 23.
[¶]Chapter 17.

termination patterns of fibers containing acetylcholine, norepinephrine, dopamine, serotonin, and histamine. This, together with consistent associations between certain transmitter systems and neurological syndromes (e.g., dopamine and Parkinson's disease, as discussed in Chapter 19), indicates that each of these four transmitters plays a distinctive role in the CNS.

There were demonstrations more than half a century ago that some neurons secrete hormones, as in the case of neurosecretory neurons of the hypothalamus that produce oxytocin and vasopressin (see Fig. 23-10). These observations were extended when, beginning in the early 1970s, the factors released by the hypothalamus to control the pituitary gland were isolated and characterized as short chains of amino acids, or peptides. Work since that time, using newer experimental techniques, has fundamentally transformed our view of the relationship between peptides and the function of the nervous system. It is now apparent that there are far more kinds of neuroactive peptides (or **neuropeptides**) in the brain than previously imagined—the number now stands at more than 100—and that most or all of them can function as neurotransmitters. For example, the 14–amino acid peptide **somatostatin** was originally described as the hypothalamic inhibiting factor that controls the secretion of growth hormone by the anterior pituitary. It was subsequently found that hormonally released somatostatin accounts for only about 10% of the somatostatin

in the brain and that this peptide is localized primarily in the synaptic endings of neurons in many different CNS locations. Another example is the 11–amino acid peptide **substance P,** originally described as a smooth muscle relaxant isolated from gut, which has been localized in the synaptic endings of some basal ganglia neurons, dorsal root ganglion cells, and other neurons. Finally, **enkephalins** are neuropeptides that play a prominent role in pain-control circuitry (see Fig. 11-21).

Some neuropeptides are widely distributed and presumably have multiple or general functions. Others have a more restricted distribution and may be associated with a specific function. For example, the octapeptide **angiotensin II** is a blood-borne hormone produced as part of the kidney's response to dehydration; it acts in the kidney and elsewhere outside the nervous system to promote water retention. Blood-borne angiotensin II also acts as a neurohormone by entering the CNS in the walls of the third ventricle and activating neurons in the subfornical organ (see Fig. 6-29). Finally, a system of neurons (including those of the subfornical organ) that apparently use angiotensin II as a transmitter orchestrate vasopressin secretion, blood pressure adjustments, and a search for water.

Neuropeptides are metabolically expensive for cells to make and transport, so they are present and effective at very low concentrations. In addition, their initial synthesis from larger precursor proteins allows neurons to get some extra mileage: the precursor may contain multiple copies of a smaller neuropeptide or copies of multiple neuropeptides with different effects.

Most or all neurons that contain a neuropeptide also contain one or more of the "classic" small-molecule transmitters. This means that there are often separate subpopulations of neurons in a CNS area, each with its own chemical signature. For example, GABA-containing neurons of the putamen that project to one part of the globus pallidus also contain enkephalin; those that project to another part of the globus pallidus also contain substance P. The functional consequences of this coexistence of transmitter substances are unknown in most cases, but it seems clear that single synapses can mediate multiple effects with different time courses and sensitivities.

Drugs, Diseases, and Toxins Can Selectively Affect Particular Parts of Individual Neurotransmitter Systems

Synaptic transmission involves a much wider array of proteins and processes than does the generation and conduction of action potentials, and there is a correspondingly enormous array of toxins, disease processes, and drugs that affect different aspects of synaptic transmission. For example, one would predict that a molecule that binds to nicotinic receptors and prevents them

Drugs, Diseases, and Toxins Can Cause Weakness by Interfering With Neuromuscular Transmission

Three conditions that cause weakness by interfering with different aspects of neuromuscular transmission (Fig. 8-24), either by preventing the release of acetylcholine or by blocking its receptors, provide instructive examples of the kinds of processes that can affect synaptic transmission in general.

Lambert-Eaton myasthenic syndrome (*myasthenia* means "muscle weakness") is an autoimmune disorder in which patients produce antibodies to the voltage-gated Ca^{2+} channels in their motor nerve terminals. As a result, less Ca^{2+} enters the nerve terminals in response to action potentials in motor nerves, fewer acetylcholine-filled vesicles release their contents, and the patient is weak. This syndrome is most commonly associated with small cell carcinoma of the lung. Apparently, antibodies produced in response to channels in the tumor cells cross-react with the voltage-gated Ca^{2+} channels of motor nerve terminals.

The bacterium *Clostridium botulinum* produces one of the most potent neurotoxins known—as little as 0.1 µg can be fatal. Botulinum toxin is taken up by presynaptic cholinergic terminals in the PNS, where it cleaves one or more of the proteins involved in the fusion of synaptic vesicles with the presynaptic membrane and prevents exocytosis of their contents. As a result, acetylcholine release is prevented, and weakness or paralysis and a variety of autonomic symptoms ensue. **Botulism*** in humans can result from eating contaminated food or from production of the toxin by *Clostridium* growing in the intestinal tract (usually of infants) or in a wound. In a striking turnabout, localized injections of botulinum toxin (these days called Botox) are now used to treat certain clinical conditions in which particular muscles or groups of muscles are tonically contracted. (Interestingly, *Clostridium tetani* produces a toxin that works by the same mechanism. However, it is first transported retrogradely along the axons of motor neurons, reaches the spinal cord, and moves into inhibitory interneurons, where it blocks the release of glycine. The resulting loss of inhibition causes the excessive muscle contractions of tetanus.)

Myasthenia gravis, by far the most common of the three disorders mentioned here, is an autoimmune disease in which patients produce antibodies to their own nicotinic receptors. Normal amounts of acetylcholine are produced, packaged, and released, but as a consequence of the decreased number of functional nicotinic receptors, acetylcholinesterase is abnormally likely to hydrolyze each acetylcholine molecule before it binds to a receptor. As a result, patients become progressively weaker with repeated muscle contractions. Treatment with acetylcholinesterase blockers helps most patients (Fig. 8-25). In more severe cases, immunosuppressive therapies or removal of antibodies from the patient's plasma may be required.

*Botulus is Latin for "sausage," and botulism was once called *sausage disease* in reference to its frequent association with the consumption of sausages.

---

from opening would cause weakness or paralysis by blocking neuromuscular transmission. This is in fact the mechanism of action of **curare,** the active ingredient of the plant extracts used for centuries on arrow tips to paralyze prey. Mutations affecting ligand-gated ion channels or other molecules involved in synaptic or neuromuscular transmission, like mutations affecting voltage-gated ion channels, can also impair neurological or neuromuscular function (Box 8-1). For example, glycine is an important neurotransmitter released by spinal cord interneurons at inhibitory synapses. Mutations of the gene that encodes glycine-gated Cl^- channels cause hyperekplexia (Greek for "excessive jumping") or "startle disease." Affected individuals are born with generally increased muscle tone, which decreases to normal in 1 to 2 years. They are left with an exaggerated version of the startle reflex that we have all experienced, as though missing an inhibitory influence normally present in the spinal cord. In response to unexpected stimuli (especially loud sounds), there is forceful blinking, grimacing, flexion of the arms, and sometimes pronounced contraction of the leg muscles, resulting in a fall. (Similarly, sublethal poisoning with strychnine, which blocks glycine-gated Cl^- channels, results in violent, generalized muscle contractions in response to minor stimuli.)

Although the plethora of transmitters, receptors, and receptor subtypes may sometimes seem like a curse of enormous proportions, it is actually a huge blessing. As we learn more about each, it becomes progressively more feasible to design pharmaceutical agents that precisely target particular neural processes (Fig. 8-26).

Gap Junctions Mediate Direct Current Flow From One Neuron to Another

Many cells in the body are electrically coupled to one another by junctions that allow the passage of not only ions but also a variety of small molecules. The morphological substrate is the **gap junction** (Fig. 8-27), a site at which the normal separation between cells is narrowed to only about 3 nm. At gap junctions, cylindrical assemblies of six transmembrane protein molecules (**connexins**) form a **connexon** that butt up against one another, so that their aqueous centers are aligned and form a continuous channel interconnecting the two cells. The central pore is larger than in the case of ion channels, allowing the easy bidirectional passage of small molecules.

Gap junctions between neurons form **electrical synapses,** allowing the direct spread of current from one neuron into another. This would seem to have considerable advantages—duplication of the presynaptic signal in the postsynaptic cell, no delay in the transmission of electrical information, and no need to synthesize vesicles and transmitters. However, the overriding disadvantage is a partial loss of the functional individuality of the coupled neurons. Chemical transmission allows neurons to be separate computational units, each one potentially doing something entirely different from its neighbor. Presumably for this reason, gap junctions are relatively rare in mammalian nervous systems. They are more common during development, probably allowing populations of cells to share metabolic information and signaling molecules. In adult nervous systems, they are often found interconnecting dendrites while located in some groups of neurons that tend to fire action potentials synchronously, and they are also found in some networks of cells designed to spread information electrotonically over long distances. Horizontal cells of the retina (see Chapter 17) are one example of the latter. The conductance of gap junctions may not be static; many can be modulated by second-messenger effects,

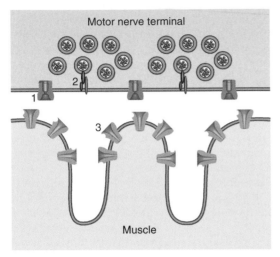

Figure 8-24 Examples of processes that can interfere with neuromuscular transmission. Blocking the entry of Ca^{2+} ions into motor nerve terminals (1), as in Lambert-Eaton myasthenic syndrome, prevents the essential signal that normally triggers acetylcholine release. Hydrolysis of one or more of the proteins required for vesicle attachment and fusion by botulinum toxin (2) also prevents acetylcholine release. Finally, blockade of nicotinic receptors on the postjunctional muscle membrane (3) by antibodies (as in myasthenia gravis) or toxins (curare and others) prevents binding of acetylcholine.

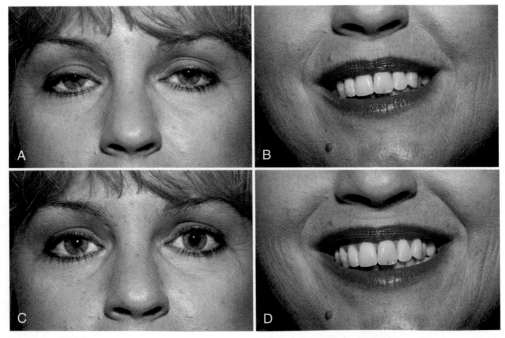

Figure 8-25 The eyes and smile of a patient with myasthenia gravis. When looking straight ahead **(A)**, her eyelids droop. Looking to either side (not shown) causes diplopia because of weakness of her eye muscles. Facial movements are also somewhat limited when she tries to smile **(B)**. Minutes after the administration of an acetylcholinesterase inhibitor (which enhances the activity of acetylcholine at the neuromuscular junction by preventing its breakdown), her eyes are open wider **(C)**, her diplopia has resolved, and her smile is much broader **(D)**.

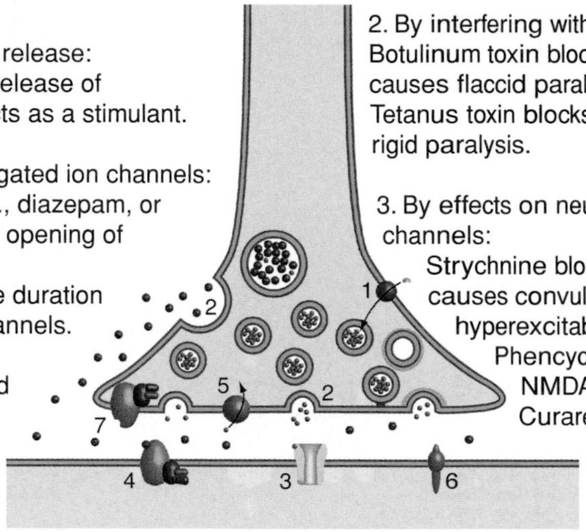

DRUGS OR TOXINS THAT ENHANCE TRANSMISSION

1. By enhancing synthesis or packaging of neurotransmitter:
L-dopa crosses the blood-brain barrier and is metabolized into dopamine, compensating for lower dopamine levels in Parkinson's disease.

2. By enhancing neurotransmitter release:
Amphetamine causes increased release of norepinephrine and dopamine, acts as a stimulant.

3. By effects on neurotransmitter-gated ion channels:
Benzodiazepine tranquilizers (e.g., diazepam, or Valium) increase the frequency of opening of GABA-gated Cl⁻ channels.
Barbiturate sedatives increase the duration of opening of GABA-gated Cl⁻ channels.

4. By effects on G protein–coupled neurotransmitter receptors:
Morphine mimics opioid peptides, binds to their receptors, causes analgesia and other effects.

5. By blocking removal of neurotransmitter:
Fluoxetine (Prozac), an antidepressant, blocks serotonin reuptake.
Cocaine blocks reuptake of norepinephrine and dopamine.

6. By blocking degradation of neurotransmitter:
Pyridostigmine (Mestinon) blocks acetylcholinesterase, is used to treat patients with myasthenia gravis.

7. By blocking retrograde signaling:
Caffeine blocks presynaptic adenosine receptors, prevents suppression of transmitter release, acts as a stimulant.

DRUGS OR TOXINS THAT DEPRESS TRANSMISSION

1. By interfering with synthesis or packaging of neurotransmitter:
Vesamicol and reserpine block transport of acetylcholine and amines, respectively, into synaptic vesicles.

2. By interfering with neurotransmitter release:
Botulinum toxin blocks release of acetylcholine, causes flaccid paralysis.
Tetanus toxin blocks release of glycine, causes rigid paralysis.

3. By effects on neurotransmitter-gated ion channels:
Strychnine blocks glycine-gated Cl⁻ channels, causes convulsions and other signs of hyperexcitability.
Phencyclidine (PCP, "angel dust") blocks NMDA receptors.
Curare (arrow tip poison) blocks skeletal muscle nicotinic receptors, causes paralysis.
Hexamethonium blocks autonomic nicotinic receptors.

4. By effects on G protein–coupled neurotransmitter receptors:
Haloperidol (Haldol), an antipsychotic, blocks some dopamine receptors.
Atropine blocks muscarinic acetylcholine receptors, causes autonomic changes.

Figure 8-26 Examples of agents that affect different aspects of synaptic transmission.

allowing some control over the coupling between neurons.

The properties of gap junction channels, like those of other channels, can be altered by mutations affecting their constituent proteins. Charcot-Marie-Tooth disease provides a striking example of a gap junction channelopathy, underscoring the importance of gap junctions for the movement of small molecules across apposed membranes. Charcot-Marie-Tooth disease is a group of disorders that are collectively the most common cause of inherited peripheral neuropathy. Affected individuals have a progressive loss of PNS axons, beginning with the longest ones, resulting in weakness, muscle atrophy, and sensory loss that begins in the feet and legs and moves into the hands. The X-linked form of the disease is caused by a mutation affecting the connexin that forms the gap junction channels of Schwann cells. Gap junctions typically interconnect adjoining cells in the nervous system and elsewhere, but in the case of Schwann cells, they join adjacent membranes of single cells in the Schmidt-Lanterman incisures and near nodes of Ranvier (Fig. 8-28; see also Figs. 1-24 and 1-25). Small molecules traveling between a Schwann cell nucleus and a myelinated axon can take a "shortcut" through these gap junctions, avoiding what would otherwise be a much longer, spiral course through Schwann cell cytoplasm. The nature of the critical chemical messengers normally traversing the gap junction shortcut is still unknown, but

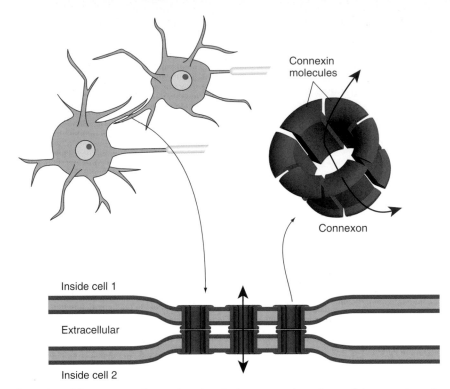

Figure 8-27 Schematic illustration of the structure of a gap junction. Each connexon is made up of six connexin molecules surrounding a central pore, allowing diffusion of small molecules (typically, but not always, in both directions).

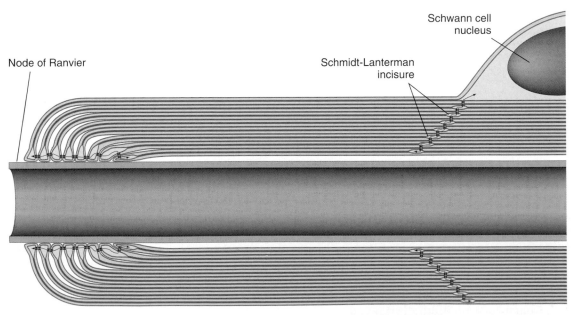

Figure 8-28 Gap junctions interconnecting parts of individual Schwann cells. These junctions are thought to allow chemical communication between the cell's nucleus, at the outside of the myelin sheath, and parts of the cell closer to the axon it ensheathes. This route circumvents what would otherwise be a much longer, spiral path. (Although not apparent in this drawing, the pockets of Schwann cell cytoplasm near the node of Ranvier are also continuous with cytoplasm near the nucleus, as shown in Fig. 1-24.)

disruption of this molecular traffic pattern is thought to cause loss of myelinated axons. Although (as in the case of other channels) the relationships between specific mutations and clinical symptoms are not yet understood in all cases, various connexin mutations are associated with defective function of the heart, reproductive organs, and receptor cells of the inner ear.

SUGGESTED READINGS

Abrams CK, et al: Mutations in connexin 32: the molecular and biophysical bases for the X-linked form of Charcot-Marie-Tooth disease. Brain Res Rev 32:203, 2000.

Agnati LF, et al: Intercellular communication in the brain: wiring versus volume transmission. Neurosci 69:711, 1995.

In this context, "wiring" means anatomically defined synapses, and "volume transmission" means diffusion of transmitters through extracellular space to receptors in nonsynaptic locations.

Alvarez VA, Sabatini BL: Anatomical and physiological plasticity of dendritic spines. Annu Rev Neurosci 30:79, 2007.

Attwell D, Barbour B, Szatkowski M: Nonvesicular release of neurotransmitter. Neuron 11:401, 1993.

There may be a little, in some special situations.

Beal MF, Martin JB: Neuropeptides in neurological disease. Ann Neurol 20:547, 1986.

Benarroch EE: Adenosine and its receptors: multiple modulatory functions and potential therapeutic targets for neurologic disease. Neurol 70:231, 2008.

Bliss TVP, Collingridge GL: A synaptic model of memory: long-term potentiation in the hippocampus. Nature 361:31, 1993.

Burnstock G: Physiology and pathophysiology of purinergic neurotransmission. Physiol Rev 87:659, 2007.

Cherington M: Clinical spectrum of botulism. Muscle Nerve 21:701, 1998.

Choi DW, Rothman SM: The role of glutamate neurotoxicity in hypoxic-ischemic neuronal death. Annu Rev Neurosci 13:171, 1990.

Clapham DE: Direct G protein activation of ion channels. Annu Rev Neurosci 17:441, 1994.

Connors BW, Long MA: Electrical synapses in the mammalian brain. Annu Rev Neurosci 27:393, 2004.

Cooper JR, Bloom FE, Roth RH: The biochemical basis of neuropharmacology, ed 8, New York, 2002, Oxford University Press.

A concise, easily readable review.

Dawson TM, Snyder SH: Gases as biological messengers: nitric oxide and carbon monoxide in the brain. J Neurosci 14:5147, 1994.

Eccles JC: The physiology of synapses, New York, 1964, Academic Press.

A review by one of the pioneers of synaptic physiology.

Edwards RH: The neurotransmitter cycle and quantal size. Neuron 55:835, 2007.

Freund TF, Katona I, Piomelli D: Role of endogenous cannabinoids in synaptic signaling. Physiol Rev 83:1017, 2003.

Guillemin R: Peptides in the brain: the new endocrinology of the neuron. Science 202:390, 1978.

Guix FX, et al: The physiology and pathophysiology of nitric oxide in the brain. Prog Neurobiol 76:126, 2005.

Hahn AF, et al: Pathological findings in the X-linked form of Charcot-Marie-Tooth disease: a morphometric and ultrastructural analysis. Acta Neuropathol 101:129, 2001.

Herkenham M: Mismatches between neurotransmitter and receptor localization in brain: observations and implications. Neuroscience 23:1, 1987.

Heuser JE: Review of electron microscopic evidence favouring vesicle exocytosis as the structural basis for quantal release during synaptic transmission. Q J Exp Physiol 74:1051, 1989.

Isaacson JS, Walmsley B: Counting quanta: direct measurement of transmitter release at a central synapse. Neuron 15:875, 1995.

Jessell TM, Kandel ER: Synaptic transmission: a bidirectional and self-modifiable form of cell-cell communication. Cell 72/Neuron 10(Suppl):1, 1993.

An overview article introducing a special issue about synaptic transmission.

Katz B: Nerve, muscle and synapse, New York, 1966, McGraw-Hill.

A lucid introduction to neurophysiology by a Nobel laureate who did much of the early work on neuromuscular transmission.

Kostyuk P, Verkhratsky A: Calcium stores in neurons and glia. Neuroscience 63:381, 1994.

A review of the elaborate mechanisms used by the nervous system to control intracellular levels of free $Ca2+$.

Lipton SA, Rosenberg PA: Excitatory amino acids as a final common pathway for neurological disorders. N Engl J Med 330:613, 1994.

Liu H, et al: Synaptic relationship between substance P and the substance P receptor: light and electron microscopic characterization of the mismatch between neuropeptides and their receptors. Proc Natl Acad Sci U S A 91:1009, 1994.

Lundberg JM, Hökfelt T: Coexistence of peptides and classical neurotransmitters. Trends Neurosci 6:325, 1983.

Marty A, Llano I: Excitatory effects of GABA in established brain networks. Trends Neurosci 28:284, 2005.

Sometimes the line between excitation and inhibition is not so clear.

Menichella DM, et al: Connexins are critical for normal myelination in the CNS. J Neurosci 23:5963, 2003.

Olney JW: Inciting excitotoxic cytocide among central neurons. In Schwartz RW, Ben-Ari Y, editors: Excitatory amino acids and epilepsy, New York, 1986, Plenum Press.

"One of my major research goals in recent years has been to answer a simple question: 'Can one CNS neuron excite another CNS neuron to death?'"

O'Neill JH, Murray NMF, Newsom-Davis J: The Lambert-Eaton myasthenic syndrome: a review of 50 cases. Brain 111:577, 1988.

Rajendra S, Schofield PR: Molecular mechanisms of inherited startle syndromes. Trends Neurosci 18:80, 1995.

Sabatini BL, Regehr WG: Timing of neurotransmission at fast synapses in the mammalian brain. Nature 384:170, 1996.

Direct measurements of the remarkable speed of transmitter release at mammalian CNS synapses.

Savtchenko LP, Rusakov DA: The optimal height of the synaptic cleft. Proc Natl Acad Sci U S A 104:1823, 2007.

Narrowing the synaptic cleft increases the concentration of transmitter released there, but it also makes it harder for current to get in. These modeling studies indicate that the observed width of 10 to 20 nm is the best compromise.

Schiavo G, Matteoli M, Montecucco C: Neurotoxins affecting neuroexocytosis. Physiol Rev 80:717, 2000.

Seki K, Perlmutter SI, Fetz EE: Sensory input to primate spinal cord is presynaptically inhibited during voluntary movement. Nat Neurosci 6:1309, 2003.

One example of a probably routine use of presynaptic inhibition: to cancel self-generated sensory inputs during voluntary movement.

Shepherd GM: The dendritic spine: a multifunctional integrative unit. J Neurophysiol 75:2197, 1996.

Siegel GJ, et al: Basic neurochemistry: molecular, cellular and medical aspects, ed 7, Burlington, Mass, 2006, Elsevier Academic Press.

Stevens CF, Tsujimoto T: Estimates for the pool size of releasable quanta at a single central synapse and for the time required to refill the pool. Proc Natl Acad Sci U S A 92:846, 1995.

Stuart G, Spruston N, Häusser M, editors: Dendrites, ed 2, New York, 2008, Oxford University Press.

Dendrites increase the surface area available for synaptic inputs, but they contribute much more than this to the computational capabilities of neurons.

von Euler US, Gaddum JH: An unidentified depressor substance in certain tissue extracts. J Physiol 72:74, 1931.

The original description of the isolation of substance P from intestine and brain. Unbeknownst to the authors, this was the first recorded isolation of a neuropeptide.

Walmsley B, Alvarez FJ, Fyffe REW: Diversity of structure and function at mammalian central synapses. Trends Neurosci 21:81, 1998.

Yuste R, Denk W: Dendritic spines as basic functional units of neuronal integration. Nature 375:682, 1995.

Technically extraordinary experiments in which Ca2+ concentration changes in individual spines are observed directly.

Sensory Receptors and the Peripheral Nervous System

The ongoing activity and output of the central nervous system (CNS) are greatly influenced, and sometimes more or less determined, by incoming sensory information. An example is our constant awareness of the position of our limbs in space and the use of this awareness in guiding movements. The basis of this incoming sensory information is an array of **sensory receptors,**[a] cells that detect various stimuli and produce **receptor potentials** in response, often with astonishing effectiveness. Rod photoreceptors, for example, can produce measurable responses to single photons (see Chapter 17), and olfactory receptors may be able to respond to single odorant molecules (see Chapter 13); auditory and vestibular receptors can respond to almost unimaginably small mechanical deflections (see Chapter 14). The physiological processes employed by sensory receptors turn out to be gratifyingly similar to those found in synapses.

This chapter considers some general principles of the anatomy and physiology of sensory receptors. The emphasis is on the general receptors of the body—the principal purveyors of sensory information to the spinal cord (see also Chapter 10). Specialized receptors, such as those of the eye, ear, mouth, and nose, are described in more detail in later chapters.

Receptors Encode the Nature, Location, Intensity, and Duration of Stimuli

There are many types of receptors on and within the human body and several different systems for classifying them. One system subdivides receptors according to the traditional five senses of vision, hearing, touch, smell, and taste. This system is too restrictive in that it does not recognize sensations such as balance, position, or pain, or sensory information from internal organs that usually does not reach consciousness. Another system distinguishes **interoceptors, proprioceptors,** and **exteroceptors.** Interoceptors monitor events within the body, such as distention of the stomach or changes in the pH of blood. Proprioceptors respond to changes in the position of the body or its parts; examples are the receptors in muscles and joint capsules. Vestibular receptors of the inner ear are commonly classified as proprioceptors because they signal movement and changes in the orientation of the head in space. Exteroceptors respond to stimuli that arise outside the body, such as the receptors

---

[a]*Receptor,* like *nucleus,* is a term with two meanings in neurobiology. A sensory receptor, as described in this chapter, is a specialized cell that conveys to the nervous system information about some stimulus. Neurotransmitter receptors, as described in Chapter 8, are molecules in postsynaptic membranes. To make matters worse, some sensory receptors receive feedback synapses and so have neurotransmitter receptors in their membranes.

involved in touch, hearing, and vision. Interoceptor-proprioceptor-exteroceptor terminology is used less commonly than in the past, partly because some receptors do not fit neatly and uniquely into one of these categories. For example, the visual system is very much involved in perception of motion and body position (i.e., proprioception), but visual receptors are exteroceptors.

Each Sensory Receptor Has an Adequate Stimulus, Allowing It to Encode the Nature of a Stimulus

A more commonly used and straightforward classification system subdivides receptors on the basis of the type of stimulus to which they are most sensitive (called the **adequate stimulus**). **Chemoreceptors** include those for smell, taste, and many internal stimuli such as pH and metabolite concentrations. **Photoreceptors** are the visual receptors of the retina. **Thermoreceptors** respond to temperature and its changes. **Mechanoreceptors,** the most varied group, respond to physical deformation. These include cutaneous receptors for touch, receptors that monitor muscle length and tension, auditory and vestibular receptors, and others. Pain receptors are a bit difficult to classify in this system because different pain receptors have varying degrees of sensitivity to mechanical, thermal, and chemical stimuli. This problem is commonly finessed by classifying pain receptors separately as **nociceptors** (from the Latin verb *nocere,* meaning "to hurt," as in noxious or obnoxious). Virtually all animals have these kinds of receptors, but this is not an exhaustive list. There are other kinds of energy, and various species have developed ways to sample them, such as magnetoreceptors used by migratory birds to help find their way, infrared receptors used by some snakes to detect warm animals nearby, and electroreceptors used by some fish to navigate.

To a first approximation, the type of receptor that is stimulated defines the nature, or **modality,** of the sensation that is experienced—you experience touch if something actually touches you or if a peripheral nerve attached to a touch receptor is stimulated electrically. Each sensory modality has a series of associated submodalities, or **qualities.** Stimuli delivered to the skin, for example, can feel like light touch, pressure, a tickle, or vibration. This roughly corresponds to the presence in the skin of multiple receptor types whose separate outputs are combined by the CNS to produce sensations that are richer and more complex—for example, sensations such as the texture of objects.

Many Sensory Receptors Have a Receptive Field, Allowing Them to Encode the Location of a Stimulus

Specific wiring patterns in ascending sensory pathways and in the cerebral cortex preserve information about the nature of a stimulus. In some sensory systems, individual receptors convey information not only about the

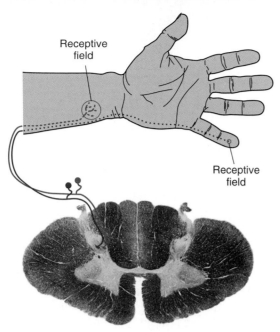

Figure 9-1 Receptive fields of two cutaneous receptors.

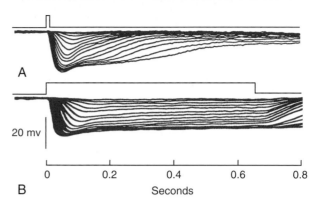

20 mv

0   0.2   0.4   0.6   0.8

B   Seconds

Figure 9-2 Intracellular recordings of the receptor potentials produced by a single cone photoreceptor in response to a series of brief **(A)** or longer **(B)** flashes, each about twice as bright as the next dimmer one. Brief, dim flashes cause brief hyperpolarizations that are graded with light intensity (vertebrate photoreceptors produce hyperpolarizing receptor potentials). Longer flashes produce sustained receptor potentials that last as long as the flashes. *(From Baylor DA, Hodgkin AL, Lamb TD: J Physiol 242:759, 1974.)*

nature of a stimulus but also about its location. That is, in addition to adequate stimuli, individual receptors may have **receptive fields,** particular areas in the periphery where application of an adequate stimulus causes them to respond. The receptive field of a cutaneous receptor, for example, is an area of skin where its receptive endings reside (Fig. 9-1). The receptive field of a retinal photoreceptor correlates to some small location in the outside world whose image falls on a particular spot on the retina where that photoreceptor is located. This preservation of spatial information in the CNS is part of the distorted maps of visual sensory stimuli (see Fig. 3-30). Even arrays of receptors with no obvious spatial domain to map may have systematic representations of some other parameter, such as the mapping of sound frequencies in the cochlea and in auditory cortex (see Fig. 14-19).

Neurons in successive levels of sensory pathways—second-order neurons, thalamic and cortical neurons—also have receptive fields, although they may be considerably more elaborate than those of the receptors. Neurons in visual cortex, for example, typically respond not to spots of light but rather to edges with particular orientations.

Receptor Potentials Encode the Intensity and Duration of Stimuli

The nature and location of a stimulus are indicated by the identities of the receptors that respond. To a great extent the intensity and duration of a stimulus are indicated by the size and duration of the receptor potentials produced—more intense stimuli produce larger

receptor potentials, and longer stimuli cause longer receptor potentials (Fig. 9-2). There is a bit more to the intensity-duration story than this, however. Some sensory systems include more sensitive and less sensitive receptors (e.g., the rods and cones of the retina), so increasing intensity may be signaled in part by the identities of the active receptors. In addition, as discussed in the next section, some sensory receptors produce only brief receptor potentials, even in response to maintained stimuli.

Most Sensory Receptors Adapt to Maintained Stimuli, Some More Rapidly Than Others

Nearly all receptors show some **adaptation,** which means they become less sensitive during the course of a maintained stimulus.[b] Those that adapt relatively little are called **slowly adapting** and are suitable receptors for such things as static position. Those that adapt a great deal typically do so quickly and are called **rapidly adapting;** they are better suited to indicate change and movement of stimuli (Fig. 9-3). Some rapidly adapting receptors (e.g., the Pacinian corpuscles shown in Fig. 9-8) do so completely and signal only the beginning and end of a stimulus; others continue to respond, but at a diminished level, throughout a stimulus. Adaptation is usually a property of one or more parts of the receptor's membrane: Ca^{2+} ions entering through transduction channels, for example, set in motion biochemical processes that decrease the sensitivity of some receptors. In addition, various accessory structures may modify the

---

[b]Nociceptors are a prominent exception. Many do not adapt to maintained stimuli, and, as discussed later in this chapter, repeated or prolonged noxious stimuli can make some nociceptors even more sensitive.

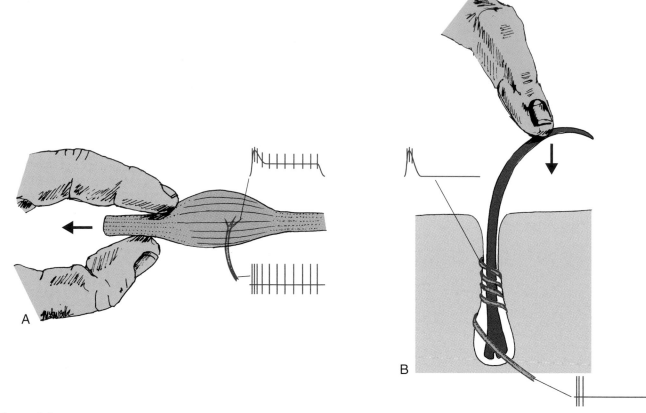

Figure 9-3 Slowly adapting versus rapidly adapting receptors. In both, a receptor potential is produced in the sensory ending and spreads to a trigger zone, initiating action potentials that spread passively back into the sensory ending. **A,** A muscle spindle continues to fire action potentials as long as the muscle is stretched. **B,** Most hair receptors fire a short burst of action potentials and are then silent, even if the bending of the hair is maintained.

physical stimulus before it reaches the sensory ending, as in the case of the multilayered capsules of Pacinian corpuscles.

Adaptation is a receptor-level process, but the CNS also has ways to regulate the sensitivity of receptors on a moment-to-moment basis. One such mechanism is the control of other structures related to receptors—for example, controlling the amount of light reaching the retina by regulating pupil size, or controlling the muscle fibers in stretch receptors (see Fig. 9-15). Another mechanism used is efferent projections from the CNS that synapse on receptor cells themselves; these are prominent in the inner ear (see Chapter 14) but occur in some other sensory systems as well.

Sensory Receptors All Share Some Organizational Features

Although their morphologies vary widely, all receptors have three general parts: a receptive area, an area rich in mitochondria (near the receptive area), and a synaptic area, where the receptor's message is passed toward or into the CNS (Fig. 9-4). The receptive area may have specializations suited to the adequate stimulus, as in the case of photoreceptors, which have an elaborately folded array of photopigment-bearing membrane; in other cases, there are no obvious specializations in this area. The area rich in mitochondria is either immediately adjacent to the receptive membrane or nearby and is presumed to supply the energy needs of the transduction process. In some receptors the synaptic area may be far removed from the other two, as in the case of a cutaneous mechanoreceptor with its receptive endings in the skin and its synaptic terminals in the spinal cord or brainstem.

Sensory Receptors Use Ionotropic and Metabotropic Mechanisms to Produce Receptor Potentials

Sensory receptors **transduce** (Latin for "lead across") some physical stimulus into an electrical signal—a receptor potential—that the nervous system can understand. Receptor potentials, like other electrical signals across neuronal membranes, are produced by the opening or closing of ion channels. (The only known exception in primates is the taste receptors that detect saltiness, as discussed in Chapter 13.) In many ways, most sensory receptors can be thought of as analogous to postsynaptic membranes, and their adequate stimuli

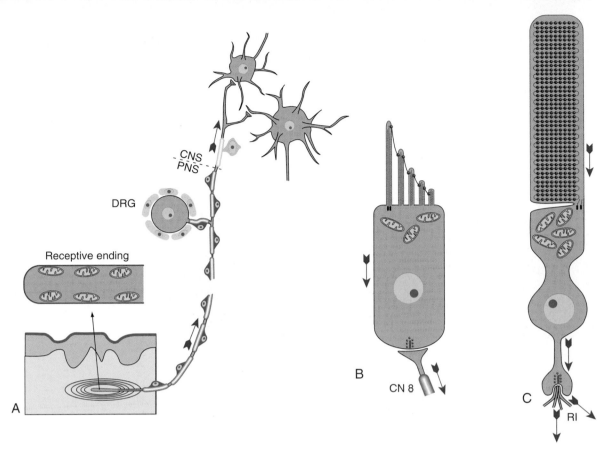

Figure 9-4 General organization of sensory receptors, as illustrated by a somatosensory receptor (Pacinian corpuscle, **A**), a hair cell of the inner ear **(B)**, and a retinal rod photoreceptor **(C).** Each has a receptive area (orange) and mitochondria nearby. The receptive ending of the Pacinian corpuscle has no obvious anatomical specializations but is surrounded by a layered capsule. The microvillar projections of the hair cell contain mechanosensitive channels (see Chapter 14), and the receptive area of the rod contains a collection of pigment-studded membranous disks (see Chapter 17). Somatosensory receptors make synapses far away in the CNS, whereas hair cells and photoreceptors make synapses nearby on peripheral endings of vestibulocochlear nerve fibers (CN 8) or on retinal interneurons (RI), respectively. DRG, dorsal root ganglion.

as analogous to neurotransmitters (Fig. 9-5). Just as postsynaptic membranes use ionotropic and metabotropic mechanisms to produce postsynaptic potentials, almost all known transduction mechanisms involve ion channels whose conductance is affected either directly by a stimulus (as in transmitter-gated ion channels) or indirectly by way of a G protein–coupled mechanism. As in the case of synapses, some sensory receptors (e.g., somatosensory mechanoreceptors) produce depolarizing receptor potentials when stimulated, and others (e.g., photoreceptors) produce hyperpolarizing receptor potentials. Auditory and vestibular receptors can produce either, depending on the details of the stimulus.

Receptors with directly gated ion channels include the somatosensory receptors discussed in this chapter, auditory and vestibular receptors, some taste receptors, and some visceral receptors. Some have channels that are directly sensitive to mechanical distortion, and others have channels directly gated by some molecule or ion or by temperature changes. Receptors with a G

protein–coupled transduction mechanism include photoreceptors, olfactory receptors, some taste receptors, and some visceral receptors.

All Sensory Receptors Produce Receptor Potentials, but Some Do Not Produce Action Potentials

Receptor potentials, like postsynaptic graded potentials, are focally produced events that spread electrotonically. If a particular sensory receptor is physically small relative to its length constant—that is, if it contacts the next cell in its neuronal pathway close to the site of transduction—the receptor potential itself can adequately modulate the rate of transmitter release at the synaptic terminal. This in turn causes a postsynaptic potential, and typically a change in action potential frequency, in the second cell (Fig. 9-6A). This is the case for many receptors, prominently including photoreceptors and auditory and vestibular receptors, all of which produce receptor potentials but no action potentials. Some receptors, however, must convey information over long distances (e.g., from a big toe to the spinal cord),

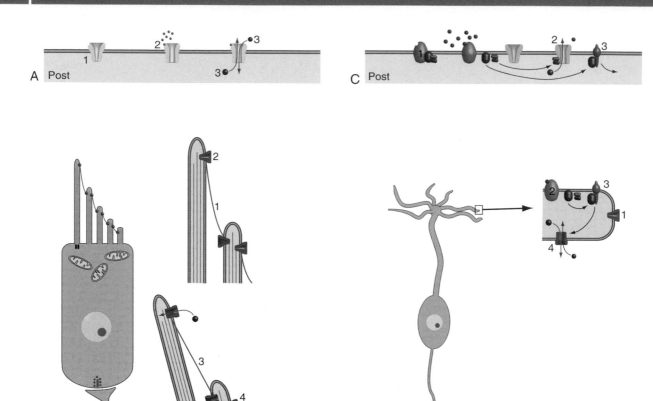

Figure 9-5 Similarities between the general mechanisms of postsynaptic potentials and receptor potentials; a vestibular receptor cell (see Chapter 14) and an olfactory receptor cell (see Chapter 13) are used as examples, but almost all receptors use mechanisms that are similar in principle. **A,** Rapid synaptic transmission involves ligand-gated (ionotropic) channels (1) that bind neurotransmitter (2) and then change permeability (3). **B,** Cochlear and vestibular hair cells have channels that are anchored to the cytoskeleton and to one another. When there is little tension (1) in the filamentous proteins interconnecting the channels, they spend much of their time closed (2). Increasing the tension (3) by deflecting the microvilli bearing the channels causes direct opening of the channels (4) and depolarizing current flow. **C,** Slow synaptic transmission involves G protein–coupled (metabotropic) receptors (1). Dissociation of the G protein in response to neurotransmitter binding may affect ion channels either directly (2) or indirectly via enzymatic cascades (3). **D,** Olfactory receptor cells contain normally closed channels (1) and G protein–coupled receptors for odorants (2). Dissociation of the G protein activates an enzyme (3, adenylate cyclase), which catalyzes the production of a second messenger (cyclic adenosine monophosphate) that in turn opens the transduction channels (4), causing a depolarizing receptor potential.

even though the receptor potential dies out within a few millimeters. In such cases, most of the receptor, beginning near the site of transduction, is capable of propagating action potentials. The action potential frequency is then modulated by the receptor potential (see Fig. 9-6B). Receptor potentials that directly cause changes in action potential frequency are also called **generator potentials.** All somatosensory receptors of the body operate in this manner, as do olfactory receptors and many visceral receptors. In vertebrates, all produce depolarizing receptor potentials, and an increased frequency of action potentials, in response to stimulation.

Somatosensory Receptors Detect Mechanical, Chemical, or Thermal Changes

Somatosensory receptors include an assortment of mechanoreceptors, thermoreceptors, and nociceptors.

All are pseudounipolar neurons with cell bodies in a dorsal root or cranial nerve ganglion, a central process that terminates in the spinal cord or brainstem, and a peripheral receptive ending in someplace like the skin, a muscle, or a joint (see Fig. 9-1). A great deal is understood about the moment-to-moment responses of many of these receptors, mostly from animal studies, but also in large part because it is possible to record from the axons of single receptors of human volunteers, using a process called **microneurography** (see Fig. 9-14C, insets).

Cutaneous Receptors Have Either Encapsulated or Nonencapsulated Endings

The skin and adjacent subcutaneous tissues are richly innervated by a wide variety of sensory endings. These endings can be divided broadly into **encapsulated** and **nonencapsulated** receptors (Table 9-1), depending on whether a capsule surrounds the ending.

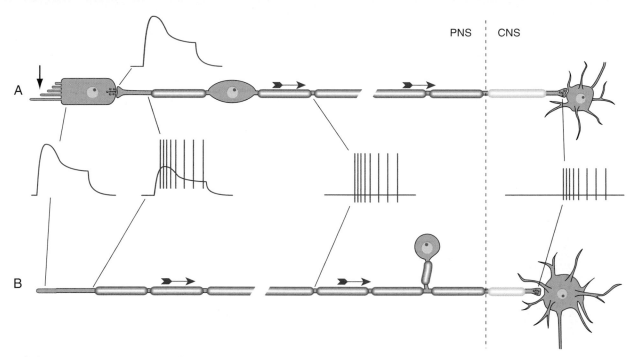

Figure 9-6 Short and long receptors, as illustrated by a hair cell of the inner ear (**A**) and a somatosensory ending (**B**). Hair cells produce a depolarizing receptor potential, but no action potentials, in response to deflection in the direction of the longest microvillar process *(arrow)*. The receptor potential spreads passively to the synaptic area of the hair cell, where it increases the release of excitatory neurotransmitter (glutamate) onto the peripheral ending of an eighth nerve fiber. The postsynaptic potential then spreads passively to the trigger zone of the nerve fiber and initiates the firing of action potentials, which are conducted to synaptic terminals in the CNS. Events in the somatosensory receptor are similar, except that no peripheral synapse is involved: the trigger zone of the peripheral nerve fiber is part of the same neuron that contains the receptive ending.

Table 9-1	Principal Types of Cutaneous Receptors			
	Capsules, Accessory Structures	**Receptors**	**Adaptation**	**Modality**
Encapsulated	Layered capsule	Pacinian corpuscle	Rapid	Vibration
		Meissner corpuscle	Rapid	Touch
	Thin capsule	Ruffini ending	Slow	Pressure
Nonencapsulated	Accessory structures	Endings around hairs	Rapid	Touch
		Merkel endings	Slow	Touch
	None	Free nerve ending	Varies	Pain, temperature, itch, touch

A bewildering variety of encapsulated receptors have been described in the past, and an equally bewildering variety of mostly eponymous names have been attached to them. However, these classifications are just variations on two common themes: receptors with layered capsules and receptors with thin capsules. This chapter describes only the best known of these. The function of the capsule is not known for all encapsulated receptors, but in at least some instances it serves as a mechanical filter, modifying mechanical stimuli before they reach the sensory ending. For example, receptors with layered capsules are rapidly adapting, due in large part to these mechanical properties of the capsules. The capsules also have barrier properties (discussed later in this chapter) that may be important in regulating the composition of the fluid surrounding the sensory endings contained within them.

Nonencapsulated receptors can be divided into two categories: **free nerve endings** and endings with **accessory structures** that are associated with the ending but do not surround it. Free nerve endings, as the name implies, are formed by branching terminations of sensory fibers in the skin, with no obvious specialization around them other than partial ensheathment by Schwann cells. Such endings are not restricted to the skin but are found throughout the body. Even though

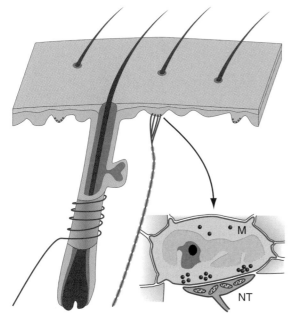

Figure 9-7 Two receptor types from hairy skin. Receptor endings wrap around hairs in a variety of configurations; a simple helical winding is shown. The inset is an enlarged drawing of a sensory nerve terminal (NT) forming a Merkel ending applied to a Merkel cell (M) in the basal layer of the epidermis. The Merkel cell is anchored among basal epidermal cells and has a prominent lobulated nucleus and dense-cored vesicles across from the sensory terminal.

microscopically they look similar to one another, many are known to be nociceptors, others thermoreceptors, and still others mechanoreceptors.

Capsules and Accessory Structures Influence the Response Properties of Cutaneous Mechanoreceptors

In addition to mechanoreceptive free nerve endings, there are five other prominent types of mechanoreceptor found in the skin and adjacent subcutaneous tissue. Two are nonencapsulated endings with accessory structures, and three are encapsulated.

Endings around hairs vary in their degree of complexity. Those around the base of a cat's whiskers are very elaborate, but those around most ordinary human body hairs are longitudinal neural processes or spiral endings that wrap around the base of the hair (Fig. 9-7). Bending the hair is presumed to deform the nonencapsulated sensory ending, distort mechanically sensitive channels, and lead to the production of a generator potential. Most hair receptors are rapidly adapting; they respond well to something brushing across the skin but not to steady pressure.[c]

The second type of nonencapsulated receptor is the **Merkel ending,** which is found in both hairy and

[c]You can easily demonstrate this yourself: bend a single hair on the back of your hand (or have someone else do it), then hold it in the bent position. You will feel it bending but almost immediately lose awareness of its new position.

glabrous skin (see Fig. 9-7). The ending is a disk-shaped expansion of a terminal of a sensory fiber, which is applied to the base of a specialized cell called a **Merkel cell.** A single fiber branches to innervate several Merkel cells, which usually occur in clusters. Each Merkel cell is situated in the basal layer of the epidermis and contains dense-cored vesicles in what looks like a synaptic ending onto the sensory terminal. This apparent synapse naturally led to the hypothesis that the Merkel cell is sensitive to deformation and uses this synapse to pass information about mechanical stimuli along to the nerve ending (which would make it the only known example of a somatosensory receptor that is not part of a dorsal root ganglion cell). However, the available evidence is inconclusive, and the role of the Merkel cell is currently uncertain. Recordings from these sensory fibers have shown that Merkel endings are slowly adapting mechanoreceptors.

Meissner corpuscles are elongated, encapsulated endings in the dermal papillae of hairless skin just beneath the epidermis, oriented with their long axis perpendicular to the surface of the skin (Fig. 9-8). The encapsulation consists of a thin outer capsule and a layered stack of Schwann cells within the capsule, with the Schwann cells oriented perpendicular to the long axis of the capsule (like a stack of pancakes). One or more myelinated fibers approach the base of the corpuscle, lose their myelin, and wind back and forth between the stacked cells within the capsule. These are rapidly adapting receptors, and it is assumed that the capsule and the layered Schwann cells within it are important in determining the degree of adaptation. Vertical pressure on a dermal papilla compresses the nerve endings between the stacked capsular cells of a Meissner corpuscle, whereas pressure on a neighboring papilla is not nearly so effective. Meissner corpuscles are abundant in the skin of fingertips, and they, along with Merkel endings, are largely responsible for our ability to perform fine tactile discriminations with our fingertips (Fig. 9-9; see also Fig. 9-18). Most animals have their own species-specific patterns of distribution of receptors, with specializations in functionally important parts of the body. Rats and cats have elaborate arrays of receptors surrounding their whiskers and large areas of somatosensory cortex devoted to their whiskers. Elephants mind their trunks. Other animals have other patterns (Box 9-1).

Pacinian corpuscles are almost as widespread as free nerve endings. They are found subcutaneously over the entire body and in numerous other connective tissue sites. They are wrapped in the ultimate expression of a layered capsule and look like an onion in cross section (see Fig. 9-8). The capsule consists of many concentric layers of very thin epithelial cells, with fluid spaces between adjacent layers. Pacinian corpuscles are also rapidly adapting, and in this case the role of the capsule

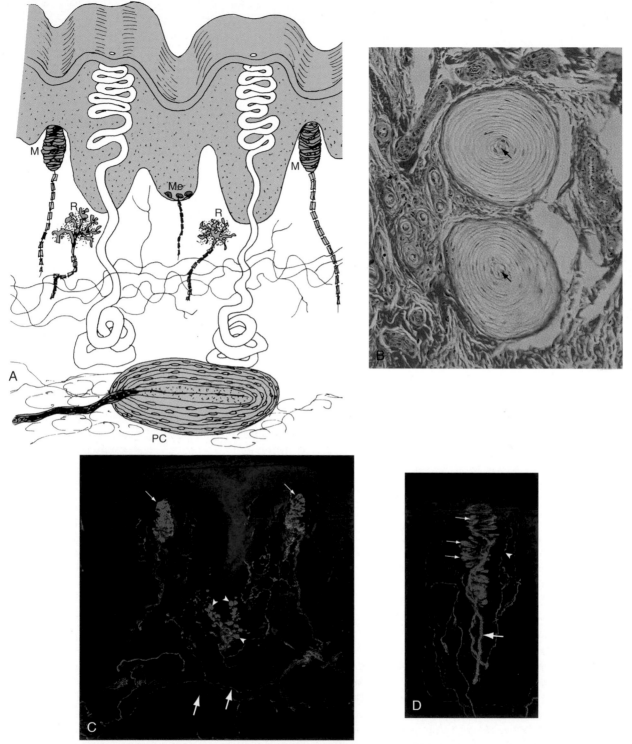

Figure 9-8 Some of the sensory endings found in glabrous skin. **A,** Schematic overview. M, Meissner corpuscle; Me, Merkel cell; PC, Pacinian corpuscle; R, Ruffini ending. **B,** Light micrograph of two Pacinian corpuscles from monkey skin, sectioned transversely. Multiple thin layers of each capsule surround a central mechanosensitive ending *(arrows)*. **C,** Section of biopsied skin from a human fingertip, stained to show epidermis (blue fluorescence), myelin (red fluorescence), and nerve fibers (green fluorescence). Myelinated and unmyelinated axons course horizontally in a dermal plexus *(thick arrows)*, giving off branches that end in Meissner corpuscles *(thin arrows)* and as Merkel endings (arrowheads). **D,** Higher-magnification view of a human Meissner corpuscle (actual size about 30 × 80 μm), stained as in **C.** A myelinated axon *(thick arrow)* enters the corpuscle, loses its myelin, and winds back and forth *(thin arrows)* between the stacked Schwann cells. Other unmyelinated fibers *(arrowhead)* head off into the epidermis to form free nerve endings. *(**B,** courtesy Dr. Nathaniel T. McMullen, University of Arizona College of Medicine. **C** and **D,** courtesy Dr. Maria Nolano, Salvatore Maugeri Foundation, Terme, Italy.)*

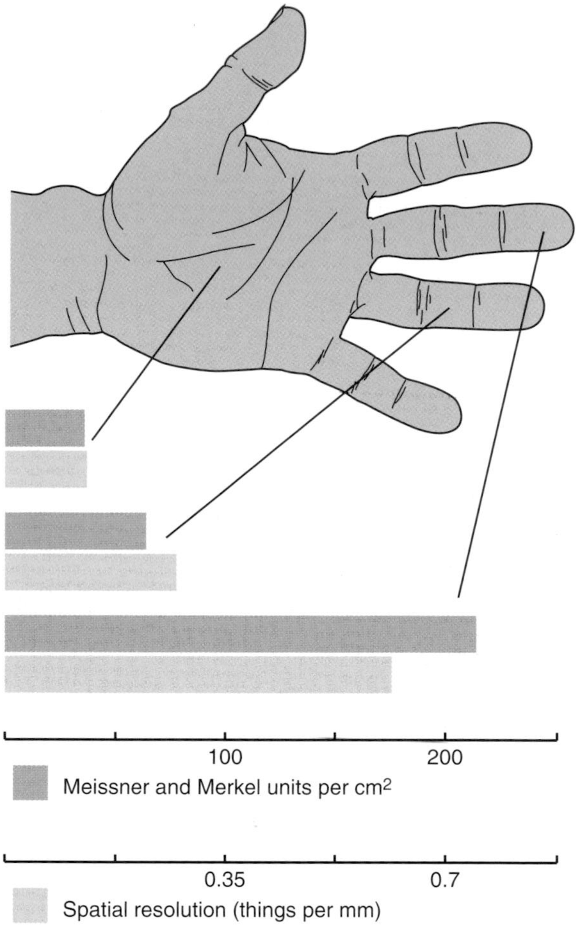

Figure 9-9 Correlation of spatial resolution and number of cutaneous receptors in different areas of the human hand. Spatial resolution (the reciprocal of the two-point discrimination threshold) was determined in psychophysical experiments by touching humans with two points and determining the minimum separation needed for them to be recognized as two separate points; this separation is less than 2 mm for fingertips but more than 8 mm for the palm of the hand. Correspondingly, there are many more Meissner corpuscles and Merkel endings per square centimeter in the fingertips than in the palm. *(Modified from Vallbo ÅB, Johansson RS: Hum Neurobiol 3:3, 1984.)*

is understood. Quickly applied forces are transmitted through the interior of the capsule and reach the ending, but maintained forces are not, as a result of the elastic properties of the capsular layers. During maintained pressure, each successive layer is slightly less deformed than its outer neighbor—imagine indenting the outermost of a series of balloons, one inflated inside another—and the ending itself is not deformed at all. These corpuscles are amazingly sensitive: much like the Merkel endings, they can respond to skin indentations as small as 1 μm.

Because Pacinian corpuscles are probably the most rapidly adapting receptors we have, they are poor receptors for pressure but good ones for the rapidly changing mechanical stimulation that we perceive as vibration. That is, a vibratory stimulus causes a steady train of

A Remarkable Somatosensory Specialization: *The Snout of the Star-Nosed Mole*

Star-nosed moles (*Condylura cristata*, Fig. 9-10A) live beneath the surface of wetlands, burrowing through the mud with large, powerful forelimbs, searching for worms and insects. Vision is not very useful in a dark environment such as this, and these moles have relatively tiny eyes. Instead, they find their prey with the help of one of the most remarkable sets of somatosensory appendages ever described. Each nostril is surrounded by a series of 11 rays (Fig. 9-10B) that are moved backward and forward as rapidly as 10 times a second as the mole searches for food. The surface of each ray is paved with a series of papillae (Fig. 9-10C and D), each about 40 μm across.

The function of these rays was a mystery for a long time. Logically, one might have suspected that they are somehow related to the sense of smell or taste, but in fact they are largely or totally devoted to somatic sensation. Each ray in cross section (Fig. 9-11A) contains a large central nerve from which smaller nerve bundles leave to innervate receptor complexes called *Eimer's organs* that underlie each of the surface papillae. Each Eimer's organ (Fig. 9-11B to E) contains an elaborate array of free nerve endings, a Merkel cell–Merkel ending complex, and an associated Pacinian-like corpuscle. The most superficial of the free nerve endings is a mere 5 μm from the mole's surface.

The numbers of Eimer's organs and the accompanying innervation density are extraordinary. The 11 rays surrounding each nostril contain a total of about 13,000 Eimer's organs, innervated by more than 50,000 nerve fibers. By comparison, a human hand, with its very highly developed somatosensory capabilities, is innervated by about 17,000 somatosensory nerve fibers. The obvious functional implication is that star-nosed moles are probably capable of amazingly subtle somatosensory discriminations, although this has not yet been tested rigorously. Certainly they devote a large proportion of their cortical processing power to these rays (see Fig. 22-11).

impulses from such an ending, so that in this sense, the receptor is "slowly adapting." It is important to understand that slowly adapting receptors, as they are conventionally defined, are simply receptors that respond best to *unchanging* stimuli. Rapidly adapting receptors, in contrast, respond best to *changing* stimuli, giving a constant output to a stimulus with constant velocity, constant acceleration, or some other temporal property.

The fifth type of cutaneous mechanoreceptor is an encapsulated receptor called a **Ruffini ending,** which

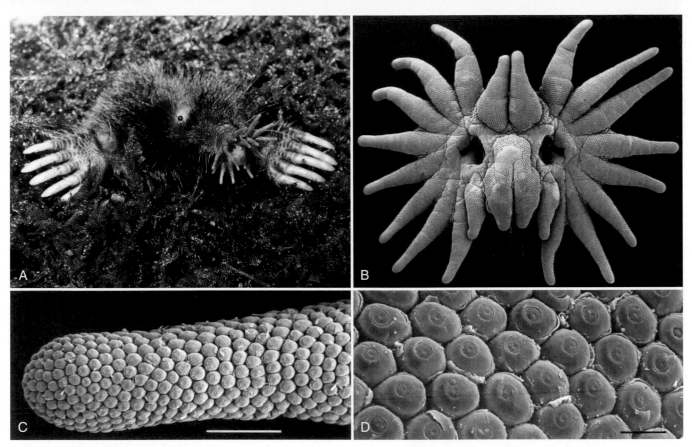

Figure 9-10 Surface anatomy of the star-nosed mole. **A,** A mole peering out from its burrow. **B** to **D,** Scanning electron micrographs at successively higher magnifications of the rays surrounding the nose. The scale marks in **C** and **D** are 250 µm and 50 µm, respectively. (**A, C,** and **D,** courtesy Dr. Kenneth C. Catania, Vanderbilt University. **B,** from Catania KC: J Comp Neurol 351:536, 1995.)

is widespread in the dermis and in subcutaneous and other connective tissue sites. It consists of a thin, cigar-shaped capsule traversed longitudinally by strands of collagenous connective tissue. A sensory fiber enters the capsule and branches profusely, so that many small processes are interspersed among the collagenous strands. This is a slowly adapting receptor and is thought to work by the squeezing of sensory terminals between strands of connective tissue when tension is applied to one or both ends of the capsule. Because collagen is not very elastic, the deformation of the endings is maintained as long as the tension is maintained, so adaptation is slow.

Nociceptors, Thermoreceptors, and Some Mechanoreceptors Have Free Nerve Endings

Nociceptors, thermoreceptors, and some mechanoreceptors are all free nerve endings; no pronounced morphological differences are seen among them with presently available techniques. Electrophysiological studies, however, have clearly differentiated among them. Some individual fibers respond selectively to gentle brushing, to cooling the skin, to warming it, or to stimuli that are perceived as painful. Unlike the majority of the sensory

receptors and their ability to adapt, nociceptors can become sensitized, resulting in more activity and relaying of pain information to the CNS. Most tissues also contain free nerve endings that normally respond poorly to essentially all stimuli but become sensitive after tissue damage or in disease states. Activation of these **silent** or **sleeping nociceptors** is thought to contribute to the pain accompanying inflammation and certain pathological processes.

The unmyelinated fibers that detect innocuous mechanical stimuli contribute little to perception of the details of such stimuli; instead, they work in the background to help generate a feeling of how pleasant they are (see Box 23-1). The temperature sensitivity of free nerve endings is the result of a series of closely related cation channels, each with a specific range of temperatures that increases its probability of opening (Fig. 9-12). Some respond to innocuous warming or cooling, others to painful heat and cold. Remarkably, the same channels have binding sites for various botanical molecules, leading to the warm and cool "taste" of chili peppers and menthol, respectively (see Chapter 13).

Some free nerve endings have axons that are small and thinly myelinated, whereas the axons of others are

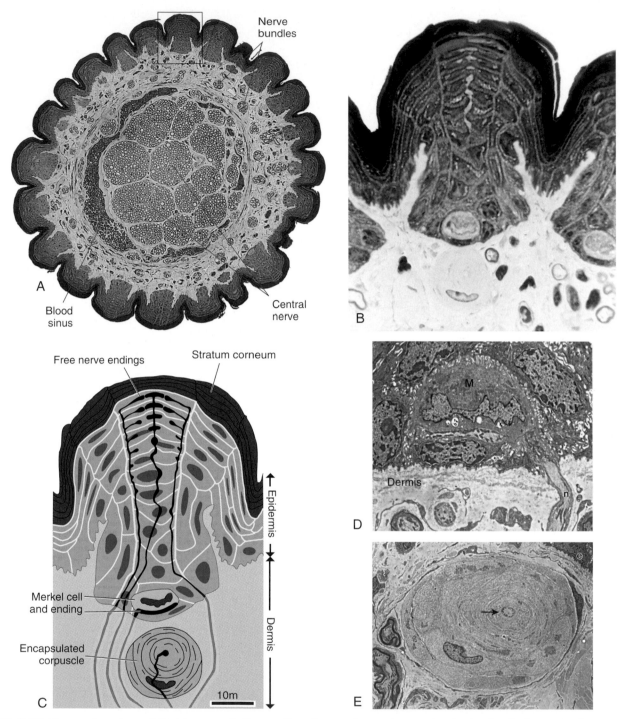

Figure 9-11 Microscopic anatomy of Eimer's organs. **A,** Cross section of one ray from a star-nosed mole, showing the large central nerve partially surrounded by a blood sinus. **B** and **C,** An Eimer's organ such as that outlined in **A** is enlarged **(B),** and its components are indicated schematically **(C).** **D,** Electron micrograph of an Eimer's organ Merkel cell (M) and the neural process (n) that innervates it. **E,** Electron micrograph of an Eimer's organ Pacinian-like corpuscle and the neural process *(arrow)* that innervates it. e, epidermal cell column at the core of the Eimer's organ. *(A and B, from Catania KC: J Comp Neurol, 351:536, 1995. **C** to **E,** from Catania KC: J Comp Neurol 365:343, 1996.)*

very small and unmyelinated. Each of these groups of free nerve endings includes some nociceptors, whose business it is to detect stimuli that have damaged tissue or threaten to do so. The adequate stimuli of nociceptors as a group include intense mechanical stimuli (e.g., pinching or cutting), noxious levels of heat or cold, and an assortment of chemicals released by damaged tissues. Individual nociceptors may respond preferentially to stimuli from just one or two of these categories, but some, referred to as **polymodal nociceptors,** respond to all three (using multiple sets of transduction molecules coexisting in single receptive endings). Polymodal

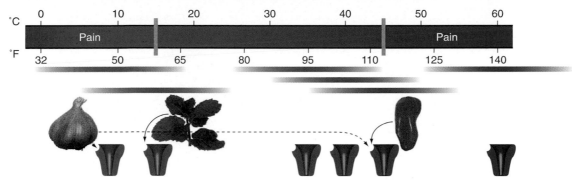

Figure 9-12 The six currently known types of temperature-sensitive channels, the range of temperatures that causes each to open, and a few examples of plants whose extracts also cause them to open. Capsaicin, the active ingredient in chili peppers, binds to the same channel that is activated by moderately painful heat, and the menthol in mint binds to a cold-sensitive channel. (The pungency of garlic seems to be at odds with garlic extracts binding to the channel that responds to painful cold; however, the same extracts may also weakly activate capsaicin-sensitive channels.)

nociceptors are relatively common among the free nerve endings with unmyelinated axons (which conduct very slowly), whereas free nerve endings with thinly myelinated axons typically are more selective.

Corresponding to the two different size classes of axons carrying nociceptive information, pain is perceived in two different stages. Most of us have verified this in unintentional experiments on ourselves. If a painful stimulus is applied abruptly—you hit your thumb with a hammer, for example—there is an initial sensation of sharp, pricking, well-localized pain (Ow!). This is followed by an aching, longer-lasting pain (Ohhh!). The initial sharp pain is carried by the more rapidly conducting, thinly myelinated fibers. For reasons explained later in the chapter, these are classified as Aδ fibers, so this phase is sometimes referred to as **delta pain** or **first pain.** The aching pain that follows (**slow pain**) is carried by the more slowly conducting, unmyelinated fibers referred to as C fibers. The many local chemicals that are released from the damaged tissue and blood vessels result in the on-going aching pain that activates these C fibers. This has been verified experimentally in human volunteers because it is possible to block different classes of nerve fibers selectively. Local anesthetics applied to peripheral nerves block unmyelinated fibers before myelinated fibers; during the period when only unmyelinated fibers are blocked, a pinprick is felt only as a sharp, brief pain. Externally applied pressure, however, blocks axons in order of size, so that myelinated fibers can be blocked while unmyelinated fibers continue to conduct. In this situation, most forms of tactile sensation disappear, and a pinprick is felt only as a dull, aching pain that is even more unpleasant than usual. The two forms of pain are processed differently within the CNS, so they may be dissociated at sites other than peripheral nerves. The aching pain due to chemicals activating unmyelinated C fibers can be attenuated by the common nonsteroidal anti-inflammatory drugs (NSAIDs) such as aspirin and ibuprofen. Understanding the nociceptors and the different types of pain can be of major clinical importance and is discussed further in subsequent chapters.

Nociceptors Have Both Afferent and Efferent Functions

All of us have had the experience of increased susceptibility to pain in injured areas of the body. Stimuli that are normally perceived as only mildly uncomfortable may become extremely painful (**hyperalgesia,** from the Greek for "excessive pain"); even normally innocuous stimuli, such as a light touch, may be painful (**allodynia,** from the Greek for "pain from something else"). Common examples include the hyperalgesia of sunburned skin, in which a friendly slap on the back becomes excruciatingly painful, and the allodynia of a sore throat, in which simply swallowing (normally nonpainful) is painful.

Some types and aspects of hyperalgesia and allodynia involve changes within the CNS, but others are mediated by events near the receptive endings themselves. Tissue injury sets in motion an array of processes collectively designed to heal and remove the injury—debris, appropriate cells proliferate, and repairs are made. Some of the signals that induce these processes come directly from the nociceptive endings in the area of injury. One well-studied example is the response to localized skin damage, such as a small burn (Fig. 9-13). Chemicals released in the damaged tissue, including K$^+$ ions from injured cells, serotonin from platelets, and assorted proteins (e.g., bradykinin, histamine) from multiple sources, **sensitize** nociceptive endings in the damaged skin, producing hyperalgesia. In addition, the area surrounding the burn becomes red (flare) and swollen (edema). The flare and edema are produced locally by an **axon reflex** that involves branches of the same nociceptors signaling pain from the injured area (see Fig. 9-13), in the only known example of a reflex that does not involve at least one synapse in the CNS. Nociceptors, like other primary afferents, release glutamate from their central terminals onto second-order neurons in the CNS, and many of them also release one or more neuropeptides at these

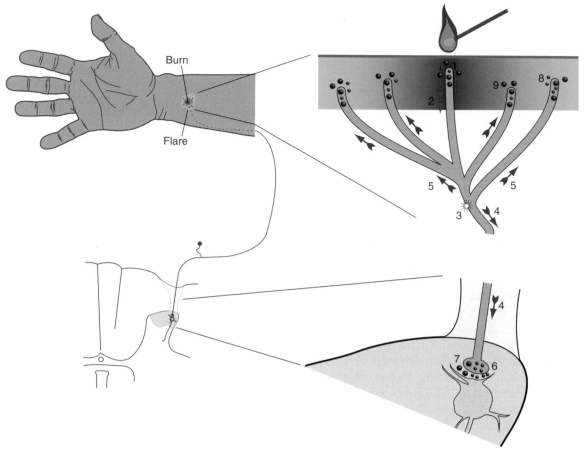

Figure 9-13 Production of flare and edema by axon reflexes. Injuring a localized area of skin (1) causes a receptor potential in nociceptive endings located there (2). If the receptor potential depolarizes the receptor's trigger zone (3) to threshold, action potentials travel in both directions, propagating toward the spinal cord (4) and spreading distally into nearby branches of the same nociceptor (5). Impulses reaching the spinal cord cause the release of glutamate (6) and neuropeptides (7) onto second-order neurons. Impulses spreading into sensory endings also cause the peripheral release of glutamate (8) and neuropeptides (9). Thus two different branches of a single neuron form the afferent and efferent limbs of the axon reflex circuit. The neuropeptides are vasoactive and cause flare and edema; the effects of peripherally released glutamate are less well understood.

synapses. Unlike other primary afferents,[d] however, nociceptors release the same neurotransmitters from their sensory endings in response to depolarization there. Hence action potentials initiated by a painful stimulus travel both centrally, toward the spinal cord or brainstem, and peripherally, invading branches of the same neuron outside the area of injury. Neuropeptides released peripherally cause dilation of arterioles (flare), leakage of plasma from venules (edema), and a host of wound-healing activities such as proliferation of skin cells and attraction of phagocytes. Nociceptive endings also contain glutamate receptors, and glutamate released peripherally may play a role in sensitization. At the same time, reorganization of the synaptic connections of noci-

ceptors in the spinal cord leads to increased pain sensitivity in areas surrounding the injury.

Pain Serves Useful Functions

Most people think that freedom from pain would be a terrific condition. However, pain has useful functions, such as warning us of damage and encouraging us to protect injured parts of the body; its absence is actually a handicap. Some rare individuals are born unable to feel pain. They characteristically have many injuries that heal poorly or remain unhealed. They may fracture bones without realizing it, have mutilated fingers and toes, or incur serious burns. The deficit may involve only the sensation of pain, but sometimes autonomic functions and other forms of sensation are involved as well. The condition takes several different forms and is often classified as congenital insensitivity to pain. Some patients have a selective loss of unmyelinated sensory fibers in their peripheral nerves; others have apparently normal nerves, so in these cases the disorder is often at

---

[d]This may not be strictly true. The sensory endings of muscle stretch receptors and at least some other mechanoreceptors have metabotropic glutamate receptors and release glutamate in response to stimulation. Little is known, however, about the normal role of this glutamate release.

a molecular level in nociceptors in which they lack a receptor to detect pain or an ion channel necessary to conduct action potentials in nociceptors.

Cutaneous Receptors Are Not Distributed Uniformly

The skin is often thought of as a uniform sensory surface varying in hairiness but basically uniform in sensitivity. This is far from true, however; some areas (e.g., the lips and fingertips) are much more densely innervated than other areas (e.g., the back). More densely innervated areas can subserve subtler tactile discrimination than less densely innervated areas because of the close packing of receptors. One way this capability can be measured is in terms of **two-point discrimination,** which refers to the minimum distance by which two stimuli can be separated and still be perceived as two stimuli. This minimum distance is less than 2 mm for the fingertips (see Fig. 9-9) but several centimeters for the back. Corresponding to this two-point discrimination ability is the capacity to localize a single stimulus accurately. We can easily detect the movement of a stimulus from one ridge to the next on a fingertip, but we are not nearly so accurate for stimuli delivered to the back of the thigh. The brain generally does a very good job of keeping us unaware of this and many other limitations in our ability to localize stimuli (Box 9-2).

Even though acuity is better in some areas than in others, many of us still tend to consider the skin a uniform sensory surface because we think we can detect the occurrence of a stimulus anywhere on it. This too is inaccurate, because receptors are discrete entities whose zones of termination in the skin may not overlap. For example, temperature sensitivity is distributed like polka dots across the skin (more densely in some areas than in others). A fine, cold probe touched to an appropriate spot on the skin elicits a sensation of coolness. The same probe touched to the skin between cold-sensitive spots may elicit only a sensation of touch. Because the skin is more or less densely innervated everywhere, there are probably no places that are insensitive to all stimuli, but a given small location is likely to be most sensitive to a particular *type* of stimulus. In real life, we are usually not stimulated by fine probes, so we are not aware that sensitivity is distributed across the skin in small, selective spots.

Receptors in Muscles and Joints Detect Muscle Status and Limb Position

Muscle, like other tissues, receives an abundant supply of free nerve endings. The function of these endings is largely unknown, but some are undoubtedly involved in muscle pain, whereas others may be chemoreceptors responsive to changes in extracellular fluid composition during muscle activity. Muscles are also supplied with two important types of encapsulated receptors: **muscle**

BOX 9-2

Perceptual Illusions: *The Nervous System Getting Fooled**

Subjectively, we usually feel as though our sensory receptors, in collaboration with the CNS, present us with a precisely accurate report of the nature, location, and intensity of stimuli. In fact, however, the nervous system economizes on receptors and neural processing, collecting only the most important subset of the data that would be required to be 100% accurate and then making an "educated guess" about the stimulus. A consequence is that the nervous system can be fooled by stimuli of certain configurations: we may misinterpret the nature, the location, or even the existence or nonexistence of a stimulus. One well-known example is our lack of awareness of the blind spot in the visual field of each eye (see Fig. 17-10), but illusions occur in all other sensory systems as well.

The sense of taste provides another example. We perceive the taste of something we are eating as localized to that bit of food, although taste actually involves the stimulation of not only taste buds but also the olfactory epithelium and of somatosensory endings inside the mouth that signal the texture of the food (see Chapter 13). So even though soluble factors such as salt and sugar are distributed widely to taste buds in various parts of the tongue, and volatile substances from the same food stimulate olfactory receptors high in the nasal cavity, we localize the taste to the site at which the food touches the tongue.

Similarly, although we feel subjectively that we can localize thermal stimuli on the skin accurately, the nervous system actually localizes the touch and uses this information to decide the position of a thermal stimulus. This forms the basis of a striking somatosensory illusion described by Green in 1977,[†] which you can easily demonstrate to yourself. Take three similar coins, put two of them in a freezer, and leave one at room temperature. After a few minutes, set all three coins in a row on a table, with the room-temperature coin in the center. Now touch the two cold coins with your index and ring fingers while simultaneously touching the room-temperature coin with your middle finger. You will experience a very compelling illusion that the room-temperature coin is just as cold as the other two coins.

*Modified in part from Bartoshuk LM, Weiffenbach JM: Chemical senses and aging. In Schneider EL, Rowe JW, editors: Handbook of the biology of aging, ed 3, San Diego, 1990, Academic Press.
[†]Green BG: Perception and Psychophysics 22:331, 1977.

spindles, which are unique to muscle, and **Golgi tendon organs,** which are similar to Ruffini endings.

Muscle Spindles Detect Muscle Length

Muscle spindles (Fig. 9-14) are long, thin stretch receptors scattered throughout virtually every striated muscle in the body. These muscle spindles sense muscle length and proprioception ("one's own" perception). They are quite simple in principle, consisting of a few small muscle fibers with a capsule surrounding the middle third of the fibers. These fibers are called **intrafusal muscle fibers** (*fusus* is Latin for "spindle," so *intrafusal* means "inside the spindle"), in contrast to the ordinary **extrafusal muscle fibers** ("outside the spindle"). The ends of the intrafusal fibers are attached to extrafusal fibers, so whenever the muscle is stretched, the intrafusal fibers are also stretched. The central region of each intrafusal fiber has few myofilaments and is noncontractile, but it does have one or more sensory endings applied to it. When the muscle is stretched, the central part of the intrafusal fiber is stretched, mechanically sensitive channels are distorted, the resulting receptor potential spreads to a nearby trigger zone, and a train of impulses ensues at each sensory ending.

Numerous specializations occur in this simple basic organization, so that in fact the muscle spindle is the most complex of the somatosensory receptors. Only three of these specializations are described here; their overall effects are to make muscle spindles adjustable and to give them a dual function, with part of each spindle being particularly sensitive to the length of the muscle in a static sense, and part being particularly sensitive to the rate at which this length changes.

1. Intrafusal muscle fibers are of two types. All are multinucleated, and the central, noncontractile region contains the nuclei. In one type of intrafusal fiber, the nuclei are lined up single file; these are called **nuclear chain fibers.** In the other type, the nuclear region is broader, and the nuclei are arranged several abreast; these are called **nuclear bag fibers.** There are typically two or three nuclear bag fibers per spindle and about twice that many chain fibers, but these numbers are variable.
2. There are also two types of sensory ending in the muscle spindle. The first type, called the **primary ending,** is formed by a single, very large nerve fiber that enters the capsule and then branches, supplying every intrafusal fiber in a given spindle (although it innervates[e] the bag fibers more heavily than the chain fibers). Each branch wraps around the central region of an intrafusal fiber, frequently in a spiral fashion, so these are sometimes called **annulospiral endings.** The second type of ending is formed by a few smaller nerve fibers that branch and primarily innervate nuclear chain fibers on both sides of the primary ending. These are the **secondary endings,** which are

sometimes referred to as **flower-spray endings** because of their appearance. Primary endings are selectively sensitive to the onset of muscle stretch but discharge at a slower rate while the stretch is maintained (see Fig. 9-14). Secondary endings are less sensitive to the onset of stretch, but their discharge rate does not decline very much while the stretch is maintained.

3. Muscle spindles also receive a motor innervation. The large motor neurons that supply extrafusal muscle fibers are called **alpha motor neurons,** whereas the smaller ones supplying the contractile portions of intrafusal fibers are called **gamma motor neurons** (or **fusimotor neurons**). Intrafusal fibers are too small and too few to contribute to the strength of a muscle, and firing all the gamma motor neurons to a muscle does not generate significant force. The function of this motor innervation is discussed in conjunction with motor control systems (Chapter 18), but a simple example indicates one of the possibilities (Fig. 9-15). Consider a muscle spindle in the biceps, and suppose that this muscle is contracted. This relieves most or all of the tension on the nuclear region of the intrafusal fibers, so the sensory endings are quite insensitive to muscle stretch that starts from this contracted state. Suppose that, at the same time, the gamma motor neurons to that spindle fire. This causes the parts of each intrafusal fiber on both sides of the nuclear region to contract. This in turn generates some tension on the nuclear region and restores its sensitivity. Thus gamma motor neurons can regulate the sensitivity of a muscle spindle so that this sensitivity can be maintained during voluntary contractions. Not surprisingly, there are two types of gamma motor neurons, one of which preferentially ends on bag fibers, the other on chain fibers.

This is just one example of feedback control by the nervous system over its sensory pathways. Such control is very common; sometimes it occurs at the level of the receptor (as in this instance), and sometimes it occurs at relay nuclei, but it occurs at one or more locations in every sensory pathway.

Golgi Tendon Organs Detect Muscle Tension

Golgi tendon organs are spindle-shaped receptors found at the junctions between muscles and tendons. They are similar to Ruffini endings in their basic organization, consisting of interwoven collagen bundles surrounded by a thin capsule (Fig. 9-16). Large sensory fibers enter the capsule and branch into fine processes that are

---

[e]The word *innervate* means "to supply with nerve endings." The nerve endings can be sensory, as in the case of these stretch-sensitive endings, or motor, as in the endings made by motor neurons on muscle fibers.

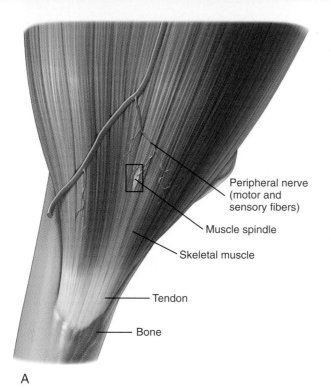

Peripheral nerve
(motor and
sensory fibers)

Muscle spindle

Skeletal muscle

Tendon

Bone

A

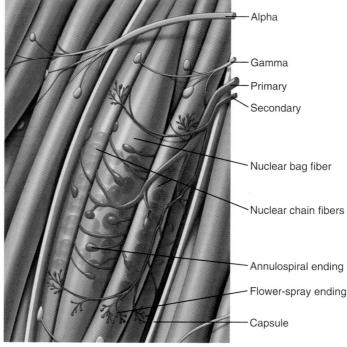

Alpha

Gamma

Primary

Secondary

Nuclear bag fiber

Nuclear chain fibers

Annulospiral ending

Flower-spray ending

Capsule

B

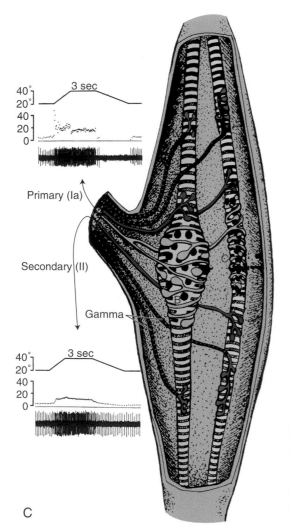

Primary (Ia)

Secondary (II)

Gamma

C

Figure 9-14 A, Diagram of a muscle spindle fiber found within the skeletal muscle that relays the sensory information of proprioception and the detection of muscle length. **B,** The intrafusal fibers of the spindle are of two types, the nuclear bag and nuclear chain fibers, both with sensory components in the middle of the fibers and contractile parts on the ends of the fibers. The nuclear bag fibers are innervated with primary (Ia) afferent fibers given the name annulospiral endings. The nuclear chain fibers may have some (Ia) afferent endings but are more abundantly innervated with primary (II) afferents given the name of flower-spray endings. The contractile parts of the intrafusal fibers are innervated by gamma motor neurons that will maintain the length of the sensory component. **C,** The upper and lower insets show the response properties of axons from primary and secondary in human finger extensors, stretched by passive bending at the metacarpophalangeal joint angle, the lower trace shows the actual potentials recorded. (**C,** *Drawing, modified from Warwick R, Williams PL, editors: Gray's anatomy, Br ed 35, Philadelphia, 1975, WB Saunders. Insets, from Edin BB, Vallbo ÅB: J Neurophysiol 63:1297, 1990.*)

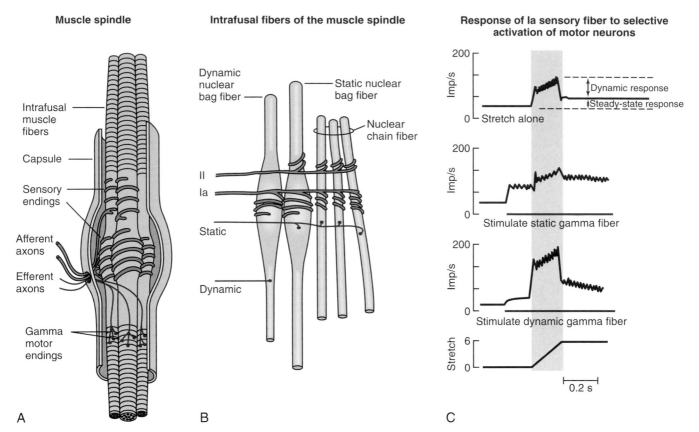

Figure 9-15 A, The main components of the muscle spindle are intrafusal muscle fibers, afferent sensory fiber endings, and efferent motor fiber endings. The intrafusal fibers are specialized muscle fibers; their central regions are not contractile. The sensory fiber endings spiral around the central regions of the intrafusal fibers and are responsive to stretch of these fibers. Gamma motor neurons innervate the contractile polar regions of the intrafusal fibers. Contraction of the intrafusal fibers pulls on the central regions from both ends and changes the sensitivity of the sensory fiber endings to stretch. **B,** The muscle spindle contains three types of intrafusal fibers: dynamic nuclear bag, static nuclear bag, and nuclear chain fibers. A single Ia sensory fiber innervates all three types of fibers, forming a primary sensory ending. A group II sensory fiber innervates nuclear chain fibers and static bag fibers, forming a secondary sensory ending. Two types of motor neurons innervate different intrafusal fibers. Dynamic gamma motor neurons innervate only dynamic bag fibers; static gamma motor neurons innervate various combinations of chain and static bag fibers. **C,** Selective stimulation of the two types of gamma motor neurons has different effects on the firing of the primary sensory endings in the spindle (the Ia fibers). Without gamma stimulation the Ia fiber shows a small dynamic response to muscle stretch and a modest increase in steady-state firing. When a static gamma motor neuron is stimulated the steady-state response of the Ia fiber increases but there is a decrease in the dynamic response. When a dynamic gamma motor neuron is stimulated, the dynamic response of the Ia fiber is markedly enhanced but the steady-state response gradually returns to its original level. *(Republished with permission from Kandel E et al: Principles of neural science, 5e, New York, 2013, McGraw-Hill.)*

inserted among the collagen bundles. Tension on the capsule along its long axis squeezes these fine processes, and the resulting distortion stimulates them. As in the case of Ruffini endings, these are slowly adapting receptors, because the collagen is nonelastic and the squeezing action is maintained as long as the tension is maintained.

For many years, Golgi tendon organs were studied physiologically by pulling on a tendon while recording from the sensory axon. When they are stimulated in this way, considerable force must be applied before a response is obtained, so it was thought that these are high-threshold receptors designed to inform the nervous system when muscle tension is reaching dangerous levels. However, the amount of tension actually applied to a tendon organ by such a stimulus is quite small: the muscle acts something like a rubber band attached to a

piece of string, and most of the tension is absorbed by the muscle. However, if tension is generated in a tendon by making its attached muscle contract, tendon organs are found to be much more sensitive and can actually respond to the contraction of just a few muscle fibers. Thus Golgi tendon organs very specifically monitor the tension generated by muscle contraction and come into play when fine adjustments in muscle tension need to be made (e.g., when handling a raw egg).

Thus the mode of action of Golgi tendon organs is quite different from that of muscle spindles (Fig. 9-17). If a muscle contracts isometrically, tension is generated across its tendons, and the tendon organs signal this; however, the muscle spindles signal nothing because muscle length has not changed (assuming that the activity of the gamma motor neurons remains unchanged). In contrast, a relaxed muscle can be stretched easily, and

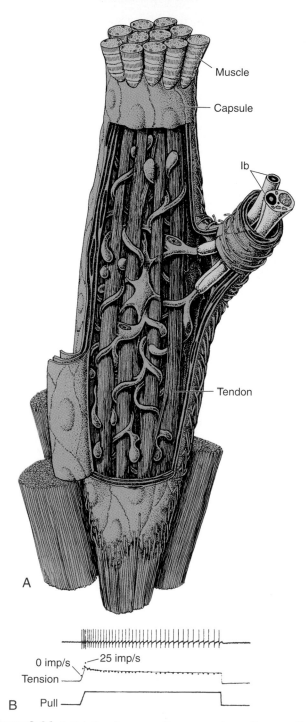

Muscle

Capsule

Ib

Tendon

A

0 imp/s   25 imp/s

Tension

B   Pull

Figure 9-16 A, Golgi tendon organ. One or more large-diameter afferent fibers enter a capsule around part of the myotendinous junction and then break up into many branches that interweave with bundles of collagen. **B,** Responses of a single afferent fiber from a Golgi tendon organ to a pull on the tendon that stretched it by 50 μm. The firing rate of the afferent, indicated by dots in the middle trace, closely tracks the tension developed in the tendon. (**A,** adapted from Krstić RV: General histology of the mammal, Berlin, 1985, Springer-Verlag. **B,** from Fukami Y, Wilkinson RS: J Physiol 265:673, 1977.)

the muscle spindles fire; the tendon organs, however, experience little tension and remain silent. A muscle, by virtue of these two types of receptors, can have its length and tension monitored simultaneously.

Joints Have Receptors

The receptors found in joints and their capsules are similar to some of those found in skin and muscle. In addition to the usual free nerve endings, there are endings equivalent to Golgi tendon organs in the ligaments and Ruffini endings and a few Pacinian corpuscles in joint capsules (Table 9-2). As might be expected from their morphology, a few joint receptors (presumably the Pacinian corpuscles) are rapidly adapting, but most are slowly adapting and respond to joint position and movement.

Muscle Spindles Are Important Proprioceptors

The identity of the receptors involved in position sense and kinesthesia (conscious awareness of movement) was a topic of debate for a long time. Muscle receptors play a major role, while joint and cutaneous receptors are of more limited importance in proprioception. If a local anesthetic is injected into the knee joint capsule of a human volunteer or into the skin of the knee, there is no loss of position sense or kinesthesia. However, if tendons of human volunteers are vibrated (through the skin), illusions of movement and altered perceptions of position are experienced at the joints where the muscles of these tendons act. A vibrating stimulus of moderate intensity should be ineffective at activating Golgi tendon organs, but it should activate muscle spindles. In particular, it should excite the primary endings because these are especially sensitive to changing stimuli. Hence it is thought that the muscle spindles but not the tendon organs are involved in these illusions and in our sense of limb position and movement. However, the tendon organs appear to contribute to our sense of the force exerted during a movement.

Visceral Structures Contain a Variety of Receptive Endings

Much less is known about visceral receptors than about the other types discussed in this chapter; they have been studied mostly in terms of their physiology and reflex effects. Most visceral receptors are supplied by thinly myelinated and unmyelinated fibers that terminate as free nerve endings with or without accessory structures, sometimes with complex branching patterns. Functionally, most of these receptors act at a subconscious level through visceral reflexes. They include (1) mechanoreceptors in the walls of hollow organs, such as the endings in the aortic arch and carotid sinus, which, when stimulated by increased arterial pressure, cause reflex vasodilation and decreased heart rate; (2) chemoreceptors, which when stimulated directly by changes in blood gases or pH (or indirectly by chemosensory cells in places such as the carotid body), cause compensating cardiovascular and respiratory changes; and (3) nociceptors, which can cause severe pain when stimulated, such as by distention of an organ or its capsule (some are silent nociceptors, sensitive only when an organ is inflamed or diseased). In some instances a single

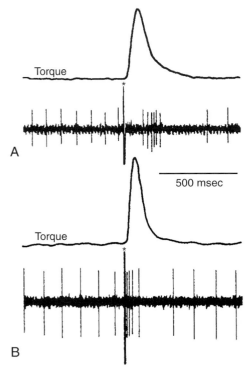

Figure 9-17 Responses of single afferents from a muscle spindle **(A)** and a Golgi tendon organ **(B)** in a human finger extensor to an electrically elicited twitch of the muscle. The spindle afferent stops firing as the muscle contracts and shortens, then fires a burst of action potentials as the muscle relaxes and lengthens. In contrast, the tendon organ afferent fires faster as the muscle contracts and increases tension on the tendon, then falls silent as the muscle relaxes and tension diminishes. The asterisk above each trace indicates the time of the shock that elicited the contraction. *(From Edin BB, Vallbo ÅB: Acta Physiol Scand 131:129, 1987.)*

visceral receptor may be able to serve as a mechanoreceptor at low discharge frequencies and a nociceptor at higher frequencies.

Particular Sensations Are Sometimes Related to Particular Receptor Types

Because we have a variety of morphologically distinct types of receptors, it was widely assumed in the past that different types are uniquely responsible for particular sensations. Certainly, the photoreceptor cells of the retina and the hair cells of the cochlea unequivocally form the basis of vision and hearing. This kind of association is true in a very general way for somatic sensation, which has been shown perhaps most elegantly in microneurography experiments on human volunteers. By recording from single nerve fibers innervating Meissner corpuscles of the fingertip, it has been found that a tiny mechanical indentation of a few micrometers, just enough to cause a single action potential in one nerve fiber, can give rise to the perception of touch. Conversely, stimulation of a fiber electrically, without touching the fingertip, also gives rise to the perception of touch. Because Meissner corpuscles are rapidly adapting, a continuous train of impulses would be expected to signify repeated touches—and subjects do in fact report a sensation of repeated, gentle tapping. In contrast, stimulation of a fiber associated with a slowly adapting Merkel ending gives rise to a sensation of maintained pressure. A train of impulses in the axon from a Pacinian corpuscle, which is very rapidly adapting, is interpreted as vibration. Some receptor types are well suited for detecting fine spatial details of tactile stimuli, whereas others are not (Fig. 9-18).

However, thinking of somatic sensation in terms of a unique, one-to-one pairing of specific receptor types and specific sensations is an oversimplification. First, there are counterexamples in which a single receptor type signals different types of stimulation, depending on the location of the receptor. For example, Ruffini endings

Table 9-2	Principal Types of Somatosensory Receptors Found in Various Tissues*		
	Free Nerve Endings With Accessory Structures	**Receptors With Layered Capsules**	**Receptors With Thin Capsules**
Hairy skin	Endings around hairs Merkel endings	Pacinian corpuscles	Ruffini endings
Glabrous skin	Merkel endings	Pacinian corpuscles Meissner corpuscles	Ruffini endings
Muscle, tendon			Muscle spindles Golgi tendon organs
Joints		Pacinian corpuscles	Ruffini endings Golgi endings

*Free nerve endings are not included because they are ubiquitous.

array of receptors is important in determining the resulting sensation. Here again, Ruffini endings provide an instructive example. Whereas touching the skin overlying a Ruffini ending causes its axon to discharge, stimulating the same axon selectively in microneurography experiments causes no sensation at all. Presumably, because any naturally occurring touch stimulates many afferents in addition to the Ruffini ending, the CNS is unable to interpret isolated activity in the latter. Similarly, causing unmyelinated nociceptors to fire in response to chemical irritants produces a sensation of pain; causing the same firing rate with mechanical stimuli (and simultaneously exciting myelinated mechanoreceptor fibers) may produce only a sensation of firm pressure. The CNS thus seems to survey all the information coming in from a given area of the body before deciding on the probable nature of a stimulus.

Peripheral Nerves Convey Information To and From the CNS

The nerve fibers innervating the receptors described thus far have their cell bodies in dorsal root ganglia adjacent to the spinal cord or, in the case of those reporting from the head, in various cranial nerve ganglia near the brainstem. The central process of each of these ganglion cells enters the CNS. Each peripheral process joins motor axons emerging from the spinal cord (or brainstem) to form spinal nerves (or cranial nerves). The formal boundary between the central and peripheral nervous systems occurs as fibers enter or leave the spinal cord or brainstem, at the point where the myelinating cells change from oligodendrocytes to Schwann cells; for now, however, we consider only those portions distal to the sensory ganglia (i.e., the wrappings and contents of spinal and cranial nerves). Some aspects of the sensory ganglia and of the sensory and motor roots of the spinal and cranial nerves are discussed in subsequent chapters.

Extensions of the Meninges Envelop Peripheral Nerves

Extensions of the meninges invest peripheral nerves with three connective tissue coverings (Fig. 9-19), each with a different function. From the outside layer in, these are the **epineurium,** the **perineurium,** and the **endoneurium** (Fig. 9-20).

The epineurium is a loose connective tissue sheath surrounding each peripheral nerve. Composed mainly of collagen and fibroblasts, it forms a substantial covering over nerve trunks, then thins to an incomplete layer around smaller branches near their terminations. The abundant longitudinally and spirally arranged collagen fibers of the epineurium are largely responsible for the

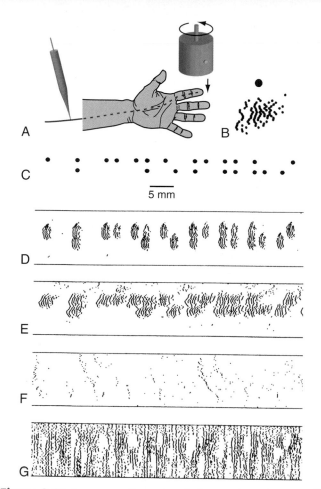

Figure 9-18 Responses of receptors in human fingertips to Braille characters. **A,** Recordings were made from single axons in the median nerve as a rotating drum swept embossed Braille characters across a fingertip. After each revolution the drum was advanced 200 μm, thereby slowly moving the Braille characters through the receptive field of the receptor whose responses were being recorded. **B,** Sample records from the fiber also shown in **E.** The upper dot indicates the size of one Braille dot relative to the size of the receptive field. Each dot in the lower swarm corresponds to a single action potential, and each horizontal row corresponds to a single revolution of the drum. **C,** An array of Braille characters swept across a fingertip while recording from an axon innervating a probable Merkel ending **(D),** Meissner corpuscle **(E),** Ruffini ending **(F),** and Pacinian corpuscle **(G).** Meissner corpuscles and especially Merkel endings are able to encode the spatial properties of the Braille characters, but Ruffini endings and Pacinian corpuscles are not. *(B to G, from Phillips JR, Johansson RS, Johnson KO: Exp Brain Res 81:589, 1990.)*

in the skin are activated by touch, but morphologically similar receptors in joint capsules are activated by changes in limb position. Another example involves free nerve endings. As noted previously, some of these respond best to temperature changes, others to mechanical stimuli, and still others to intense, tissue-damaging stimuli. Second, few situations dealing with mechanical stimuli such as touch and movement involve only one receptor type. The microneurography experiments just cited were performed under carefully controlled laboratory conditions, and it seems likely that under ordinary circumstances the overall pattern of activity in an

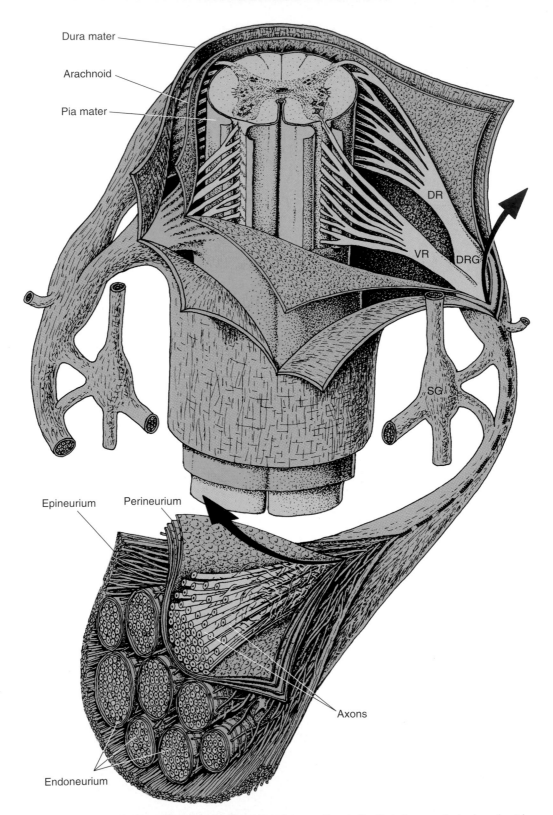

Dura mater

Arachnoid

Pia mater

DR

VR DRG

SG

Epineurium   Perineurium

Axons

Endoneurium

Figure 9-19 Continuity of spinal meninges and the sheaths of peripheral nerves. The continuity between spinal subarachnoid space and extracellular space within nerve fascicles is indicated by the *arrow* emerging from both the cut end of the nerve and the vicinity of a dorsal root ganglion (DRG). The pia mater is reflected from the exit zone of the ventral rootlets for clarity. DR, dorsal root; SG, sympathetic ganglion; VR, ventral root. *(Adapted from Krstić RV: General histology of the mammal, Berlin, 1985, Springer-Verlag.)*

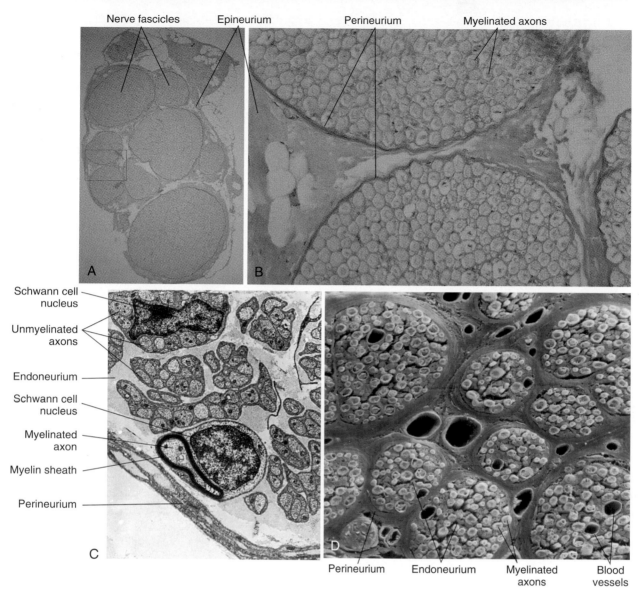

Figure 9-20 Wrappings of peripheral nerves. **A,** Light micrograph of a peripheral nerve, showing its several bundles (fascicles) of nerve fibers and its ensheathment by epineurium. **B,** The outlined area in **A** is enlarged, showing the perineurial sheath around nerve fascicles and the extension of epineurium between fascicles. **C,** Electron micrograph of part of one fascicle from another nerve, showing part of the perineurium surrounding myelinated and unmyelinated axons, and endoneurium between nerve fibers. **D,** Scanning electron micrograph of a freeze-fractured preparation of peripheral nerve. (**A** and **B,** courtesy Dr. Nathaniel T. McMullen, University of Arizona College of Medicine. **C,** from Moran DT, Rowley JC III: Visual histology, Philadelphia, 1988, Lea and Febiger. **D,** from Kessel RG, Kardon RH: Tissues and organs: a text-atlas of scanning electron microscopy, San Francisco, 1979, WH Freeman.)

considerable tensile strength of peripheral nerves. The epineurium is continuous centrally with the dura mater. Peripherally, it usually ends near the termination of a nerve fiber, but it also contributes to the capsule of some encapsulated endings.

The perineurium, continuous with the arachnoid and lying within the epineurium, is a layer of thin, concentrically arranged cells with interspersed collagen. Adjacent perineurial cells are connected to one another by tight junctions that effectively isolate the epineurial spaces from the endoneurial spaces around peripheral nerve fibers. In addition, the endothelial cells of capillaries within the perineurium are connected to one another by tight junctions. Thus functional equivalents of the arachnoid barrier and the blood-brain barrier persist in the peripheral nervous system (PNS) as a **blood-nerve barrier.** The perineurium continues as the capsule of many endings, including Pacinian and Meissner corpuscles, muscle spindles, and Golgi tendon organs. However, at other places, such as near neuromuscular junctions, the perineurium is open-ended, allowing the endoneurial space around nerve fibers to communicate with the general extracellular space of the body. This is of clinical importance because certain toxins (e.g., tetanus) and viruses (e.g., polio, herpes simplex) can gain access to the nervous system at these sites.

The endoneurium is the loose connective tissue within the perineurium, continuing into nerve fascicles and surrounding individual fibers. In at least some species, these individual endoneurial sheaths are compact enough that they may help direct the regrowth of nerve fibers after injury.

The Diameter of a Nerve Fiber Is Correlated With Its Function

Peripheral nerve fibers come in a wide range of diameters; some are myelinated, others are not. There is some correlation between the size of a fiber and its function, so it has proven useful to subdivide them. Unfortunately, there are two major classification systems, and neither is used universally for all fibers.

The first system is based on conduction velocity. Larger fibers conduct action potentials faster than do smaller fibers. If the compound action potential of a peripheral nerve—the summated action potentials generated by all the individual axons in the nerve—is recorded extracellularly at some distance from the site at which the nerve was stimulated electrically, the fast impulses reach the recording electrode before the slower ones. Conduction velocities (and axonal diameters) are not distributed in a bell-shaped curve but rather in a curve with several peaks. Therefore the remotely recorded compound action potential has several peaks corresponding to these favored conduction velocities. Three deflections can be easily demonstrated and have been named **A, B,** and **C.** The fibers responsible for the A deflection (the **A fibers**) are the myelinated sensory and motor fibers. **B fibers** are myelinated visceral fibers, both preganglionic autonomic fibers and some visceral afferents. **C fibers** are unmyelinated. The A deflection is complex and was subdivided into α, β, γ, and δ peaks (α being the fastest). Although the β and γ peaks as originally described were probably recording artifacts, the terminology has become established in the literature and is still commonly used. Thus **Aα** fibers are the largest and most rapidly conducting myelinated fibers, and **Aδ** are the smallest and slowest of the A group. The slowest conducting fibers of the body are the C fibers (Table 9-3).

The second classification system is based on direct microscopic measurement of axonal diameters. In this system myelinated fibers are categorized as group **I, II,** or **III** in order of decreasing size. Unmyelinated fibers are group **IV.**

Portions of both systems are still used (Fig. 9-21). Most commonly the letter system is used for myelinated efferent fibers and the roman numeral system for myelinated afferents. Unmyelinated fibers are usually referred to as *C fibers* but may be called *group IV.* The sizes, conduction velocities, and functional correlates involved in

---

Table 9-3 — **Classification of Peripheral Nerve Fibers**

Roman Numeral Classification	Diameter (mm)	Letter Classification	Conduction Velocity (m/sec)	Myelinated?	Structures Innervated
Ia*	12-20	—	70-120	Yes	Muscle spindle primary endings
Ib*	12-20	—	70-120	Yes	Golgi tendon organs
—	12-20	α	70-120	Yes	Efferents to extrafusal muscle fibers
II	6-12+	Aβ+	30-70	Yes	Other encapsulated endings and endings with accessory structures: Meissner corpuscles, Merkel endings, muscle spindle secondary endings, etc.
—	2-10	γ	10-50	Yes	Efferents to intrafusal muscle fibers
III	1-6	Aδ	5-30	Yes	Some nociceptors (sharp pain) Most cold receptors Most hair receptors Some visceral receptors
—	<3	B	3-15	Yes	Preganglionic autonomic efferents
IV	<1.5	C	0.5-2	No	Most nociceptors (dull, aching pain) Most warmth receptors Itch receptors Some touch receptors Some visceral receptors Postganglionic autonomic efferents

*Data from carefully studied peripheral nerves of cats. Muscle afferents in primates, including humans, probably conduct more slowly, up to only about 80 m/sec.

+Some afferents in nonmuscle nerves, particularly joint afferents, range up to 17 μm in diameter. Some investigators refer to these larger fibers, in the 12- to 17-μm range, as Aα and call those in the 6- to 12-μm range Aβ. Others refer to all nonmuscle afferents larger than 6 μm as Aβ.

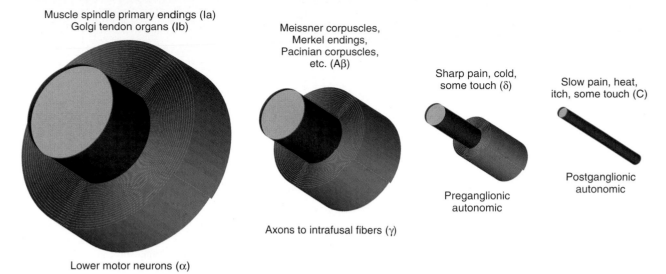

Muscle spindle primary endings (Ia)
Golgi tendon organs (Ib)

Meissner corpuscles,
Merkel endings,
Pacinian corpuscles,
etc. (Aβ)

Sharp pain, cold,
some touch (δ)

Slow pain, heat,
itch, some touch (C)

Postganglionic
autonomic

Preganglionic
autonomic

Axons to intrafusal fibers (γ)

Lower motor neurons (α)

Figure 9-21 Relative sizes of PNS axons and myelin sheaths. The major afferent functions or receptors associated with each size class are indicated above each one, along with commonly used terminology; major efferent functions and terminology are indicated below.

both systems are listed in Table 9-3 for reference purposes.

The commonly used terminology for efferent fibers is fairly simple. The large axons innervating the extrafusal fibers of skeletal muscle are in the Aα category, and the smaller axons innervating intrafusal muscle fibers are in the Aγ category. The "A" is commonly dropped, and these are simply called α and γ **motor neurons.** Preganglionic autonomic axons are usually called just that but are occasionally referred to as *B fibers.*

Myelinated afferents are slightly more complicated. The largest fibers, group I, are found only in muscle nerves; some form the primary endings of muscle spindles, and others innervate Golgi tendon organs. To distinguish between them, spindle primary fibers are called **Ia** and tendon organ fibers are called **Ib.** Group II, corresponding to Aβ fibers, is quite diverse and includes the fibers that form the secondary endings of muscle spindles and those that form all the encapsulated receptors of skin and joints. Group III consists of small myelinated afferents that form free nerve endings and includes mechanoreceptors, cold-sensitive thermoreceptors, and the nociceptors responsible for fast pain. Group III corresponds to Aδ, so these fibers are often referred to as δ **fibers.**

SUGGESTED READINGS

Allt G, Lawrenson JG: The blood-nerve barrier: enzymes, transporters and receptors—a comparison with the blood-brain barrier. Brain Res Bull 52:1, 2000.

Bewick GS, Reid B, Banks RW: Autogenic modulation of mechanoreceptor excitability by glutamate release from synaptic-like vesicles: evidence from the rat muscle spindle primary sensory ending. J Physiol 562:381, 2005.

Block SM: Biophysical principles of sensory transduction. In Corey DP, Roper SD, editors: Sensory transduction, New York, 1992, Rockefeller University Press.

An interesting discussion of the physical limits on the transduction process in sensory receptors.

Burgess PR, et al: Signaling of kinesthetic information by peripheral sensory receptors. Annu Rev Neurosci 5:171, 1982.

Caterina MJ, Gold MS, Meyer RA: Molecular biology of nociceptors. In Hunt S, Koltzenburg M, editors: The neurobiology of pain, Oxford, 2005, Oxford University Press.

Cervero F, Laird JMA: Understanding the signaling and transmission of visceral nociceptive events. J Neurobiol 61:45, 2004.

Cox JJ, et al: An SCN9A channelopathy causes congenital inability to experience pain. Nature 444:894, 2006.

Dhaka A, Viswanath V, Patapoutina A: TRP ion channels and temperature sensation. Annu Rev Neurosci 29:135, 2006.

Dow RR, Shinn SL, Ovalle WK, Jr: Ultrastructural study of a blood-muscle spindle barrier after systematic administration of horseradish peroxidase. Am J Anat 157:375, 1980.

Dyson C, Brindley GS: Strength-duration curves for the production of cutaneous pain by electrical stimuli. Clin Sci 30:237, 1966.

Direct production of both sharp, pricking pain and slow, burning pain by small electrical stimuli.

Gandevia SC, McCloskey DI: Joint sense, muscle sense, and their combination as position sense, measured at the distal interphalangeal joint of the middle finger. J Physiol 260:387, 1976.

Clever experiments taking advantage of an anatomical quirk of the middle finger. This finger can be positioned in such a way that muscles and their receptors are functionally disengaged from its terminal phalanx, so the position sense of the distal interphalangeal joint can be measured both with and without a contribution from muscle receptors.

Ghabriel MN, Jennings KH, Allt G: Diffusion barrier properties of the perineurium: an in vivo ionic lanthanum tracer study. Anat Embryol 180:237, 1989.

Goodwin GM, McCloskey DI, Matthews PBC: The contribution of muscle afferents to kinaesthesia shown by vibration induced illusions of movement and by the effects of paralysing joint afferents. Brain 95:705, 1972.

The paper that sparked the reinvestigation of the role of muscle spindles in our sense of position and movement. It contains a skeptical review of the earlier literature on this topic and several simple but interesting experiments.

Halata Z, Grim M, Baumann KI: Friedrich Sigmund Merkel and his Merkel cell, morphology, development, and physiology: review and new results. Anat Rec 271A:225, 2003.

Hallin RG, Torebjörk HE: Studies on cutaneous A and C fiber afferents, skin nerve blocks and perception. In Zotterman Y, editor: Sensory functions of the skin of primates, Elmsford, NY, 1976, Pergamon Press.

A description of experiments involving recording from the radial nerve; the experimenter notes afferent fiber activity in response to stimulation, and the experimentee reports his sensations, all during selective block of A fibers by pressure or of C fibers by a local anesthetic.

Houk J, Henneman E: Responses of Golgi tendon organs to active contraction of the soleus muscle of the cat. J Neurophysiol 30:466, 1967.

Experiments demonstrating that tendon organs are really highly sensitive receptors when responding to muscle contraction.

Hunt CC: Mammalian muscle spindle: peripheral mechanisms. Physiol Rev 70:643, 1990.

Iggo A: Sensory receptors in the skin of mammals and their sensory functions. Rev Neurol 141:599, 1985.

Jami L: Golgi tendon organs in mammalian skeletal muscle: functional properties and central actions. Physiol Rev 72:623, 1992.

Jänig W, Koltzenburg M: On the function of spinal primary afferent fibres supplying colon and urinary bladder. J Autonom Nerv Sys 30:S89, 1990.

Single receptors in cats that apparently can signal both normal fullness and painful distention.

Johnson KO, Yoshioka T, Vega-Bermudez F: Tactile functions of mechanoreceptive afferents innervating the hand. J Clin Neurophysiol 17:539, 2000.

A review of elegant experiments exploring the functions of Meissner, Merkel, Pacinian, and Ruffini endings.

Kenshalo DR, Gallegos ES: Multiple temperature-sensitive spots innervated by single nerve fibers. Science 158:1064, 1967.

Kinkelin I, Stucky CL, Koltzenburg M: Postnatal loss of Merkel cells, but not of slowly adapting mechanoreceptors in mice lacking the neurotrophin receptor p75. Eur J Neurosci 11:3963, 1999.

Relatively recent evidence that Merkel cells are not necessary for the mechanical sensitivity of Merkel endings.

Klede M, Handwerker HO, Schmelz M: Central origin of secondary mechanical hyperalgesia. J Neurophysiol 90:353, 2003.

Indications that flare arises from axon reflexes, but tenderness in areas surrounding an injury results from changes in the spinal cord.

Kruger L: The functional morphology of thin sensory axons: some principles and problems. In Kumazawa T, Kruger L, Mizumura K, editors: The polymodal nociceptor—a gateway to pathological pain, Amsterdam, 1996, Elsevier.

Data and speculations on the efferent roles of nociceptors.

Kucenas S, et al: CNS-derived glia ensheath peripheral nerves and mediate motor root development. Nature Neurosci 11:143, 2008.

Recent evidence that the perineurium may be formed, at least in part, by glial cells that migrate out from the CNS.

Landau W, Bishop GH: Pain from dermal, periosteal, and fascial endings and from inflammation: electrophysiological study employing differential nerve block. Arch Neurol Psychiatry 69:490, 1953.

The volunteers in this case were the authors themselves, who, with admirable fortitude, studied the effects of pressure blocks and local anesthetics on the pain caused by needles, bee stings, and other obnoxious stimuli.

Macefield G, Gandevia SC, Burke D: Conduction velocities of muscle and cutaneous afferents in the upper and lower limbs of human subjects. Brain 112:1519, 1989.

Evidence that human muscle afferents may not conduct as rapidly as those of cats and other experimental animals, and that they may be no faster than large-diameter cutaneous afferents.

Macpherson LJ, et al: The pungency of garlic: activation of TRPA1 and TRPV1 in response to allicin. Curr Biol 15:929, 2005.

TRPA1 is cold sensitive; TRPV1 is heat and capsaicin sensitive.

Mano T, Iwase S, Toma S: Microneurography as a tool in clinical neurophysiology to investigate peripheral neural traffic in humans. Clin Neurophysiol 117:2357, 2006.

McCloskey DI, et al: Sensory effects of pulling or vibrating exposed tendons in man. Brain 106:21, 1983.

Heroic experiments in which one of the investigators had the tendon of his own extensor hallucis longus transected and then pulled on.

McMahon SB, Koltzenburg M: Wall and Melzack's textbook of pain, ed 5, Edinburgh, 2005, Churchill Livingstone.

Munger BL, et al: A re-evaluation of the cytology of cat Pacinian corpuscles. I. The inner core and clefts. Cell Tissue Res 253:83, 1988.

Nagasako EM, Oaklander AL, Dworkin RH: Congenital insensitivity to pain: an update. Pain 101:213, 2003.

Nolano M, et al: Quantification of myelinated endings and mechanoreceptors in human digital skin. Ann Neurol 54:197, 2003.

A series of beautiful micrographs similar to those in Figure 9-8C and D.

Ochoa J, Torebjörk E: Sensations evoked by intraneural microstimulation of single mechanoreceptor units innervating the human hand. J Physiol 342:633, 1983.

Schmelz M, et al: Specific C-receptors for itch in human skin. J Neurosci 17:8003, 1997.

Schoultz TW, Swett JE: The fine structure of the Golgi tendon organ. J Neurocytol 1:1, 1972.

Shanthaveerappa TR, Bourne GH: Perineural epithelium: a new concept of its role in the integrity of the peripheral nervous system. Science 154:1464, 1966.

Torre V, et al: Transduction and adaptation in sensory receptor cells. J Neurosci 15:7757, 1995.

A nice discussion of unifying themes in the transduction mechanisms used by different kinds of receptors.

Vallbo ÅB, Johansson RS: Properties of cutaneous mechanoreceptors in the human hand related to touch sensation. Hum Neurobiol 3:3, 1984.

Good review of the properties of skin receptors, as determined by recordings from individual sensory axons of human volunteers.

Vallbo ÅB, et al: Somatosensory, proprioceptive, and sympathetic activity in human peripheral nerves. Physiol Rev 59:919, 1979.

Vallbo Å, et al: A system of unmyelinated afferents for innocuous mechanoreception in the human skin. Brain Res 628:301, 1993.

Van Hees J, Gybels J: C nociceptor activity in human nerve during painful and nonpainful skin stimulation. J Neurol Neurosurg Psychiatry 44:600, 1981.

Direct demonstration that a given level of activity in the axon of a nociceptor may be interpreted as pain in some situations but not in others.

Voets T, et al: Sensing with TRP channels. Nat Chem Biol 1:85, 2005.

A nice, succinct review of the role of this family of channels in temperature and other sensations.

Wessberg J, et al: Receptive field properties of unmyelinated tactile afferents in the human skin. J Neurophysiol 89:1567, 2003.

Zelená J: Nerves and mechanoreceptors, London, 1994, Chapman and Hall.

Zylka MJ, et al: Topographically distinct epidermal nociceptive circuits revealed by axonal tracers targeted to Mrgprd. Neuron 45:17, 2005.

Although C nociceptors are usually treated as a more or less uniform population, there may in fact be multiple types, each with its own chemical identity and pattern of connections.

Spinal Cord

The spinal cord is the traditional starting point for a detailed consideration of the central nervous system (CNS). It is a uniformly organized part of the CNS and one of the simplest (in a relative sense), but many principles of cord function also apply to other levels of the nervous system. At the same time, the spinal cord is extraordinarily important in the day-to-day activities we tend not to think about. In it reside all the motor neurons supplying the muscles we use to move our bodies around, as well as major populations of autonomic efferents. It also receives all the sensory input from the body and some from the head and performs the initial processing operations on most of this input.

The Spinal Cord Is Segmented

An adult human spinal cord appears surprisingly small on first inspection, being only about 42 to 45 cm long and about 1 cm in diameter at its widest point. It weighs only about 35 g, so one could be mailed for just two stamps. It is anatomically segmented—not obviously, like an earthworm, but in terms of the nerve roots attached to it (Fig. 10-1). A continuous series of **dorsal** (i.e., posterior) **rootlets** enter the cord in a shallow longitudinal groove (the **posterolateral sulcus**) on its posterolateral surface, and a continuous series of **ventral** (i.e., anterior) **rootlets** leaves from the poorly defined **anterolateral sulcus.** The dorsal and ventral rootlets from discrete sections of the cord coalesce to form **dorsal** and **ventral roots (also known as posterior and anterior roots, respectively),** which in turn join to form **spinal nerves** (Fig. 10-2). Each dorsal root bears a **dorsal root ganglion (also called spinal ganglion)** just proximal to the junction between dorsal and ventral roots; it contains the cell bodies of the primary sensory neurons whose processes travel through that particular spinal nerve. The dorsal root ganglia originate from the neural crest cells and have extensions into the periphery (a peripheral process) and a central process that grows back into the posterior aspect of the spinal cord to make connections with other neurons. A portion of the cord that gives rise to a spinal nerve constitutes a **segment.** There are 31 segments in a human

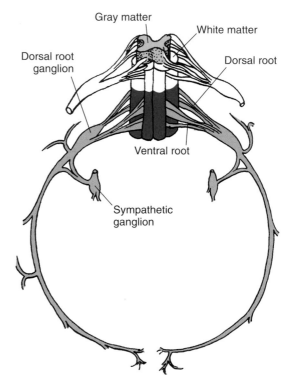

Figure 10-1 Segmentation of the spinal cord. The portion in color, giving rise to a single spinal nerve on each side, represents a single segment. *(From Mettler FA: Neuroanatomy, ed 2, St. Louis, 1948, Mosby.)*

spinal cord: 8 **cervical,** 12 **thoracic,** 5 **lumbar,** 5 **sacral,** and 1 **coccygeal.**

The spinal cord itself, stripped of its dorsal (posterior) and ventral (anterior) rootlets, gives no obvious sign of segmentation. Rather, it is a continuous column with two enlargements that ends caudally in the pointed **conus medullaris** (Fig. 10-3). The two enlargements occur in those regions of the cord that supply the upper and lower extremities and therefore contain increased numbers of motor neurons and interneurons. The limits of the enlargements are not distinct, but the **cervical enlargement,** which supplies the upper extremities, is conventionally considered to extend from the fifth cervical to the first thoracic segment (C5 to T1), inclusive. The **lumbar** (or **lumbosacral**) **enlargement,** which supplies the lower extremities, extends from the second lumbar to the third sacral segment (L2 to S3).

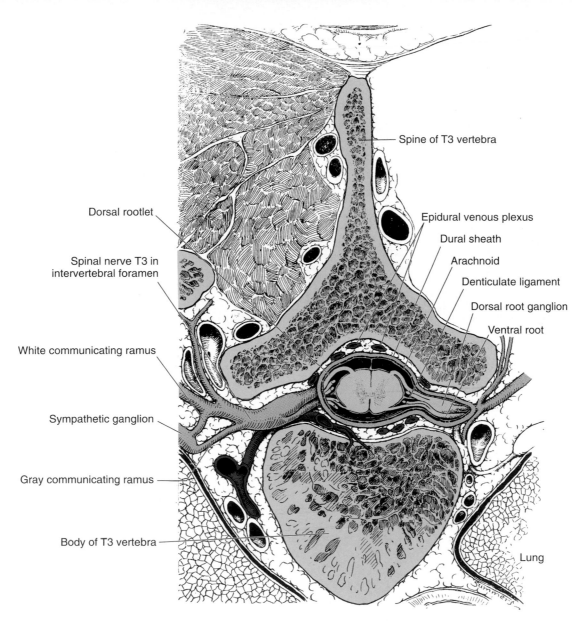

Figure 10-2 A section through the third thoracic vertebra and the spinal cord at that level, showing the relationship between the cord and surrounding vertebrae. *(From Mettler FA: Neuroanatomy, ed 2, St. Louis, 1948, Mosby.)*

Each Spinal Cord Segment Innervates a Dermatome

As the neural tube closes, the adjacent mesoderm also segments, here into a series of somites (see Fig. 2-3) that will give rise to skin, muscle, and bone. Each spinal nerve retains its relationship with a somite during development, with the result that spinal cord segments are related systematically to areas of skin, to muscles, and in some instances to bones (e.g., vertebrae). Hence each spinal nerve (except C1, which typically has only a rudimentary dorsal root) innervates a single **dermatome** (Fig. 10-4). This dermatomal arrangement is particularly apparent in the trunk, where pairs of dermatomes form bands that encircle the chest and abdomen; outgrowth

of limb buds during development makes the dermatomal arrangement somewhat more complex in the upper and lower extremities.[a] Similarly, the innervation of skeletal muscles is related systematically to spinal segments (Table 10-1).

Knowledge of the segmental innervation of muscles and cutaneous areas (Table 10-2) can be extremely helpful in diagnosing the site of damage in or near the

---

[a]Dermatomes are generally not demarcated from one another as abruptly as Figure 10-4 seems to indicate. When neighboring areas of skin are innervated by consecutive spinal segments (e.g., T6 and T7), the territories innervated by the two segments overlap considerably. However, when neighboring areas of skin are innervated by nonconsecutive segments (e.g., C4 and T2 dermatomes), the overlap between the two territories is limited.

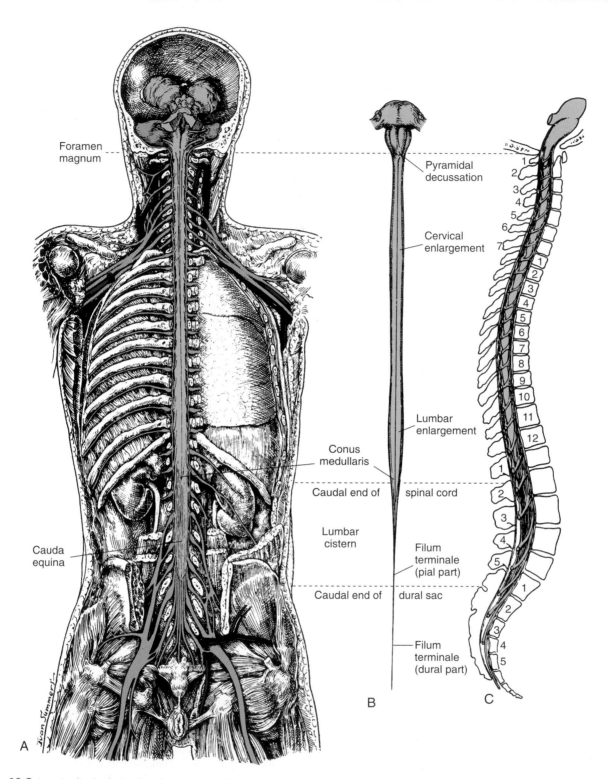

Foramen
magnum

Pyramidal
decussation

Cervical
enlargement

Lumbar
enlargement

Conus
medullaris

Caudal end of   spinal cord

Lumbar
cistern

Filum
terminale
(pial part)

Cauda
equina

Caudal end of   dural sac

Filum
terminale
(dural part)

A

B

C

Figure 10-3 Longitudinal relationships between spinal cord and vertebral column. **A,** Posterior surface of a spinal cord within a vertebral canal dissected from the back. **B,** How the anterior surface of the same spinal cord would look after removal of dura, arachnoid, and spinal nerves. **C,** Spinal cord exposed from the lateral direction, showing that the cord ends at about the L1-L2 level and spinal nerves travel progressively longer distances in the cauda equina to reach their exits from the vertebral canal. (See Video 10-1.) *(From Mettler FA: Neuroanatomy, ed 2, St. Louis, 1948, Mosby.)*

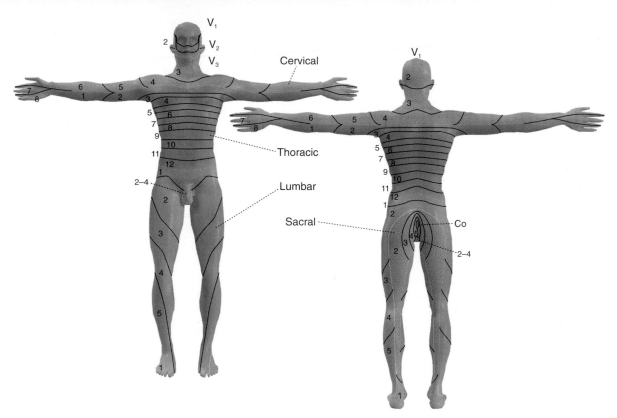

Figure 10-4 Cutaneous territories innervated by spinal nerves (dermatomes) and the trigeminal nerve (V₁, V₂, V₃). Co, coccygeal segment. *(Based on Bonica JJ: Applied anatomy relevant to pain. In Bonica JJ, editor: The management of pain, ed 2, Philadelphia, 1990, Lea & Febiger.)*

Table 10-1	Innervation of Major Muscles	
Movement	**Peripheral Nerve (Muscle)**	**Cord Segment***
Arm		
Abduction	Suprascapular (supraspinatus)	**C5**, C6
	Axillary (deltoid)	**C5**, C6
Elbow		
Flexion	Musculocutaneous (brachialis, biceps)	C5, **C6**
	Radial (brachioradialis)	C5, **C6**
Extension	Radial (triceps)	C6, **C7**, C8
Wrist		
Flexion	Median, ulnar	C6, **C7**, C8
Extension	Radial	C5, **C6, C7**, C8
Hand		
Finger movements	Median, radial, ulnar	C7, **C8**, T1
Thumb movements	Median, radial, ulnar	C7, **C8**, T1
Hip		
Flexion	Lumbar spinal nerves, femoral (iliopsoas)	L1, **L2**, L3
Extension	Inferior gluteal (gluteus maximus)	L5, **S1**, S2
Knee		
Flexion	Sciatic (hamstrings)	**L5, S1**, S2
Extension	Femoral (quadriceps)	L2, **L3, L4**
Ankle		
Dorsiflexion	Sciatic → peroneal (tibialis anterior)	**L4**, L5
Plantar flexion	Sciatic → tibial (gastrocnemius)	**S1**, S2

*Major segments indicated in **bold.**

Table 10-2	Dermatomal Levels of Clinical Importance*	
Cutaneous Area		**Cord Segment**
Upper arm (lateral surface)		C5
Thumb and lateral forearm		C6
Middle finger		C7
Little finger		C8
Nipple		T4
Umbilicus		T10
Big toe		L5
Heel		S1
Back of the thigh		S2

*See Figure 10-4 for additional details.

spinal cord. For example, compression of a dorsal root can cause pain in its dermatome, allowing pain caused by root compression to be differentiated from pain caused by peripheral nerve damage. In addition, the highest level of a sensory or motor deficit may allow deductions about the segmental level of a suspected spinal cord lesion (see Fig. 10-31).

The Spinal Cord Is Shorter Than the Vertebral Canal

The spinal cord approaches its adult length before the vertebral canal does. Until the third month of fetal life, both grow at about the same rate, and the cord fills the canal. Thereafter the body and the vertebral column grow faster than the spinal cord does, so that at the time of birth the spinal cord ends at the third lumbar vertebra. A small additional amount of differential growth in the vertebral column occurs subsequent to this, and by a few months of age the cord ends at about the level of the first lumbar vertebra. However, the spinal nerves still exit through the same intervertebral foramina as they did early in development, and each dorsal root ganglion remains at the level of the appropriate foramen. Proceeding from cervical to sacral levels, the dorsal and ventral roots become progressively longer because they have longer and longer distances to travel before reaching their sites of exit from the vertebral canal (see Fig. 10-3A). The **lumbar cistern,** from the end of the spinal cord at vertebral level L1-L2 to the end of the dural sheath at vertebral level S2, is filled with this collection of dorsal and ventral roots, collectively referred to as the **cauda equina** (Latin for "horse's tail"; Fig. 10-5E and F). Hence a needle carefully inserted into the lumbar cistern will pass harmlessly among nerve roots, allowing safe sampling of cerebrospinal fluid.

Each of the first seven cervical nerves leaves the vertebral canal *above* the corresponding vertebra; for instance, the first cervical nerve leaves between the occiput and the first cervical vertebra (the atlas), the second leaves between the first and second cervical vertebrae (the atlas and the axis), and so on. However, because there are only seven cervical vertebrae, the eighth cervical nerve leaves between the seventh cervical and first thoracic vertebrae, and each of the subsequent nerves leaves *below* the corresponding vertebra.

The meningeal coverings of the spinal cord are described in Chapter 4 (see Fig. 4-13). The cord is suspended within an arachnoid-lined dural tube by the denticulate ligaments (Fig. 10-6A), which are extensions of the pia-arachnoid, similar to but more substantial than arachnoid trabeculae. In addition, the caudal end of the cord is anchored to the end of the dural tube by the **filum terminale** (see Fig. 10-6B), an extension of the pial covering of the conus medullaris. The filum terminale then acquires a dural outer layer and in turn is anchored to the coccyx.

All Levels of the Spinal Cord Have a Similar Cross-Sectional Structure

In cross section the spinal cord consists of a roughly H-shaped area of gray matter that floats like a butterfly in a surround of white matter. The gray matter can be divided into **horns** and the white matter into **funiculi** (from the Latin *funiculus,* meaning "string") (Fig. 10-7). The spinal cord is, to a great extent, a longitudinally organized structure, even though it is most conveniently studied in cross section. For example, the posterior gray horns are continuous cell columns rather than a series of discrete nuclei, and at any given level the posterior horn cells interact with cells from many other levels.

In addition to the posterolateral and anterolateral sulci, several other longitudinal grooves indent the cross-sectional outline of the cord (see Fig. 10-7). The deep **anterior median fissure** extends almost to the center of the cord; at the apex of this fissure, only a thin zone of white matter (the **anterior white commissure**[b]) and a thin zone of gray matter separate the central canal from subarachnoid space. The **posterior median sulcus** is much less distinct, but a glial septum extends from it all the way to the gray matter surrounding the central canal. Therefore the two sides of the spinal cord can communicate with each other only through a narrow band of neural tissue near the central canal. Because the fibers of some ascending pathways cross the midline in the spinal cord, this small area where crossing occurs may be clinically important in diseases affecting the center of the cord (see Fig. 10-32). Finally, at cervical and upper thoracic levels, a **posterior intermediate sulcus** is found. Another glial septum projects from this sulcus, partially subdividing each posterior funiculus.

---

[b]"White" to distinguish it from the much larger anterior commissure of the cerebrum (see Figs. 3-15 and 3-20).

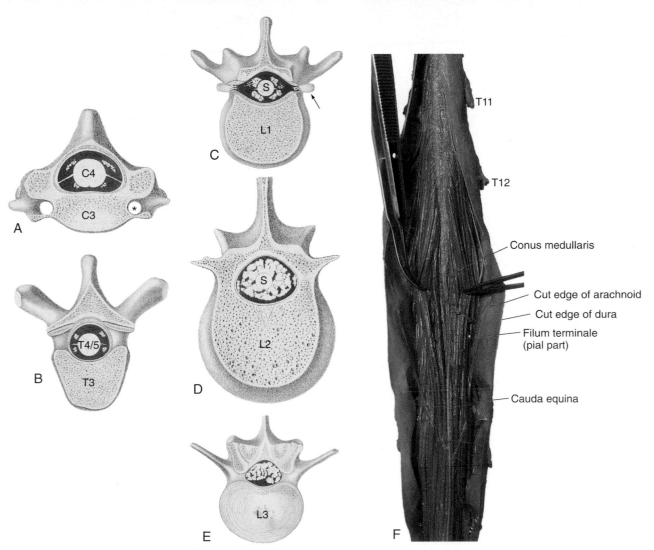

Figure 10-5 Formation of the cauda equina. **A** to **E,** Cross sections from progressively more caudal levels of a vertebral column in which the sub-arachnoid space was filled with dyed gelatin (C3, T3, L1, L2, and L3 vertebrae, respectively). The C3 and T3 vertebrae encase spinal cord segments C4 and T4-T5, each adjacent to the dorsal and ventral roots of these segments and suspended by denticulate ligaments. The L1 and L2 vertebrae encase the sacral spinal cord (S) together with a collection of dorsal and ventral roots from lumbar and sacral segments. By the level of the L3 vertebra, the spinal cord has ended and only the cauda equina remains. **F,** Actual-size view of the caudal end of the spinal cord and the cauda equina, seen from the posterior side after the arachnoid and dura were spread apart. *Asterisk* in **A,** foramen for the vertebral artery; *arrow* in **C,** spinal nerve emerging from the intervertebral foramen. (**A** to **E,** from Key A, Retzius G: Studien in der anatomie des nervensystems und des bindegewebes, vol 1, Stockholm, 1875, Norstad. **F,** courtesy Dr. Norman Koelling, University of Arizona College of Medicine. Adapted from Nolte J, Angevine JB Jr: The human brain in photographs and diagrams, ed 3, St. Louis, 2007, Mosby.)

The Spinal Cord Is Involved in Sensory Processing, Motor Outflow, and Reflexes

Afferent fibers enter the cord via the dorsal (posterior) roots[c] and then end almost exclusively on the ipsilateral side of the CNS. They may reach their site of termination either by synapsing on neurons in the ipsilateral gray matter of the spinal cord or by ascending directly and uncrossed to relay nuclei in the medulla. The relay cells in the spinal gray matter or the medulla then project their axons through defined sensory pathways to more rostral structures. In subsequent discussions of these sensory pathways, it may sometimes sound as if a particular primary afferent synapses on only one relay cell and sends its information into only one pathway. However, it is important to realize that each primary afferent fiber gives rise to many branches feeding into more than one ascending sensory pathway as well as into local reflex circuits (see Fig. 3-27). It is estimated, for example, that a single Ia afferent from a muscle spindle

---

[c]The Bell-Magendie law, a long-standing neuroanatomical tenet, states that the dorsal root contains only primary afferent fibers and the ventral root only efferent fibers of various sorts. However, a small percentage of ventral root fibers are in fact finely myelinated or unmyelinated primary afferents. Ventral root afferents may be at least partially responsible for the persistence or the return of pain after the dorsal roots have been sectioned. In addition, as discussed in Chapter 9, at least some primary afferents (nociceptive C fibers) in the dorsal roots have efferent functions as well.

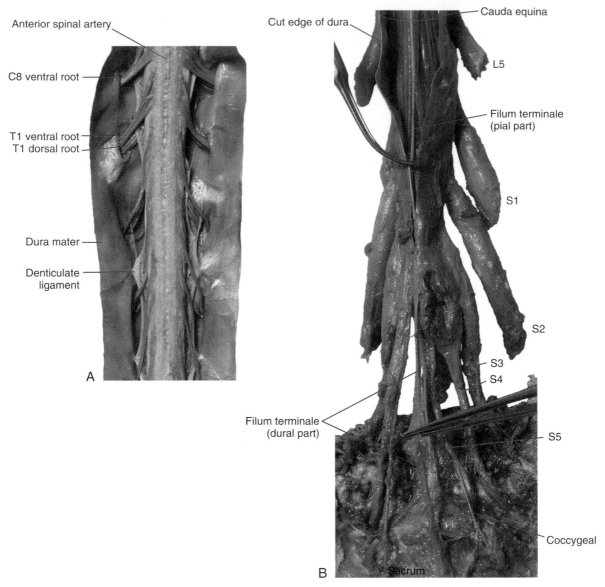

Anterior spinal artery

C8 ventral root

T1 ventral root
T1 dorsal root

Dura mater

Denticulate
ligament

A

Cut edge of dura

Cauda equina

L5

Filum terminale
(pial part)

S1

S2

S3
S4

Filum terminale
(dural part)

S5

Coccygeal

B Sacrum

Figure 10-6 Meningeal suspension of the spinal cord. **A,** Anterior surface of the lower cervical and upper thoracic cord, revealed by cutting open the spinal dural sheath. **B,** Posterior view of the filum terminale traveling among the roots of the cauda equina, emerging from the spinal dural sheath, and crossing the sacrum on its way to an anchor point on the coccyx. *(Courtesy Dr. Norman Koelling, University of Arizona College of Medicine. Adapted from Nolte J, Angevine JB Jr: The human brain in photographs and diagrams, ed 3, St. Louis, 2007, Mosby.)*

may give rise to 500 or more branches within the spinal cord.

The motor neurons that innervate skeletal muscles are located in the anterior horns, and many preganglionic autonomic neurons are located in the intermediate gray matter of some segments. The axons of these motor neurons leave the cord in the ventral (anterior) roots. Activity in these neurons is modulated by local reflex circuits and by pathways that descend through the spinal white matter from the cerebral cortex and from various brainstem and diencephalic nuclei.

Certain specified afferent inputs cause stereotyped motor outputs, called **reflexes,** such as the familiar

knee-jerk reflex. Many of these involve neural circuitry that is wholly contained within the spinal cord; several examples are discussed later in this chapter.

Spinal Gray Matter Is Regionally Specialized

The Posterior Horn Contains Sensory Interneurons and Projection Neurons

The posterior horn consists mainly of interneurons whose processes remain within the spinal cord and of projection neurons whose axons collect into long, ascending sensory pathways. This area of gray matter contains two prominent parts, the **substantia gelatinosa**

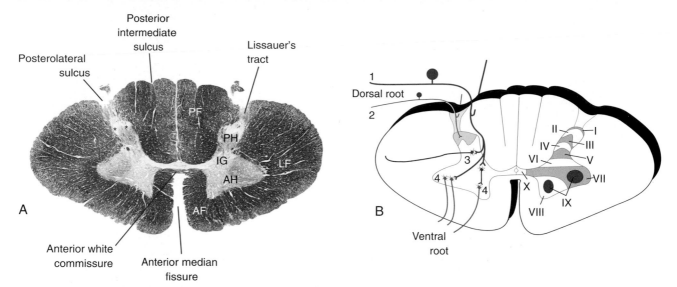

Figure 10-7 General cross-sectional anatomy of the spinal cord, represented in this case by the eighth cervical segment. **A,** Cross section of C8. **B,** Laminae of Rexed are indicated on the right, and the general kinds of cells and connections in these different areas are indicated on the left. Large-diameter, heavily myelinated afferents (1) enter medially through the posterior funiculus, whereas small-diameter afferents (2) enter laterally near the substantia gelatinosa. This corresponds to the way tactile and proprioceptive information is processed, relative to pain and temperature information. These afferents then contact interneurons (3) and, in some cases, motor neurons (4) directly. AF, anterior funiculus; AH, anterior horn; IG, intermediate gray matter; LF, lateral funiculus; PF, posterior funiculus; PH, posterior horn; asterisks indicate the substantia gelatinosa.

and the **body** of the posterior horn, both present at all spinal levels.

The substantia gelatinosa is a distinctive region of gray matter that caps the posterior horn (Fig. 10-8). In myelin-stained preparations this region looks pale compared with the rest of the gray matter because it deals mostly with finely myelinated and unmyelinated sensory fibers that carry pain and temperature information. Between the substantia gelatinosa and the surface of the cord is a relatively pale-staining area of white matter called **Lissauer's tract.**[d] This tract stains more lightly than the rest of the white matter because it contains the finely myelinated and unmyelinated fibers with which the substantia gelatinosa deals.

The body of the posterior horn consists mainly of interneurons and projection neurons that transmit various types of somatic and visceral sensory information. In this respect it functionally overlaps parts of the intermediate gray matter.

---

[d]Lissauer's tract is an unusual case in which an eponym is becoming more commonly used rather than fading away. For many years Lissauer's tract was also known by the descriptive term **dorsolateral fasciculus.** However, as described elsewhere in this and the next chapter, the dorsal part of the lateral funiculus is now known to contain some distinctively important ascending and descending pathways. As a result, many now refer to the latter area of spinal white matter as the **dorsolateral fasciculus** or **funiculus.** To avoid ambiguity, Lissauer's tract is probably best referred to by its eponymous name.

The Anterior Horn Contains Motor Neurons

The anterior horn contains the cell bodies of the large motor neurons that supply skeletal muscle (Fig. 10-9). These alpha motor neurons, also referred to as **lower motor neurons,**[e] are the only means by which the nervous system can exercise control over body movements, whether voluntary or involuntary; a number of different parts and pathways of the nervous system can influence these lower motor neurons, but they alone can elicit muscle contraction. Destruction of the lower motor neurons supplying a muscle or interruption of their axons therefore causes complete paralysis of that muscle. Lower motor neuron lesions cause paralysis of a type called **flaccid paralysis,** indicating that the muscle is limp and uncontracted. Reflex contractions can no longer be elicited, and the muscle slowly atrophies (owing to a lack of trophic factors normally delivered to it by motor axons; see Chapter 24). This occurs, for example, in poliomyelitis (a viral disease that attacks the motor neurons of the anterior horn) and in injuries in which ventral roots are damaged.

Alpha motor neurons occur in longitudinally oriented, cigar-shaped groups, each group innervating an individual muscle. Hence in cross sections they appear to be arranged in clusters (Fig. 10-10), separated from one another by areas of interneurons; the clusters that

---

[e]They are also referred to simply as **anterior horn cells,** even though other cell types also live in the anterior horn.

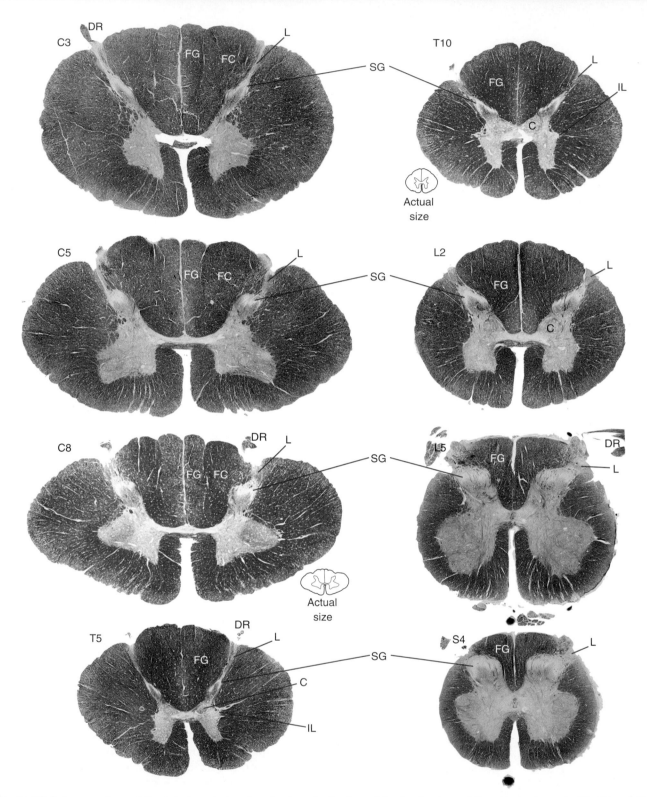

Figure 10-8 Cross sections of the spinal cord at various levels; note the large lateral extensions of the anterior horns in C5, C8, and L5. C, Clarke's nucleus; DR, dorsal root; FC, fasciculus cuneatus; FG, fasciculus gracilis; IL, intermediolateral cell column; L, Lissauer's tract; SG, substantia gelatinosa.

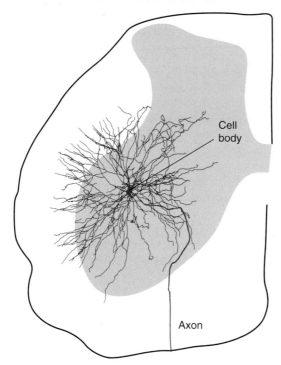

Figure 10-9 A single motor neuron from the lumbar spinal cord of an adult cat. A marker substance (horseradish peroxidase) was injected from the intracellular tip of a microelectrode, and the neuron was subsequently reconstructed from a series of sections. The extent and complexity of the dendritic trees of real neurons are obviously different from those of the "cartoon" neurons in most of the diagrams in this book. *(Modified from Ulfhake B et al: J Comp Neurol 278:69, 1988.)*

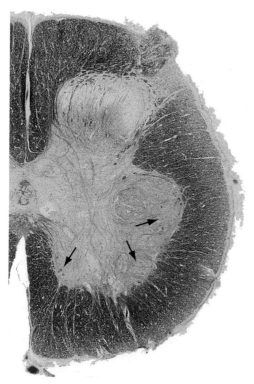

Figure 10-10 Clusters of motor neurons *(arrows)* in the anterior horn at S4.

innervate axial muscles are medial to those that innervate limb muscles. In the cervical and lumbar enlargements, which innervate the limbs, the anterior horns are enlarged laterally to accommodate the additional motor neurons (see Fig. 10-8). Smaller gamma motor neurons are interspersed with alpha motor neurons in all such groups. They innervate the intrafusal muscle fibers of muscle spindles, so they are also referred to as **fusimotor neurons.**

Two columns of motor neurons in the anterior horn of the cervical cord are recognized as separate entities. The **spinal accessory nucleus** extends from the caudal medulla to about C5. The axons of these motor neurons emerge from the lateral surface of the spinal cord just posterior to the denticulate ligament as a separate series of rootlets that form the accessory nerve (see Fig. 3-17). The **phrenic nucleus,** containing the motor neurons that innervate the diaphragm, is located in the medial portion of the anterior horn in segments C3 to C5. This makes injuries to the upper cervical spinal cord a matter of grave concern, because destruction of the descending pathways that control the phrenic nucleus and other respiratory motor neurons renders a patient unable to breathe.

The Intermediate Gray Matter Contains Autonomic Neurons

The gray matter that is intermediate to the anterior and posterior horns has some characteristics of both and also contains the spinal preganglionic autonomic neurons. In addition, at some levels it includes a distinctive region called **Clarke's nucleus.**

The preganglionic sympathetic neurons for the entire body lie in segments T1 through L3, most of them located in a column of cells called the **intermediolateral cell column,** which forms a pointy lateral horn on the spinal gray matter (see Fig. 10-8). Their axons leave through the ventral roots. Cells in a corresponding location in segments S2 to S4 constitute the **sacral parasympathetic nucleus** but do not form a distinct lateral horn. Their axons leave through the ventral roots and synapse on the postganglionic parasympathetic neurons for the pelvic viscera.

The **posterior thoracic nucleus** (i.e., Clarke's nucleus or the nucleus dorsalis of Clarke) is a rounded collection of large cells located on the medial surface of the base of the posterior horn from about T1 to L2. It is particularly prominent at lower thoracic levels (see Fig. 10-8). This is an important relay nucleus for the transmission of information to the cerebellum and may also play a role in forwarding proprioceptive information from the leg to the thalamus. Because of its prominent role in sensory processing, it is treated as part of the posterior horn.

The remainder of the intermediate gray matter is a collection of various projection neurons, sensory

Table 10-3	Important Subdivisions of Spinal Cord Gray Matter		
Nucleus	**Levels**	**Lamina**	**Function**
Marginal zone	All	I	Some spinothalamic tract cells
Substantia gelatinosa	All	II	Modulate transmission of pain and temperature information
Body of posterior horn	All	III-VI	Sensory processing
Clarke's nucleus	T1-L2	VII	Posterior spinocerebellar tract cells
Intermediolateral column	T1-L3	VII	Preganglionic sympathetic neurons
Sacral parasympathetic nucleus	S2-S4	VII	Preganglionic parasympathetic neurons → pelvic viscera
Accessory nucleus	Medulla-C5	IX	Motor neurons → sternocleidomastoid and trapezius
Phrenic nucleus	C3-C5	IX	Motor neurons → diaphragm

interneurons, and interneurons that synapse on motor neurons.

Spinal Cord Gray Matter Is Arranged in Layers

In 1952, Rexed devised a system for subdividing the gray matter of the cat's spinal cord into layers, or laminae. The same system has since been applied to the cords of other mammals, including humans (see Fig. 10-7B). **Lamina I** (also called the **marginal zone**) is a thin layer of gray matter that covers the substantia gelatinosa, **lamina II** is the substantia gelatinosa, and **laminae III** through **VI** are the body of the posterior horn; **lamina VII** roughly corresponds to the intermediate gray matter (including Clarke's nucleus) but also includes large extensions into the anterior horn; **lamina VIII** comprises some of the interneuronal zones of the anterior horn, whereas **lamina IX** consists of the clusters of motor neurons embedded in the anterior horn; **lamina X** is the zone of gray matter surrounding the central canal.

This terminology has proved useful for experimental anatomists and physiologists because the histological differences among the laminae correspond to functional differences (Table 10-3). For example, the functional dichotomy between large- and small-diameter peripheral nerve fibers is maintained to a great extent in the patterns of termination of these fibers in the spinal gray matter: there are prominent (though not exclusive) terminations of pain and temperature afferents in laminae I and II, tactile afferents from cutaneous nerves in lamina III, and Ia muscle spindle afferents in laminae VI, VII, and IX.

Reflex Circuitry Is Built Into the Spinal Cord

A reflex is an involuntary, stereotyped response to a sensory input. All reflex pathways, other than axon reflexes (see Fig. 9-13), therefore must involve at least a receptor structure and associated afferent neuron (with its cell body in a dorsal root ganglion or some other sensory ganglion) and an efferent neuron (with its cell body within the CNS). With the exception of the **stretch reflex,** all reflexes involve one or more interneurons as well.

Reflexes range from the simple ones described in this chapter (which serve as a useful introduction to neural integration and are the basis for common clinical tests) to neural subroutines so complex that calling them "reflexes" seems an oversimplification. For example, a cat with its spinal cord transected at thoracic levels can, under certain conditions, perform coordinated walking movements with its hindlimbs. If its hindfeet are placed on a moving treadmill, the gait changes in a predictable fashion with the speed of the treadmill, from alternating stepping movements at low speeds to galloping movements (in which both legs move together in phase) at higher speeds.

Muscle Stretch Leads to Excitation of Motor Neurons

All skeletal muscles (except perhaps some muscles in the head) contract to at least some extent in response to being stretched. The reflex arc responsible for this contraction utilizes the simplest possible route through the CNS because it involves only two neurons and a single intervening synapse. It is therefore sometimes referred to as the **monosynaptic reflex** or the **myotatic reflex** (from two Greek words meaning "muscle stretch"). The afferent limb of the arc is a Ia afferent with its associated muscle spindle primary ending. Central processes of the Ia afferent make synapses within the spinal cord directly on the alpha motor neurons that innervate the muscle containing the stimulated spindle (Fig. 10-11).

The stretch reflex is commonly used for clinical testing purposes. Tapping the patellar tendon, as in the familiar **knee-jerk reflex,** stretches the quadriceps slightly. Ia endings in quadriceps muscle spindles are excited and in turn excite quadriceps alpha motor neurons; these cause the quadriceps to contract, completing the reflex. Similarly, tapping the Achilles tendon stretches the gastrocnemius slightly, thereby causing a reflex contraction. Testing a variety of stretch reflexes can provide valuable clinical information about the integrity not only of peripheral nerves but also of predictable spinal cord segments (Table 10-4). Because stretch reflexes are usually elicited by tapping a tendon, they are often referred to as **deep tendon reflexes** (sometimes abbreviated as **DTRs**). Even though the reflex is studied in this manner, the responsible receptors are in the muscles attached to the tapped tendons.

Stretch reflexes are thought to be important for the constant automatic corrections performed during movements and postures (although other reflexes may be more important for this function). For example, when standing still and upright, a person sways to and fro a bit. Each time that person sways in one direction, muscles are stretched and the resulting reflex contraction helps return him or her toward the desired position.

Muscle Tension Can Lead to Inhibition of Motor Neurons

Stimulation of a Ib fiber from a Golgi tendon organ has an effect that varies, depending on the position and activity of the limb at the time of stimulation. It sometimes has an effect opposite to that of stimulating a Ia

fiber: the alpha motor neurons that innervate the muscle connected to that tendon organ are inhibited. This effect is a form of **autogenic inhibition** and involves an inhibitory interneuron between the afferent and efferent fibers (Fig. 10-12). Under other circumstances (e.g., stimulating a tendon organ attached to a weight-supporting muscle), excitation of the motor neurons can result (again, through an interneuron).

The normal role of reflexes mediated by Golgi tendon organs is not yet completely understood. It was thought for a time that autogenic inhibition initiated by these receptors is protective in nature, preventing muscles from developing excess tension. However, in view of the great sensitivity of tendon organs to actively generated tension, it is clear that this reflex is activated long before hazardous levels are reached. Therefore it is now thought that Golgi tendon organs contribute to fine adjustments in the force of muscle contraction during ordinary motor activities and that other receptors initiate additional forms of autogenic inhibition at higher tension levels.

Clinically, autogenic inhibition may be manifested in a phenomenon called the **clasp-knife response.** In

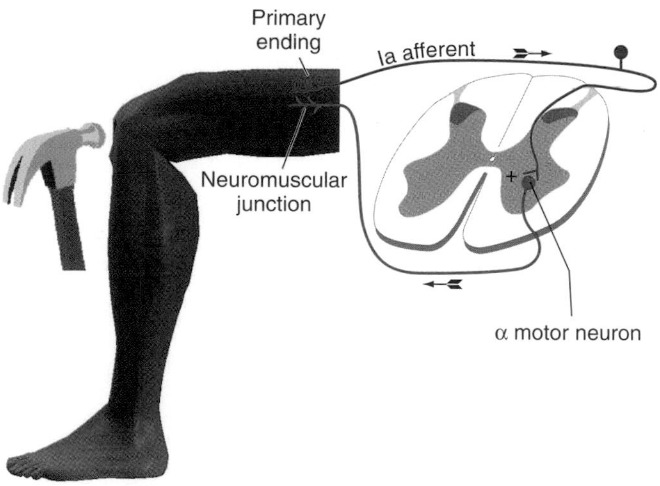

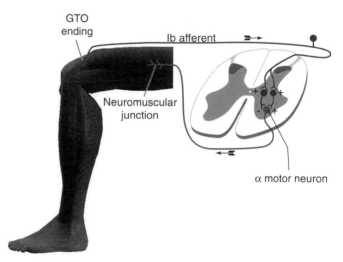

Figure 10-11 Stretch reflex. Striking the patellar tendon activates muscle spindle primary endings, which then monosynaptically excite alpha motor neurons that innervate the stretched muscle.

Figure 10-12 Reflex connections of Golgi tendon organs. Contraction of a muscle activates the Golgi tendon organ (GTO) in its attached tendon. Under some conditions, the Ib afferents then activate inhibitory interneurons that inhibit the motor neurons to that muscle (autogenic inhibition). Under other conditions, the opposite effect is noted, mediated by excitatory interneurons.

Table 10-4	Deep Tendon Reflexes Commonly Tested Clinically		
Reflex	**Muscle Involved**	**Principal Cord Segment**	**Peripheral Nerve**
Biceps	Biceps brachii	C5	Musculocutaneous
Brachioradialis	Brachioradialis	C6	Radial
Triceps	Triceps brachii	C7	Radial
Knee-jerk (patellar)	Quadriceps femoris	L4	Femoral
Ankle-jerk (Achilles)	Gastrocnemius, soleus	S1	Tibial

certain pathological conditions that follow damage to descending motor pathways, the resistance of muscles to manipulation is greatly increased. Thus one would have considerable difficulty flexing the leg of an individual with such a condition. If sufficient force is applied, however, the leg slowly flexes until at some point all resistance suddenly disappears and the leg collapses in flexion, like a clasp knife snapping shut. This collapse of resistance was once attributed to autogenic inhibition initiated by Golgi tendon organs, but here too, other receptors play the major role.

Painful Stimuli Elicit Coordinated Withdrawal Reflexes

Whereas stretch reflexes and autogenic inhibition are initiated by muscle or tendon receptors and primarily involve the muscle stretched or tensed, the **flexor reflex** is initiated by cutaneous receptors and involves a whole limb. A familiar example is withdrawal from a painful stimulus; after accidentally touching something painfully hot or sharp, we automatically remove the offended hand from that vicinity by flexing the arm to which it is attached.

The flexor reflex pathways in the spinal cord are normally held in a somewhat inhibited state by descending influences from the brainstem, so that only noxious stimuli result in a strong reflex. If these descending influences are removed, either surgically in experimental animals or as a result of some pathological condition, reflex flexion can result from harmless tactile stimulation. This indicates that most or all cutaneous receptors feed into the pathway, but ordinarily only nociceptors have a powerful enough influence to cause a reflex withdrawal.

Because the flexor reflex involves an entire limb, its pathway must spread over several spinal segments to include the motor neurons innervating all the various flexor muscles of that limb. This spreading occurs in two ways. First, all primary afferent fibers bifurcate on entering the spinal cord, and their processes then extend one or more segments in both rostral and caudal directions. Second, the flexor pathway includes at least one interneuron, which itself may have processes extending over several segments (Fig. 10-13).

Although this reflex is usually called the **flexor reflex,** the term **withdrawal reflex** is also used and is perhaps more appropriate. The reflex is not an all-or-none phenomenon for a given limb; rather, it shows different patterns, depending on which portion of the limb is stimulated (each pattern being appropriate to withdraw the stimulated area). It would be imprudent to flex a lower extremity when a painful stimulus was applied to the anterior surface of the thigh because this would drive the thigh into the stimulus. In such a situation, it would make much more sense to activate the extensors, which

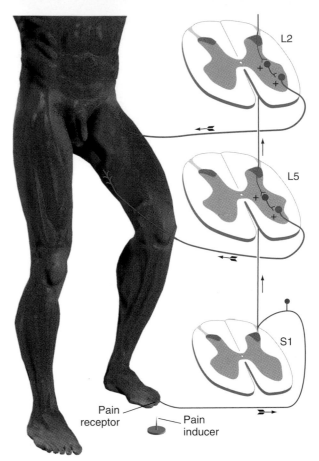

Figure 10-13 Flexor reflex. This reflex involves several segments, and all connections are polysynaptic. In the example shown, a nociceptive fiber from the foot enters the spinal cord at S1 and activates (through at least one interneuron) motor neurons to iliopsoas and hamstring muscles.

is in fact what happens. Modification of the reflex response so that it reflects the area being stimulated is called **local sign.**

Reflexes Are Accompanied by Reciprocal and Crossed Effects

So far, this has been a simplified description of reflex circuits, including only the most direct and dominant motor effects. However, these reflexes also include weaker influences on other muscles of the same limb and even of contralateral limbs.

It would clearly be easier to shorten a stretched muscle if the motor neurons to its synergists were excited and those to its antagonists inhibited. This **reciprocal inhibition** does occur and is a general principle in all reflexes: reflex activity in a given muscle produces similar activity in its ipsilateral synergists and the opposite activity in its ipsilateral antagonists (Fig. 10-14). Thus the standard tap on the patellar tendon causes not only excitation of quadriceps motor neurons but also inhibition

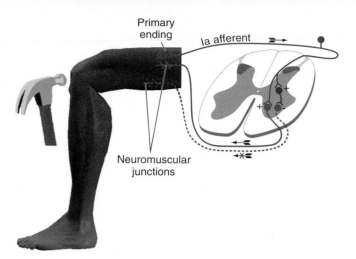

Figure 10-14 Reciprocal inhibition. Striking the patellar tendon initiates a stretch reflex, as in Figure 10-11. It also causes inhibition, through an interneuron, of the motor neurons to the antagonist hamstring muscles.

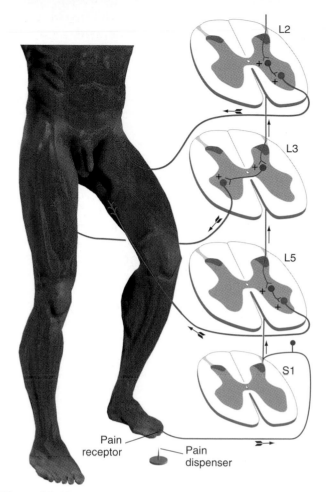

Figure 10-15 Crossed extension. Stepping on a tack initiates a flexor reflex, as in Figure 10-13. It also causes excitation, through an interneuron, of the contralateral antagonist muscles. In this case, contraction of the contralateral quadriceps helps the leg with the nonpunctured foot to support the body.

(through an interneuron) of motor neurons to the hamstring muscles. If one extensor muscle of the thigh were selectively stretched, its motor neurons would be monosynaptically excited, as would those of all the other thigh extensors. After stimulation of a Golgi tendon organ the pattern may be just the reverse: if tension is applied to the patellar tendon during certain phases of a movement, the quadriceps is inhibited and the hamstring muscles are excited, both actions occurring through interneurons. Finally, the flexor reflex is accompanied by inhibition of the extensors of that limb.

The **crossed effects** in reflex actions are most easily understood with reference to the flexor reflex (Fig. 10-15). If the only effect of stepping on a tack with the left foot were withdrawal of the left leg, the maladaptive behavior of falling over and possibly landing on the tack might follow. This is avoided by a simultaneous and opposite pattern of activity in the contralateral limb; as the left leg flexes and withdraws, the right leg extends and is thus better able to support the body. Similar observations have been made after stimulation of muscle spindles and Golgi tendon organs, although the effects on contralateral antagonists are not pronounced.

These crossed effects may be the basic building blocks for more complex subroutines, such as those for the coordinated stepping movements referred to earlier. Individual interneurons receive multiple inputs and can participate in tendon organ–mediated reflexes, withdrawal reflexes, and more complex movements.

Reflexes Are Modifiable

The preceding discussion makes it sound as though reflexes are fixed and unchangeable, a function of only the type and magnitude of the stimulus. This is largely an illusion created by the way in which reflexes are tested, with relaxed patients in static postures; the sensitivity of reflex arcs in fact varies substantially, depending on the functional requirements of the nervous system at any given time. The stretch reflex, for example, must be variable, or we would be unable to sit: sitting should stretch the quadriceps just as tapping the patellar tendon does, in which case reflex contraction of the quadriceps would be expected to make us stand up again. Gamma motor neurons play a key role here. During the act of sitting, the gamma motor neurons to quadriceps muscle spindles decrease their firing rate. This decreases the excitability of the quadriceps spindles just enough so that they do not respond to the stretch imposed by sitting. The activities of the alpha and gamma motor neuron populations are generally coordinated during movements; this is discussed in more detail in Chapter 18.

In addition to generally suppressing or enhancing reflexes during different behavioral states, the CNS adjusts the sensitivity of individual reflex arcs from moment to moment in response to different postures or during different parts of a task. For example, during normal walking each leg alternates between a stance phase, in which it supports the body and then pushes off, and a swing phase, in which the foot is lifted off the ground and moved forward. The foot is dorsiflexed during the swing phase, keeping the toes clear of the ground. This dorsiflexion stretches the soleus. The monosynaptic stretch reflex involving the soleus is almost completely suppressed specifically during this phase of the step cycle, preventing it from contracting, extending the foot, and possibly causing the toes to contact the ground. Reflex responses to something touching the sole of the foot can reverse direction, depending on the phase of the step cycle during which the touch occurs (Fig. 10-16A). Similarly, the withdrawal reflex in response to a painful stimulus is automatically enhanced or suppressed, depending on the postural support role being played by that limb at the moment of the stimulus (see Fig. 10-16B). Some of these adjustments to reflex sensitivity are accomplished by circuitry built into the spinal cord, whereas others depend on pathways descending from the brainstem.

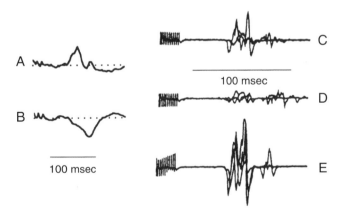

Figure 10-16 Moment-to-moment changes in the sensitivity of reflexes. **A** to **E** show the mass electrical activity (electromyogram) of a foot flexor (tibialis anterior) recorded from the skin surface. **A** and **B** show average responses to 20 or more stimuli; **C** to **E** show three superimposed single responses. In **A** and **B**, innocuous electrical stimuli delivered to the ipsilateral posterior tibial nerve as the subject walked on a treadmill caused somatic sensations in the sole of the foot and reflex changes in the electrical activity of the muscle. A stimulus delivered during the swing phase (mimicking something touching the sole) caused increased activity of the muscle **(A)**, but a stimulus delivered as the heel touched down caused decreased activity **(B)**. A painful electrical stimulus delivered to the sole of one foot caused some ipsilateral contraction and foot flexion when the subject stood on both legs **(C)**, much less when standing on the leg whose foot was stimulated **(D)** and much more when standing on the other leg **(E)**. *(A and B, from De Serres SJ, Yang JF, Patrick SK: J Physiol 488:249, 1995. C to E, from Rossi A, Decchi B: J Physiol 481:521, 1994.)*

Ascending and Descending Pathways Have Defined Locations in the Spinal White Matter

The nerve fibers in the white matter of the spinal cord are of three general types:
1. Long, ascending fibers projecting to the thalamus, the cerebellum, or assorted brainstem nuclei.
2. Long, descending fibers projecting from the cerebral cortex or from several brainstem nuclei to the spinal gray matter.
3. Shorter **propriospinal** fibers interconnecting different spinal cord levels, such as the fibers responsible for the coordination of flexor reflexes.

Fibers having similar connections typically band together, forming the various tracts of the spinal cord. Propriospinal fibers mostly remain in a thin shell surrounding the gray matter called the **propriospinal tract** or **fasciculus proprius** (the Latin word *fasciculus* means "little bundle"). In primates, descending tracts are found primarily in the lateral and anterior funiculi; ascending tracts are found in all three funiculi.

A great many ascending and descending tracts have been described, largely on the basis of their origins and terminations; the function of some is unknown. This chapter includes descriptions of the largest and best-known tracts descending from the cerebral cortex or ascending to the cerebellum or the thalamus. Consideration of several other tracts is deferred until subsequent chapters, where the structures in which they arise or terminate are discussed.

As mentioned previously, there is a tendency to think of individual primary afferents as performing a single function (e.g., either participating in a particular reflex arc or transmitting information to a single ascending tract). Single fibers are drawn that way in textbooks for convenience and clarity, but in fact, each primary afferent probably participates in one or more reflex arcs and also in one or more ascending tracts. In a similar way, there is a tendency to think of particular sensory functions as uniquely associated with particular tracts (e.g., pain with one tract and touch with another), so that damage to an ascending tract should result in total loss of some sensory function. This is not the case, and most kinds of sensory information reach the thalamus and the cerebellum by more than one route. Why this is so and the consequences in an intact nervous system are not understood, but one result is that the loss of a single tract can often be compensated for, to a surprising extent, by the remaining tracts.

The following section describes the principal pathways by which somatic sensory information reaches the thalamus and the cerebellum. Information that reaches the thalamus is relayed to the cerebral cortex and perceived consciously. Information that reaches the cerebellum is used in the regulation of movements; we are not consciously aware of cerebellar activity.

The Posterior Column–Medial Lemniscus System Conveys Information About Touch and Limb Position

The term *posterior column* refers to the entire contents of a posterior funiculus, exclusive of its share of the propriospinal tract. The posterior columns consist mainly of ascending collaterals of large myelinated primary afferents carrying impulses from various kinds of mechanoreceptors (although substantial numbers of second-order fibers and unmyelinated fibers are also included). This has traditionally been considered the major pathway by which information from low-threshold cutaneous, joint, and muscle receptors reaches the cerebral cortex.

Spinal primary afferent fibers of all diameters and degrees of myelination have their cell bodies in ipsilateral dorsal root (spinal) ganglia (Fig. 10-17). As each dorsal (posterior) rootlet enters the spinal cord, its fibers segregate themselves into a **medial** and a **lateral division** (Fig. 10-18). The medial division contains large-diameter, heavily myelinated afferents, whereas the lateral division contains small-diameter, finely myelinated or unmyelinated afferents. Fibers of the medial division enter the posterior column and ascend toward the brainstem, giving off numerous collaterals to deeper laminae of the spinal gray matter. Many reach the caudal

medulla before making their final synapse. Caudal to T6, each posterior column is an undivided bundle called **fasciculus gracilis** (the Latin word *gracilis* means "slender"). Rostral to T6, fibers may leave fasciculus gracilis, but few if any are added. Afferents entering rostral to T6 accumulate in a second bundle, roughly triangular in shape and lateral to the fasciculus gracilis, called **fasciculus cuneatus** (the Latin word *cuneus* means "wedge"). A glial partition (the **posterior intermediate septum**) extends inward to partially separate the two.

At each successive spinal level, fibers entering the posterior columns add on laterally to those already present (Fig. 10-19). A lamination results, with layers of fibers from sacral levels most medial and layers from cervical levels most lateral. This sort of arrangement, in which particular portions of the body are represented in particular regions of a pathway or nucleus, is called **somatotopic** organization and is characteristic of most sensory and motor pathways.

Those posterior column fibers that reach the brainstem synapse in **nucleus gracilis** or **nucleus cuneatus** (the **posterior column nuclei**) in the caudal medulla. Second-order fibers arising in these nuclei cross the midline and form the **medial lemniscus** (the Greek word *lemniskos* means "ribbon"), a flattened, ribbon-shaped bundle of fibers that proceeds rostrally through the brainstem and terminates in the thalamus (see Fig. 10-19). Third-order fibers arising in the thalamus (specifically in the **ventral posterolateral nucleus** of the thalamus, or VPL) ascend through the internal capsule

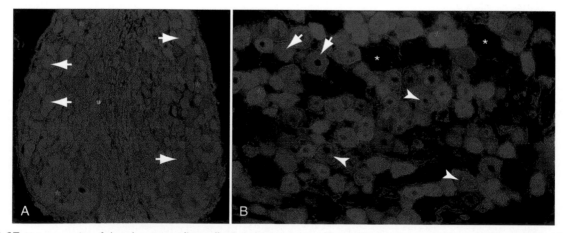

Figure 10-17 Heterogeneity of dorsal root ganglion cells. **A,** Low-power view of a single dorsal root ganglion double-labeled with fluorescent antibodies. Green and yellow-green fluorescence *(arrows)* is seen primarily in large neurons and indicates a neurofilament protein concentrated in myelinated axons and their parent cell bodies. Orange fluorescence *(blue asterisks)* is seen primarily in small neurons and indicates an intermediate filament protein concentrated in unmyelinated axons and their parent cell bodies. Similarly labeled nerve fibers run vertically through the ganglion on their way out. **B,** Higher power view of a dorsal root ganglion double-labeled with fluorescent antibodies. Orange fluorescence indicates the presence of a membrane receptor (for nerve growth factor) characteristic of nociceptors, green fluorescence indicates the presence of another cell surface molecule characteristic of neurons with unmyelinated axons, and yellow fluorescence indicates the presence of both markers. Hence in this image, orange neurons *(arrows)* presumably give rise to thinly myelinated nociceptive fibers, yellow neurons *(blue asterisks)* to unmyelinated nociceptive fibers, and green neurons *(arrowheads)* to unmyelinated thermoreceptive or mechanoreceptive fibers. Unlabeled areas *(white asterisks)* are large cell bodies that give rise to heavily myelinated axons that end peripherally in skin, muscle, and joints. *(From Molliver DC et al: J Comp Neurol 361:404, 1995.)*

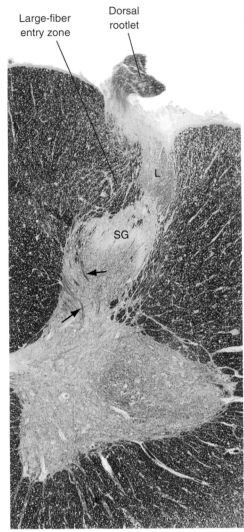

Large-fiber entry zone   Dorsal rootlet

Figure 10-18 Dorsal root entry zone, using C8 as an example. Small-diameter fibers enter the cord laterally and join Lissauer's tract (L) before terminating in the substantia gelatinosa (SG) and other superficial laminae of the posterior horn. Large-diameter fibers enter the spinal cord through the medial division, forming a large-fiber entry zone medial to Lissauer's tract and joining the posterior columns. Collaterals of many of these fibers sweep over the medial surface of the posterior horn *(arrows)* to reach deeper laminae. *(From Nolte J, Angevine JB Jr: The human brain in photographs and diagrams, ed 3, St. Louis, 2007, Mosby.)*

to synapse mainly in the primary somatosensory cortex of the postcentral gyrus.

Information About the Location and Nature of a Stimulus Is Preserved in the Posterior Column–Medial Lemniscus System

When the primary afferents of the posterior columns terminate in the posterior column nuclei, they maintain their somatotopic organization. Fibers from sacral levels terminate in the most medial portions of nucleus gracilis, and fibers from cervical levels terminate in the most lateral portions of nucleus cuneatus. A somatotopic arrangement is found throughout the rest of this pathway, so that information from sacral segments travels through a particular part of the medial lemniscus, projects to a particular portion of VPL, and proceeds to a particular region of the postcentral gyrus. This does not mean that the sacral-to-cervical sequence remains along a medial-to-lateral line throughout the pathway, but rather that sacral information remains adjacent to lumbar information but segregated from cervical information at all points along the way to somatosensory cortex. It may be easier to keep track of the somatotopic arrangement of the pathway at different levels if you envision it as an actual map of the body (a **homunculus,** Latin for "little person"), with sacral and lumbar levels corresponding to the legs, thoracic to the trunk, and cervical to the arms and neck. Viewed in this way, the homunculus is lying down, with its feet toward the midline, up to the level of the posterior column nuclei. Its subsequent gyrations are described in Chapter 11.

Details about the nature and time course of a stimulus are also preserved in this pathway. Some individual neurons of the posterior column nuclei receive sufficiently powerful excitatory input from individual posterior column fibers that information is transmitted faithfully to the medial lemniscus (Fig. 10-20A). Similar transmission at subsequent thalamic and cortical levels results in a remarkably precise representation of certain peripheral stimuli in somatosensory cortex (see Fig. 10-20B to D).

Damage to the Posterior Column–Medial Lemniscus System Causes Impairment of Proprioception and Discriminative Tactile Functions

As might be expected from the types of afferents contained in the posterior columns, this pathway carries information important for the conscious appreciation of touch, pressure, and vibration and of joint position and movement. However, because input from cutaneous receptors also reaches the cortex by other routes, damage to the posterior columns causes impairment, but not abolition, of tactile perception. Complex discrimination tasks are more severely affected than is the simple detection of stimuli.[f] Other functions, such as proprioception and kinesthesia, are classically considered to be totally lost after posterior column destruction. The result is a distinctive type of **ataxia** (incoordination of movement); the brain is unable to direct motor activity properly without sensory feedback about the current position of parts of the body (see Fig. 18-9). This ataxia is particularly pronounced when the patient's eyes are closed, preventing visual compensation.

[f]For this reason, whereas posterior column function is commonly tested clinically by touching a vibrating tuning fork to the surface of the body, a more effective test is having a patient try to identify a pattern drawn on the skin.

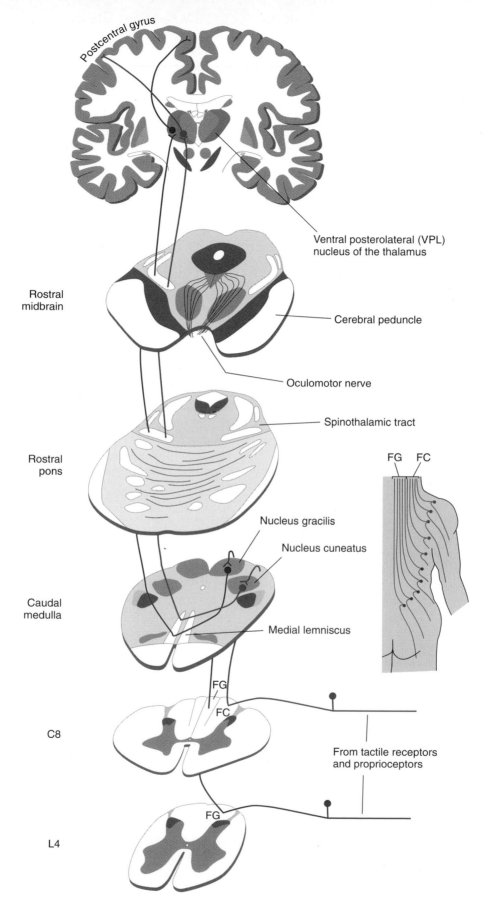

Figure 10-19 Posterior column–medial lemniscus pathway. Primary afferents carrying tactile and proprioceptive information synapse in the posterior column nuclei of the ipsilateral medulla. The axons of second-order cells then cross the midline, form the medial lemniscus, and ascend to the ventral posterolateral (VPL) nucleus of the thalamus. Third-order fibers then project to the somatosensory cortex of the postcentral gyrus. A somatotopic arrangement of fibers is present at all levels. The beginnings of this somatotopic arrangement, as a lamination of fibers in the posterior columns, is indicated in the inset to the right. FC, fasciculus cuneatus; FG, fasciculus gracilis. *(Inset, redrawn from Mettler FA: Neuroanatomy, ed 2, St. Louis, 1948, Mosby.)*

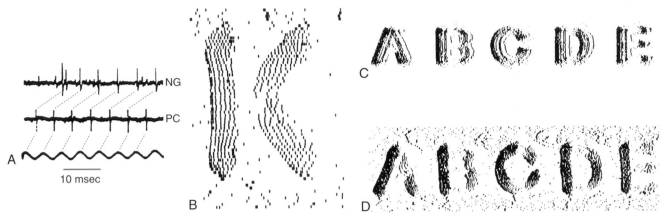

Figure 10-20 Preservation of spatial information in the posterior column–medial lemniscus pathway. **A,** One-to-one transmission from the posterior columns to the posterior column nuclei. A small probe vibrating at 200 Hz (lower trace) and moving less than 2 μm was applied to the skin of a cat's hindlimb while simultaneous recordings were made from a Pacinian corpuscle (PC) afferent in fasciculus gracilis and from a neuron on which it synapsed in nucleus gracilis (NG). Each oscillation caused a spike in the primary afferent. The first of these caused a pair of spikes in the postsynaptic neuron, after which there was a faithful one-to-one coupling between spikes in the primary afferent and the postsynaptic neuron. **B to D,** Responses of a probable Merkel afferent **(C)** and a neuron in somatosensory cortex **(B, D)** as a rotating drum swept embossed letters across a monkey's fingertip. After each revolution the drum was advanced 200 μm, thereby slowly moving the letters through the receptive field of the receptor whose responses were being recorded. One part of such a record, obtained as the letter K was swept across the fingertip, is shown enlarged in **B,** in which each small tick mark corresponds to the occurrence of a single action potential; for additional details on this technique, see Figure 9-18. (**A,** from Ferrington DG, Rowe MJ, Tarvin RPC: J Physiol 386:293, 1987. **B** to **D,** from Phillips JR, Johnson KO, Hsaio SS: Proc Natl Acad Sci U S A 85:1317, 1988.)

The posterior columns provide a particularly instructive example of the notion that sensory information travels in multiple pathways, so that damage to a single pathway seldom causes a total loss of function. Classic views in which the posterior columns were seen as the pathway responsible for fine tactile discrimination and kinesthesia were based mostly on clinical observations. However, selective lesions of the posterior columns are rare. For example, any process impinging on the posterior columns, such as a tumor, would probably affect the adjacent posterior horns and roots, as well as ascending pathways in the posterior part of the lateral funiculus. Tabes dorsalis, a disease process seen in the late stages of neurosyphilis, was traditionally regarded as typifying posterior column damage. Tabetic patients show all the symptoms one would expect if the classic view were correct: their two-point discrimination and vibratory sense are impaired; their senses of movement and position are impaired, and they have great difficulty walking unless they can watch their limbs; if they try to stand erect with their eyes closed and their feet together, they sway and may fall if not supported (**Romberg's sign**). Consistent with this, there is pronounced degeneration in the posterior columns. However, there is also degeneration of dorsal (posterior) root fibers, particularly the heavily myelinated fibers of the medial division, so mechanoreceptive input to all spinal pathways is affected to some extent.

If the posterior columns of a monkey are selectively transected surgically, there is severe impairment initially. The animal has great difficulty coordinating the affected limbs and tends to neglect and not use them. Over a period of months, a remarkable recovery ensues, particularly if the animal is encouraged to use those limbs. After this recovery process, movement and coordination appear nearly normal, tactile threshold is normal, and two-point discrimination and position sense are only slightly impaired. What remains permanently impaired is the ability to use somatosensory information for more complex tasks, for example, judging the shape of an object pressed against the skin (**stereognosis**) or the direction or speed of a stimulus moving across the skin.

The Spinothalamic Tract Conveys Information About Pain and Temperature

Pain is a complex sensation, in that a noxious stimulus leads not only to the perception of where it occurred but also to things such as a rapid increase in level of attention, emotional reactions, autonomic responses, and a greater likelihood that the event and its circumstances will be remembered. Corresponding to this complexity, multiple pathways convey nociceptive information rostrally from the spinal cord. One of them (the **spinothalamic tract**) is analogous to the posterior column–medial lemniscus pathway. It reaches VPL and nearby nuclei of the thalamus and is involved in the awareness and localization of painful stimuli. The others convey nociceptive information to a variety of other sites in the thalamus, reticular formation, and limbic system that subserve the other aspects of pain. These tracts (including the

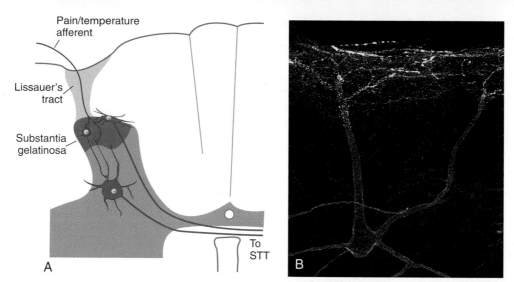

Figure 10-21 A, Origin of the spinothalamic tract (STT) from the posterior horn, both from neurons on the surface of the substantia gelatinosa (lamina I) and from deeper neurons. Transmission to these deeper tract cells is modulated by small neurons of the substantia gelatinosa, reflecting inputs from large-diameter afferents and from descending pain-control pathways (discussed in Chapter 11). The details of the mechanisms involved in these interactions are not fully understood; other parts of the posterior horn are also involved. **B,** A single spinothalamic tract neuron from the spinal cord of a rat, demonstrated by staining receptors for substance P (a neuropeptide released by many nociceptors) using a fluorescent antibody technique. The cell body of the neuron is located in lamina III, but its dendrites extend into more superficial layers where nociceptive fibers terminate. (**B,** from Mantyh PW et al: Science 268:1629, 1995.)

spinothalamic tract) travel together in the spinal cord and are referred to collectively as the **anterolateral pathway,** reflecting their location in the anterior half of the lateral funiculus.

Nociceptive, thermoreceptive, and some mechanoreceptive fibers enter the spinal cord in the lateral division of the dorsal root and project branches into the posterior horn. There they synapse in its superficial laminae (Fig. 10-21A) on neurons of lamina I, on neurons of deeper laminae whose dendrites project dorsally into the substantia gelatinosa (see Fig. 10-21B), and on small interneurons of the substantia gelatinosa, which in turn convey this information to neurons in other laminae. These second- and third-order cells of the pain and temperature pathways then send their axons across the midline with a slight rostral inclination to form the anterolateral pathway (Fig. 10-22). The tract occupies most of the anterior half of the lateral funiculus. New fibers join the anterolateral pathway at its anteromedial edge, so that this system, like the posterior columns, is somatotopically organized. Fibers from the most caudal segments occupy its most posterolateral portion, and those from more rostral segments occupy more anteromedial portions (see Fig. 10-22).

The anterolateral pathway can be subdivided on the basis of the origin, destination, and probable function of the fibers. Most of the direct spinothalamic fibers arise from laminae I and V and project to their own parts of VPL and adjoining nuclei of the thalamus in a somatotopic pattern similar to that of the medial lemniscus. They are thought to have a special role in the conscious

awareness of the nature of a painful stimulus (e.g., burning, stinging, aching) and the details of its location, and they are also one alternative pathway by which mechanoreceptive input reaches the thalamus and cerebral cortex. Cortical areas of termination are more widespread than those from the posterior column–medial lemniscus pathway, reaching not just the postcentral gyrus but also the insula and other areas. This reflects the multiple levels of conscious awareness of painful stimuli. A second subset of spinothalamic fibers, arising mainly from the intermediate gray matter, projects to different parts of the thalamus (intralaminar and other nuclei) without a somatotopic arrangement. Many of the latter projections are indirect, following a polysynaptic course through the reticular formation, which makes up much of the core of the brainstem (see Chapter 11), so they are more properly called **spinoreticular** fibers. This system is more likely to be important for changes in level of attention in response to pain. In addition, a collection of **spinomesencephalic** fibers, also arising mainly from laminae I and V, plays an important role in intrinsic pain-control mechanisms (discussed in Chapter 11). Finally, there are nociceptive projections to autonomic control regions of the spinal cord and brainstem, and **spinohypothalamic** fibers that reach the hypothalamus directly. All these spinothalamic, spinoreticular, spinomesencephalic, and spinohypothalamic fibers are intermingled with or adjacent to one another in the spinal cord.

The role of the substantia gelatinosa in the transmission of pain information is still not completely

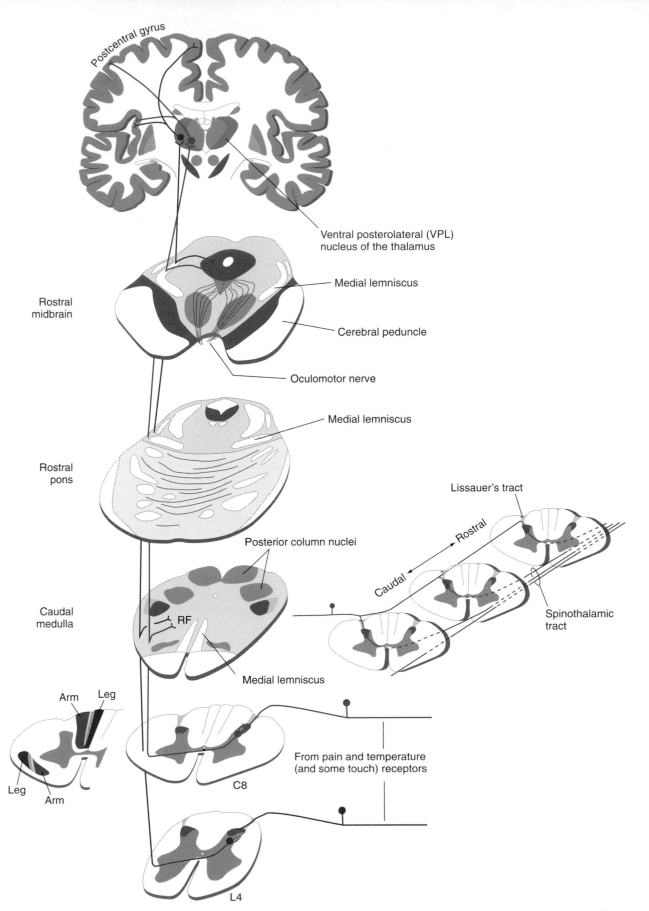

Figure 10-22 Spinothalamic tract. Pain, temperature, and some touch and pressure afferents end in the posterior horn. Second- or higher-order fibers cross the midline, form the spinothalamic tract, and ascend to the ventral posterolateral (VPL) nucleus of the thalamus (and also to other thalamic nuclei not shown). Thalamic cells then project to the somatosensory cortex of the postcentral gyrus, to the insula, and to other cortical areas (also not shown). Along their course through the brainstem, spinothalamic fibers give off many collaterals to the reticular formation (RF). The inset to the left shows the lamination of fibers in the posterior columns and the spinothalamic tract in a leg–lower trunk–upper trunk–arm sequence. The inset to the right shows the longitudinal formation of the spinothalamic tract. Primary afferents ascend several segments in Lissauer's tract before all their branches terminate; fibers crossing to join the spinothalamic tract do so with a rostral inclination. As a result, a cordotomy incision at any given level will spare most of the information entering the contralateral side of the spinal cord at that level, and to be effective, the incision must be made several segments rostral to the highest dermatomal level of pain.

understood. Anatomically it consists of large numbers of small cells among which many unmyelinated afferents terminate. Several populations of these small neurons have been identified based on their neurotransmitter content, but very few from any category give rise to long ascending axons. Rather, they appear to be involved in multiple ways in regulating the access of pain and temperature information to the projection neurons of the anterolateral pathway, either by conveying such information or by participating in processes that suppress or enhance the perception of pain (discussed in Chapter 11).

Damage to the Anterolateral System Causes Diminution of Pain and Temperature Sensations

Although the spinothalamic tract carries some tactile and pressure information, a great deal also travels in the posterior column system, so destruction of the spinothalamic tract causes no significant tactile deficit. There are, however, several types of sensation, in addition to pain and temperature, subserved more or less predominantly by the spinothalamic tract. These are itch (and probably tickle) sensations, pressure sensations from bladder and bowel, and sexual sensations. However, with the exception of itch (and possibly tickle), this information is carried bilaterally, so unilateral damage generally results in little dysfunction. This seems to be a particularly elegant example of the providence of nature.

The spinothalamic tract is, however, the principal pathway for somatic pain sensations, and its destruction produces contralateral analgesia. An operation to destroy the tract (called **cordotomy**) is sometimes performed on patients suffering from intractable pain. This operation consists of cutting the lateral funiculus from the denticulate ligament to the line of ventral rootlets. The cut is usually made several segments rostral to the highest dermatomal level of pain, for two reasons (see Fig. 10-22). First, collaterals of primary afferents may ascend one or more segments in Lissauer's tract before synapsing, so input from these is spared if the cut is made at the highest dermatomal level of pain. Second, the axons that form the spinothalamic tract cross the midline with a rostral inclination, so a cut at any given level spares fibers that arise contralaterally at that level because they join the tract rostral to the cut.

Cordotomy provides prompt contralateral analgesia; however, analogous to the recovery following posterior column damage, the analgesia is seldom permanent. After a varying interval (generally several months), the patient's pain usually returns. The reason is not known, but it may be the increasing efficacy of a few uncrossed fibers in the contralateral spinothalamic tract, of additional spinothalamic fibers located more dorsally in the lateral funiculus, or of a limited number of pain fibers in other pathways. Visceral pain is much less affected by cordotomy; recent evidence indicates that much of this information travels instead in the posterior columns, through axons that originate from neurons near the central canal (lamina X). These fibers travel in the most medial part of the fasciculus gracilis and near the posterior intermediate septum between the fasciculus gracilis and fasciculus cuneatus, on their way to synapses in the posterior column nuclei. The medial lemniscus then conveys both touch-position and visceral pain signals to the thalamus.

Additional Pathways Convey Somatosensory Information to the Thalamus

Additional routes for the transmission of tactile and proprioceptive (and, to a lesser extent, pain) information have also been described. One such route consists of nonprimary afferents, fibers with their cell bodies in the posterior horn that nevertheless project to the posterior column nuclei. Some of these travel within the posterior columns, but others travel in the posterior part of the lateral funiculus. The latter route seems to be particularly important for conveying proprioceptive information from the leg to nucleus gracilis.

Another alternative route is the **spinocervical tract.** Primary afferents conveying information from hair receptors, some other tactile receptors, and some nociceptors synapse on projection neurons in the body of the posterior horn. These projection neurons send their axons ipsilaterally through the posterior part of the lateral funiculus as the spinocervical tract. The spinocervical tract then terminates in the small **lateral cervical nucleus,** which is embedded in the lateral funiculus of the first two cervical segments. The axons of neurons in the lateral cervical nucleus then cross the midline, join the medial lemniscus as it forms in the caudal medulla, and ascend to VPL.

The size and importance of these alternative pathways in the lateral funiculus are not known for humans, although both are known to exist in monkeys. The acute and chronic effects of posterior column damage, for example, leave little doubt that the posterior columns are ordinarily involved in a major way in kinesthesia and tactile sensation. However, the degree of recovery that occurs also leaves little doubt that much of this information reaches the thalamus by additional routes. One of these additional routes is undoubtedly the ascending fibers in the posterior part of the lateral funiculus, bound for the posterior column nuclei or the lateral cervical nucleus. These fibers lie near the surface of the cord and can be transected without damaging the lateral corticospinal tract. Such a lesion by itself has no particular effects, but when added to a posterior column lesion, it makes the effects of the latter much more severe and prolonged.

Table 10-5	Major Spinocerebellar Tracts		
	Posterior Spinocerebellar Tract	**Anterior Spinocerebellar Tract**	**Cuneocerebellar Tract**
Origin	Clarke's nucleus (T1-L2/3)	Spinal border cells (T12-L5)	Lateral cuneate nucleus (medulla)
Body part represented	Trunk, lower extremity	Trunk, lower extremity	Trunk, upper extremity
Major inputs	Mechanoreceptors in muscles, joints, skin	Mechanoreceptors, movement-related interneurons	Mechanoreceptors in muscles, joints, skin
Midline crossing	None	Once in cord, again in cerebellum	None
Peduncle used to enter cerebellum	Inferior	Superior	Inferior

Spinal Information Reaches the Cerebellum Both Directly and Indirectly

The spinal cord is an important source of information used by the cerebellum in the coordination of movement (discussed in greater detail in Chapter 20). This information reaches the cerebellar cortex and nuclei both directly, by way of **spinocerebellar tracts,** and indirectly, by way of relays in brainstem nuclei (described further in Chapters 11 and 20). A number of spinocerebellar tracts have been described, some representing the upper extremity and others the lower extremity. Only three have been well characterized (Table 10-5, see Fig. 10-23).

The Posterior Spinocerebellar Tract and Cuneocerebellar Tract Convey Proprioceptive Information

Collaterals of posterior column fibers conveying tactile, pressure, and proprioceptive information (mainly the latter, from muscle spindles and Golgi tendon organs) synapse on neurons of Clarke's nucleus. These then send their axons into the lateral funiculus of the same side, forming the **posterior (dorsal) spinocerebellar tract** (see Fig. 10-23). This tract, a curved band of fibers extending from the dorsal (posterior) root entry zone to the denticulate ligament, lies at the surface of the spinal cord. Fibers in the tract project ipsilaterally to medial zones of the cerebellum (the vermis and adjoining areas) through the **inferior cerebellar peduncle.** Collaterals of some of these fibers end in the nucleus gracilis, providing an important route by which nonprimary afferents transmit proprioceptive information from the leg to the posterior column–medial lemniscus system. Because Clarke's nucleus does not exist caudal to about L2, neither does the posterior spinocerebellar tract. However, afferents from segments caudal to L2 ascend to that level in fasciculus gracilis to synapse in Clarke's nucleus. This probably explains why Clarke's nucleus is so large at

upper lumbar and lower thoracic levels (see Fig. 10-8), because at these levels it has a substantial backlog of afferent input to process.

The posterior spinocerebellar tract is principally concerned with the ipsilateral leg. Most spinocerebellar-type afferents that enter in cervical and upper thoracic segments—those representing the arm, for example—do not project to Clarke's nucleus. Rather, they travel in fasciculus cuneatus to an analogous nucleus in the medulla, called the **lateral (or external) cuneate nucleus** because it is located just lateral to nucleus cuneatus (see Figs. 11-9 and 11-10). Axons of these cells form the **cuneocerebellar tract,** which also projects ipsilaterally to the vermis and adjoining areas of the cerebellum through the inferior cerebellar peduncle.

The Anterior Spinocerebellar Tract Conveys More Complex Information

Cells on the lateral surface of the lumbar anterior horn (called *spinal border cells*) give rise to the **anterior (ventral) spinocerebellar tract.** Although this tract is also concerned primarily with the leg, it differs from the posterior spinocerebellar tract in three important respects. First, inputs to these projection neurons are more complex. They come not only from group I muscle afferents (mainly Golgi tendon organs) but also from a wide variety of cutaneous receptors, from spinal interneurons, and from fibers of descending tracts. As a result, activity in anterior spinocerebellar tract neurons is related more to attempted movement than simply to sensory signals. Second, the tract is crossed at the level of the spinal cord, in contrast to the posterior spinocerebellar tract, which ascends uncrossed to an ipsilateral termination in the cerebellum. Finally, the anterior spinocerebellar tract takes a roundabout route to the cerebellum (Fig. 10-23). It ascends as far as the rostral pons, then turns caudally and enters the cerebellum via the **superior cerebellar peduncle.** There, most of its fibers recross the midline before ending in the vermis and

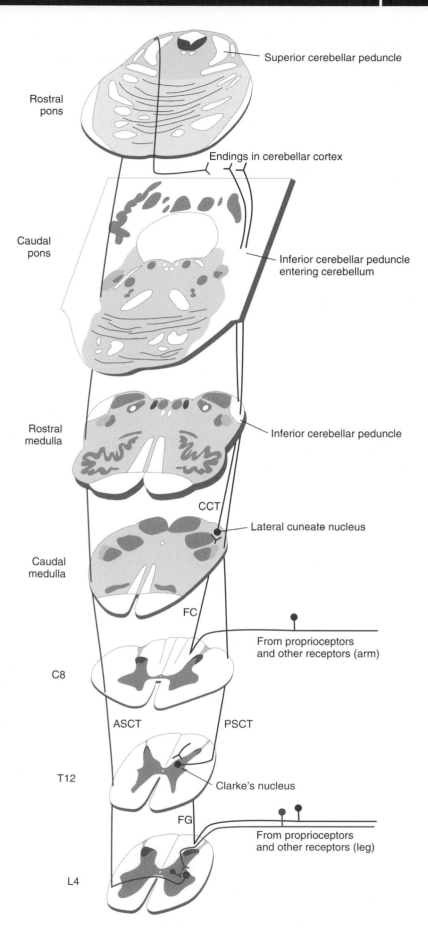

Figure 10-23 Spinocerebellar and cuneocerebellar tracts. Mechanoreceptive afferents from the lower extremity ascend through fasciculus gracilis (FG) to reach Clarke's nucleus, whose cells give rise to the ipsilateral posterior spinocerebellar tract (PSCT), which enters the inferior cerebellar peduncle and ends ipsilaterally in the vermis of the anterior lobe. A larger variety of afferents end on other cells of the spinal gray matter, whose axons form the contralateral anterior spinocerebellar tract (ASCT); this tract ascends to the pons, loops over the superior cerebellar peduncle, and recrosses in the vermis of the anterior lobe. Mechanoreceptive afferents from the upper extremity ascend to the medulla in the fasciculus cuneatus (FC) and end in the lateral cuneate nucleus (analogous to Clarke's nucleus); these cells give rise to the cuneocerebellar tract (CCT), which enters the inferior cerebellar peduncle and ends ipsilaterally in the vermis of the anterior lobe. The rostral spinocerebellar tract is not shown.

adjoining areas of the anterior lobe, so they too ultimately end in the cerebellum on the side ipsilateral to their origin.

A presumed forelimb equivalent of the anterior spinocerebellar tract, called the **rostral spinocerebellar tract,** originates from the posterior horn of lower cervical segments, ascends uncrossed, and enters the cerebellum via both inferior and superior cerebellar peduncles. Little is known of its properties, and it is mentioned here mainly for reasons of symmetry.

Clinically detectable deficits can seldom be attributed to spinocerebellar damage, partially because the spinocerebellar tracts are rarely if ever affected in isolation. Even in the family of inherited diseases referred to as the *spinocerebellar atrophies,* other areas of the cord are always affected as well. For example, the most common type of spinocerebellar atrophy is Friedreich's ataxia. This inherited disorder is characterized by loss of coordination, which is consistent with cerebellar damage, but also by other impairments not consistent with cerebellar damage, such as disturbed tactile sensation and proprioception and loss of reflexes. Correspondingly, widespread damage is found in and around the spinal cord, affecting not only the posterior spinocerebellar tracts but also the posterior columns and some dorsal root fibers. If the spinocerebellar tracts were selectively affected, one would not expect any sensory changes at all because the cerebellum and its connections are not directly involved with sensation.

Descending Pathways Influence the Activity of Lower Motor Neurons

The alpha and gamma motor neurons of the anterior horn are regulated in a variety of ways by supraspinal centers. Some of these centers are located in the brainstem and are discussed in later chapters. The major descending outflow is from the cerebral cortex, particularly the precentral gyrus. This **corticospinal** system is dealt with at greater length in Chapter 18, but a few basic concepts are introduced here.

The Corticospinal Tracts Mediate Voluntary Movement

The **lateral corticospinal tract** (Fig. 10-24), also known as the **pyramidal tract** (because of its course through a pyramid of the medulla), is a large, crossed, descending tract that contains approximately 85% of fibers from the contralateral pyramid that cross in the pyramidal decussation. In the spinal cord, this tract is located in the posterior half of the lateral funiculus, medial to the posterior spinocerebellar tract. Its fibers originate in the cerebral cortex (in the precentral gyrus and nearby areas); descend through the internal capsule, cerebral peduncle, basal pons, and medullary pyramid; decussate at the spinomedullary junction; and end in the anterior horn or intermediate gray matter. They terminate on the

motor neurons of the anterior horn or, more often, on smaller interneurons that in turn synapse on these motor neurons. Surprisingly, and in contrast to sensory tracts, no anatomical evidence has yet been found for a somatotopic arrangement of the fibers in this tract below the level of the midbrain.[g]

Fibers of the corticospinal tract and motor axons of the ventral (anterior) root have distinctly different, though obviously interrelated, roles in the generation of movement. Alpha motor neurons (and the ventral [anterior] root fibers to which these neurons give rise) contact striated muscle directly and are called **lower motor neurons.** They are also sometimes called the **final common pathway** of the motor system because, as noted earlier, they are the only means by which the nervous system can exercise control over body movements. Interruption of the lower motor neurons supplying a muscle causes flaccid paralysis and, eventually, atrophy of the muscle.

Neurons with axons that descend from the cerebral cortex or brainstem and end on lower motor neurons, either directly or by way of an interneuron, are called **upper motor neurons.**[h] An upper motor neuron lesion caused by corticospinal damage has very different effects from those of a lower motor neuron lesion (Table 10-6). Characteristically, the muscles involved show hyperactive reflexes. Their resting tension is increased (i.e., they are **hypertonic**), and there is paralysis or weakness (**paresis**), particularly of fine voluntary movements. This complex of symptoms is referred to as **spastic paralysis.** A number of pathological reflexes are associated with upper motor neuron lesions. The best known is Babinski's sign—dorsiflexion of the big toe and fanning of the others in response to firmly stroking the sole of the foot.[i]

The 15% or so of the fibers in each pyramid that do not cross in the pyramidal decussation continue into the anterior funiculus (located adjacent to the anterior median fissure) as the **anterior corticospinal tract** (see Fig. 10-24). These fibers terminate on motor neurons or interneurons in medial portions of the anterior horn or intermediate gray matter, so they preferentially affect the activity of motor neurons for axial muscles. Many of them cross in the anterior white commissure before synapsing, but some do not. Most anterior corticospinal

---

[g]Nevertheless, damage arising in the center of the cervical spinal cord is often associated with bilateral weakness that is more pronounced in the arms than in the legs. This has led to the longstanding clinical teaching that the fibers of the lateral corticospinal tract are arranged somatotopically, with those destined for more caudal cord levels located more laterally. It has been suggested that this apparent discrepancy may simply reflect the greater importance of this tract for arm movement than for leg movement.

[h]Some use this term in a more restricted sense to refer only to corticospinal neurons.

[i]Babinski's sign is either present or not present; it is not "positive" or "negative."

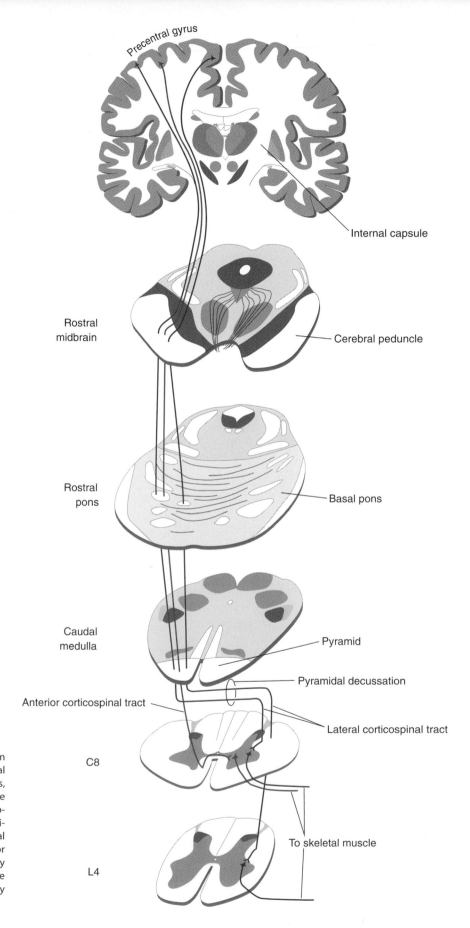

Precentral gyrus

Internal capsule

Rostral midbrain

Cerebral peduncle

Rostral pons

Basal pons

Caudal medulla

Pyramid

Pyramidal decussation

Anterior corticospinal tract

Lateral corticospinal tract

C8

L4

To skeletal muscle

Figure 10-24 Corticospinal tracts. Fibers from the precentral gyrus and other nearby cortical areas descend through the cerebral peduncles, pons, and medullary pyramids; most cross in the pyramidal decussation to form the lateral corticospinal tract. Those that do not cross in the pyramidal decussation form the anterior corticospinal tract; most of these fibers cross in the anterior white commissure before ending in the spinal gray matter. Most corticospinal fibers do not synapse directly on motor neurons; they are drawn that way here for simplicity.

Table 10-6	**Effects of Upper and Lower Motor Neuron Damage**	
	Lower Motor Neuron Damage	**Upper Motor Neuron Damage**
Strength	Decreased	Decreased
Muscle tone	Decreased	Increased
Stretch reflexes	Decreased	Increased
Atrophy	Severe	Mild
Other signs	Fasciculations* Fibrillations[†]	Clonus[‡] Pathological reflexes (e.g., Babinski's sign)

*Spontaneous contractions of groups of muscle fibers, visible through the skin as small twitches.
[†]Spontaneous contractions of individual muscle fibers, not grossly visible but apparent in electrical recordings.
[‡]A rapid series of alternating muscle contractions in response to sudden stretch.

tract fibers end in cervical and thoracic segments, so they may have a special role in the control of neck and shoulder muscles. However, damage to this tract typically does not result in obvious weakness, perhaps partly because of the bilateral distribution of fibers from the contralateral tract. Strictly speaking, the term *pyramidal tract* refers to the combination of lateral and anterior corticospinal tracts.

The Autonomic Nervous System Monitors and Controls Visceral Activity

The goings-on of our cardiac and smooth muscles and our glands proceed, for the most part, without conscious supervision—indeed, in spite of attempts at conscious supervision. For instance, we automatically digest food, regulate our heartbeat, sweat when appropriate, and divert blood to active muscles. Because of the relative automaticity of such functions, the afferents and efferents that innervate these organs are referred to as the **autonomic nervous system.**[j]

The autonomic nervous system has three subdivisions: the **sympathetic, parasympathetic,** and **enteric nervous systems.** Although less well known than the other two, the enteric nervous system perhaps best exemplifies the concept of automatic, self-regulating function. It consists of two interconnected plexuses (the **myenteric plexus** [of Auerbach] and the **submucosal plexus** [of Meissner]), including sensory neurons, interneurons, and visceral motor neurons, in the walls of the

[j]The autonomic nervous system as originally defined consists only of visceral efferents. However, most now use the term to include visceral afferents as well.

alimentary canal; all these neurons and their processes lie entirely outside the CNS. The plexuses are quite extensive, containing an estimated 10^8 neurons, a number comparable to the number of neurons in the entire spinal cord. The enteric nervous system accounts for the observation that near-normal, coordinated gut motility persists even in the total absence of connections between the gut and the CNS. The normally present sympathetic and parasympathetic connections between the gut and the CNS allow for modulation of this motility.

The sympathetic and parasympathetic divisions of the autonomic nervous system have a more familiar organization. Similar to the somatic portions of the nervous system considered thus far, there are visceral sensory fibers, ascending visceral sensory pathways, visceral reflex arcs, and descending pathways that control the activity of visceral motor neurons (Fig. 10-25); systematic maps are common, in which clusters of visceral motor neurons or second-order visceral sensory neurons deal with individual organs. One fundamental difference is that sympathetic and parasympathetic efferents originating in the CNS do not reach their targets directly; rather, a two-neuron chain is involved (Fig. 10-26). The first neuron, referred to as a **preganglionic neuron,** has its cell body in the CNS. Its axon terminates in a peripheral ganglion on the second neuron, termed a **postganglionic neuron.**[k] Preganglionic fibers are thinly myelinated (group B), whereas postganglionic fibers are unmyelinated (accounting for many of the C fibers in peripheral nerves). Sympathetic ganglia are located relatively near the CNS; parasympathetic ganglia are located near the organs they innervate (Fig. 10-27). Although functionally different autonomic neurons release distinctive cocktails of neurotransmitters, the sympathetic and parasympathetic nervous systems also differ in the major neurotransmitter used by their postganglionic neurons (see Fig. 10-27). The preganglionic neurons of both systems liberate acetylcholine onto the postganglionic neurons, where it acts on nicotinic receptors. Postganglionic parasympathetic neurons also release acetylcholine onto their targets, in this case affecting muscarinic receptors. Most postganglionic sympathetic neurons, in contrast, release norepinephrine (a prominent exception is the sympathetic innervation of sweat glands, which is cholinergic). Other differences between the sympathetic and parasympathetic systems are reviewed briefly in the following sections, and the higher order CNS systems that control them are discussed in Chapter 23.

[k]Although the axons of these neurons are indeed postganglionic, there is a bit of a logical inconsistency in calling the neurons themselves postganglionic (because they live in an autonomic ganglion). For this reason, many have begun to refer to these neurons as autonomic ganglion cells.

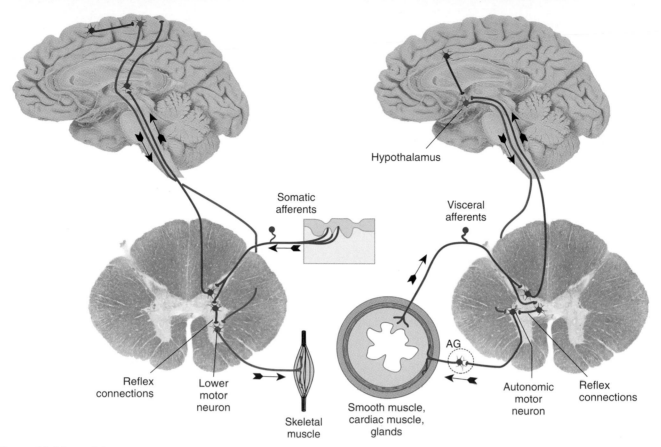

Somatic afferents

Hypothalamus

Visceral afferents

Reflex connections   **Lower motor neuron**   **Skeletal muscle**   **Smooth muscle, cardiac muscle, glands**   **AG**   **Autonomic motor neuron**   **Reflex connections**

Figure 10-25 Parallels between somatic and autonomic parts of the nervous system. Both involve specialized afferents and efferents, reflex connections, and ascending and descending pathways to and from higher levels of the CNS. In the case of the sympathetic and parasympathetic systems, however, the hypothalamus rather than the thalamus receives much of the ascending information, and the hypothalamus rather than the cerebral cortex is a major source of descending pathways. In addition, sympathetic and parasympathetic transmission to the periphery involves an intermediate synapse in an autonomic ganglion (AG).

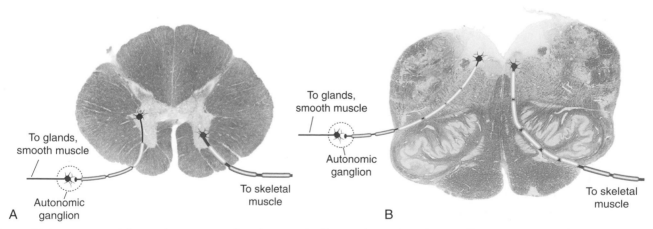

To glands, smooth muscle

To glands, smooth muscle

Autonomic ganglion

To skeletal muscle

Autonomic ganglion

To skeletal muscle

A   **B**

Figure 10-26 One major difference between somatic and autonomic efferents. The myelinated axons of lower motor neurons leave the spinal cord through ventral roots **(A),** or leave the brainstem through cranial nerves **(B),** and reach skeletal muscle directly. The autonomic system, in contrast, uses a two-neuron path. The thinly myelinated axons of preganglionic neurons leave through ventral roots or cranial nerves and end on postganglionic neurons in autonomic ganglia outside the CNS. Unmyelinated axons of postganglionic neurons then innervate smooth muscle, cardiac muscle, and glands.

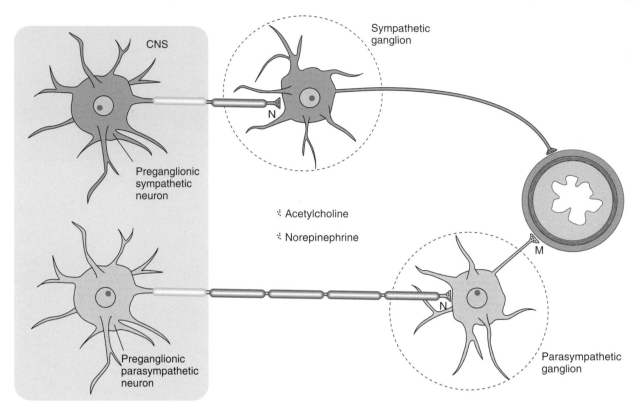

Figure 10-27 Major differences between the sympathetic and parasympathetic systems. The axons of preganglionic sympathetic neurons end in ganglia relatively close to the spinal cord, whereas those of preganglionic parasympathetic neurons travel a longer distance and reach ganglia near the innervated organ. The preganglionic neurons of both systems use acetylcholine as a neurotransmitter, but at the synapses of postganglionic neurons, the parasympathetic system uses acetylcholine and the sympathetic system typically uses norepinephrine. M, muscarinic synapse; N, nicotinic synapse.

Preganglionic Parasympathetic Neurons Are Located in the Brainstem and Sacral Spinal Cord

Preganglionic parasympathetic fibers originate from neurons in two widely separated parts of the CNS—the brainstem and the sacral spinal cord (Fig. 10-28). They travel in sacral spinal nerves or in certain cranial nerves (III, VII, IX, and, most important, X, as discussed further in Chapter 12) to ganglia in or near their targets. Postganglionic neurons in these peripheral parasympathetic ganglia then innervate the target organ. The degree of divergence is traditionally considered to be smaller in parasympathetic than in sympathetic ganglia. This, together with the location of parasympathetic ganglia in individual organs, makes it possible for the parasympathetic system to exert restricted, localized control. Sympathetic activation, in contrast, can be more widespread. (The amount of divergence in both systems, however, varies from organ to organ. Just as finely controlled skeletal muscles are innervated by relatively large numbers of lower motor neurons [see Chapter 18], the postganglionic parasympathetic and sympathetic neurons for finely controlled organs receive inputs from relatively large numbers of preganglionic neurons.)

The parasympathetic (or **craniosacral**) outflow goes almost exclusively to thoracic, abdominal, and pelvic viscera and to some important cranial targets (see Fig. 10-28). There are, for example, no parasympathetic fibers to the limbs. In a general sense, the parasympathetic system enhances energy storage. Activation of parasympathetic nerves causes decreased cardiac output and blood pressure, increased peristalsis in the gut, and salivation, as well as pupillary constriction and bladder contraction. Visceral afferents traveling with sacral spinal nerves and with cranial nerves IX and X are appropriate for these functions, carrying information about blood pressure and chemistry and fullness of the bladder and gastrointestinal tract. Cranial nerves VII, IX, and X also carry information from taste buds, obviously relevant to energy intake.

Preganglionic Sympathetic Neurons Are Located in Thoracic and Lumbar Spinal Segments

Preganglionic sympathetic fibers originate from neurons in the thoracic and upper two or three lumbar segments (see Fig. 10-28). Thus this division of the autonomic nervous system is also referred to as the **thoracolumbar outflow.** The preganglionic fibers travel in spinal nerves to ganglia relatively close to the spinal cord. Some of these ganglia form an interconnected **sympathetic chain** just distal to the dorsal root ganglia (see Figs. 10-1

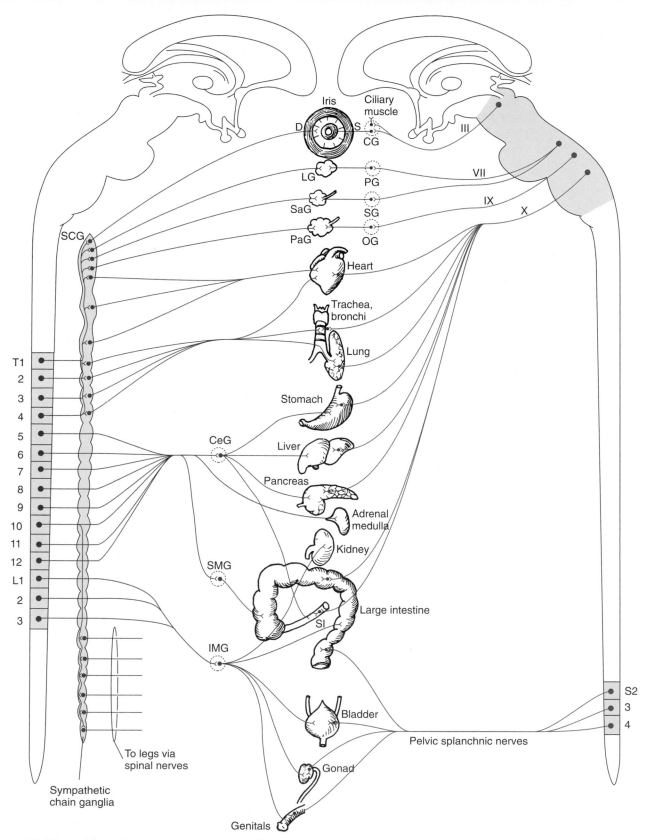

Figure 10-28 Origin and distribution of sympathetic (left) and parasympathetic (right) efferents. Postganglionic neurons that live in sympathetic chain ganglia and project to the body wall and upper extremity are omitted from the diagram to avoid excessive complexity; their axons travel in spinal nerves in a way analogous to that indicated for the lower extremity supply. Although the cranial nerves have distinct and separate parasympathetic contents, there is substantial overlap in the contents of ventral roots S2 to S4. CeG, celiac ganglion; CG, ciliary ganglion; D, pupillary dilator; IMG, inferior mesenteric ganglion; LG, lacrimal gland; OG, otic ganglion; PaG, parotid gland; PG, pterygopalatine ganglion; S, pupillary sphincter; SaG, submandibular and sublingual salivary glands; SCG, superior cervical ganglion; SG, submandibular ganglion; SMG, superior mesenteric ganglion. *(Modified from Mettler FA: Neuroanatomy, ed 2, St. Louis, 1948, Mosby.)*

and 10-2), whereas others, referred to as **prevertebral ganglia,** are a little farther away. The major exception is the adrenal medulla, which is directly innervated by preganglionic sympathetic fibers. The adrenal medulla develops from neural crest cells and, similar to postganglionic sympathetic neurons, its cells secrete norepinephrine (and epinephrine as well); it can therefore be thought of as a displaced sympathetic ganglion.

Sympathetic fibers are more widely distributed than parasympathetic fibers, reaching all parts of the body. Preganglionic fibers exit the spinal cord in thoracic and upper lumbar ventral (anterior) roots and then travel from the spinal nerves to the sympathetic chain via **white communicating rami** (see Fig. 10-2), so called because the preganglionic fibers are myelinated and hence white; only spinal nerves T1 to L2-L3 have white rami. Some end in sympathetic chain ganglia at that or another level, from which unmyelinated postganglionic fibers rejoin spinal nerves via **gray communicating rami;** all spinal nerves include gray rami and postganglionic sympathetic fibers. Other preganglionic fibers continue through the chain without synapsing and reach prevertebral ganglia. Postganglionic fibers destined for the head, heart, airways, body wall, and limbs originate in sympathetic chain ganglia, whereas those destined for abdominal and pelvic viscera originate in prevertebral ganglia.

Generally, the sympathetic system prepares us for situations in which energy needs to be expended. Activation of sympathetic fibers increases heart rate, decreases peristalsis, and diverts blood from the gut to skeletal muscles. Because of the widespread distribution of postganglionic sympathetic fibers and because sympathetic stimulation causes the adrenal medulla to secrete epinephrine and norepinephrine into the circulation, sympathetic activation can produce widespread and relatively long-lasting effects. On a moment-to-moment basis, however, restricted sympathetic activity can affect selected organs or parts of the body.

Although in some instances, such as effects on gut motility and heart rate, the sympathetic and parasympathetic systems have opposite effects, in other instances one or the other is unopposed or both act cooperatively (Table 10-7). For example, sweat glands and limb vasculature receive only sympathetic innervation, but the parasympathetic system is the dominant influence in control of the pupil and the bladder. The two systems cooperate in male sexual function, with erection mediated primarily by parasympathetic fibers and ejaculation by sympathetic fibers.

Visceral Distortion or Damage Causes Pain That Is Referred to Predictable Dermatomes

Visceral afferent fibers, with their cell bodies in T1 to L2 or L3 spinal ganglia, accompany sympathetic efferents in spinal nerves. Similarly, visceral afferents with cell bodies in S2 to S4 spinal ganglia or certain cranial nerve ganglia accompany parasympathetic efferents. Most of these afferents carry information that subserves visceral reflexes and does not reach consciousness, such as data about vascular tone. Others, primarily in sympathetic nerves, carry messages about distortion or inflammation of visceral organs, which are interpreted as pain. Visceral pain is different from somatic pain in that it is poorly localized to the diseased organ and commonly is **referred** to an area of the body surface. The area to which the pain is referred corresponds to the dermatome innervated by the spinal segment to which the visceral afferents project. Thus the heart is supplied by visceral afferents that enter the cord in upper thoracic segments, and coronary artery disease is associated with pain referred to the left side of the chest and part of the left arm (angina pectoris). The basis of this referred pain is the convergence of visceral and somatic pain fibers in a given dorsal (posterior) root on the same spinothalamic tract cells reached by somatic pain fibers, leading to the brain interpreting spinothalamic tract impulses as pain in the somatic region. The functional utility of such an arrangement is not clear, but knowledge of typical patterns of referred pain is important clinically (Table 10-8).

A Longitudinal Network of Arteries Supplies the Spinal Cord

The arterial supply of the spinal cord comes from the vertebral arteries and from branches, ultimately from the thoracic and abdominal aorta, called **radicular arteries.** Each vertebral artery gives rise to an **anterior spinal artery;** the two anterior spinal arteries fuse to form a single midline vessel—the longest artery in the body—that courses along the anterior median fissure of the spinal cord (Fig. 10-29). The vertebral or posterior inferior cerebellar artery of each side also gives rise to a **posterior spinal artery,** which proceeds along the line of attachment of the dorsal (posterior) rootlets. The posterior spinal arteries and the midline anterior spinal artery supply upper cervical levels with blood from the vertebral arteries. Below this, all three spinal arteries form a more or less continuous series of anastomoses with radicular arteries for the length of the cord. The spinal arteries are too small to convey blood from the vertebral arteries to all spinal levels; beginning with lower cervical segments, the cord depends on these radicular arteries for its survival. One particular radicular artery, present at about spinal cord level T12 in most individuals, is called the **great radicular artery** (or **artery of Adamkiewicz**) and may provide the entire arterial supply for the lumbosacral spinal cord.

The anterior spinal artery, which is usually a continuous vessel for the length of the spinal cord, gives rise

Table 10-7 | Principal Physiological Effects of Autonomic Activity

Structure or System	PSN	Sympathetic Effect	PPN*	Parasympathetic Effect
Head				
Pupillary sphincter			E-W	Contract (miosis)
Pupillary dilator	T1-T3	Contract (mydriasis)		
Superior tarsal muscle	T1-T3	Contract (lid elevation)		
Ciliary muscle			E-W	Contract (accommodation)
Lacrimal gland	T1-T3	Slightly ↑ secretion	SSN	↑ Secretion
Salivary glands	T1-T3	Slightly ↑ secretion, ↑ viscosity	ISN, SSN	↑ Secretion, ↓ viscosity
Pineal gland	T1-T3	↑ Melatonin synthesis		
Respiratory System				
Bronchial muscles	T1-T5	Relax	DMNX	Contract
Cardiovascular System				
Heart rate and output	T1-T5	↑	NA	↓
Arteries (skeletal muscle)	T1-L3	Constrict or dilate†		
Arteries (skin)	T1-L3	Constrict		
Arteries (viscera)	T1-L3	Constrict	DMNX	Dilate
Gastrointestinal System				
Motility	T6-L3	↓	DMNX‡	↑
Sphincters	T6-L3	Contract	DMNX‡	Relax
Secretion	T6-L3	↓	DMNX‡	↑
Gallbladder	T6-T9	Relax	DMNX	Contract
Urogenital System				
Bladder detrusor	T12-L2	Relax	S2-S4	Contract
Bladder sphincter (internal)	T12-L2	Contract	S2-S4	Relax
Seminal vesicles, vas deferens	T10-L1	Contract (during ejaculation)		
Penile/clitoral arteries	T10-L1	Dilate or constrict§	S2-S4	Dilate (erection)
Skin				
Sweat glands	T1-L3	↑ Secretion‖		
Piloerector muscles	T1-L3	Contract (goose bumps)		
Adrenal Medulla	T8-L1	↑ Secretion		

*Brainstem sites containing preganglionic parasympathetic neurons are discussed in Chapter 12.
†Effect depends on conditions of stimulation. Most postganglionic sympathetic fibers to skeletal muscle arteries cause constriction, but there are some cholinergic vasodilator fibers. In addition, sympathetic activation of the adrenal medulla causes skeletal muscle vasodilation in response to circulating catecholamines.
‡Spinal segments S2-S4 provide the preganglionic parasympathetic neurons for the digestive tract below the left colic flexure.
§Depends on conditions. Sympathetically induced vasoconstriction mediates detumescence, but sympathetic activity has also been implicated in psychogenic erection.
‖Postganglionic sympathetic fibers to sweat glands are atypical in that they are cholinergic.
DMNX, dorsal motor nucleus of the vagus (in the medulla); E-W, Edinger-Westphal nucleus (in the midbrain); ISN, inferior salivary nucleus (in the medulla); NA, nucleus ambiguus (in the medulla); PPN, location of preganglionic parasympathetic neurons; PSN, location of preganglionic sympathetic neurons; SSN, superior salivary nucleus (in the pons).

to a series of hundreds of central and circumferential branches (see Fig. 10-29) that supply the anterior two thirds of the spinal cord, including the base of the posterior horn and a variable portion of the lateral corticospinal tract (Fig. 10-30). The posterior spinal arteries may subdivide into longitudinal branches medial and lateral to the dorsal (posterior) roots (see Fig. 10-29) and are really more of a plexiform network of small arteries. Collectively they supply the posterior columns, substantia gelatinosa, dorsal (posterior) root entry zone, and a variable portion of the lateral corticospinal tract.

Venous drainage is by a series of six irregular, plexiform channels: one each along the anterior and posterior midlines, and one along the line of attachment of the dorsal (posterior) and ventral (anterior) rootlets of each side. These are drained by **radicular veins,** which in turn empty into the **epidural venous plexus.**

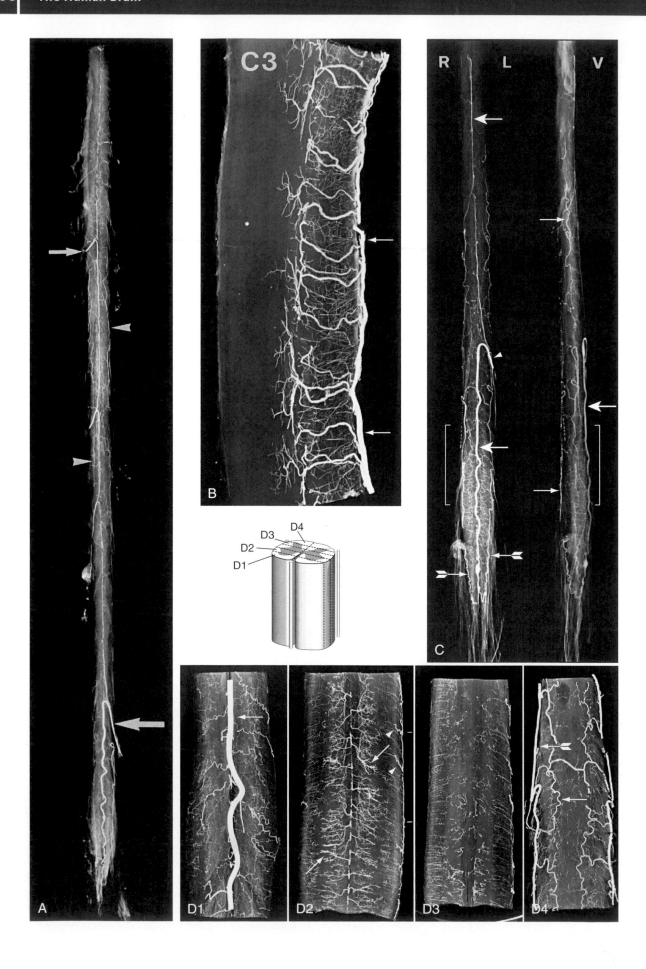

Table 10-8	Typical Patterns of Referred Pain

Organ Damaged	Dermatomes in Which Pain May Be Felt
Diaphragm	C3-C4
Heart	T1-T4 (mainly left)
Stomach	T6-T9 (mainly left)
Gallbladder	T7-T8 (right)
Duodenum	T9-T10
Appendix	T10 (right)
Reproductive organs	T10-T12
Kidney, ureter	L1-L2

Spinal Cord Damage Causes Predictable Deficits

Long-Term Effects of Spinal Cord Damage Are Preceded by a Period of Spinal Shock

Spinal cord transection eventually leads to spastic (upper motor neuron) paralysis below the level of damage. This is preceded, however, by a stage of **spinal shock** that may last for weeks, characterized by more or less completely flaccid paralysis and areflexia. Deep tendon reflexes then begin to return and finally become hyperactive. Lesser degrees of spinal shock may occur even in cases of contusion of the spinal cord, in which total or near-total recovery can be expected. The mechanism of spinal shock is incompletely understood, but the whole sequence of events is thought to be a consequence of interruption of fibers from the brainstem and cerebrum descending to spinal cord motor neurons and interneurons. In addition to corticospinal tracts, there are a number of other descending influences, some facilitatory and some inhibitory. Spinal shock would thus be caused by the sudden loss of a collection of descending influences whose net effect is facilitatory. Multiple mechanisms contribute to the transition from spinal shock to spasticity. Early on, spinal cord neurons probably upregulate their complements of transmitter receptors and become abnormally sensitive. Later stages of the transition are thought to involve the formation of new synaptic connections. The degeneration of the endings of descending fibers leaves vacant synaptic sites at various places on motor neurons and interneurons, adjacent to intact reflex connections. Multiplication of these reflex connections to fill up the vacated sites would be expected to increase the sensitivity and magnitude of reflexes.

Spinal shock followed by long-term hyperreflexia affects autonomic functions as well. Cervical spinal cord injury leads to a brief initial period of hypertension, caused by the release of epinephrine and norepinephrine from the adrenal medulla. This is followed by the autonomic equivalent of spinal shock, in which sympathetic (and sacral parasympathetic) activity is greatly reduced. Cardiovascular manifestations include hypotension and bradycardia, as a result of diminished sympathetic outflow from thoracic segments. Over a longer time, spinal sympathetic (and sacral parasympathetic) reflexes become hyperactive, and **autonomic dysreflexia** commonly develops. Noxious stimuli (e.g., bladder catheterization) that would normally cause a moderate sympathetic response lead instead to massive vasoconstriction and potentially life-threatening hypertension.

The Side and Distribution of Deficits Reflect the Location of Spinal Cord Damage

Partial lesions of the spinal cord are (fortunately) much more common than complete transections. Complete transection of one side of the cord (hemisection), though rare, results in an instructive complex of symptoms called the **Brown-Séquard syndrome** (Fig. 10-31). After a period of spinal shock (particularly prominent in those areas subserved by the damaged portion of the cord), spastic paralysis develops below the level of the lesion and ipsilateral to it because of interruption of the lateral corticospinal tract. Tactile, vibratory, and position senses are disturbed ipsilaterally below the level of the lesion because of interruption of the posterior column. There is loss of pain and temperature sensation *contralateral* to the lesion, beginning one or two segments caudal to the level of the lesion, as a result of interruption of the spinothalamic tract. This is one of many examples of **crossed findings,** that is, some symptoms referable to one side of the head or body and others to the other side, which may seem strange and inexplicable unless one

Figure 10-29 Arterial supply of the spinal cord, demonstrated in a beautiful series of angiograms obtained after postmortem injection of barium sulfate and gelatin. **A,** Anterior view, showing the anterior spinal artery joined by a large radicular artery at C7 *(small arrow)* and by the great radicular artery of Adamkiewicz *(large arrow)* at T11. Parts of posterior spinal arteries *(arrowheads)* can also be seen. **B,** Midsagittal view at C3 showing the anterior spinal artery *(arrows)* giving rise to many branches that run posteriorly through the anterior median fissure to reach central regions of the cord. **C,** Anterior and lateral (V, ventral) views of the thoracic and lumbosacral portions of a spinal cord, showing the anterior *(large arrows)* and posterior *(small arrows)* spinal arteries and the artery of Adamkiewicz *(arrowhead)*. Near the cauda equina, anastomoses *(tailed arrows)* typically interconnect the anterior and posterior spinal arteries in a kind of miniature circle of Willis. **D,** Vertical slices of the bracketed region in **C,** showing the anterior spinal artery *(arrow,* **D1**), its branches to central regions of the cord *(arrows,* **D2**), branches from circumferential anterior-posterior arterial interconnections that feed parts of the cord closer to the surface (**D3** and *arrowheads,* **D2**), and posterior spinal arteries medial and lateral to the dorsal root entry zone *(arrow* and *tailed arrow,* **D4**). *(From Thron AK: Vascular anatomy of the spinal cord, Vienna, 1988, Springer-Verlag.)*

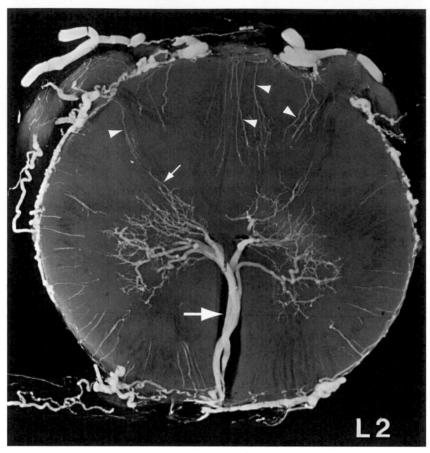

Figure 10-30 Microangiogram of a cross section at L2. Branches *(large arrow)* of the anterior spinal artery run posteriorly through the anterior median fissure to reach central regions of the cord. Branches of circumferential connections between the anterior and posterior spinal arteries supply parts of the cord closer to the surface. Branches *(arrowheads)* of the posterior spinal artery supply the posterior columns and share with anterior spinal branches *(small arrow)* in the supply of the posterior horn. *(From Thron AK: Vascular anatomy of the spinal cord, Vienna, 1988, Springer-Verlag.)*

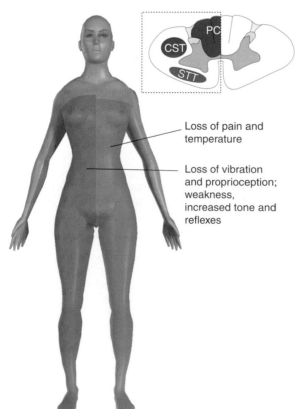

Loss of pain and temperature

Loss of vibration and proprioception; weakness, increased tone and reflexes

Figure 10-31 Brown-Séquard syndrome. Damage to the outlined area of the spinal cord (in this example at C8) would affect the indicated tracts, causing ipsilateral spastic paralysis and loss of fine touch and proprioception, and contralateral loss of pain and temperature beginning one or more segments below the level of damage. CST, corticospinal tract; PC, posterior column; STT, spinothalamic tract.

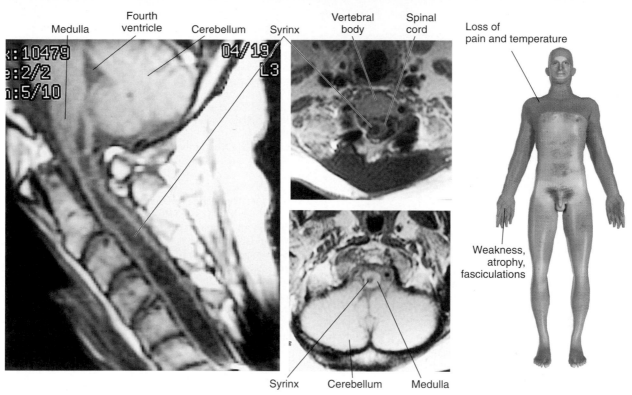

Figure 10-32 Syringomyelia. A 39-year-old man was thrown from the bed of a pickup truck in a motor vehicle accident, sustaining vertebral fractures at T5-T6 and C4-C5. About 2 years later he began to notice progressive weakness and atrophy of his hand muscles. Magnetic resonance imaging revealed a central cavity in his spinal cord (syringomyelia), extending into the caudal medulla. The cavity is somewhat irregular in shape, and damage is more extensive at some levels than at others. Typical findings in such a case would be a band of bilateral loss of pain and temperature sensation (extending into the distribution of the trigeminal nerve, in a pattern explained in Chapter 12) and weakness and atrophy at levels where the damage extends into the anterior horns (in this case, at lower cervical levels). *(Magnetic resonance images, courtesy Dr. Raymond F. Carmody, University of Arizona College of Medicine.)*

understands the anatomical sites at which different pathways cross the midline.

Syringomyelia (*syrinx* is Greek for "tube," as in syringe) is a disease of the central part of the spinal cord in which a tubelike enlargement of the central canal develops, typically at lower cervical or upper thoracic levels (Fig. 10-32). As the syrinx enlarges, surrounding neural tissue is destroyed. The first damage is to fibers crossing through the limited available area around the central canal (see Fig. 10-7A). The next area damaged is usually the anterior horn. The result is a distinctive combination of loss of pain and temperature sensation bilaterally over the arms and shoulders (as a result of the damage to crossing fibers) and weakness and atrophy of the muscles of the hands (as a result of anterior horn damage). Of course, if the syrinx occurred at a different spinal level, the symptoms would be referred to a correspondingly different part of the body.

SUGGESTED READINGS

Andrew D, Craig AD: Spinothalamic lamina I neurons selectively sensitive to histamine: a central neural pathway for itch. Nat Neurosci 4:72, 2001.

Appel NM, Elde RP: The intermediolateral cell column of the thoracic spinal cord is comprised of target-specific subnuclei: evidence from retrograde transport studies and immunohistochemistry. J Neurosci 8:1767, 1988.

Applebaum ML, et al: Organization and receptive fields of primate spinothalamic tract neurons. J Neurophysiol 38:572, 1975.

Basbaum AI: Conduction of the effects of noxious stimulation by short-fiber multisynaptic systems of the spinal cord in the rat. Exp Neurol 40:699, 1973.
  A series of experiments showing that rats can learn to avoid painful stimuli even after hemisection of both sides of the spinal cord, which should transect the long ascending fibers of both sides.

Bosco G, Poppele RE: Representation of multiple kinematic parameters of the cat hindlimb in spinocerebellar activity. J Neurophysiol 78:1421, 1997.

Briner RP, et al: Evidence for unmyelinated sensory fibers in the posterior columns in man. Brain 111:999, 1988.

Brown AG: The spinocervical tract. Prog Neurobiol 17:59, 1981.

Calne DB, Pallis CA: Vibratory sense: a critical review. Brain 89:723, 1966.
  Interesting reading, with a review of old clinical observations.

Cervero F, Iggo A: The substantia gelatinosa of the spinal cord: a critical review. Brain 103:717, 1980.

Cervero F, Morrison JFB, editors: Visceral sensation. Prog Brain Res 67:1986.

Chung K, Coggeshall RE: Unmyelinated primary afferent fibers in dorsal funiculi of cat sacral spinal cord. J Comp Neurol 238:365, 1985.

Coggeshall RE: Law of separation of function of the spinal roots. Physiol Rev 60:716, 1980.

Collins WF, Nulsen FE, Randt CT: Relation of peripheral nerve fiber size and sensation in man. Arch Neurol 3:381, 1960.
Postcordotomy abolition of the painful consequences of controlled electrical stimulation of the sural nerve.

Craig AD: Pain mechanisms: labeled lines versus convergence in central processing. Annu Rev Neurosci 26:1, 2003.

Creed RS, et al: Reflex activity of the spinal cord (reprinted with annotations by DPC Lloyd), New York, 1972, Oxford University Press.

Critchley E, Eisen A, editors: Spinal cord disease: basic science, diagnosis and management, London, 1997, Springer-Verlag.

Crock HV, Yoshizawa H: The blood supply of the vertebral column and spinal cord in man, New York, 1977, Springer-Verlag.

Davidoff RA: The dorsal columns. Neurology 39:1377, 1989.
A good review of the complications lurking in this seemingly simple pathway.

Ditunno JF, et al: Spinal shock revisited: a four-phase model. Spinal Cord 42:383, 2004.

Furness JB: The enteric nervous system, Oxford, 2006, Blackwell Publishing.

Garrett JR: The proper role of nerves in salivary secretion: a review. J Dental Res 66:387, 1987.

Gibbins I: Peripheral autonomic pathways. In Paxinos G, Mai JK, editors: The human nervous system, ed 2, San Diego, 2004, Elsevier Academic Press.

Gillilan LA: The arterial blood supply of the human spinal cord. J Comp Neurol 110:75, 1958.

Gillilan LA: Veins of the spinal cord. Neurology 20:860, 1970.

Giuliano F, Rampin O: Neural control of erection. Physiol Behav 83:189, 2004.

Glees P, Soler J: Fibre content of the posterior column and synaptic connections of nucleus gracilis. Z Zellforsch 36:381, 1951.
Documents the fact that, at least in cats, only about 25% of the fibers that enter the posterior columns reach the posterior column nuclei; the rest end within the spinal cord.

Ha H: Cervicothalamic tract in the rhesus monkey. Exp Neurol 33:205, 1971.

Hosobuchi Y: The majority of unmyelinated afferent axons in human ventral roots probably conduct pain. Pain 8:167, 1980.

Ikoma A, et al: The neurobiology of itch. Nat Rev Neurosci 7:535, 2006.

Jänig W: The integrative action of the autonomic nervous system: neurobiology of homeostasis, Cambridge, 2006, Cambridge University Press.

Keswani NH, Hollinshead WH: Localization of the phrenic nucleus in the spinal cord of man. Anat Rec 125:683, 1956.

Kiehn O: Locomotor circuits in the mammalian spinal cord. Ann Rev Neurosci 29:279, 2006.

Kuhn RA: Functional capacity of the isolated human spinal cord. Brain 73:1, 1950.
A careful study of the course of events after complete transection of the spinal cord, particularly spinal shock and its gradual fading.

Laird JMA, Schaible H-G: Visceral and deep somatic pain. In Hunt S, Koltzenburg M, editors: The neurobiology of pain, Oxford, 2005, Oxford University Press.

Levi ADO, Tator CH, Bunge RP: Clinical syndromes associated with disproportionate weakness of the upper versus the lower extremities after spinal cord injury. Neurosurgery 38:179, 1996.
A review of the evidence that the corticospinal tract, surprisingly, is not somatotopically organized in the lower brainstem and the spinal cord.

Liddell EGT, Sherrington C: Reflexes in response to stretch (myotatic reflexes). Proc R Soc Lond B 96:212, 1924.

Macdonald A, et al: Level of termination of the spinal cord and the dural sac: a magnetic resonance study. Clin Anat 12:149, 1999.

Matthews PBC: The 1989 James A. F. Stevenson memorial lecture. The knee jerk: still an enigma. Can J Physiol Pharmacol 68:347, 1990.

Melzack R, Wall PD: Pain mechanisms: a new theory. Science 150:971, 1965.
A seminal paper in which the modulating effect of the substantia gelatinosa on pain transmission was proposed in a scheme called the "gate control theory" of pain. Although apparently wrong in some of its details, the gate control theory has been very influential on pain research since 1965.

Mense S: Structure-function relationships in identified afferent neurones. Anat Embryol 181:1, 1990.
A review of elegant demonstrations of how single primary afferents with known functions end in precisely defined patterns in the spinal cord.

Miller S, van der Meché FGA: Coordinated stepping of all four limbs in the high spinal cat. Brain Res 109:395, 1976.

Morin F: A new spinal pathway for cutaneous impulses. Am J Physiol 183:245, 1955.
The original physiological description of the spinocervical tract.

Nathan PW, Smith MC: The location of descending fibres to sympathetic preganglionic vasomotor and sudomotor neurons in man. J Neurol Neurosurg Psychiatry 50:1253, 1987.

Nathan PW, Smith MC, Cook AW: Sensory effects in man of lesions of the posterior columns and of some other afferent pathways. Brain 109:1003, 1986.
"The total evidence from all the relevant cases shows that the major pathway subserving every kind of mechanoreception is in the posterior third of the cord."

Nathan PW, Smith MC, Deacon P: The corticospinal tracts in man: course and location of fibres at different segmental levels. Brain 113:303, 1990.

Nauta HJW, et al: Punctate midline myelotomy for the relief of visceral cancer pain. J Neurosurg (Spine 2) 92:125, 2000.
Direct evidence from human surgical procedures that fibers subserving pelvic visceral pain travel near the midline in the posterior columns.

Norrsell U: Behavioral studies of the somatosensory system. Physiol Rev 60:327, 1980.

Novy J, et al: Spinal cord ischemia: clinical and imaging patterns, pathogenesis, and outcomes in 27 patients. Arch Neurol 63:1113, 2006.

Nudo RJ, Masterton RB: Descending pathways to the spinal cord: a comparative study of 22 mammals. J Comp Neurol 277:53, 1988.

Palecek J, Paleckova V, Willis WD: The roles of pathways in the spinal cord lateral and dorsal funiculi in signaling nociceptive somatic and visceral stimuli in rats. Pain 96:297, 2002.

Perl ER: Effects of muscle stretch on excitability of contralateral motoneurones. J Physiol 145:193, 1959.

Petras JM: Spinocerebellar tract neurons in the rhesus monkey. Brain Res 130:146, 1977.

Pratt CA: Evidence of positive force feedback among hindlimb extensors in the intact standing cat. J Neurophysiol 73:2578, 1995.
Conditions under which Golgi tendon organs cause excitatory reflex effects.

Rexed B: The cytoarchitectonic organization of the spinal cord in the cat. J Comp Neurol 96:415, 1952.

Rossi A, Decchi B: Flexibility of lower limb reflex responses to painful cutaneous stimulation in standing humans: evidence of load-dependent modulation. J Physiol 481:521, 1994.

Routal RV, Pal GP: A study of motoneuron groups and motor columns of the human spinal cord. J Anat 195:211, 1999.

Routal RV, Pal GP: Location of the spinal nucleus of the accessory nerve in the human spinal cord. J Anat 196:263, 2000.

Rustioni A, Hayes NL, O'Neill SO: Dorsal column nuclei and ascending afferents in macaques. Brain 102:95, 1979.
An account of the nonprimary afferents ascending to nuclei gracilis and cuneatus in the posterior columns and the posterior part of the lateral funiculus.

Rymer WZ, Houk JC, Craggo PE: Mechanisms of the clasp-knife reflex studied in an animal model. Exp Brain Res 37:93, 1979.

Physiological experiments suggesting that Golgi tendon organs cannot entirely account for the clasp-knife reflex and that group III and IV muscle afferents may be involved.

Sandrini G, et al: The lower limb flexion reflex in humans. Prog Neurobiol 77:353, 2005.

Schoenen J, Faull RLM: Spinal cord: cyto- and chemoarchitecture. In Paxinos G, Mai JK, editors: The human nervous system, ed 2, San Diego, 2004, Elsevier Academic Press.

Smith MC, Deacon P: Topographical anatomy of the posterior columns of the spinal cord in man: the long ascending fibers. Brain 107:671, 1984.

Snyder R: The organization of the dorsal root entry zone in cats and monkeys. J Comp Neurol 174:47, 1977.

Takahashi Y, Takahashi K, Moriya H: Mapping of dermatomes of the lower extremities based on an animal model. J Neurosurg 82:1030, 1995.

Tamaki N, Batzdorf U, Nagashima T, editors: Syringomyelia: current concepts in pathogenesis and management, Berlin, 2001, Springer.

Thron AK: Vascular anatomy of the spinal cord: neuroradiological investigations and clinical syndromes, Vienna, 1988, Springer-Verlag.

Truex RC, et al: The lateral cervical nucleus of cat, dog and man. J Comp Neurol 139:93, 1970.

Tubbs RS, et al: Clinical anatomy of the C1 dorsal root, ganglion, and ramus: a review and anatomical study. Clin Anat 20:618, 2007.

Vierck CJ, Jr: Alterations of spatio-tactile discrimination after lesions of primate spinal cord. Brain Res 58:69, 1973.

Some speculations on how primates compensate for loss of a posterior column, plus experiments to show the much greater deficits caused by damage to both a posterior column and the posterior part of the ipsilateral lateral funiculus.

Vierck CJ, Jr, Luck MM: Loss and recovery of reactivity to noxious stimuli in monkeys with primary spinothalamic cordotomies, followed by secondary and tertiary lesions of other cord sectors. Brain 102:233, 1979.

Wall PD, Noordenbos W: Sensory functions which remain in man after complete transection of dorsal columns. Brain 100:641, 1977.

A description of the surprising sensory capabilities left in two unfortunate patients after transection of all but one anterior quadrant of the cord. "We conclude that patients with dorsal column lesions do not lose one or more of the classical primary modalities of sensation but lose an ability to carry out tasks where they must simultaneously analyze spatial and temporal characteristics of the stimulus."

Wang FB, Holst M-C, Powley TL: The ratio of pre- to postganglionic neurons and related issues in the autonomic nervous system. Brain Res Rev 21:93, 1995.

The traditional account of more divergence in the sympathetic system than in the parasympathetic system is an oversimplification.

Weaver TA, Walker AE: Topical arrangement within the spinothalamic tract of the monkey. Arch Neurol Psychiatry 46:877, 1941.

White JC, Sweet WH: Pain and the neurosurgeon: a forty year experience, Springfield, Ill, 1969, Charles C Thomas.

Willis WD, Jr, Coggeshall RE: Sensory mechanisms of the spinal cord, vol 1, Primary afferent neurons and the spinal dorsal horn, vol 2, Ascending sensory tracts and their descending control, ed 3, New York, 2004, Kluwer.

A well-written, thoroughly documented review of the literature.

Willis WD, Jr, et al: Projections from the marginal zone and deep dorsal horn to the ventrobasal nuclei of the primate thalamus. Pain 92:267, 2001.

Wilson DA, Prince JR: MR imaging determination of the location of the normal conus medullaris throughout childhood. AJR Am J Roentgenol 152:1029, 1989.

Xu Q, Grant G: Course of spinocerebellar axons in the ventral and lateral funiculi of the spinal cord with projections to the anterior lobe: an experimental anatomical study in the cat with retrograde tracing techniques. J Comp Neurol 345:288, 1994.

Yang JF, Stein RB: Phase-dependent reflex reversal in human leg muscles during walking. J Neurophysiol 63:1109, 1990.

Zehr EP, Stein RB: What functions do reflexes serve during human locomotion? Prog Neurobiol 58:185, 1999.

Organization of the Brainstem

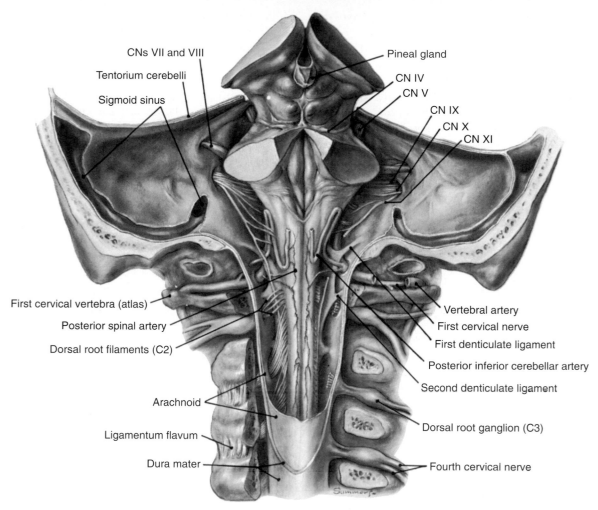

Figure 11-1 Posterior view of the brainstem and rostral spinal cord. The cerebellum and cerebral hemispheres have been removed. *(From Mettler FA: Neuroanatomy, ed 2, St. Louis, 1948, Mosby.)*

The spinal cord continues rostrally into the brainstem (Fig. 11-1), which performs spinal cord–like functions for the head. The brainstem contains the lower motor neurons for the muscles of the head and does the initial processing of general afferent information concerning the head. However, it does much more than this, reflecting in large part the additional functions of the cranial nerves attached to it, as well as some distinctive built-in brainstem functions.

The Brainstem Has Conduit, Cranial Nerve, and Integrative Functions

Brainstem activities may be divided (not very cleanly) into three general types: **conduit functions, cranial nerve functions,** and **integrative functions.**

The need for conduit functions is apparent: the only way for ascending tracts to reach the thalamus or cere-bellum, or for descending tracts to reach the spinal cord, is by passing through the brainstem. Many of these tracts, however, are not straight-through affairs, and identifi-able relay nuclei in the brainstem are frequently involved.

The cranial nerves contain not only the head's equivalent of spinal nerve fibers but also those involved in the special senses of olfaction, sight, hearing, equilibrium, and taste (Table 11-1). The olfactory and optic nerves project directly to the telencephalon and diencephalon, respectively, the accessory nerve originates in the cervical spinal cord, while the others are connected to the brainstem. Thus a wide assortment of sensory and motor nuclei related to cranial nerve function can be found at various brainstem levels.

A number of integrative functions are organized at the level of the brainstem, such as complex motor pat-terns, multiple aspects of respiratory and cardiovascular activity, and even some regulation of the level of con-sciousness itself. Much of this is accomplished by the

reticular formation, which forms the central core of the brainstem.

These three general types of activity are far from mutually exclusive. For example, ascending pathways to the thalamus arise not only in the spinal cord but also from cranial nerve nuclei; the latter therefore contribute to both conduit and cranial nerve functions. However, this parcellation does provide a useful framework on which to organize a treatment of the brainstem. It is difficult to learn about this portion of the nervous system all at once, so it is presented here in several parts. This chapter describes the overall anatomy of the brainstem and presents a series of sections showing the locations of some prominent nuclei and major ascending and descending tracts. The next three chapters describe the central connections of cranial nerves III to XII, and Chapter 15 presents a similar series of sections, labeled in more detail, with summary descriptions of the contents of various tracts and nuclei.

Table 11-1	Highly Simplified Overview of Cranial Nerve Functions*	
Cranial Nerve	**Main Sensory Function**	**Main Motor Function**
I	Smell	—
II	Sight	—
III	—	Eye movements, pupil and lens function
IV	—	Eye movements
V	Facial sensation	Chewing
VI	—	Eye movements
VII	Taste	Facial expression
VIII	Hearing, equilibrium	—
IX	Taste	Swallowing
X	Thoracic and abdominal viscera; chemoreceptive and baroreceptor	Speech, swallowing; thoracic and abdominal viscera
XI	—	Head and shoulder movements
XII	—	Tongue movements

*For more details, see Table 12-2 and Chapters 12 to 14.

The Medulla, Pons, and Midbrain Have Characteristic Gross Anatomical Features

Each of the three major subdivisions of the brainstem—medulla, pons, and midbrain (Fig. 11-2)—has a characteristic set of surface features. As explained in subsequent sections, knowledge of these surface features can help make sense of the internal organization of the brainstem.

The Medulla Includes Pyramids, Olives, and Part of the Fourth Ventricle

The medulla is vaguely scoop-shaped (see Fig. 11-2). The "handle" corresponds to the **caudal** or **closed** portion, containing a central canal continuous with that of the spinal cord. The open portion of the scoop corresponds to the **rostral** or **open medulla,** in which the central canal expands into the fourth ventricle. The apex of the V-shaped caudal fourth ventricle, where it narrows into the central canal, is called the **obex** (Fig. 11-3A).

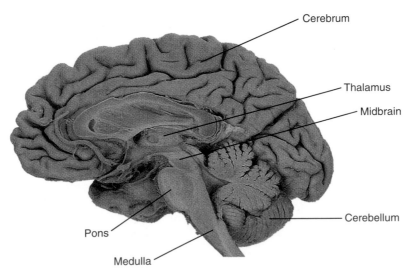

Figure 11-2 The major subdivisions of the brainstem. (See Video 11-1.)

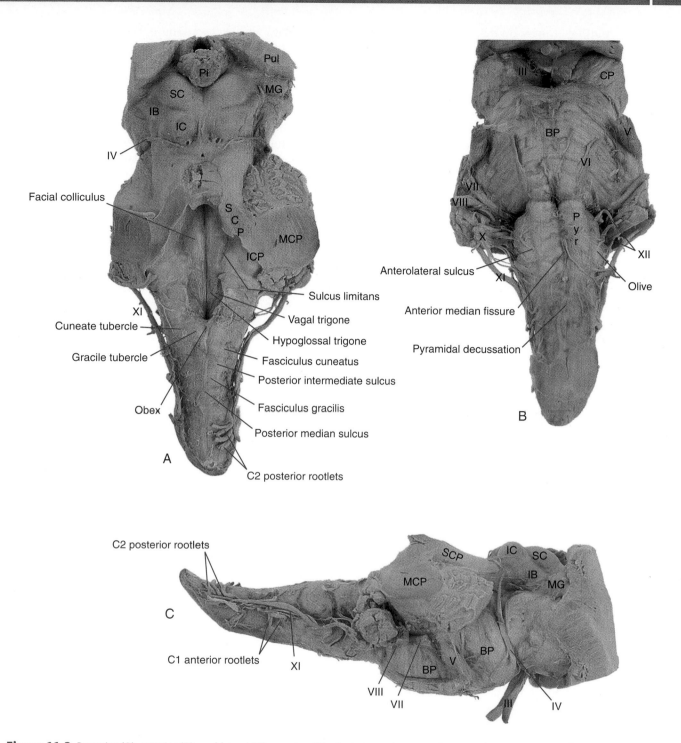

Figure 11-3 Posterior **(A)**, anterior **(B)**, and lateral **(C)** aspects of the brainstem, shown at about 1.3 times actual size, after the cerebellum and cerebrum were removed. Cranial nerves are indicated by roman numerals. BP, basal pons; CP, cerebral peduncle; IB, brachium of the inferior colliculus; IC, inferior colliculus; ICP, inferior cerebellar peduncle; MCP, middle cerebellar peduncle; MG, medial geniculate nucleus; Pi, pineal gland; Pul, pulvinar; Pyr, pyramid; SC, superior colliculus; SCP, superior cerebellar peduncle. *(Courtesy Grant Dahmer, University of Arizona College of Medicine. Modified from Nolte J, Angevine JB Jr: The human brain in photographs and diagrams, ed 3, St Louis, 2007, Mosby.)*

The longitudinal grooves on the surface of the spinal cord continue into the medulla; they are well-delineated inferiorly, gradually becoming more obscure as one moves rostrally. They divide the surface of the caudal medulla and part of the rostral medulla into a series of columns (see Fig. 11-3). The anterior median fissure is briefly interrupted by the **pyramidal decussation** at the junction between spinal cord and brainstem, but then it continues rostrally to the edge of the pons, separating the two pyramids (see Fig. 11-3B). Proceeding around posteriorly, the anterolateral sulcus marks the other side of the pyramid. The rootlets of the hypoglossal nerve (CN XII) emerge from this sulcus, mainly in the rostral medulla. In the rostral medulla, the column posterior to the hypoglossal rootlets is enlarged to form an oval swelling called the **olive.** The rootlets of the glossopharyngeal (CN IX) and vagus (CN X)[a] nerves emerge from a shallow lateral groove posterior to the olive. The posterolateral sulcus also continues into the medulla; the area between it and the line of rootlets of cranial nerves IX and X (which in the spinal cord would overlie the posterolateral [Lissauer's] tract and the posterior horn) overlies the **spinal tract of the trigeminal nerve.** As explained in the next chapter, the spinal tract of the trigeminal nerve is the head's equivalent of the posterolateral tract. Finally, the posterior columns continue into the medulla. Fasciculus cuneatus, adjacent to the posterolateral sulcus, extends rostrally to a small swelling called the **cuneate tubercle,** which marks the site of nucleus cuneatus. Fasciculus gracilis, adjacent to the midline, extends rostrally to a similar small swelling called the **gracile tubercle,** which marks the site of nucleus gracilis.

If the cerebellum is removed (as it has been in Fig. 11-3), one can peer down on the floor of the fourth ventricle. Here too, various grooves and elevations signify the presence of underlying nuclei. The sulcus limitans can often be followed rostrally along the floor of the ventricle into the pons (see Fig. 11-3A). As in the embryonic spinal cord, it is a line of separation between motor nuclei (now medial to it) and sensory nuclei (now lateral to it; see Figs. 2-10 and 12-1). The portion of the medulla and pons in the floor of the ventricle, lateral to the sulcus limitans, is mostly occupied by vestibular nuclei and is referred to as the **vestibular area.** The area medial to the sulcus limitans overlies a series of motor nuclei, three of

which make visible elevations. In the medulla, the hypoglossal nucleus and the dorsal motor nucleus of the vagus make small triangular swellings, appropriately called the **hypoglossal** and **vagal trigones.** Farther rostrally, in the pons, is another elevation called the **facial colliculus.** This elevation is not caused by an underlying motor nucleus of the facial nerve, as one might surmise from its name. Rather, it is the location of the abducens nucleus; fibers destined for the facial nerve loop over it at this location on their way out of the brainstem (see Figs. 12-6 and 12-7).

The Pons Includes the Basal Pons, Middle Cerebellar Peduncles, and Part of the Fourth Ventricle

The pons is dominated by the massive, transversely oriented structure on its anterior surface from which it derives its name (Figs. 11-3 and 11-4). *Pons* is the Latin word for "bridge," and this portion of it (called the **basal pons**) looks like a bridge interconnecting the two cerebellar hemispheres. It is not, however, a direct interconnection. Rather, many of the fibers descending in each cerebral peduncle synapse in scattered nuclei of the ipsilateral half of the basal pons. These nuclei in turn project their fibers across the midline, after which they funnel into the **middle cerebellar peduncle (brachium pontis**[b]**)** and finally enter the cerebellum (see Fig. 11-12).

The trigeminal nerve (CN V) joins the brainstem at a midpontine level, and three others connect along the groove between the basal pons and the medulla (see Fig. 11-3). The abducens nerve (CN VI) is the smallest and most medially located of these three, exiting where the pyramid emerges from the basal pons. The facial nerve (CN VII) is farther lateral and consists of two parts: a larger and more medial **motor root** and a smaller **sensory root** (sometimes referred to as the **intermediate nerve** [see Fig. 3-17B]). The vestibulocochlear nerve (CN VIII) is slightly lateral to the facial nerve and also has two parts: a **vestibular division** and a more lateral **cochlear division.**

The superior cerebellar peduncle (**brachium conjunctivum**[c]) forms much of the roof of the fourth ventricle in the pons. It emerges from the cerebellum, moves toward the midline and the brainstem, and enters the latter near the junction between the pons and midbrain.

---

[a]The glossopharyngeal, vagus, and accessory nerves travel together through the jugular foramen, and the most caudal vagal filaments were long thought to join the accessory nerve briefly along this course. For this reason, the caudal vagal filaments were spoken of as the *cranial part of the nerve.* Careful dissections have shown, however, that this is not the case: all the filaments leaving the caudal medulla run directly into the vagus nerve, and the fibers emerging from the lateral surface of the upper cervical cord form the accessory nerve. There is no cranial part of the accessory nerve.

---

[b]*Brachium* is the Latin word for "arm" and is used neuroanatomically to refer to some prominent bands of white matter extending from or to an area of gray matter. In this case the brachium pontis—literally the "arm of the pons"—extends posteriorly from the pons to reach the cerebellum.

[c]Latin for "joined-together arm," named for the path taken by the two peduncles as they enter the brainstem and decussate (see Fig. 20-22A).

At this same junction, the trochlear nerve (CN IV) emerges from the posterior surface of the brainstem. The superior cerebellar peduncle is covered in the rostral pons by a flattened band of fibers called the **lateral lemniscus,** which forms part of the ascending auditory system and terminates in the inferior colliculus.

The Midbrain Includes the Superior and Inferior Colliculi, the Cerebral Peduncles, and the Cerebral Aqueduct

The midbrain is characterized by four bumps (the paired superior and inferior colliculi) on its posterior surface and by the large cerebral peduncles on its anterior

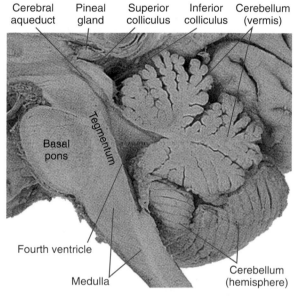

Figure 11-4 Medial surface of the right half of a hemisected brain, showing major features of the brainstem and cerebellum. *(Courtesy Grant Dahmer, University of Arizona College of Medicine. Modified from Nolte J, Angevine JB Jr: The human brain in photographs and diagrams, ed 3, St. Louis, 2007, Mosby.)*

surface. The oculomotor nerve (CN III) emerges from the interpeduncular fossa between the peduncles.

The **brachium of the inferior colliculus** (usually shortened to **inferior brachium**) is a broad, low ridge extending rostrally from the inferior colliculus. This is a continuation of the ascending auditory pathway, projecting from the inferior colliculus to the thalamic relay nucleus for hearing (the **medial geniculate nucleus**).

The Internal Structure of the Brainstem Reflects Surface Features and the Position of Long Tracts

At any given brainstem level rostral to the obex, three general areas can be identified in cross section (Fig. 11-5): (1) the area posterior to the ventricular space, (2) the area anterior to the ventricular space, and (3) large structures "appended" to the anterior surface of the brainstem. (In the caudal medulla the central canal is surrounded by structures, including some that are anterior to the ventricular space at more rostral levels.)

The only place where the portion posterior to the ventricular space contains a substantial amount of neural tissue is the midbrain. This region is called the **tectum** (Latin for "roof") and consists of the superior and inferior colliculi. In the pons and rostral medulla, the fourth ventricle is covered posteriorly by the superior and inferior medullary vela (and, of course, the cerebellum).

The area anterior to the ventricular space is called the **tegmentum** (Latin for "covering"). The tegmentum contains most of the structures described in this and the next three chapters: the reticular formation, cranial nerve nuclei and tracts, pathways ascending from the spinal cord, and some descending pathways.

The structures appended to the anterior surface of the brainstem contain fibers descending from the cerebral cortex to the spinal cord, to certain cranial nerve

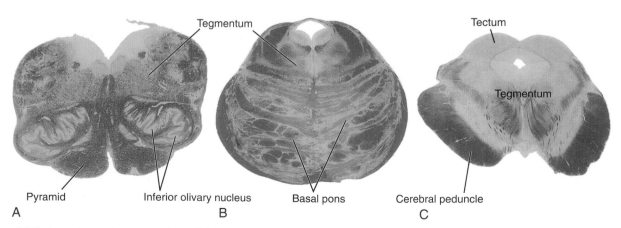

Figure 11-5 General areas in cross sections of the brainstem, as seen in the rostral medulla **(A),** pons **(B),** and midbrain **(C).** The tegmentum is prominent at all levels, the tectum only in the midbrain. Anteriorly appended structures include the pyramids and inferior olivary nuclei of the rostral medulla, the basal pons, and the cerebral peduncles and substantia nigra of the rostral midbrain.

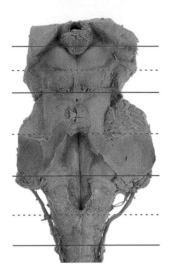

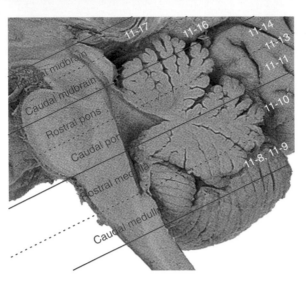

Figure 11-6 Transverse planes defining the subdivisions of the brainstem and the planes of sections shown elsewhere in this chapter. In brief: (1) the medulla contains the pyramids, together with part of the central canal, in its caudal half and part of the fourth ventricle in its rostral half; (2) the pons contains the basal pons and part of the fourth ventricle; (3) the midbrain contains cerebral peduncles and the aqueduct, together with the inferior colliculi in the caudal midbrain and the superior colliculi in the rostral midbrain.

nuclei, or to pontine nuclei (which in turn project to the cerebellum). These appended structures primarily include the large fiber bundles of the cerebral peduncles, the basal pons, and the pyramids of the medulla.

Although the brainstem is derived embryologically from a serial array of vesicles, in adults it no longer possesses an organization quite so neat (see Fig. 11-4). For example, the basal pons usually extends rostrally to a point anterior to the tectum of the midbrain, and the pineal gland and part of the thalamus extend posteriorly so far that they overlap the tectum of the midbrain. Because the most instructive way to study the brainstem is to consider a series of parallel sections through it (all perpendicular to its long axis), we will ignore minor inconveniences such as the intrusion of the basal pons under the midbrain and have used, for purposes of the following discussion, reference transverse planes (Fig. 11-6) that subdivide the brainstem into six parts: caudal and rostral medulla, **caudal** and **rostral pons,** and **caudal** and **rostral midbrain.**

The following discussion points out major brainstem structures at these levels and the locations of tracts that begin or end in the spinal cord. The next three chapters deal with the cranial nerves and their tracts and nuclei. Finally, as noted previously, the material of all four chapters is integrated in a series of more extensively labeled sections in Chapter 15.

The Corticospinal Tract and Anterolateral System Have Consistent Locations Throughout the Brainstem[d]

The three major longitudinal pathways (corticospinal tract, posterior columns, and spinothalamic tract) that

[d]This discussion was modified from Nolte J, Angevine JB Jr: *The human brain in photographs and diagrams,* ed 3, St Louis, 2007, Mosby.

were followed through the spinal cord in Chapter 10 can be followed systematically through the brainstem, as indicated in Figure 11-7. Two of the three stay in more or less the same location throughout the brainstem. Corticospinal axons travel in the most anterior part of the brainstem, traversing the cerebral peduncle, basal pons, and medullary pyramid. At the spinomedullary junction, most of the axons in the pyramids decussate at the junction between the medulla and the spinal cord and form the lateral corticospinal tracts. The spinothalamic tracts (lateral and anterior), of the anterolateral system (along with spinoreticular, spinotectal or spinomesencephalic, and spinohypothalamic tracts), are in or near the anterolateral corner of the tegmentum at all levels of the brainstem, similar to its position in the spinal cord. The posterior columns terminate in the posterior column nuclei (nucleus gracilis and nucleus cuneatus) of the medulla. Efferent fibers from these nuclei decussate in the medulla to form the medial lemniscus, which reaches the thalamus. The medial lemniscus starts out near the midline and then moves progressively more laterally, rotating nearly 180 degrees as it proceeds rostrally through the brainstem.

The Medial Lemniscus Forms in the Caudal Medulla

The caudal (closed) medulla extends from the caudal edge of the pyramidal decussation (where the medulla becomes continuous with the spinal cord) to the obex, which marks the caudal end of the fourth ventricle.

The caudal medulla (Figs. 11-8 and 11-9) looks somewhat like the spinal cord. Part of the anterior horn is still present caudally (see Fig. 11-8), as are structures similar to the posterolateral (Lissauer's) tract and part of the posterior horn. The latter two are actually the **spinal tract** and **spinal nucleus of the trigeminal nerve.** These

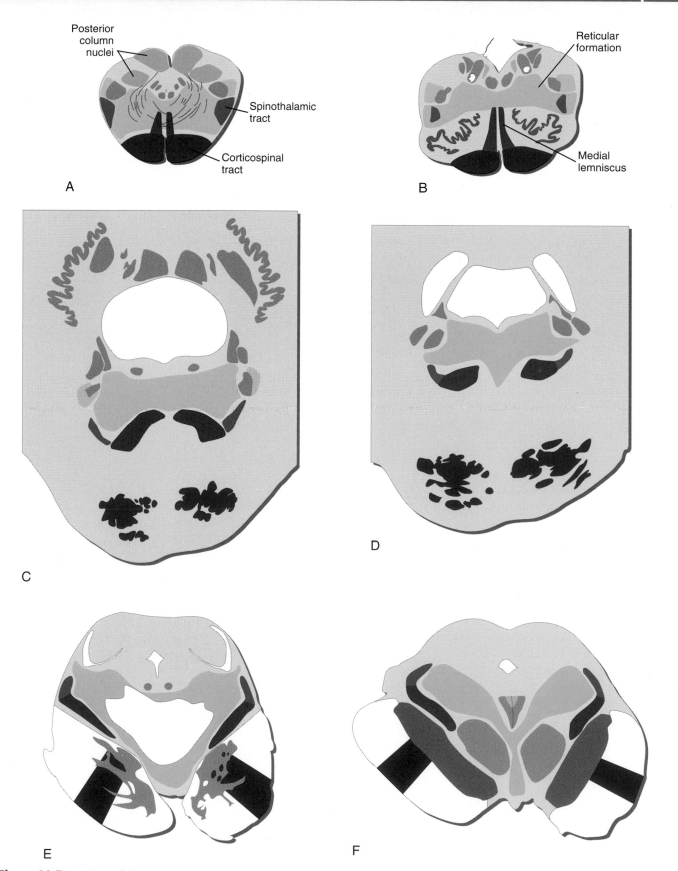

Figure 11-7 Locations of the corticospinal tract, medial lemniscus, spinothalamic tract, and reticular formation in the caudal and rostral medulla **(A, B),** caudal pons and midpons **(C, D),** and caudal and rostral midbrain **(E, F).** *(Modified from Nolte J, Angevine JB Jr: The human brain in photographs and diagrams, ed 3, St. Louis, 2007, Mosby.)*

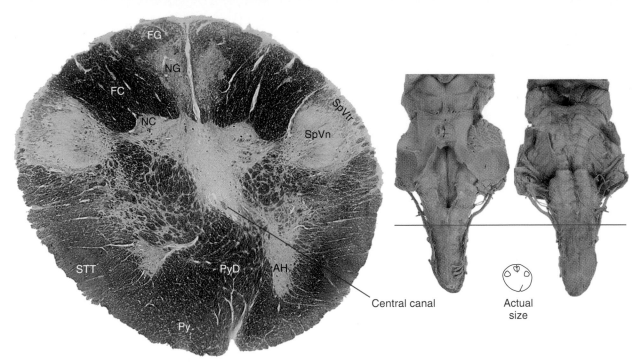

Figure 11-8 Caudal medulla near the spinomedullary junction, at the level of the pyramidal decussation. Actual size: 11 mm wide × 10 mm from anterior to posterior. AH, anterior horn (contains the accessory nucleus at this level); FC, fasciculus cuneatus; FG, fasciculus gracilis; NC, nucleus cuneatus; NG, nucleus gracilis; Py, pyramid; PyD, pyramidal decussation; SpVn, spinal trigeminal nucleus; SpVtr, spinal trigeminal tract; STT, spinothalamic tract.

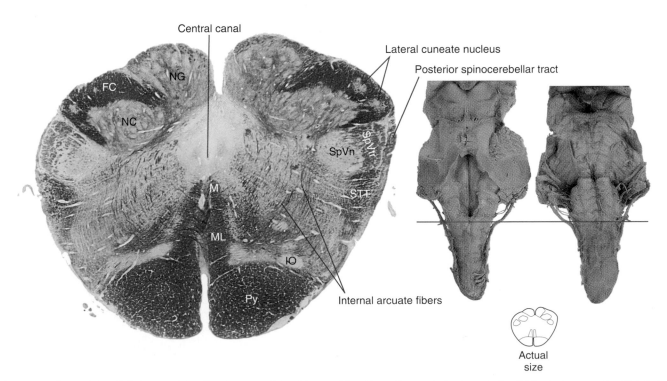

Figure 11-9 Caudal medulla, just caudal to the obex. Actual size: 12 mm wide × 10 mm from anterior to posterior. FC, fasciculus cuneatus; IO, inferior olivary nucleus (a small portion of the inferior olivary nucleus, a landmark of the rostral medulla, extends into the caudal medulla); M, medial longitudinal fasciculus; ML, medial lemniscus; NC, nucleus cuneatus; NG, nucleus gracilis; Py, pyramid; SpVn, spinal trigeminal nucleus; SpVtr, spinal trigeminal tract; STT, spinothalamic tract.

are the head's equivalent of the posterolateral tract and the substantia gelatinosa (i.e., they deal with pain, temperature, and some tactile information, as discussed in Chapter 12).

Fasciculi gracilis and cuneatus continue into the caudal medulla but are gradually replaced by the posterior column nuclei (nucleus gracilis and nucleus cuneatus). Nucleus cuneatus begins and ends a bit rostral to nucleus gracilis, so even in Figure 11-9, part of fasciculus cuneatus is still present. Postsynaptic fibers leave these two nuclei in an anterior direction and arch across the midline to form the contralateral medial lemniscus, a vertically oriented band of fibers (see Fig. 11-9). These decussating fibers are part of the collection of **internal arcuate fibers** often referred to as the **sensory decussation.** Throughout the medulla, the medial lemniscus is organized so that fibers representing cervical segments are most posterior (i.e., as though the homunculus were standing upright in these cross sections).

Adjacent to nucleus cuneatus and embedded in fasciculus cuneatus is the **lateral** (or **external**) **cuneate nucleus** (see Fig. 11-9). This is the upper extremity equivalent of the posterior thoracic (Clarke's) nucleus, and the axons of these cells join the posterior spinocerebellar tract in the inferior cerebellar peduncle at a slightly more rostral level.

The spinothalamic tract is one of several that are not as compact or heavily myelinated as the medial lemniscus and therefore cannot be distinguished as clearly in myelin-stained sections. However, this tract stays in more or less the same location (the anterolateral portion of the tegmentum) during its passage through the brainstem, at least until it reaches the rostral midbrain. As it ascends rostrally, it flattens out and becomes more distinguishable, and is often referred to as the spinal lemniscus.

The prominent pyramids (see Fig. 11-9) and their decussation (see Fig. 11-8) are located most anteriorly in the caudal medulla. Each pyramid consists of corticospinal fibers that originated in ipsilateral cerebral cortex and are (mostly) bound for the contralateral anterior horn.

Most of the area traversed by internal arcuate fibers in Figure 11-9 is **reticular formation.** A casual observer looking at this region in photographs such as these would not see much. This is, to a first approximation, what distinguishes the reticular formation from the rest of the brainstem; the posterior column nuclei, for example, *look* like nuclei, whereas the reticular formation just looks like the uniform neural tissue filling the gaps between identifiable structures, forming a central core throughout the brainstem tegmentum (see Fig. 11-7). In fact, however, the reticular formation is organized—but on a microscopic level, as discussed briefly later in this chapter.

The Rostral Medulla Contains the Inferior Olivary Nucleus and Part of the Fourth Ventricle

The rostral (open) medulla, as defined here, extends from the obex to the rostral wall of the lateral recess, where the inferior cerebellar peduncle turns posteriorly to enter the cerebellum. The rostral medulla (Fig. 11-10) no longer looks much like the spinal cord, partly because the walls of the embryonic neural tube have been pushed outward to form the floor of the fourth ventricle (see Fig. 2-10).

The caudal boundary (the obex) is approximately coincident with the caudal edge of the **inferior olivary nucleus,** a prominent structure that is responsible for the appearance of the olive as a surface swelling (see Fig. 11-3). The inferior cerebellar peduncle is located posterolaterally at these levels and grows progressively larger as it continues rostrally. Fibers can be seen leaving the medially facing mouth (or **hilus**) of the inferior olivary nucleus, arching across the midline, and joining the contralateral inferior cerebellar peduncle. These too are internal arcuate fibers. More and more are added at progressively more rostral levels of the medulla, increasing the size of the peduncle.

Medial to the inferior olivary nucleus is the medial lemniscus, which still has the shape of a flattened band with a posterior-anterior axis. Anterior to the medial lemniscus is the pyramid. Fascicles of the hypoglossal nerve (CN XII) (see Figs. 11-3 and 11-10) emerge lateral to the pyramid in the groove between it and the inferior olivary nucleus. Posterior to the medial lemniscus, near the floor of the fourth ventricle, is a small but distinctive bundle of fibers that can be followed all the way to the midbrain. This is the **medial longitudinal fasciculus (MLF),** which is involved in coordinating head and eye movements.

The spinothalamic tract remains in the anterolateral portion of the tegmentum, just above the inferior olivary nucleus, as does the anterior spinocerebellar tract. The posterior spinocerebellar tract moves posteriorly and joins the inferior cerebellar peduncle.

The Caudal Pons Is Attached to the Cerebellum by the Middle Cerebellar Peduncle

The caudal pons (Fig. 11-11), as defined here, extends from the rostral wall of the lateral recess of the fourth ventricle to the rostral edge of the middle cerebellar peduncle (i.e., the caudal pons is physically connected to the cerebellum in cross sections). In the caudal pons the inferior olivary nucleus ends, and the inferior cerebellar peduncle bends posteriorly and enters the cerebellum (see Fig. 11-15). The MLF is in the same relative position as it was previously, adjacent to the midline and the floor of the fourth ventricle.

As the inferior olivary nucleus ends, the medial lemniscus assumes a more oval shape, as though it had

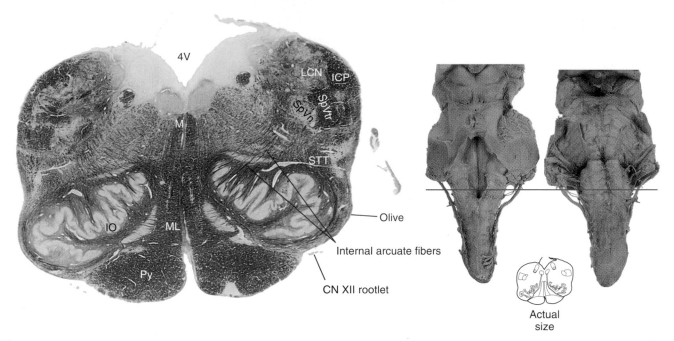

Figure 11-10 Rostral medulla, just rostral to the obex. Actual size: 16 mm wide × 12 mm from anterior to posterior. 4V, fourth ventricle; ICP, inferior cerebellar peduncle; IO, inferior olivary nucleus; LCN, lateral cuneate nucleus; M, medial longitudinal fasciculus; ML, medial lemniscus; Py, pyramid; SpVn, spinal trigeminal nucleus; SpVtr, spinal trigeminal tract; STT, spinothalamic tract.

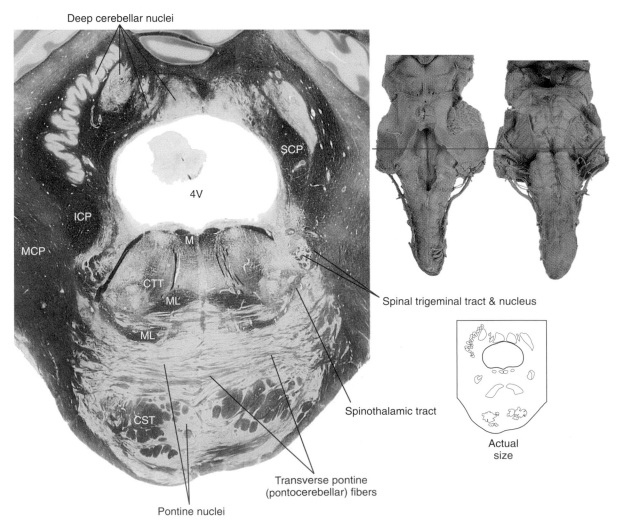

Figure 11-11 Caudal pons, at the level of the facial colliculus. Actual size: 23 mm wide × 30 mm from anterior to posterior. CST, corticospinal tract; CTT, central tegmental tract; 4V, fourth ventricle; ICP, inferior cerebellar peduncle; M, medial longitudinal fasciculus; MCP, middle cerebellar peduncle; ML, medial lemniscus; SCP, superior cerebellar peduncle.

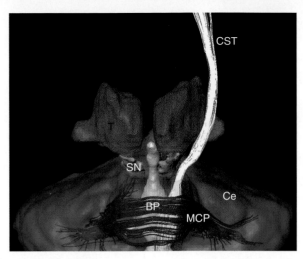

Figure 11-12 Diffusion tensor image of an anterior-posterior view of the basal pons (BP), showing the course of corticospinal tract (CST) through the pons and of transverse pontine fibers as they funnel into the middle cerebellar peduncle (MCP). (This imaging technique does not demonstrate neuronal cell bodies, and the reconstructed transverse pontine fibers look as though they extend from one side of the cerebellum to the other. In fact, each of these fibers originates from pontine nuclei on one side and extends to the contralateral half of the cerebellum.) Ce, cerebellum; SN, substantia nigra; T, thalamus. *(From Mori S et al: MRI atlas of human white matter, Amsterdam, 2005, Elsevier.)*

previously been held upright against the midline. Now the homunculus starts slumping down slowly into a horizontal position, with its feet directed laterally.

The pyramidal tract becomes dispersed in the basal pons, which contains bundles of longitudinally oriented fibers, bundles of transversely oriented fibers, and **pontine nuclei** scattered among these bundles. Some of the longitudinally oriented fibers are those of the pyramidal tract (Fig. 11-12). Most of the others are **corticopontine fibers;** these fibers originate in many areas of the cerebral cortex and terminate on ipsilateral pontine nuclei. Fibers arising in the pontine nuclei cross the midline and form the massive middle cerebellar peduncle (brachium pontis).

The spinothalamic tract and the anterior spinocerebellar tract remain in the anterolateral portion of the tegmentum. Spinoreticular fibers, also part of the anterolateral system of fibers, terminate medial to the direct spinothalamic fibers in the reticular formation throughout the brainstem, as do collaterals of direct spinothalamic fibers.

The Superior Cerebellar Peduncle Joins the Brainstem in the Rostral Pons

The rostral pons extends from the rostral edge of the middle cerebellar peduncle to the beginning of the cerebral aqueduct, so it includes parts of the basal pons and fourth ventricle but has no physical connection with the cerebellum. The trigeminal nerve (CN V) is attached to the brainstem at a midpontine level (Fig. 11-13), and the trochlear nerve (CN IV) emerges at the pons-midbrain junction (see Fig. 11-3). The MLF is visible throughout the rostral pons, as is the basal pons (Fig. 11-14). The fourth ventricle narrows as the plane of section approaches the cerebral aqueduct, and the superior cerebellar peduncle (brachium conjunctivum) becomes apparent in the wall of the ventricle. This is the major outflow from the cerebellum, projecting to the thalamus and to other structures (Fig. 11-15).

The medial lemniscus gradually takes on a more flattened profile, now with a medial-lateral axis, and assumes a transverse orientation at the junction between the basal pons and the pontine tegmentum. As in the caudal pons, the homunculus is arranged so that its feet are most lateral. As the medial lemniscus moves laterally, it approaches the spinal lemniscus; from there through the midbrain, the two are adjacent. The corticospinal tract travels through the rostral pons as a series of longitudinally oriented bundles of fibers, accompanied by more numerous corticopontine bundles.

The anterior spinocerebellar tract moves posteriorly onto the surface of the superior cerebellar peduncle (see Fig. 11-13). From there it turns caudally and enters the cerebellum, traveling "backward" along the peduncle.

The Superior Cerebellar Peduncles Decussate in the Caudal Midbrain

The caudal midbrain is marked by the presence of the inferior colliculi. It extends from the point of emergence of the trochlear nerve to the groove between the inferior and superior colliculi. The fourth ventricle has narrowed into the cerebral aqueduct (Fig. 11-16), the superior cerebellar peduncles sink deeper into the midbrain tegmentum and begin to decussate, and the MLF continues on its usual course. The basal pons protrudes rostrally under the tegmentum of the caudal midbrain. The inferior colliculus, a major component of the ascending auditory pathway discussed in Chapter 14, is (literally) a prominent nuclear mass. Medial to it, encircling the aqueduct, is a particularly pale-staining region of gray matter called, appropriately enough, the **periaqueductal gray.** The periaqueductal gray is part of an important descending pain-control system discussed later in this chapter.

The medial lemniscus is still a flattened band of fibers, now curving a bit posteriorly, and the spinal lemniscus is posterior to it near the surface of the brainstem. The adjacent locations position the two tracts to terminate in overlapping regions of the posterior thalamus. In the caudal midbrain, the basal pons gives way to a **cerebral peduncle** on each side, through which corticospinal and corticopontine fibers travel.

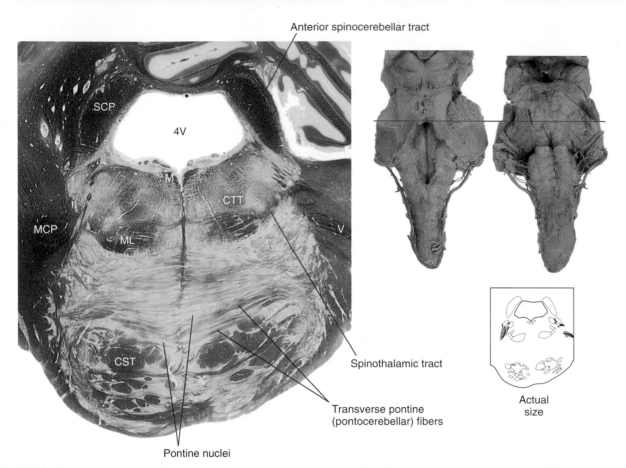

Figure 11-13 Midpons, at the level of the trigeminal nerve. Actual size: 21 mm wide × 26 mm from anterior to posterior. CST, corticospinal tract; CTT, central tegmental tract; 4V, fourth ventricle; M, medial longitudinal fasciculus; MCP, middle cerebellar peduncle; ML, medial lemniscus; SCP, superior cerebellar peduncle; V, trigeminal nerve fibers.

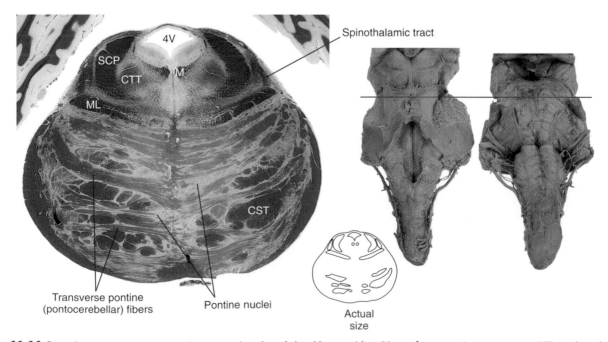

Figure 11-14 Rostral pons, near the pons-midbrain junction. Actual size: 23 mm wide × 20 mm from anterior to posterior. CST, corticospinal tract; CTT, central tegmental tract; 4V, fourth ventricle; M, medial longitudinal fasciculus; ML, medial lemniscus; SCP, superior cerebellar peduncle.

The Rostral Midbrain Contains the Red Nucleus and Substantia Nigra

The rostral midbrain contains the superior colliculi (Fig. 11-17) and extends from the intercollicular groove to the **posterior commissure.** At this level the MLF is ending,

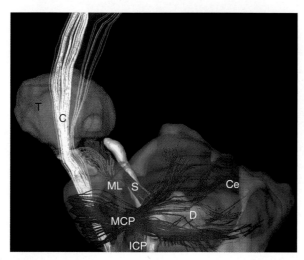

Figure 11-15 Diffusion tensor image of a lateral view of the brainstem, showing the course of the superior cerebellar peduncle (S) from the deep cerebellar nuclei (D) toward the thalamus (T), as well as the courses of some other major fiber bundles. C, corticospinal tract; Ce, cerebellum; ICP, inferior cerebellar peduncle; MCP, middle cerebellar peduncle; ML, medial lemniscus. *(From Mori S et al: MRI atlas of human white matter, Amsterdam, 2005, Elsevier.)*

decussation of the superior cerebellar peduncles is complete, and in their place a large **red nucleus** becomes visible on each side. Some fibers from the contralateral half of the cerebellum end there, but most continue on to the thalamus. Anterior to the red nucleus is the **substantia nigra** (pale in myelin-stained preparations but dark in unstained or cell-stained preparations; see Fig. 19-20). The pigmented cells characteristic of the dorsal part of the substantia nigra use dopamine for their neurotransmitter and end profusely among neurons of the putamen and caudate nucleus, providing one example of the chemically coded systems discussed later in this chapter. The loss of this particular dopamine system results in Parkinson's disease (see Chapter 19).

Anterior to the substantia nigra is a massive bundle of fibers commonly referred to as the cerebral peduncle.[e] This bundle consists principally of descending corticopontine, corticospinal, and corticobulbar fibers. The oculomotor nerve (CN III) emerges into the space between the cerebral peduncles (the interpeduncular

---

[e]Strictly speaking, the term *cerebral peduncle* refers to all of the midbrain anterior to the superior colliculus, and the term **basis pedunculi** ("base of the peduncle") or **crus cerebri** ("leg of the cerebrum") refers to the massive fiber bundle in the anterior part of the peduncle. However, in common usage, *basis pedunculi, crus cerebri,* and *cerebral peduncle* have become more or less interchangeable, all referring to the fiber bundle.

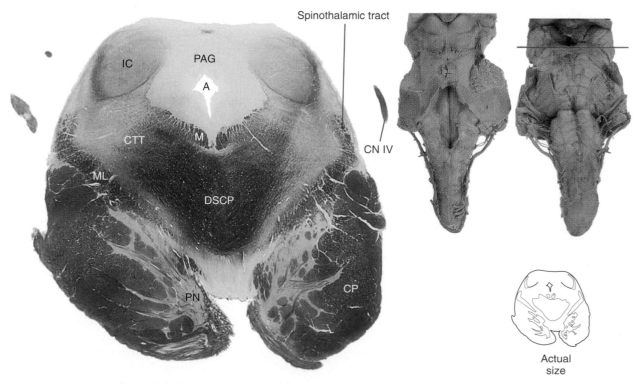

Figure 11-16 Caudal midbrain, at the level of the inferior colliculus. Actual size: 20 mm wide × 20 mm from anterior to posterior. A, cerebral aqueduct; CP, cerebral peduncle; CTT, central tegmental tract; DSCP, decussation of the superior cerebellar peduncles; IC, inferior colliculus; M, medial longitudinal fasciculus; ML, medial lemniscus; PAG, periaqueductal gray; PN, pontine nuclei.

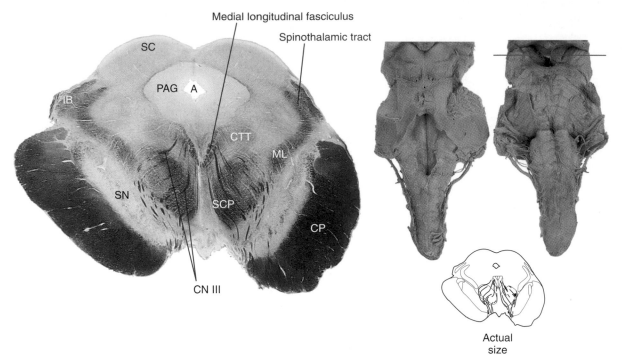

Figure 11-17 Rostral midbrain, at the level of the superior colliculus. Actual size: 26 mm wide × 20 mm from anterior to posterior. A, cerebral aqueduct; CP, cerebral peduncle; CTT, central tegmental tract; IB, brachium of the inferior colliculus; ML, medial lemniscus; PAG, periaqueductal gray; SC, superior colliculus; SCP, superior cerebellar peduncle (at this level, crossed and entering the red nucleus); SN, substantia nigra.

fossa). Several parts of the diencephalon (the pineal gland and some thalamic nuclei) hang back over and alongside the rostral midbrain.

At rostral midbrain levels, the medial lemniscus and the spinothalamic tract form a continuous curved band of fibers. Spinomesencephalic fibers (sometimes referred to as the **spinotectal tract**) that have accompanied the spinothalamic tract through the brainstem terminate in the periaqueductal gray, adjacent regions of the reticular formation, and certain portions of the superior colliculus.

The Reticular Core of the Brainstem Is Involved in Multiple Functions

The reticular formation is an apparently (but not actually) diffusely organized area that forms the central core of the brainstem (see Fig. 11-7). It has been likened to a hot dog surrounded by a bun of discrete tracts and nuclei.[f] The reason it appears to be diffusely organized is twofold.

1. Its pattern of connectivity is characterized by a great deal of convergence and divergence, so that a single cell may respond to several different sensory modalities or to stimuli applied practically anywhere on the body.

2. Although it is involved in several quite separate functions, the areas involved in these functions overlap considerably, almost as though several nuclei had been scrambled together and dispersed along the brainstem while their constituent cells retained their original connections.

At most levels of the brainstem, the reticular formation can be divided into three longitudinal zones arranged in a medial-to-lateral sequence. The **raphe nuclei** (from the Greek word *rhaphe,* meaning "seam," referring to the midline seam of the brainstem) are thin plates of neurons in and immediately adjacent to the sagittal plane. The **medial zone,** alongside the midline raphe nuclei, contains a mixture of large and small neurons and is the source of most of the long ascending and descending projections from the reticular formation. Some of the neurons in the medial zone of the rostral medullary reticular formation are so large that this area is referred to as the **gigantocellular reticular nucleus.** Finally, the **lateral zone,** which is particularly prominent in the rostral medulla and caudal pons, is primarily concerned with cranial nerve reflexes and visceral functions. These reticular zones have been further subdivided into a series of nuclei based on histology, connections, and function, although such nuclei cannot be distinguished easily in conventionally prepared sections such as those shown in this chapter.

Many reticular neurons have extensive and complex axonal projections. They may innervate multiple levels of the spinal cord, send numerous collaterals to the

[f]Dr. Michael Earnest, personal communication, 1974.

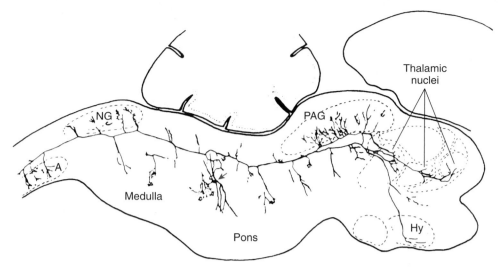

Figure 11-18 Drawing of a Golgi-stained parasagittal section from the brain of a young rat. The single stained cell *(small green arrow)* in the pontine reticular formation has an axon that bifurcates and ends in wide areas of the CNS, reaching the anterior horn of the spinal cord (A), nucleus gracilis (NG), periaqueductal gray (PAG), hypothalamus (Hy), thalamus, and multiple levels of the reticular formation. If one cell has projections this extensive, imagine the complexity of the reticular formation as a whole. *(From Scheibel ME, Scheibel AB: Structural substrates for integrative patterns in the brainstem reticular core. In Jasper HH et al, editors: Reticular formation of the brain, Boston, 1958, Little, Brown.)*

brainstem and diencephalon, or even have bifurcating axons that give rise to both ascending and descending connections (Fig. 11-18). Some reticular neurons with distinctive neurochemical characteristics (described later in this chapter) project directly to the cerebral cortex; these are an exception to the usual pattern of transmission through the thalamus on the way to the cortex. Reticular neurons also have large fields of dendrites, sometimes spreading out in a plane perpendicular to the long axis of the brainstem, that allow them to receive synaptic inputs from ascending sensory pathways, descending cortical axons, and a variety of other sources. A look at the processes of a single reticular neuron in a single plane (see Fig. 11-18) should demonstrate why the reticular formation has been a tremendously difficult area of the brain to study; still, some progress has been made.

The Reticular Formation Participates in the Control of Movement Through Connections With Both the Spinal Cord and the Cerebellum

Two **reticulospinal tracts** arise from the medial zone of the pontine and the rostral medullary reticular formation. Fibers from the pons descend near the ipsilateral MLF and travel through the anterior funiculus in the spinal cord (Fig. 11-19). Those from the medulla descend bilaterally, but mostly uncrossed, in the anterior part of the lateral funiculus. The reticulospinal tract is a major alternative route (to the pyramidal tract) by which spinal motor neurons are controlled, both influencing motor neurons directly and regulating the sensitivity of spinal reflex arcs. For example, tonic inhibition of flexor reflexes originates in the reticular formation, with the result that

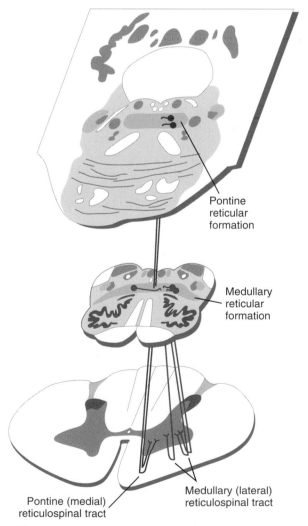

Figure 11-19 Medullary and pontine reticulospinal tracts.

only noxious stimuli can normally evoke such a reflex. Reticulospinal neurons receive projections from many areas, including the basal nuclei, vestibular nuclei, and substantia nigra. Input from widespread areas of the cerebral cortex, particularly the somatosensory and motor cortex, is especially important. Most of these descending fibers travel to their reticular terminations in the **central tegmental tract** (see Figs. 11-11, 11-13, 11-14, 11-16, and 11-17). This is a complex tract that passes through the reticular formation containing afferents to and efferents from the reticular formation, as well as descending projections from the red nucleus to the inferior olivary nucleus (see Fig. 20-23).

The reticulospinal tracts carry descending motor commands generated within the reticular formation. Just as the spinal cord contains the basic neural machinery for simple (and some not so simple) reflexes, so the reticular formation contains the neural machinery for considerably more complex patterns of movement. A cat whose brainstem has been surgically separated from its diencephalon can, after a recovery period, walk and run spontaneously, properly right itself if tipped over, and assume a variety of complex postures. There have been cases of human infants born without cerebral hemispheres who were nevertheless capable of apparently normal yawning, stretching, suckling, and orienting behavior. Beyond its more traditionally described role in gross movements, such as in postural adjustments and locomotion, more recent studies suggest that the reticular formation also has a role in fine, dexterous movements of the hand. Finally, certain reticular regions are closely related to the cerebellum and its motor control functions. A fairly discrete collection of cells in the medullary reticular formation called the **lateral reticular nucleus** can often be resolved adjacent to the spinothalamic tract in conventionally prepared brainstem sections. It extends rostrally to midolivary levels and caudally into the caudal medulla, receiving direct spinoreticular fibers and collaterals of spinothalamic fibers and projecting to the cerebellum. It also receives input from the red nucleus, so it is more than just a somatosensory relay to the cerebellum. Collections of reticular neurons near the medullary midline, collectively called the **paramedian reticular nucleus,** also project to the cerebellum. Afferents to the paramedian nucleus arise in the cerebellum and in other locations, including the cerebral cortex. Finally, the **reticular tegmental nucleus,** located between the medial lemnisci in the rostral pons, receives inputs from the cerebral cortex and other sites and projects to the cerebellum.

The Reticular Formation Modulates the Transmission of Information in Pain Pathways

It is a common experience that we are able to focus attention on particular sensory modalities at some times and ignore them (with varying success) at others. This is particularly evident in the case of noxious stimuli, which are experienced as more painful or less painful depending on an individual's circumstances. The classic example of reduced experience of pain is soldiers wounded in battle, who nevertheless continue to function and are not nearly as distressed as one would expect. The nervous system has several pain-control pathways available, some of which suppress and some of which facilitate the experience of pain. The reticular formation typically plays a prominent role in these pathways, as illustrated by one well-studied pain-suppression system.

Electrical stimulation (through implanted electrodes) of the periaqueductal gray of the midbrain of rats causes an analgesia so profound that major surgery can be performed without the aid of an anesthetic. Similar stimulation of the periaqueductal gray of humans can ameliorate intractable pain. This effect is a selective stimulation-produced analgesia, diminishing pain without substantially affecting other somatosensory modalities such as touch. The periaqueductal gray receives information about the level of noxious stimulation through spinomesencephalic fibers (part of the anterolateral system, also known as spinotectal fibers); it also receives inputs from the hypothalamus and several cortical areas, presumably related to behavioral state and relevant to decisions about whether to activate this pain-control system (Fig. 11-20). Efferents from the periaqueductal gray then project to one of the raphe nuclei (**nucleus raphe magnus**) of the rostral medulla and caudal pons and to

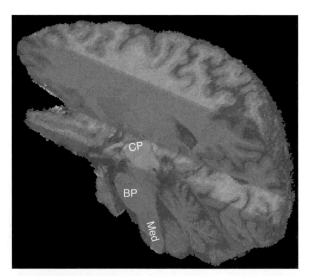

Figure 11-20 Activation of descending pain control by conscious efforts to suppress pain. In this cutaway three-dimensional magnetic resonance imaging (MRI) reconstruction with superimposed functional MRI data, blood flow can be seen to increase in a small area in the periaqueductal gray (orange) when a painfully hot stimulus (vs. a warm stimulus) was applied to normal subjects. When the same subjects were asked to distract themselves and not pay attention to the painful stimuli, blood flow in this region increased even more, and the stimuli were perceived as less unpleasant. BP, basal pons; CP, cerebral peduncle; Med, medulla. (*Courtesy Dr. Irene Tracey, Oxford University.*)

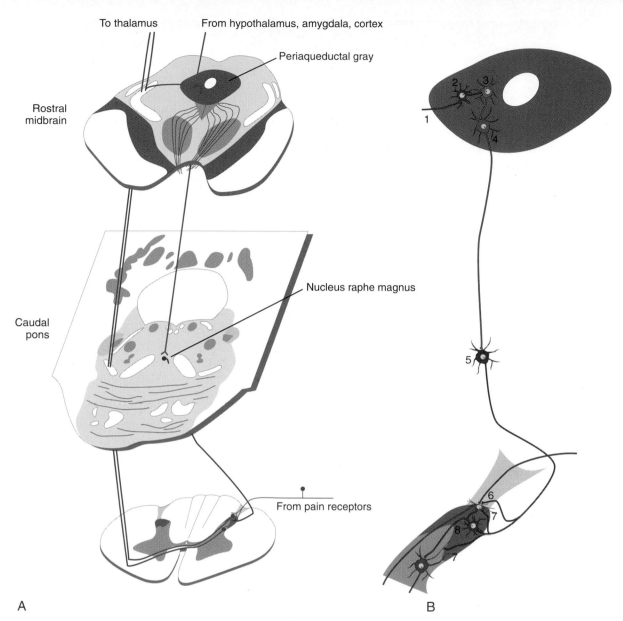

Figure 11-21 A, The periaqueductal gray–raphe nuclei pathway, one of several pain-control systems. Microinjection of opiates into either the periaqueductal gray or the posterior horn of the spinal cord elicits analgesia. **B,** Serotonin-containing neurons of the nucleus raphe magnus (5) and nearby reticular neurons, when stimulated by projection neurons of the periaqueductal gray (4), inhibit pain transmission by presynaptically inhibiting nociceptive primary afferents (6) and by inhibiting spinothalamic tract neurons either directly (7) or by making excitatory synapses on inhibitory, enkephalin-containing interneurons (8) in the substantia gelatinosa. The system can be activated by spinomesencephalic and other inputs (1) that stimulate periaqueductal, enkephalin-containing inhibitory interneurons (2). These in turn inhibit inhibitory interneurons (3) that ordinarily suppress this pain-control pathway. (Microinjection of opiates into the vicinity of the nucleus raphe magnus also causes analgesia, implying that control circuitry involving enkephalin-containing interneurons is present there as well, but this is not indicated for reasons of simplicity.)

adjacent areas of the medullary reticular formation. These areas in turn project to superficial laminae of the posterior horn via a pathway that travels through the posterior part of the lateral funiculus (Fig. 11-21), suppressing the transmission of pain information by spinothalamic neurons.

Opium and its derivatives, especially morphine, have long been used for pain control, and one way they work is by activating the periaqueductal gray–raphe nucleus pain-control system at multiple levels. Opiate receptors

are found in abundance in the periaqueductal gray, nucleus raphe magnus, and superficial laminae of the posterior horn. Microinjection of opiates at any of these three sites causes analgesia, and the analgesia induced by stimulation of the periaqueductal gray is blocked by opiate antagonists. (Opiate receptors are also found at a number of other sites in the central nervous system [CNS], presumably accounting for some of the other effects of morphine and related drugs.) The endogenous ligands for opiate receptors are various opioid peptides—in this

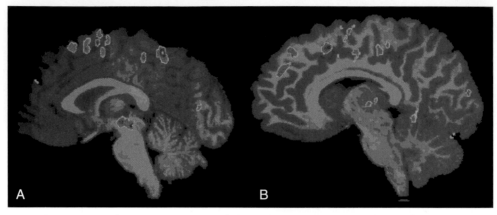

Figure 11-22 Positron emission tomography images in parasagittal planes, demonstrating increased blood flow in the midbrain reticular formation (**A**) and intralaminar nuclei of the thalamus (**B**) as a subject engages in an attention-demanding task (pressing a key as quickly as possible after a visual or somatosensory stimulus). The plane in **A** is about 2 mm from the midline, and that in **B** is about 9 mm from the midline; areas of increased blood flow are indicated in red and yellow. *(From Kinomura S et al: Science 271:512, 1996.)*

pathway, **enkephalin** and **endorphin.** Small enkephalin-containing inhibitory interneurons are involved in suppressing transmission by spinothalamic tract neurons at the level of the spinal cord (see Fig. 11-21).

The Reticular Formation Contains Autonomic Reflex Circuitry

A great deal of visceral information reaches the reticular formation, which programs appropriate responses to environmental changes and projects to the autonomic nuclei of the brainstem and spinal cord. Centers controlling inspiration, expiration, and the normal rhythm of breathing have been identified physiologically in the medulla and pons. Other centers controlling heart rate and blood pressure have been identified in the medullary reticular formation. These are in many ways comparable to the previously mentioned pattern generators in the reticular formation for various kinds of complex movements.

The hypothalamus also gives rise to numerous fibers concerned with autonomic regulation. Many of those involved in sympathetic control traverse the brainstem near the spinothalamic tract and reach the intermediolateral cell column of the spinal cord (mostly uncrossed). Interruption of the descending sympathetic pathway causes ipsilateral **Horner's syndrome,** which refers to a combination of miosis (small pupil), ptosis (drooping eyelid), and enophthalmos (recession of the eyeball; this is more apparent than real). Horner's syndrome may be accompanied by flushing and lack of sweating in ipsilateral skin of the face and part of the body.

The Reticular Formation Is Involved in the Control of Arousal and Consciousness

Ascending projections from the reticular formation terminate in the thalamus, subthalamus, hypothalamus, basal nuclei, and cerebral cortex itself. The functions of many of these are poorly understood, but those to the thalamus and cortex seem to be particularly important. Neurons in the reticular formation of the midbrain and rostral pons collect information about multiple sensory modalities—for example, information about pain via spinoreticular fibers—and project to the intralaminar nuclei of the thalamus. The intralaminar nuclei in turn project to widespread areas of the cortex, causing heightened arousal in response to sensory stimuli or attention-demanding tasks (Fig. 11-22). This pathway collaborates with monoamine-containing reticular projections (described in the next section) in modulating the activity of the cerebral cortex. The reticulothalamic and monoamine projections are essential for the maintenance of a normal state of consciousness, and bilateral damage to neurons of the midbrain reticular formation and fibers passing through it results in prolonged coma. This is an astounding notion: a normal, intact cerebrum is incapable of functioning in a conscious manner by itself; sustaining input from the brainstem reticular formation is required. The portion of the reticular formation that provides this input is known as the **ascending reticular activating system** (ARAS). It is important to understand that the ARAS is defined by physiological criteria; it is not synonymous with the anatomically defined reticular formation but rather is a portion of it. Modulation of the ARAS has a basic role in the sleep-wakefulness cycle, as discussed in Chapter 22.

Some Brainstem Nuclei Have Distinctive Neurochemical Signatures

Most of the connections discussed thus far in this book are quite precise, obviously designed to convey a particular type of information from one part of the nervous system to another. Some neurons of the reticular

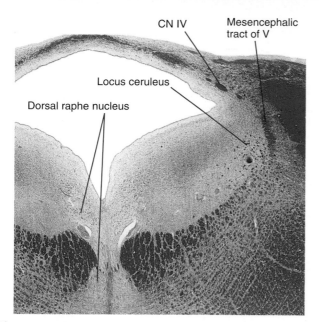

CN IV   Mesencephalic tract of V

Locus ceruleus

Dorsal raphe nucleus

Figure 11-23 Section through the rostral pons showing the locus ceruleus. One of the serotonin-containing raphe nuclei can also be seen. (The mesencephalic tract of the trigeminal nerve is discussed in Chapter 12.) This figure is an enlargement of part of the section shown in Figure 11-14.

formation are an exception, projecting to multiple areas in a way consistent with a general alerting function (see Fig. 11-18). An extreme example of such widely distributed connections is provided by brainstem neurons that contain biogenic amine neurotransmitters (norepinephrine, dopamine, and serotonin) and by hypothalamic histamine-containing neurons (see Fig. 22-31). Similarly configured neurons that contain acetylcholine are found primarily in the telencephalon, although some are also present in the reticular formation.

Neurons of the Locus Ceruleus Contain Norepinephrine

CNS neurons containing norepinephrine (called **noradrenergic** neurons, from the synonym **noradrenaline** for norepinephrine) are found only in the pons and medulla. Most are located in the **locus ceruleus** (Latin for "blue spot"), a collection of pigmented cells located near the floor of the fourth ventricle (Fig. 11-23). The pigmented neurons contain neuromelanin, accounting for the blue-black appearance of the locus ceruleus in unstained brain tissue. The remainder of the noradrenergic neurons are located in lateral parts of the medullary reticular formation, in some nuclei associated with cranial nerves (the solitary nucleus and the dorsal motor nucleus of the vagus; see Chapter 12), and in a few other sites (Fig. 11-24). Collectively, these noradrenergic neurons innervate virtually the entire CNS. Ascending fibers, many of which travel through the central tegmental tract, reach

the thalamus, hypothalamus, limbic forebrain structures, and cerebral cortex. All areas of the cerebral cortex appear to receive some noradrenergic innervation, but that to the somatosensory cortex is particularly dense. Descending fibers project to other parts of the brainstem and to all spinal levels, and some travel through the superior cerebellar peduncle to reach the cerebellum. Despite the diverse nature of these projections, there is some anatomical specificity in their pattern. For example, the locus ceruleus provides most of the output to the cerebral cortex, whereas the lateral reticular formation provides most of the output to the spinal cord.

As might be expected from the extensive pattern of these terminations, activation of noradrenergic neurons and pathways results in widespread effects in other areas of the CNS. Some hints about the possible functions of this system are provided by the response patterns of neurons in the locus ceruleus. These cells are nearly silent electrically during sleep, become somewhat active during wakefulness, and are most active in situations that are startling or call for watchfulness. Hence the locus ceruleus and other noradrenergic neurons may play a role in maintaining attention and vigilance.

Neurons of the Substantia Nigra and Ventral Tegmental Area Contain Dopamine

Most **dopaminergic** neurons are mesencephalic, located in dorsal portions of the substantia nigra (the **compact part** of the substantia nigra) and in the medially adjacent **ventral tegmental area** (Fig. 11-25), and they project rostrally in three partially overlapping streams of fibers. The first, a massive projection from the substantia nigra to the caudate nucleus and putamen, is discussed in Chapter 19. These fibers are referred to either as **nigrostriatal,** because the caudate and putamen together constitute the **striatum,** or as **mesostriatal,** reflecting their origin in the midbrain (mesencephalon). **Mesolimbic** and **mesocortical** fibers originate primarily in the ventral tegmental area and travel to a variety of forebrain destinations, including the cerebral cortex and limbic structures such as the amygdala (Fig. 11-26). As in the case of the locus ceruleus, the cortical projections are extensive but nonuniform; in this instance, frontal (including motor) and limbic areas are emphasized. The nigrostriatal projection and the mesocortical projection to motor cortex are both consistent with the idea that the dopaminergic system is involved in the initiation of movement and that its disruption is instrumental in the movement deficits seen in Parkinson's disease. However, the extensive dopaminergic projections to other frontal cortical areas and limbic structures suggest that this system is also involved in motivation and cognition. Consistent with this, there is evidence that imbalances in the dopamine system may play a role in certain forms of mental illness. Interestingly, many drugs of abuse

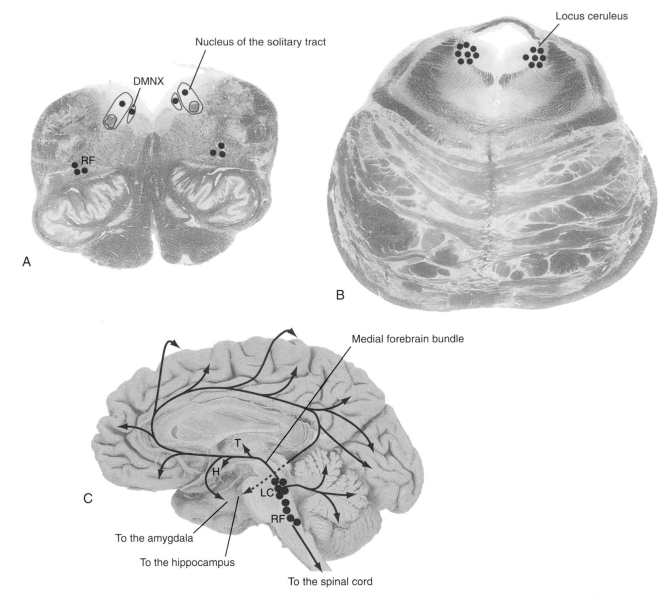

Figure 11-24 Locations of noradrenergic neurons in the rostral medulla **(A)** and rostral pons **(B)**, and a schematic indication of their widespread CNS projections **(C)**. DMNX, dorsal motor nucleus of the vagus; H, hypothalamus; LC, locus ceruleus; RF, reticular formation; T, thalamus. *(Modified from Nolte J, Angevine JB Jr: The human brain in photographs and diagrams, ed 3, St. Louis, 2007, Mosby.)*

directly or indirectly cause dopamine release in limbic forebrain structures, suggesting that the mesolimbic projection is involved in whatever it is that makes some things pleasurable.

Additional dopaminergic neurons are found in the retina (see Fig. 1-6D), the olfactory bulb, and the hypothalamus (where dopamine participates in the control of prolactin secretion and in other hypothalamic functions).

Neurons of the Raphe Nuclei Contain Serotonin

Serotonergic neurons are found at most levels of the brainstem, concentrated in the raphe nuclei (see Fig. 11-23). Like the noradrenergic neurons described earlier,

they innervate virtually all parts of the CNS (Fig. 11-27); serotonergic innervation is in fact even more extensive and profuse. Projections from the rostral raphe nuclei reach the forebrain, providing a cortical innervation that is most dense in sensory and limbic areas. Caudal raphe nuclei provide most of the projection to the cerebellum, brainstem, and spinal cord.

The firing rates of both serotonergic and noradrenergic neurons fluctuate with sleep and wakefulness, suggesting that both play a role in modulating the general activity levels of the CNS. However, there are differences in the cortical layers and areas emphasized by these two transmitters, indicating that their roles are at least somewhat different. For example, it has been proposed that the serotonin system is more important for determining

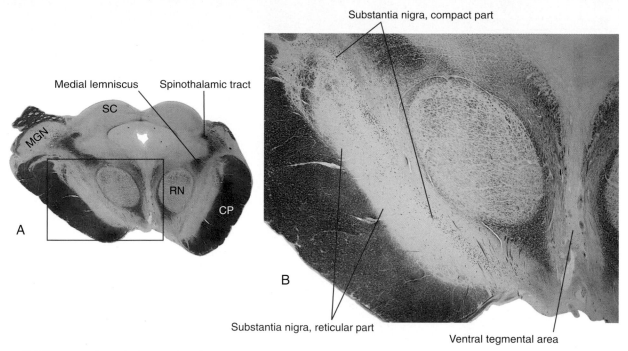

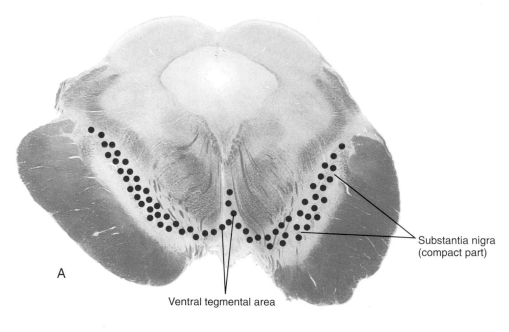

Figure 11-25 Section through the rostral midbrain showing the locations of dopaminergic neurons. The area outlined in **A** is enlarged in **B.** The compact part of the substantia nigra contains pigmented, dopaminergic neurons; the reticular part, as discussed in Chapter 19, has a different pattern of connections with the basal nuclei. CP, cerebral peduncle; MGN, medial geniculate nucleus; RN, red nucleus; SC, superior colliculus.

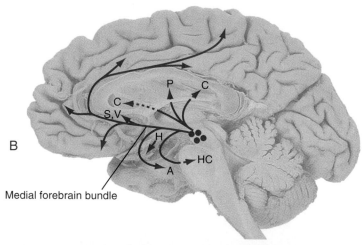

Figure 11-26 Locations of dopaminergic neurons in the midbrain **(A),** and a schematic indication of their widespread CNS projections **(B).** A, amygdala; C, caudate nucleus; H, hypothalamus; HC, hippocampus; P, putamen; S, septal nuclei (see Chapter 23); V, ventral striatum (the area of fusion between the putamen and the caudate nucleus; see Chapter 19). *(Modified from Nolte J, Angevine JB Jr: The human brain in photographs and diagrams, ed 3, St. Louis, 2007, Mosby.)*

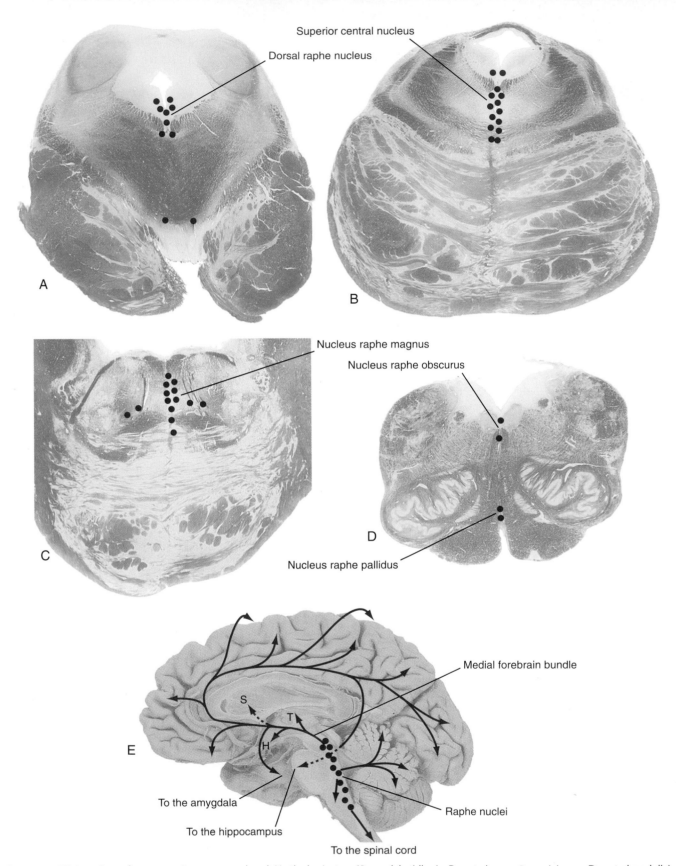

Figure 11-27 Locations of serotonergic neurons and nuclei in the brainstem (**A,** caudal midbrain; **B,** rostral pons; **C,** caudal pons; **D,** rostral medulla), and a schematic indication of their widespread CNS projections **(E).** Names of individual raphe nuclei are indicated for reference purposes. H, hypothalamus; S, septal nuclei (see Chapter 23); T, thalamus. *(Modified from Nolte J, Angevine JB Jr: The human brain in photographs and diagrams, ed 3, St. Louis, 2007, Mosby.)*

the overall level of arousal, and the norepinephrine system is more important for phasic changes in the level of attention. In addition, the serotonin system has at least one other important role—as part of the descending pain-control system described earlier.

Neurons of the Rostral Brainstem and Basal Forebrain Contain Acetylcholine

Acetylcholine plays an especially prominent role in the peripheral nervous system (PNS) as the transmitter released by alpha and gamma motor neurons, preganglionic autonomic neurons, and postganglionic parasympathetic neurons. The distribution of CNS neurons that use it, however, is more restricted. **Cholinergic** neurons (Fig. 11-28) are concentrated in parts of the reticular formation and in the **basal forebrain,** and there are also some large cholinergic interneurons in the caudate nucleus and putamen. The physiological action of acetylcholine is different at central and peripheral endings, depending on the interaction at either nicotinic or muscarinic receptors. As discussed in Chapter 8, nicotinic receptors (ion channels) mediate brief and spatially precise excitatory events, whereas muscarinic receptors (G protein–coupled) have slower and more diffuse effects.

Basal forebrain is a loosely used term that refers approximately to the area at and near the inferior surface of the telencephalon, between the hypothalamus and the orbital cortex. The basal forebrain reaches the surface of the brain in the anterior perforated substance and extends superiorly into limbic regions near the rostrum of the corpus callosum. The connections and function of this portion of the telencephalon have been notoriously difficult to unravel; partly as a result of this difficulty, the area beneath the anterior commissure was long referred to somewhat oxymoronically as the **substantia innominata** (literally, the "stuff with no name"). One prominent component of the substantia innominata, the **basal nucleus** (of **Meynert**), is the major collection of forebrain cholinergic neurons. Neurons of the basal nucleus, together with some from related nearby nuclei, blanket the cerebral cortex, hippocampus, and amygdala with cholinergic endings. These widespread projections suggest that the basal nucleus is also involved in general regulation of the level of forebrain activity, and there is considerable evidence that these cholinergic neurons (together with cholinergic projections from the reticular formation to the thalamus) play a critical role in the sleep-wakefulness cycle and in some forms of learning and memory.

Neurochemical Imbalances Are Involved in Certain Forms of Mental Illness

Many of the drugs used to treat neurological and psychiatric disorders are known to have effects at synapses involving particular neurotransmitters. For example, phenothiazine derivatives (e.g., chlorpromazine [Thorazine]) and related drugs used as antipsychotics in the treatment of schizophrenia block dopamine receptors, suggesting that the mesolimbic and mesocortical projections may be involved in this disorder. Similarly, drugs commonly used as antidepressants enhance the effectiveness of transmission at norepinephrine and serotonin synapses by inhibiting their reuptake into the presynaptic neuron. Observations like these, coupled with our current ability to map out the cells, axons, and synaptic endings that use a neurotransmitter, have contributed to a better understanding of these disorders and to the development of more effective drugs for their treatment. Although there are few disorders in which malfunction of a single neurotransmitter system accounts for all findings, there are increases in examples in which one transmitter plays a major role.

Alzheimer's disease is a devastating and sadly common illness characterized by extensive neuronal atrophy (particularly in the cerebral cortex and hippocampus), memory loss, personality changes, and, ultimately, profound dementia. In patients with Alzheimer's disease, there is a dramatic loss of acetylcholine in the cortex and hippocampus and a corresponding loss of neurons in the basal nucleus and nearby cholinergic cell groups. Such findings have led to a variety of treatments, including acetylcholine replacement therapy, and more recently, the dual use of cholinesterase inhibitors and NMDA-receptor antagonists. None of the currently available treatments has yet proved to be as effective as researchers and patients are hoping for.

The Brainstem Is Supplied by the Vertebral-Basilar System

The brainstem depends almost entirely on the vertebral-basilar system for its blood supply. The vertebral and basilar arteries travel along the anterior surface of the brainstem (Fig. 11-29), giving rise to a series of circumferential arteries (e.g., the superior cerebellar artery) that wrap around some level of the brainstem on their way to a final area of distribution. As a result, the brainstem supply is a series of wedge-shaped territories (Fig. 11-30), with anterior and medial areas supplied mostly by perforating branches of the vertebral and basilar arteries, and lateral and posterior areas supplied by perforating branches of the circumferential arteries. This shows up in brainstem stroke syndromes, in which medial or lateral areas are often affected selectively (see Figs. 12-29 and 12-30).

The caudal medulla has a supply much like that of the spinal cord. Anterolateral portions are supplied by the anterior spinal artery, small branches of the vertebral artery, or both. Posterolateral portions are supplied by

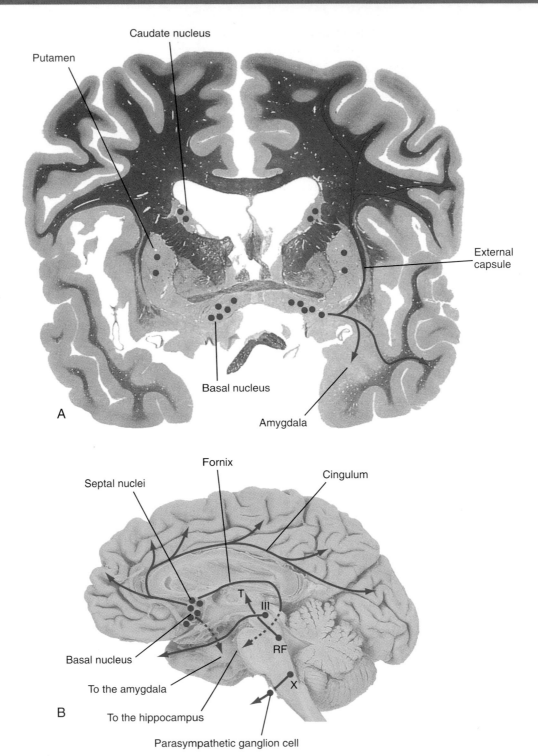

Figure 11-28 Locations of cholinergic neurons in the forebrain **(A)**, and a schematic indication of their widespread CNS projections and the locations of other cholinergic neurons **(B)**. III, oculomotor nucleus (representing motor neurons in general); RF, reticular formation; T, thalamus; X, dorsal motor nucleus of the vagus (representing preganglionic autonomic neurons in general). *(Modified from Nolte J, Angevine JB Jr: The human brain in photographs and diagrams, ed 3, St. Louis, 2007, Mosby.)*

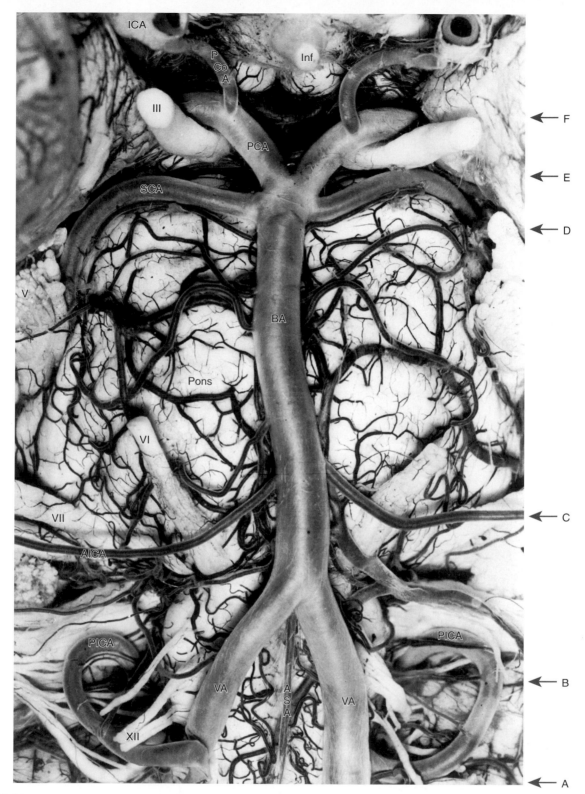

Figure 11-29 Anterior surface of a human brainstem, after its arteries were injected with a mixture of gelatin and India ink. Arteries of the vertebral-basilar system can be seen clearly, overlying the various divisions of the brainstem. By considering where different vessels and branches leave the vertebral-basilar system, one can imagine the vascular supply of each brainstem level; the arrows on the right indicate the levels for which vascular territories are charted in Figure 11-30. Cranial nerves are indicated by roman numerals. *AICA,* anterior inferior cerebellar artery; *ASA,* anterior spinal artery; *BA,* basilar artery; *ICA,* internal carotid artery; *Inf,* infundibular stalk; *PCA,* posterior cerebral artery; *PCoA,* posterior communicating artery; *PICA,* posterior inferior cerebellar artery; *SCA,* superior cerebellar artery; *VA,* vertebral artery. *(From Duvernoy HM: Human brainstem vessels, ed 2, New York, 1999, Springer-Verlag.)*

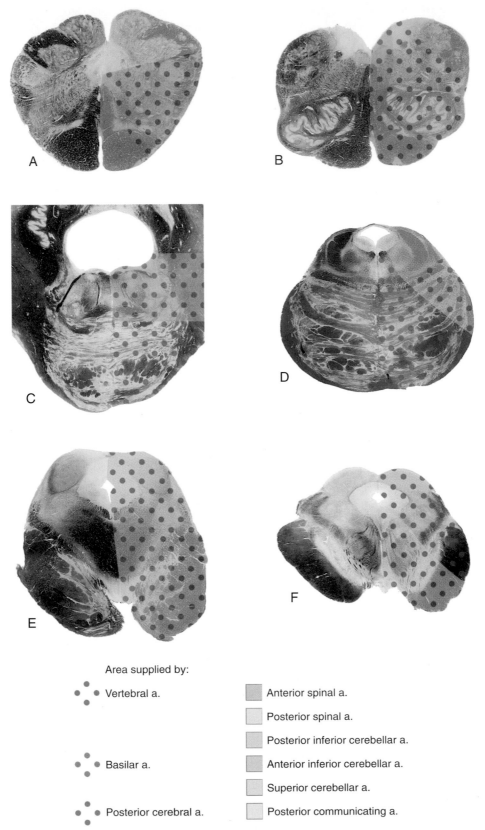

Area supplied by:

Vertebral a.

Basilar a.

Posterior cerebral a.

Anterior spinal a.

Posterior spinal a.

Posterior inferior cerebellar a.

Anterior inferior cerebellar a.

Superior cerebellar a.

Posterior communicating a.

Figure 11-30 Approximate arterial supply of various brainstem levels; corresponding levels of an intact brainstem are indicated in Figure 11-29. Although there is variability from one individual to another, different vertebral-basilar branches, or combinations of these branches, typically supply wedge-shaped areas at each brainstem level. The zones of damage in brainstem strokes frequently correspond to these wedge-shaped areas.

the posterior spinal artery, small branches of the posterior inferior cerebellar artery (PICA), or both. The rostral medulla receives a varying supply. Anterior and medial structures, such as the pyramid and the medial lemniscus, depend on some combination of vertebral branches and the anterior spinal artery. Lateral and posterior structures, such as the spinothalamic tract and the inferior cerebellar peduncle, depend on the branches of the vertebral artery, the PICA, and, to a lesser extent, the posterior spinal artery.

Most of the pons is supplied by unnamed **paramedian** and **circumferential** branches of the basilar artery. The anterior inferior cerebellar artery and the superior cerebellar artery contribute branches to the middle and superior cerebellar peduncles and to posterior and lateral portions of the pontine tegmentum.

The supply of the midbrain is chiefly from the posterior cerebral artery, with some contribution from the basilar and superior cerebellar arteries caudally. In addition, the anterior choroidal artery and the posterior communicating artery may send branches to the cerebral peduncle.

SUGGESTED READINGS

Baker KG, et al: The human locus coeruleus complex: an immuno-histochemical and three-dimensional reconstruction study. Exp Brain Res 77:257, 1989.

Beecher HR: Pain in men wounded in battle. Ann Surg 123:96, 1946.
A fascinating paper showing that wounds we would expect to be terribly painful may not be, depending in part on the circumstances surrounding the incurrence of the injury.

Berridge CW, Waterhouse BD: The locus coeruleus-noradrenergic system: modulation of behavioral state and state-dependent cognitive processes. Brain Res Rev 42:33, 2003.

Bianchi AL, Denavit-Saubié M, Champagnat J: Central control of breathing in mammals: neuronal circuitry, membrane properties, and neurotransmitters. Physiol Rev 75:1, 1995.

Brozoski TJ, et al: Cognitive deficit caused by regional depletion of dopamine in prefrontal cortex of rhesus monkey. Science 205:929, 1979.

Caplan LR: Posterior circulation disease: clinical findings, diagnosis, and management, Cambridge, 1996, Blackwell Science.
An extensive review of the vascular anatomy and symptoms involved in brainstem strokes.

Carlsson A, Falck B, Hillarp N-Å: Cellular localization of brain monoamines. Acta Physiol Scand 56(Suppl):196, 1962.
The first systematic mapping of monoamine-containing neurons in the CNS, using a histochemical technique that makes them fluorescent.

Carrive P, Morgan MM: Periaqueductal gray. In Paxinos G, Mai JK, editors: The human nervous system, ed 2, San Diego, 2004, Elsevier Academic Press.
It does a lot more than participate in pain control.

Cooper JR, Bloom FE, Roth RH: The biochemical basis of neuropharmacology, ed 8, New York, 2003, Oxford University Press.

Craig AD, Serrano LP: Effects of systemic morphine on lamina I spinothalamic tract neurons in the cat. Brain Res 636:233, 1994.

Duvernoy HM: Human brain stem vessels, ed 2, Berlin, 1999, Springer-Verlag.

Engberg I, Lundberg A, Ryall RW: Reticulospinal inhibition of transmission in reflex pathways. J Physiol 194:201, 1968.

Fields HL, Basbaum AI, Heinricher MM: Central nervous system mechanisms of pain modulation. In McMahon S, Koltzenburg M: Wall and Melzack's textbook of pain, ed 5, Edinburgh, 2006, Churchill Livingstone.

Fillenz M: Noradrenergic neurons, New York, 1990, Cambridge University Press.

Foote SL, Morrison JH: Extrathalamic modulation of cortical function. Annu Rev Neurosci 10:67, 1987.
A review of direct cortical input from fiber systems containing norepinephrine, dopamine, serotonin, and acetylcholine.

Gaspar P, et al: Catecholamine innervation of the human cerebral cortex as revealed by comparative immunohistochemistry of tyrosine hydroxylase and dopamine-beta-hydroxylase. J Comp Neurol 279:249, 1989.

Grant SJ, Aston-Jones G, Redmond DE, Jr: Responses of primate locus coeruleus neurons to simple and complex sensory stimuli. Brain Res Bull 21:401, 1988.

Hasselmo ME: The role of acetylcholine in learning and memory. Curr Opin Neurobiol 16:710, 2006.

Hobson JA, Brazier MAB, editors: The reticular formation revisited: specifying function for a nonspecific system, International Brain Research Organization monograph series, vol 6, New York, 1980, Raven Press.

Hornung J-P: The human raphe nuclei and the serotonergic system. J Chem Neuroanat 26:331, 2003.

Hosobuchi Y, Adams JE, Linchitz R: Pain relief by electrical stimulation of the central gray matter in humans and its reversal by naloxone. Science 197:183, 1977.
Evidence that the analgesia caused by stimulation of the periaqueductal gray has properties in common with morphine analgesia.

Huang X-F, Paxinos G: Human intermediate reticular zone: a cyto- and chemoarchitectonic study. J Comp Neurol 360:571, 1995.
The anatomy of the part of the reticular formation most closely related to autonomic control mechanisms.

Hughes J: Isolation of an endogenous compound from the brain with pharmacological properties similar to morphine. Brain Res 88:295, 1975.
The original discovery of enkephalins.

Hyman SE, Malenka RC, Nestler EJ: Neural mechanisms of addiction: the role of reward-related learning and memory. Annu Rev Neurosci 29:565, 2006.
"A central role for dopamine."

Jacobs BL: Single-unit activity of locus ceruleus neurons in behaving animals. Prog Neurobiol 27:183, 1986.

Jacobs BL, Azmitia EC: Structure and function of the brain serotonin system. Physiol Rev 72:165, 1992.

Kinomura S, et al: Activation by attention of the human reticular formation and thalamic intralaminar nuclei. Science 271:512, 1996.

Kuhar MJ, Pert CB, Snyder SH: Regional distribution of opiate receptor binding in monkey and human brain. Nature 245:447, 1973.

Lachman N, Acland RD, Rosse C: Anatomical evidence for the absence of a morphologically distinct cranial root of the accessory nerve in man. Clin Anat 15:4, 2002.

Le Moal M, Simon H: Mesocorticolimbic dopaminergic network: functional and regulatory roles. Physiol Rev 71:155, 1991.

Loewy AD, Araujo JC, Kerr FWL: Pupillodilator pathways in the brain stem of the cat: anatomical and electrophysiological identification of a central autonomic pathway. Brain Res 60:65, 1973.

Luiten PGM, et al: The course of paraventricular hypothalamic efferents to autonomic structures in medulla and spinal cord. Brain Res 329:374, 1985.

Mayer DJ, Price DD, Rafii A: Antagonism of acupuncture analgesia in man by the narcotic antagonist naloxone. Brain Res 121:368, 1977.

A provocative paper providing initial evidence that acupuncture works by somehow causing the release of enkephalins.

Mesulam M-M, Geula C: Nucleus basalis (Ch 4) and cortical cholinergic innervation in the human brain: observations based on the distribution of acetylcholinesterase and choline acetyltransferase. J Comp Neurol 275:216, 1988.

Mesulam M-M, et al: Human reticular formation: cholinergic neurons of the pedunculopontine and laterodorsal tegmental nuclei and some cytochemical comparisons to forebrain cholinergic neurons. J Comp Neurol 281:611, 1989.

Mitani A, et al: Descending projections from the gigantocellular tegmental field in the cat: cells of origin and their brainstem and spinal cord trajectories. J Comp Neurol 268:546, 1988.

Mufson EJ: Human cholinergic basal forebrain: chemoanatomy and neurologic dysfunction. J Chem Neuroanat 26:233, 2003.

Naidich TP, et al: Duvernoy's atlas of the human brain stem and cerebellum: high-field MRI, surface anatomy, internal structure, vascularization and 3 D sectional anatomy, New York, 2008, Springer.

Newman DB, Ginsberg CY: Brainstem reticular nuclei that project to the thalamus in rats: a retrograde tracer study. Brain Behav Evol 44:1, 1994.

Nieuwenhuys R: Chemoarchitecture of the brain, Berlin, 1985, Springer-Verlag.

Nygren L-G, Olson L: A new major projection from locus coeruleus: the main source of noradrenergic nerve terminals in the ventral and dorsal columns of the spinal cord. Brain Res 132:85, 1977.

Olszewski J, Baxter D: Cytoarchitecture of the human brainstem, Philadelphia, 1954, JB Lippincott.

Paxinos G, Huang X-F: Atlas of the human brainstem, San Diego, 1995, Academic Press.

Pearson J, et al: Human brainstem catecholamine neuronal anatomy as indicated by immunocytochemistry with antibodies to tyrosine hydroxylase. Neuroscience 8:3, 1983.

Peterson BW: The reticulospinal system and its role in the control of movement. In Barnes CD, editor: Brainstem control of spinal cord function, Orlando, Fla, 1984, Academic Press.

Raina P, et al: Effectiveness of cholinesterase inhibitors and memantine for treating dementia: Evidence review for a clinical practice guideline. Ann Intern Med 148:379, 2008.

Reynolds DV: Surgery in the rat during electrical analgesia induced by focal brain stimulation. Science 164:444, 1969.
The original demonstration of stimulation-induced analgesia.

Saper CB, Chelimsky TC: A cytoarchitectonic and histochemical study of nucleus basalis and associated cell groups in the normal human brain. Neuroscience 13:1023, 1984.

Saper CB, et al: Direct hypothalamo-autonomic connections. Brain Res 117:305, 1976.

Savoiardo M, et al: The vascular territories in the cerebellum and brainstem: CT and MR study. AJNR Am J Neuroradiol 8:199, 1987.

Schwartz J-C, et al: Histaminergic transmission in the mammalian brain. Physiol Rev 71:1, 1991.
One more amine neurotransmitter, this one prominent in hypothalamic neurons.

Soteropoulos DS, et al: Cells in the monkey ponto-medullary reticular formation modulate their activity with slow finger movements. J Phys 590(16):4011, 2012.

Steriade M, McCarley RW: Brain control of wakefulness and sleep, ed 2, New York, 2005, Springer.
A recent, extensive review of the structure, connections, and electrophysiology of the reticular formation.

Torack RM, Morris JC: The association of ventral tegmental area histopathology with adult dementia. Arch Neurol 45:497, 1988.

Tracey DJ, Stone J, Paxinos G, editors: Neurotransmitters in the human brain. In Advances in behavioral biology, vol 43, New York, 1995, Plenum Press.

Tracey I, Mantyh PW: The cerebral signature for pain perception and its modulation. Neuron 55:377, 2007.

Tracey I, et al: Imaging attentional modulation of pain in the periaqueductal gray in humans. J Neurosci 22:2748, 2002.
The experiments depicted in Figure 11-20.

Whitehouse PJ, et al: Alzheimer's disease and senile dementia: loss of neurons in the basal forebrain. Science 215:1237, 1982.

Willis WD, Haber LH, Martin RF: Inhibition of spinothalamic tract cells and interneurons by brain stem stimulation in the monkey. J Neurophysiol 40:968, 1977.

Willner P, Scheel-Kruger J: The mesolimbic dopamine system: from motivation to action, New York, 1991, John Wiley & Sons.

Woolf NJ: Cholinergic systems in mammalian brain and spinal cord. Prog Neurobiol 37:475, 1991.

Cranial Nerves and Their Nuclei

The caudal medulla looks somewhat similar to the spinal cord, but this similarity seems to disappear at more rostral levels of the brainstem. One of the complicating factors is the arrangement of the tracts and nuclei associated with cranial nerves III to XII. These tracts and nuclei appear discouragingly intricate on first inspection, but there is a common way of systematizing the cranial nerves so that their central connections make sense. This involves categorizing the tracts and nuclei according to the kinds of afferent and efferent fibers contained within each nerve (often referred to as the **functional components** of each nerve).

Cranial Nerve Nuclei Have a Generally Predictable Arrangement

Spinal nerves contain sensory and motor fibers. A given axon entering or leaving the spinal cord can be placed in one of the following four categories:

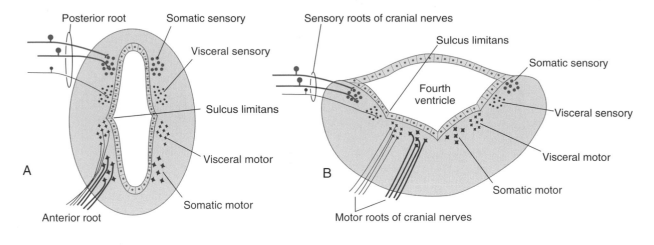

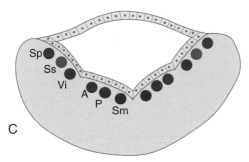

Figure 12-1 Arrangement of cranial nerve nuclei in the brainstem. **A,** Arrangement of the general afferent and efferent cell columns in the embryonic spinal cord. **B,** Movement of these columns to the floor of the fourth ventricle in the embryonic rhombencephalon. **C,** Further subdivision of these cell columns, showing the "ideal" locations of the cranial nerve nuclei, corresponding to the six functional categories of cranial nerve fibers: A, preganglionic autonomic (visceral motor); P, pharyngeal motor; Sm, somatic motor; Sp, special sensory; Ss, somatic sensory; Vi, visceral sensory.

1. **Somatic sensory** fibers convey information from receptive endings for pain, temperature, and mechanical stimuli in somatic structures such as skin, muscles, and joints.
2. **Visceral sensory** fibers convey information from receptive endings in visceral structures such as the walls of blood vessels or of the digestive tract.
3. **Visceral motor** fibers are preganglionic autonomic axons.
4. **Somatic motor** fibers innervate skeletal muscle (i.e., they are the axons of alpha and gamma motor neurons).

By and large the cell bodies on which spinal afferents synapse and the cell bodies of spinal efferent fibers are located in portions of the spinal gray matter are predictable from its embryological development (Fig. 12-1A). The sulcus limitans separates the alar plate (which develops into the posterior horn) from the basal plate (which develops into the anterior horn). Within both the alar and the basal plates, cells concerned with visceral function tend to be located nearer the sulcus limitans. This is shown most clearly in the adult central nervous system (CNS) by the location of the cell bodies of visceral motor neurons in the intermediolateral cell column. So for each of the four spinal axon categories there is a corresponding column of cells in the spinal gray matter. The

somatic sensory and motor columns extend the length of the cord; the visceral sensory and motor columns are found at spinal levels T1 to L2-L3 and S2 to S4.

The Sulcus Limitans Intervenes Between Motor and Sensory Nuclei of Cranial Nerves

Axons from all four categories found in spinal nerves are also found in various cranial nerves, where they take care of the same functions for the head. However, some cranial nerves contain axons from additional categories, reflecting specialized structures and functions associated with the head. Thus there are **special sensory** fibers that, in the case of the cranial nerves attached to the brainstem, are related to the special senses of hearing and equilibrium.[a] In addition, motor axons in certain cranial nerves innervate striated muscles in and near the head and neck in humans and other mammals. Such muscles develop from the pharyngeal arches, known as

---

[a]The cranial nerve fibers conveying information from taste buds are often considered special afferents as well—special visceral afferents—but, as discussed in this and the next chapter, they have connections similar in many ways to those of other visceral afferents. Hence in this account all visceral afferents are treated as one category.

Table 12-1 **Categories of Nerve Fibers in Cranial Nerves of the Brainstem**

	Structures Innervated	Cranial Nerves*
Sensory		
Somatic	Skin, muscles, joints of the head	V
Visceral	Cranial, thoracic, abdominal viscera	X
		VII, IX
	Taste buds	
Special	Inner ear	VIII
Motor†		
Somatic	Extraocular muscles	III, IV, VI
	Tongue muscles	XII
Visceral	Parasympathetic ganglia for cranial, thoracic, and abdominal viscera	X
Pharyngeal	Jaw muscles	V
	Facial muscles	VII
	Laryngeal and pharyngeal muscles	X
		V, VII
	Middle ear muscles	XI
	Sternocleidomastoid, trapezius	

*Principal cranial nerves only. Smaller contributions that may nevertheless be clinically important (e.g., parasympathetics for the pupil in cranial nerve III) are not indicated here but are included in Table 12-2.

†Does not include the efferents in cranial nerve VIII (described in Chapter 14) that innervate the receptor cells of the inner ear, which do not fit comfortably into any of these categories.

branchial or gill arches in fishes. Pharyngeal arch derived musculature include the muscles of the larynx, pharynx, jaw, and face. Functionally and histologically, pharyngeal arch derived musculature is identical to ordinary skeletal muscle, but the motor neurons for such muscles have a distinctive location in the brainstem, different from that of ordinary somatic motor neurons. In recognition of their special development and location, they are classified as a separate category, here called **pharyngeal motor neurons.**[b] Hence there are six different categories of nerve fibers in the cranial nerves attached to the brainstem (Table 12-1).

As in the case of the spinal cord, the locations of the cell bodies where cranial nerve afferents terminate or cranial nerve efferents originate can be predicted, to

[b]Because muscles derived from the pharyngeal arches tend to be concentrated around the mouth at a junction between visceral and somatic areas, the motor fibers that innervate them were historically referred to as special visceral efferent fibers. This classification is somewhat confusing (particularly because the sensory fibers from these muscles are called somatic afferent fibers), so it is not used here.

some extent, from the embryology of the brainstem. The walls of the neural tube spread apart in the medulla and pons to form the floor of the fourth ventricle (see Fig. 2-10). The sulcus limitans runs longitudinally along the floor of the adult ventricle (see Fig. 11-3A), still separating sensory alar plate derivatives (now lateral) from motor basal plate derivatives (now medial) (see Fig. 12-1B). As in the case of the spinal cord, cells concerned with visceral functions are usually located nearer the sulcus limitans.

Ideally the cell columns subserving the special components of the cranial nerves would be located adjacent to those for the corresponding general components, as indicated in Figure 12-1C. The actual arrangement in the adult brainstem is not quite as simple as in this idealized diagram, for two principal reasons. First, the cell columns of the brainstem are not continuous like those of the spinal cord; rather, they are interrupted and form a series of nuclei located at longitudinal levels roughly corresponding to the attachment points of the cranial nerves. As a result, all components are seldom present in a given transverse plane (Fig. 12-2; see also Fig. 15-2). Second, in a few instances, portions of a cell column migrate away from their expected locations (Fig. 12-3). For example, most pharyngeal motor neurons are located in the anterolateral part of the tegmentum rather than in the floor of the ventricle adjacent to other efferent neurons. The actual locations of cranial nerve nuclei in the rostral medulla are shown in Figure 12-3; also indicated are the functional types of fibers in each of the cranial nerves of the brainstem. (This is only meant to be a convenient summary; not all cranial nerves project to or originate from the rostral medulla.)

It can be seen from Figure 12-3 that no cranial nerve contains axons from all six categories. If the compositions of all the nerves are tabulated (as in Table 12-2), it becomes apparent that there are three types of cranial nerves. Some nerves (III, IV, VI, XI and XII) contain motor axons for ordinary skeletal muscle and little or nothing else, so they may be referred to as **somatic motor nerves.** Others (I, II, and VIII) contain special sensory fibers and little or nothing else. The remaining nerves (V, VII, IX, and X) are somewhat more complex and typically contain several components; all innervate pharyngeal arch musculature, they are called **branchiomeric nerves**, owing to the older nomenclature that refers to their development in the region of the gill (branchial) arches in fish.

A presentation of the cranial nerves involves too much material for one comfortable sitting, so it is spread out over several chapters. The remainder of this chapter is divided into two more or less distinct sections, discussing first the somatic motor nerves and then most components of the branchiomeric nerves. Chapter 13 discusses the chemical senses of taste and smell subserved by some brainstem cranial nerves and the olfactory nerve. Chapter 14 deals with the eighth nerve, the

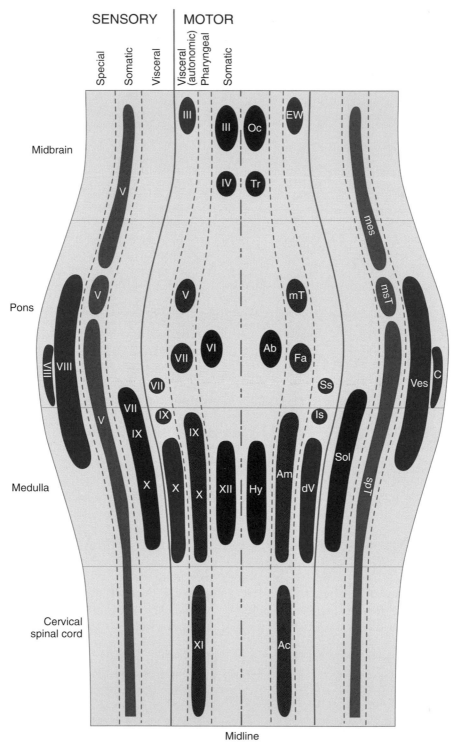

Figure 12-2 Longitudinal arrangement of functional types of cranial nerve nuclei in the brainstem, indicating their derivation from cell columns. Names of nuclei are indicated on the right, and the principal cranial nerves associated with each nucleus are indicated on the left by roman numerals. This diagram summarizes the way in which the medial-lateral location of a nucleus suggests its function, and its location along the longitudinal extent of the brainstem suggests the cranial nerve with which it is associated. Ab, abducens nucleus; Ac, accessory nucleus; Am, nucleus ambiguus; C, cochlear nuclei; dV, dorsal motor nucleus of the vagus; EW, Edinger-Westphal; Fa, facial motor nucleus; Hy, hypoglossal nucleus; Is, inferior salivary nucleus; mes, mesencephalic nucleus ; msT, main sensory nucleus; mT, trigeminal motor nucleus; Oc, oculomotor nucleus; Sol, nucleus of the solitary tract; spT, spinal trigeminal nucleus; Ss, superior salivary nucleus; Tr, trochlear nucleus; Ves, vestibular nuclei. *(Modified from Nieuwenhuys R et al: The human central nervous system: a synopsis and atlas, ed 3, New York, 1988, Springer-Verlag.)*

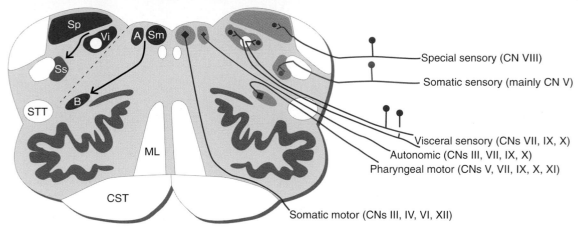

Figure 12-3 Drawing of a section through the rostral medulla of an adult brain, showing the actual medial-lateral arrangement of cranial nerve (CN) nuclei. On the left the nuclei corresponding to the six functional categories are indicated. On the right the cranial nerves containing each of these fiber types are indicated; cranial nerves I and II are not included, nor are some minor components such as the few somatic sensory fibers in cranial nerve VII. Not all of the nerves listed actually emerge at this brainstem level; they are included here for summary purposes. A, preganglionic autonomic (visceral motor); CST, corticospinal tract; ML, medial lemniscus; Sm, somatic motor; Sp, special sensory; Ss, somatic sensory; STT, spinothalamic tract; Vi, visceral sensory.

special sensory nerve subserving hearing and equilibrium. (The remaining special sensory nerve, the optic nerve, is an outgrowth of the diencephalon and is really a tract of the CNS. It is considered separately in Chapter 17.) Finally, as mentioned previously, Chapter 15 contains a series of brainstem sections with labels and summary descriptions indicating the locations and contents of cranial nerve nuclei and other important brainstem structures.

Cranial Nerves III, IV, VI, XI, and XII Contain Somatic Motor Fibers

The somatic motor nerves are the simplest of the cranial nerves because each contains fibers of only one category (except for cranial nerve III, which has a small but important complement of preganglionic parasympathetic fibers).[c] The nuclei of origin of all these nerves are located adjacent to the midline near the cerebral

aqueduct or the floor of the fourth ventricle, as would be expected from their embryological origins.

The Oculomotor Nerve (III) Innervates Four of the Six Extraocular Muscles

Cranial nerve III supplies the levator palpebrae superioris (the principal elevator of the eyelid); medial, superior and inferior recti; and the inferior oblique. The fibers originate in the wedge-shaped **oculomotor nucleus,** which is located at the anterior edge of the periaqueductal gray in the rostral midbrain (Fig. 12-4). They then proceed anteriorly and arch through the midbrain tegmentum in bundles that join to form the nerve just as they emerge into the interpeduncular fossa.

The oculomotor nucleus actually consists of a series of longitudinal cell columns, or subnuclei, much like the columns of spinal cord motor neurons that supply individual muscles. The column supplying the levator palpebrae superioris is located in the midline and innervates this muscle bilaterally. The column supplying the superior rectus projects to the contralateral eye. The columns supplying the medial rectus, inferior oblique, and inferior rectus all project to the ipsilateral eye. Finally, a column containing preganglionic parasympathetic neurons, known as the **accessory oculomotor** (Edinger-Westphal) **nucleus,** straddles the midline and projects to the ipsilateral ciliary ganglion. The ciliary ganglion in turn innervates the pupillary sphincter and the ciliary muscle.

The partly crossed–partly uncrossed nature of the oculomotor nerve is a curious fact but one of limited clinical significance. This is because the oculomotor nuclei of the two sides are so close to each other that a

---

[c]Tongue and extraocular muscles, like almost all skeletal muscles, contain muscle spindles and other proprioceptors, but cranial nerves III, IV, VI, and XII have no sensory ganglia. Lingual proprioceptive fibers probably originate from upper cervical spinal ganglia and the sensory ganglia of cranial nerves V, IX, or X, then join the hypoglossal nerve along their course to the tongue; their central projections reach the spinal trigeminal nucleus and other brainstem sites. The function of these lingual proprioceptors is largely unknown, but they are assumed to be important for the fine control of tongue movements. Those from the extraocular muscles travel in cranial nerves III, IV, and VI within the orbit, then join the ophthalmic division of the trigeminal nerve for the rest of their course to the brainstem. Eye muscle proprioceptors may play a role in depth perception or its development.

Table 12-2 Contents of the Cranial Nerves

Nerve	Axon Categories	CNS Origin or Termination	Peripheral Origin or Termination
I (olfactory)	Sp	Olfactory bulb	Olfactory epithelium
II (optic)	Sp	Lateral geniculate nucleus, superior colliculus, hypothalamus	Retinal ganglion cells
III (oculomotor)*	Sm	Oculomotor nucleus	Superior, inferior, medial recti; inferior oblique; levator palpebrae superioris
	A	Accessory oculomotor nucleus (part of the oculomotor nucleus)	Pupillary sphincter, ciliary muscle†
IV (trochlear)	Sm	Trochlear nucleus	Superior oblique
V (trigeminal)	Ss	Spinal and main sensory nuclei	Skin, deep tissues, and dura mater of the head
		Mesencephalic nucleus	Muscle spindles and other mechanoreceptors
	P	Trigeminal motor nucleus	Muscles of mastication, tensor tympani, and a few others
VI (abducens)	Sm	Abducens nucleus	Lateral rectus
VII (facial)	Ss	Spinal trigeminal nucleus	Skin of the outer ear
	Vi	Nucleus of the solitary tract	Taste buds of anterior two thirds of the tongue; some mucous membranes of the nasopharynx
	A	Superior salivary nucleus	Submandibular and sublingual salivary glands, nasal and palatine glands, lacrimal glands†
	P	Facial motor nucleus	Muscles of facial expression, stapedius
VIII (vestibulocochlear)	Sp	Cochlear and vestibular nuclei	Organ of Corti, cristae of semicircular ducts, maculae of utricle and saccule
IX (glossopharyngeal)	Ss	Spinal trigeminal nucleus	Skin of the outer ear
	Vi	Nucleus of the solitary tract	Taste buds of the posterior third of the tongue; carotid body and sinus
		Nucleus of the solitary tract, spinal trigeminal nucleus	Mucous membranes of the posterior third of the tongue, nasal and oral pharynx, and middle ear
	A	Inferior salivary nucleus	Parotid gland†
	P	Nucleus ambiguus	Pharynx (stylopharyngeus)
X (vagus)	Ss	Spinal trigeminal nucleus	Skin of the outer ear
	Vi	Nucleus of the solitary tract	Taste buds of the epiglottis and esophagus
		Nucleus of the solitary tract, spinal trigeminal nucleus	Thoracic and abdominal viscera; mucous membranes of the larynx and laryngeal pharynx
	A	Dorsal motor nucleus	Thoracic and abdominal viscera†
	P	Nucleus ambiguus	Larynx and pharynx
XI (accessory)	P	Accessory nucleus (cervical cord)	Sternocleidomastoid, trapezius
XII (hypoglossal)	Sm	Hypoglossal nucleus	Tongue muscles

The three types of cranial nerves are indicated by shading. Somatic motor nerves have no shading, special sensory nerves have light shading, and nerves serving muscles derived from pharyngeal arches have darker shading.
*Most conveniently considered as one of the somatic motor nerves, despite the clinically important autonomic component.
†Final destination after synapse in a parasympathetic ganglion.
A, autonomic (visceral motor); P, pharyngeal motor; Sm, somatic motor; Sp, special sensory; Ss, somatic sensory; Vi, visceral sensory.

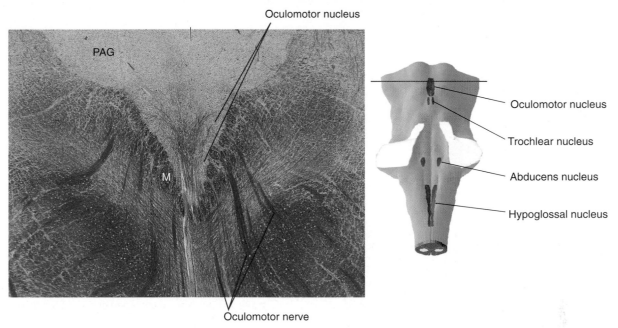

Figure 12-4 Section through the rostral midbrain showing the oculomotor nucleus. This figure is an enlargement of part of the section shown in Figure 11-17. The oculomotor nucleus is actually a tight cluster of subnuclei, each of which innervates a different muscle. M, medial longitudinal fasciculus; PAG, periaqueductal gray.

central lesion in this vicinity is likely to damage both nuclei. However, once a given oculomotor nerve emerges from the brainstem, it supplies only ipsilateral muscles, so a lesion of the third nerve, or of fibers curving through the midbrain tegmentum on their way to the third nerve, affects only one eye. Therefore the dissociated findings of paralysis of the superior rectus on one side and of other extraocular muscles on the opposite side are rarely encountered.

Damage to one oculomotor nerve causes a series of deficits (see Fig. 12-31B to E). The eye ipsilateral to the lesion deviates laterally because the medial rectus is now paralyzed and the lateral rectus is unopposed. This is called **lateral strabismus,** indicating that the eyes are misaligned because one of them deviates laterally from midposition. As a result, the patient complains of **diplopia** (double vision) and is unable to move the affected eye medially; vertical movements are also impaired because of paralysis of the superior and inferior recti and the inferior oblique. The ipsilateral levator palpebrae superioris is paralyzed, so **ptosis** occurs. In addition, the pupillary sphincter and ciliary muscle are nonfunctional. The pupil on the affected side is dilated (**mydriasis**) as a result of the now-unopposed pupillary dilator, and it does not constrict in response to light.[d] The lens cannot be focused for near vision; allowing the lens to "round up" for near vision is known as **accommodation.**

Along the course of the oculomotor nerve from brainstem to orbit, the preganglionic parasympathetic fibers from the accessory oculomotor nucleus travel in a superficial location within the nerve and are therefore especially susceptible to external pressures. A dilated pupil, unresponsive to light, may be the first clinically detectable sign of something pressing on the third nerve.

Because ptosis and pupils of unequal size accompany Horner's syndrome, one might think that this syndrome could be confused with third nerve damage. However, in Horner's syndrome the ptosis is on the same side as a nonfunctional pupillary dilator, hence on the same side as the *smaller* pupil. In contrast, the ptosis caused by third nerve damage is on the same side as a nonfunctional pupillary sphincter, hence on the same side as the *larger* pupil. Also, the ptosis caused by third nerve damage is more pronounced and is usually accompanied by defective eye movements and lateral strabismus.

The Trochlear Nerve (IV) Innervates the Superior Oblique

Cranial nerve IV, the trochlear nerve, supplies the superior oblique and is named for the sling of connective tissue (the *trochlea*—Latin for "pulley") through which the tendon of the superior oblique passes (see Fig. 21-2). Its cell bodies of origin are located in the contralateral **trochlear nucleus.** This is a small nucleus (because it has only one small muscle to supply) located at the level of the inferior colliculus, where it indents the medial longitudinal fasciculus (MLF) (Fig. 12-5). Fibers leaving

[d]Both pupils normally constrict when light is shone into either eye. This is the pupillary light reflex, which is discussed further in Chapter 17.

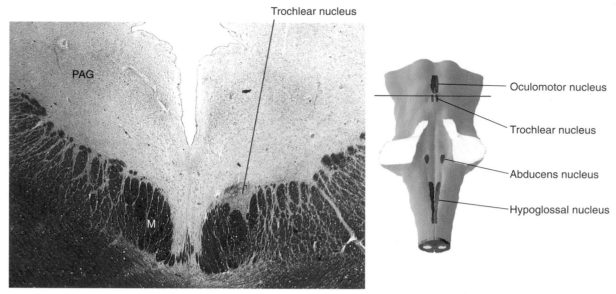

Figure 12-5 Section through the caudal midbrain showing the trochlear nucleus. This figure is an enlargement of part of the section shown in Figure 11-16. M, medial longitudinal fasciculus; PAG, periaqueductal gray.

the nucleus turn caudally in the periaqueductal gray, then arch posteriorly to decussate and leave the brainstem at the pons-midbrain junction. The trochlear nerve is thus unique in two respects: it is the only cranial nerve attached to the posterior surface of the brainstem and the only one to originate entirely from a contralateral nucleus.[e]

Damage to the trochlear nerve results in much less drastic and noticeable deficits than does damage to either the oculomotor or the abducens nerve. The superior oblique helps move the eye downward and laterally, so attempted movement in these directions (typically when reading or descending stairs) may cause diplopia.

The Abducens Nerve (VI) Innervates the Lateral Rectus

Cranial nerve VI, the abducens nerve, supplies the lateral rectus, which abducts the eye (hence the name of the nerve). The fibers originate from the ipsilateral **abducens nucleus,** which is located in the caudal pons beneath the floor of the fourth ventricle (Fig. 12-6).

Medial to this nucleus are two bundles of fibers. The more medial of the two is the MLF. Between the MLF and the abducens nucleus are motor fibers of the facial nerve, which take an unusual course in leaving the brainstem. They originate in the facial motor nucleus (see Figs. 12-6 and 12-24), which is located in the anterolateral part of the pontine tegmentum at about the same level as the abducens nucleus. The facial fibers travel posteromedially, wrap around the abducens nucleus, and turn anteriorly to exit from the brainstem (Fig. 12-7). The place where these fibers wrap around the abducens nucleus is called the **internal genu of the facial nerve.**[f] The abducens nucleus, together with the internal genu, is responsible for the **facial colliculus** in the floor of the fourth ventricle (see Fig. 11-3A).

The Abducens Nucleus Also Contains Interneurons That Project to the Contralateral Oculomotor Nucleus

Damage to the abducens nerve causes a **medial strabismus** (i.e., the affected eye deviates medially) as a result of the action of the now-unopposed medial rectus. The individual may be able to move the affected eye from the adducted position to midposition (but not past it) by relaxing its medial rectus (Fig. 12-8A). Damage to the abducens nucleus causes the same deficit, but with a significant addition: the ipsilateral eye will not abduct past midposition, and the contralateral eye will not *adduct* past midposition (see Fig. 12-8B; see also Fig. 12-10C). This is called **lateral gaze paralysis,** and it occurs because the abducens nucleus contains not only

---

[e]As discussed by Zee (Ann Neurol 4:384, 1978), this may reflect an adaptation to maintain certain relationships between head movements and eye movements. Eye movements are discussed in more detail in Chapter 21, but consider the following example: tilting your head toward your left shoulder evokes a reflex counterrotation of your eyes. The principal muscles that need to contract in this counterrotation are the left superior oblique and superior rectus, and the right inferior oblique and inferior rectus. Because fibers to the superior oblique and superior rectus cross before leaving the brainstem, all the lower motor neurons needed for this counterrotation are located on the right side of the brainstem.

---

[f]"Internal" to distinguish it from the bend in the peripheral course of the facial nerve at the level of the geniculate ganglion.

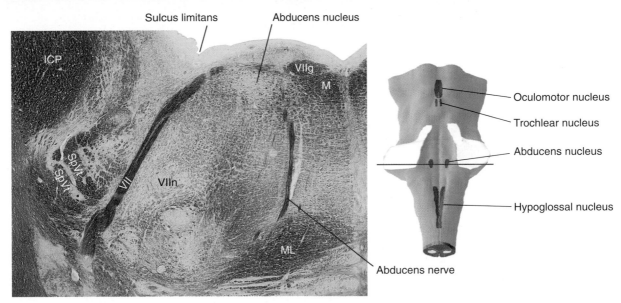

Figure 12-6 Section through the caudal pons showing the abducens nucleus and fibers of the facial nerve cut at different points along their course. The rounded elevation in the floor of the fourth ventricle between the midline and the sulcus limitans is the facial colliculus (see Fig. 11-3A). This figure is an enlargement of part of the section shown in Figure 11-11. ICP, inferior cerebellar peduncle; M, medial longitudinal fasciculus; ML, medial lemniscus; SpVt, spinal trigeminal tract; VII, facial nerve; VIIg, internal genu of the facial nerve; VIIn, facial motor nucleus.

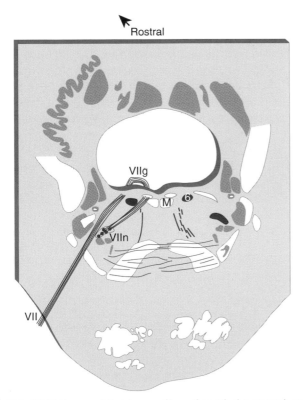

Figure 12-7 Course of facial nerve fibers through the internal genu. M, medial longitudinal fasciculus; 6, abducens nucleus; VII, facial nerve; VIIg, internal genu of the facial nerve; VIIn, facial motor nucleus.

lateral rectus motor neurons but also an approximately equal number of **internuclear neurons** with axons that ascend through the MLF.

The function of the MLF in lateral gaze becomes apparent if you consider that both eyes normally work together: when we look to one side, for example, one lateral rectus and the contralateral medial rectus contract simultaneously. The pathway that interconnects the abducens, trochlear, and oculomotor nuclei to make these sorts of movements possible is the MLF. Vertical movements and the higher centers that direct coordinated eye movements are discussed in Chapter 21, but for purely horizontal movements, the crucial interconnecting fibers are those that arise from the internuclear neurons in the abducens nucleus (Fig. 12-9). These cells send their axons across the midline as they emerge from the abducens nucleus; they then join the contralateral MLF and ascend to the oculomotor nucleus. There they make excitatory synapses on medial rectus motor neurons. Simultaneous firing of abducens motor neurons and internuclear neurons thus results in coordinated lateral gaze.

Damage to one MLF removes this excitatory influence from medial rectus motor neurons, so the eye ipsilateral to the lesion fails to move medially past midposition during attempted horizontal gaze (see Fig. 12-8C). Because both abducens nuclei are intact, full lateral movements of both eyes are still possible. In addition, although the affected medial rectus fails to contract during attempted horizontal gaze, it still functions normally when used without the opposite lateral rectus (i.e., during convergence). This condition has the ponderous but logical name **internuclear ophthalmoplegia**[g] (often abbreviated as INO).

---

[g]Literally, "paralysis of the eye caused by damage between the nuclei."

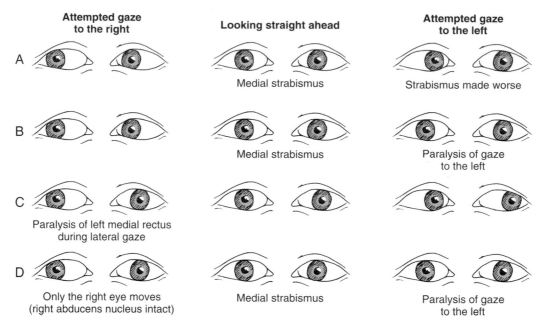

Attempted gaze to the right   **Looking straight ahead**   **Attempted gaze to the left**

A

Medial strabismus   Strabismus made worse

B

Medial strabismus   Paralysis of gaze to the left

C

Paralysis of left medial rectus during lateral gaze

D

Only the right eye moves (right abducens nucleus intact)   Medial strabismus   Paralysis of gaze to the left

Figure 12-8 Deficits of horizontal gaze after damage to the abducens–MLF system at the sites indicated in Figure 12-9. **A,** Abducens palsy resulting from damage to the left abducens nerve. **B,** Lateral gaze paralysis resulting from damage to the left abducens nucleus. **C,** Internuclear ophthalmoplegia resulting from damage to the left MLF. **D,** "One-and-a-half" (combination of **B** and **C**) resulting from damage to the left abducens nucleus and MLF. In all these situations, convergence, which does not depend on abducens-oculomotor interconnections, is preserved.

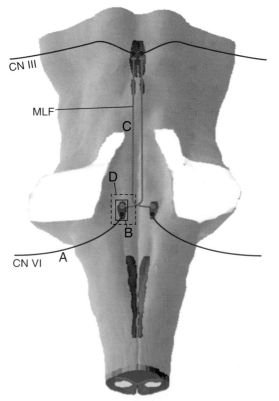

Figure 12-9 Connections between abducens and oculomotor nuclei involved in lateral gaze. Lesions labeled **A, B, C,** and **D** would cause the eye movement deficits indicated in Figure 12-8A to D.

Another eye movement disorder, clinically called a **one-and-a-half,** is rarely seen but is nevertheless instructive. It is caused by damage in the vicinity of the abducens nucleus and is characterized by the patient's inability to move either eye toward the side of the lesion in lateral gaze, or to move the eye on the side of the lesion in gaze toward the opposite side (see Fig. 12-8D). Thus, of the two directions of horizontal gaze (right and left), only half of one is intact. This is caused by destruction of one abducens nucleus plus destruction of fibers from the contralateral internuclear neurons as they join the MLF on the side of the lesion. The nearby internal genu of the facial nerve may also be affected (Fig. 12-10).

The Accessory Nerve (XI) Innervates Neck and Shoulder Muscles

Cranial nerve XI consists of fibers that originate from the very caudal medulla and the anterior horn of the upper five cervical spinal cord segments, exit just posterior to the denticulate ligament, and innervate the sterno-cleidomastoid and the trapezius. Earlier descriptions of the accessory nerve included the most caudal filaments leaving nucleus ambiguus as a cranial root of this nerve, because they were thought to travel with other accessory nerve fibers for a short distance before transferring to the vagus nerve in the jugular foramen. However, careful dissections have revealed that all motor fibers destined for laryngeal and pharyngeal muscles usually enter cranial nerve X (or IX) directly, so none of them is included in the account of cranial nerve XI in this book.

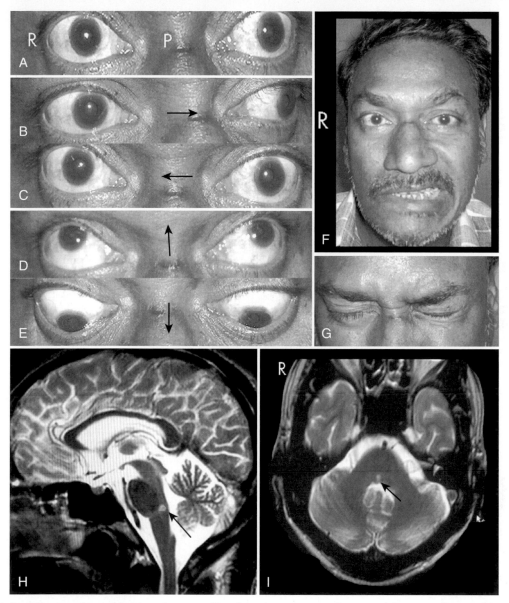

Figure 12-10 Horizontal gaze palsy and facial weakness resulting from damage centered on one abducens nucleus. In this case, "a 52 year old man . . . presented with sudden onset of binocular diplopia on looking to the left side [and] right facial weakness." There was a slight medial strabismus when he looked straight ahead **(A)**. Examination of his eye movements revealed an inability of either eye to move past midposition during attempted gaze to the right **(C),** consistent with damage to the right abducens nucleus. When he tried to look to the left, his left eye abducted (intact left abducens nucleus) but his right eye stopped near midposition **(B;** internuclear ophthalmoplegia, from damage to the axons of left internuclear neurons as they entered the right medial longitudinal fasciculus). Vertical gaze **(D, E)** was unaffected. Weakness of the right side of his face, consistent with damage to fibers of the facial nerve as they loop around the abducens nucleus, was apparent when he tried to bare his teeth **(F)** or close his eyes tightly **(G).** This unusual combination of a one-and-a-half plus seventh nerve palsy is sometimes referred to as an *eight-and-a-half syndrome.* T2-weighted magnetic resonance imaging scans in sagittal **(H)** and axial **(I)** planes revealed a small infarct *(arrows)* at precisely the location of the right abducens nucleus. *(From Nandhagopal R, Krishnamoorthy SG: J Neurol Neurosurg Psychiatry 77:463, 2006.)*

The Hypoglossal Nerve (XII) Innervates Tongue Muscles

Cranial nerve XII enters the tongue from below and supplies its intrinsic muscles and most of its extrinsic muscles (*hypoglossal* is Greek for "under the tongue"). The fibers originate in the ipsilateral **hypoglossal nucleus,** which extends from the caudal medulla through most of the rostral medulla (Fig. 12-11). This nucleus is situated adjacent to the midline just beneath the floor of the fourth ventricle and forms an elevation there called the **hypoglossal trigone.** Hypoglossal axons proceed anteriorly and emerge as a series of rootlets in the groove between the pyramid and the olive (see Fig. 11-3).

Damage to the hypoglossal nerve causes weakness of one side of the tongue and, because this is a lower motor neuron lesion, atrophy of that side of the tongue. This weakness is most easily demonstrated by asking the

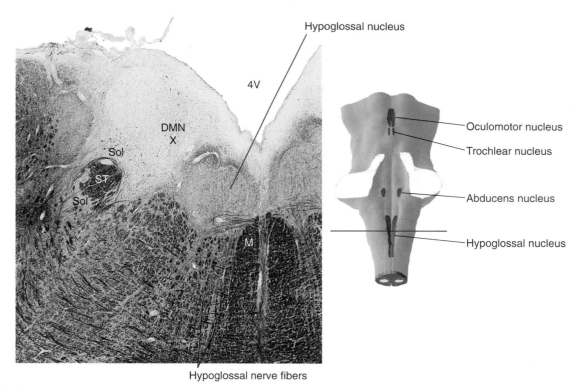

Hypoglossal nucleus

4V

DMN X

Sol

ST

Sol

M

Oculomotor nucleus

Trochlear nucleus

Abducens nucleus

Hypoglossal nucleus

Hypoglossal nerve fibers

Figure 12-11 Section through the rostral medulla showing the hypoglossal nucleus and other cranial nerve nuclei. This figure is an enlargement of part of the section shown in Figure 11-10. DMNX, dorsal motor nucleus of the vagus; 4V, fourth ventricle; M, medial longitudinal fasciculus; Sol, nucleus of the solitary tract; ST, solitary tract.

patient to protrude his or her tongue; the tongue deviates toward the side of the lesion (i.e., toward the weak side). Bilateral hypoglossal lesions may cause difficulties in both speaking and eating.

Branchiomeric Nerves Contain Axons From Multiple Categories

The branchiomeric nerves all innervate striated muscle of branchial (pharyngeal) arch origin (i.e., they all contain pharyngeal motor fibers). In spite of this, each has one function with which it is principally associated: the trigeminal nerve (V) is the major general sensory nerve for the head; the facial nerve (VII) is the motor nerve for facial expression; the glossopharyngeal nerve (IX) is the most important conveyor of taste and pharyngeal sensations; the vagus nerve (X) carries the parasympathetic outflow to the thoracic and abdominal viscera.

The Trigeminal Nerve (V) Is the General Sensory Nerve for the Head

With respect to somatic sensory innervation, cranial nerve V (Figs. 12-12 and 12-13) and its connections are to the head what the posterior roots and spinal cord are to the body. That is, the trigeminal system is ultimately

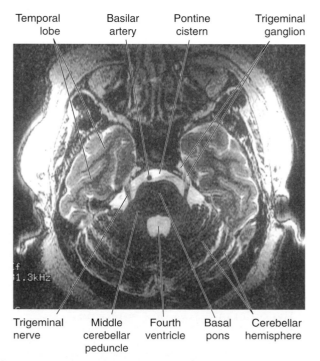

Temporal lobe   Basilar artery   Pontine cistern   Trigeminal ganglion

Trigeminal nerve   Middle cerebellar peduncle   Fourth ventricle   Basal pons   Cerebellar hemisphere

Figure 12-12 Axial (horizontal) magnetic resonance image at a mid-pontine level, showing the trigeminal nerve. *(Courtesy Dr. Raymond F. Carmody, University of Arizona College of Medicine.)*

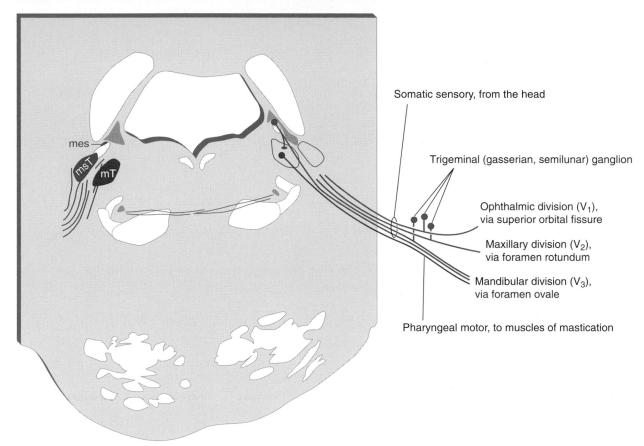

Figure 12-13 Fiber types in the trigeminal nerve and their peripheral destinations. mes, mesencephalic nucleus of the trigeminal; msT, trigeminal main sensory nucleus; mT, trigeminal motor nucleus.

responsible for the transmission of tactile, proprioceptive, and pain and temperature information from the head to the cerebral cortex, cerebellum, and reticular formation. The primary afferent fibers are distributed peripherally in the three divisions for which the trigeminal nerve was named (*trigeminal* is Latin for "born three at a time"), the **ophthalmic (V$_1$), maxillary (V$_2$), and mandibular (V$_3$)** divisions, in the pattern shown in Figure 12-14.

Three sensory nuclei are associated with trigeminal afferents, connected in ways homologous to spinal cord systems (Table 12-3). They form a long, almost continuous column of cells that extends from the rostral midbrain to the upper cervical spinal cord. The **main** (chief, principal) **sensory nucleus** (Fig. 12-15) forms an enlargement in this column in the midpons, slightly lateral to the **trigeminal motor nucleus.** The **spinal nucleus** extends caudally from this level, and the very slender **mesencephalic nucleus** extends rostrally (all the way into the midbrain, as its name implies). The main sensory and spinal nuclei are involved in processing somatosensory information, with different longitudinal levels specialized for different aspects of the processing. The mesencephalic nucleus, in contrast, is notable primarily

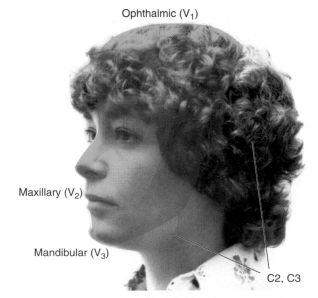

Figure 12-14 Peripheral distribution of the ophthalmic, maxillary, and mandibular branches of the trigeminal nerve. Not indicated is the innervation of the outer ear, at the junction between V$_3$ and the C2-C3 territory, by cranial nerves VII, IX, and X.

Table 12-3	Homologous Structures in Spinal and Trigeminal Systems	
	Spinal Cord	**Trigeminal System**
Touch, Proprioception		
Primary afferents (cell bodies)	Spinal ganglia	Trigeminal ganglion, mesencephalic nucleus
Primary afferents (central processes)	Posterior columns	Entering trigeminal fibers
Second-order neurons	Posterior column nuclei	Main sensory nucleus
Ascending pathway	Medial lemniscus	Medial lemniscus, posterior trigeminothalamic
Destination	VPL	VPM
Pain, Temperature		
Primary afferents (cell bodies)	Spinal ganglia	Trigeminal ganglion
Primary afferents (central processes)	Posterolateral tract (Lissauer's tract)	Spinal tract
Second-order neurons	Posterior horn	Spinal nucleus (caudal nucleus)
Ascending pathway	Spinothalamic tract	Spinothalamic tract
Destination	VPL and others	VPM and others
Pathways to the Cerebellum		
Second-order neurons	Intermediate gray	Spinal nucleus (interpolar and oral nuclei)
Reflexes		
Stretch reflex components	Spinal ganglion cells, anterior horn motor neurons	Mesencephalic nucleus cells, trigeminal motor neurons
Withdrawal reflex interneurons	Intermediate gray	Blink reflex: spinal nucleus (interpolar and oral nuclei)

VPL, ventral posterolateral nucleus; VPM, ventral posteromedial nucleus.

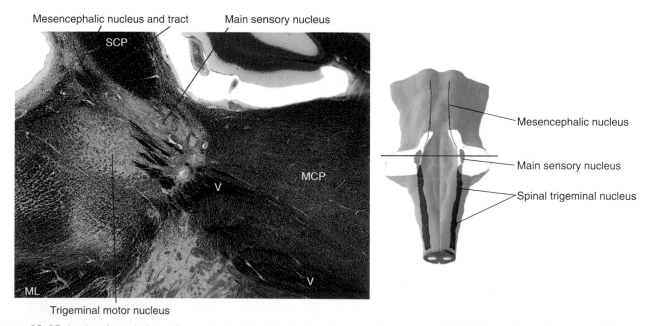

Figure 12-15 Section through the midpons showing the trigeminal motor and main sensory nuclei. This figure is an enlargement of the section shown in Figure 11-13. MCP, middle cerebellar peduncle; ML, medial lemniscus; SCP, superior cerebellar peduncle; V, trigeminal nerve fibers.

as an anatomical aberration; it is essentially a bit of the **trigeminal ganglion** located within the CNS rather than in the periphery. The cells of the mesencephalic nucleus are pseudounipolar neurons (homologous to spinal ganglion cells), and their myelinated processes collect in a bundle, called the **mesencephalic trigeminal tract,**

adjacent to the nucleus (see Fig. 12-15). The peripheral processes of these fibers are distributed through the trigeminal nerve to muscle spindles in the muscles of mastication and some mechanoreceptors of the gums, teeth, and hard palate. The central processes have connections similar to those of more conventional large-diameter trigeminal afferents with cell bodies in the trigeminal ganglion.

The Main Sensory Nucleus Receives Information About Touch and Jaw Position

The main sensory nucleus of the trigeminal nerve, located near the motor nucleus, is the trigeminal homologue of the posterior column nuclei. Thus it is primarily concerned with discriminative tactile and proprioceptive sensations and receives large-diameter, heavily myelinated tactile afferents. Unlike in the spinal cord, it gives rise to two ascending pathways to the thalamus. One, the **anterior trigeminothalamic tract,** is the expected collection of fibers that cross the midline, join the medial lemniscus adjacent to the representation of cervical dermatomes, and terminate in the **ventral posteromedial (VPM) nucleus** of the thalamus, adjacent to the ventral posterolateral (VPL) nucleus (Fig. 12-16; see also Fig. 12-21). The other is an uncrossed projection from the posteromedial portion of the main sensory nucleus, where the oral cavity is represented (a part of the nucleus that does not project through the medial lemniscus). This is called the **posterior trigeminothalamic tract;** it travels through the posteromedial part of the brainstem tegmentum and ends in its own separate portion of VPM, thus the oral cavity is represented bilaterally in the thalamus. The significance of this tract being uncrossed is not clear; it may well owe to the importance of what we choose to ingest, as it relates to survival of the individual. However, it does end alongside the ascending taste pathway (see Chapter 13), which is also uncrossed; hence intraoral sensations from one side of the mouth are processed in adjacent areas of the thalamus.

The Spinal Trigeminal Nucleus Receives Information About Pain and Temperature

Primary afferent fibers reach the spinal trigeminal nucleus by turning caudally as they enter the pons and joining the **spinal trigeminal tract,** which is just lateral to the nucleus. Both nucleus and tract extend caudally to about the third cervical segment of the spinal cord (hence their name), with the nucleus gradually blending with the posterior horn and the tract gradually blending with the posterolateral tract, which also allows fibers to ascend or descend as appropriate.

The spinal trigeminal nucleus has been subdivided into three regions on the basis of its histology. The most caudal part, extending from the spinal cord to the obex, is the **caudal nucleus.** The most rostral part, extending from the main sensory nucleus to about the pontomedullary junction, is the **oral nucleus.** Between these two is the **interpolar nucleus** in the rostral medulla. Differences exist among these nuclei in terms of the types of afferents that terminate at each level and the types of secondary connections made from each level. The

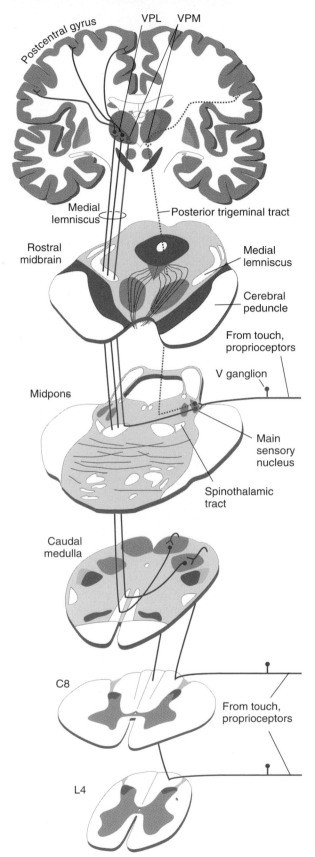

Figure 12-16 Ascending trigeminal pathways from the main sensory nucleus. VPL, ventral posterolateral nucleus; VPM, ventral posteromedial nucleus.

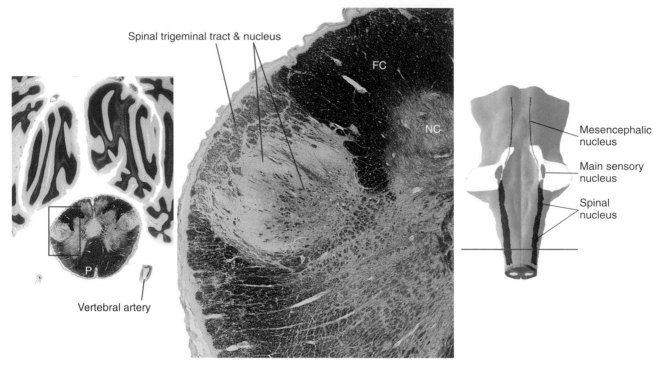

Figure 12-17 Section through the caudal medulla, where the spinal trigeminal tract and nucleus have an appearance much like that of the posterolateral tract and the posterior horn in the spinal cord. At levels rostral to the obex (see Fig. 11-11), the spinal trigeminal tract and nucleus do not have this appearance. FC, fasciculus cuneatus; NC, nucleus cuneatus; P, pyramid.

functional correlates of these differences are incompletely understood for the oral and interpolar nuclei, but the caudal nucleus is known to be particularly important for the processing of pain and temperature information from the head.[h] This fits nicely with its appearance (Fig. 12-17): the caudal nucleus looks much like the posterior horn of the spinal cord, with a cap of cells resembling the substantia gelatinosa.

Small-diameter trigeminal afferents conveying pain and temperature information descend through the spinal trigeminal tract and synapse in the caudal nucleus. Second-order neurons of the caudal nucleus, homologous to spinothalamic tract neurons, give rise to a crossed ascending pain pathway—the posterior trigeminothalamic tract, that terminates in VPM (Fig. 12-18). So the principal difference between spinal and trigeminal somatosensory projections to the thalamus lies in the position of the second-order neurons (Fig. 12-19). Trigeminal pain information also reaches the thalamus indirectly (via relays in the reticular formation) in a manner thought to be similar to spinoreticulothalamic projections.

---

[h]The only exception is pain in the teeth and other intraoral structures, which is processed partly in more rostral portions of the spinal trigeminal nucleus—the interpolar nucleus and possibly the oral nucleus as well.

Different parts of the ipsilateral half of the face are represented systematically in different parts of the caudal spinal trigeminal nucleus (Fig. 12-20). At all levels of the spinal tract, mandibular division fibers are most posterior, ophthalmic division fibers most anterior, and maxillary division fibers in between. The primary afferents retain this arrangement as they terminate in the medially adjacent spinal nucleus, so that neurons in anterior parts of the caudal nucleus, for example, respond to areas of the face in the ophthalmic distribution. Some pain fibers from all three divisions of the trigeminal nerve reach the upper cervical spinal cord, but most end at various levels in the caudal medulla. There is a somatotopic arrangement in this rostral-caudal distribution of endings as well, so that in each trigeminal division pain fibers representing areas near the center of the face end near the obex, whereas fibers representing areas toward the back of the head end in the upper cervical cord. This seemingly peculiar arrangement makes sense, because it allows for a smooth transition from spinal levels processing cutaneous information from the back of the head to brainstem levels processing similar cutaneous information from the face. That is, the trigeminal fibers ending in the cervical cord wind up overlapping spinal fibers that represent adjacent areas of skin (see Fig. 12-14). This gives rise to a characteristic pattern of sensory loss, sometimes referred to clinically as an **onion-skin distribution,** when the spinal

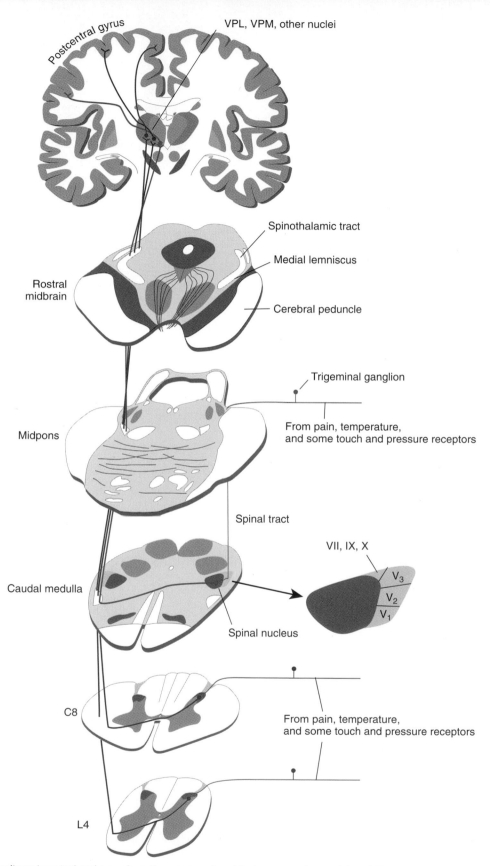

Figure 12-18 Ascending trigeminal pathways from the spinal nucleus. The inset near the caudal medulla section indicates the arrangement within the spinal trigeminal tract of fibers from the three subdivisions of the trigeminal nerve, as well as those from cranial nerves VII, IX, and X that innervate the outer ear and some mucous membranes of the head and neck. (Trigeminal pain information, like pain information from the body, also projects to other parts of the thalamus and cortex not indicated in this figure.) VPL, ventral posterolateral nucleus; VPM, ventral posteromedial nucleus.

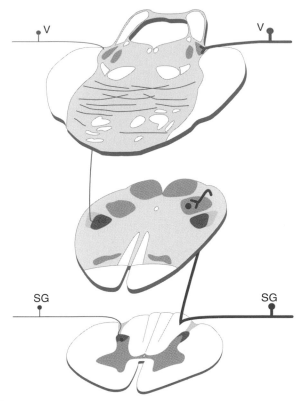

Figure 12-19 Locations of second-order neurons for pain-temperature pathways and for touch-proprioceptive pathways. (Primary afferents with cell bodies in the mesencephalic nucleus are not indicated, but they contact second-order neurons in much the same way as do large-diameter fibers with cell bodies in the trigeminal ganglion.) SG, spinal ganglion; V, trigeminal ganglion.

trigeminal tract is damaged; the farther caudally a lesion is located, the larger the area surrounding the mouth that is spared from sensory loss. Conversely, destructive lesions ascending from the spinal cord into the brainstem (such as a syrinx expanding upward from the cervical spinal cord) can cause sensory loss that starts at the back of the head and converges on the mouth (see Fig. 10-32).

Abnormalities in the trigeminal system manifest themselves clinically in a number of syndromes involving head pain. **Trigeminal neuralgia** (also called **tic douloureux**) is a prominent example. This condition is characterized by brief attacks of excruciating pain, usually less than a minute in duration, in the distribution of one (or sometimes more than one) division of the trigeminal nerve. Between attacks, there are no significant sensory abnormalities. There is frequently a "trigger zone" in the involved area, where tactile stimulation may precipitate an attack. Most cases appear to be caused by compression of the trigeminal nerve by a blood vessel or tumor, resulting in demyelination and spontaneous activity in trigeminal nerve fibers; subsequent changes in the sensory nuclei where these fibers terminate are likely to be involved as well. Trigeminal neuralgia can be

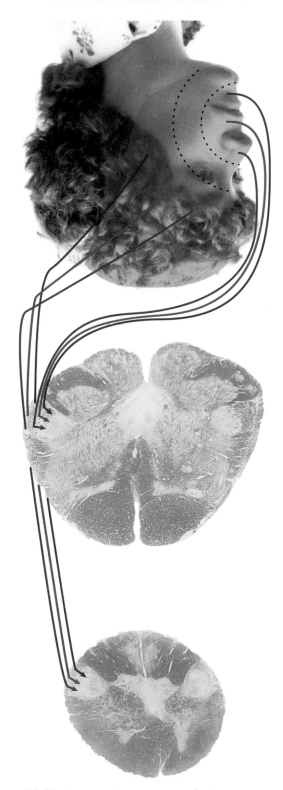

Figure 12-20 Somatotopic arrangement of pain-temperature afferents and their endings in the spinal trigeminal system.

treated pharmacologically, but a number of surgical treatments are available if necessary. These include sectioning the involved nerve root and destroying or mechanically disturbing the trigeminal ganglion. The destructive procedures have a serious disadvantage, in that the patient loses all tactile sensibility, in addition to pain, in the area. A more complex and rarely performed operation (but one that avoids this problem) is to section the spinal trigeminal tract slightly caudal to the obex, thus removing the afferent input to the caudal nucleus. Tactile sensibility remains intact, and the corneal blink reflex is usually preserved. The fact that this operation abolishes pain sensation over one entire half of the face is a major piece of evidence that the caudal part of the spinal trigeminal nucleus deals with pain and that afferents from all three divisions of the trigeminal nerve extend at least into the caudal medulla.

Remaining parts of the spinal trigeminal nucleus (the interpolar and oral nuclei) are heavily involved in the remaining functions homologous to somatic functions of the spinal cord. Some project fibers to the cerebellum (through the inferior cerebellar peduncle), and some carrying tactile information project to the contralateral VPM. These are presumably similar to spinocerebellar fibers and to the tactile component of the spinothalamic tract, respectively. There are also reflex connections within the brainstem involving the reticular formation and other cranial nerve nuclei. One of these, the corneal reflex, is of considerable clinical and practical importance and is discussed in conjunction with the facial nerve (see Fig. 12-25). The relative contributions of the three portions of the spinal nucleus to these various functions are not completely understood.

The Trigeminal Motor Nucleus Innervates Muscles of Mastication

There is also a pharyngeal motor nucleus, the **trigeminal motor nucleus,** associated with cranial nerve V. It innervates the muscles of the first pharyngeal arch, which consist mainly of the muscles of mastication (masseter, temporalis, medial and lateral pterygoid). They also include the tensor tympani, tensor palati, mylohyoid, and the anterior belly of digastric. The nucleus is located in the midpons at the level of attachment of the trigeminal nerve to the brainstem (see Fig. 12-15). Fibers arising in the trigeminal motor nucleus emerge as a separate motor root and are distributed peripherally with the mandibular division.

Trigeminal motor neurons form the efferent limb of the **jaw-jerk reflex.** Stretching the masseter, typically by a downward tap on the chin, causes it to contract (bilaterally) in a reflex fashion. This is a monosynaptic reflex basically similar to spinal stretch reflexes. The afferent limb is a mesencephalic trigeminal neuron whose peripheral process innervates a masseter muscle spindle and whose central process synapses on a trigeminal motor neuron (Fig. 12-21). The amplitude of the jaw-jerk reflex is typically minor, but, like other stretch reflexes, it is enhanced after upper motor neuron damage; this can be useful clinically in determining the longitudinal level of damage in the CNS.

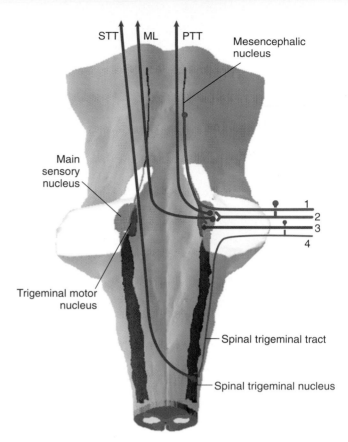

Figure 12-21 Major connections of the trigeminal nerve. 1, Peripheral branches of mesencephalic trigeminal neurons, on their way to innervate masseter spindles and other mechanoreceptors. 2, Tactile afferents. 3, Axons of trigeminal motor neurons, on their way to muscles of mastication. 4, Pain-temperature afferents. PTT, posterior trigeminothalamic tract; ML, medial lemniscus; STT, spinothalamic tract.

The Facial (VII), Glossopharyngeal (IX), and Vagus (X) Nerves All Contain Somatic and Visceral Sensory, Visceral Motor, and Pharyngeal Motor Fibers

Cranial nerves VII, IX, and X all contain fibers belonging to several different categories (Fig. 12-22), with the relative importance of each category varying. All three play a comparatively minor role in somatic sensation, whereas the vagus nerve is very important for visceral sensory and motor functions, and both the facial and vagus nerves contain large numbers of pharyngeal motor fibers.

All three nerves contain somatic sensory fibers from the skin around the ear. The somatic afferent fibers of nerves VII, IX, and X all enter the spinal trigeminal tract and thereafter behave like trigeminal afferents. They are the most posteromedial fibers in the spinal tract and occupy a position adjacent to those from the mandibular division of nerve V (see Fig. 12-18).

Nerves VII, IX, and X also contain visceral sensory fibers, some from visceral structures and some from

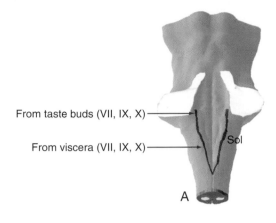

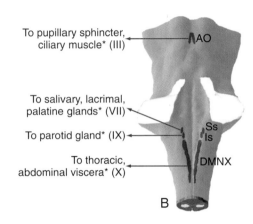

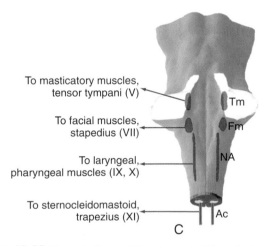

Figure 12-22 Visceral afferent **(A)**, autonomic **(B)**, and pharyngeal motor **(C)** components of cranial nerves VII, IX, X, and XI. Ac, accessory nucleus; AO, accessory oculomotor nucleus; DMNX, dorsal motor nucleus of the vagus; Fm, facial motor nucleus; Is, inferior salivary nucleus; NA, nucleus ambiguus; Sol, nucleus of the solitary tract; Ss, superior salivary nucleus; Tm, trigeminal motor nucleus. *Final destination after a synapse in a parasympathetic ganglion.

ents (the **nucleus of the solitary tract,** or the **solitary nucleus**) and looks isolated in cross section. Both tract and nucleus extend throughout the rostral medulla and into the caudal medulla and caudal pons. The nucleus of the solitary tract is the major visceral sensory nucleus of the brainstem. Its further connections related to autonomic control and to conveying taste information to places such as the cerebral cortex are discussed in Chapters 23 and 13, respectively.

The Facial Nerve (VII) Innervates Muscles of Facial Expression

Most of the fibers of the facial nerve (Figs. 12-23 and 12-24) are pharyngeal motor, innervating muscles derived from the second pharyngeal arch. These are the muscles of facial expression and the stapedius, a small muscle in the middle ear. Primarily, the nucleus of origin of all these fibers, the **facial motor nucleus,** is located in the anterolateral tegmentum of the caudal pons (see Fig. 12-6). The peculiar course of these fibers, through the internal genu of the facial nerve, is shown in Figure 12-7.

The facial motor nucleus is involved in a reflex of considerable functional and clinical importance—the **corneal blink reflex** (Fig. 12-25). If either cornea is touched by a foreign object (in testing situations, typically a wisp of cotton), both eyes automatically blink. Sensory innervation of the cornea is by way of the ophthalmic division of the trigeminal nerve—the afferent limb of the reflex. The afferents enter the spinal trigeminal tract and synapse on interneurons in the spinal trigeminal nucleus, mostly rostral to the obex. The spinal trigeminal interneurons then project bilaterally via relays in the reticular formation to motor neurons of the facial motor nucleus, which form the efferent limb. (Some corneal afferents also project to the main sensory nucleus, which then projects to the ipsilateral facial nucleus. This uncrossed component of the blink reflex is brief and relatively small, but it can be recorded electrically [see Fig. 12-25B].) Thus, by touching each cornea in turn and observing the resulting blinks, it is possible to test, in a crude fashion, the integrity of both trigeminal nerves, both facial nerves, and some of their central connections.

Other components of the facial nerve are somatic sensory fibers from the skin of the outer ear; a small collection of visceral sensory fibers that innervates parts of the nasal cavity and soft palate; visceral afferents from taste buds on the anterior two thirds of the tongue (see Chapter 13); and preganglionic parasympathetic fibers for the submandibular and sublingual salivary glands, nasal and palatine glands, and lacrimal gland. The parasympathetic fibers originate from a scattered group of cells called the **superior salivary nucleus,** located in the reticular formation near the internal genu of the facial nerve.

taste buds. The visceral sensory fibers from all three nerves enter a discrete bundle called the **solitary tract** (see Fig. 12-11). This bundle received its name as a result of its unusual appearance: it is a collection of afferents surrounded by the nucleus of termination of these affer-

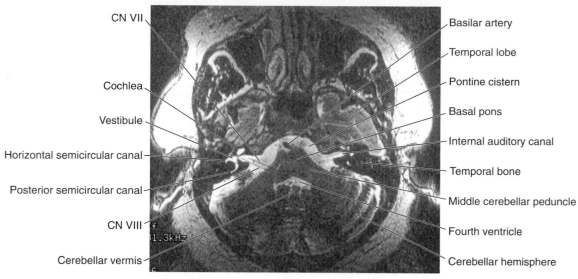

Figure 12-23 Axial (horizontal) magnetic resonance image just above the pontomedullary junction, showing the facial and vestibulocochlear nerves leaving the brainstem and entering the internal auditory canal. *(Courtesy Dr. Raymond F. Carmody, University of Arizona College of Medicine.)*

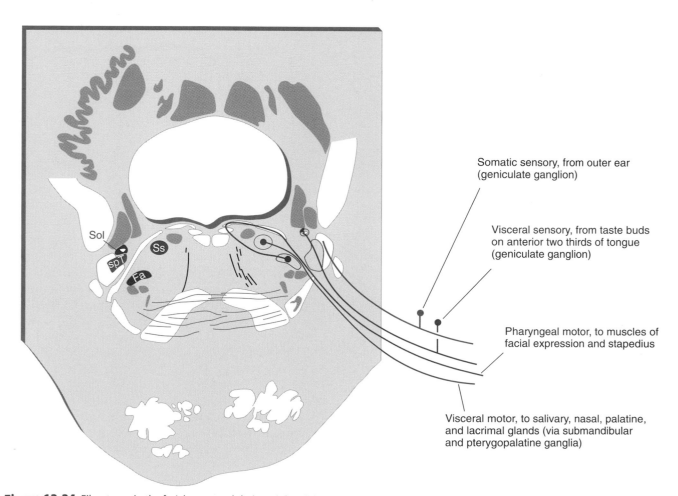

Figure 12-24 Fiber types in the facial nerve and their peripheral destinations. *Fa,* facial motor nucleus; *Sol,* nucleus of the solitary tract; *spT,* spinal trigeminal tract; *Ss,* superior salivatory nucleus.

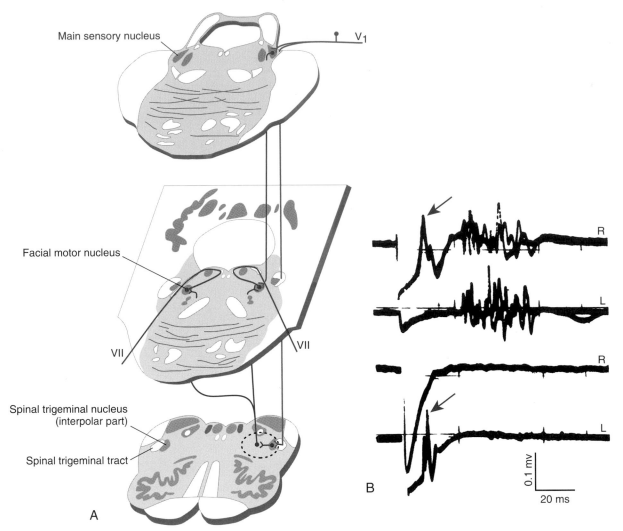

Figure 12-25 A, Connections involved in the blink reflex. **B,** Electrical activity of the orbicularis oculi during a comparable blink reflex elicited by electrical stimulation of the supraorbital nerve in a patient with an infarct in the left lateral medulla (the area outlined by a dashed line in **A**). The upper two traces show the normal responses of the right (R) and left (L) orbicularis oculi after stimulation of the right supraorbital nerve; there is a brief ipsilateral contraction *(arrow)* mediated by connections involving the main sensory nucleus, followed by a more prolonged bilateral contraction mediated by the spinal trigeminal nucleus. Stimulating the left supraorbital nerve (lower two traces) elicits a normal fast ipsilateral response *(arrow)* but no later response on either side. *(**B,** from Ongerboer de Visser BW, Kuypers HGJM: Brain 101:285, 1978.)*

Upper Motor Neuron Damage Affects the Upper and Lower Parts of the Face Differently

Pyramidal system upper motor neurons originating in the cortex of the frontal lobe supply motor nuclei of the cranial nerves, much as corticospinal fibers supply alpha motor neurons of the spinal cord. These upper motor neurons are called **corticobulbar neurons** (*bulbar* is a loosely used term referring to just the medulla in some applications and to the medulla, pons, and midbrain in others); their axons accompany the corticospinal tract until they reach the brainstem levels of the nuclei they innervate.

As described in more detail in Chapter 18, corticobulbar fibers originate in the head and face portions of the maps in the precentral gyrus and nearby areas of cortex and generally project bilaterally to the somatic and branchial (pharyngeal) motor nuclei of the cranial nerves, or to nearby areas of the reticular formation (see Fig. 18-18). This bilateral innervation corresponds to the way the muscles of both sides of the head and neck are typically used simultaneously (e.g., pharyngeal muscles during swallowing). The major exception to this pattern involves the muscles of facial expression. The lower motor neurons of each facial motor nucleus project to ipsilateral muscles, so damage to this nucleus or to the facial nerve itself causes weakness of the entire ipsilateral half of the face (see Fig. 12-10). As in the case of other cranial nerve motor nuclei, corticobulbar fibers originating from some motor cortical areas reach motor neurons for the upper part of the face bilaterally (presumably corresponding to the way we typically blink both eyes or wrinkle both sides of the forehead simultaneously). In contrast, and more like the projection of corticospinal fibers to finger motor neurons, corticobulbar projections to the motor neurons for facial muscles below the eye are predominantly crossed; this presumably corresponds to the way we can move one side of the mouth independently of the other. The consequence of this pattern is that a lesion of motor cortex or corticobulbar fibers on one side produces weakness that is most prominent in the lower facial muscles of the opposite side (Fig. 12-26). This is a clinical mainstay for distinguishing facial weakness resulting from a supranuclear lesion from that resulting from a nuclear or root lesion. Interestingly, innervation of the lower face originating in limbic cortices may remain intact, thus an individual may lose the ability to voluntarily smile, yet can still respond involuntarily to a joke with a smile. The limbic

innervation of facial musculature is more pronounced for the lower face, making movements of the mouth more responsive to emotion relative to the rest of the face.

The Glossopharyngeal Nerve (IX) Conveys Information From Intraoral Receptors

The glossopharyngeal nerve (Fig. 12-27) contains a number of visceral sensory fibers, among them afferents from the carotid body, carotid sinus, mucous membranes lining the middle ear cavity and walls of the pharynx, and mucous membranes and taste buds of the posterior third of the tongue. The extensive involvement of the glossopharyngeal nerve with intraoral sensation accounts for its name (*glossopharyngeal* is Greek for "tongue and throat"). Many of these visceral sensory fibers enter the solitary tract and synapse in the nucleus of the solitary tract. However, clinical evidence (described shortly) indicates that the fibers conveying information about pain from the pharynx and posterior part of the tongue (or at least collaterals of these fibers) enter the spinal trigeminal tract and terminate in the spinal trigeminal nucleus. The same may be true of those fibers subserving tactile and temperature sensations; in addition, glossopharyngeal afferents probably reach the part of the main sensory nucleus concerned with intraoral sensation. This fits with common experience: even though the pharynx is technically a visceral structure, it "feels" like a somatic structure because of the way we can localize and discriminate stimuli applied there. Thus

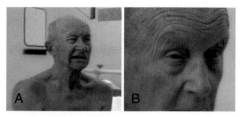

Figure 12-26 Selective weakness of lower facial muscles after corticobulbar damage. This patient suffered a stroke that resulted in weakness of his left hand (not shown) and the left side of his face. When he tried to bare his teeth **(A)**, weakness of left lower facial muscles was apparent. However, he could raise his eyebrows symmetrically **(B)**.

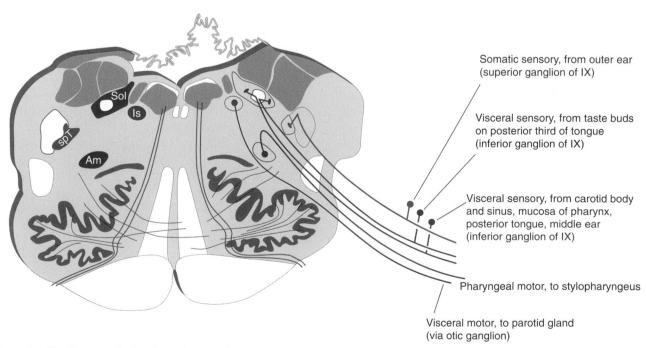

Somatic sensory, from outer ear
(superior ganglion of IX)

Visceral sensory, from taste buds
on posterior third of tongue
(inferior ganglion of IX)

Visceral sensory, from carotid body
and sinus, mucosa of pharynx,
posterior tongue, middle ear
(inferior ganglion of IX)

Pharyngeal motor, to stylopharyngeus

Visceral motor, to parotid gland
(via otic ganglion)

Figure 12-27 Fiber types in the glossopharyngeal nerve and their peripheral destinations. Am, nucleus ambiguus; Is, inferior salivary nucleus; Sol, nucleus of the solitary tract; spT, spinal trigeminal nucleus.

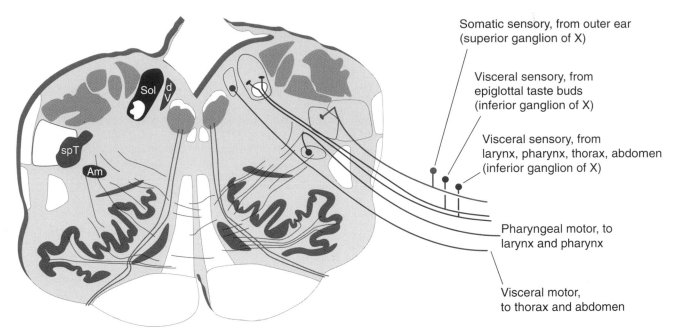

Somatic sensory, from outer ear
(superior ganglion of X)

Visceral sensory, from
epiglottal taste buds
(inferior ganglion of X)

Visceral sensory, from
larynx, pharynx, thorax, abdomen
(inferior ganglion of X)

Pharyngeal motor, to
larynx and pharynx

Visceral motor,
to thorax and abdomen

Figure 12-28 Fiber types in the vagus nerve and their peripheral destinations. Am, nucleus ambiguus; dV, dorsal motor nucleus of the vagus; Sol, nucleus of the solitary tract; spT, spinal trigeminal nucleus.

it is not surprising that the afferents involved should enter the trigeminal system.

Other components of the glossopharyngeal nerve are somatic sensory fibers from the middle ear cavity; a small group of preganglionic parasympathetic fibers for the parotid gland, arising from scattered cells in the reticular formation of the rostral medulla collectively called the **inferior salivary nucleus;** and pharyngeal motor fibers for the stylopharyngeus, a small muscle that helps elevate the pharynx during swallowing and speaking. The latter efferents, together with vagal motor neurons for the other laryngeal and pharyngeal muscles, arise from cells in the aptly named **nucleus ambiguus.** This nucleus is located in the anterolateral medullary tegmentum just posterior to and roughly coextensive with the inferior olivary nucleus (see Fig. 12-27), but its cells are scattered to the extent that it is difficult to distinguish in myelin-stained sections.

Glossopharyngeal neuralgia is similar in many ways to trigeminal neuralgia; it is rare but particularly distressing. The attacks of pain usually begin in the posterior tongue or the walls of the pharynx and radiate to the vicinity of the ear. One reason this condition is so distressing is that the trigger zone is often on the tongue or pharyngeal wall, and attacks may be set off by simply swallowing or talking. Pharmacological relief is usually available, but in rare cases when it is not, the posteromedial portion of the spinal trigeminal tract can be transected in the caudal medulla (see Fig. 12-18, inset). The fact that this surgical procedure is effective provides evidence that the involved pain fibers (technically visceral afferents) travel in the spinal trigeminal tract.

The Vagus Nerve (X) Is the Principal Parasympathetic Nerve

Cranial nerve X, the vagus nerve, is the most widely distributed of the cranial nerves (*vagus* is Latin for "wandering," as in vagabond—fibers of the vagus nerve wander throughout the thoracic and abdominal cavities). The vagus has components and connections similar to, partially overlapping, but more extensive than those of the glossopharyngeal nerve (compare Figs. 12-27 and 12-28). A major collection of preganglionic parasympathetic fibers travels in the vagus nerve to thoracic and abdominal viscera generally. Most of these arise in the **dorsal motor nucleus of the vagus,** which is the principal parasympathetic nucleus of the brain. It is located in the floor of the fourth ventricle, just lateral to the hypoglossal nucleus (see Fig. 12-11) and underlying an elevation in the floor of the fourth ventricle called the **vagal trigone.**

The vagus also contains a large collection of visceral sensory fibers innervating the thoracic and abdominal viscera, including pressure receptors and chemoreceptors of the aortic arch, as well as those from the taste buds of the epiglottis and soft palate. Most vagal visceral sensory fibers enter the solitary tract and terminate in caudal portions of the nucleus of the solitary tract. Some vagal afferents innervating the larynx, esophagus, and lower pharynx, like similar fibers from the glossopharyngeal nerve, are thought to enter the spinal trigeminal tract and terminate in the spinal trigeminal nucleus.

Vagal pharyngeal motor fibers arise in nucleus ambiguus and innervate most of the striated muscles of the

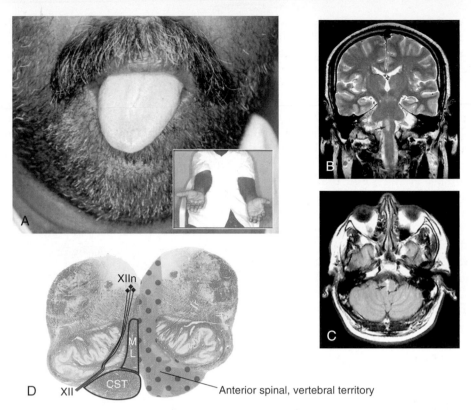

Figure 12-29 Medial medullary syndrome. In this case, "a 60 year old man . . . sought neurological consultation for sudden onset of numbness over the left side of the body." Examination revealed deficits in tactile sensation on the left side of his body and weakness of the right side of his tongue (**A**). There was slight weakness of his left arm and leg; when he held both arms outstretched, the left arm drifted downward and rotated inward (pronator drift; inset, **A**). T2-weighted magnetic resonance imaging scans in coronal (**B**) and axial (**C**) planes revealed a small infarct in the medial part of the right rostral medulla. **D,** Vascular territory involved in the medial medullary syndrome (right side of the figure), and the structures whose damage would account for the resulting symptoms and signs (left side of the figure). CST, corticospinal tract; ML, medial lemniscus; XII, hypoglossal nerve; XIIn, hypoglossal nucleus. (**A** to **C,** from Nandhagopal R, Krishnamoorthy SG, Srinivas D: J Neurol Neurosurg Psychiatry 77:215, 2006.)

larynx and pharynx. A clinically useful (though unpleasant for the patient) reflex is the **gag reflex.** Touching the wall of one side of the pharynx in a normal individual elicits a bilateral response. The afferent limb is via the glossopharyngeal nerve, whereas the efferent limb is almost entirely via the vagus. The central connections are not entirely clear and may involve the spinal trigeminal tract and nucleus, the solitary tract and nucleus, or both, in addition to nucleus ambiguus. Nevertheless the gag reflex, like the blink reflex, can be used to test two cranial nerves (in this case, IX and X) and some of their central connections.

The only other component of the vagus nerve is a small collection of somatic sensory fibers from the skin of the outer ear.

Brainstem Damage Commonly Causes Deficits on One Side of the Head and the Opposite Side of the Body

The Brown-Séquard syndrome (see Fig. 10-31), which follows hemisection of the spinal cord, demonstrates the possibility of crossed or **alternating** syndromes in which some symptoms are referred to one side of the body and others to the opposite side. In the brainstem, most pathways descending to the spinal cord are contralateral to the side on which they terminate, and most pathways ascending from the spinal cord are contralateral to the side on which they arise. However, all the exiting cranial nerves are ipsilateral to the side they innervate.[i] In addition, almost all the cranial nerve nuclei deal with ipsilateral structures (i.e., those containing second-order sensory neurons receive uncrossed primary afferents, and almost all of those containing lower motor neurons project to ipsilateral muscles). As a result, alternating syndromes, in which long-tract symptoms are referred to one side and cranial nerve symptoms to the other side, are the hallmark of brainstem lesions. For example, consider the effects of a lesion involving the medial portion of one side of the rostral medulla (Fig. 12-29),

[i]Even in unusual cases, such as efferents to the superior rectus and superior oblique, the crossing occurs within the brainstem, near the cell bodies of origin.

which could be caused by occlusion of a branch of one vertebral or anterior spinal artery. The symptoms of the resulting **medial medullary syndrome** include contralateral hemiparesis (damage to the pyramid), contralateral tactile and kinesthetic deficits (damage to the medial lemniscus), and ipsilateral paralysis with eventual atrophy of the tongue muscles (damage to the hypoglossal nucleus or exiting hypoglossal nerve). This syndrome is also referred to as **alternating hypoglossal hemiplegia.**

More lateral damage at the same brainstem level (which can be caused by occlusion of branches of one vertebral or posterior inferior cerebellar artery) results in the **lateral medullary** (or **Wallenberg's**) **syndrome** (Fig. 12-30). The damaged structures may include the spinothalamic tract, spinal trigeminal tract, nucleus ambiguus, and descending sympathetic fibers. Symptoms of such damage are loss of pain and temperature sensations over the contralateral body (with relative sparing of tactile sensation), loss of pain and temperature sensations over the ipsilateral face, hoarseness and difficulty in swallowing (as a result of paralysis of ipsilateral laryngeal and pharyngeal muscles), and ipsilateral Horner's syndrome. The inferior cerebellar peduncle and adjacent vestibular nuclei are often included in the lesion, resulting in vertigo, abnormal eye movements, and ipsilateral cerebellar deficits such as ataxia (see Fig. 14-34).

A final example involves a lesion of the cerebral peduncle on one side of the rostral midbrain (Fig. 12-31), as might result from occlusion of a penetrating branch of one posterior cerebral artery. This damages descending corticospinal fibers, causing contralateral spastic paralysis; it also damages one oculomotor nerve, causing ipsilateral ptosis, pupillary dilation, and lateral strabismus. This symptom complex is called **Weber's syndrome.** Posterior extension of the damage into the midbrain tegmentum could result in contralateral ataxia

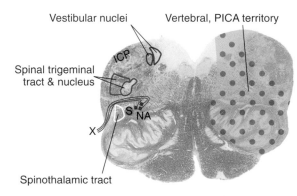

Figure 12-30 Vascular territory involved in the lateral medullary syndrome (right side of figure), and the structures whose damage would account for the resulting symptoms and signs (left side of figure). ICP, inferior cerebellar peduncle; NA, nucleus ambiguus; PICA, posterior inferior cerebellar artery; S, descending sympathetic fibers; X, vagus nerve.

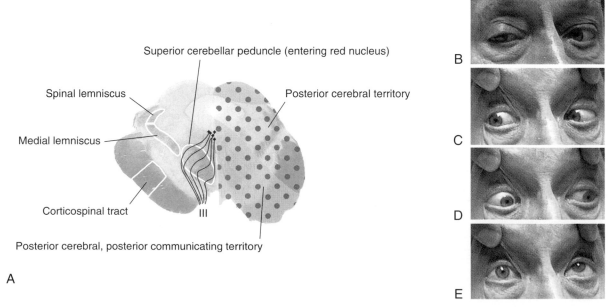

Figure 12-31 A, Vascular territory typically involved in the various midbrain syndromes (right side of figure), and the structures whose damage would account for the resulting symptoms and signs (left side of figure). **B to E,** Eye movements of a patient with vascular damage in the right rostral midbrain. At rest **(B)** he had ptosis on the right, and his eyes deviated to the right (a way to minimize the diplopia caused by a weak right medial rectus). Gaze to the right **(C)** was preserved, but during attempted gaze to the left **(D)** his right eye failed to adduct fully. Weakness of right eye muscles was also apparent when he attempted to look up **(E).** Downward gaze was better preserved, and his pupils were equal in size and reactive to light, indicating that not all the bundles of oculomotor fibers arching through the midbrain tegmentum were affected. The patient also had slight weakness of his left arm and leg, Babinski's sign on the left, and ataxia of his left arm and leg. He recovered completely over a period of about a week.

(crossed superior cerebellar peduncle) and somatosensory deficits (medial lemniscus, spinothalamic tract).

SUGGESTED READINGS

Beckstead RM, Morse JR, Norgren R: The nucleus of the solitary tract in the monkey: projections to the thalamus and brain stem nuclei. J Comp Neurol 190:259, 1980.

Beckstead RM, Norgren R: An autoradiographic examination of the central distribution of the trigeminal, facial, glossopharyngeal and vagal nerves in the monkey. J Comp Neurol 184:455, 1979.

Berthoud H-R, Neuhuber WL: Functional and chemical anatomy of the afferent vagal system. Autonom Neurosci 85:1, 2000.

Bogousslavsky J, Meienberg O: Eye-movement disorders in brainstem and cerebellar stroke. Arch Neurol 44:141, 1987.
A comprehensive review.

Brodal A: Central course of afferent fibers for pain in facial, glossopharyngeal and vagus nerves. Arch Neurol Psychiatry 57:292, 1947.

Brodal A: Neurological anatomy in relation to clinical medicine, ed 3, New York, 1981, Oxford University Press.

Gan R, Noronha A: The medullary vascular syndromes revisited. J Neurol 242:195, 1995.
A review of the medial and lateral medullary syndromes and their variants.

Gauthier JM, Mommay D, Vercher JL: Ocular muscle proprioception and visual localization of targets in man. Brain 113:1857, 1990.
The use we make of information from the proprioceptors in extraocular muscles has long been a mystery; it is not crucial for guiding eye movements. This paper presents one possibility.

Goodwin GM, Luschei ES: Effects of destroying spindle afferents from jaw muscles on mastication in monkeys. J Neurophysiol 37:967, 1974.
In summary, not much effect at all. The physiological significance of the mesencephalic nucleus remains obscure.

Hirata H, et al: A novel class of neurons at the trigeminal subnucleus interpolaris/caudalis transition region monitors ocular surface fluid status and modulates tear production. J Neurosci 24:4224, 2004.
A nice demonstration of the longitudinal distribution of functions in trigeminal sensory nuclei.

Hopkins DA, Armour JA: Brainstem cells of origin of physiologically identified cardiopulmonary nerves in the rhesus monkey (Macaca mulatta). J Auton Nerv Syst 68:21, 1998.

Huang X-F, Törk I, Paxinos G: Dorsal motor nucleus of the vagus nerve: a cyto- and chemoarchitectonic study in the human. J Comp Neurol 330:158, 1993.

Jones EG, Schwark HD, Callahan PA: Extent of the ipsilateral representation in the ventral posterior medial nucleus of the monkey thalamus. Exp Brain Res 63:310, 1986.

Kobayashi Y, Matsumura G: Central projections of primary afferent fibers from the rat trigeminal nerve labeled with isolectin B4-HRP. Neurosci Lett 217:89, 1996.
Isolectin B4 injected into the trigeminal ganglion selectively labels small-diameter primary afferents, and this study demonstrates nicely the somatotopic arrangement of their terminations in the spinal trigeminal nucleus.

Kunc Z: Treatment of essential neuralgia of the 9th nerve by selective tractotomy. J Neurosurg 23:494, 1965.
Clinical evidence regarding the location of glossopharyngeal pain fibers in the spinal trigeminal tract of humans.

Kwon J-H, et al: Isolated superior rectus palsy due to contralateral midbrain infarction. Arch Neurol 60:1633, 2003.

Lachman N, Acland RD, Rosse C: Anatomical evidence for the absence of a morphologically distinct cranial root of the accessory nerve in man. Clin Anat 15:4, 2002.

Leblanc A: Encephalo-peripheral nervous system, Berlin, 2004, Springer-Verlag.
A beautifully illustrated account of the peripheral courses of the cranial nerves and their appearance in clinical images.

Love S, Coakham HB: Trigeminal neuralgia: pathology and pathogenesis. Brain 124:2347, 2001.

Lowe AA: The neural regulation of tongue movements. Prog Neurobiol 15:295, 1980.

Manger PR, Woods TM, Jones EG: Representation of face and intra-oral structures in area 3b of macaque monkey somatosensory cortex. J Comp Neurol 371:513, 1996.

Matsumoto S, et al: A sensory level on the trunk in lower lateral brainstem lesions. Neurology 38:1515, 1988.
Clinical evidence about the course of projections from the spinal trigeminal nucleus to the thalamus.

McCrea RA, Strassman A, Highstein SM: Morphology and physiology of abducens motoneurons and internuclear neurons intracellularly injected with horseradish peroxidase in alert squirrel monkeys. J Comp Neurol 243:291, 1986.

McRitchie DA, Törk I: The internal organization of the human solitary nucleus. Brain Res Bull 31:171, 1993.

Mizuno N, Nomura S: Primary afferent fibers in the glossopharyngeal nerve terminate in the dorsal division of the principal sensory trigeminal nucleus. Neurosci Lett 66:338, 1986.

Morecraft RJ, et al: Cortical innervation of the facial nucleus in the non-human primate: a new interpretation of the effects of stroke and related subtotal brain trauma on the muscles of facial expression. Brain 124:176, 2001.

Nandhagopal R, Krishnamoorthy SG: Eight-and-a-half syndrome. J Neurol Neurosurg Psychiatry 77:463, 2006.

Nandhagopal R, Krishnamoorthy SG, Srinivas D: Medial medullary infarction. J Neurol Neurosurg Psychiatry 77:215, 2006.

Nazruddin, et al: The cells of origin of the hypoglossal afferent nerves and central projections in the cat. Brain Res 490:219, 1989.

Nurse CA: Neurotransmission and neuromodulation in the chemosensory carotid body. Autonom Neurosci 120:1, 2005.

Ohya A: Responses of trigeminal subnucleus interpolaris neurons to afferent inputs from deep oral structures. Brain Res Bull 29:773, 1992.

Olszewski J: On the anatomical and functional organization of the spinal trigeminal nucleus. J Comp Neurol 92:401, 1950.

Ongerboer de Visser BW: Afferent limb of the human jaw reflex: electrophysiologic and anatomic study. Neurology 32:563, 1982.

Porter JD: Brainstem terminations of extraocular muscle primary afferent neurons in the monkey. J Comp Neurol 247:133, 1986.

Porter JD, Guthrie BL, Sparks DL: Innervation of monkey extraocular muscles: localization of sensory and motor neurons by retrograde transport of horseradish peroxidase. J Comp Neurol 218:208, 1983.

Proctor GB, Carpenter GH: Regulation of salivary gland function by autonomic nerves. Autonom Neurosci 133:3, 2007.

Rokx JTM, Jüch PJW, van Willigen JD: Arrangements and connections of mesencephalic trigeminal neurons in the rat. Acta Anat 127:7, 1986.

Rushton JG, Stevens JC, Miller RH: Glossopharyngeal (vago-glossopharyngeal) neuralgia: a study of 217 cases. Arch Neurol 38:201, 1981.

Smith RL: Axonal projections and connections of the principal sensory trigeminal nucleus in the monkey. J Comp Neurol 163:347, 1975.

Steindler DA: Trigeminocerebellar, trigeminotectal and trigeminothalamic projections: a double retrograde axonal tracing study in the mouse. J Comp Neurol 237:155, 1985.

Stewart WA, King RB: Fiber projections from the nucleus caudalis of the spinal trigeminal nucleus. J Comp Neurol 121:271, 1963.

Strassman AM, Potrebic S, Maciewicz RJ: Anatomical properties of brainstem trigeminal neurons that respond to electrical stimulation of dural blood vessels. J Comp Neurol 346:349, 1994.

A possible explanation of the pattern of referred pain in response to dural irritation.

Tamai Y, Iwamoto M, Tsujimoto T: Pathway of the blink reflex in the brainstem of the cat: interneurons between the trigeminal nuclei and the facial nucleus. Brain Res 380:19, 1986.

Torvik A: The ascending fibers from the main trigeminal sensory nucleus. Am J Anat 100:1, 1957.

Waite PME, Ashwell KWS: Trigeminal sensory system. In Paxinos G, Mai JK, editors: The human nervous system, ed 2, San Diego, 2004, Elsevier Academic Press.

Walker AE: The origin, course and terminations of the secondary pathways of the trigeminal nerve in primates. J Comp Neurol 71:59, 1939.

Wall M, Wray SH: The one-and-a-half syndrome—a unilateral disorder of the pontine tegmentum: a study of 20 cases and review of the literature. Neurology 33:971, 1983.

Young RF: Effect of trigeminal tractotomy on dental sensation in humans. J Neurosurg 56:812, 1982.

Tractotomy near the obex causes facial analgesia but no change in dental pain.

Young RF, Perryman KM: Neuronal responses in rostral trigeminal brain-stem nuclei of macaque monkeys after chronic trigeminal tractotomy. J Neurosurg 65:508, 1986.

Evidence that dental pain is processed rostral to the obex, and facial pain caudal to the obex, in the spinal trigeminal nucleus.

Younge BR: Analysis of trochlear nerve palsies: diagnosis, etiology and treatment. Mayo Clin Proc 52:11, 1977.

Zee DS: The organization of the brainstem ocular motor subnuclei. Ann Neurol 4:384, 1978.

Speculation on why the motor axons to the superior oblique and superior rectus cross.

The Chemical Senses of Taste and Smell

13

Dating back to their origins in some primordial sea, living cells have shared an ability to respond to chemicals, at a minimum detecting and absorbing nutrients. Neurons detect chemicals at synapses, but some cells in or closely associated with the nervous system go beyond this, specializing in the detection of certain classes of chemicals adjacent to their membranes and using this information to affect autonomic function, behavior, or perception. These cells fall into four general categories[a]: (1) the myriad visceral chemoreceptors that work in the background, mostly inaccessible to conscious awareness, keeping track of the concentrations of oxygen, glucose, neuroactive hormones, and other substances; (2) **gustatory receptor cells,** or **taste receptor cells,** that mediate the sense of taste; (3) **olfactory receptor neurons** that mediate the sense of smell; and (4) chemosensitive endings, such as some trigeminal endings in mucous membranes, that mediate what has been termed the **common chemical sense**—sensations such as the heat of chili peppers, the sting of ammonia, or the coolness of menthol. The visceral chemoreceptors monitor internal chemical composition, and the other three monitor external chemistry, whether of local air or of substances being considered for ingestion.

---

[a]Most animals have a fifth category—pheromone receptors—but, as discussed in Box 13-1, the role of this system in humans is reduced and is not well understood.

Taste, smell, and the common chemical sense, like all the other senses of which we are consciously aware, have both rewarding and warning functions. In this case, the chemical senses are the basis not only of the enjoyment of a meal or a glass of wine but also of the detection of things such as spoiled food or smoke from a fire.

The Perception of Flavor Involves Gustatory, Olfactory, Trigeminal, and Other Inputs

The term *taste* as used in this book is synonymous with the **gustatory** sense, the set of sensations engendered by stimulating taste buds. We commonly assume that this is the same thing as the total sensation we perceive when eating or drinking, but such integrated sensations of **flavor** are actually the result of the combination of at least three different kinds of input: (1) direct chemical stimulation of taste buds, (2) stimulation of olfactory receptors by vapors from food (see Fig. 13-8), and (3) stimulation of chemical-sensitive and somatosensory free nerve endings of the trigeminal and other nerves in the mucous membranes of the oral and nasal cavities. The latter sets of endings respond to qualities such as the pungency, spiciness, temperature, and texture of food. We have difficulty appreciating the subtleties of foods and beverages using just our taste buds, and people with deficits in their sense of olfaction complain that things "taste" bland.

Although gustation, olfaction, and the common chemical sense are emphasized in this chapter, the full perception of flavor with all its nuances requires the integration of multiple inputs. Somatosensory aspects of flavor perception, for example, are more important than we usually realize. Some things "taste" better hot; others taste better cold. Some foods are designed to be chewy (e.g., some candies); others are expected to be tender or crunchy.[b] Vision also comes into play; the appearance of food affects not just our anticipation of it but also its palatability. Even the visceral chemoreceptors of which we are usually unaware come into play, as in the common experience of something tasting much better when one is really hungry. The **orbital cortex** of the frontal lobe is a major site where these multiple factors are combined (see Fig. 13-21), giving the overall sensation about food and drink.

Taste Is Mediated by Receptors in Taste Buds Innervated by Cranial Nerves VII, IX, and X

Despite the somewhat limited role played by the sense of taste in the perception of flavor, receptor cells in the

[b]My favorite example of the importance of texture is raw oysters, which some find appealing and others find appalling.

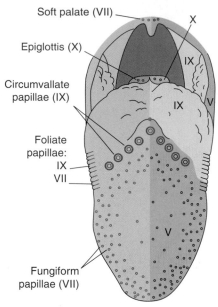

Figure 13-1 Distribution and innervation of taste buds (left), and innervation of the epithelium of the oral cavity (right). The trigeminal nerve (V) subserves general sensation (and the common chemical sense) from the anterior two thirds of the tongue, and the glossopharyngeal nerve (IX) has a similar function for the posterior third of the tongue. The innervation of the soft palate is indicated as being trigeminal, but it also receives a contribution from the facial nerve. Similarly, the innervation of the oropharynx is indicated as being glossopharyngeal, but it also receives a contribution from the vagus nerve.

taste buds of the oral cavity encode some basic aspects of the probable nutritional value of food.

The Tongue Is Covered by a Series of Papillae, Some of Which Contain Taste Buds

The tongue is mostly muscle, but its surface is covered by a series of bumps and folds called **papillae** (Fig. 13-1). Most are small conical projections called filiform papillae not involved in taste but in the movement of food in the mouth. However, **fungiform, foliate,** and **circumvallate** papillae contain taste buds (Fig. 13-2). About 200 to 300 fungiform ("mushroom-shaped") papillae are scattered across the surface of the anterior two thirds of the tongue, concentrated on the tip and sides. Typical fungiform papillae contain three to five taste buds. Foliate ("leaflike") papillae are the most posterior of a series of about 20 folds on the sides of the posterior tongue; each has 100 to 150 taste buds in its walls. Finally, a series of eight to nine circumvallate ("surrounded by a wall") or **vallate** papillae are arranged in a V-shaped line two thirds of the way back along the dorsal surface of the tongue. Each circumvallate papilla is surrounded by a deep groove in the lingual epithelium (see Fig. 13-2A), with about 250 taste buds located in the walls of the groove. Hence, even though the circumvallate papillae are few in number, they contain nearly half of the 5000 taste buds found on an average tongue.

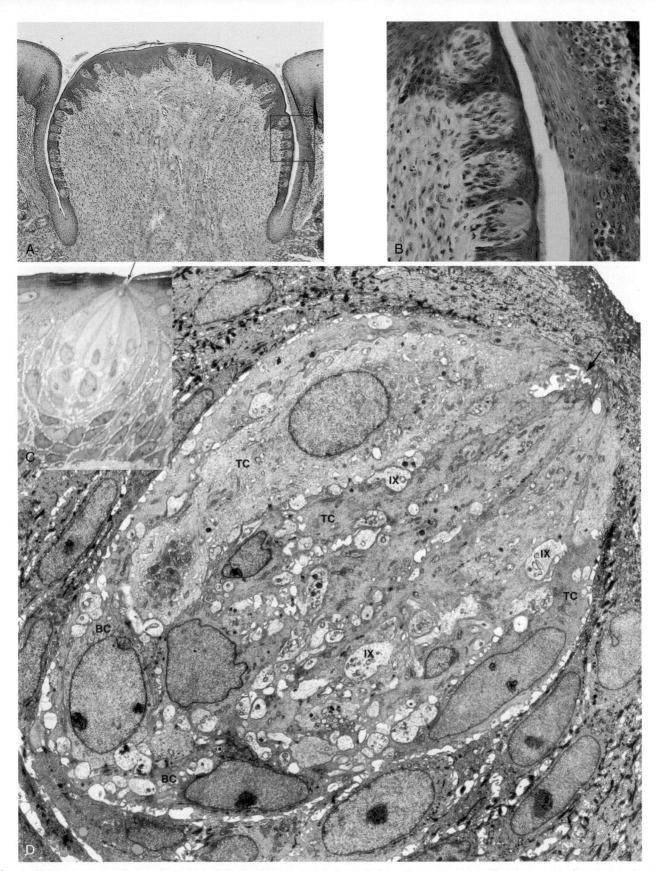

Figure 13-2 Morphology of taste buds. **A,** Section of a single circumvallate papilla from the tongue of a cat. **B,** Enlargement of the area outlined in **A.** Individual taste buds *(arrows)* can be seen just beneath the surface of the papilla. **C,** Light micrograph of a section through the center of a single taste bud from a human fungiform papilla, showing the taste pore *(arrow).* **D,** Electron micrograph of a taste bud from a human circumvallate papilla. The section is not quite through the middle of the taste bud, but the arrow indicates the apex where the taste pore would open in a nearby section. The principal cellular elements are taste cells (TC) of various categories and basal cells (BC). Discrete synapses of the receptor cells onto afferent fibers cannot be seen easily in this micrograph, but numerous glossopharyngeal nerve processes (IX) are apparent. *(**A** and **B,** courtesy Dr. Nathaniel T. McMullen, University of Arizona College of Medicine. **C** and **D,** courtesy Pamela Eller, University of Colorado Health Sciences Center.)*

Although an "average" tongue contains about 5000 taste buds, the numbers of both papillae and taste buds are surprisingly variable. For example, among normal, healthy individuals, some have as many as 100 times more taste buds in their fungiform papillae than others do. This is presumably the basis of the 100-fold variation in threshold concentration for various substances among normal individuals.

Taste buds are usually associated with the tongue, but they are also distributed widely, although in smaller numbers, over the palate and pharynx.[c] The pharyngeal and palatal taste buds are probably more important for swallowing and for reflex responses to good or bad tastes than for conscious awareness of taste.

Taste Receptor Cells Are Modified Epithelial Cells With Neuron-Like Properties

Each taste bud is an ovoid structure containing about 100 spindle-shaped epithelial cells modified as **taste cells.** Some of these are supporting cells with glial properties, and the rest are taste receptor cells (see Fig. 13-2B to D). Taste receptor cells have microvillar processes that extend through a small opening, the **taste pore,** where they are exposed to chemical stimuli. At the deep end of the taste bud, the receptor cells communicate with visceral sensory fibers from the facial, glossopharyngeal, and vagal nerves (Fig. 13-3). Some make typical chemical synapses, releasing adenosine triphosphate (ATP) and probably other transmitters onto these afferent endings; others use a less conventional communication method, releasing ATP directly into extracellular space, where it diffuses to the same afferent endings. Fibers from the facial nerve innervate the taste buds of fungiform and anterior foliate papillae and the palate; fibers from the glossopharyngeal nerve innervate those of circumvallate and most foliate papillae and the pharynx; a few vagal fibers innervate those of the epiglottis and esophagus (Fig. 13-4).

Taste receptor cells differentiate from the surrounding lingual epithelium and subsequently depend on chemical interactions with the gustatory nerves for their continued existence; denervation of an area of tongue causes degeneration of its taste buds. Despite their epithelial origin, taste receptor cells have some very neuron-like properties: they contain transduction machinery in their apical membranes and produce receptor potentials in response to appropriate taste stimuli. Some make typical chemical synapses on the peripheral

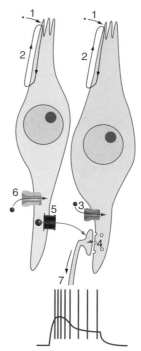

Figure 13-3 Communication from taste receptor cells to peripheral endings of facial, glossopharyngeal, and vagal nerve fibers. Tastant molecules activate the transduction machinery in the apical microvilli of taste receptor cells (1) and cause the production of depolarizing receptor potentials (2). In some receptor cells, this depolarization causes entry of Ca^{2+} through voltage-gated Ca^{2+} channels (3), release of adenosine triphosphate (ATP) onto a peripheral nerve ending (4), and increased firing of the nerve fiber (7). In others, depolarization causes the direct release of ATP onto nearby nerve endings through a Ca^{2+}-independent mechanism in which gap junction channels, instead of forming a connection with another cell, connect to extracellular space and allow ATP to spill out (5). Large depolarizations are required to open these channels, and voltage-gated Na^+ channels (6) apparently provide the needed amplification of the receptor potential.

endings of gustatory nerves, and others produce action potentials when sufficiently depolarized by a receptor potential.[d] However, unlike almost all neurons, taste receptor cells have a limited life span. Each lives only a week or two before being replaced by differentiation of **basal cells,** which migrate in from the surrounding epithelium and wait, as their name implies, near the base of the taste bud.

Taste Receptor Cells Utilize a Variety of Transduction Mechanisms to Detect Sweet, Salty, Sour, and Bitter Stimuli

The four basic taste qualities traditionally recognized are sweet, salty, sour, and bitter, but there are others. For

---

[c]Different species of animals often adapt to their environments by utilizing elaborate configurations of the same receptor cells used by other species. An example is the star-nosed mole (see Box 9-1). Taste buds provide another example: fish have taste buds on the external surface of their bodies, allowing them to "taste" the water through which they swim. A single channel catfish may have 100,000 external taste buds—20 times as many as an entire human tongue.

[d]The role of these action potentials was a puzzle for a long time, because taste receptor cells are small enough for receptor potentials to spread electrotonically to their sites of communication with nerve endings. It is now thought that this large voltage change is required to open gap junction hemichannels and allow ATP to escape (see Fig. 13-3).

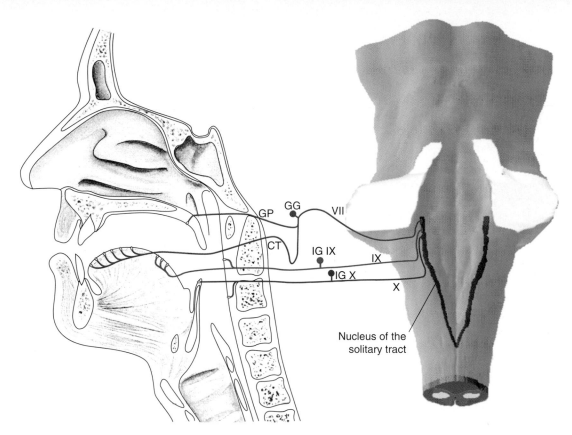

Figure 13-4 Innervation of taste buds in different parts of the oral cavity by the facial (VII), glossopharyngeal (IX), and vagus (X) nerves. The central processes of all three terminate in rostral parts of the nucleus of the solitary tract. CT, chorda tympani nerve; GG, geniculate ganglion; GP, greater petrosal nerve; IG IX, inferior ganglion of the glossopharyngeal nerve (petrosal ganglion); IG X, inferior ganglion of the vagus nerve (nodose ganglion). *(Drawing of hemisected head, modified from Parker CA: A guide to diseases of the nose and throat and their treatment, New York, 1906, Longmans, Green.)*

example, the flavor-enhancing effect of glutamate (as in monosodium glutamate, or MSG) is a separate taste in its own right. This taste is often referred to as *umami,* which is Japanese for "delicious," and it is based on taste receptor cells specifically sensitive to glutamate. Other receptor cells may be selectively sensitive to fats and other components of **tastants.** Although some areas of the tongue are somewhat more sensitive to certain taste qualities—the tip to sweet, the sides to salt and sour, and posterior portions to bitter—all parts of the tongue are sensitive to all kinds of tastants. Corresponding to these multiple taste qualities, taste receptor cells utilize multiple methods to transduce chemical stimuli into electrical signals (Fig. 13-5). Some are epithelial mechanisms adapted for use in taste transduction, and others are familiar ligand-gated or G protein–coupled mechanisms. Transduction processes include the following:

1. The transduction process for sodium chloride (NaCl), the prototypical salty stimulus, is ultimately simple. No receptor molecules are involved: cation channels in the apical membranes of taste receptor cells allow inward movement of Na^+ ions, depolarizing the cell (see Fig. 13-5A). Some of these channels are selective for Na^+, reflecting the dietary importance of NaCl;

others are nonselective, accounting for the salty taste of compounds such as potassium chloride (KCl).

2. Acids taste sour, but not in a way that is related in a simple way to the pH of saliva. Weak organic acids (e.g., acetic acid in vinegar) taste more sour than a hydrochloric acid (HCl) solution of the same pH. Corresponding to this, there are at least two different transduction mechanisms for acidic solutes (see Fig. 13-5B). Weak organic acids diffuse across the receptor cell apical membrane, dissociate, acidify the cytoplasm, and initiate the opening of cation channels. Stronger acids depolarize receptor cells by acting as the ligand that opens pH-sensitive cation channels.

3. Sweet compounds and glutamate, in contrast, bind to G protein–coupled receptor molecules that, through a second messenger cascade, cause cation channels to open in other parts of the cell (see Fig. 13-5C).

4. Bitter tastes, typical of many toxic substances, serve a protective function and are usually avoided by humans and other animals.[e] Bitter-sensitive taste

---

[e]Although many people learn to enjoy the bitterness of things such as the caffeine in coffee, the quinine in tonic water, and the hops in beer.

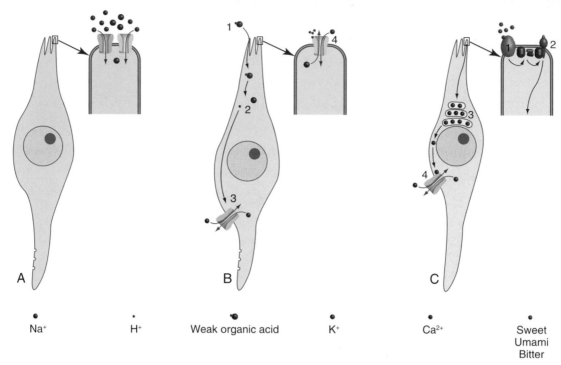

Na⁺ H⁺ Weak organic acid K⁺ Ca²⁺ Sweet Umami Bitter

Figure 13-5 Transduction mechanisms used by taste receptor cells. **A,** Increased extracellular Na⁺ concentration moves the Na⁺ equilibrium potential in a positive direction, and Na⁺ ions (salty taste) flow directly through open Na⁺ channels; increased extracellular concentrations of other cations also cause depolarization via open nonselective cation channels. **B,** Weak organic acids (sour taste) diffuse across receptor cell membranes in an undissociated state (1), then acidify the cytoplasm (2). Intracellular acidity causes cation channels to open (3). The extracellular protons from stronger acids cause pH-sensitive cation channels to open (4). **C,** The transduction process for sweet and bitter substances and glutamate (umami) is more convoluted. All bind to different G protein–coupled receptors (1) on different taste receptor cells. Dissociation of the G protein from one of these receptors activates an enzyme, phospholipase Cβ2 (2), whose products (inositol trisphosphate and diacylglycerol) lead to the release of Ca²⁺ from internal stores (3) and the opening of Ca²⁺-gated cation channels (4).

receptor cells use another set of about 30 different G protein–coupled receptors, allowing them to be depolarized by a broad range of chemicals. Using the same second messenger cascade as sweet- and umami-sensitive receptors, they too release ATP onto afferent endings (see Figs. 13-3 and 13-5C).

Second-Order Gustatory Neurons Are Located in the Nucleus of the Solitary Tract

Chemosensory information reaches consciousness as the perception of flavor, but in its role in autonomic responses and the acquisition of food, it has much closer ties to the hypothalamus and limbic system than do other senses. The second-order neurons that mediate the involvement of taste in all these connections are located in the nucleus of the solitary tract (see Fig. 12-11). The nucleus of the solitary tract, the principal visceral sensory nucleus of the brainstem, receives (via the solitary tract) gustatory afferents as well as the other visceral sensory fibers mentioned in Chapters 12 and 23. However, the gustatory fibers and chemosensitive trigeminal fibers end separately in lateral and rostral portions of the solitary nucleus (see Fig. 13-4).

Second-order taste fibers do two things (Fig. 13-6). Some participate in reflex activities, such as salivation, swallowing,[f] and coughing, by way of cranial nerve motor nuclei. Others, like fibers in most sensory systems, project to the cerebral cortex by way of the thalamus. In this case, however, the projection is uncrossed. Fibers travel through the ipsilateral central tegmental tract to the most medial part of the ventral posteromedial (VPM) nucleus, where they end adjacent to the uncrossed fibers of the dorsal trigeminal tract (see Fig. 12-16). This medial part of VPM then projects to gustatory cortex, which is located in the insula and the medial surface of the frontal operculum, near the base of the central sulcus. Gustatory cortex projects in turn to orbital cortex of the frontal lobe (see Fig. 13-21), where taste information is integrated with olfactory and other information, and to the amygdala, through which taste information reaches the hypothalamus and the limbic system. (In most mammals,

---

[f]Swallowing usually is not thought of as a reflex activity, but its success depends greatly on sensory input from the oral cavity. For example, try to swallow multiple times in succession, as rapidly as you can, with an empty mouth. Compare this maximum rate to the rate that can be achieved when drinking a beverage.

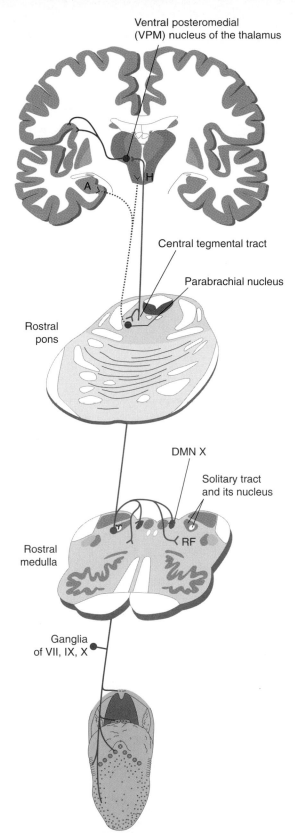

Ventral posteromedial (VPM) nucleus of the thalamus

Central tegmental tract

Parabrachial nucleus

Rostral pons

DMN X

Solitary tract and its nucleus

Rostral medulla

RF

Ganglia of VII, IX, X

Figure 13-6 Taste pathways in the CNS. Second-order neurons feed into reflexes both by direct projections (e.g., to the nearby dorsal motor nucleus of the vagus [DMN X]) and by connections with the reticular formation (RF). The projection from the parabrachial nucleus to the hypothalamus (H) and amygdala (A) is dashed because, although it is present in most mammals, its existence in primates is doubtful.

taste information reaches the hypothalamus and amygdala more directly, through a projection from the parabrachial nuclei[g] of the pontine reticular formation, which also distribute nociceptive information and information from visceral structures. The gustatory portion of this set of functions appears to have been lost in primates.)

Information About Taste Is Coded, in Part, by the Pattern of Activity in Populations of Neurons

Sensory systems such as somatic sensation and vision depend on the receipt of information about specific aspects of a stimulus, highly organized in space and time (see Figs. 3-30, 10-20, and 17-35). Activity in many of the neurons in these systems signals the occurrence of a particular kind of event—particularly its location, as is evident in the detailed topographic maps in places such as somatosensory, visual, and motor cortex (see Figs. 3-30 and 17-29). In contrast, the nervous system also uses combinations of inputs to interpret stimuli, as in the case of Ruffini endings that are involved in the sense of touch but produce no sensation when stimulated in isolation (see Chapter 9). Taste and olfaction also utilize this combinatorial type of processing. Taste stimuli are widely dispersed in the mouth during chewing, and odorants fill the nose during breathing, so spatial localization is less important and we actually use the *touching* of the tongue by a piece of food to localize it (see Box 9-2). Instead, the gustatory and olfactory systems together are faced with the task of coding the identities of many thousands of different chemicals, both singly and in mixtures. In principle, this could be accomplished by having many thousands of different receptor types, each particularly sensitive to one chemical ("labeled-line" coding). An alternative strategy is to code the identity of a stimulus in terms of the pattern of activity in a large population of neurons with multiple sensitivities ("across-fiber" coding). Although this might seem like a cumbersome way to do things, it is actually an efficient system for encoding information about a large variety of potential stimuli using a relatively small number of neurons, similar in principle to using just three kinds of cones as the basis for perceiving hundreds of hues (see Chapter 17).

The gustatory system uses a combination of labeled-line and across-fiber coding; the relative importance of the two strategies is still debated. Taste receptor cells apparently contain in their apical membranes only one of the transduction mechanisms shown in Figure 13-5, but at every subsequent level of the gustatory system individual cells respond to more than one kind of tastant.

[g]So called because they partially surround the superior cerebellar peduncle (brachium conjunctivum) as it traverses the rostral pons (see Fig. 23-11B).

Gustatory nerve fibers branch and innervate multiple taste buds that may even be located in multiple papillae, and ATP released by an assortment of taste receptor cells reaches each afferent ending. As a result, each responds to more than one tastant, although one kind of sensitivity usually predominates for any given nerve fiber. This "tuning" corresponds to the relative sensitivities of different areas of the tongue: most facial nerve (chorda tympani) fibers are maximally sensitive to sweet or salty stimuli, and most glossopharyngeal fibers to sour or bitter stimuli. Second-order neurons in the nucleus of the solitary tract are more broadly tuned (Fig. 13-7A), although there is still some selectivity. By the time gustatory information reaches higher cortical levels, specific features of a taste stimulus have been extracted, and neurons with particular chemical sensitivities are found (see Fig. 13-7B).

Olfaction Is Mediated by Receptors That Project Directly to the Telencephalon

The other principal player in conscious chemical sensation, the olfactory system, is specialized to detect volatile chemicals or **odorants** drawn into the nasal cavity (Fig. 13-8). Odorants arriving during breathing or sniffing feel subjectively like samples of the outside world, whereas those wafting into it from the oropharynx during eating are referred to the mouth and contribute to the flavor of whatever is being eaten. Although the olfactory sense is relatively less important for visually oriented species like humans than for many other animals, it has very impressive capabilities nonetheless. Humans are able to distinguish thousands of different odors—for trained sniffers, perhaps as many as 10,000 or more—some at remarkably low concentrations. Most mammals, and many other animals as well, also have another set of specialized chemoreceptors to detect specific chemicals produced by other members of their species. However, the **vomeronasal organ** of adult humans is rudimentary; any remaining chemical communication by **pheromones** (Box 13-1) in humans is probably mediated by olfactory receptors.

The Axons of Olfactory Receptor Neurons Form Cranial Nerve I

The olfactory system begins peripherally with the **olfactory epithelium,** a pigmented, yellowish patch of cells that occupies about 1 to 2 cm² of the roof and adjacent walls of the nasal cavity on each side. Each patch of olfactory epithelium consists of about 3 million receptor cells interspersed with supporting cells and the ducts of small glands (called **Bowman's glands**). Sensory endings of trigeminal nerve fibers are also found in the olfactory epithelium. The trigeminal endings are

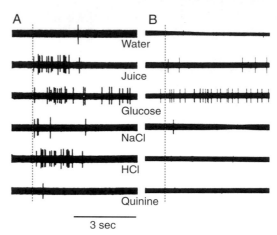

Figure 13-7 Responses of single gustatory neurons in the nucleus of the solitary tract (**A**) and the orbital cortex (**B**) of monkeys to tastants applied at the time indicated by the vertical dashed lines. The brainstem neuron responds to multiple tastants (but not all of them), whereas the cortical neuron is more selective. (**A,** from Scott TR et al: J Neurophysiol 55:182, 1986. **B,** from Rolls ET, Yaxley S, Sienkiewicz ZJ: J Neurophysiol 64:1055, 1990.)

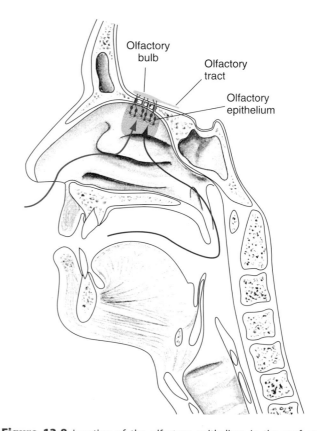

Figure 13-8 Location of the olfactory epithelium in the roof and lateral wall of the nasal cavity. The olfactory epithelium continues across the roof of the cavity into a patch of similar size on the nasal septum. Odorants can reach this epithelium either through the nostrils (orthonasally) or by way of the oropharynx (retronasally). (Modified from Parker CA: A guide to diseases of the nose and throat and their treatment, New York, 1906, Longmans, Green.)

BOX 13-1

Communication by Pheromones in Humans?

We usually think of communication between individuals in terms of signals detected by the visual, auditory, and somatosensory systems, but animals also use chemicals to communicate with one another. Some of these signals are clearly olfactory and more or less obvious—ants laying down trails of formic acid for other ants to follow, or a skunk warning a potential predator—but others are more subtle and may produce no conscious sensation. Rather, they work by inducing an "urge" to do something or a "mood" conducive to some kind of behavior. In contrast to hormones, which are chemicals produced by an animal that have effects on the tissues and organs of that animal at very low concentrations, pheromones (Greek for "to transfer stimulation") are chemicals produced by an animal that have specific effects on other individuals of the same species, also at very low concentrations. The first pheromone identified was a long-chain alcohol called *bombykol,* a sex attractant produced by female moths that can be detected by males at the extraordinarily low level of 1 part in 10^{17}. Male moths use this sensitivity to fly long distances up bombykol concentration gradients, anticipating that they may encounter a female moth.

Communication by pheromones is widespread among animals, including mammals, and often centers around reproductive behaviors. Pheromones in the urine of male rodents, for example, affect the onset of puberty in females, the timing of estrous cycles, and even the likelihood of implantation of fertilized ova; the vaginal secretions of female rodents stimulate the mating behavior of males. Some behavioral responses to chemical messages are mediated by the olfactory system, but in terrestrial vertebrates, many of the receptors for pheromones are located in the tubular vomeronasal organ, named for its location beneath the surface of the cartilaginous part of the nasal septum (one on each side) near the vomer (see Fig. 13-9). Pheromones enter the vomeronasal organ through an aperture at the surface of the nasal septum and reach receptor neurons in the walls of the organ. Vomeronasal receptors, like olfactory receptors, are bipolar neurons with a chemosensitive

dendrite and a long, thin axon. However, they differ in having chemosensitive microvilli (rather than cilia) at the luminal surface of the vomeronasal organ and in using an entirely different set of G protein–coupled receptor molecules. The axons of vomeronasal receptors form the vomeronasal nerve, which projects to the accessory olfactory bulb, a distinctive area on the dorsomedial surface of the main olfactory bulb. The accessory olfactory bulb projects not to the olfactory targets indicated in Figure 13-17 but to a part of the amygdala closely related to the hypothalamus. Because pheromonal inputs reach limbic structures so directly, it is thought that they act at a subconscious level to influence mood and behavior.

The extent to which humans communicate by pheromones has long been a matter of debate. There have been numerous anecdotal reports (but few controlled studies) of changes in human mood or outlook allegedly induced by airborne chemical messages, undetectable consciously as odors, from other humans. There are also indications that chemicals produced by others can influence some aspects of human reproductive function. For example, early reports that the menstrual cycles of women living in the same house or dormitory room tend to become synchronized have been confirmed and analyzed in more detail: axillary secretions collected from women, though seemingly odorless, can lengthen or shorten the menstrual cycles of other women, depending on the phase of the cycle during which the secretions are collected. Not surprisingly, there is considerable commercial interest in substances that can be added to cosmetics or fragrances to influence perceived sexual attractiveness.

The anatomical and physiological basis of human pheromonal responses has also been a contentious subject. Vomeronasal organs and accessory olfactory bulbs are present in human fetuses, but they degenerate more or less completely by childhood. It now appears that any remaining pheromonal functions in humans have been taken over by the main olfactory epithelium and olfactory bulb.

responsible for the noxious sensation (not really one of smell) elicited by irritants such as concentrated ammonia. The olfactory receptor neurons, unlike taste receptor cells, are true neurons. Each olfactory receptor is a small bipolar neuron with a single slender dendrite emerging from one end of its cell body and an axon emerging from the other end (Fig. 13-10). The dendrite extends to a bulbous termination, the **olfactory vesicle,** from which a series of 10 to 30 immotile cilia spread out over the surface of the epithelium in a layer of mucus secreted by the supporting cells and Bowman's glands.

Odorants diffuse across the mucous layer, either directly or bound to an **odorant-binding protein** in the mucus, and stimulate the chemosensitive cilia of the olfactory receptors.

The unmyelinated axons of the olfactory receptors are among the thinnest (only 0.2 μm in diameter) and the most slowly conducting (0.1 m/sec) axons in the entire nervous system. They collect into a series of about 20 small bundles, the **olfactory fila** (from the Latin *filum,* meaning "thread"), which pass through the holes in the cribriform plate of the ethmoid bone (Fig. 13-11) and

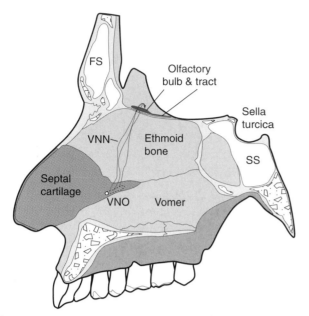

Figure 13-9 Location of the vomeronasal organ (VNO). The course of the vomeronasal nerve (VNN) is portrayed by analogy to other mammals, although there is little or no trace of it in adult humans. In other mammals, it passes through the nasal septum and through the cribriform plate to reach the accessory olfactory bulb on the dorsomedial surface of the main olfactory bulb. (The nasal septum has an anterior cartilaginous part and a posterior part formed from two thin bones, the vomer and the perpendicular plate of the ethmoid bone.) FS, frontal sinus; SS, sphenoidal sinus.

end in the **olfactory bulb.** Collectively the olfactory fila make up the first cranial nerve.

Olfactory receptors are unusual among mammalian neurons in that, like taste receptor cells, they are replaced throughout life. Individual receptors have a life span of a month or two, and new receptors arise from undifferentiated basal cells of the olfactory epithelium. The particular **olfactory receptor protein** made by a newly formed receptor gives it a chemical identity that helps its axon find its way to the proper synaptic sites in the olfactory bulb.

Olfactory Receptor Neurons Utilize a Large Number of G Protein–Coupled Receptors to Detect a Wide Range of Odors

Distinguishing 10,000 different odors is no mean feat. This is much greater than the number of tones we can hear or colors we can see, and it is accomplished by having many kinds of olfactory receptor neurons. Mice, for example, make about 1000 different but closely related olfactory receptor proteins. Each olfactory receptor neuron manufactures only one of these proteins, so mice have about 1000 different kinds of olfactory receptor neurons. We also have 1000 or so genes for olfactory receptor proteins, but about two thirds of them are inactive; even so, humans wind up with about 300 different kinds of olfactory receptor neurons. In contrast to the

situation in taste receptor cells, however, all these olfactory receptor neurons apparently use the same transduction mechanism. Olfactory receptor proteins are coupled to G proteins and are structurally similar to other G protein–coupled receptors, such as postsynaptic receptor molecules and rhodopsin in retinal photoreceptors (see Chapter 17). Each olfactory receptor protein binds an array of odorants—an array that overlaps but is somewhat different from the array bound by other olfactory receptor proteins. This extraordinary diversity of receptor proteins presumably reflects the antiquity and evolutionary importance of olfaction: upward of 1% of our entire genome is devoted to the specification of olfactory receptor proteins.

The second messenger cascade set in motion by the binding of an appropriate odorant causes the opening of cation channels (Fig. 13-12). The channels are permeable not just to Na^+ and K^+ but also to Ca^{2+}, and the resulting Ca^{2+} influx causes the opening of Ca^{2+}-gated Cl^- channels. In most neurons, opening Cl^- channels causes hyperpolarization—this is the basis of the inhibitory postsynaptic potentials produced by γ-aminobutyric acid (GABA) acting at $GABA_A$ receptors—but olfactory receptor neurons pump in enough Cl^- that the intracellular and extracellular concentrations of this ion are about equal to each other. Because the resulting Cl^- equilibrium potential is about 0 mV (see Equation 7-15 in Chapter 7), opening Cl^- channels causes depolarization of an olfactory receptor neuron and amplifies the receptor potential. The depolarization spreads to the trigger zone of the receptor neuron and, if large enough, initiates action potentials (Fig. 13-13). The receptor potential soon adapts in most olfactory receptor neurons, even if the odorant concentration remains constant. This is part of the basis for the common experience of the rapidly fading perception of maintained odors.

Olfactory Information Bypasses the Thalamus on Its Way to the Cerebral Cortex

The olfactory bulb develops as an outgrowth from the telencephalon. As a result, the olfactory nerve is unique, in that it reaches the ipsilateral cerebral hemisphere and does so directly, without a relay in the thalamus. However, the thalamus is part of subsequent stages of olfactory circuitry.

The Olfactory Nerve Terminates in the Olfactory Bulb

Animals that depend heavily on their sense of smell (called **macrosmatic** animals; from the Greek *osme,* meaning "odor") have a well-developed central olfactory apparatus, including a neatly laminated olfactory bulb (Fig. 13-14). In **microsmatic** humans, this lamination is not as apparent, and the olfactory bulb is relatively small and poorly developed. Its most prominent cell type is the

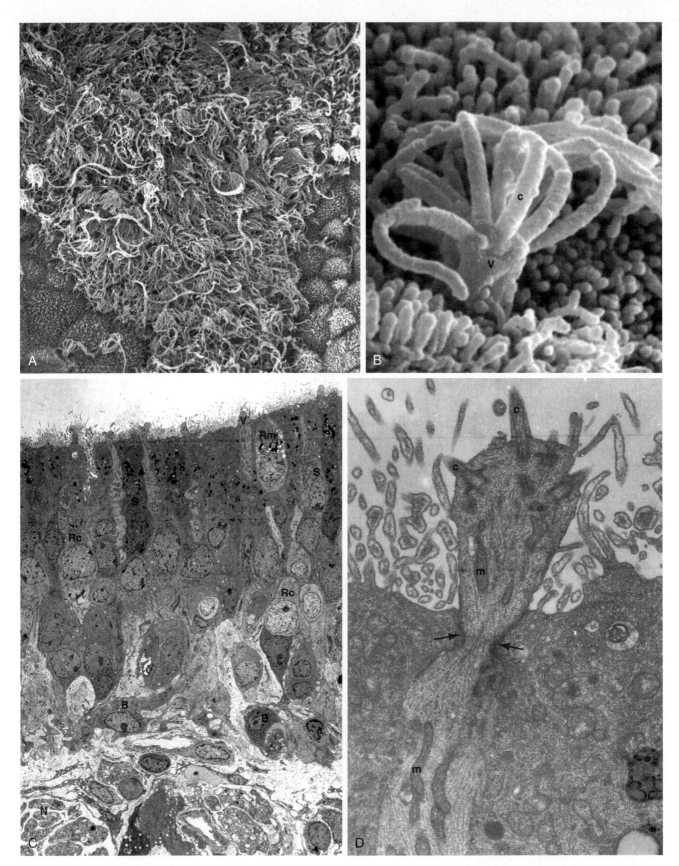

Figure 13-10 Human olfactory epithelium. **A,** Low-power scanning electron micrograph showing the mucosal surface of the epithelium, covered by a feltwork of chemosensory cilia. This area is at the edge of the olfactory epithelium, and nonsensory cells with short microvilli form the adjacent epithelium. **B,** Higher-power view showing chemosensory cilia (c) emerging from a single olfactory vesicle (V). **C,** Transmission electron micrograph showing ciliated receptor cells (Rc), supporting cells (S), olfactory vesicles (V), and basal cells (B). The receptor cell on the right (Rm) is of a second type that has microvillar rather than ciliary processes; these are much less numerous than the ciliated receptor cells and are poorly understood. Deep to the basal cells, axons of olfactory receptors (N) begin to form olfactory fila. **D,** Higher-magnification micrograph of an olfactory vesicle showing emerging chemosensory cilia (c) and abundant mitochondria (m) in and near the vesicle. Junctional complexes *(arrows)* separate the mucous layer from the extracellular spaces of the olfactory epithelium. *(A and B, courtesy Dr. Edward E. Morrison, Auburn University College of Veterinary Medicine. C and D, courtesy Pamela Eller, University of Colorado Health Sciences Center.)*

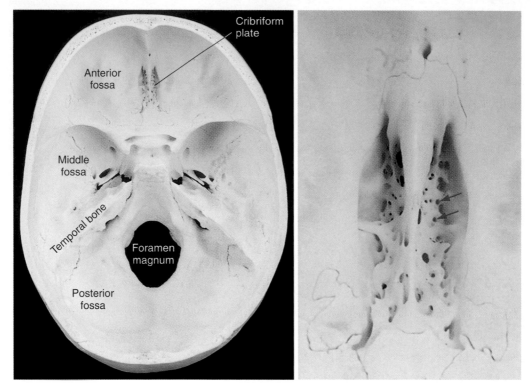

Figure 13-11 Cribriform plate of the ethmoid bone, as seen from inside a human skull. Olfactory fila pass through small holes *(arrows)* in the plate to reach the olfactory bulb.

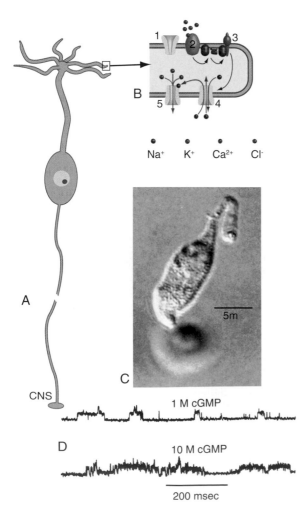

Figure 13-12 Chemosensory transduction in olfactory receptor cells. **A,** The tip of one chemosensory cilium from the olfactory receptor neuron is shown schematically and enlarged in **B. B,** Olfactory receptor cells contain normally closed cation channels (1) and G protein–coupled receptors for odorants (2). Dissociation of G protein activates an enzyme, adenylate cyclase (3), which catalyzes the production of a second messenger (cyclic AMP), which in turn opens the transduction channels (4), causing a depolarizing receptor potential. The transduction channels are permeable not just to Na^+ and K^+ but also to Ca^{2+}, and the resulting Ca^{2+} influx causes Cl^- channels to open (5). Cl^- efflux through these channels accounts for as much as 80% of the depolarizing current flow. **D,** Individual channels can be seen opening and closing during application of cyclic GMP (which can substitute for cyclic AMP), using patch-clamp electrodes applied to single, isolated human olfactory receptor neurons **(C).** *(C and D, from Thüraüf N et al: Eur J Neurosci 8:2080, 1996.)*

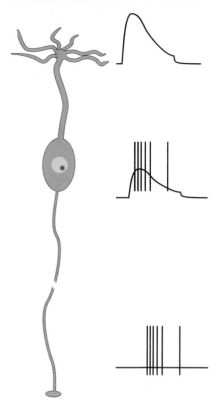

Figure 13-13 Transmission of electrical information in olfactory receptor neurons. Receptor potentials produced in chemosensory cilia in response to odorants spread passively through the cell body to the axon initial segment. Action potentials generated there are propagated along the axon and reach synaptic endings in the olfactory bulb.

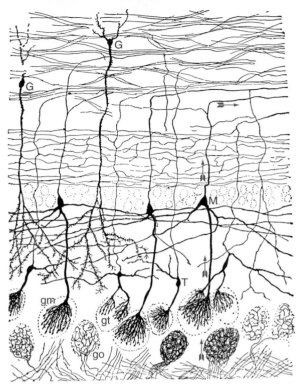

Figure 13-15 Glomeruli and neurons of the olfactory bulb. For clarity, most glomeruli in this drawing contain only one type of neural process: axon terminals of olfactory receptor neurons (go), dendrites of mitral cells (gm), or dendrites of tufted cells (gt). In reality, each glomerulus contains all of these, together with processes of interneurons. G, granule cells; M, mitral cells; T, tufted cells. *(From Ramón y Cajal S: Histologie du système nerveux de l'homme et des vertébrés, Paris, 1909, 1911, Maloine.)*

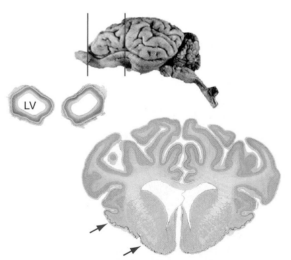

Figure 13-14 Coronal sections through the olfactory bulbs (left) and frontal lobes (right) of a white-tailed deer, both at about 1.25 times actual size. The olfactory bulbs are so large that the lateral ventricles (LV) extend into them, and olfactory cortex *(arrows)* covers most of the base of the cerebrum. *(From www.brainmuseum.org, courtesy Dr. Wally Welker; supported by NSF grant 0131028.)*

mitral cell, which has a triangular cell body and was named for its fancied resemblance to a bishop's miter. A mitral cell is configured like a typical cortical pyramidal cell in reverse (compare Figs. 13-15 and 1-4E): an axon emerges from the pointed side of the pyramid and moves toward the interior of the bulb to enter the **olfactory tract,** whereas a dendrite emerges from the broad side, descends to the surface of the bulb, and receives contacts from the incoming axons of olfactory receptors (CNI). These dendrites spread out in large spherical arborizations 100 to 200 μm in diameter called **glomeruli.** The axons of all the hundreds of olfactory receptor neurons that express a given receptor protein converge on just one or two of these glomeruli (Fig. 13-16), providing another stage of amplification of the olfactory signal. Hence different odorants activate different sets of glomeruli in patterns that systematically map out the chemical properties of odorants across the surface of the olfactory bulb. The olfactory bulb also contains interneurons (many of them called **granule cells** here, as in other regions of the CNS) and a collection of **tufted cells,** which are smaller than mitral cells but like mitral cells also send their dendrites into the glomeruli and their

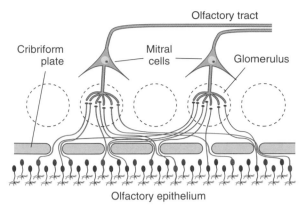

Figure 13-16 Sorting of olfactory nerve fibers among glomeruli of the olfactory bulb. Olfactory receptors of different types—each type characterized by its receptor protein and a restricted range of odor sensitivities (represented here by different colors)—are intermingled in a given area of olfactory epithelium. The axon terminals of any given type all converge on one or two glomeruli (which in reality would contain thousands of axon terminals and the dendrites of up to dozens of mitral and tufted cells).

axons into the olfactory tract. The olfactory bulb, like other sensory relays in the CNS, also receives a contingent of efferent fibers that are assumed to regulate or tune its sensitivity in some way. Some are norepinephrine and serotonin inputs from the locus ceruleus and raphe nuclei, similar to those received by other CNS areas. Most, however, arise from the **anterior olfactory nucleus,** a collective name for clusters of cells scattered all along the olfactory tract, or from olfactory areas of cerebral cortex.

The Olfactory Bulb Projects to Olfactory Cortex

Axons of mitral and tufted cells proceed caudally in the olfactory tract, giving off collaterals to cells of the anterior olfactory nucleus along the way. Fibers from the anterior olfactory nucleus then project back through the olfactory tracts to both olfactory bulbs (Fig. 13-17); crossing fibers do so through the anterior part of the

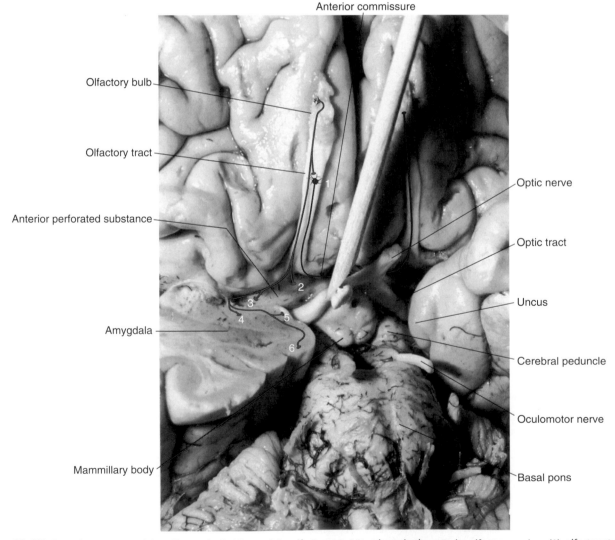

Figure 13-17 Central projections of the olfactory bulb. Fibers of the olfactory tract terminate in the anterior olfactory nucleus (1), olfactory tubercle (2), piriform cortex (3), part of the amygdala (4), periamygdaloid cortex (5), and a small anterior portion of the parahippocampal gyrus (6)—specifically, a part of the entorhinal cortex (described further in Chapter 24).

anterior commissure. At the posterior end of the orbital frontal cortex, where the olfactory tract attaches to the base of the brain, some of its fibers end in the **anterior perforated substance.** (This area forms a distinct elevation called the **olfactory tubercle** in many animals. It is not very obvious in humans but is often referred to as the *olfactory tubercle* anyway.) Remaining fibers curve laterally as the **lateral olfactory tract** (Fig. 13-18), the principal central projection pathway for the olfactory system.

The lateral olfactory tract travels along the edge of the anterior perforated substance, near the surface of an unusually thin layer of cerebral cortex. When it reaches the lateral border of the anterior perforated substance, it curves up onto the surface of the temporal lobe in the vicinity of the uncus, and its remaining fibers disperse and terminate. Along this course from the olfactory bulb, fibers of the olfactory tract end in two general places (see Fig. 13-17): the primary olfactory cortex and a small portion of the amygdala. The

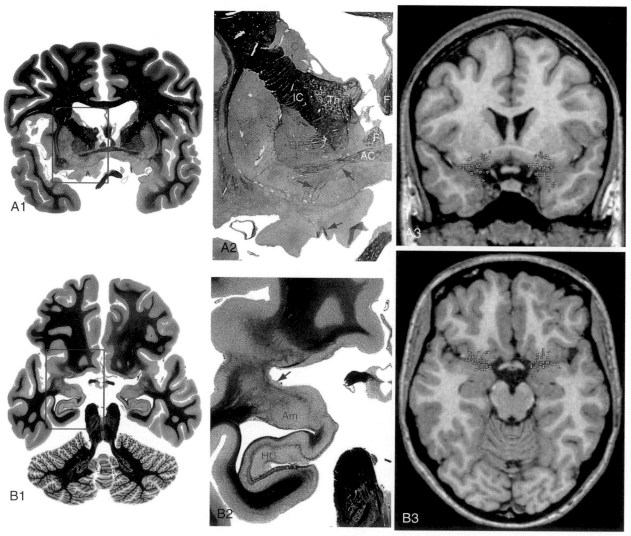

Figure 13-18 Course of the lateral olfactory tract, shown in coronal **(A)** and axial **(B)** planes. **A,** Near the site where the olfactory tract *(blue arrow)* attaches to the base of the brain, fibers *(green arrows)* that arise in the anterior olfactory nucleus leave and move toward the anterior commissure (or arrive from the contralateral anterior olfactory nucleus). **B,** Just beyond the attachment point shown in **A,** the lateral olfactory tract *(blue arrow)* moves laterally onto the surface of the temporal lobe, headed for piriform cortex *(red arrow)* and other targets indicated in Figure 13-17. **A3** and **B3** are magnetic resonance images in comparable planes; the dots indicate the sites where increased activity in response to odorants was found in 23 different functional imaging (PET and fMRI) studies. The correspondence between the areas of activation and the olfactory structures indicated in **A2** and **B2** is apparent. AC, anterior commissure; Am, amygdala; C, caudate nucleus; F, fornix; GP, globus pallidus; HC, hippocampus; IC, internal capsule; P, putamen; Th, thalamus. *(**A3** and **B3,** courtesy Dr. Jelena Djordjevic, Montreal Neurological Institute, McGill University. Adapted from Djordjevic J, Jones-Gotman M: Olfaction and the temporal lobes. In Brewer WJ, Castle D, Pantelis C, editors: Olfaction and the brain, Cambridge, 2006, Cambridge University Press.)*

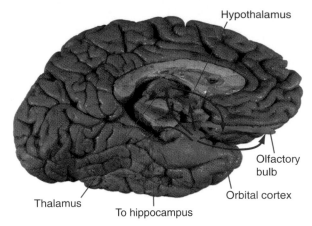

Figure 13-19 Projections of the primary olfactory cortex.

primary olfactory cortex consists of the cortex adjacent to the lateral olfactory tract (called **piriform cortex**), an area of cortex covering part of the amygdala (**periamygdaloid cortex**), and a small anterior region of the parahippocampal gyrus. In addition, the anterior olfactory nucleus and olfactory tubercle have a cortex-like structure in many animals and are often included as part of the primary olfactory cortex. These primary receiving sites for olfactory information project in turn to the hypothalamus, to limbic structures such as the hippocampus and the rest of the amygdala, and to the thalamus (Fig. 13-19).

Olfactory Information Reaches Other Cortical Areas Both Directly and Via the Thalamus

The olfactory system is unique, in that no thalamic relay is interposed between receptors and cerebral cortex. However, in this case, the initial cortical destination is a distinctive, thin area of cortex (called **paleocortex,** for reasons explained in Chapter 22). The thalamus does become involved in the pathway from the olfactory bulb to the olfactory association cortex. One such area is located posteriorly on the orbital surface of the frontal lobe, extending onto the anterior insula (adjacent to gustatory cortex). The primary olfactory cortex sends information to this cortical area primarily through direct projections but also through a relay in the thalamus (the **dorsomedial nucleus;** see Chapter 16). The net result of this sequence of connections is that olfactory receptor neurons, like taste buds, wind up represented in the ipsilateral cerebral hemisphere. Hence the chemical senses are at the opposite end of the spectrum from the somatosensory and motor systems, in which a given part of the body is represented primarily in the contralateral cerebral hemisphere. Other sensory systems are somewhere in between, as in the partly crossed–partly uncrossed representation of each ear (see Chapter 14) and eye (see Chapter 17).

Neurons of the olfactory bulb and primary olfactory cortex, like neurons in early stages of the gustatory system, respond to multiple odorants. Neurons of olfactory association cortex, like those of gustatory association cortex, are more likely to respond only to selected stimuli.

Conductive and Sensorineural Problems Can Affect Olfactory Function

Although our sense of smell is exquisitely sensitive and allows some remarkable discriminations, it is less well developed in humans (and less important in everyday life) than in many other species. Someone deprived of the sense of smell (i.e., rendered **anosmic**) by disease or injury is likely to complain less of olfaction loss than of a taste disorder. However, testing olfaction can sometimes provide useful diagnostic clues. For example, tumors growing at the base of the skull beneath the orbital surface of the frontal lobe can become quite large before they cause any symptoms other than unilateral anosmia.

Two general kinds of processes can disrupt the sense of smell: processes that prevent odorants from reaching the olfactory epithelium (**conductive** olfactory deficit) and processes that damage olfactory receptor neurons or parts of the olfactory CNS (**sensorineural** olfactory deficit). Conductive olfactory deficits can be caused by things such as nasal polyps, septal deviation, and inflammation. Sensorineural olfactory deficits are most commonly a consequence of head injuries or neurodegenerative conditions such as Parkinson's or Alzheimer's disease. The olfactory fila may be torn loose from the olfactory bulb as a consequence of head trauma and be unable to regrow through a scarred cribriform plate, or olfactory areas at the base of the brain may be damaged by slight movement of the brain across the base of the skull. In addition, for unknown reasons, some patients suffer permanent damage to olfactory receptor neurons after a severe upper respiratory infection. Patients with anosmia of sensorineural origin are likely to have an intact common chemical sense and be able to perceive a range of volatile substances, such as ammonia and menthol, most but not all of which are irritating.[h]

Conversely, *excess* activity in olfactory structures can also cause disturbances. Piriform cortex has been directly identified as functionally important olfactory cortex in humans because electrical stimulation there causes olfactory sensations. Clues pointing in this direction were provided in the 19th century by British

---

[h]Hence these substances are *not* useful for testing olfaction, and common odorants such as coffee are used instead.

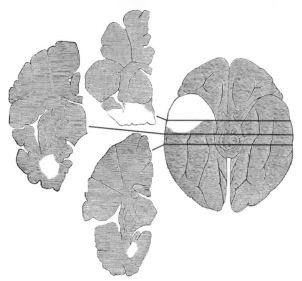

Figure 13-20 A classic case of uncinate seizures. A 53-year-old woman began to have spells during which she had hallucinations of a small woman "who was rather agreeable and was always flitting about the kitchen; she always saw the same woman in every paroxysm. She never thought it was anything but a vision, but was very worried about it." At the same time she would have illusions of very unpleasant odors, variously described as "burning dirty stuff" or a "nasty dreadful smell," and a feeling of suffocation. Between the seizures, her sense of smell was intact bilaterally. Subsequently she developed weakness and somatosensory changes on the left side and died. At autopsy "a tumour the size of a tangerine orange" was found that occupied the indicated parts of her brain. *(Adapted from Hughlings Jackson J, Beevor CE: Brain 12:346, 1889.)*

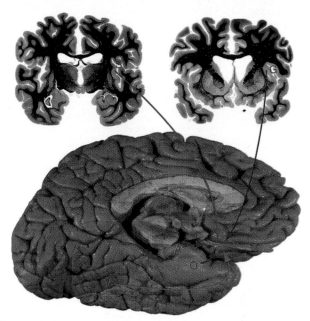

Figure 13-21 Convergence in orbital cortex of projections from gustatory cortex (G) in the anterior insula, piriform cortex (O), somatosensory association areas (S) in the posterior insula, visual association areas (V) in the inferior temporal lobe, and limbic structures such as the amygdala (A).

neurologist Hughlings Jackson, who noted that seizures originating in the vicinity of the uncus may begin with an illusion of smell or taste, most often an unpleasant one (Fig. 13-20). The seizure may go on to include motor phenomena such as chewing movements or smacking of the lips and alterations of consciousness such as a "dreamy state" or a feeling of déjà vu. Seizures of this type are still known as **uncinate seizures.**

Multiple Flavor-Related Signals Converge in Orbital Cortex

Gustatory and olfactory cortices project to the orbital surface of the frontal lobe (Fig. 13-21), parts of which serve as an association cortex for flavor. The same areas receive converging inputs that convey somatosensory and visual information, and some neurons there respond to the smell, taste, texture, or sight of a particular kind of food. Orbital neurons have an important role in signaling the reward value of foods and beverages. An individual neuron, for example, may respond in the same way as a neuron in gustatory cortex when an animal is hungry, but respond much less vigorously when the same animal is satiated.

SUGGESTED READINGS

Axel R: The molecular logic of smell. Sci Am 273:154, 1995.

Barlow LA, Chien C-B, Northcutt RG: Embryonic taste buds develop in the absence of innervation. Development 122:1103, 1996.

Beckstead RM, Morse JR, Norgren R: The nucleus of the solitary tract in the monkey: projections to the thalamus and brain stem nuclei. J Comp Neurol 190:259, 1980.

Beckstead RM, Norgren R: An autoradiographic examination of the central distribution of the trigeminal, facial, glossopharyngeal and vagal nerves in the monkey. J Comp Neurol 184:455, 1979.

Beidler LM, Smallman RL: Renewal of cells within taste buds. J Cell Biol 27:263, 1965.

Brewer WJ, Castle D, Pantelis C, editors: Olfaction and the brain, Cambridge, 2006, Cambridge University Press.

Buck L, Axel R: A novel multigene family may encode odorant receptors: a molecular basis for odor recognition. Cell 65:175, 1991.
    The initial description of the very large family of genes now known to code olfactory receptor proteins.

Chandrashekar J, et al: The receptors and cells for mammalian taste. Nature 444:288, 2006.

Collings VB: Human taste response as a function of locus of stimulation on the tongue and soft palate. Percep Psychophys 16:169, 1974.

Deems DA, et al: Smell and taste disorders: a study of 750 patients from the University of Pennsylvania Smell and Taste Center. Arch Otolaryngol Head Neck Surg 117:519, 1991.
    Although 66% of the patients complained of a taste deficit, less than 4% actually had one.

DeSimone JA, Lyall V: Taste receptors in the gastrointestinal tract. III. Salty and sour taste: sensing of sodium and protons by the tongue. Am J Physiol G1005:2006.

Doty RL, editor: Handbook of olfaction and gustation, ed 2, New York, 2003, Marcel Dekker.

An extensive review of both basic and clinical aspects of the chemical senses.

Doty RL, et al: Olfactory dysfunction in patients with head trauma. Arch Neurol 54:1131, 1997.

Eichenbaum H, et al: Selective olfactory deficits in case H.M. Brain 106:459, 1983.

H.M. is a famous patient who had the anterior parts of both temporal lobes removed. A severe memory impairment resulted, as discussed in Chapter 24. In addition, he lost the ability to identify odors, even though his ability to detect odors was unimpaired.

Finger TE: Solitary chemoreceptor cells in the nasal cavity serve as sentinels of respiration. Proc Natl Acad Sci U S A 100:8981, 2003.

An example of a widely distributed population of additional receptors related to taste receptor cells.

Finger TE, Silver WL, Restrepo D: Neurobiology of taste and smell, ed 2, New York, 2000, John Wiley & Sons.

A review of the comparative anatomy and physiology of the chemical senses.

Finger TE, et al: ATP signaling is crucial for communication from taste buds to gustatory nerves. Science 310:1495, 2005.

Gonzalez C, et al: Carotid body chemoreceptors: from natural stimuli to sensory discharges. Physiol Rev 74:829, 1994.

One example of the array of chemoreceptors of which we are not consciously aware.

Graziadei PPC, Monti Graziadei GA: Neurogenesis and neuron regeneration in the olfactory system of mammals. I. Morphological aspects of differentiation and structural organization of the olfactory sensory neurons. J Neurocytol 8:1, 1979.

Henkin RI, Christiansen RL: Taste localization on the tongue, palate and pharynx of normal man. J Appl Physiol 22:316, 1967.

Höfer D, Püschel B, Drenkhahn D: Taste receptor–like cells in the rat gut identified by expression of α-gustducin. Proc Natl Acad Sci U S A 93:6631, 1996.

The same transduction mechanisms used by taste receptor cells may be used for local signaling by cells in the intestinal wall.

Hughlings Jackson J, Beevor CE: Case of tumour of the right temporo-sphenoidal lobe bearing on the localisation of the sense of smell and on the interpretation of a particular variety of epilepsy. Brain 12:346, 1889.

Imfeld TM, Schroeder HE: Palatal taste buds in man: topographical arrangement in islands of keratinized epithelium. Anat Embryol 185:259, 1992.

Jean A: Brainstem control of swallowing: neuronal network and cellular mechanisms. Physiol Rev 81:871, 2001.

Johnson BA, Leon M: Chemotopic odorant coding in a mammalian olfactory system. J Comp Neurol 503:1, 2007.

Lalonde ER, Eglitis JA: Number and distribution of taste buds on the epiglottis, pharynx, larynx, soft palate and uvula in a human newborn. Anat Rec 140:91, 1961.

Landis BN, et al: Transient hemiageusia in cerebrovascular lateral pontine lesions. J Neurol Neurosurg Psychiatry 77:680, 2006.

The relationship between the side of the damage and the side of the deficit varies in the few reported human cases of gustatory disturbance. The experimental literature, however, consistently shows the pathway to be uncrossed.

Lawrence C: Dysgeusia ("cognate, dis-gusting"). Lancet 348:1102, 1996.

A first-person account of the distorted and disagreeable sensations that can accompany diminution of taste.

Liberles SD, Buck LB: A second class of chemosensory receptors in the olfactory epithelium. Nature 442:645, 2006.

Receptors for trace amines that play a role in social signaling.

McCabe C, Rolls ET: Umami: a delicious flavor formed by convergence of taste and olfactory pathways in the human brain. Eur J Neurosci 25:1855, 2007.

Glutamate by itself is not particularly delicious, but when paired with food odors, it enhances their pleasantness and increases the activity of orbital cortex.

McRitchie DA, Törk I: The internal organization of the human solitary nucleus. Brain Res Bull 31:171, 1993.

Michlig S, Damak S, Le Coutre J: Claudin-based permeability barriers in taste buds. J Comp Neurol 502:1003, 2007.

Miller IJ, Jr: Variation in human fungiform taste bud densities among regions and subjects. Anat Rec 216:474, 1986.

Miller IJ, Jr, Reedy FE, Jr: Variations in human taste bud density and taste intensity perception. Physiol Behav 47:1213, 1990.

Mombaerts P, et al: Visualizing an olfactory sensory map. Cell 87:675, 1996.

Technically elegant experiments providing a visual demonstration of the convergence of a multitude of olfactory neurons with the same putative receptor protein onto just two glomeruli.

Moran DT, et al: The fine structure of the olfactory mucosa in man. J Neurocytol 11:721, 1982.

Morrison EE, Costanzo RM: Morphology of the human olfactory epithelium. J Comp Neurol 297:1, 1990.

Morrot G, Brochet F, Dubourdieu D: The color of odors. Brain Lang 79:309, 2001.

The words used to describe the aromas of a glass of wine depend more on the color of the wine than on its actual bouquet.

Nakamura T, Gold GH: A cyclic nucleotide-gated conductance in olfactory receptor cilia. Nature 325:442, 1987.

These data suggest a remarkable similarity between the mechanisms of olfactory and visual transduction and indicate considerable conservation of sensory transduction mechanisms.

Plassman H, et al: Marketing actions can modulate neural representations of experienced pleasantness. Proc Natl Acad Sci U S A 105:1050, 2008.

If you think a wine is expensive, it tastes better and there's more activity in orbital cortex.

Porter J, et al: Mechanisms of scent-tracking in humans. Nat Neurosci 10:27, 2007.

We can do it. And just as comparisons between the two eyes or ears are important for localizing sights and sounds, internostril comparisons play a role.

Price JL: Olfactory system. In Paxinos G, Mai JK, editors: The human nervous system, ed 2, San Diego, 2004, Elsevier Academic Press.

Pritchard TC, Norgren R: Gustatory system. In Paxinos G, Mai JK, editors: The human nervous system, ed 2, San Diego, 2004, Elsevier Academic Press.

Reisert J, et al: Mechanism of the excitatory Cl− response in mouse olfactory receptor neurons. Neuron 45:553, 2005.

Rolls ET, Baylis LL: Gustatory, olfactory, and visual convergence within the primate orbitofrontal cortex. J Neurosci 14:5437, 1994.

Romanov RA, et al: Afferent neurotransmission mediated by hemichannels in mammalian taste cells. EMBO J 26:657, 2007.

The unconventional mechanism of ATP release from most taste receptor cells.

Roquier S, Blancher A, Giorgi D: The olfactory receptor gene repertoire in primates and mouse: evidence for reduction of the functional fraction in primates. Proc Natl Acad Sci U S A 97:2870, 2000.

Schiffman SS: Taste and smell losses in normal aging and disease. JAMA 278:1357, 1997.

Schul R, Slotnick BM, Dudai Y: Flavor and the frontal cortex. Behav Neurosci 110:760, 1996.

Scott TR, et al: Gustatory responses in the nucleus tractus solitarius of the alert cynomolgus monkey. J Neurophysiol 55:182, 1986.

Shepherd GM, Greer CA: Olfactory bulb. In Shepherd GM, editor: The synaptic organization of the brain, ed 5, New York, 2003, Oxford University Press.

Simon SA, et al: The neural mechanisms of gustation: a distributed processing code. Nat Rev Neurosci 7:890, 2006.

Slotnick BM, Kaneko N: Role of mediodorsal thalamic nucleus in olfactory discrimination learning in rats. Science 214:91, 1981.

Small DM, et al: Differential neural responses evoked by orthonasal versus retronasal odorant perception in humans. Neuron 47:593, 2005.

Stern K, McClintock MK: Regulation of ovulation by human pheromones. Nature 392:177, 1998.

Stone LM, et al: Taste receptor cells arise from local epithelium, not neurogenic ectoderm. Proc Natl Acad Sci U S A 92:1916, 1995.

Tegoni M, et al: Mammalian odorant binding proteins. Biochim Biophys Acta 1482:229, 2000.

Wansink B, Payne CR, North J: Fine as North Dakota wine: sensory expectations and the intake of companion foods. Physiol Behav 90:712, 2007.

Another nice example of the interaction of multiple factors in determining flavor: where you think a wine comes from influences not just how much you enjoy the wine but also the taste of whatever you eat with it.

Wysocki CJ, Preti G: Facts, fallacies, fears, and frustrations with human pheromones. Anat Rec 281A:1201, 2004.

Xu F, et al: Simultaneous activation of mouse main and accessory olfactory bulbs by odors or pheromones. J Comp Neurol 489:491, 2005.

Zhang Z, et al: The transduction channel TRPM5 is gated by intracellular calcium in taste cells. J Neurosci 27:5777, 2007.

Hearing and Balance: The Eighth Cranial Nerve

14

Hearing and balance are very different senses functionally, but they begin peripherally in very similar ways. The eighth cranial nerve carries two special sensory components, one in a **cochlear division** and one in a **vestibular division.** Both divisions innervate elaborate end-organs containing specialized mechanoreceptors (called **hair cells** because of their appearance), but accessory structures in the end-organs specialize the two divisions to respond to different types of mechanical stimuli. The cochlear division carries information about sound, whereas the vestibular division signals position and movement of the head.

Auditory and Vestibular Receptor Cells Are Located in the Walls of the Membranous Labyrinth

The structures innervated by the eighth nerve are embedded in the temporal bone (Figs. 14-1 and 14-2), where the receptor cells form parts of the walls of a convoluted, membranous tube that is suspended within the bony structure of the temporal bone (Fig. 14-3).

The Membranous Labyrinth Is Suspended Within the Bony Labyrinth, a Cavity in the Temporal Bone

The walls of the bony structure are formed by the hardest bone in the body—the petrous ("like a rock") portion of the temporal bone. Because the structure consists of so many twists and turns, it is called the **bony labyrinth.** The coiled **cochlea** (Latin for "snail shell") extends anteriorly from an enlargement called the **vestibule,** to which three **semicircular canals** are attached. The **membranous labyrinth,** the membranous tube suspended within the bony labyrinth, generally follows the same contours (see Fig. 14-3). Hence there is a **cochlear duct** within the bony cochlea and a **semicircular duct** within each semicircular canal. However, the vestibule contains two enlargements of the membranous labyrinth, the **utricle** (to which the semicircular ducts attach) and the **saccule** (which is connected to the cochlear duct and to the utricle).

The bony labyrinth is filled with **perilymph,** which is similar in composition to cerebrospinal fluid (CSF) and therefore to extracellular fluid generally (i.e., low K^+ concentration and high Na^+ concentration—about 5 and 140 mM, respectively). The subarachnoid space around the brain is actually continuous with the perilymphatic space of the bony labyrinth through a tiny canal in the temporal bone (the cochlear aqueduct). The membranous labyrinth, in contrast, is filled with **endolymph,** a very peculiar fluid that is more like intracellular fluids in ionic composition (K^+ concentration about 150 mM, Na^+ concentration about 1 to 2 mM). As might be expected from this difference in fluid composition, the membranous labyrinth is a continuous, closed system in which every part communicates with every other part (like CSF in the ventricles). A system of tight junctions joins some

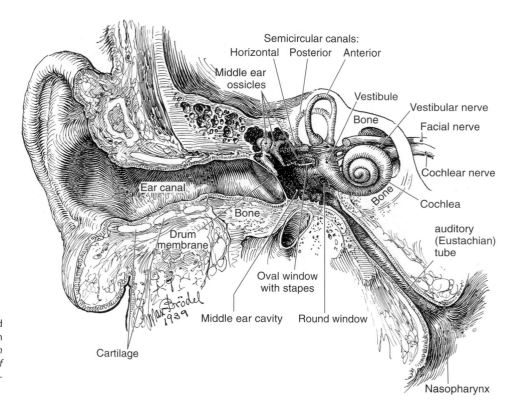

Figure 14-1 The outer, middle, and inner ears, showing the bony labyrinth embedded in the temporal bone. *(From Brödel M: Three unpublished drawings of the anatomy of the human ear, Philadelphia, 1946, WB Saunders.)*

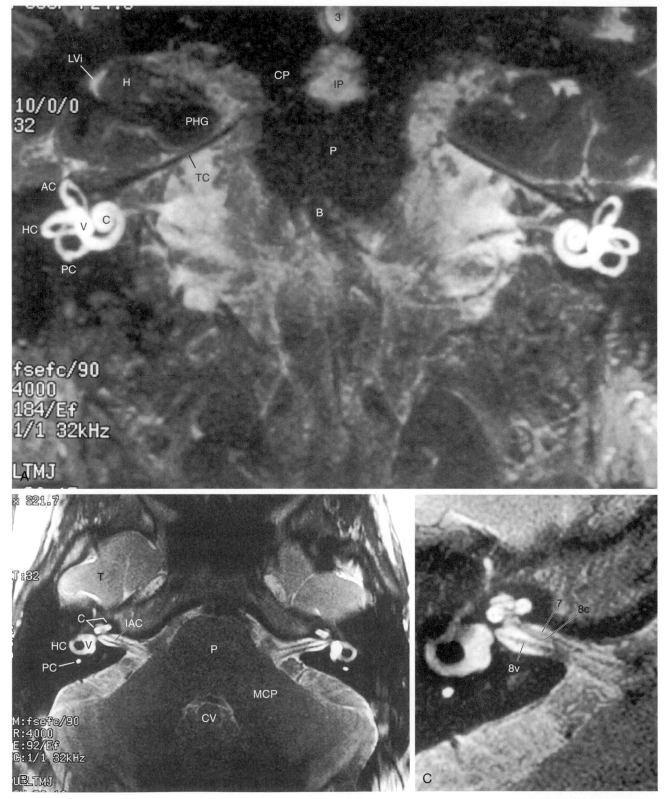

Figure 14-2 Magnetic resonance images of the labyrinth, shown in coronal **(A)** and axial **(B)** views and an enlargement **(C)** of the latter. Notice in **A** the proximity of the medial temporal lobe (parahippocampal gyrus [PHG]) to the cerebral peduncle (CP) as the brainstem passes through the notch in the tentorium cerebelli (TC). 3, third ventricle; 7, facial nerve; 8c, vestibulocochlear nerve (cochlear division); 8v, vestibulocochlear nerve (vestibular division); AC, anterior semicircular canal; B, basilar artery; C, cochlea; CV, cerebellar vermis (protruding into the fourth ventricle); H, hippocampus; HC, horizontal semicircular canal; IAC, internal auditory canal; IP, interpeduncular cistern; LVi, lateral ventricle (inferior horn); MCP, middle cerebellar peduncle; P, pons; PC, posterior semicircular canal; T, temporal lobe; TC, tentorium cerebelli; V, vestibule. (*Courtesy Dr. Ric Harnsberger, University of Utah College of Medicine.*)

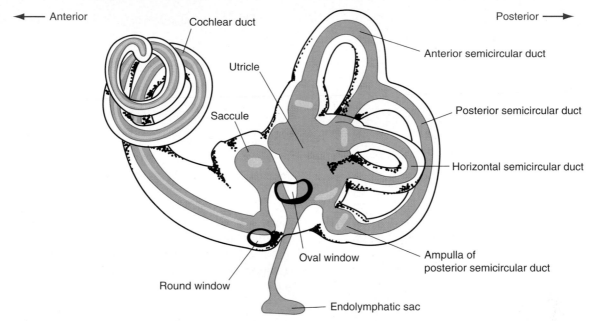

Figure 14-3 Membranous labyrinth of the left ear as seen through an outline of the bony labyrinth. Pale green areas indicate the locations of patches or strips of hair cells in the wall of the membranous labyrinth. The endolymphatic sac is located beneath the dura on the surface of the temporal bone. It contains no receptor cells but rather is a site of absorption of endolymph. *(Modified from Warwick R, Williams PLW, editors: Gray's anatomy, Br ed 35, Philadelphia, 1973, WB Saunders.)*

cells in the walls of the membranous labyrinth, forming a diffusion barrier between endolymph and perilymph. The receptor cells of the labyrinth (hair cells) form part of this diffusion barrier; as discussed later in this chapter, the resulting voltage and concentration gradients across parts of their membranes are important in the transduction process.

Endolymph Is Actively Secreted, Circulates Through the Membranous Labyrinth, and Is Reabsorbed

Endolymph is produced continuously by specialized epithelial cells called stria vascularis in one wall of the cochlear duct and in several other locations in the membranous labyrinth, using an active pumping mechanism that results in a positive electrical potential inside the membranous labyrinth. Endolymph seems to have a path of circulation and reabsorption reminiscent of that of CSF. The semicircular ducts communicate with the utricle, and the cochlear duct communicates with the saccule. The ducts interconnecting the utricle and saccule meet in a Y-shaped junction through which endolymph can enter the **endolymphatic duct,** leave the labyrinth, and reach the **endolymphatic sac** in the dura covering the temporal bone, where some of it is reabsorbed. Just as obstruction of CSF flow causes expansion of the ventricles and neurological symptoms, obstruction of endolymph flow was naturally thought to cause ballooning of the membranous labyrinth and otological symptoms. **Ménière's disease** is characterized by transient attacks of vertigo, nausea, and hearing loss

accompanied by ringing in the ears (**tinnitus**); its defining anatomical feature is swelling of the membranous labyrinth (referred to as **endolymphatic hydrops**), usually attributed to endolymphatic blockage. Some cases of hydrops are asymptomatic, however, and there are occasional cases of patients with Ménière's symptoms but no hydrops. Although there are probably multiple causes of Ménière's disease, in many cases the hydrops is likely to be a secondary result of some still unknown process that disrupts fluid secretion in the membranous labyrinth and damages hair cells.

Auditory and Vestibular Receptors Are Hair Cells

Hair cells of the labyrinth were named for the array of a hundred or so specialized microvilli that project as a bundle from one end of the cell into the endolymphatic interior of the membranous labyrinth (Fig. 14-4); the other end of each hair cell synapses on peripheral processes of eighth nerve fibers, which in turn convey auditory and vestibular information to the central nervous system (CNS). Hair cell microvilli, somewhat illogically referred to as **stereocilia,** are arranged asymmetrically: they are lined up in graduated rows, so that the tallest are toward one side of the hair cell. Adjacent to the tallest stereocilia of each hair cell in the semicircular ducts, utricle, and saccule is a single true cilium, the **kinocilium.** Cochlear hair cells have kinocilia that degenerate during fetal development, indicating that these processes play no essential role in the transduction process;

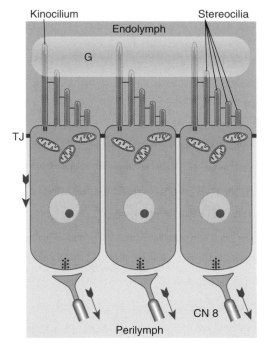

Figure 14-4 Schematic view of typical hair cells. Tight junctions (TJ) near the microvillar end of the cells join them to one another or to neighboring supporting cells, forming part of the diffusion barrier between endolymph and perilymph (see Figs. 14-5 and 14-12). Hence each hair cell is bathed partly in endolymph and partly in perilymph. The kinocilium (when present) and the tallest stereocilia are inserted into a gelatinous mass (G) that couples each hair bundle to mechanical forces. Transduction channels are located near the tips of the stereocilia, and arrows indicate the direction of information flow. CN, cranial nerve.

Table 14-1 **Locations and Functions of Hair Cells**

Location of Hair Cells	Part of Labyrinth	Gelatinous Material	Stimulus Transduced
Organ of Corti	Cochlea	Tectorial membrane	Sound
Cristae	Semicircular ducts	Cupula	Angular acceleration
Maculae	Utricle, saccule	Otolithic membrane	Linear acceleration

the hair cells, between the hair cells and neighboring supporting cells. Because perilymph is continuous with the CSF of subarachnoid space, marker substances introduced into cisterna magna infiltrate the sensory epithelia of the labyrinth and surround the hair cells, stopping only at the array of tight junctions (Fig. 14-5). Hence the stereocilia and the apical surfaces of hair cells are exposed to endolymph, whereas other surfaces of the hair cells, and the nerve fibers they contact, are bathed in perilymph (see Fig. 14-9E).

Hair Cells Have Mechanosensitive Transduction Channels

Stereocilia are packed full of cross-linked actin filaments (Fig. 14-6C), which makes them rigid. In response to mechanical deformation they do not bend but rather pivot at their bases, where they are attached to the hair cell. Various linking molecules interconnect neighboring stereocilia, so the whole hair bundle moves as a unit in response to mechanical stimuli. Some of these links are symmetrical, connecting a given stereocilium to all of its neighbors. In addition, fine filamentous connections called **tip links** extend from the tip of each stereocilium to its next tallest neighbor (see Fig. 14-6). Tip links have a special role in the transduction process, which (at least in a conceptual sense) is remarkably straightforward (Fig. 14-7). A mechanically gated cation channel is located at one or both ends of each tip link and is normally open part of the time. Deflecting the hair bundle toward the tallest stereocilia stretches the tip links, increasing the probability of channel opening. The channels are permeable to most small cations, and because K^+ ions are the most abundant cations in endolymph, they flow down the electrical gradient from the positive endolymph into the negative interior of the hair cells. The resulting inward K^+ current depolarizes the hair cells,[a] causing the opening of voltage-gated Ca^{2+}

kinocilia may instead be important for establishing the anatomical asymmetry of hair cells or for some mechanical connections of the hair cells in which they persist.

Hair cells are grouped into six discrete clusters in different parts of the labyrinth (Table 14-1; see also Fig. 14-3), and fundamental aspects of the arrangement of each cluster are the same. The stereocilia of the hair cells (and the kinocilium, when present) protrude into the endolymphatic space inside the membranous labyrinth, where the tips of the kinocilium and the tallest stereocilia are usually embedded in a specialized mass of gelatinous material, one for each cluster of hair cells. Movement of the gelatinous mass relative to the hair cells causes deflection of stereocilia, which in turn causes a receptor potential through a transduction mechanism described later.

In sections through the labyrinth (see Fig. 14-9), hair cells and associated structures often appear to be bathed in the endolymph that fills the membranous labyrinth. If this was the case, however, eighth nerve fibers reaching the bases of hair cells would also be passing through endolymph. Endolymph has such a high K^+ concentration that standard nerve fibers could not work in its presence. In fact, the real barrier between endolymph and perilymph is a series of tight junctions near the tops of

[a]Increased K^+ conductance in typical neurons causes K^+ efflux and hyperpolarization, reflecting the fact that the K^+ equilibrium potential is typically around −90 mV. However, because of the high K^+ concentration in endolymph, the K^+ equilibrium potential across the membranes of stereocilia is about 0 mV.

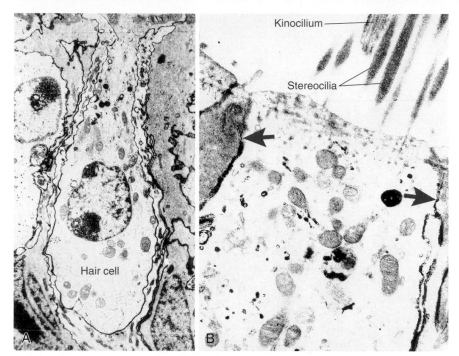

Figure 14-5 Part of the membranous labyrinth of a guinea pig after a tracer substance (horseradish peroxidase) had been injected into cisterna magna. **A,** Electron micrograph of the saccular macula; dark reaction product outlines all the cellular elements of the macula. **B,** Higher-magnification micrograph of the apical end of the hair cell shown in **A;** reaction product fills extracellular space up to, but not beyond, junctional complexes *(arrows)* that separate the perilymphatic and endolymphatic spaces. *(Courtesy Dr. David L. Asher.)*

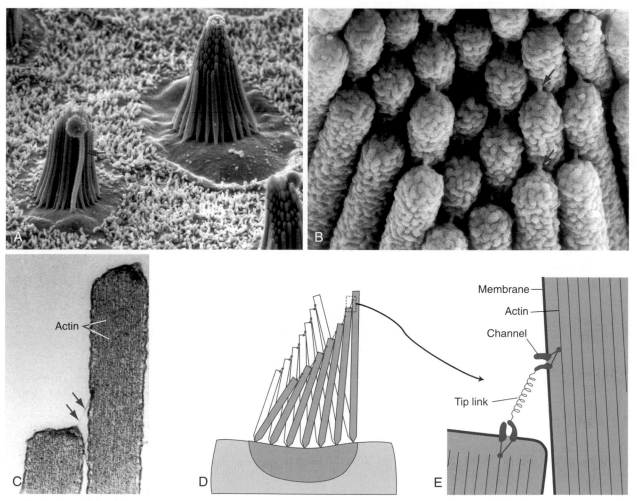

Figure 14-6 Stereocilia and tip links. **A,** Scanning electron micrograph of the tops of hair cells in the saccule of a bullfrog, showing the graduated arrays of stereocilia extending from each. Adjacent to the tallest stereocilia is the single kinocilium *(arrow)*, which has a characteristic bulbous tip in this species. **B,** Higher-magnification micrograph of a group of stereocilia. Each stereocilium is connected to its next taller neighbor by a filamentous tip link *(arrows)*. **C,** Longitudinal transmission electron micrograph through parts of two stereocilia, showing the actin filaments filling them and the tip link *(arrows)* interconnecting them. **D,** Apparent mechanism of action of stereocilia and tip links. Deflecting the hair bundle toward the tallest stereocilia stretches the tip links. **E,** This stretch increases the probability of cation channels at one or both ends of the tip links being open. *(Courtesy Drs. David Corey and G. M. G. Shepherd, Howard Hughes Medical Institute, Harvard Medical School.)*

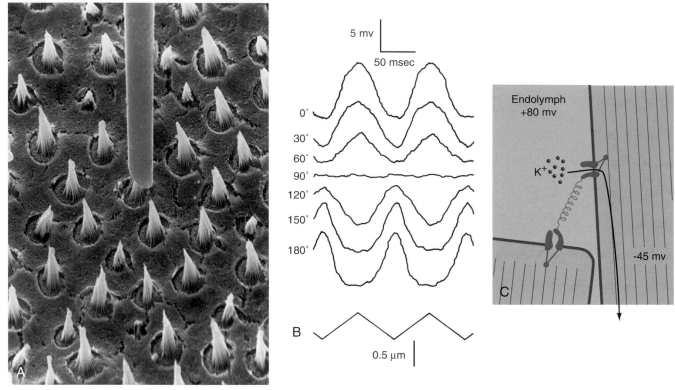

Figure 14-7 Transduction in hair cells. The otolithic membrane (see Fig. 14-27) was removed from the macula of a bullfrog's saccule. **A,** A glass micropipette was slipped over a bundle of stereocilia and used to wiggle it in various directions. **B,** Receptor potentials were simultaneously recorded using a second micropipette (not shown). The bottom trace indicates the time course of 0.5-μm movements, and the traces above show the dependence of the resulting receptor potentials on the direction of deflection. Movement toward the kinocilium (0 degrees) produces a depolarizing receptor potential; movement away (180 degrees) produces a hyperpolarizing receptor potential. Movement perpendicular to the plane of the tip links (90 degrees) has no effect on the hair cell. **C,** Stretching a tip link opens cation channels in the stereocilia. Even though the K^+ concentration in endolymph is about the same as that inside the stereocilia, the positive endolymphatic potential and the negative membrane potential of the hair cell combine to form a large electrical driving force that moves K^+ ions through these open cation channels. (*A and B, from Shotwell SL, Jacobs R, Hudspeth AJ: Ann N Y Acad Sci 374:1, 1981.* **C,** *modified from a drawing provided by Drs. David Corey and G. M. G. Shepherd, Howard Hughes Medical Institute, Harvard Medical School.*)

channels and increased release of transmitter onto eighth nerve endings. The excitatory transmitter (probably glutamate) then causes an increased firing frequency in the eighth nerve fibers. Deflecting the hair bundle in the opposite direction decreases the tension on the tip links; the transduction channels close, baseline K^+ current stops, the hair cells hyperpolarize, and transmitter release and firing rate diminish. Deflecting the hair bundle in a perpendicular direction (i.e., parallel to the rows of stereocilia) has no effect on the tip links and so does not cause a receptor potential.

Subtle Differences in the Physical Arrangements of Hair Cells Determine the Stimuli to Which They Are Most Sensitive

Hair cells in all parts of the labyrinth use the same basic transduction mechanism, initiated by movement of a gelatinous mass and deflection of stereocilia. The critical variable in different parts of the labyrinth is the physical coupling between the gelatinous masses and the stereocilia. This is the key: variations in the way these gelatinous masses are made up and arranged, and the way different parts of the membranous labyrinth are suspended mechanically, set up some hair cells to respond to sound, others to head movement, and still others to head position.

The Cochlear Division of the Eighth Nerve Conveys Information About Sound

The auditory system faces a basic mechanical problem: the sound vibrations that it must detect are propagated in air, whereas the auditory receptor cells (like other elements of the nervous system) live in a fluid-filled environment. Water is harder to move than air, and nearly all the sound energy incident on a simple air-water interface is reflected. Fluids in small channels like the labyrinth are even harder to move, with the result that if the auditory receptor organ (the **organ of Corti**) and its fluid surroundings were mechanically coupled to the outside world by a simple membrane, it would receive no more than 0.1% of the sound energy that fell on the membrane. One major task of the air-filled **outer** and **middle ears** (see Fig. 14-1) is therefore to transfer sound as efficiently as possible to the fluid-filled **inner ear.**

The Outer and Middle Ears Convey Airborne Vibrations to the Fluid-Filled Inner Ear

The outer ear is basically a complicated funnel consisting of the **auricle** (or **pinna**) and the **external auditory meatus** or **canal;** it conducts sound to the **tympanic membrane.** Sound-induced vibrations are then transferred along a chain of three small bones, or **ossicles,** that traverse the middle ear cavity (an air-filled cavity in the temporal bone). The handle of the **malleus** is attached to the medial surface of the tympanic membrane, so movements of this membrane are transferred directly to the malleus. The malleus in turn is attached to the **incus,** which is attached to the **stapes,** so sound-induced vibrations eventually reach the oval-shaped footplate of the stapes. The footplate of the stapes occupies a hole in the temporal bone called the **oval window;** on the other side of the oval window is the perilymph-filled vestibule of the bony labyrinth. The vestibule leads directly to the cochlea, which contains the organ of Corti. Thus, vibration of the tympanic membrane ultimately results in movement of the fluids of the inner ear.

The chain of middle ear ossicles acts as a lever system with a small mechanical advantage, so a given force at the tympanic membrane results in a slightly greater force at the footplate of the stapes. More importantly, the active, or moving, area of the tympanic membrane is about 15 times that of the footplate of the stapes. The net result of the mechanical advantage and the size difference is that stapedial vibrations have a much greater force *per unit area* of the footplate; this force is sufficient to move the perilymph, and more than 60% of the sound energy incident on the tympanic membrane is successfully transferred to the inner ear. Hence the middle ear apparatus acts as a transformer, much as an electrical transformer alters the voltage and current of a source to better match the requirements of a particular circuit. The effectiveness of this system is quite extraordinary. At a threshold of 3000 Hz (the frequency to which we are most sensitive) the tympanic membrane moves a distance somewhat less than the diameter of a single hydrogen atom.[b] By the time such a threshold vibration of the tympanic membrane reaches the

cochlear hair cells, it deflects their stereocilia through an angle of only about 0.003 degree. Bending the Empire State Building through an angle of 0.003 degree would deflect its top by less than an inch.[c] From this threshold we can hear over a 10 million–fold range of sound pressure levels before sounds become painfully loud. (Because it is cumbersome to keep track of all the zeros in such large numbers, a logarithmic **decibel** scale, as described in Box 14-1, is used to express sound pressure levels.) In addition, although human hearing is most sensitive at about 3000 Hz, the frequency range of human hearing in healthy young adults extends from about 20 to 20,000 Hz (Fig. 14-8). All this is accomplished with a surprisingly small number of nerve fibers: in contrast to the million or so axons in an optic nerve, there are only about 30,000 fibers in a human cochlear nerve. Somehow, the CNS analyzes the information carried by these 30,000 fibers, enabling us to detect and interpret the myriad sounds of nature, music, and human language.

Two tiny muscles attached to the middle ear bones modulate the transmission of vibrations to the inner ear. One, the **tensor tympani,** is attached to the handle of the malleus; when it contracts, it increases the tension on the tympanic membrane and decreases the transmission of vibrations through the ossicular chain. The other muscle, the **stapedius,** is attached to the neck of the stapes; it too decreases the transmission of vibrations when it contracts. The tensor tympani receives motor innervation from the trigeminal nerve and the stapedius from the facial nerve; both muscles are involved in certain auditory reflexes (described later).

The Cochlea Is the Auditory Part of the Labyrinth

The auditory part of the inner ear, like the vestibular part, consists of a portion of the endolymph-filled membranous labyrinth suspended within a portion of the perilymph-filled bony labyrinth.

The bony part is the cochlea, which coils through 2¾ turns from its relatively broad **base** to its **apex.** (The cochlea lies on its side in the temporal bone, with its base facing medially and posteriorly [see Fig. 14-26], but for the sake of simplicity, it is usually discussed as though it sits upright on its base.) The cochlea has a core of spongy bone called the **modiolus,** from which the **osseous spiral lamina** projects like the threads of a screw (Fig. 14-9). A winding cavity within the modiolus parallels the spiral lamina and houses the **spiral ganglion,** which contains the cell bodies of the auditory primary afferent fibers. The central processes of these cells collect at the base of the cochlea to form the

---

[b]This is as sensitive as an ear can usefully be made. Under ideal conditions in a very quiet setting, blood can be heard flowing through the vessels near the ear. If ears were much more sensitive, we would be distracted by hearing noise generated by air molecules colliding with the tympanic membrane.

[c]An Americanization of an Eiffel Tower analogy presented by A. J. Hudspeth in *Nature* 341:397, 1989.

BOX 14-1

The Frequency and Intensity Range of Human Hearing

Because the range of sound levels over which we have useful hearing is so vast, a logarithmic scale has been devised to indicate the volume of one sound relative to some standard. The unit in this scale as originally defined is the **bel,** named for Alexander Graham Bell, the inventor of the telephone:

$$\text{intensity (in bels)} = \log\frac{I}{I_0} \quad [14\text{-}1]$$

where I is the intensity of the sound in question and I_0 is a reference intensity (usually the threshold for normal hearing).

Bels are big units, representing large changes in sound intensities, so tenths of bels, or **decibels (dB),** are used instead:

$$\text{intensity (in dB)} = 10\log\frac{I}{I_0} \quad [14\text{-}2]$$

In practice, it is much easier to measure the pressure level of a sound than its intensity. Because intensity is proportional to the square of the pressure, decibels are 20 times the log of the pressure ratio (seemingly contrary to the implication of the term *deci*bel):

$$dB = 10\log\frac{I}{I_0} = 10\log\frac{P^2}{P_0^2} = 20\log\frac{P}{P_0} \quad [14\text{-}3]$$

where P is the pressure of the sound in question and P_0 is a reference pressure (usually the threshold for normal hearing).

So a sound pressure level 10 million times greater than threshold is 140 dB above threshold (see Fig. 14-8):

$$20\log\frac{10^7}{1} = 20\times 7 = 140\,dB \quad [14\text{-}4]$$

Multiple mechanical properties of the outer, middle, and inner ears collaborate to determine the sensitivity of ears to sounds of various frequencies. The combined result of all these factors is that we are most sensitive in the 1000- to 3000-Hz range important for spoken language, somewhat less sensitive at higher frequencies, and much less sensitive at lower frequencies (see Fig. 14-8).

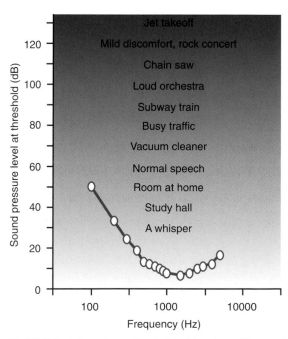

Figure 14-8 Variation of the threshold of hearing with sound frequency, expressed as decibels relative to the threshold sound pressure level at the most effective frequency. The decibel levels of a variety of sounds are indicated on the same scale. Exposure to sounds of 90 dB or greater for periods of less than 8 hours can cause permanent cochlear damage. *(Courtesy Dr. Theodore J. Glattke, University of Arizona.)*

cochlear division of the eighth nerve; the peripheral processes pass in bundles through a series of canals in the osseous spiral lamina to innervate the auditory receptors.

The cochlear duct (the auditory portion of the membranous labyrinth) is firmly anchored to the bony labyrinth in such a way that the duct is triangular in cross section (see Fig. 14-9C). One corner of the triangle is attached to the osseous spiral lamina, and the other two corners are attached to the outer wall of the bony cochlea. The result is that the cochlear duct and osseous spiral lamina act as a partition between two perilymphatic spaces (except at the apex of the cochlea, where perilymph can pass from one space to the other through a small opening called the **helicotrema** [Greek for "the hole in the spiral"]). The perilymphatic space above the cochlear duct is called **scala vestibuli** because it is directly continuous with the perilymph of the vestibule. The space below the cochlear duct is called **scala tympani** because it ends blindly at the **round window membrane** (also called the **secondary tympanic membrane**). The space enclosed by the cochlear duct is filled with endolymph and is called **scala media.** Each of the three walls of the cochlear duct has a different structure (see Fig. 14-9D). The thin **vestibular** (or **Reissner's**) **membrane** borders scala vestibuli and probably serves mainly as a diffusion barrier between the endolymph and perilymph, playing no great role in the mechanical properties of the cochlea. The **spiral ligament,**

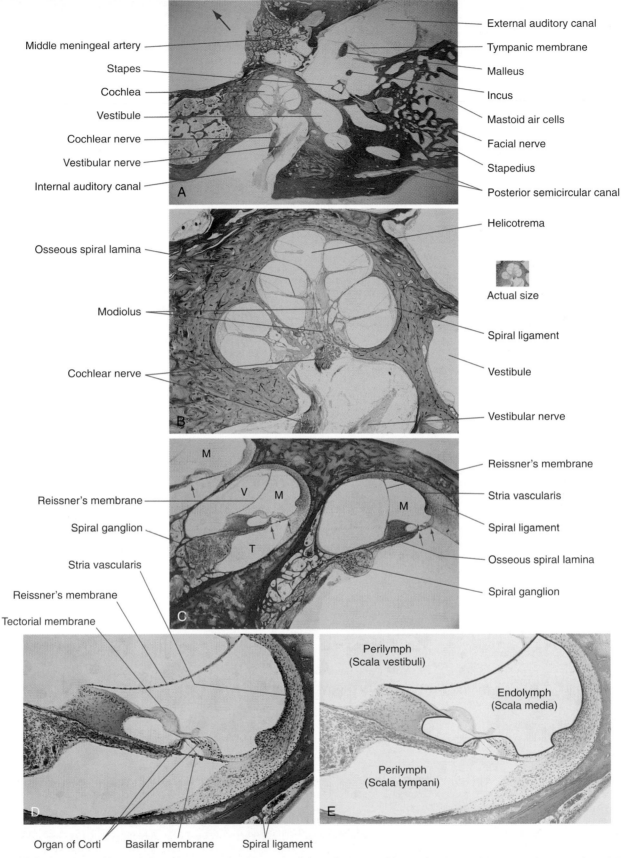

Figure 14-9 The temporal bone and cochlea. **A,** Horizontal section of the right temporal bone of a 39-year-old woman, shown at about 2.5 times actual size. The section was rotated slightly counterclockwise so that the orientation of the cochlea would correspond to that in other parts of the figure; anterior is indicated by the *arrow*. **B,** Enlarged view of the cochlea in **A. C,** One side of another human cochlea, cutting through scala media (M) three times; the basal turn is toward the lower right, the apical turn toward the upper left. The width of the basilar membrane *(arrows)* increases progressively going from the base to the apex. T, scala tympani; V, scala vestibuli. **D** and **E,** Enlargement of scala media from the middle turn of the section in **C.** The blue line in **E** indicates the location of the band of junctional complexes that restrict diffusion between endolymph and perilymph. *(A and B, courtesy Dr. David L. Asher. C to E, courtesy Dr. Allen L. Bell, University of New England College of Osteopathic Medicine.)*

thickened periosteal tissue adhering to the inner surface of the bony cochlea, forms the second wall. It includes on its endolymph-facing surface the **stria vascularis,** a specialized secretory epithelium that produces most of the endolymph in the membranous labyrinth. Finally, the **basilar membrane** spans the gap between the edge of the osseous spiral lamina and the spiral ligament, completing the "floor" of the cochlear duct and separating scala media from scala tympani.

Vibrations reaching the stapes footplate are transferred to the perilymph of the vestibule, adjacent to scala vestibuli. Although perilymph is incompressible, the round window membrane is elastic, allowing these vibrations to enter the labyrinth. When the stapes footplate moves inward, the round window membrane bulges out; when the footplate moves outward, the membrane is drawn inward. In the process, small quantities of perilymph are displaced within the cochlea. Most of this energy passes directly from scala vestibuli to scala tympani, deforming the cochlear duct (Fig. 14-10). The cochlear duct contains the auditory receptors, and this deformation stimulates some of them. Static pressure changes and vibrations of very low frequency simply move a little perilymph through the helicotrema and do not deform the cochlear duct.

Traveling Waves in the Basilar Membrane Stimulate Hair Cells in the Organ of Corti, in Locations That Depend on Sound Frequency

Three basic parameters that must be encoded by the auditory system during its initial analysis of a sound are the intensity, frequency, and location of the stimulus. The intensity of a sound, like intensity in other sensory systems, is coded by the rate of action potential firing in populations of nerve fibers and by the numbers of nerve fibers responding. Frequency is indicated largely by the particular part of the organ of Corti that is most active, through a mechanism described shortly. Analysis of the location of a sound, as discussed later in this chapter, depends heavily on a comparison of sounds reaching the two ears and so is accomplished in the CNS.

The organ of Corti (Figs. 14-11 and 14-12) is a strip of hair cells and supporting cells about 35 mm long that rests on the basilar membrane. The hair cells are arranged in two groups: a single row of about 3500 **inner hair cells** near the edge of the osseous spiral lamina and a band of about 15,000 **outer hair cells** three to five cells wide, directly above the flexible basilar membrane. The two groups are separated by a perilymphatic space called the **tunnel of Corti,** through which the peripheral processes

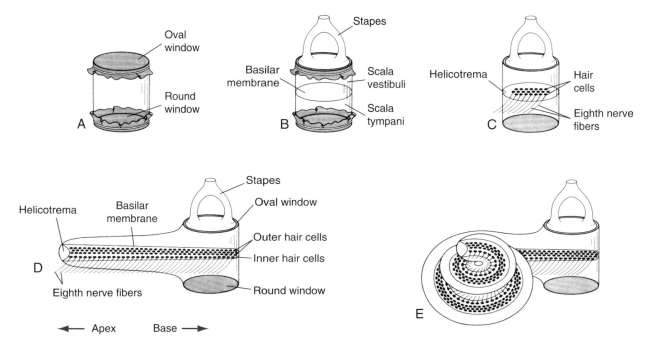

Figure 14-10 Building a cochlea, step by step. **A,** The bony cochlea is represented by a rigid cylinder; its contents of perilymph, cochlear duct, and endolymph by fluid; and the oval and round windows by two elastic membranes; pushing on one of the membranes displaces some fluid and causes the other membrane to bulge out. **B,** Added are a piston-like stapes to push or pull on the oval window and an interposed, elastic basilar membrane (representing scala media). Now, pushing on the stapes displaces not only the round window membrane but also the basilar membrane. **C,** Hair cells are added to the basilar membrane, and a helicotrema connects the scala vestibuli and scala tympani. Pushing quickly on the stapes still displaces both the basilar and round window membranes, but a steady push or pull causes perilymph to move slowly through the helicotrema and allows the basilar membrane to resume its initial position. **D,** Stretching out the basilar membrane and making it narrower near the oval and round windows provides an array of hair cells coupled to sections of the basilar membrane with differing resonant frequencies. **E,** Coiling up the elongated cochlea completes the model. *(Redrawn from Kiang NYS: Stimulus representation in the discharge patterns of auditory neurons. In Tower DB, editor: The nervous system, vol 3, New York, 1975, Raven Press.)*

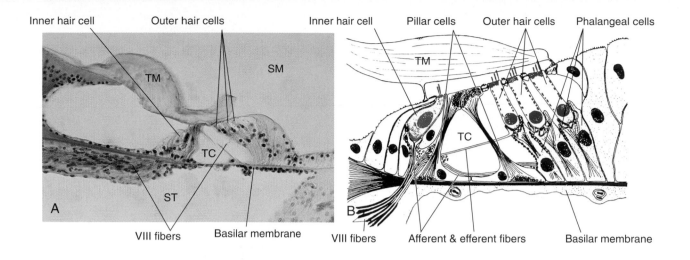

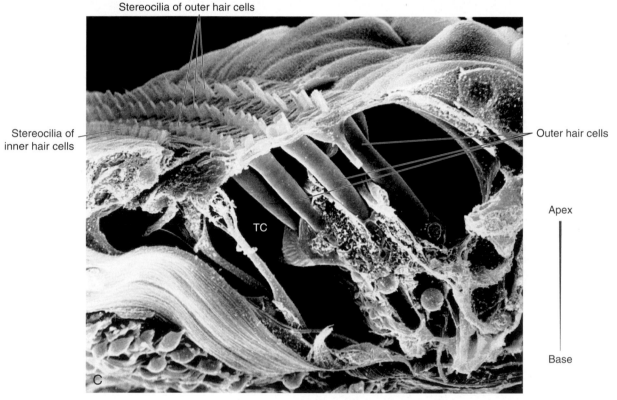

Figure 14-11 Structure of the organ of Corti. **A,** Light micrograph of a human organ of Corti (enlarged from Fig. 14-9D). **B,** Drawing of a cross section of the organ of Corti. Of the several types of supporting cells in the organ of Corti, two in particular make major contributions to its mechanical stability. The pillar cells produce microtubule-filled processes (see Fig. 14-12A) that frame the tunnel of Corti (TC). The phalangeal cells (Deiters' cells) form cup-shaped, microtubule-filled structures that support the outer hair cells (see Fig. 14-12B); thin processes of these cells also extend to the tops of the outer hair cells, where their platelike expansions fill the spaces between outer hair cells, forming the reticular lamina. **C,** Scanning electron micrograph of the organ of Corti of a guinea pig. The tectorial membrane has been removed, and the stereocilia of the three rows of outer hair cells can be seen protruding into scala media; normally these stereocilia would be embedded in the tectorial membrane. No inner hair cells are present in this view, but their stereocilia can also be seen protruding into scala media. To the right of **C,** the actual size of an unrolled basilar membrane is shown. SM, scala media; ST, scala tympani; TM, tectorial membrane. *(A, courtesy Dr. Allen L. Bell, University of New England College of Osteopathic Medicine. B, from Northern JL: Hearing disorders, ed 2, Boston, 1984, Little, Brown. C, from Bredberg G: In Evans EF, Wilson JP, editors: Psychophysics and physiology of hearing, New York, 1977, Academic Press.)*

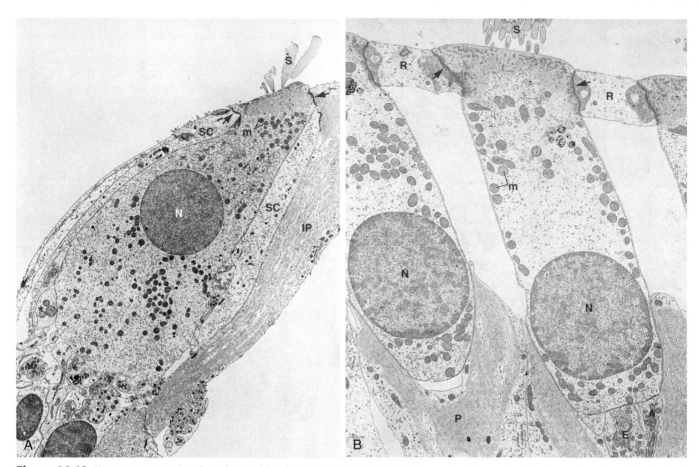

Figure 14-12 Electron micrographs of monkey cochlear hair cells. **A,** Inner hair cells have a flask-shaped cell body, round nucleus (N), abundant mitochondria (m), and the expected tuft of stereocilia (S) protruding into scala media. The cell body is flanked by supporting cells (SC), and at its base the cell makes synaptic contacts with endings of eighth nerve fibers (*). Nearby, a microtubule-filled process of a special kind of supporting cell, an inner pillar cell (IP), forms one side of the tunnel of Corti. Junctional complexes *(arrows)* near the apex of the inner hair cell separate the endolymph of scala media from the perilymph in the rest of the organ of Corti. **B,** Outer hair cells also have abundant mitochondria (m) and round nuclei (N), but their cell bodies are cylindrical and exposed directly to perilymph-filled extracellular spaces. The bases of the cells form synaptic contacts with both afferent (A) and efferent (E) nerve endings and are supported by cup-shaped, microtubule-rich processes of phalangeal cells (P). Thin processes (not seen in this section) of the phalangeal cells end as platelike expansions attached by junctional complexes *(arrows)* to the tops of the outer hair cells, forming the reticular lamina (R) that mechanically supports the top of this part of the organ of Corti. *(From Kimura RS: Sensory and accessory epithelia of the cochlea. In Friedmann I, Ballantyne J, editors: Ultrastructural atlas of the inner ear, London, 1984, Butterworths.)*

of eighth nerve fibers must pass on their way to the outer hair cells. The stereocilia of the outer hair cells are inserted into the gelatinous **tectorial membrane,** so that vibration of the basilar membrane causes oscillations of the hairs and therefore oscillation of the membrane potential of the hair cells. The stereocilia of the inner hair cells, in contrast, are not attached to the tectorial membrane; these hair cells apparently are stimulated directly by endolymph squirting back and forth through the narrow space between their tops and the tectorial membrane.

A pressure pulse delivered to scala vestibuli by movement of the stapes causes a **traveling wave** of deformation to move along the basilar membrane (Fig. 14-13A and B), much as waves spread from the site of a pebble dropped into a body of water. However, because the mechanical properties of the basilar membrane vary progressively along its length, the traveling wave reaches

its peak amplitude at a location that depends on the frequency of the stimulus. The basilar membrane is about 100 μm wide and relatively stiff at the base of the cochlea, and about 500 μm wide and relatively floppy at the apex (see Fig. 14-11, inset). The entire basilar membrane, from the base to the apex of the cochlea, responds to intense low-frequency sounds, but closer to threshold it is driven most effectively by sounds of progressively higher frequencies as one moves from the apex to the base of the cochlea (see Fig. 14-13C). Because the organ of Corti (which contains the auditory receptor cells) rests on the basilar membrane, different receptor cells respond best to sounds of different frequencies.[d] Individual eighth nerve fibers respond to a broad range of

---

[d]Low frequencies vibrate large extents of the basilar membrane and additional information about low frequencies is provided by multiple eighth nerve fibers all firing in phase with the sound wave.

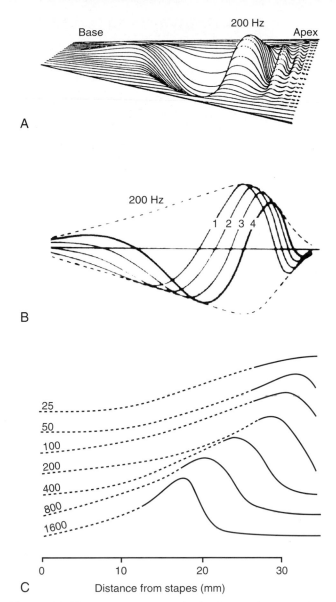

Figure 14-13 Traveling waves in the basilar membrane. **A,** Three-dimensional representation of the displacement of a model basilar membrane at one instant in time during the traveling wave in response to a 200-Hz vibration. (The amplitude of the displacement is greatly exaggerated for clarity.) **B,** The displacements seen along the longitudinal midline of a human basilar membrane at a series of successive instants (1 to 4) in response to a 200-Hz tone. The *dashed* lines show the envelope of the displacements over time. Individual traveling waves move from the base to the apex of the cochlea, but their envelope has a maximum at one point along the length of the basilar membrane. **C,** The envelopes of the traveling waves produced by tones of successively higher frequency peak progressively closer to the base of the cochlea. (**A,** *from Tonndorf J: J Acoust Soc Am 32:238, 1960.* **B** *and* **C,** *redrawn from von Békésy G: Experiments in hearing, New York, 1960, McGraw-Hill.)*

frequencies when the sound is intense but are sharply tuned to a narrow range of frequencies at threshold (see Fig. 14-15). This mechanical tuning of the basilar membrane is the beginning of a **tonotopic organization** within the auditory system, analogous to the somatotopic organization of the somatosensory system and the

retinotopic organization of the visual system; in this case, particular frequencies are mapped in an orderly fashion onto particular areas of relay nuclei and auditory cortex of the temporal lobe (see Fig. 14-19).

Cochlear implants take advantage of this tonotopic organization of the basilar membrane and its overlying hair cells. Some common forms of deafness are caused by processes that either damage cochlear hair cells or prevent their normal development, leaving eighth nerve endings intact. In such cases, it is often possible to provide substantial auditory function by threading an array of electrodes through the round window membrane and into scala tympani, so that different electrodes in the array are located near different points along the basilar membrane. A small microphone and associated electronics can then be used to analyze the sound frequencies of auditory stimuli, break them down into different frequency bands, and stimulate endings of eighth nerve fibers at tonotopically appropriate levels. In many cases, such direct stimulation of cochlear nerve fibers makes nearly normal speech perception possible. Deaf infants who receive cochlear implants often develop speech that is indistinguishable from that of infants with normal hearing.

Inner Hair Cells Are Sensory Cells; Outer Hair Cells Are Amplifiers

Hints about the roles played by the inner and outer hair cells are provided by their patterns of innervation (Fig. 14-14; see also Fig. 14-21). Even though there are many more outer than inner hair cells, about 90% to 95% of all cochlear nerve fibers receive their entire input from single inner hair cells. A single inner hair cell typically synapses on about 10 different auditory afferents. This is the beginning of the remarkably economical use of neurons in peripheral parts of the auditory system: in contrast to the 100 million photoreceptors per retina and the 3 million olfactory receptors per nostril, the output of each cochlea starts out as the output of a relatively minuscule population of 3500 inner hair cells. The remaining 5% to 10% of the auditory afferents branch repeatedly, and each innervates many outer hair cells.

Outer hair cells do something completely different. The function of the small population of afferents that innervate them is largely unknown but not critical. However, the sensitivity of individual cochlear nerve fibers (conveying information from inner hair cells) at their preferred frequencies is much greater than can be accounted for by the mechanical tuning of different parts of the basilar membrane—greater by more than a thousand-fold for some fibers (Fig. 14-15A). This means that some active process must add energy to the vibration of the basilar membrane in the area of maximum amplitude of the traveling wave (see Fig. 14-15B). The source of this added energy is the outer hair cells, which use the energy in their receptor potentials to change

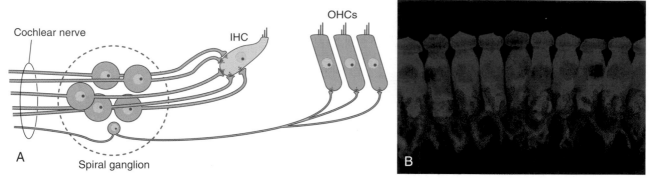

Figure 14-14 Innervation of cochlear hair cells by sensory endings. **A,** Most spiral ganglion cells send afferent terminals to individual inner hair cells (IHC). A few smaller cells send branched endings to multiple outer hair cells (OHCs). **B,** Three-dimensional reconstructions built from double immuno-fluorescence micrographs, demonstrating the sensory innervation of mouse inner hair cells. Inner hair cells (green fluorescence), each about 10 μm across, were stained with an antibody against calretinin, a calcium-binding protein found in these cells. Staining afferent endings (red fluorescence) with a different antibody specific for these endings reveals numerous sensory terminals at the base of each hair cell. **(B,** courtesy Dr. Sonja Pyott, University of North Carolina–Wilmington, and Dr. Richard W. Aldrich, University of Texas at Austin.)

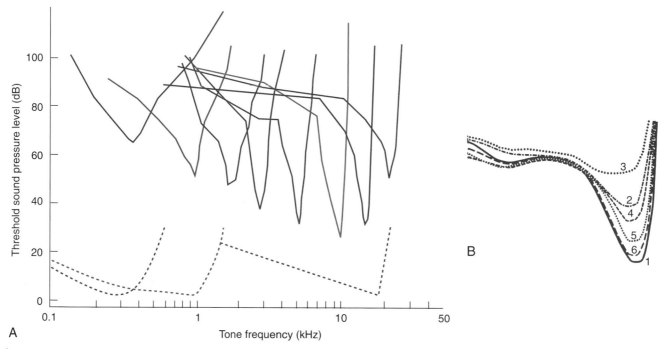

Figure 14-15 Tuning of the frequency response of individual cochlear nerve fibers by a combination of the mechanical properties of the basilar membrane and an active amplification mechanism. **A,** Threshold versus frequency plots for eight different guinea pig cochlear nerve fibers. Each responds over a range that extends far into the low frequencies if sound is loud, but has a much narrower range of maximum sensitivity. The dotted curves at the bottom show the expected mechanical tuning of the basilar membrane (on an arbitrary scale); all three lack the sharply tuned portion of the curves demonstrated for cochlear nerve fibers. **B,** The tuning curve of a single eighth nerve fiber of a cat before (1) and during (2, 3) instillation of a metabolic inhibitor (potassium cyanide) into the inner ear. The sharply tuned portion of the tuning curve is lost, indicating that it depends on some active metabolic process. After washing out the cyanide, the sharp tuning is regained (4 to 6). **(A,** redrawn from Evans EF: J Physiol 226:263, 1972. **B,** from Evans EF, Klinke R: J Physiol 242:129P, 1974.)

length (Fig. 14-16). Near threshold, these mechanical oscillations amplify basilar membrane vibrations, in turn increasing the mechanical stimulation of the inner hair cells and increasing the magnitude of their receptor potentials. Consistent with this, certain ototoxic drugs that selectively destroy the outer hair cells cause the auditory threshold to rise by a factor of 10^3 to 10^4 (a hearing loss of 60 to 80 dB).

If motion of the outer hair cells can enhance the vibration of the basilar membrane, it might be expected that these vibrations could travel backward through the perilymph and middle ear ossicles to vibrate the tympanic membrane slightly. A vibrating tympanic membrane would behave like a tiny loudspeaker, producing sound. This sound can in fact be recorded as **otoacoustic emissions** (Fig. 14-17). For several milliseconds after the

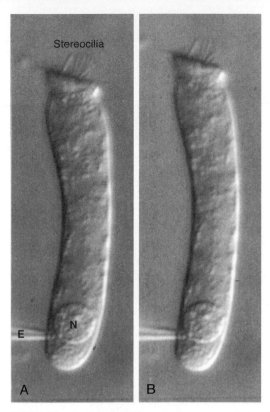

Figure 14-16 Electrically induced length changes in an isolated outer hair cell from a guinea pig. A microelectrode was used to depolarize **(A)** and hyperpolarize **(B)** the cell, causing it to shorten and lengthen. E, electrode; N, nucleus. *(Courtesy Dr. Matthew Holley, University of Sheffield.)*

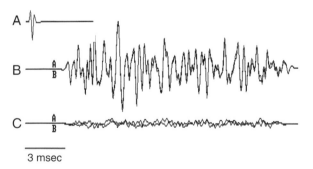

3 msec

Figure 14-17 Otoacoustic emissions. In response to 82-dB clicks **(A)** delivered to the right ear, that ear emits sound of about 19-dB sound pressure level for about 15 msec **(B).** In contrast, a similar click delivered to the same patient's left ear elicits no otoacoustic emissions **(C)**, indicating damage to the middle ear apparatus or outer hair cells. Both **B** and **C** show superimposed average responses to two series of 1000 clicks (A and B), demonstrating how reproducible the response is. *(Courtesy Dr. Theodore J. Glattke, University of Arizona.)*

arrival of a brief sound ("click") at the ear, a sensitive microphone in the external auditory canal can detect faint sounds, up to about 20 dB, emitted by the ear itself. These are sounds coming from the resulting vibrations of the tympanic membrane in response to the outer hair cells amplifying the initial "click" input. Because the production of otoacoustic emissions requires a normal

middle ear, as well as inner ear function up to and including the outer hair cells, it is now the basis of important audiological tests. Measuring otoacoustic emissions is particularly useful to screen for hearing problems in newborns.

Auditory Information Is Distributed Bilaterally in the CNS

Auditory primary afferents, whose cell bodies are located in the spiral ganglion of the modiolus, enter the brainstem at the pontomedullary junction. There each fiber bifurcates and sends one branch to the **dorsal cochlear nucleus** and one branch to the **ventral cochlear nucleus.** These cochlear nuclei form a continuous band of cells that covers the dorsal and lateral aspects of the inferior cerebellar peduncle (Fig. 14-18, lower inset).

Sensory systems characteristically analyze multiple aspects of a stimulus, such as the color and brightness of a visual stimulus or the shape and texture of a somatosensory stimulus. Similarly, the auditory system analyzes things such as the frequency (perceived as pitch), intensity, and location of a sound. Some aspects of this auditory analysis are initiated in the cochlea and involve a fairly straightforward CNS pathway (see Fig. 14-18), but determining the location of a sound source involves additional processing at the level of the brainstem.

Some fibers from the cochlear nuclei (mainly from the dorsal cochlear nucleus) loop over the top of the inferior cerebellar peduncle, cross the midline with a rostral inclination, and join the **lateral lemniscus,** the major ascending auditory pathway of the brainstem. The lateral lemniscus is somewhat diffuse as it forms in the caudal pons, but in the rostral pons it forms a flattened band (the Greek word *lemniskos* means "ribbon") on the lateral surface of the tegmentum. A smaller number of axons leaving the cochlear nuclei do not cross the midline but instead join the ipsilateral lateral lemniscus; hence each lateral lemniscus carries some information from both ears. Rather than heading straight for the thalamus, virtually all fibers of the lateral lemniscus terminate in the inferior colliculus. The inferior colliculus then projects bilaterally through the **brachium** (Latin for "arm") **of the inferior colliculus** (or **inferior brachium**), which travels along the surface of the brainstem to the **medial geniculate nucleus,** a portion of the thalamus that protrudes in a posterior direction, overlapping the midbrain. Fibers from the medial geniculate nucleus project tonotopically (Fig. 14-19) to the primary auditory cortex, located in the **transverse temporal gyri (of Heschl)** on the superior surface of the temporal lobe, mostly buried in the lateral sulcus (see Fig. 14-18, upper inset).

A much larger number of fibers leave the ventral cochlear nucleus and pass beneath the inferior cerebellar peduncle. Some join the lateral lemniscus of each

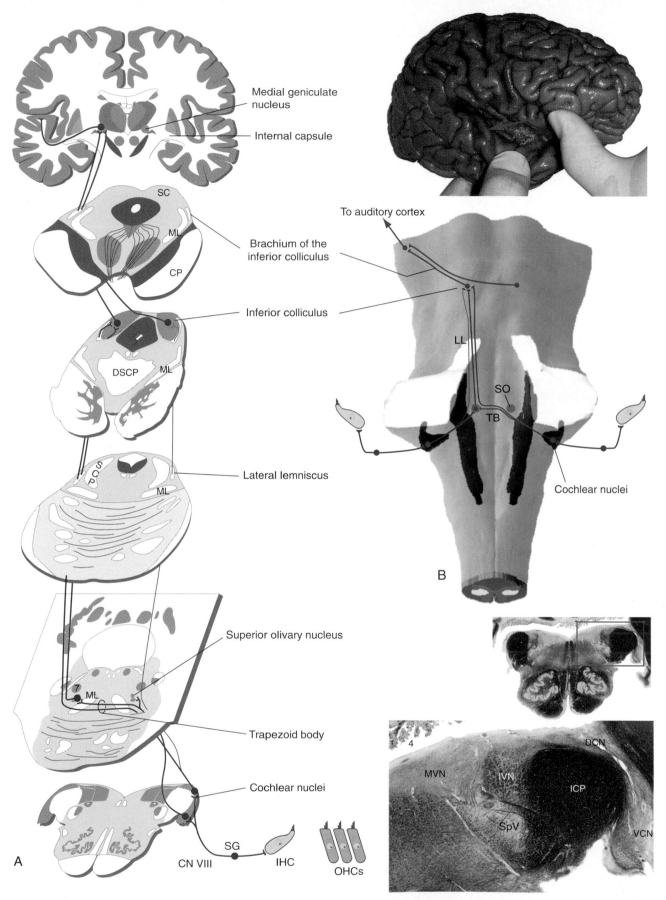

Figure 14-18 The ascending auditory pathway, as seen in a series of cross sections **(A)** showing the projections emanating from one cochlea and in a three-dimensional reconstruction **(B)** showing the way both ears are represented in each lateral lemniscus. Fibers representing one ear are shown in bright blue; fibers representing both ears in dark blue. The lower inset shows a dorsolateral quadrant of the brainstem at the pontomedullary junction. The upper inset shows the location of primary auditory cortex *(arrow)* in the transverse temporal (Heschl's) gyrus (or in the more anterior gyrus, in cases like this one with two gyri). 4, fourth ventricle; 7, facial motor nucleus; CP, cerebral peduncle; DCN, dorsal cochlear nucleus; DSCP, decussation of the superior cerebellar peduncles; ICP, inferior cerebellar peduncle; IHC, inner hair cell; IVN, inferior vestibular nucleus (see Fig. 14-29); LL, lateral lemniscus; ML, medial lemniscus; MVN, medial vestibular nucleus (see Fig. 14-29); OHC, outer hair cell; SC, superior colliculus; SCP, superior cerebellar peduncle; SG, spiral ganglion; SO, superior olivary nucleus; SpV, spinal trigeminal nucleus; TB, trapezoid body; VCN, ventral cochlear nucleus.

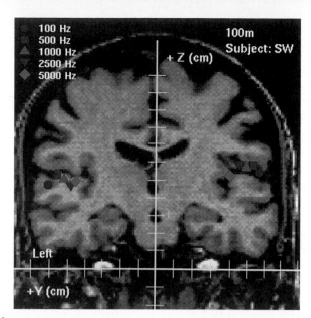

Figure 14-19 Tonotopic mapping in human primary auditory cortex, demonstrated by applying 500-msec tone bursts at five different sound frequencies to one ear while mapping the magnetic field changes produced by neuronal current flow in primary auditory cortex. *(Adapted from Cansino S, Williamson SJ, Karron D: Brain Res 663:38, 1994.)*

side and proceed to the inferior colliculus. Many, however, are involved in sound localization and end in the **superior olivary nucleus,** at the rostral end of the facial motor nucleus in the pons. There are two general strategies that can be used to localize sounds coming from the left or the right, and the superior olivary complex contains a medial and a lateral subnucleus corresponding to these two strategies. A sound coming from the left reaches the left ear slightly before it reaches the right ear. In addition, because the head creates a "shadow" for high-frequency sounds, the sound may be a little bit more intense at the left ear. Sound localization can therefore be accomplished by comparing the time of arrival and the intensity of a sound at the two ears.[e] The time-of-arrival comparison, which is begun in the medial superior olive, is more effective for low frequencies and for terrestrial animals with relatively large heads

(like humans). Humans have a correspondingly large medial superior olive and small lateral superior olive. Fibers from the ventral cochlear nuclei of both sides converge on the medial superior olive of each side, providing the anatomical substrate for binaural comparison. Crossing from one cochlear nucleus to the contralateral superior olivary nucleus occurs in the **trapezoid body,** a large collection of second-order fibers that pass through and ventral to the medial lemnisci.[f] Each superior olivary nucleus then projects through the lateral lemniscus to the ipsilateral inferior colliculus.

Each lateral lemniscus thus conveys information from both ears, because the cochlear nuclei project bilaterally and because the superior olive receives bilateral input. One consequence is that damage to the auditory pathway at any level rostral to the cochlear nuclei does not cause deafness in either ear. Rather, it causes problems with localizing sounds and may cause difficulties in separating sounds from background noise.

Activity in the Ascending Auditory Pathway Generates Electrical Signals That Can Be Measured From the Scalp

A brief sound causes a series of electrical waves, in the nanovolt range, that can be recorded from the surface of the head. The signals are so small that they are normally buried in background electrical noise, but when the same brief stimulus is presented many times and the responses are averaged; the waves can be measured reproducibly. Early peaks of the waveform represent electrical activity in the eighth nerve arriving at the cochlear nuclei, and later peaks represent combined activity at successive sites in the auditory pathway. Because this pathway extends from the pontomedullary junction to the temporal lobes, abnormalities in the **brainstem auditory evoked response** can be helpful in localizing lesions (Fig. 14-20).

Efferents Control the Sensitivity of the Cochlea

The sensitivity of all sensory systems is monitored and regulated by the CNS, often resulting in a reflex as seen with a deep tendon reflex in the somatosensory system. This reflex always involves control of synaptic transmission at various CNS sites, and in some sensory systems it also involves effects on the receptor organs themselves. Examples of the latter include projections to intrafusal muscle fibers (see Fig. 9-14) and to the pupillary sphincter (see Fig. 17-39). The auditory system also uses this strategy by controlling both middle ear muscles and hair cells themselves.

---

[e]This method works well for determining the horizontal position of a sound but is of little help in telling up from down or front from behind. Some animals (e.g., owls) have one ear located higher than the other, so that even sounds in the sagittal plane affect the two ears differently. Most animals with symmetrically placed ears (e.g., cats and dogs) can create interaural differences by moving one or the other auricle or by cocking their heads. Humans take advantage of the fact that sounds coming from different directions in the sagittal plane are distorted in characteristic ways by the auricle. For example, high frequencies are attenuated more by the auricle when coming from behind the head than when coming from in front. The CNS apparently compares what something sounds like to what it ought to sound like and uses this comparison to help determine elevation.

---

[f]Historically, the term *trapezoid body* was used to refer to the trapezoid-shaped area of the brainstem containing both the medial lemnisci and the crossing auditory fibers. The term is now used in a functional sense, referring only to the crossing auditory fibers.

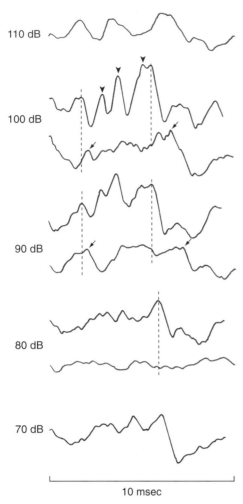

Figure 14-20 Brainstem auditory evoked responses to sounds presented to the right (red traces) or left (blue traces) ear of a 42-year-old man who complained of hearing loss in his left ear. Sounds in the right ear elicited a response with a series of well-defined peaks *(arrowheads, dashed lines)* at normal latencies. Using two of these peaks as reference points *(dashed lines)*, it can be seen that the corresponding peaks elicited by sounds in the left ear *(arrows)* were smaller and delayed. This patient had an acoustic neuroma (see Fig. 14-22D). *(Courtesy Dr. Theodore J. Glattke, University of Arizona.)*

Middle Ear Muscles Contract in Response to Loud Sounds

As noted earlier, contraction of the stapedius stiffens the ossicular chain and alters the transmission of vibrations. When a loud sound enters one ear, both stapedius muscles contract as part of an **acoustic reflex;** an individual with a damaged facial nerve may complain that sounds are too loud in the ipsilateral ear (a condition known as **hyperacusis**). The pathway involved is from one ventral cochlear nucleus to both superior olivary nuclei and from there to both facial motor nuclei. It is possible to test this reflex arc in a useful clinical procedure. When the stapedius contracts, less low-frequency sound energy incident on the eardrum is transferred along the ossicular chain, and more is reflected back

from the eardrum. By measuring changes in the amount of a test sound reflected back from one eardrum after a loud sound is introduced into the ipsilateral or contralateral ear, the acoustic reflex can be analyzed quantitatively.

The physiological function of the acoustic reflex is a matter of some dispute. The traditional view is that it protects the inner ear from damage caused by excessively loud sounds. Clearly this works only for continuous noise, because a brief loud sound (e.g., a gunshot) would damage the ear before the stapedius could contract. However, no continuous noise of sufficient intensity to activate the reflex exists in nature, except near large waterfalls. A second view of the reflex is that it helps the inner ear extract meaningful sounds from noisy backgrounds. Stapedial contraction selectively impedes the transmission of *low frequencies* and so can selectively reduce the effects of low-frequency noise.

The function of the tensor tympani in auditory processes is less clear. This muscle too is activated bilaterally in some individuals in response to a loud sound in one ear, but only if the sound is extremely loud. However, the tensor tympani contracts bilaterally in response to something touching the face, in response to startling stimuli (auditory or not), and before speech production or chewing; it may have a role in filtering out self-generated noise. The tensor tympani muscle is innervated by the mandibular (V_3) division of the trigeminal nerve.

Different Sets of Efferents Control Outer Hair Cells and the Afferent Endings on Inner Hair Cells

Some neurons of the superior olivary nucleus have axons that, rather than projecting through the lateral lemniscus, join the vestibular division of the eighth nerve. Near the cochlea, these fibers transfer to the cochlear division and then project to the organ of Corti. Just as inner and outer hair cells have different patterns of afferent innervation (see Fig. 14-14), they are also affected in distinctive ways by different sets of **olivocochlear** neurons (Fig. 14-21). Those from the lateral superior olive end on the afferent nerve endings at the bases of inner hair cells, primarily in the ipsilateral cochlea; their role in normal hearing is not understood.[g] Efferents from the medial superior olive instead project bilaterally to outer hair cells, where they make inhibitory synapses. These medial olivocochlear neurons form the efferent limb of a reflex that suppresses the contractility of outer hair cells in the presence of *high-frequency* noise, including the frequencies important for speech perception (see Fig. 14-21C).

---

[g]The *afferent* fibers innervating outer hair cells are unmyelinated and have small diameters. In this sense they are similar to the afferents that convey nociceptive signals, and there is some evidence that their signals initiate reflex responses by the lateral olivocochlear neurons that help protect inner hair cell synapses from noise-induced damage.

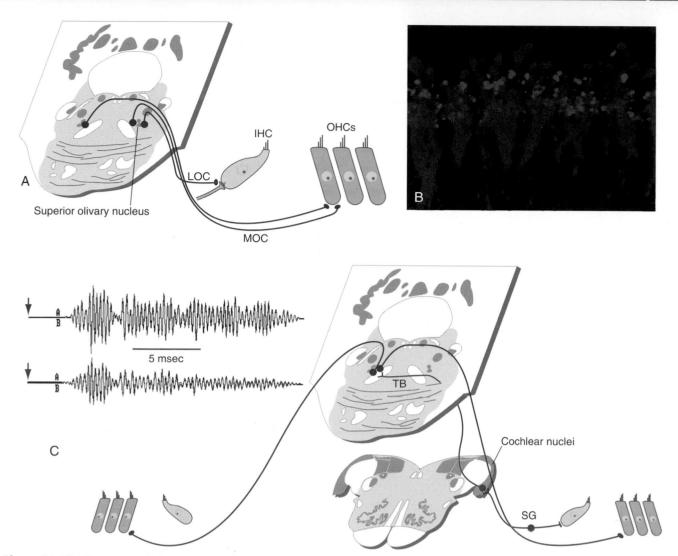

Figure 14-21 Efferent control of cochlear hair cells. **A,** The pattern of efferent innervation of inner and outer hair cells. **B,** Three-dimensional reconstructions built from double immunofluorescence micrographs, demonstrating the efferent innervation of mouse inner hair cell afferents. Afferent endings (red fluorescence) were stained as in Figure 14-14B. A second antibody (green fluorescence) to synapsin, a protein involved in transmitter release, reveals numerous efferent terminals applied to the afferent endings. **C,** Circuitry of the medial olivocochlear reflex and its effects. The upper trace shows a normal otoacoustic emission in response to clicks in an otherwise quiet room. The lower trace shows the reduced otoacoustic emission in response to the same clicks while broadband noise about as loud as a whisper was delivered to the contralateral ear. Arrows indicate the time of the clicks. IHC, inner hair cell; LOC, lateral olivocochlear efferent; MOC, medial olivocochlear efferent; OHCs, outer hair cells; SG, spiral ganglion; TB, trapezoid body. (**B,** courtesy Dr. Sonja Pyott, University of North Carolina–Wilmington, and Dr. Richard W. Aldrich, University of Texas at Austin. Traces in **C,** courtesy Dr. Theodore J. Glattke, University of Arizona.)

The resulting reduction in the inner hair cell responses to noise means that more of their response range can be devoted to detecting other sounds, such as speech, in the presence of background noise. Hence the stapedius and medial olivocochlear reflexes may have complementary roles, enhancing the ability of the auditory system to discriminate sounds in the presence of low-frequency and high-frequency noise, respectively. The same medial olivocochlear neurons receive inputs from the inferior colliculus and probably play a role in modulating the sensitivity of the organ of Corti during changes in attention.

Conductive and Sensorineural Problems Can Affect Hearing

Basic aspects of hearing can be tested simply by measuring an individual's thresholds for hearing a series of pure tones of different frequencies, presented either through earphones (**air conduction**) or by way of a vibrator applied to the mastoid process or forehead (**bone conduction**). Plotting threshold sound levels for each frequency, relative to the average thresholds for a normal population of young subjects, yields an **audiogram** (Fig. 14-22A).

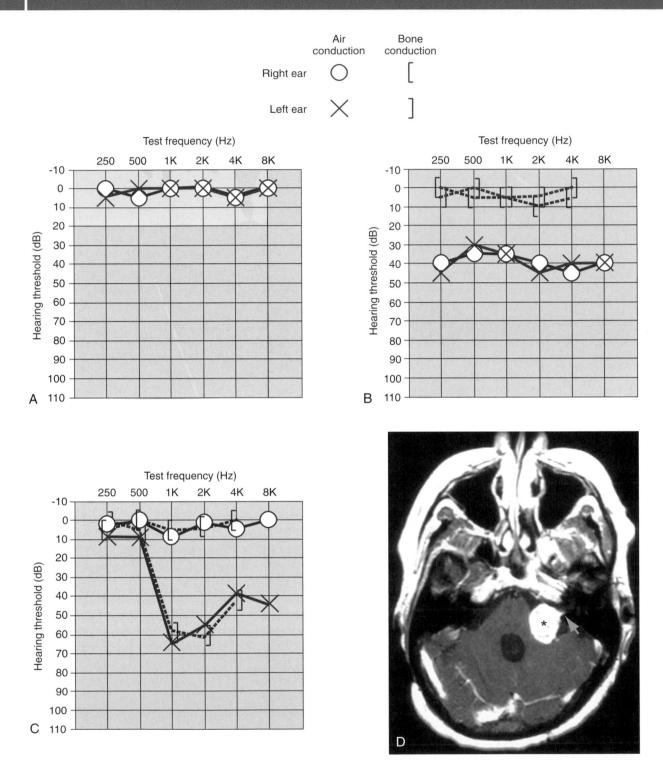

Figure 14-22 Normal and abnormal audiograms. **A,** Normal audiogram obtained with an audiometer, which compensates for the frequency dependence shown in Figure 14-8. Only the results obtained by air conduction are shown; although hearing by air conduction is normally more sensitive than hearing by bone conduction, the audiometric procedure compensates for the difference. Hence curves for hearing by bone conduction would normally be more or less superimposed on those for hearing by air conduction. Readings displaced downward from this level would indicate hearing loss (i.e., that a greater than normal sound pressure level was required for hearing at that frequency). **B,** Audiometric results for a patient with bilateral conductive hearing loss caused by chronic otitis media (middle ear infection). Hearing by bone conduction is normal, but hearing by air conduction is impaired. **C,** Audiometric results for the patient described in Figure 14-20. Hearing in the right ear is normal, but thresholds for the left ear are elevated whether air conduction or bone conduction is used. **D,** Magnetic resonance image of a 67-year-old woman with an acoustic neuroma. The tumor (*) presses against the left side of the brainstem and extends laterally *(arrow)* into the internal auditory canal. Although commonly called acoustic neuromas, these tumors are more properly referred to as vestibular schwannomas, because they usually arise from Schwann cells in the vestibular division of the eighth nerve. (*A to C, courtesy Dr. Theodore J. Glattke, University of Arizona. D, courtesy Dr. Raymond F. Carmody, University of Arizona College of Medicine.*)

Just as in the case of olfaction, two general kinds of processes can cause loss of hearing: processes that prevent sound from reaching the labyrinth (**conductive** hearing loss), and processes that damage hair cells, cochlear nerve fibers, or the cochlear nuclei (**sensorineural** hearing loss).[h] Comparing audiograms obtained by air conduction and bone conduction can often help distinguish between the two. Hearing normally by air conduction requires normal function of the outer, middle, and inner ears. Hence hearing loss measured by air conduction could be the result of damage at any of these sites. Hearing by bone conduction, in contrast, involves direct transmission of vibrations from the skull to the fluids of the inner ear, bypassing the outer and middle ears.[i] Hence hearing loss measured by bone conduction indicates a sensorineural problem. Someone who hears normally by bone conduction but not by air conduction (see Fig. 14-22B) is therefore likely to have a conductive hearing loss. Typical causes are accumulation of fluid in the middle ear as a result of infection, or bony growths that impede vibration of the middle ear ossicles (otosclerosis). In contrast, someone with hair cell damage (e.g., from ototoxic drugs such as the aminoglycoside antibiotics like gentamicin) or cochlear nerve damage (e.g., from an acoustic neuroma) would have comparable hearing losses measured by either air or bone conduction (see Fig. 14-22C).

The Vestibular Division of the Eighth Nerve Conveys Information About Linear and Angular Acceleration of the Head

One universal task for living creatures is keeping track of their orientation relative to the outside world. Mobile creatures have the added task of adjusting their orientation in response to self-generated or externally imposed movements. Vertebrates developed an adaptation to meet these needs long ago. All jawed vertebrates have basically similar vestibular labyrinths, featuring three semicircular canals on each side of the head together with two or more **otolithic organs.** In every case the three semicircular canals are approximately orthogonal

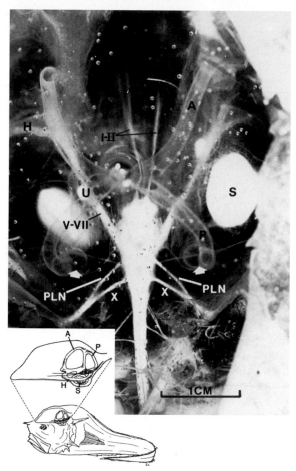

Figure 14-23 Striking illustration of the arrangement of vertebrate semicircular canals. Acanthonus armatus (drawn at the bottom left) is a species of small, deep-water fish that has particularly large semicircular canals and a particularly tiny brain. The photograph is a view into the cranial cavity from above; the orthogonally arranged anterior (A), posterior (P), and horizontal (H) semicircular canals can be seen clearly. The large otoliths of the utricle (U) and especially the saccule (S) are also evident. Each saccular otolith weighed about four times as much as the fish's entire brain. I, II, V, VII, and X are cranial nerves. The posterior lateral line nerve (PLN) innervates sensory receptors along the fish's side. *(Modified from Fine ML, Horn MH, Cox B: Proc R Soc Lond B 230:257, 1987.)*

to one another, with one in a roughly horizontal plane and the other two in more or less vertical planes (Figs. 14-23 and see 14-26). The vestibular portion of the human bony labyrinth consists of a central area called the **vestibule** and three semicircular canals—**horizontal, anterior,** and **posterior**—that are attached to the vestibule (see Figs. 14-1 and 14-2). Within each semicircular canal is a semicircular duct,[j] which is the corresponding part of the membranous labyrinth. Within the vestibule are the two otolithic organs—the utricle and the

---

[h]Because damage to the auditory pathway at levels rostral to the cochlear nuclei does not cause substantial hearing loss in either ear, sensorineural hearing loss in one ear implies damage to the cochlea, eighth nerve, or cochlear nuclei. More sophisticated tests are required to assess changes in hearing resulting from damage at more rostral sites.

[i]Most conventional hearing aids deliver amplified sound through the air conduction route. Selected patients, however, are better treated with bone-attached hearing aids. These involve a titanium screw attached to the mastoid process, a vibrating transducer snapped onto a fixture on the external end of the screw, and the direct delivery of vibrations via bone conduction.

---

[j]Although technically the term *semicircular canal* designates a part of the bony labyrinth, it is often used interchangeably to refer to either a bony semicircular canal or a membranous semicircular duct.

saccule—each a dilation of the membranous labyrinth. The semicircular ducts and otolithic organs are suspended within the bony labyrinth rather than being stretched across it like the cochlear duct. Pressure changes caused by movement of the stapes are therefore equally distributed throughout the perilymph surrounding the vestibular parts of the membranous labyrinth and do not deform them, except in certain unusual pathological conditions.

Receptors in the Semicircular Ducts Detect Angular Acceleration of the Head

Each semicircular duct communicates at both ends with the utricle. At one end of each duct is a dilation called an **ampulla.** Each ampulla contains a **crista,** a transversely oriented ridge of tissue covered by supporting cells and sensory hair cells (Fig. 14-24). As in other parts of the labyrinth, each hair cell bears a graduated array of stereocilia (here accompanied by a kinocilium) embedded in a gelatinous mass. In this case the gelatinous mass, called a **cupula,** covers the crista and extends across the ampulla as a partition. All the hair cells of a given crista are aligned with their kinocilia facing in the same direction, so deflection of the cupula in one direction causes the afferents that innervate that crista to increase their firing rate, and deflection in the opposite direction causes them to decrease their firing rate. The hair cells of the horizontal canal have their kinocilia facing the utricle, so deflecting the cupula of this canal toward the utricle causes an increased firing rate. In contrast, the hair cells of the anterior and posterior canals have their kinocilia facing away from the utricle.[k]

The most straightforward way to deflect a cupula is to rotate its semicircular duct about an axis perpendicular to it (like a wheel on an axle). As such rotation begins, the endolymph lags behind because of inertia; this motion of duct and endolymph relative to each other deflects the cupula and stimulates the hair cells (Fig. 14-25A). However, as the rotation continues, the endolymph "catches up" because of factors such as the elasticity of the cupula and friction between the endolymph and the wall of the duct, and the stimulation ceases (see Fig. 14-25B). At the end of the rotation, the endolymph continues to move for a short time (again, because of inertia), and the cupula bulges in the opposite direction (see Fig. 14-25C). Thus each semicircular canal responds best to *changes* in the speed of rotation in a particular plane (i.e., angular acceleration). Because

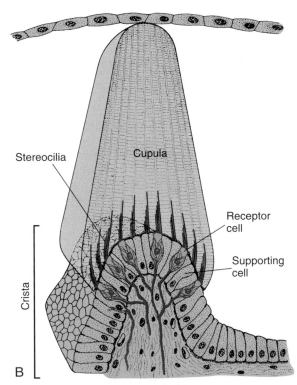

Figure 14-24 Two views of the interior of an ampulla. **A,** Arrangement of the cupula as a diaphragm across the endolymph-filled ampulla. Rotation in an appropriate plane causes endolymph to push against the cupula and deform it, which in turn causes deflection of hair cell stereocilia. **B,** Enlargement of a crista and cupula, showing the relationship of hair cells, their bundles of stereocilia, and the cupular diaphragm. (**A,** *modified from Melvill Jones G, Milsum JH: IEEE Trans Biomed Eng 12:54, 1965.* **B,** *modified from Wersäll J: Acta Otolaryngol Suppl 126:1, 1956.*)

---

[k]As in the cochlea, the vestibular division of the eighth nerve does its job with a small number of axons—only about 1600 per semicircular duct.

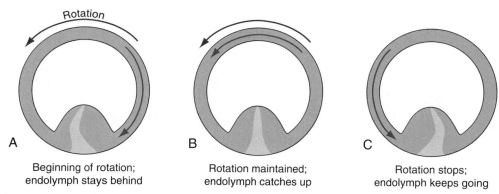

Rotation

A — Beginning of rotation; endolymph stays behind

B — Rotation maintained; endolymph catches up

C — Rotation stops; endolymph keeps going

Figure 14-25 Relative movement of semicircular ducts, endolymph, and cupula at the beginning of rotation **(A)**, during maintained rotation **(B)**, and at the end of rotation **(C)**.

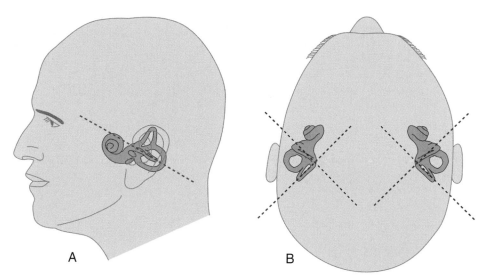

A   B

Figure 14-26 Orientation of different parts of the labyrinth, as seen from the left **(A)** and from above **(B)**. (The labyrinth is enlarged relative to the head for clarity.)

the three semicircular canals are arranged in roughly orthogonal planes (Fig. 14-26), and because most head movements have a rotational component, movement in any direction can be detected. The fact that the semicircular canals cannot detect maintained rotation is not a great disadvantage because we usually do not experience maintained rotation (except on amusement park rides).

The relative orientations of the three semicircular canals (see Fig. 14-26) dictate which canals work together. The horizontal canal, as its name implies, is roughly horizontal (actually, it is tilted backward about 30 degrees), whereas the anterior and posterior canals are roughly vertical. However, the anterior and posterior canals are also arranged at an angle of about 45 degrees to the sagittal plane. The anterior canal of one side is therefore parallel to the posterior canal of the other side, so movements that affect one will affect the other. Thus the horizontal canals of the two sides form a functional pair, whereas the anterior canal of one side forms a functional pair with the posterior canal of the other side.

Receptors in the Utricle and Saccule Detect Linear Acceleration and Position of the Head

There are no cristae in the utricle and saccule, but each has in its wall a patch of supporting cells and hair cells called a **macula.** The utricular macula, lying at the bottom of the utricle, is roughly horizontal (i.e., stereocilia pointing toward the sky) when the head is in an upright position. The saccular macula is on the medial wall of the saccule and is roughly vertical (i.e., stereocilia pointing laterally). The sensory hairs of the macular receptors are also embedded in a gelatinous membrane similar in composition to the cupula and tectorial membrane. However, in the case of each macula, the gelatinous substance also contains minute crystals of calcium carbonate called **otoconia** or **otoliths**[l] and so is

---

[l]Technically speaking, the very small crystals in the human otolithic membrane are *otoconia* (Greek for "ear dust"), whereas the somewhat larger concretions of some other vertebrates are *otoliths* (Greek for "ear stones"). However, the two terms are often used interchangeably.

Surface of hair cell   Tip of kinocilium   Bundle of stereocilia   Otoconia

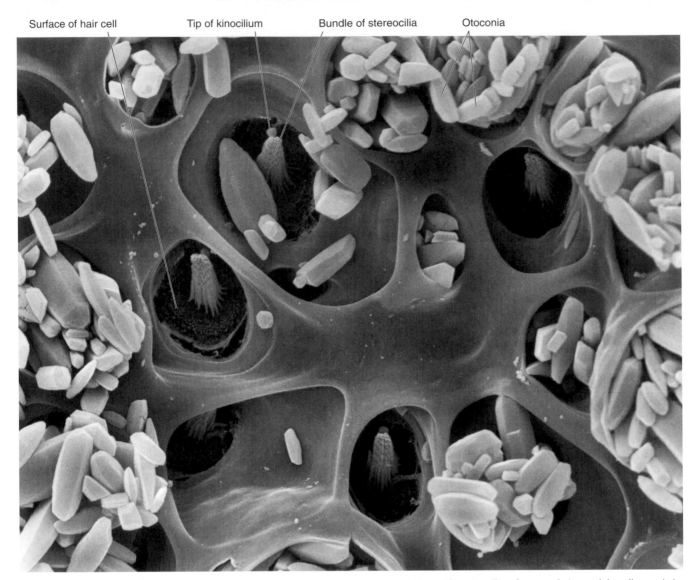

Figure 14-27 Scanning electron micrograph of the otolithic membrane of the saccule of a bullfrog. Bundles of sensory hairs, each bundle consisting of a single kinocilium and numerous stereocilia, can be seen projecting from individual hair cells into holes in the otolithic membrane. These holes are enlarged as a result of preparation for electron microscopy; in life the hair bundles are inserted directly into the otolithic membrane. *(From Corey DP, Hudspeth AJ: Biophys J 26:499, 1979.)*

called an **otolithic membrane** (Fig. 14-27), from which the otolithic organs get their name. The otoconia make the otolithic membrane denser than endolymph, so the membrane flops around and stays flopped when the position of the head changes. This stimulates the hair cells, which then signal the new position of the head. In this case the macula is responding to the force of gravity, but it responds equally well to other linear accelerating forces, such as those experienced in elevators and automobiles.

Because its macula is in a horizontal plane, the utricle is most sensitive to linear acceleration with a component in this plane (i.e., forward-backward or side to side) and to tilts beginning from a head-upright position; vertical acceleration does not deflect its bundles of stereocilia. The saccule, in contrast, is more sensitive to linear

acceleration with a component in the sagittal plane (i.e., forward-backward or up-down) and to tilts beginning from a head-sideways position. The hair cells of a given macula are arranged with their kinocilia facing in multiple directions (Fig. 14-28), so any tilt stimulates some cells more than others. The result is that each different head position causes a unique pattern of activity in the few thousand eighth nerve fibers that innervate the utricle and saccule.

Vestibular Primary Afferents Project to the Vestibular Nuclei and the Cerebellum

Vestibular primary afferents have their cell bodies in the **vestibular** (or **Scarpa's**) **ganglion** in the internal auditory canal. Their peripheral processes receive input from the

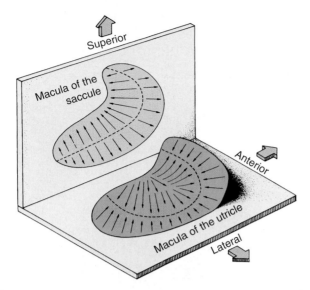

Figure 14-28 Orientation of hair cells in the utricle and saccule (of the right labyrinth in this diagram). *Arrows* in each macula point in the direction of the kinocilium of the hair cells in that vicinity (i.e., the direction in which deflection would cause depolarization). The *dashed line* in each macula indicates the location of the **striola,** a specialized zone at which the orientations of the hair cells switch direction. In the utricle, kinocilia are oriented toward the striola; in the saccule, they are oriented away from it. *(Modified from Barber HO, Stockwell CW: Manual of electronystagmography, St. Louis, 1976, Mosby.)*

hair cells of the semicircular ducts, utricle, and saccule. Their central processes enter the brainstem at the pontomedullary junction. Some proceed directly to the cerebellum, passing through the **juxtarestiform body,** which is located on the medial edge of the inferior cerebellar peduncle. They end in the **nodulus** and nearby areas, as discussed in more detail in Chapter 20. Most primary vestibular afferents, however, end in the vestibular nuclei of the rostral medulla and caudal pons (Fig. 14-29).

Four vestibular nuclei have been distinguished on the basis of their histology and connections: the **inferior, medial, lateral,** and **superior vestibular nuclei.** Each individual semicircular canal and otolithic organ has its own pattern of termination in the vestibular nuclei, and each vestibular nucleus has its own pattern of secondary connections. For the sake of simplicity, these patterns are mostly ignored in this account, and the vestibular nuclear complex is treated as one big nucleus.

Other inputs to the vestibular nuclei include projections from the cerebellum (by way of the juxtarestiform body), the spinal cord, the contralateral vestibular nuclei (see Fig. 14-29), and some small brainstem nuclei that convey information about things moving in peripheral parts of the visual field. The cerebellar projections arise directly from the flocculonodular lobe and indirectly from other cerebellar areas, as discussed further in Chapter 20. Input from the spinal cord makes sense, because it would be difficult to adjust posture properly in response to movement or tilt without knowledge of

the current orientation of the body. A small amount of this information travels with the posterior spinocerebellar tract as direct spinovestibular fibers, but most of it reaches the vestibular nuclei indirectly via relays in the cerebellum or reticular formation. Similarly, visual inputs help sort out whether images are moving across the retina because of head movement or object movement. Finally, the left and right halves of the vestibular system normally function together as a coordinated pair, and the vestibular nuclei of the two sides are extensively interconnected.

The Vestibular Nuclei Project Primarily to the Spinal Cord, Cerebellum, and Nuclei of Cranial Nerves III, IV, and VI

The connections of the vestibular nuclei are varied and widespread but are largely predictable in view of their function. We use the vestibular system principally to regulate posture and to coordinate eye and head movements; the anatomical substrates of these functions are connections with the spinal cord and with the motor nuclei of the extraocular muscles. The cerebellum is also involved in both these functions, so there are substantial interconnections between it and the vestibular nuclei. We also have a conscious awareness of movement through space, and there is a corresponding vestibular projection through the thalamus to cerebral cortex. Finally, there are connections between the vestibular nuclei and visceral nuclei of the brainstem and spinal cord; these mediate things such as cardiovascular adjustments when standing up or lying down, and they can have powerful autonomic effects (as anyone who has been seasick can attest).

Secondary fibers arising in the vestibular complex (see Fig. 14-29) project to (1) parts of the cerebellum, mainly the vermis and flocculonodular lobe (again, via the juxtarestiform body); (2) the thalamus; (3) the spinal cord, in the lateral and medial vestibulospinal tracts; (4) the motor nuclei of the extraocular muscles; and (5) the vestibular apparatus. (This is in addition to the previously mentioned projections to the reticular formation and the contralateral vestibular nuclei.)

Vestibular projections to the thalamus, and from there to the cerebral cortex, have been a matter of some controversy. Secondary vestibular fibers reach the thalamus bilaterally—some by traveling with the auditory fibers of the lateral lemniscus, and others by traversing the reticular formation near the medial longitudinal fasciculus (MLF). The thalamic relay is in inferior parts of the thalamus, near and including the ventral posterolateral nucleus. Several cortical areas receive vestibular information from the thalamus; their relative roles are not completely understood. One is located in the parietal lobe at the junction between the intraparietal and postcentral sulci, and another is in the depths of the central

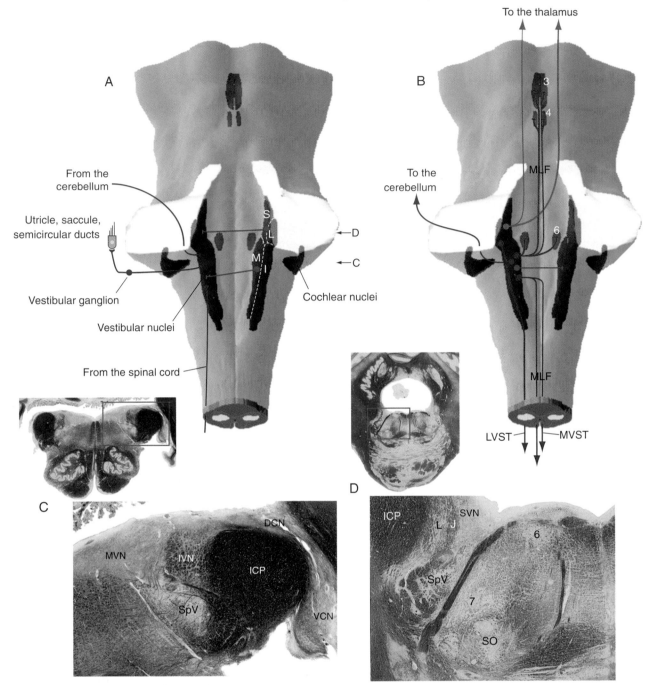

Figure 14-29 Inputs to **(A)** and outputs from **(B)** the vestibular nuclei; not shown in **A** are inputs from small accessory optic nuclei in the midbrain. C and D in **A** refer to the planes of the brainstem cross sections in **C** and **D,** showing the vestibular nuclei. 3, oculomotor nucleus; 4, trochlear nucleus; 6, abducens nucleus; 7, facial motor nucleus; DCN, dorsal cochlear nucleus; I and IVN, inferior vestibular nucleus; ICP, inferior cerebellar peduncle; J, juxtarestiform body; L, lateral vestibular nucleus; LVST, lateral vestibulospinal tract; M and MVN, medial vestibular nucleus; MLF, medial longitudinal fasciculus; MVST, medial vestibulospinal tract; S and SVN, superior vestibular nucleus; SO, superior olivary nucleus; SpV, spinal trigeminal nucleus; VCN, ventral cochlear nucleus.

sulcus; both are near the portion of the postcentral gyrus where the head is represented. This makes sense, because the somatosensory cortex of the postcentral gyrus is concerned with conscious appreciation of body position. Another cortical area, which may be most directly concerned with vestibular information, is in a posterior part of the insula near auditory cortex (Fig. 14-30).

Vestibulospinal Fibers Influence Antigravity Muscles and Neck Muscles

The **lateral vestibulospinal tract** arises in the lateral vestibular nucleus, travels through the ventral part of the lateral funiculus (near the spinothalamic tract), and sends excitatory projections to the motor neurons for antigravity muscles at all ipsilateral spinal levels. This is the principal route by which the vestibular system brings about postural changes to compensate for tilts and movements of the body. If as a child (or an adult) you ever spun yourself around until you felt dizzy and then proceeded to stagger, you have experienced the effects of exaggerated activity in your lateral vestibulospinal tract.

The **medial vestibulospinal tract** arises mainly in the medial vestibular nucleus and reaches both sides of the cervical spinal cord by projecting caudally through the MLF. It is responsible for stabilizing head position as we walk around or when our heads move in space in other ways, and for coordinating head movements with eye movements.

The Vestibular Nuclei Participate in the Vestibuloocular Reflex

The most critical function of the vestibular system is not to mediate awareness of movement or to adjust posture,

but rather to help generate eye movements that compensate for head movements in order to keep the fovea fixed on an object. Retinal photoreceptors, as discussed in Chapter 17, use a second-messenger transduction process that is relatively slow, and clear vision of images that move across the retina is impossible. The nervous system, as described further in Chapter 21, works hard to keep images from moving around on the retina.

Many secondary vestibular fibers project directly through the MLF and through the adjacent reticular formation to the motor neurons of the oculomotor, trochlear, and abducens nuclei. These serve as the interneuronal connections of the **vestibuloocular reflex** (VOR), by which gaze can stay fixed on an object even though the head is moving or being moved. One might think that this is a form of visual tracking, but the reflex is faster than visual tracking[m] and works even in the dark in those with normal vestibular systems. Individuals with bilateral vestibular damage can keep images stable on their retinas only during slow head movements (Fig. 14-31). This is because the vestibular division of cranial nerve VIII forms the afferent limb of the VOR. Each semicircular canal has connections via the vestibular nuclei that are appropriate to cause eye deviation in its own plane. This is most easily understood in the case of the horizontal canal. Imagine starting to spin to the left about a vertical axis. This would cause the cupula of the left horizontal canal to bulge toward the utricle, hence

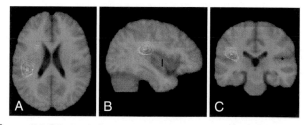

Figure 14-30 Cortical area in the posterior insula and parietal operculum activated by cold caloric stimulation of the horizontal semicircular duct (see Fig. 14-33C), shown in axial **(A)**, sagittal **(B)**, and coronal **(C)** planes. These results from positron emission tomography scans show areas where blood flow increased in normal subjects but not in six patients whose contralateral facial and vestibulocochlear nerves had been severed during surgery for removal of a tumor. *, lateral sulcus; I, insula. *(From Emri M et al: Cortical projection of peripheral vestibular signaling. J Neurophysiol 89:2639, 2003. Used with permission.)*

---

[m]You can easily demonstrate this to yourself by comparing the speeds of visual tracking and the VOR. Move this text back and forth in front of you while reading, keeping your head still, and note the speed (the maximum speed of visual tracking) at which it becomes blurred. Now hold the text still and continue to read while wagging your head back and forth, using the VOR to stabilize your gaze. It should be apparent that the VOR is capable of much higher velocities.

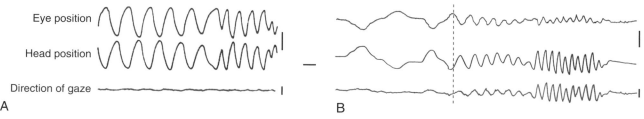

Figure 14-31 Normal and abnormal vestibuloocular reflexes. The surface of the cornea is electrically positive relative to the back of the eye, so deviation of an eye toward a nearby electrode causes the electrode to become more positive relative to a reference electrode. This is used clinically to record eye movements. These traces show the position of the eyes in the horizontal plane (blue), the position of the same individual's head (red), and the sum of these two positions (green), which corresponds to the net direction in which the individual is looking. By convention, an upward deflection indicates movement to the right. **A,** A normal individual moved her head back and forth while trying to maintain her gaze fixed on a stationary target. Notice that as her head moves in one direction, her eyes move through an equal but opposite angle, so the direction of gaze does not change. This is the normal vestibuloocular reflex. **B,** A patient with bilateral loss of vestibular hair cells (caused by ototoxicity of the streptomycin used to treat her pneumonia) attempts to do the same thing. At the slow head velocities at the beginning of the recording, she was able to use visual feedback to generate compensatory eye movements. However, once head velocity reached about 50 degrees/sec *(dashed line)*, the lack of a vestibuloocular reflex made it impossible to generate large enough compensatory eye movements. As a result, the direction of gaze began to oscillate in phase with head movement, and the patient had a disturbing visual illusion of the world moving. All vertical scale marks correspond to 40 degrees, and the horizontal scale mark corresponds to 1 second. *(Redrawn from Atkin A, Bender MB: Arch Neurol 19:559, 1968.)*

depolarizing the hair cells of this canal and increasing the firing rate of the eighth nerve fibers that innervate them. Excitatory connections with the left vestibular nuclei and from there to the right abducens nucleus result in deviation of both eyes to the right (Fig. 14-32), compensating for the rotation. Other combinations of semicircular canals and extraocular muscles are similarly straightforward, although more difficult to visualize. For example, rotating forward and to the right in the plane of the right anterior canal causes contraction of the right superior rectus and left inferior oblique, which in turn causes compensatory elevation and rotation of both eyes. As in the case of spinal reflexes, VOR circuitry includes inhibitory connections to the motor neurons for antagonist muscles.

A VOR is not always a good thing to have, and like the stretch reflex and other reflexes, it is modifiable. For example, we do a lot of looking around by using head movements in combination with eye movements. Unless the VOR were suppressed during the part of a gaze shift mediated by head turning, a counter-rotation of the eyes would be generated, and the direction of gaze would not change. Another example is compensating for the effects of eyeglasses, which change the relationship between head movement and the movement of images across the retina. All this is addressed by the flocculus, which adjusts the gain of the VOR as necessary. In fact, the degree of plasticity of this reflex, as discussed further in Chapter 20, is quite remarkable: in some experimental situations it can actually reverse direction.

Nystagmus Can Be Physiological or Pathological

During head rotations that are too large to be compensated for by the VOR, the reflex is periodically interrupted by very rapid eye movements in the opposite direction (Fig. 14-33). The resulting back-and-forth eye movements, with a slow phase in one direction and a fast phase in the other, are a form of **nystagmus** (from a Greek word meaning "to nod off," referring to the way a sleepy person's head sags slowly and then snaps back upright when trying to stay awake). The eye movements of nystagmus may be horizontal, vertical, or torsional; they may have a faster component in one direction, or the movements in both directions may have the same speed. Nystagmus of certain types is a normal physiological response to stimulation of the vestibular or visual system, but spontaneous or exaggerated nystagmus is characteristic of some kinds of neuropathology (Fig. 14-34).

An example of normal physiological nystagmus is the one just described—horizontal nystagmus, with a fast component in one direction, induced by rotation. In this case the nystagmus is named for the direction of rapid movement (e.g., if the eyes move slowly to the right and then rapidly back to the left, it would be called **nystagmus to the left,** or **left-beating nystagmus**). Left-beating

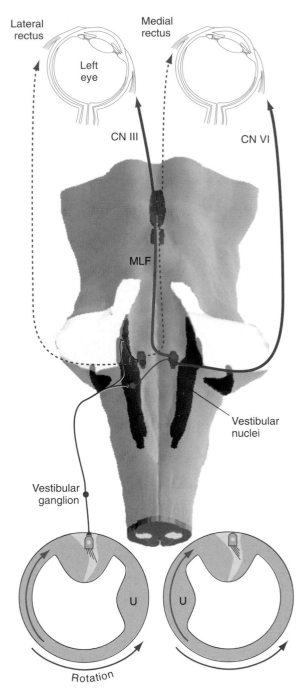

Figure 14-32 Pathway of the vestibuloocular reflex underlying the response to rotation to the left. Excitation of the left horizontal semicircular duct causes increased contraction of the right lateral rectus and left medial rectus, by way of excitatory interneurons (green) in the left vestibular nuclei; simultaneously, motor neurons for the left lateral rectus and right medial rectus (the antagonist muscles) are inhibited, by way of inhibitory interneurons (red). Notice that this rotation also causes bulging of the cupula of the right horizontal semicircular canal away from the utricle (U), thus hyperpolarizing the hair cells of this canal. Although its connections are not shown in this figure, this would have a complementary effect (i.e., less inhibition of motor neurons for the right lateral rectus and left medial rectus, less excitation of motor neurons for the left lateral rectus and right medial rectus). MLF, medial longitudinal fasciculus.

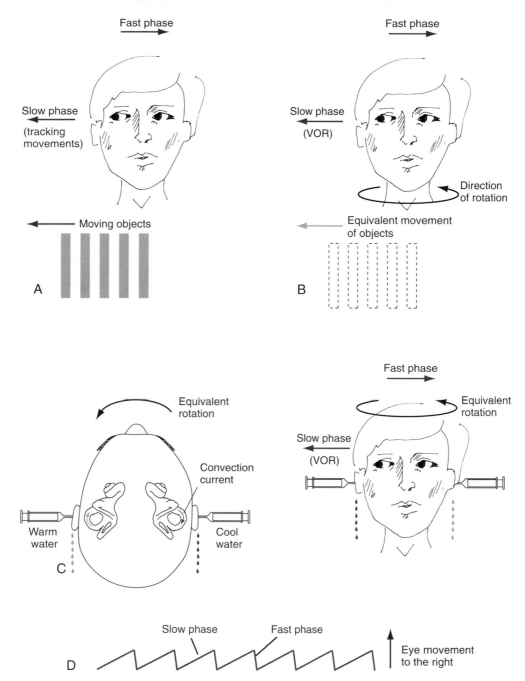

Figure 14-33 Three different ways to cause nystagmus with its fast phase to the left. **A,** Movement of a series of objects to an individual's right causes slow tracking eye movements to the right, followed by rapid "reset" movements to the left. **B,** Rotation to the left is equivalent, as far as retinal image movement is concerned, to movement of objects to the right. The result is nystagmus to the left, as in **A.** If the individual's eyes are open, visual movement continues throughout the rotation, and the nystagmus may persist. If the eyes are closed, the nystagmus is mediated only by the vestibular system and is transient. The direction of nystagmus reverses at the end of rotation in either condition. **C,** Warm water instilled into the left ear (or cool water in the right) causes the same movement of endolymph in the left (or right) horizontal semicircular duct as does the rotation in **B.** Again, the result is nystagmus to the left. **D,** Idealized electrical recording of horizontal nystagmus with its fast phase to the left.

nystagmus is seen at the beginning of rotation to the left (see Figs. 14-32 and 14-33B), ensuring a stable image on the retina except during the brief "reset" movements of the fast phase. When the rotation stops, the cupula is deflected in the opposite direction for a little while (see Fig. 14-25C), fooling the brainstem into thinking that the direction of rotation has reversed, and a brief period of right-beating **postrotatory nystagmus** ensues. The response during sustained rotation, when there is no cupular deflection (see Fig. 14-25B), depends on the conditions of illumination. In the dark or with the subject's eyes closed, nystagmus would cease. Yet with visual input, for reasons explained later, left-beating nystagmus might continue throughout the rotation.

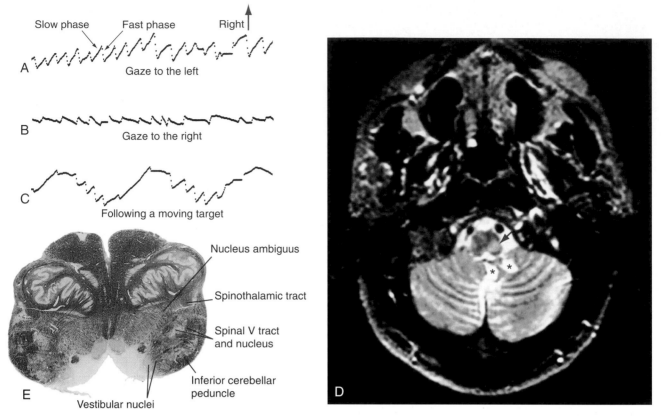

Figure 14-34 Pathological nystagmus caused by brainstem damage. A 62-year-old man developed the abrupt onset of vertigo and nausea. He was found to have spontaneous nystagmus to the left that increased when he looked to the left **(A)** and changed to right-beating nystagmus when he looked to the right **(B).** Smooth tracking of moving targets was severely impaired when the target moved to the left **(C)** because his nystagmus was accentuated by gaze in this direction. He also had signs of left-sided cerebellar damage (see Chapter 20): intention tremor on the left, incoordination of the left arm on finger-to-nose testing, and slight left dysdiadochokinesia. He was markedly off balance and could hardly sit up because of nausea that worsened with movement of his head. **D,** T2-weighted axial magnetic resonance image shows increased signal intensity in the left lateral medulla *(arrow)* and left paramedian cerebellum *(asterisks),* both areas supplied by the posterior inferior cerebellar artery (see Fig. 11-30). **E,** A section of the rostral medulla in a plane similar to **D.** In this case of lateral medullary (or Wallenberg's) syndrome, damage to the vestibular nuclei, inferior cerebellar peduncle, and cerebellum produced the findings described. Other structures likely to be damaged in such a case (and the resulting deficits) include the spinal trigeminal tract and nucleus (ipsilateral facial analgesia), spinothalamic tract (analgesia of the contralateral side of the body), and nucleus ambiguus (hoarseness, ipsilateral palatal and pharyngeal weakness). In addition, damage to fibers descending from the hypothalamus to the intermediolateral cell column of the spinal cord could cause ipsilateral Horner's syndrome. *(Courtesy Dr. Terry Fife, St. Joseph's Hospital and Regional Medical Center and University of Arizona College of Medicine.)*

The same movement of endolymph that underlies nystagmus at the beginning and end of rotation can be produced by instilling cool or warm water into a subject's ear, causing endolymphatic convection currents that in turn induce nystagmus. Consider an individual whose head is tilted back about 60 degrees, bringing the horizontal semicircular canals into a vertical plane. Warm water instilled into the left ear causes the endolymph in the left horizontal canal to warm and rise, causing a convection current of endolymph in a clockwise direction (viewed from the top of the head). This movement of endolymph relative to the canal is the same movement that is produced at the onset of rotation of the individual to the left (see Fig. 14-33C), and the response of this single semicircular canal is sufficient to cause nystagmus to the left. This is called **caloric nystagmus,** and its mechanism is the same as that of rotationally induced vestibular nystagmus.[n] Endolymph movement in the same direction can be induced in the contralateral ear by instilling cool water (see Fig. 14-33C).

Finally, because the whole purpose of vestibular nystagmus is to keep images from moving on the retina, it is not surprising that a similar pattern of eye movements can be elicited by moving visual stimuli. Consider the reflex eye movements that might occur if you

---

[n]This gravitational model seems so logical that it has been accepted without much question since 1908, when caloric nystagmus was first described. The era of space flight has allowed demonstrations that caloric nystagmus can be elicited in orbiting astronauts, who are experiencing nearly zero gravity. However, its properties under these conditions are somewhat different from normal, and the current consensus is that caloric nystagmus is mostly the result of convection currents and partly the result of a direct thermal effect of some sort.

were sitting in a rapidly moving train, vaguely watching regularly spaced telephone poles fly by. Your eyes would slowly follow a particular pole toward the rear of the train and then flick back toward the front of the train to find a new pole to fixate on. In the case of an individual seated on the right side of the train, this would constitute nystagmus to the left (see Fig. 14-33A). Because it is induced by moving visual stimuli, this is called **optokinetic nystagmus** (OKN). Fortunately, it is not necessary to use trains and telephone poles to demonstrate OKN clinically; a rotating striped drum or a moving piece of striped cloth usually suffices. OKN accounts for the continued nystagmus during sustained rotation if the lights are on.

The pathway involved in vestibular nystagmus primarily involves the MLF for connections rostral to the abducens nucleus. The slow phase is simply a reflection of direct VOR connections from the vestibular nuclei to the abducens, trochlear, and oculomotor nuclei. The fast phase, like fast eye movements in general (see Chapter 21), requires timing signals that originate from the reticular formation. One consequence is that a comatose patient with depressed function of the reticular formation, but with an otherwise intact brainstem, may show only the slow phase of caloric nystagmus—that is, caloric stimulation produces only a tonic deviation of the eyes in the direction of the slow phase of the expected nystagmus. Abnormalities of this conjugate deviation can therefore be of value in determining the location of structural damage in the brainstem of a comatose patient. Turning the head of a comatose individual from side to side can elicit similar conjugate lateral eye movements. The movements in this case are those appropriate to keep both eyes pointed in the same forward direction relative to the trunk (e.g., head movement to the right causes eye movements to the left). These are called **doll's head eye movements** (or the **oculocephalic reflex**) and generally represent no more than a VOR that is normally suppressed when a conscious individual moves head and eyes to one side simultaneously to look at something. The afferent limb of the oculocephalic reflex probably also includes proprioceptors of the neck, because some reflex movement can still be elicited from patients with nonfunctional labyrinths.

At the termination of rotation to the left, nystagmus with its fast phase to the right is seen in a normal individual, as discussed earlier. In addition, trying to point at something while the eyes are closed results in deviation of the arm to the left; this is called **past pointing.** There is also a tendency to fall to the left when walking. The lateral vestibulospinal tract ordinarily is quite important in directing the changes in muscle tone that correspond to the postural changes involved in balance; postrotatory past pointing and a tendency to fall are a result of exaggerated activity in this tract. Similarly, a patient with diminished output from one labyrinth is likely to complain of balance problems and to veer to the ipsilateral side while walking forward with eyes closed.

Conditions That Make the Cupula Sensitive to Gravity Cause Nystagmus and Illusions of Movement

A normal cupula has the same density as its endolymphatic surroundings, so gravity causes no movement of the cupula relative to its crista, and the semicircular ducts are insensitive to head position. Conditions that change the relative densities of cupula and endolymph would be expected to make the semicircular ducts gravity sensitive, resulting in illusions of movement in response to certain orientations of the head. This is the commonly accepted explanation for the positionally dependent **vertigo** (illusions of movement) and nystagmus seen during and after excessive alcohol consumption (Fig. 14-35). As blood alcohol levels rise, alcohol initially leaves the capillaries and infiltrates the cupulae, making them less dense than surrounding endolymph. During this period, holding the head in a position that allows cupular deflection by attempted flotation causes nystagmus. This lasts for several hours, until the alcohol concentrations of cupulae and endolymph equilibrate and the nystagmus stops. Subsequently, after blood alcohol levels drop, alcohol leaves the cupulae first. This makes them *more* dense than endolymph and causes several hours of positionally dependent nystagmus in the opposite direction.

Age or trauma can cause detachment of otoconia in the utricle, allowing them to enter a semicircular duct. There they can move to and fro in response to gravity, causing a "plunger" effect that results in transient movement of endolymph against the cupula of that duct. The posterior duct is most often affected (presumably because of its position partially below the utricle; see Fig. 14-3), with the result that head movements with a component in the plane of this canal (typically by tilting the head or rolling over in bed) cause brief episodes of vertigo and nystagmus. This syndrome is called **benign paroxysmal positional vertigo**—benign because in most patients the otoconia work their way out of the semicircular duct and the symptoms vanish. For patients with persistent symptoms, a series of positioning maneuvers can usually speed the return of the otoconia to the utricle.

Efferents Control the Sensitivity of Vestibular Hair Cells

There are no muscles comparable to the stapedius that can affect vestibular function, but there are efferent projections to the hair cells. Small groups of neurons in the reticular formation lateral to the abducens nucleus project bilaterally through the eighth nerve (vestibular division) and end on the vestibular hair cells or their afferent endings. The most common hypothesis regarding the function of vestibular efferents is that they can

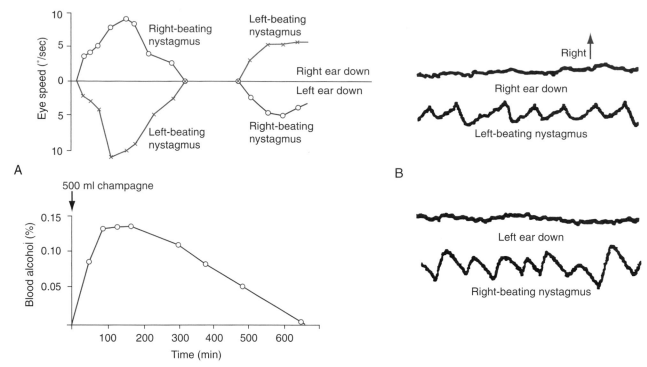

Figure 14-35 Induction of nystagmus by alteration of the relative density of the cupula and endolymph. **A,** During the period of peak blood alcohol levels after ingestion of half a liter of champagne, placing the head in a right-ear-down position (parts of the curve above the horizontal axis) causes nystagmus with its fast phase to the right; a left-ear-down position causes nystagmus with its fast phase to the left. As blood alcohol levels drop, alcohol levels in the cupulae and endolymph equilibrate; the nystagmus ceases, followed by a period in which the nystagmus reverses direction. **B,** Ingestion of heavy water (deuterium oxide), which is more dense than normal cupulae and endolymph, has the opposite effect. Before drinking heavy water, the subject has no nystagmus in either head position (upper trace of each pair). Thirty minutes after drinking 200 mL of heavy water, the subject has left-beating nystagmus when the right ear faces down and right-beating nystagmus when the left ear faces down (lower trace of each pair). (**A,** redrawn from Aschan G, Bergstedt M: Acta Otolaryngol Suppl 330:15, 1975. **B,** from Money KE, Myles WS: Nature 247:404, 1974.)

compensate for self-generated head movements. For example, the horizontal semicircular canals receive the same stimulation whether you rotate your head or someone begins to rotate the chair in which you are sitting. However, the reflex postural adjustments to the two rotations are quite different. If the efferent system compensated for the hair cell response to self-generated rotation, the reflex postural adjustments would be eliminated. There is experimental evidence that this may be the case in some species, but the afferents from primate semicircular ducts respond in the same way to active and passive head movements, and the role of human vestibular efferents is presently unknown.

Position Sense Is Mediated by the Vestibular, Proprioceptive, and Visual Systems Acting Together

The vestibular system is not the only source of information about the position and motion of the head in space. The visual system also plays a major role and, in most situations, is actually dominant. Most of us have experienced an illusion of movement when we were stationary and a nearby large object (such as a train on the next track) moved. Because vestibular signals provide no information about the position of the *body*, additional inputs are required for tasks such as reaching with a hand for a seen object. Much of the additional information is provided by mechanoreceptors in the neck that detect the orientation of the head relative to the body. If the first three cervical dorsal roots of a monkey are anesthetized bilaterally, severe disorientation results, involving not only eye-hand coordination but also such basic activities as walking and climbing.

Vestibular, visual, and somatosensory inputs are normally combined seamlessly to produce our sense of orientation and movement. The combining begins at the level of the vestibular nuclei, where somatosensory, visual, and vestibular inputs all converge. If one of the three systems is defective, the remaining two are adequate for most functions. For example, humans can compensate reasonably well for total loss of vestibular function, as long as visual cues are available. However, loss of two of the three systems is disabling. This is the basis of **Romberg's sign,** the greatly increased swaying and loss of balance caused by closing the eyes in a patient with defective vestibular or somatosensory function.

SUGGESTED READINGS

Ashmore J: Cochlear outer hair cell motility. Physiol Rev 88:173, 2008.

Baloh RW, Honrubia V: Clinical neurophysiology of the vestibular system, ed 3, New York, 2001, Oxford University Press.

Barmack NH: Central vestibular system: vestibular nuclei and posterior cerebellum. Brain Res Bull 60:511, 2003.

Bender MB, Feldman M: Visual illusions during head movement in lesions of the brain stem. Arch Neurol 17:354, 1967.
An interesting discussion of what happens if a patient's vestibular apparatus is damaged so that it is impossible to tell whether movement of a visual image is caused by head movement or motion in the outside world.

Boyle R: Activity of medial vestibulospinal tract cells during rotation and ocular movement in the alert squirrel monkey. J Neurophysiol 70:2176, 1993.

Bracchi F, et al: Multiday recordings from the primary neurons of the statoreceptors of the labyrinth of the bullfrog. Acta Otolaryngol Suppl 334:1975.
Technically astonishing experiments in which continuous recordings were made from single utricular primary afferents of a bullfrog aboard a rocket that blasted off and put the frog in orbit for a few days.

Brandt T, Daroff RB: The multisensory physiological and pathological vertigo syndromes. Ann Neurol 7:195, 1980.
Stimulation or dysfunction of the vestibular, visual, or somatosensory systems can cause illusions of movement.

Brandt TH, Dieterich M: The vestibular cortex: its locations, functions, and disorders. Ann N Y Acad Sci 871:293, 1999.

Bredberg G, Ades HW, Engström H: Scanning electron microscopy of the normal and pathologically altered organ of Corti. Acta Otolaryngol Suppl 301:3, 1972.
Pretty pictures from a variety of mammals.

Brindley GS: How does an animal that is dropped in a nonupright posture know the angle through which it must turn in the air so that its feet point to the ground? J Physiol 180:20P, 1965.
Briefly, it remembers which way was up when it was dropped. The paper is not much longer than its title.

Büttner-Ennever JA, Gerrits NM: Vestibular system. In Paxinos G, Mai JK, editors: The human nervous system, ed 2, San Diego, 2004, Elsevier Academic Press.

Cohen LA: Role of eye and neck proprioceptive mechanisms in body orientation and motor coordination. J Neurophysiol 24:1, 1961.

Couloigner V, Sterkers O, Ferrary E: What's new in ion transports in the cochlea? Pflugers Arch Eur J Physiol 453:11, 2006.

Cullen KE, Minor LB: Semicircular canal afferents similarly encode active and passive head-on-body rotations: implications for the role of vestibular efference. J Neurosci 22:RC226, 2002.

Darrow KN, Maison SF, Liberman MC: Selective removal of lateral olivocochlear efferents increases vulnerability to acute acoustic injury. J Neurophysiol 97:1775, 2007.

de Jong PTVM, et al: Ataxia and nystagmus induced by injection of local anesthetics in the neck. Ann Neurol 1:240, 1977.

Dieterich M, Brandt TH, Fries W: Otolith function in man: results from a case of otolith Tullio phenomenon. Brain 112:1377, 1989.
A remarkable case of a patient whose stapes footplate popped through the oval window, where it could push against the utricle. Loud sounds subsequently caused nystagmus and loss of balance.

Emri M, et al: Cortical projection of peripheral vestibular signaling. J Neurophysiol 89:2639, 2003.

Felix H, et al: Morphological features of human Reissner's membrane. Acta Otolaryngol 113:321, 1993.

Fernández C, Goldberg JM, Abend WK: Response to static tilts of peripheral neurons innervating otolith organs of the squirrel monkey. J Neurophysiol 35:978, 1972.

Fine ML, Horn MH, Cox B: Acanthonus armatus, a deep-sea teleost fish with a minute brain and large ears. Proc R Soc Lond B 230:257, 1987.
"Acanthonus armatus, a deep-water benthopelagic fish, has, per unit body weight, the smallest brain and largest semicircular canals of any known teleost and possibly any vertebrate.".

Fray JP, Puria S, Steele CR: The discordant eardrum. Proc Natl Acad Sci U S A 103:19743, 2005.
Every little detail about the shape, orientation, and makeup of the tympanic membrane contributes to auditory function.

Friedmann I, Ballantyne J, editors: Ultrastructural atlas of the inner ear, London, 1984, Butterworth.

Giraud AL, et al: Auditory efferents involved in speech-in-noise intelligibility. Neuroreport 8:1779, 1997.

Goldberg JM, Fernández C: Efferent vestibular system in the squirrel monkey: anatomical location and influence on afferent activity. J Neurophysiol 43:986, 1980.

Graf W, Baker R: The vestibuloocular reflex of the adult flatfish. I. Oculomotor organization. II. Vestibulooculomotor connectivity. J Neurophysiol 54:887, 900, 1985.
Flatfish (e.g., flounder) start out like any other fish, then wind up with both eyes on one side of their body, but their semicircular canals do not change. This is the story of CNS changes that compensate for the mismatch.

Guinan JJ, Jr: Olivocochlear efferents: anatomy, physiology, function, and the measurement of efferent effects in humans. Ear Hear 27:589, 2006.

Highstein SM, Fay RR, Popper AN: The vestibular system, New York, 2004, Springer-Verlag.

Jenkins WM, Masterton RB: Sound localization: effects of unilateral lesions in the central auditory system. J Neurophysiol 47:987, 1982.

Kemp DT: Stimulated acoustic emissions from within the human auditory system. J Acoust Soc Am 64:1386, 1978.
The original description of evoked otoacoustic emissions, which were once known as "Kemp echoes."

Klinke R, Schmidt CL: Efferent influence on the vestibular organ during active movements of the body. Pflugers Arch 318:325, 1970.
Clever experiments giving a hint about a goldfish's use of the efferent fibers in its vestibular nerve.

Kulesza RJ, Jr: Cytoarchitecture of the human superior olivary complex: medial and lateral superior olive. Hear Res 225:80, 2007.

Lee D, Lishman R: Vision in movement and balance. New Scientist 65:59, 1975.
A popularized but fascinating account of how easy it is to confuse one's position sense by presenting conflicting visual and vestibular inputs.

Liberman MC, Guinan JJ, Jr: Feedback control of the auditory periphery: anti-masking effects of middle ear muscles vs olivocochlear efferents. J Commun Disord 31:471, 1998.

Lidén G, Peterson JL, Harford ER: Simultaneous recording of changes in relative impedance and air pressure during acoustic and non-acoustic elicitation of the middle-ear reflexes. Acta Otolaryngol Suppl 263:208, 1970.

Living without a balancing mechanism. N Engl J Med 246:458, 1952.
A firsthand account by an anonymous physician of the remarkable compensation we can achieve after bilateral damage to the vestibular apparatus.

Lopez I, et al: Estimation of the number of nerve fibers in the human vestibular endorgans using unbiased stereology and immunohistochemistry. J Neurosci Meth 145:37, 2005.

Mahoney T, Vernon J, Meikle M: Function of the acoustic reflex in discrimination of intense speech. Arch Otolaryngol 105:119, 1979.

Middlebrooks JC, Green DM: Sound localization by human listeners. Annu Rev Psychol 42:135, 1991.

Minor LB: Clinical manifestations of superior semicircular canal dehiscence. Laryngoscope 115:1717, 2005.

A hole in the temporal bone in the floor of the middle cranial fossa, near the superior semicircular canal, makes this canal sensitive to sound.

Møller AR: Hearing: anatomy, physiology, and disorders of the auditory system, ed 2, San Diego, 2004, Elsevier Academic Press.

Moore JK, Lanthicum FH, Jr: Auditory system. In Paxinos G, Mai JK, editors: The human nervous system, ed 2, San Diego, 2004, Elsevier Academic Press.

Naitoh Y, et al: Projections of the individual vestibular end-organs in the brain stem of the squirrel monkey. Hear Res 87:141, 1995.

Nin F, et al: The endocochlear potential depends on two K^+ diffusion potentials and an electrical barrier in the stria vascularis of the inner ear. Proc Natl Acad Sci U S A 105:1751, 2008.

Osterhammel P, Terkildsen K, Zilstorff K: Vestibular habituation in ballet dancers. Adv Otorhinolaryngol 17:158, 1970.

How do people who rotate for a living do it?

Papsin BC, Gordon KA: Cochlear implants for children with severe-to-profound hearing loss. New Engl J Med 357:2380, 2007.

Raphael Y, Altschuler RA: Structure and innervation of the cochlea. Brain Res Bull 60:397, 2003.

Robinette MS, Glattke TJ: Otoacoustic emissions: clinical applications, ed 3, New York, 2007, Thieme Medical Publishers.

Robles L, Ruggero MA: Mechanics of the mammalian cochlea. Physiol Rev 81:1305, 2001.

Ryan A, Dallos P: Effect of absence of cochlear outer hair cells on behavioral auditory threshold. Nature 253:44, 1975.

Scharf B, Magnan J, Chays A: On the role of the olivocochlear bundle in hearing: 16 case studies. Hearing Res 103:101, 1997.

Semaan MT, Alagramam KN, Megerian CA: The basic science of Ménière's disease and endolymphatic hydrops. Curr Opin Otolaryngol 13:301, 2005.

Shaw MD, Baker R: The locations of stapedius and tensor tympani motoneurons in the cat. J Comp Neurol 216:10, 1983.

Simpson JI, Graf W: Eye-muscle geometry and compensatory eye movements in lateral-eyed and frontal-eyed animals. Ann N Y Acad Sci 374:20, 1981.

Pitching to one side or the other requires vertical compensatory eye movements in rabbits but torsional eye movements in humans, even though both species have semicircular canals arranged similarly. This fascinating paper provides an explanation.

Spoendlin H: The innervation of the organ of Corti. J Laryngol Otol 81:717, 1967.

Spoendlin H, Schrott A: Analysis of the human auditory nerve. Hear Res 43:25, 1989.

Tjellstrom A, Hakansson B: The bone-anchored hearing aid: design principles, indications, and long-term clinical results. Otolaryngol Clin North Am 28:53, 1995.

Tran Ba Huy P, Toupet M: Otolith function and disorders, Basel, 2001, Karger.

Vollrath MA, Kwan KY, Corey DP: The micromachinery of mechanotransduction in hair cells. Ann Rev Neurosci 30:339, 2007.

von Baumgarten R, et al: Effects of rectilinear acceleration and optokinetic and caloric stimulations in space. Science 225:208, 1984.

Von Békésy G: Experiments in hearing, New York, 1960, McGraw-Hill.

A large collection of clever and skillful experiments by the grand master of auditory physiology.

Yates BJ: Vestibular influences on the autonomic nervous system. Ann N Y Acad Sci 781:458, 1996.

Atlas of the Human Brainstem[a]

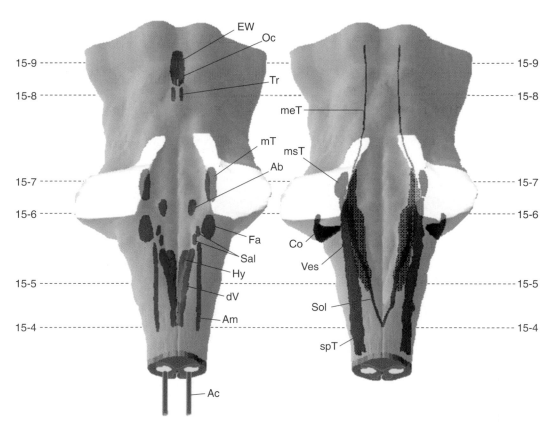

15

This series of five chapters on the functional anatomy of the brainstem concludes here, with a summary of

[a]Parts of this chapter were modified from Nolte J, Angevine JB Jr: The human brain in photographs and diagrams, ed 4, St. Louis, 2013, Mosby.

the principal contents of the brainstem at each level (Figs. 15-1 to 15-3), a series of transverse sections of the brainstem (Figs. 15-4 to 15-9), and brief descriptions of structures that are indicated in these sections.

Figure 15-1 Three-dimensional reconstructions of the brainstem, with motor (left) and sensory (right) cranial nerve nuclei indicated. Dashed lines indicate the planes of the sections shown in Figures 15-4 to 15-9. Ab, abducens nucleus; Ac, accessory nucleus; Am, nucleus ambiguus; Co, cochlear nuclei; dV, dorsal motor nucleus of the vagus; EW, Edinger-Westphal nucleus; Fa, facial motor nucleus; Hy, hypoglossal nucleus; meT, mesencephalic nucleus of the trigeminal; msT, trigeminal main sensory nucleus; mT, trigeminal motor nucleus; Oc, oculomotor nucleus; Sal, salivary nuclei; Sol, nucleus of the solitary tract; spT, spinal trigeminal nucleus; Tr, trochlear nucleus; Ves, vestibular nuclei.

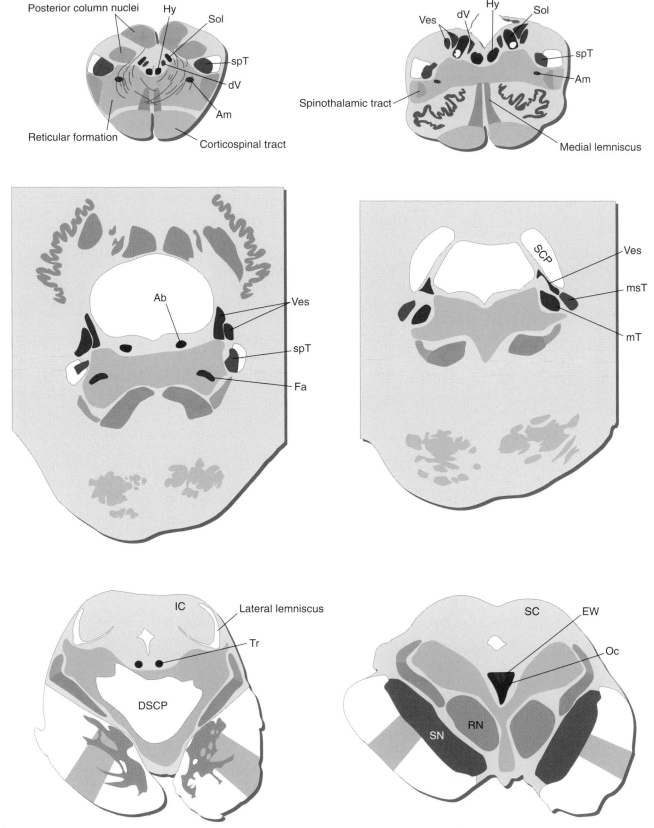

Figure 15-2 Schematic views of the transverse sections of the brainstem shown photographically in Figures 15-4 to 15-9, each enlarged to about three times its actual size. Major tracts and cranial nerve nuclei are indicated. DSCP, decussation of the superior cerebellar peduncles; IC, inferior colliculus; RN, red nucleus; SC, superior colliculus; SCP, superior cerebellar peduncle; SN, substantia nigra; other abbreviations as in Figure 15-1. *(Modified from Nolte J, Angevine JB Jr: The human brain in photographs and diagrams, ed 3, St. Louis, 2007, Mosby.)*

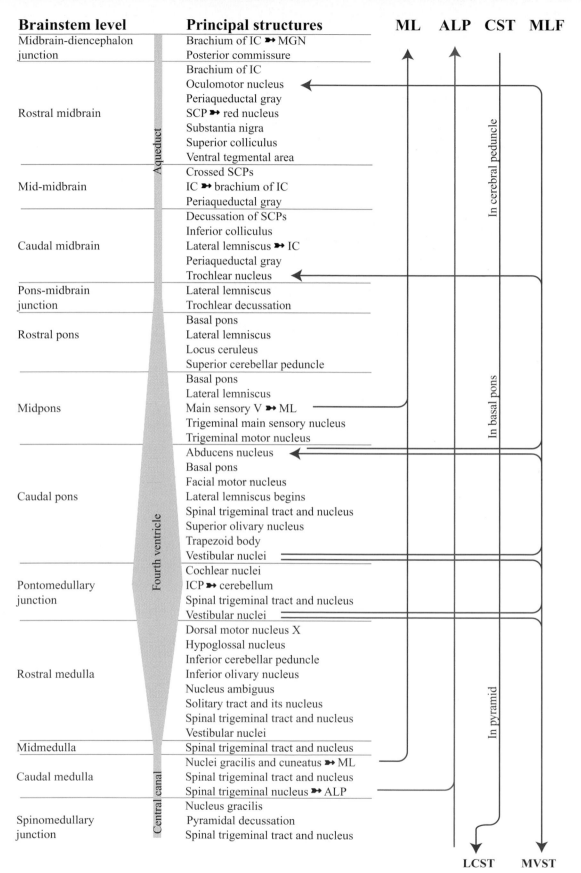

Brainstem level	Principal structures	ML	ALP	CST	MLF
Midbrain-diencephalon junction	Brachium of IC ➥ MGN				
	Posterior commissure				
Rostral midbrain	Brachium of IC				
	Oculomotor nucleus				
	Periaqueductal gray				
	SCP ➥ red nucleus				
	Substantia nigra				
	Superior colliculus				
	Ventral tegmental area				
Mid-midbrain	Crossed SCPs				
	IC ➥ brachium of IC				
	Periaqueductal gray				
Caudal midbrain	Decussation of SCPs				
	Inferior colliculus				
	Lateral lemniscus ➥ IC				
	Periaqueductal gray				
	Trochlear nucleus				
Pons-midbrain junction	Lateral lemniscus				
	Trochlear decussation				
Rostral pons	Basal pons				
	Lateral lemniscus				
	Locus ceruleus				
	Superior cerebellar peduncle				
Midpons	Basal pons				
	Lateral lemniscus				
	Main sensory V ➥ ML				
	Trigeminal main sensory nucleus				
	Trigeminal motor nucleus				
Caudal pons	Abducens nucleus				
	Basal pons				
	Facial motor nucleus				
	Lateral lemniscus begins				
	Spinal trigeminal tract and nucleus				
	Superior olivary nucleus				
	Trapezoid body				
	Vestibular nuclei				
Pontomedullary junction	Cochlear nuclei				
	ICP ➥ cerebellum				
	Spinal trigeminal tract and nucleus				
	Vestibular nuclei				
Rostral medulla	Dorsal motor nucleus X				
	Hypoglossal nucleus				
	Inferior cerebellar peduncle				
	Inferior olivary nucleus				
	Nucleus ambiguus				
	Solitary tract and its nucleus				
	Spinal trigeminal tract and nucleus				
	Vestibular nuclei				
Midmedulla	Spinal trigeminal tract and nucleus				
Caudal medulla	Nuclei gracilis and cuneatus ➥ ML				
	Spinal trigeminal tract and nucleus				
	Spinal trigeminal nucleus ➥ ALP				
Spinomedullary junction	Nucleus gracilis				
	Pyramidal decussation				
	Spinal trigeminal tract and nucleus				

Aqueduct — Fourth ventricle — Central canal

In cerebral peduncle — In basal pons — In pyramid

LCST   MVST

Figure 15-3 Principal structures at different brainstem levels. Only the levels containing the major parts of structures are indicated. Many structures extend a short distance into adjacent levels (e.g., the nucleus of the solitary tract extends a bit into athe caudal medulla and caudal pons). Raphe nuclei and other elements of the reticular formation are not indicated but are present at all brainstem levels. ALP, anterolateral pathway; CST, corticospinal tract; IC, inferior colliculus; ICP, inferior cerebellar peduncle; LCST, lateral corticospinal tract; MGN, medial geniculate nucleus; ML, medial lemniscus; MLF, medial longitudinal fasciculus; MVST, medial vestibulospinal tract; SCP, superior cerebellar peduncle.

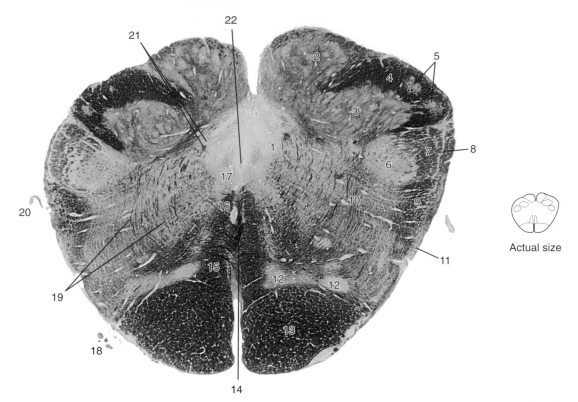

Actual size

Figure 15-4 Caudal medulla (close to the level of the obex). Actual size: 12 mm wide × 10 mm from anterior to posterior.

1. Dorsal motor nucleus of the vagus. The caudal end of the nucleus of origin of most preganglionic parasympathetic neurons for thoracic and abdominal viscera.
2. Nucleus gracilis. Site of termination of fasciculus gracilis and the origin of the leg portion of the medial lemniscus.
3. Nucleus cuneatus. Site of termination of fasciculus cuneatus and the origin of the arm portion of the medial lemniscus.
4. Fasciculus cuneatus. Uncrossed primary afferents, carrying tactile and proprioceptive information from the arm.
5. Lateral cuneate nucleus. Arm equivalent of Clarke's nucleus. Proprioceptive primary afferents travel through fasciculus cuneatus to reach the lateral cuneate nucleus, which then gives rise to uncrossed cuneocerebellar fibers that enter the cerebellum through the inferior cerebellar peduncle.
6. Spinal trigeminal nucleus (caudal nucleus). Site of termination of part of the spinal trigeminal tract, and the origin of part of the anterolateral pathway. At this level, the nucleus has the appearance of the spinal posterior horn, has a component similar to the substantia gelatinosa, and processes pain and temperature information.
7. Spinal trigeminal tract. Primary afferents from the ipsilateral side of the face, at this level conveying information about pain and temperature.
8. Posterior spinocerebellar tract. Uncrossed fibers from Clarke's nucleus, carrying proprioceptive information from the leg that will reach the ipsilateral half of the cerebellar vermis and adjoining areas through the inferior cerebellar peduncle.
9. Anterolateral pathway. Mostly crossed fibers from the spinal posterior horns and intermediate gray, conveying pain and temperature information to the thalamus (spinothalamic tract), reticular formation, and midbrain.
10. Location of nucleus ambiguus. Lower motor neurons for laryngeal and pharyngeal muscles and preganglionic parasympathetic neurons for the heart.
11. Anterior spinocerebellar tract. Crossed fibers from lumbosacral spinal gray matter, carrying proprioceptive and other information from the leg. This tract stays in approximately the same position until

the rostral pons, where it moves over the surface of the superior cerebellar peduncle (see Fig. 15-7) and turns posteriorly into the cerebellum.
12. Inferior olivary nucleus (medial accessory nucleus). The inferior olivary complex gives rise to climbing fibers that end in the contralateral half of the cerebellum (see Chapter 20). Those from the accessory nuclei project mainly to the vermis and flocculus, those from the principal inferior olivary nucleus to the cerebellar hemisphere.
13. Pyramid. Corticospinal fibers from the ipsilateral precentral gyrus and adjacent areas of cerebral cortex.
14. Raphe nuclei. Widely projecting serotonergic neurons that collectively blanket the central nervous system (CNS). Those in caudal brainstem levels such as this project mainly to the spinal cord.
15. Medial lemniscus, the principal ascending pathway for tactile and proprioceptive information. Originates in the contralateral posterior column nuclei and terminates in the thalamus (ventral posterolateral nucleus [VPL]).
16. Medial longitudinal fasciculus (MLF). At this level, the fibers of the medial vestibulospinal tract.
17. Hypoglossal nucleus. Lower motor neurons for the ipsilateral half of the tongue.
18. Hypoglossal nerve fibers, on their way to the muscles of the ipsilateral half of the tongue.
19. Internal arcuate fibers, crossing from nuclei gracilis and cuneatus to form the medial lemniscus, the principal ascending pathway for tactile and proprioceptive information.
20. Fibers of the vagus nerve, on their way to muscles of the ipsilateral half of the larynx and pharynx. These caudal filaments of the vagus were formerly considered separately as the cranial part of the accessory nerve, but they all actually join the vagus directly.
21. Solitary tract and its nucleus. Primary afferents conveying visceral information from cranial nerves VII, IX, and X (and some chemosensory information from the trigeminal nerve) travel through the solitary tract to reach the surrounding nucleus of the solitary tract. Only information from viscera reaches this caudal level.
22. Central canal. Merges rostrally with the fourth ventricle and caudally with the central canal of the spinal cord.

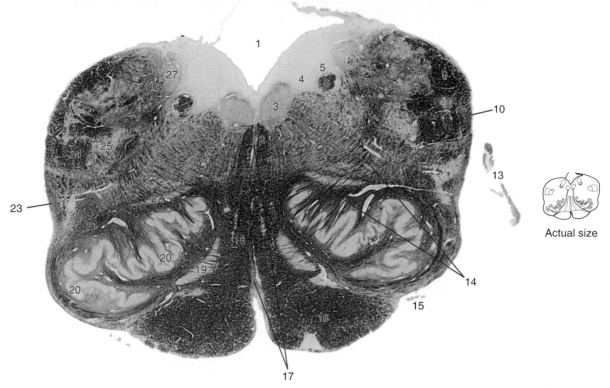

Figure 15-5 Rostral medulla. Actual size: 16 mm wide × 12 mm from anterior to posterior.

1. Fourth ventricle.
2. Medial longitudinal fasciculus (MLF). At this level, the fibers of the medial vestibulospinal tract.
3. Hypoglossal nucleus. Lower motor neurons for the ipsilateral half of the tongue.
4. Dorsal motor nucleus of the vagus. Most of the preganglionic parasympathetic neurons for thoracic and abdominal viscera.
5. Nucleus of the solitary tract. Site of termination of the visceral primary afferents in the solitary tract.
6. Solitary tract. Primary afferents conveying visceral information from cranial nerves VII, IX, and X (and some chemosensory information from the trigeminal nerve) to the surrounding nucleus of the solitary tract.
7. Nucleus cuneatus. Site of termination of fasciculus cuneatus and the origin of the arm portion of the medial lemniscus.
8. Lateral cuneate nucleus. Arm equivalent of Clarke's nucleus. Proprioceptive primary afferents travel through fasciculus cuneatus to reach the lateral cuneate nucleus, which then gives rise to uncrossed cuneocerebellar fibers that enter the cerebellum through the inferior cerebellar peduncle.
9. Inferior cerebellar peduncle. By the time it enters the cerebellum, it contains crossed olivocerebellar fibers, the uncrossed posterior spinocerebellar tract, vestibulocerebellar fibers, trigeminocerebellar fibers, and other cerebellar afferents.
10. Posterior spinocerebellar tract entering the inferior cerebellar peduncle. Uncrossed fibers from Clarke's nucleus, carrying proprioceptive information from the leg to the ipsilateral half of the cerebellar vermis.
11. Location of nucleus ambiguus. Lower motor neurons for laryngeal and pharyngeal muscles and preganglionic parasympathetic neurons for the heart.
12. Anterolateral pathway. Mostly crossed fibers from the spinal posterior horns and intermediate gray, conveying pain and temperature information to the thalamus (spinothalamic tract), reticular formation, and midbrain.
13. Vagus nerve (cranial nerve X).
14. Internal arcuate fibers. At this level, olivocerebellar fibers that cross the midline, join the inferior cerebellar peduncle, and end in the cerebellar cortex as climbing fibers.
15. Hypoglossal nerve fibers, on their way to the muscles of the ipsilateral half of the tongue.
16. Pyramid. Corticospinal fibers from the ipsilateral precentral gyrus and adjacent areas of cerebral cortex.
17. Raphe nuclei. Serotonergic neurons that at this level are one source of descending pain-control fibers to the spinal cord.
18. Medial lemniscus, the principal ascending pathway for tactile and proprioceptive information. Originates in the contralateral posterior column nuclei and terminates in the thalamus (VPL).
19. Inferior olivary nucleus (medial accessory nucleus). The inferior olivary complex gives rise to climbing fibers that end in the contralateral half of the cerebellum (see Chapter 20). Those from the accessory nuclei project mainly to the vermis and flocculus; those from the principal inferior olivary nucleus project to the cerebellar hemisphere.
20. Inferior olivary nucleus (principal nucleus). The inferior olivary complex gives rise to climbing fibers that end in the contralateral half of the cerebellum (see Chapter 20). Those from the accessory nuclei project mainly to the vermis and flocculus; those from the principal inferior olivary nucleus project to the cerebellar hemisphere.
21. Fibers of the central tegmental tract reaching the inferior olivary nucleus.
22. Inferior olivary nucleus (dorsal accessory nucleus). The inferior olivary complex gives rise to climbing fibers that end in the contralateral half of the cerebellum (see Chapter 20). Those from the accessory nuclei project mainly to the vermis and flocculus; those from the principal inferior olivary nucleus project to the cerebellar hemisphere.
23. Anterior spinocerebellar tract. Crossed fibers from lumbosacral spinal gray matter, carrying proprioceptive and other information from the leg. This tract stays in approximately the same position until the rostral pons, where it moves over the surface of the superior cerebellar peduncle (see Fig. 15-7) and turns posteriorly into the cerebellum.
24. Spinal trigeminal tract. Primary afferents from the ipsilateral side of the face, including those on their way to the caudal nucleus conveying information about pain and temperature.
25. Spinal trigeminal nucleus (interpolar nucleus). Some primary afferents of the spinal trigeminal tract, including those carrying information about dental pain, end here.
26. Inferior vestibular nucleus with bundles of vestibular primary afferents running through it.
27. Medial vestibular nucleus. Site of origin of the medial vestibulospinal tract (among other connections).

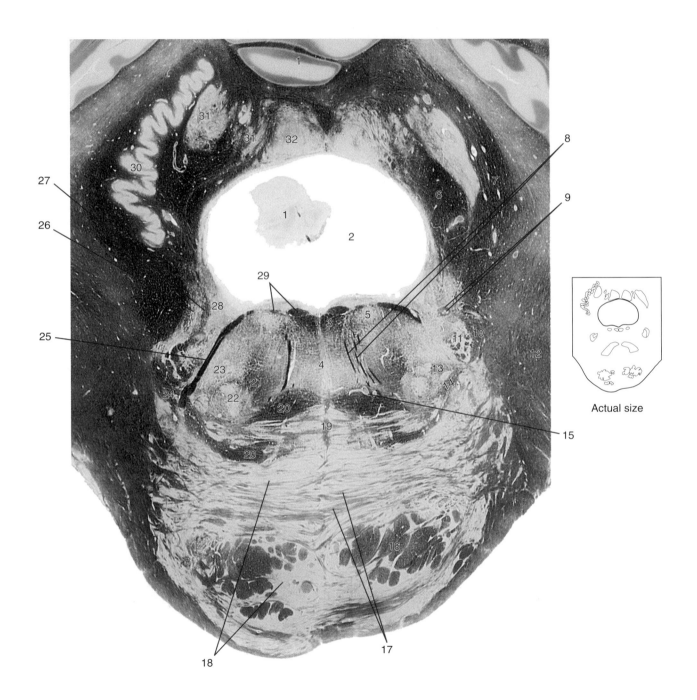

Actual size

Figure 15-6 Caudal pons. Actual size: 23 mm wide × 30 mm from anterior to posterior. (See Video 15-1.)

1. Vermis of the cerebellum. The zone of cerebellar cortex straddling the midline.
2. Fourth ventricle.
3. Medial longitudinal fasciculus (MLF). At this level, fibers from vestibular nuclei and abducens interneurons, active in coordinating eye movements.
4. Raphe nuclei. Widely projecting serotonergic neurons that collectively blanket the CNS. Those in intermediate brainstem levels such as this are one source of descending pain-control fibers to the spinal cord; they also project to other brainstem levels and the cerebellum.
5. Abducens nucleus. Contains the lower motor neurons for the ipsilateral lateral rectus and the interneurons that project through the contralateral MLF to medial rectus motor neurons.
6. Superior cerebellar peduncle. Fibers from the deep cerebellar nuclei to the contralateral red nucleus and thalamus (ventral lateral nucleus [VL]).
7. Inferior cerebellar peduncle entering the cerebellum. Contains crossed olivocerebellar fibers, the uncrossed posterior spinocerebellar tract, vestibulocerebellar fibers, trigeminocerebellar fibers, and other cerebellar afferents.
8. Abducens nerve fibers, on their way to the ipsilateral lateral rectus.
9. Solitary tract and its nucleus. Primary afferents conveying visceral information from cranial nerves VII, IX, and X (and some chemosensory information from the trigeminal nerve) travel through the solitary tract to reach the surrounding nucleus of the solitary tract. Only gustatory information reaches this rostral level.
10. Spinal trigeminal tract. Primary afferents from the ipsilateral side of the face, including those on their way to the caudal nucleus conveying information about pain and temperature.
11. Spinal trigeminal nucleus (oral nucleus). Some primary afferents of the spinal trigeminal tract, particularly those carrying tactile information, end here.
12. Middle cerebellar peduncle. Fibers from contralateral pontine nuclei that end as mossy fibers (see Chapter 20) in all areas of cerebellar cortex.
13. Lateral lemniscus. Ascending auditory fibers from the cochlear and superior olivary nuclei, representing both ears.
14. Anterolateral pathway. Mostly crossed fibers from the spinal posterior horns and intermediate gray, conveying pain and temperature information to the thalamus (spinothalamic tract), reticular formation, and midbrain.
15. Errant avian.
16. Corticospinal, corticobulbar, and corticopontine fibers, from ipsilateral cerebral cortex.
17. Pontocerebellar fibers, from pontine nuclei of one side to the opposite middle cerebellar peduncle.
18. Pontine nuclei. Source of pontocerebellar fibers that cross the midline and form the middle cerebellar peduncle.
19. Trapezoid body. Crossing auditory fibers, primarily from the ventral cochlear nucleus.
20. Medial lemniscus. The principal ascending pathway for tactile and proprioceptive information. Originates in the contralateral posterior column nuclei, terminates in the thalamus (VPL).
21. Central tegmental tract. Descending fibers from the red nucleus to the inferior olivary nucleus, together with fibers to and from different levels of the reticular formation.
22. Superior olivary nucleus. First site of convergence of fibers representing the two ears and the source of many of the fibers of the lateral lemniscus.
23. Facial motor nucleus. Lower motor neurons for ipsilateral muscles of facial expression.
24. Anterior spinocerebellar tract. Crossed fibers from lumbosacral spinal gray matter, carrying proprioceptive and other information from the leg. This tract stays in approximately the same position until the rostral pons, where it moves over the surface of the superior cerebellar peduncle (see Fig. 15-7) and turns posteriorly into the cerebellum.
25. Facial nerve fibers. Most of them are on their way to ipsilateral muscles of facial expression.
26. Lateral vestibular nucleus, source of the lateral vestibulospinal tract.
27. Juxtarestiform body. Fibers of the inferior cerebellar peduncle interconnecting the vestibular nuclei and cerebellum.
28. Superior vestibular nucleus.
29. Internal genu of the facial nerve. Facial nerve fibers, most of them on their way to ipsilateral muscles of facial expression.
30. Dentate nucleus. The deep nucleus connected to lateral parts of the cerebellar hemisphere and the source of most of the fibers in the superior cerebellar peduncle.
31. Interposed nucleus. The deep cerebellar nucleus connected to medial parts of the cerebellar hemisphere.
32. Fastigial nucleus. The deep cerebellar nucleus connected to the vermis and flocculus.

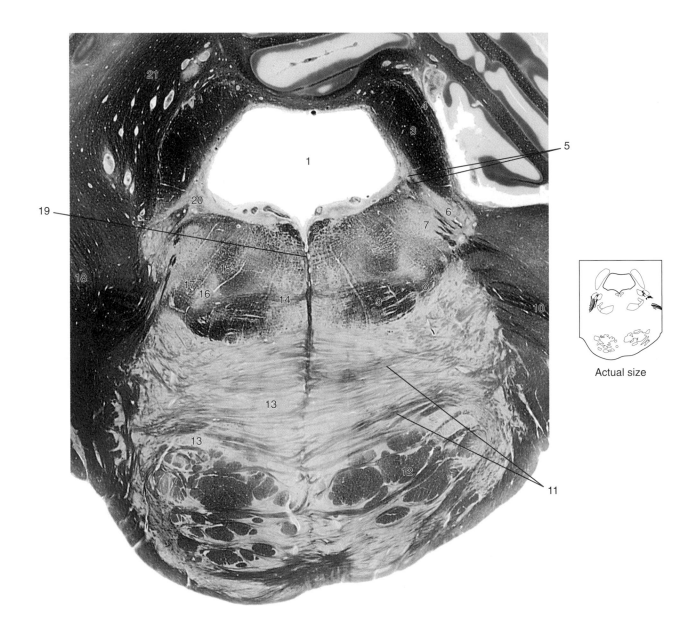

Actual size

Figure 15-7 Midpons. Actual size: 21 mm wide × 26 mm from anterior to posterior.

1. Fourth ventricle.
2. Medial longitudinal fasciculus (MLF). At this level, the fibers are from vestibular nuclei and abducens interneurons and are active in coordinating eye movements.
3. Superior cerebellar peduncle. Fibers from the deep cerebellar nuclei to the contralateral red nucleus and thalamus (VL).
4. Anterior spinocerebellar tract. Crossed fibers from lumbosacral spinal gray matter, carrying proprioceptive and other information from the leg.
5. Mesencephalic trigeminal tract and nucleus. Processes of primary afferent cell bodies in the mesencephalic trigeminal nucleus travel through the tract, leave the brainstem, and innervate mechanoreceptors in and around the mouth.
6. Trigeminal main sensory nucleus. Site of termination of large-diameter trigeminal afferents; site of origin of the uncrossed dorsal trigeminal tract and of part of the contralateral medial lemniscus.
7. Trigeminal motor nucleus. Lower motor neurons for ipsilateral muscles of mastication.
8. Anterolateral pathway. Mostly crossed fibers from the spinal posterior horns and intermediate gray, conveying pain and temperature information to the thalamus (spinothalamic tract), reticular formation, and midbrain.
9. Medial lemniscus. The principal ascending pathway for tactile and proprioceptive information. Originates in the contralateral posterior column nuclei and trigeminal main sensory nucleus, terminates in the thalamus (VPL).
10. Trigeminal nerve. Somatosensory (and some chemosensory) fibers from the ipsilateral half of the head; efferents to ipsilateral muscles of mastication.
11. Pontocerebellar fibers, from pontine nuclei of one side to the opposite middle cerebellar peduncle.
12. Corticospinal, corticobulbar, and corticopontine fibers from ipsilateral cerebral cortex.
13. Pontine nuclei. Source of pontocerebellar fibers that cross the midline and form the middle cerebellar peduncle.
14. Trapezoid body. Crossing auditory fibers, primarily from the ventral cochlear nucleus.
15. Central tegmental tract. Descending fibers from the red nucleus to the inferior olivary nucleus, together with fibers to and from different levels of the reticular formation.
16. Superior olivary nucleus. First site of convergence of fibers representing the two ears and the source of many of the fibers of the lateral lemniscus.
17. Lateral lemniscus. Ascending auditory fibers from the cochlear and superior olivary nuclei, representing both ears.
18. Middle cerebellar peduncle. Fibers from contralateral pontine nuclei that end as mossy fibers (see Chapter 20) in all areas of cerebellar cortex.
19. Raphe nuclei. Widely projecting serotonergic neurons that collectively blanket the CNS. Those in rostral brainstem levels such as this project mainly to the cerebrum and cerebellum.
20. Superior vestibular nucleus.
21. Inferior cerebellar peduncle entering the cerebellum. Contains crossed olivocerebellar fibers, the uncrossed posterior spinocerebellar tract, vestibulocerebellar fibers, trigeminocerebellar fibers, and other cerebellar afferents.

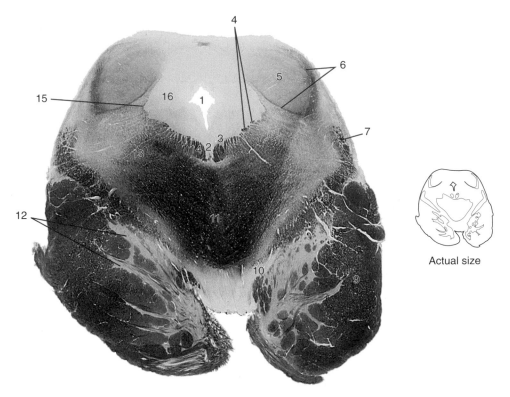

Actual size

Figure 15-8 Caudal midbrain. Actual size: 20 mm wide × 20 mm from anterior to posterior.

1. Cerebral aqueduct.
2. Raphe nuclei. Widely projecting serotonergic neurons that collectively blanket the CNS. Those in rostral brainstem levels such as this project mainly to the cerebrum.
3. Trochlear nucleus. Lower motor neurons for the contralateral superior oblique muscle.
4. Trochlear nerve fibers, on their way to the contralateral superior oblique (after crossing in the trochlear decussation at the pons-midbrain junction).
5. Inferior colliculus. Site of termination of the lateral lemniscus and site of origin of the brachium of the inferior colliculus, which carries auditory information to the medial geniculate nucleus.
6. Lateral lemniscus ending in the inferior colliculus, the next stop in the central auditory pathway.
7. Anterolateral pathway. Mostly crossed fibers from the spinal posterior horns and intermediate gray, conveying pain and temperature information to the thalamus (spinothalamic tract), reticular formation, and midbrain.
8. Medial lemniscus. The principal ascending pathway for tactile and proprioceptive information. Originates in the contralateral posterior column nuclei and trigeminal main sensory nucleus, terminates in the thalamus (VPL).

9. Cerebral peduncle, at the junction between the caudal midbrain and the basal pons. Descending corticospinal, corticobulbar, and corticopontine fibers from ipsilateral cerebral cortex.
10. Substantia nigra. The very caudal end of the compact part, containing dopaminergic neurons whose axons terminate in the caudate nucleus and putamen (see Chapter 19).
11. Decussation of the superior cerebellar peduncles. Fibers from the deep cerebellar nuclei to the contralateral red nucleus and thalamus (VL).
12. Pontine nuclei. Source of pontocerebellar fibers that cross the midline and form the middle cerebellar peduncle.
13. Central tegmental tract. Descending fibers from the red nucleus to the inferior olivary nucleus, together with fibers to and from different levels of the reticular formation.
14. Medial longitudinal fasciculus (MLF). At this level, the fibers are from vestibular nuclei and abducens interneurons and are active in coordinating eye movements.
15. Mesencephalic trigeminal tract. Processes of cell bodies in the adjacent mesencephalic trigeminal nucleus that innervate mechanoreceptors in and around the mouth.
16. Periaqueductal gray. Site of origin of the descending pain-control pathway that relays in the nucleus raphe magnus (among other connections).

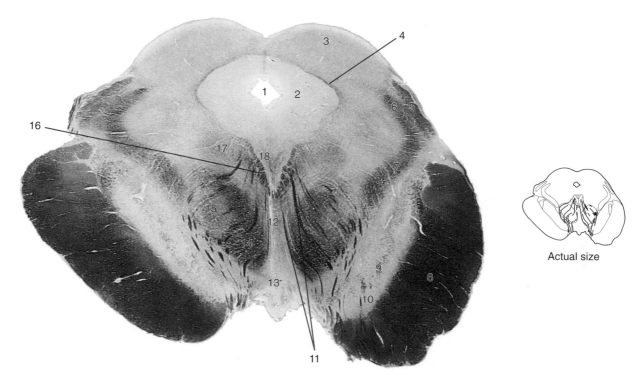

Actual size

Figure 15-9 Rostral midbrain. Actual size: 26 mm wide × 20 mm from anterior to posterior.

1. Cerebral aqueduct.
2. Periaqueductal gray. Site of origin of the descending pain-control pathway that relays in the nucleus raphe magnus (among other connections).
3. Superior colliculus. Involved in visual attention and eye movements, and the site of termination of most fibers of the superior brachium.
4. Mesencephalic trigeminal tract. Processes of cell bodies in the adjacent mesencephalic trigeminal nucleus that innervate mechanoreceptors in and around the mouth.
5. Brachium of the inferior colliculus. Ascending auditory fibers on their way from the inferior colliculus to the medial geniculate nucleus.
6. Anterolateral pathway. Mostly crossed fibers from the spinal posterior horns and intermediate gray, conveying pain and temperature information to the thalamus (spinothalamic tract), reticular formation, and midbrain.
7. Medial lemniscus. The principal ascending pathway for tactile and proprioceptive information. Originates in the contralateral posterior column nuclei and trigeminal main sensory nucleus, terminates in the thalamus (VPL).
8. Cerebral peduncle. Descending corticospinal, corticobulbar, and corticopontine fibers from ipsilateral cerebral cortex.
9. Substantia nigra (compact part). Dopaminergic neurons whose axons terminate in the caudate nucleus and putamen (see Chapter 19).
10. Substantia nigra (reticular part). Site of termination of fibers from the caudate nucleus and putamen and site of origin of fibers to

the thalamus, superior colliculus, and reticular formation (see Chapter 19).

11. Oculomotor nerve fibers. Axons of lower motor neurons and preganglionic parasympathetic neurons for the ipsilateral medial, superior, and inferior recti; inferior oblique; levator palpebrae; pupillary sphincter; and ciliary muscle.
12. Raphe nuclei. Widely projecting serotonergic neurons that collectively blanket the CNS. Those in rostral brainstem levels such as this project mainly to the cerebrum.
13. Ventral tegmental area. Dopaminergic neurons whose axons terminate in limbic and frontal cortical sites.
14. Crossed superior cerebellar peduncle entering the red nucleus. Fibers from the contralateral deep cerebellar nuclei, on their way to the red nucleus and thalamus (VL).
15. Red nucleus. Receives inputs from the contralateral deep cerebellar nuclei via the superior cerebellar peduncle and projects primarily to the inferior olivary nucleus via the central tegmental tract.
16. Medial longitudinal fasciculus (MLF). At this level the fibers are from vestibular nuclei and abducens interneurons and are active in coordinating eye movements.
17. Central tegmental tract. Descending fibers from the red nucleus to the inferior olivary nucleus, together with fibers to and from different levels of the reticular formation.
18. Oculomotor nucleus. Lower motor neurons for the ipsilateral medial and inferior recti and inferior oblique, the contralateral superior rectus, and the levator palpebrae of both sides; preganglionic parasympathetic neurons for the pupillary sphincter and the ciliary muscle.

The Thalamus and Internal Capsule: Getting to and from the Cerebral Cortex

The diencephalon, mostly hidden from view between the cerebral hemispheres (Fig. 16-1A), constitutes only about 2% of the central nervous system (CNS) by weight. Nevertheless, it has widespread and important connections, and the great majority of sensory, motor, and limbic pathways involve a stop in the diencephalon. Most motor and limbic pathways also involve telencephalic structures that are discussed in later chapters, so this chapter provides only a general overview of the connections of diencephalic nuclei. These connections are discussed in more detail in terms of functional systems in subsequent chapters, and a series of sections demonstrating major structures of both the diencephalon and the telencephalon is provided in Chapter 25. Nearly all the connections between the cerebral cortex and subcortical structures, prominently including the diencephalon, travel through the internal capsule, so an overview of this structure is provided here as well.

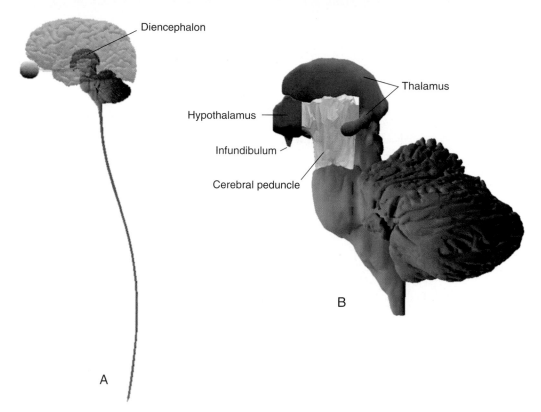

Figure 16-1 Three-dimensional reconstructions of the diencephalon. **A,** The entire CNS, showing the diencephalon (green) almost completely surrounded by the cerebral hemispheres. **B,** The diencephalon, brainstem, and cerebellum, with the cerebral hemispheres removed.

The Diencephalon Includes the Epithalamus, Subthalamus, Hypothalamus, and Thalamus

The diencephalon (see Fig. 16-1B) is conventionally divided into four parts, each of which includes the term *thalamus* (from a Greek word meaning "inner chamber") as part of its name.[a] These parts are (1) the **epithalamus,** which includes the **pineal gland** and a few nearby neural structures, (2) the **dorsal thalamus,** which is usually referred to simply as the **thalamus,** (3) the **subthalamus,** and (4) the **hypothalamus.**

The only part of the diencephalon that can be seen on an intact brain is the inferior surface of the hypothalamus (see Figs. 3-16 and 3-17), which includes the **mammillary bodies** and the **infundibular stalk.** However, the entire medial surface of the diencephalon, much of which forms each wall of the third ventricle, can be seen on a hemisected brain (Fig. 16-2). Superiorly, the diencephalon borders the body of the lateral ventricle; inferiorly, it is exposed to subarachnoid space; laterally, it is bordered by the internal capsule (Fig. 16-3). The caudal boundary of the diencephalon is a plane through

the posterior commissure; the rostral boundary is the anterior commissure. These rostral and caudal boundaries are approximate and somewhat arbitrary and are used only for purposes of discussion, as they are functionally continuous with bordering structures.

As a consequence of the cephalic flexure, the axis of the diencephalon is inclined about 80 degrees with respect to the axis of the brainstem (see Fig. 3-1). This means that sections cut in a plane similar to that used in the last few chapters (i.e., perpendicular to the long axis of the brainstem) are at a peculiar angle to the diencephalon. Therefore, in this and subsequent chapters, sections cut in axial and coronal planes are shown (see Fig. 16-1).[b]

The Epithalamus Includes the Pineal Gland and the Habenular Nuclei

The **pineal gland** is a midline, unpaired structure situated just rostral to the superior colliculi. It resembles a

---

[a]A few other structures, most notably the globus pallidus, are derived embryologically from the diencephalon but usually are not considered part of it in discussions of the adult brain.

[b]The axial sections are oriented with the anterior portion at the top of the picture, because this is the way computed tomography scans and magnetic resonance images are conventionally oriented. One result, which can sometimes cause confusion, is that anterior parts of the brainstem are situated toward the top of the picture; this is upside down relative to the way the brainstem is pictured in Chapters 11 to 15.

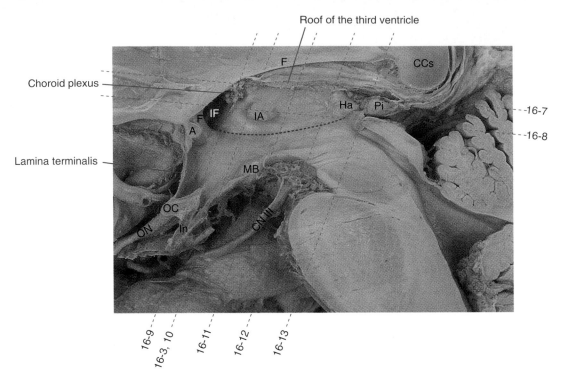

Roof of the third ventricle

Choroid plexus

Lamina terminalis

Figure 16-2 Close-up photograph of the medial surface of a hemisected brain, illustrating parts of the diencephalon and some surrounding structures. The dashed red line indicates the hypothalamic sulcus, separating the thalamus above it from the hypothalamus below it. The dashed blue lines indicate the approximate planes of section of other figures in this chapter. A, anterior commissure; CCs, splenium of the corpus callosum; CN III, oculomotor nerve; F, fornix; Ha, habenula; IA, interthalamic adhesion; IF, interventricular foramen; In, infundibular stalk; MB, mammillary body; OC, optic chiasm; ON, optic nerve; Pi, pineal gland. *(Modified from Nolte J, Angevine JB Jr: The human brain in photographs and diagrams, ed 3, St. Louis, 2007, Mosby.)*

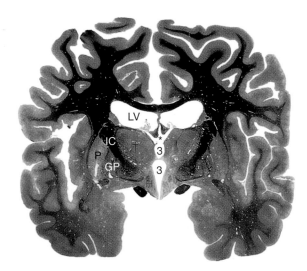

Figure 16-3 Spaces and structures bordering the thalamus (T) and hypothalamus (H), as seen in a coronal section. (The thin roof of the third ventricle that would normally separate this ventricle from the transverse cerebral fissure has been torn away.) *, transverse cerebral fissure; 3, third ventricle; GP, globus pallidus; IC, internal capsule; LV, lateral ventricle; P, putamen.

pinecone in shape, which is how it got its name. Because each of us has only one pineal gland, which is located deep within the brain, it was once thought that this organ might be the seat of the soul. This now seems unlikely, because pineal tumors do not cause the changes one would expect to find with distortion of the soul; rather, these tumors compress the midbrain and cause the changes one would expect to see with distortion of this part of the brainstem. Early findings may include hydrocephalus (because the aqueduct gets squeezed shut) and various deficits in eye movements and pupillary reactions (because of damage to the oculomotor and trochlear nuclei and pathways ending in them). In addition, pineal tumors may cause changes in sexual development, giving a clue to at least one of its possible functions. The pineal arises as an evagination from the roof of the diencephalon; in fish, amphibians, and many reptiles, it contains photoreceptor cells similar to retinal cones. In these species it is suspected of monitoring day length and season and participating in the regulation of circadian and circannual rhythms (although there are probably other functions as well). The pineal gland of birds and mammals contains no photoreceptors and consists of a collection of secretory cells (**pinealocytes**), some glial cells, and a rich vascular network. Nevertheless, it still receives a light-regulated input by way of a circuitous pathway that begins in the retina and, after one or more relays in the hypothalamus, reaches the intermediolateral cell column of the spinal cord. Preganglionic sympathetic fibers from the spinal cord then synapse on postganglionic neurons of the superior cervical ganglion, which in turn send their axons to the pineal.

The mammalian pineal is an endocrine gland involved in seasonal cycles (e.g., reproductive cycles) and other functions and has no known neural output. Instead it secretes a hormone derived from serotonin, called **melatonin,** at relatively high rates during darkness. In many species melatonin has an antigonadotropic effect, and light, by way of the neural pathway just described, causes a decrease in melatonin production. As days get longer in the spring, melatonin production declines, which in turn causes an increase in gonadal function. This system is of considerable importance in mammals with prominent seasonal sexual cycles, but its effects in humans are not as clear. It has been reported, however, that nonparenchymal pineal tumors, which presumably destroy pinealocytes, tend to be associated with precocious puberty, as though the production of some antigonadotropic substance had been halted. The converse has been reported as well—that parenchymal pineal tumors tend to be associated with hypogonadism. These tumors are relatively rare, however, and in humans the pineal is probably more important in the regulation of circadian rhythms, including sleep-wake cycles (see Chapter 22). The routine clinical importance of the pineal arises from the fact that after the age of about 17 years, calcareous concretions accrue in it. This makes it opaque to x-rays and hence a useful radiological landmark (Fig. 16-4). Because it normally lies in the midline, slight shifts in pineal position can be indicative of expanding masses of various types.

The pineal gland is attached to the diencephalon by a stalk. Caudally at the base of the stalk is the posterior commissure; rostrally is a small swelling on each side called a **habenula** (see Figs. 16-2 and 16-12). Underlying each habenula are the **habenular nuclei.** Each habenula receives one major input bundle, the **stria medullaris** ("white stripe") **of the thalamus,** and gives rise to one major output bundle with the awesome name of **habenulointerpeduncular tract** (or **fasciculus retroflexus**). The habenulointerpeduncular tract, as its name implies, extends from the habenula to the **interpeduncular nucleus,** located between the cerebral peduncles, and to other parts of the midbrain reticular formation. The fibers of the stria medullaris originate in the globus pallidus and some limbic structures, so the pathway through the habenula is one route through which the basal nuclei and limbic system can influence the brainstem reticular formation. The habenula has been shown to regulate the release of the biogenic amines from the brainstem reticular formation and is thought to play a role in assigning "reward value" to stimuli. In other words the habenula nuclei will send messages to the dopamine and serotonin cells of the brainstem, increasing their activity based on how well an individual "enjoyed" a certain stimulus. In addition, studies have shown that the lack of activity of the habenula and its

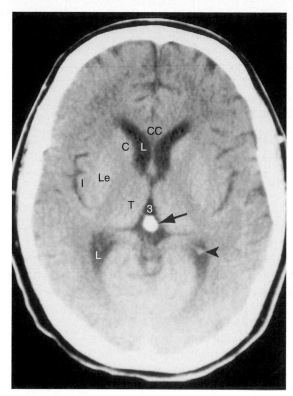

Figure 16-4 Uncontrasted computed tomography (CT) scan of a normal 58-year-old man. Calcium deposits in the pineal gland *(arrow)* and in the glomus (the enlarged region of choroid plexus in the atrium of the lateral ventricle, *arrowhead*) make them x-ray dense and hence apparent on CT scans, even without contrast. 3, third ventricle; C, caudate nucleus; CC, corpus callosum; I, insula; L, lateral ventricle; Le, lenticular nucleus; T, thalamus. *(Courtesy Dr. Raymond F. Carmody, University of Arizona College of Medicine.)*

projections to the brainstem reticular formation may play a role in depression.

The Subthalamus Includes the Subthalamic Nucleus and the Zona Incerta

Parts of the midbrain tegmentum continue into the diencephalon as the subthalamus. This area is completely surrounded by neural tissue and is located inferior to the thalamus, lateral to the hypothalamus, and medial to the cerebral peduncle and internal capsule (see Figs. 16-11 and 16-12). The subthalamus contains rostral portions of the red nucleus and substantia nigra and is traversed by somatosensory pathways on their way to the thalamus, as well as by several pathways involving the cerebellum and basal nuclei (the latter pathways are discussed in Chapters 19 and 20). In addition, the subthalamus contains the **subthalamic nucleus** and **zona incerta** (see Fig. 16-11). The subthalamic nucleus is a lens-shaped, biconvex structure located just medial and superior to parts of the cerebral peduncle and internal capsule. This nucleus is interconnected with the basal nuclei, as discussed in Chapter 19. The zona incerta is a small mass of gray matter intervening between the subthalamic nucleus and the thalamus. It appears to be a rostral continuation of the midbrain reticular formation and has very widespread connections (including direct projections to the cerebral cortex), although its function is largely unknown.

The Thalamus Is the Gateway to the Cerebral Cortex

The thalami are a pair of large, egg-shaped, nuclear masses with a posterior appendage (Figs. 16-1B and 16-5); together they make up about 80% of the diencephalon. Each thalamus extends anteriorly to the interventricular foramen, superiorly to the transverse cerebral fissure and the floor of the lateral ventricle, and inferiorly to the hypothalamic sulcus; posteriorly it overlaps the midbrain (see Fig. 16-13). The thalamus is part of a remarkably large number of pathways; all sensory pathways (other than olfaction) relay in the thalamus, and many of the anatomical circuits used by the cerebellum, basal nuclei, and limbic structures also involve thalamic relays. These various systems utilize more or less separate portions of the thalamus, which has therefore been subdivided into a series of nuclei.

Thalamic nuclei can be distinguished from one another both by their topographical locations within the thalamus and by the patterns of their inputs and outputs.

The Thalamus Has Anterior, Medial, and Lateral Divisions, Defined by the Internal Medullary Lamina

The topographical organization of the thalamus is shown in Figure 16-6 and Table 16-1. A thin, curved sheet of myelinated fibers, the **internal medullary lamina,** divides most of the thalamus into medial and lateral groups of nuclei (Figs. 16-7 and 16-8). Anteriorly, the internal medullary lamina splits and encloses an anterior group of nuclei, usually referred to collectively as the **anterior nucleus,** which borders on the interventricular foramen. The medial group similarly contains a single large nucleus, the **dorsomedial (DM) nucleus** (also commonly called the medial dorsal [MD] nucleus).

The lateral group of nuclei composes the bulk of the thalamus and is further subdivided into a dorsal tier and a ventral tier. The dorsal tier consists of the **lateral dorsal (LD) nucleus** (see Fig. 16-11), the **lateral posterior (LP)**

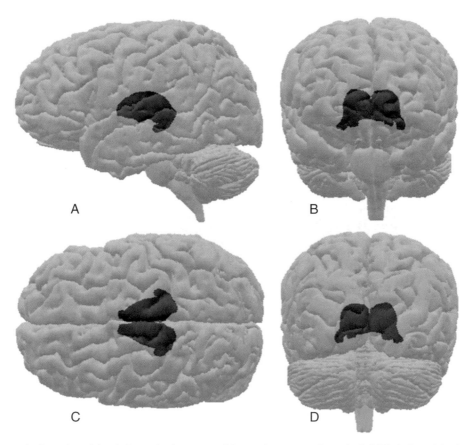

A

B

C

D

Figure 16-5 Location and orientation of the thalamus in the center of the cerebrum, seen from the left **(A)**, in front **(B)**, above **(C)**, and behind **(D)**.

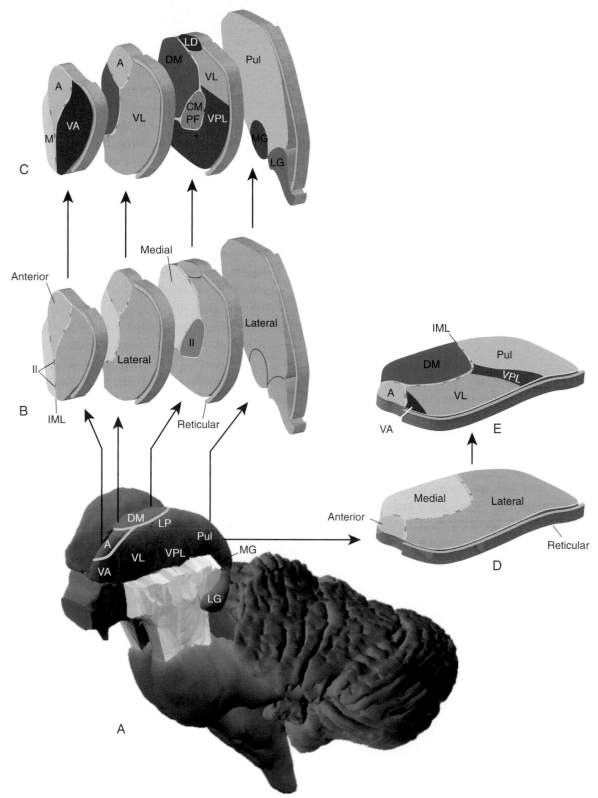

Figure 16-6 Topographical subdivisions of the thalamus. **A,** Lateral view of the left thalamus as seen from slightly above and in front. The reticular nucleus has been removed; ordinarily it would cover the entire lateral surface. **B** and **C,** Same view as **A,** but exploded into four pieces to show the internal arrangement of topographical subdivisions **(B)** and the major nuclei of each subdivision **(C).** The most anterior sliced surface corresponds approximately to Figure 16-9; the most posterior sliced surface corresponds approximately to Figure 16-13. **D** and **E,** A horizontal slab corresponding approximately to Figure 16-7 showing the internal arrangement of topographical subdivisions **(D)** and the major nuclei of each subdivision **(E).** *, ventral posteromedial nucleus; A, anterior nucleus; CM, centromedian nucleus (the largest intralaminar nucleus); DM, dorsomedial nucleus; Il, intralaminar nuclei; IML, internal medullary lamina; LD, lateral dorsal nucleus; LG, lateral geniculate nucleus; LP, lateral posterior nucleus; M, midline nuclei; MG, medial geniculate nucleus; PF, parafascicular nucleus; Pul, pulvinar; VA, ventral anterior nucleus; VL, ventral lateral nucleus; VPL, ventral postero-lateral nucleus.

Table 16-1	Topographical Subdivisions of the Thalamus and Their Principal Nuclei	
Subdivision	**Principal Nuclei**	**Common Abbreviation**
Anterior division	Anterior	
Medial division	Dorsomedial (medial dorsal)	DM (MD)
Lateral division	Dorsal tier	
	Lateral dorsal	LD
	Lateral posterior pulvinar	LP
	Ventral tier	
	Ventral anterior	VA
	Ventral lateral	VL
	Ventral posterior	VP
	Ventral posterolateral	VPL
	Medial geniculate	MGN
	Lateral geniculate	LGN
Intralaminar nuclei	Centromedian	CM
	Parafascicular	PF
	Others	
Reticular nucleus	Reticular nucleus	

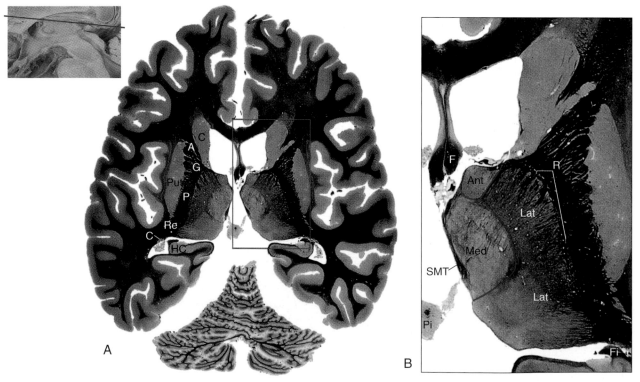

Figure 16-7 Topographical subdivisions of the thalamus, as seen in a horizontal section at the level of the stria medullaris of the thalamus (SMT). **A,** The entire section shown at about 60% actual size. **B,** Enlargement of the area indicated in **A,** showing the demarcation of anterior (Ant), medial (Med), and lateral (Lat) divisions by the internal medullary lamina (drawn in red). The lateral surface of the thalamus is covered by the reticular nucleus (R). A, anterior limb of the internal capsule; C, caudate nucleus (the head of the caudate anteriorly and the tail of the caudate posteriorly); F, fornix; Fi, fimbria (fibers associated with the hippocampus that will join the fornix); G, genu of the internal capsule; HC, hippocampus; P, posterior limb of the internal capsule; Pi, pineal gland; Put, putamen; Re, retrolenticular part of the internal capsule. *(Modified from Nolte J, Angevine JB Jr: The human brain in photographs and diagrams, ed 3, St. Louis, 2007, Mosby.)*

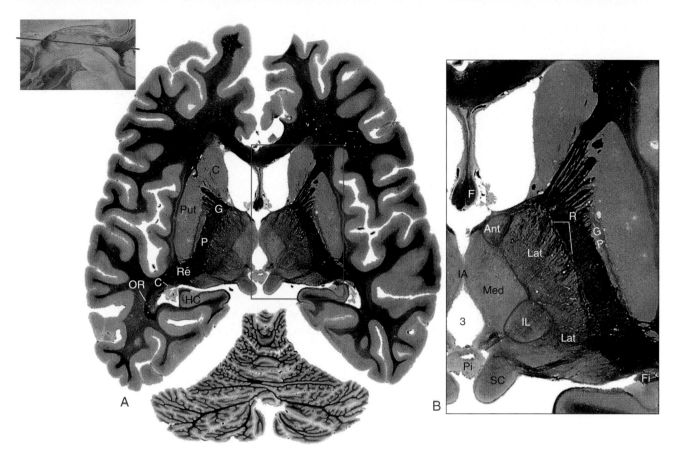

Figure 16-8 Topographical subdivisions of the thalamus, as seen in a horizontal section at a midthalamic level. **A,** The entire section shown at about 60% actual size. **B,** Enlargement of the area indicated in **A,** showing the demarcation of anterior (Ant), medial (Med), lateral (Lat), and intralaminar (IL) divisions by the internal medullary lamina (drawn in red). The lateral surface of the thalamus is covered by the reticular nucleus (R). 3, third ventricle; C, caudate nucleus (the head of the caudate anteriorly and the tail of the caudate posteriorly); F, fornix; Fi, fimbria (fibers associated with the hippocampus that will join the fornix); G, genu of the internal capsule; GP, globus pallidus; HC, hippocampus; IA, interthalamic adhesion (location of midline nuclei); OR, optic radiation (fibers on their way from the thalamus to visual cortex); P, posterior limb of the internal capsule; Pi, pineal gland; Put, putamen; Re, retrolenticular part of the internal capsule; SC, superior colliculus. *(Modified from Nolte J, Angevine JB Jr: The human brain in photographs and diagrams, ed 3, St. Louis, 2007, Mosby.)*

nucleus (see Fig. 16-12), and the large **pulvinar** (see Fig. 16-13). The lateral posterior nucleus is continuous with the pulvinar; both nuclei have similar connections, so the two together are sometimes referred to as the **pulvinar-LP complex.** The bulk of the ventral tier consists of three nuclei arranged in an anterior-posterior sequence: the **ventral anterior (VA) nucleus** (Fig. 16-9), the **ventral lateral (VL) nucleus** (Figs. 16-10 and 16-11), and the **ventral posterior (VP) nucleus** (Figs. 16-11 and 16-12). The ventral posterior nucleus is customarily subdivided into the **ventral posterolateral (VPL) nucleus** and the **ventral posteromedial (VPM) nucleus.** VPL is the somatosensory relay nucleus for the body, and VPM serves the same function for the head. VA and VL are involved in motor control circuits that include the cerebellum and basal nuclei. The **lateral geniculate nucleus** (visual system) and **medial geniculate nucleus** (auditory system) are located posterior to these ventral tier nuclei and inferior to the pulvinar, and they protrude posteriorly alongside the midbrain (Fig. 16-13).

Intralaminar Nuclei Are Embedded in the Internal Medullary Lamina

The internal medullary lamina splits at other locations within the thalamus and encloses additional groups of cells collectively called the **intralaminar nuclei.** The two largest of these are the **centromedian (CM)** and **parafascicular (PF) nuclei** (see Fig. 16-12). The centromedian nucleus is a relatively large, round nucleus located medial to VPL/VPM. The parafascicular nucleus is located medial to the centromedian nucleus and received its name from the fact that the habenulointerpeduncular tract (fasciculus retroflexus) passes through it.

The Thalamic Reticular Nucleus Partially Surrounds the Thalamus

The lateral surface of each thalamus is covered by a second curved sheet of myelinated fibers called the **external medullary lamina,** a layer where fibers sort themselves out on their way into and out of the

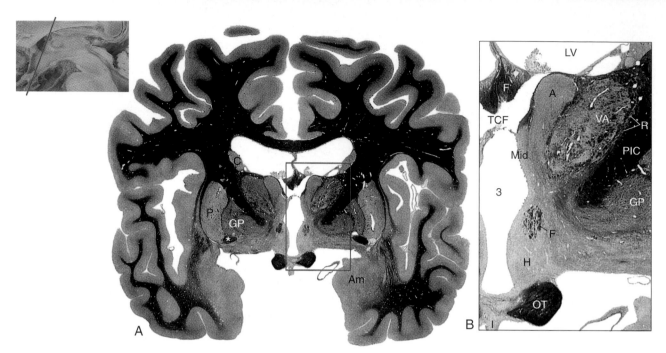

Figure 16-9 Coronal section through the anterior thalamus, near the interventricular foramen. **A,** The entire section shown at about 80% actual size. **B,** Enlargement of the area indicated in **A,** showing the anterior (A), midline (Mid), reticular (R), and ventral anterior (VA) nuclei. 3, third ventricle; *, anterior commissure (just before its fibers turn medially and cross the midline); Am, amygdala; C, caudate nucleus; F, fornix; GP, globus pallidus; H, hypothalamus; I, infundibulum; LV, lateral ventricle; OT, optic tract; P, putamen; PIC, posterior limb of the internal capsule; TCF, transverse cerebral fissure.

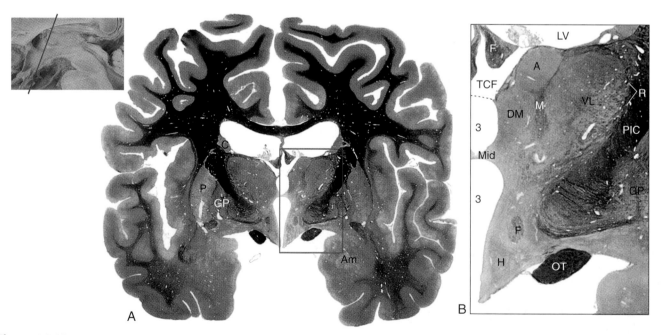

Figure 16-10 Coronal section through the anterior thalamus. **A,** The entire section shown at about 80% actual size. **B,** Enlargement of the area indicated in **A,** showing the anterior (A), dorsomedial (DM), midline (Mid), reticular (R), and ventral lateral (VL) nuclei. 3, third ventricle; Am, amygdala; C, caudate nucleus; F, fornix; GP, globus pallidus; H, hypothalamus; LV, lateral ventricle; M, mammillothalamic tract (entering the anterior nucleus); OT, optic tract; P, putamen; PIC, posterior limb of the internal capsule; TCF, transverse cerebral fissure. *(Modified from Nolte J, Angevine JB Jr: The human brain in photographs and diagrams, ed 3, St. Louis, 2007, Mosby.)*

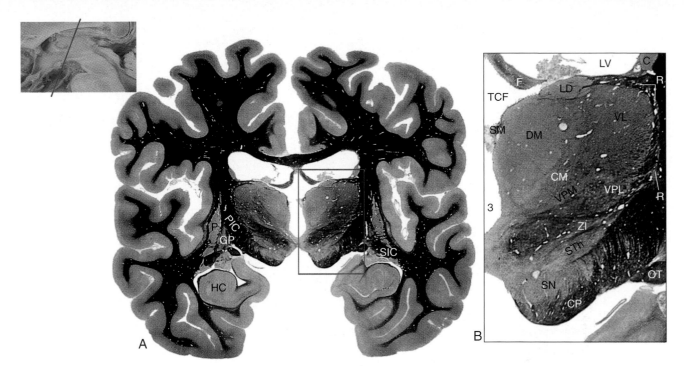

Figure 16-11 Coronal section through the midthalamus. **A,** The entire section shown at about 80% actual size. **B,** Enlargement of the area indicated in **A,** showing the centromedian (CM), dorsomedial (DM), lateral dorsal (LD), reticular (R), ventral lateral (VL), ventral posterolateral (VPL), and ventral posteromedial (VPM) nuclei. 3, third ventricle; C, caudate nucleus; CP, cerebral peduncle; F, fornix; GP, globus pallidus; HC, hippocampus; LV, lateral ventricle; OT, optic tract; P, putamen; PIC, posterior limb of the internal capsule; SIC, sublenticular part of the internal capsule; SM, stria medullaris of the thalamus; SN, substantia nigra; STh, subthalamic nucleus; TCF, transverse cerebral fissure; ZI, zona incerta. *(Modified from Nolte J, Angevine JB Jr: The human brain in photographs and diagrams, ed 3, St. Louis, 2007, Mosby.)*

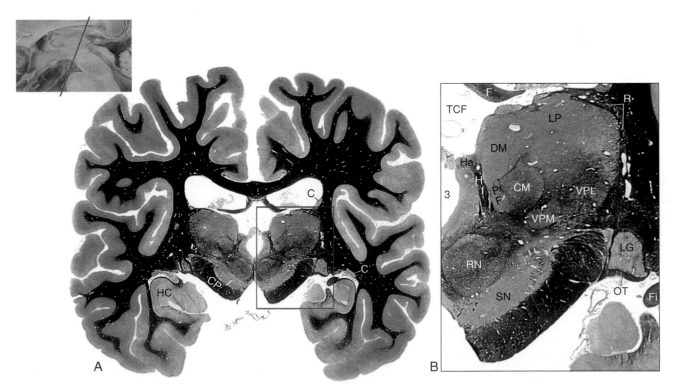

Figure 16-12 Coronal section through the posterior thalamus. **A,** The entire section shown at about 80% actual size. **B,** Enlargement of the area indicated in **A,** showing the centromedian (CM), dorsomedial (DM), lateral geniculate (LG), lateral posterior (LP), reticular (R), ventral posterolateral (VPL), and ventral posteromedial (VPM) nuclei. 3, third ventricle; C, caudate nucleus; CP, cerebral peduncle; F, fornix; Fi, fimbria (fibers associated with the hippocampus that will join the fornix); Ha, habenula; HC, hippocampus; HI, habenulointerpeduncular tract; OT, optic tract (entering the lateral geniculate nucleus); RN, red nucleus; SN, substantia nigra; TCF, transverse cerebral fissure. *(Modified from Nolte J, Angevine JB Jr: The human brain in photographs and diagrams, ed 3, St. Louis, 2007, Mosby.)*

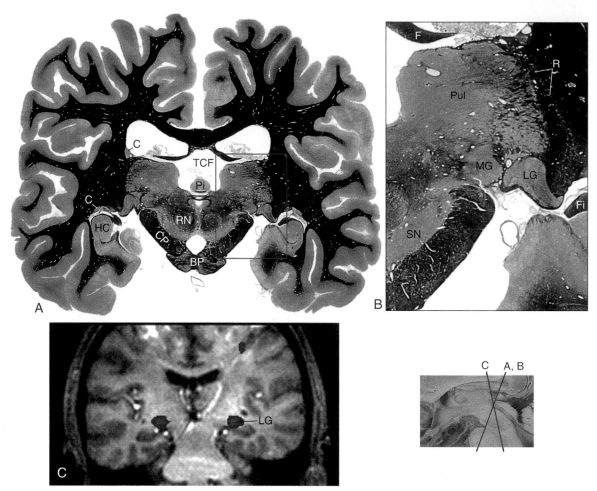

Figure 16-13 Coronal section through the posterior thalamus. **A,** The entire section shown at about 80% actual size. **B,** Enlargement of the area indicated in **A,** showing the lateral geniculate (LG), medial geniculate (MG), and reticular (R) nuclei and the pulvinar (Pul). **C,** Functional magnetic resonance imaging data from a subject watching a red and black checkerboard in which the squares reversed color 8 to 10 times per second, superimposed on a T1-weighted coronal slice at a level similar to that shown in **A.** The stimulus activates not only occipital cortex above and below the calcarine sulcus (see Fig. 6-21C) but also the lateral geniculate nucleus (LG). The inset at the bottom right shows the relative planes of section in **A, B,** and **C.** BP, basal pons; C, caudate nucleus; CP, cerebral peduncle; F, fornix; Fi, fimbria (fibers associated with the hippocampus that will join the fornix); HC, hippocampus; Pi, pineal gland; RN, red nucleus; SN, substantia nigra; TCF, transverse cerebral fissure. (**A** and **B,** *modified from Nolte J, Angevine JB Jr: The human brain in photographs and diagrams, ed 3, St. Louis, 2007, Mosby.* **C,** *from Chen W et al: Magn Reson Med 39:89, 1998.*)

thalamus. The thin shell of cells that intervenes between the external medullary lamina and the internal capsule is the **thalamic reticular nucleus**[c] (see Figs. 16-7 to 16-13). The reticular nucleus seems to be continuous inferiorly with the zona incerta (see Fig. 16-11), but this continuity is of no apparent functional significance.

Midline Nuclei Cover the Ventricular Surface of Each Thalamus

An additional layer of cells, essentially a rostral continuation of parts of the periaqueductal gray, covers portions of the medial surface of the thalamus. These cells

constitute the **midline nuclei** of the thalamus (separate and distinct from the dorsomedial nucleus). The midline nuclei of the two sides fuse in the interthalamic adhesion. The interthalamic adhesion is absent in 20% to 30% of humans.

Patterns of Input and Output Connections Define Functional Categories of Thalamic Nuclei

Thalamic nuclei are often thought of as simply pipelines through which information flows to the cerebral cortex, and for much of the time, this is a reasonable approximation of what they do. The thalamus also has a second role, however, which is presumably the reason for its continued existence. Successive stages in most neural pathways participate in transforming information or extracting features. For example, neurons at different

---

[c]Both the thalamic reticular nucleus and the brainstem reticular formation were named for their reticulated appearance, but they are distinct from each other in terms of anatomical location and patterns of connections.

levels of the retina and of visual cortical areas have different receptive fields—some emphasizing color, others emphasizing contrast or movement (see Chapter 17). In thalamic neurons, however, substantial changes in receptive fields do not develop. Rather, the thalamus is the site where decisions are implemented about which information should reach the cerebral cortex accurately for further processing. This general role is reflected in the physiological properties of thalamic neurons, and the particular type of information passed along by any given thalamic nucleus is a function of its input and output connections.

All Thalamic Nuclei (Except the Reticular Nucleus) Are Variations on a Common Theme

Developmentally, the thalamic reticular nucleus is not really part of the thalamus, and it has distinctive anatomical and physiological properties. It is nevertheless considered part of the thalamus because of its location and its extensive involvement in thalamic function, as described later in this chapter. All other thalamic nuclei are a mixture of projection neurons, whose axons provide the output from the thalamus, and small inhibitory interneurons that use γ-aminobutyric acid (GABA) as a neurotransmitter (Fig. 16-14A). Projection neurons account for 75% or more of the neurons in most thalamic nuclei, although the relative proportions of projection neurons and interneurons vary in different nuclei.

Inputs to the thalamus can be divided into two broad categories, referred to here as **specific inputs** and **regulatory inputs** (see Fig. 16-14A). Specific inputs are those conveying the information that a given thalamic nucleus may pass on accurately to the cerebral cortex (and, for some nuclei, to additional sites). The medial lemniscus, for example, is a specific input to VPL, and the optic tract is a specific input to the lateral geniculate nucleus. Regulatory inputs are those that contribute to decisions about the form in which information leaves a thalamic nucleus. The sources of regulatory inputs are broadly similar from one thalamic nucleus to another: most come from the cerebral cortex (mainly the cortical area to which a given thalamic nucleus projects), some come from the thalamic reticular nucleus, and the remainder include diffuse cholinergic, noradrenergic, serotonergic, and dopaminergic endings from the brainstem reticular formation. Although thalamic nuclei are usually thought of primarily in terms of their specific inputs, these are in fact greatly outnumbered by their regulatory inputs—a reflection of the distinctive role of the thalamus. This is nicely illustrated by the lateral geniculate nucleus, in which fewer than 10% of the synapses on projection neurons come from optic tract fibers and half or more come from visual cortex.

Distinctive patterns of outputs and specific inputs allow thalamic nuclei (other than the reticular nucleus)

to be grouped into three categories. **Relay nuclei** receive well-defined bundles of specific input fibers and project to particular functional areas of the cerebral cortex (see Fig. 16-14B); their role is to deliver information from particular functional systems to appropriate cortical areas. **Association nuclei** were originally named because they project to cortical areas traditionally referred to as *association areas* (see Chapter 22), but they have characteristic patterns of inputs as well. They receive their major contingent of specific inputs from the cerebral cortex itself (see Fig. 16-14C), and some from a variety of subcortical structures as well. Although the precise role of thalamic association nuclei is not understood, they are likely important in the distribution and gating of information *between* cortical areas. Finally, the **intralaminar** and **midline nuclei** seem to have a special role in the function of the basal nuclei and limbic system, although the details are not understood. Their specific inputs come from a wide array of sites, prominently including parts of the basal nuclei and limbic system, and they project not only to areas of cerebral cortex but also, and even more prominently, to parts of the basal nuclei and limbic system (see Fig. 16-14D).

Thalamic Projection Neurons Have Two Physiological States

The function of the thalamus as a gateway to the cerebral cortex depends on a combination of ion channels in its projection neurons that allows these neurons to function in two distinctly different physiological states. Projection neurons that are slightly depolarized are in a **tonic mode** and behave like typical neurons described elsewhere in this book. Slight additional depolarization causes a train of action potentials, and slight hyperpolarization causes their cessation (Fig. 16-15A and B). Neurons in the tonic mode can faithfully transmit to the cortex information that reaches them via specific inputs, using trains of action potentials whose frequency is a function of input magnitude.[d] Projection neurons hyperpolarized beyond the tonic range enter a **burst mode,** characterized by the availability of special voltage-gated Ca^{2+} channels (T-type VGCa2 channels). Slight depolarization of a neuron in the burst mode causes transient opening of the T-type voltage-gated Ca^{2+} channels, followed by their inactivation (similar to but slower than the opening and closing of voltage-gated Na^+ channels that underlies action potentials). The transient influx of

---

[d]Most specific inputs to the thalamus use glutamate as a neurotransmitter and act on glutamate-gated ion channels of thalamic relay neurons, with the result that increased input activity causes faster firing. Inputs from the basal nuclei, as described further in Chapter 19, use GABA as a neurotransmitter. The details of the physiological consequences of this unusual, apparently inhibitory, input are not yet known.

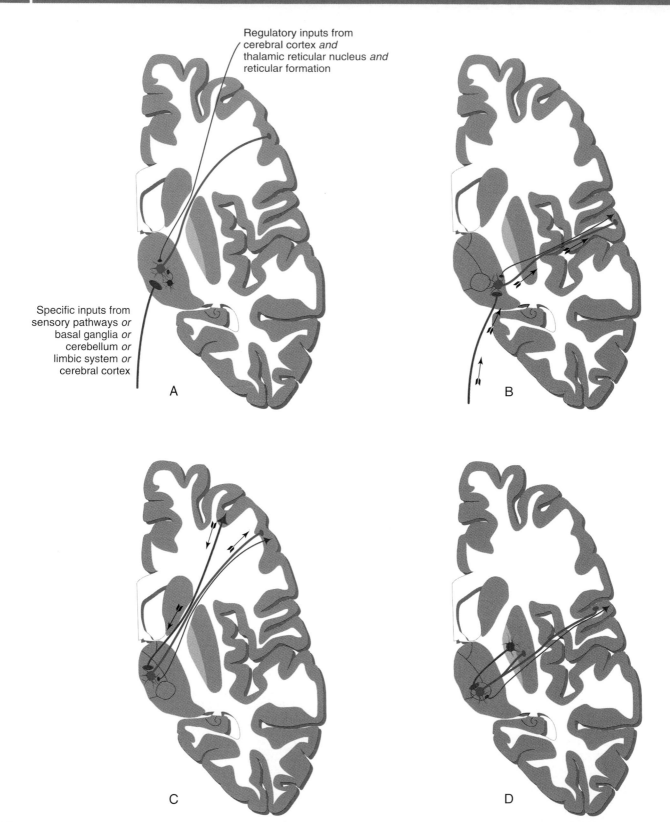

Regulatory inputs from
cerebral cortex *and*
thalamic reticular nucleus *and*
reticular formation

Specific inputs from
sensory pathways *or*
basal ganglia *or*
cerebellum *or*
limbic system *or*
cerebral cortex

A

B

C

D

Figure 16-14 Functional organization of the thalamus. **A,** Overview of the contents and connections of thalamic nuclei (except the reticular nucleus), shown in a schematic axial section through one cerebral hemisphere. Thalamic nuclei contain projection neurons (green) and inhibitory interneurons (red) in varying proportions, although the projection neurons are always in the majority. Axons of projection neurons reach the cerebral cortex (and, depending on the nucleus, other sites as well). Each nucleus receives a small but characteristic set of specific inputs (blue), usually from one principal source. Each nucleus also receives an array of large numbers of regulatory inputs (purple), most prominently from the cortical area to which it projects. **B,** Relay nuclei receive specific inputs from subcortical pathways (e.g., the medial lemniscus) and project to a well-defined functional area of cortex. **C,** Association nuclei receive major specific inputs from association cortex (e.g., prefrontal cortex) and project to related association areas. **D,** Intralaminar and midline nuclei receive distinctive sets of specific inputs (typically from basal ganglia or limbic structures) and project not only to the cerebral cortex but also to basal ganglia or limbic structures.

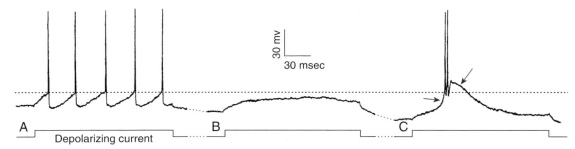

Figure 16-15 Effects of membrane potential on the physiological state of a projection neuron from the lateral geniculate nucleus of a cat. Three depolarizing current pulses of the same magnitude were injected into the neuron, starting from three different membrane potential levels; the threshold for the initiation of action potentials is indicated by the dotted red line. **A,** Starting from −55 mV, the voltage-gated Ca^{2+} channels are inactive, and depolarization initiates a train of action potentials. **B,** Starting from −60 mV, the voltage-gated Ca^{2+} channels are still inactive, but the depolarization is insufficient to bring the membrane to threshold. **C,** Starting from −70 mV, the voltage-gated Ca^{2+} channels are active, and the depolarization causes them to open and then inactivate and close; the Ca^{2+} influx causes an additional slow, depolarizing wave *(arrows)* sufficient to initiate a brief burst of action potentials. *(Modified from Sherman SM, Guillery RW: J Neurophysiol 76:1367, 1996.)*

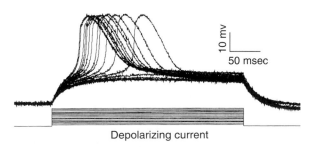

Figure 16-16 All-or-none depolarizing waves caused by the opening of voltage-gated Ca^{2+} channels in a lateral geniculate relay neuron of a cat. The neuron was treated with tetrodotoxin, to block Na^+ action potentials, and hyperpolarized to −87 mV so that voltage-gated Ca^{2+} channels were deinactivated ("reset") and available. Successively larger pulses of depolarizing current (lower traces) were then applied. Once threshold was reached, successively larger pulses each caused an all-or-none depolarizing wave, similar to an action potential but smaller and much slower. *(From Zhan XJ et al: J Neurophysiol 81:2360, 1999.)*

Ca^{2+} ions while the channels are open causes a depolarizing wave sufficient to trigger a burst of Na^+-based action potentials (Figs. 16-15C and 16-16). The duration of the inactivation of the voltage-gated Ca^{2+} channels is 100 msec or longer, so bursts of action potentials can occur only a few times per second. Neurons in this mode are very sensitive, because a small depolarization can trigger a burst. They are unable to transmit information about specific inputs accurately, however, because of the low frequency of bursts.

The functional mode of a thalamic projection neuron at any given moment is determined largely by its regulatory inputs. Focusing attention, whether on a stimulus, a task, or a thought, presumably involves placing the appropriate thalamic projection neurons in the tonic mode. The burst mode, in contrast, may have more than one function. During most phases of sleep, projection neurons are in the burst mode, dominated by rhythmic waves of depolarization and unable to transmit accurate

information about their specific inputs. Even during wakefulness, however, many projection neurons are also in the burst mode. In this case, the amplification provided by the voltage-gated Ca^{2+} channels may make these neurons particularly sensitive to the occurrence of an event, even though they would be unable to participate in the analysis of its details. It has been suggested that neurons in this state during wakefulness may serve a "lookout" function.

There Are Relay Nuclei for Sensory, Motor, and Limbic Systems

Relay nuclei and their connections are indicated in Figures 16-17 and 16-18 and Table 16-2. They include the sensory relay nuclei (VPL/VPM and the geniculate nuclei) and several others as well, because parts of the motor and limbic systems also have thalamic relays. VL and VA are the motor relay nuclei, receiving the superior cerebellar peduncle and various outputs from the basal nuclei and projecting to motor areas of cortex. The anterior nucleus is the principal relay nucleus for the limbic system, receiving the **mammillothalamic tract** (see Fig. 16-10) and projecting to the cingulate gyrus. The mammillothalamic tract, as its name implies, arises in the mammillary body. The cingulate gyrus is a prominent component of the limbic lobe (see Fig. 3-13). The way this pathway fits into the limbic system as a whole is detailed in Chapter 24. LD also projects to the cingulate gyrus; in this and other ways, it closely resembles the anterior nucleus. Therefore, in spite of the fact that a discrete input tract does not end in LD, it is treated here as a relay nucleus functionally related to the anterior nucleus.

As a general rule, the cerebral cortex is more important for the proper functioning of sensory systems in humans than it is in other mammals. For example, cats deprived of somatosensory cortex or visual cortex retain a significant portion of their previous somatosensory or

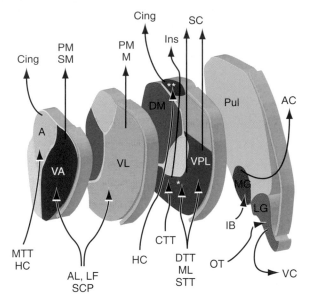

Figure 16-17 Major specific inputs to and outputs from relay nuclei. Thalamic nuclei: *, ventral posteromedial nucleus; **, lateral dorsal nucleus; A, anterior nucleus; DM, dorsomedial nucleus; LG, lateral geniculate nucleus; MG, medial geniculate nucleus; Pul, pulvinar; VA, ventral anterior nucleus; VL, ventral lateral nucleus; VPL, ventral posterolateral nucleus. Input pathways and structures: AL, ansa lenticularis (see Chapter 19); CTT, central tegmental tract; DTT, dorsal trigeminal tract; HC, hippocampus; IB, brachium of the inferior colliculus; LF, lenticular fasciculus (see Chapter 19); ML, medial lemniscus; MTT, mammillothalamic tract; OT, optic tract; SCP, superior cerebellar peduncle (see Chapter 20); STT, spinothalamic tract. Cortical destinations: AC, auditory cortex; Cing, cingulate gyrus; Ins, insula; M, primary motor cortex (precentral gyrus); PM, premotor cortex (see Chapter 18); SC, somatosensory cortex; SM, supplementary motor area (see Chapter 18); VC, visual cortex.

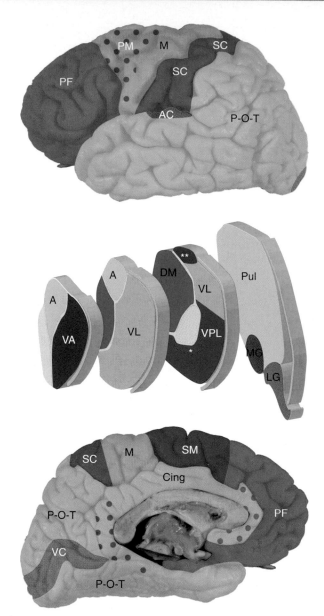

Figure 16-18 Principal cortical projection areas of relay and association nuclei. The major thalamic nucleus associated with each cortical area is indicated by the color coding, but projection areas are not nearly as exclusive as this figure implies. The pulvinar, for example, also projects to visual cortex and to parts of prefrontal cortex; these inputs are simply overshadowed by those from the lateral geniculate and dorsomedial nuclei, respectively. PF, prefrontal cortex; P-O-T, parietal-occipital-temporal association cortex; other abbreviations as in Figure 16-17.

visual capabilities, and rats treated similarly retain even more. Nevertheless, it is sometimes claimed that sensory stimuli, particularly somatosensory stimuli, "enter consciousness" in humans at the level of the thalamus. When the somatosensory cortex in humans is destroyed, the remaining awareness of stimuli is very crude, consisting mainly of an ability to recognize the fact of being touched or receiving a painful stimulus. The ability to localize the stimulus or to discriminate its intensity is severely impaired. These conclusions are based mainly on studies of humans who sustained damage to one parietal lobe, but it seems doubtful that the remaining sensory capabilities are in fact a result of consciousness at the level of the thalamus ipsilateral to the lesion. In most cases the remaining capabilities are probably the result of activity in other, undamaged, ipsilateral cortical areas and of slight bilaterality in the function of the contralateral thalamus and parietal lobe.

The Dorsomedial Nucleus and Pulvinar Are the Principal Association Nuclei

There are two great areas of association cortex in human brains (Fig. 16-18). One is the **prefrontal cortex,** anterior

to the motor areas of the frontal lobe. The second is the **parietal-occipital-temporal association cortex,** occupying the area surrounded by the primary somatosensory, visual, and auditory cortices. Corresponding to these two areas are two large association nuclei or nuclear complexes (see Fig. 16-18).

The dorsomedial nucleus is interconnected with the prefrontal cortex and is involved in prefrontal functions such as affect and foresight, as described in Chapters 22

Table 16-2	Specific Inputs to and Cortical Outputs From Thalamic Relay and Association Nuclei		
Type	**Nucleus**	**Specific Inputs**	**Cortical Output**
Relay	Anterior	Mammillothalamic tract, hippocampus	Cingulate gyrus
	Lateral dorsal (LD)	Hippocampus	Cingulate gyrus
	Ventral anterior, ventral lateral (VA/VL)*	Basal nuclei, cerebellum	Motor areas
	Ventral posterolateral (VPL)	Medial lemniscus (body), spinothalamic tract (body)	Somatosensory cortex
	Ventral posteromedial (VPM)	Medial lemniscus (face), spinothalamic tract (face) Central tegmental tract (taste)	Somatosensory cortex Insula
	Medial geniculate (MGN)	Brachium of the inferior colliculus	Auditory cortex
	Lateral geniculate (LGN)	Optic tract	Visual cortex
Association	Dorsomedial† (DM)	Prefrontal cortex, olfactory and limbic structures	Prefrontal cortex
	Lateral posterior (LP)	Parietal lobe	Parietal lobe
	Pulvinar	Parietal, occipital, and temporal lobes	Parietal, occipital, and temporal lobes

*Basal nuclei outputs go mostly to VA and cerebellar outputs mostly to VL, but the two are considered together as a combined motor relay nucleus in this account.

†Also commonly referred to as the medial dorsal (MD) nucleus.

and 23. Bilateral damage to the dorsomedial nucleus or to its connections with the frontal lobe has somewhat similar effects to damage to the prefrontal cortex itself. Major inputs to the dorsomedial nucleus, in addition to those from prefrontal cortex, come from various elements of the limbic system, such as the amygdala.

The pulvinar-LP complex is interconnected with the parietal-occipital-temporal association cortex. The major inputs to this complex, aside from those arising in association cortex, come from parts of the visual system. The pulvinar is the largest nucleus in the human thalamus and is better developed in humans than in any other mammal. One would expect that a nucleus this large and this highly developed would have an important, well-defined function. However, the role of the pulvinar (and of LP) is still largely unknown. There are hints that it may be involved in some aspects of visual perception or attention, and there are occasional reports of language deficits after damage to it, but in general, no distinctive syndrome and no obvious sensory deficits follow damage to the pulvinar-LP complex.

Intralaminar Nuclei Project to Both the Cerebral Cortex and the Basal Nuclei

The midline and intralaminar nuclei were long considered to form a nonspecific system that projects to widespread areas of the cerebral cortex and produces general changes in cortical function. However, even though the connections of these nuclei do not have the point-to-point precision seen with relay nuclei, there is a considerable degree of specificity. The inputs to these nuclei as a group are from diverse sources, including multiple cortical areas, basal nuclei, cerebellum, brainstem reticular formation, and spinothalamic and spinoreticulothalamic fibers. However, each nucleus has a specific pattern of inputs. Similarly, as a group, the midline and intralaminar nuclei have widespread projections to multiple cortical areas, basal nuclei, and limbic structures, but each individual nucleus has its own specific pattern of projections. For example, the centromedian nucleus projects to the putamen and to motor cortex, whereas the parafascicular nucleus projects to the caudate nucleus and to prefrontal cortex. As described in Chapter 19, the basal nuclei participate in a series of parallel anatomical circuits through the thalamus and cerebral cortex, each loop involving a different motor, cognitive, or affective function. Although the details and the functional implications are far from understood, it seems likely that individual midline and intralaminar nuclei affect particular circuits of the basal nuclei or limbic system. Because the basal nuclei and limbic system collectively affect most cortical

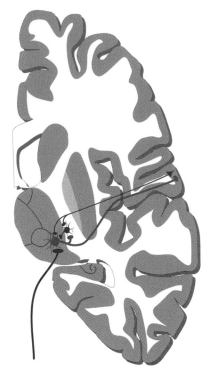

Figure 16-19 Connection pattern of the thalamic reticular nucleus. Most or all axons entering or leaving the thalamus, except for specific inputs (blue), give off collaterals to neurons of the reticular nucleus (red). Each small area of the reticular nucleus in turn sends inhibitory projections to a restricted area of the thalamus.

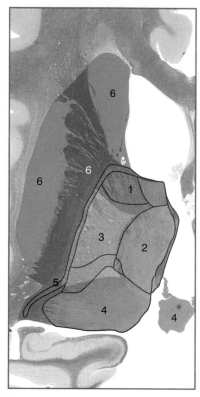

Figure 16-20 Areas of arterial supply of the thalamus and internal capsule. The thalamus is supplied by the tuberothalamic branch of the posterior communicating artery (1) and by a series of perforating branches of the posterior cerebral artery: paramedian branches (2), posterior choroidal arteries (4), and other lateral perforating branches (3) sometimes referred to as thalamogeniculate arteries. The internal capsule is mostly supplied by the anterior choroidal artery (5) and by lenticulostriate branches of the middle cerebral artery (6), which also supply large parts of the putamen and caudate nucleus.

functions, collective changes in the activity of the midline and intralaminar nuclei would be expected to have the widespread effects traditionally ascribed to these nuclei.

The Thalamic Reticular Nucleus Projects to Other Thalamic Nuclei and Not to the Cerebral Cortex

The thalamic reticular nucleus, unlike all other thalamic nuclei, has no projections to the cerebral cortex. Rather, the reticular nucleus is a sheet of neurons that receive inputs from the cortex and from thalamic projection neurons and send inhibitory (GABA) projections back to the thalamus (Fig. 16-19). Inspection of Figures 16-7 to 16-13 reveals that axons traveling from thalamus to cortex or from cortex to thalamus must traverse the reticular nucleus. As they do so, these fibers give off collaterals to the reticular nucleus. For example, the portion of the reticular nucleus adjacent to VPL/VPM receives convergent inputs from somatosensory fibers on their way to the postcentral gyrus, and from regulatory fibers on their way from the postcentral gyrus to VPL/VPM. The output of each portion of the reticular nucleus goes to that thalamic nucleus from which it receives its input. This makes the reticular nucleus an important source of regulatory input to the thalamus.

Small Branches of the Posterior Cerebral Artery Provide Most of the Blood Supply to the Thalamus

Inspection of a hemisected brain (see Fig. 6-10) reveals that the anterior and middle cerebral arteries and their branches near the cerebral arterial circle are anterior to most of the thalamus. The blood supply of the thalamus is therefore mostly from small perforating branches of the posterior cerebral artery and the nearby posterior communicating artery (Fig. 16-20; see also Fig. 6-22). The pattern of supply is consistent enough that thalamic strokes often affect predictable sets of nuclei. A branch of the posterior communicating artery (the **tuberothalamic artery**) supplies anterior regions (anterior nucleus, VA). **Paramedian** branches from the short segment of the posterior cerebral artery within the cerebral arterial circle supply DM as well as the subthalamus. More lateral branches of the posterior cerebral artery, from outside the cerebral arterial circle, take care of the rest. The posterior choroidal arteries, on their way to the roof of the third ventricle, supply posterior regions (pulvinar, LGN, MGN), and other lateral perforating branches (sometimes called **thalamogeniculate arteries**) supply VL and VPL/VPM. Finally, the anterior choroidal artery often sends a few small branches to the subthalamus and to ventral regions of the thalamus, particularly the lateral geniculate nucleus.

Damage to the thalamus most often occurs as a result of vascular accidents, typically involving the thalamogeniculate or paramedian arteries. The damage frequently involves other structures in addition to the thalamus (e.g., the adjacent internal capsule), and a large collection of deficits with far-reaching consequences can result from relatively small lesions in this area. Damage more or less restricted to the posterior thalamus can cause a characteristic type of dysesthesia that is somewhat similar to trigeminal neuralgia, in that paroxysms of intense pain may be triggered by somatosensory stimuli. The pain may spread to involve one entire half of the body and is usually resistant to analgesic drugs. In addition, those stimuli that do not cause a pain attack may be perceived abnormally; their intensity (and even their modality) may be distorted, and they may seem unusually uncomfortable or pleasant. Similar syndromes of **central pain** develop in some patients after damage almost anywhere along the anterolateral pathway; this particular variety, because of the site of damage, is called **thalamic pain.** The cause of thalamic pain is still not fully understood, but lesions that cause it almost always involve VPL/VPM. Hence it is thought that selective damage to the spinothalamic fibers that end in VPL/VPM, with sparing of the spinothalamic and spinoreticulothalamic fibers that end in other nuclei, may result in imbalances or plastic changes in thalamic activity. Extensive damage to the posterior thalamus also causes total (or near total) loss of somatic sensation in the contralateral head and body. After a period of time, some appreciation of painful, thermal, and gross tactile stimuli usually returns. Functions customarily associated with the medial lemniscus tend to be more severely and permanently impaired. Discriminative tactile sensibility may be abolished, position sense may be greatly impaired, and a sensory type of ataxia (resulting from the loss of proprioception) may persist. The combination of thalamic pain, hemianesthesia, and sensory ataxia, all contralateral to a posterior thalamic lesion, is called the **thalamic syndrome.** It is often accompanied by mild and transient paralysis (a result of damage to corticospinal fibers in the adjacent internal capsule) and by various types of residual involuntary movements (a result of damage to nearby basal ganglia).

Interconnections Between the Cerebral Cortex and Subcortical Structures Travel Through the Internal Capsule

The many thalamocortical and corticothalamic fibers just described need a route by which to travel from their origins to their destinations. This route is provided by the **internal capsule,** a compact bundle of fibers in the cleft (Fig. 16-21) between the lenticular nucleus (laterally) and the thalamus and head of the caudate nucleus (medially). Almost all the neural traffic to and from the cerebral cortex passes through the internal capsule. As Figures 16-7 and 16-8 indicate, the internal capsule is in a convenient location for fibers entering or leaving the thalamus. In addition to these fibers, others descend from the cortex through the internal capsule and then through the cerebral peduncle to reach pontine nuclei (**corticopontine fibers**), motor nuclei of cranial nerves and other brainstem sites (**corticobulbar fibers**), and spinal cord motor neurons and interneurons (**corticospinal fibers**). Still other fibers project from the cerebral cortex through the internal capsule to additional subcortical targets, such as various parts of the basal nuclei (e.g., the putamen and the caudate nucleus). All these fibers fan out as the **corona radiata** just above the internal capsule and mingle with other fiber bundles interconnecting different cortical areas in the **centrum semiovale** of each hemisphere (Fig. 16-22).

The three-dimensional shape of the internal capsule is a bit difficult to visualize, but the beautiful dissections and reconstructions shown in Figure 16-23 should help. The internal capsule is a continuous sheet of fibers that forms the medial boundary of the lenticular nucleus and then continues around posteriorly and inferiorly to partially envelop this nucleus. Inferiorly, many of the fibers in the internal capsule funnel down into the cerebral peduncle. Superiorly, they all fan out into the corona radiata and travel through the centrum semiovale to reach their cortical origins or destinations. Thus the entire fiber system is shaped like a trumpet with a large notch cut out of its bell; the flared-out bell corresponds to the region where the fibers of the internal capsule spread out to form the corona radiata, and the notch corresponds to the location where this continuous sheet of fibers is interrupted in an intact brain by the lateral sulcus. The narrowest part of the trumpet corresponds to the cerebral peduncle, and in an intact brain the lenticular nucleus sits where a mute would sit in a trumpet.

The Internal Capsule Has Five Parts

The internal capsule is divided into five regions on the basis of the relationship of each part to the lenticular nucleus (see Figs. 16-7 and 16-8). The **anterior limb** is the portion between the lenticular nucleus and the head of the caudate nucleus. The **posterior limb** is the portion between the lenticular nucleus and the thalamus. The **genu** is the portion at the junction of the anterior and posterior limbs. Because this junction occurs at the anterior end of the thalamus, the genu is adjacent to the interventricular foramen (at the anterior

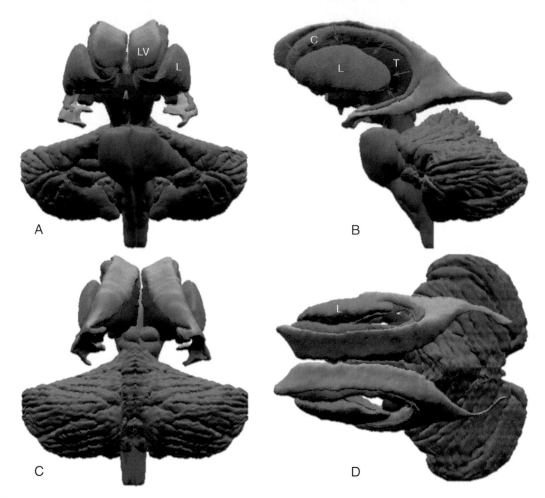

Figure 16-21 Three-dimensional reconstruction of the diencephalon, basal ganglia, lateral ventricles (LV), brainstem, and cerebellum, seen from in front **(A),** the left side **(B),** the rear **(C),** and above **(D).** The cleft through which the internal capsule passes, bounded by the thalamus (T) and the head of the caudate nucleus (C) medially and the lenticular nucleus (L) laterally, is indicated by *arrows* in **B** but is apparent in all four views. Notice in **B** and **D** how the cleft curves around behind the lenticular nucleus and dips under its posterior end.

end of the thalamus) and to the venous angle (see Fig. 6-32). The **retrolenticular part** is the portion posterior to the lenticular nucleus. The **sublenticular part** is the portion inferior to the lenticular nucleus. The demarcation of the anterior and posterior limbs is distinct at the genu, but the transition from the posterior limb to the retrolenticular part to the sublenticular part is gradual, and dividing lines between these portions are somewhat arbitrary. Because the internal capsule is a continuous, curved sheet of fibers, it is not possible to see all of its parts in any one section, regardless of the plane of the section. The first four parts mentioned here can be seen in a single horizontal section (see Figs. 16-7 and 16-8), but to get a clear idea of the sublenticular part, coronal (see Fig. 16-11) or sagittal sections are necessary.

By and large, the contents of each portion of the internal capsule can be inferred from its anatomical location (Figs. 16-24 and 16-25). Major components are as follows:

1. The anterior limb contains the fibers interconnecting the anterior nucleus and the cingulate gyrus, and most of those interconnecting the dorsomedial nucleus and prefrontal cortex. Also included are some of the fibers projecting from the frontal lobe to ipsilateral pontine nuclei (**frontopontine fibers**).

2. The posterior limb contains fibers interconnecting VA and VL with motor areas of cortex. It also contains the corticospinal and corticobulbar fibers and the somatosensory fibers projecting from VPL/VPM to the postcentral gyrus. For many years, the corticospinal tract was thought to be located in the anterior portion of the posterior limb near the genu. For most of their course, however, these fibers are actually located in the posterior third of the posterior limb adjacent to the somatosensory projections

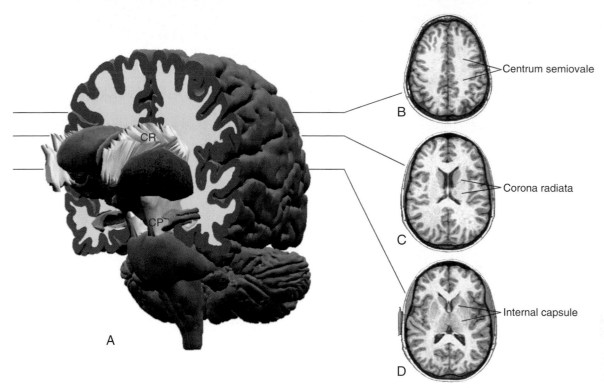

Figure 16-22 A, Three-dimensional reconstruction of the internal capsule emerging above its cleft as the corona radiata (CR), and of part of it emerging below the cleft as the cerebral peduncle (CP). **B to D,** Axial magnetic resonance images at three different levels of this fiber system. (See Video 16-1.) (*B to D, courtesy Dr. Elena M. Plante, University of Arizona. From Nolte J, Angevine JB Jr: The human brain in photographs and diagrams, ed 3, St. Louis, 2007, Mosby.*)

(Fig. 16-26). Corticobulbar fibers to motor nuclei of cranial nerves are located anterior to corticospinal fibers, closer to the genu but still well back in the posterior limb.

3. The genu is a transition zone between the anterior and posterior limbs and contains some frontopontine fibers and more fibers interconnecting the dorsomedial nucleus and prefrontal cortex.

4. The retrolenticular part of the internal capsule contains most of the fibers interconnecting the thalamus with posterior portions of the cerebral hemisphere. These include the fibers passing in both directions between parietal and occipital association areas and the pulvinar-LP complex. They also include part of the **optic radiation,** the large collection of visual system fibers projecting from the lateral geniculate nucleus to the banks of the calcarine sulcus (see Fig. 17-28). The portion of the optic radiation in the retrolenticular part of the internal capsule ends in the superior bank of the calcarine sulcus. As explained in the next chapter, these are the fibers conveying information from inferior portions of the visual fields. Finally, the retrolenticular part contains additional corticopontine fibers, principally from the parietal lobe.

5. The sublenticular part of the internal capsule is continuous with the retrolenticular part and contains the remainder of the optic radiation (i.e., those fibers ending in the inferior bank of the calcarine sulcus and carrying information about superior visual fields), as well as interconnections between temporal association areas and the pulvinar. The sublenticular part also contains the **auditory radiation,** whose fibers pass laterally from the medial geniculate nucleus, dip under the lenticular nucleus, and then turn superiorly to end in the transverse temporal gyri (see Fig. 14-18A).

Small Branches of the Middle Cerebral Artery Provide Most of the Blood Supply to the Internal Capsule

The blood supply of the internal capsule is from two principal sources: the **lenticulostriate arteries** and the **anterior choroidal artery** (see Fig. 16-20). The lenticulostriate (or **lateral striate**) arteries are the collection of fine perforating branches of the proximal portion of the middle cerebral artery, and they supply most of the anterior limb, genu, and posterior limb (see Fig. 6-7). The anterior limb also receives part of its supply from

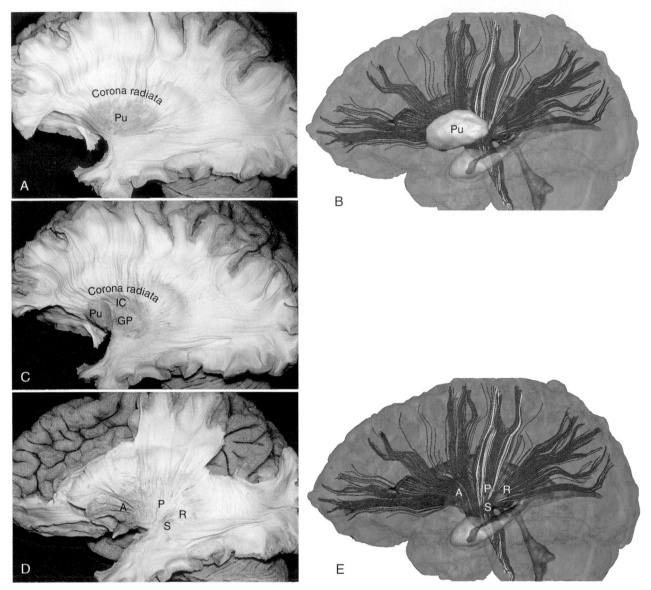

Figure 16-23 Sequential dissection of the left cerebral hemisphere from its lateral aspect, either physically (**A, C,** and **D**) or by means of diffusion tensor imaging (**B** and **E**; see Box 5-1), to reveal the internal capsule. **A,** After removing most of the temporal lobe and the insula, the surface of the putamen (Pu) can be seen, with fibers traveling above it through the corona radiata. **B,** Parts of the caudate nucleus (green) and thalamus (yellow) are visible on the other side of the cleft containing the internal capsule. **C,** Removing part of the putamen reveals the sheet of white matter covering the medial surface of the globus pallidus (GP). Now fibers of the internal capsule (IC) can be seen moving into or out of the corona radiata. **D** and **E,** Removing the globus pallidus and the rest of the putamen reveals the depression where the lenticular nucleus used to be, bordered by the anterior (A) and posterior (P) limbs, retrolenticular part (R), and sublenticular part (S) of the internal capsule. (*A, C, and D, from Kawashima M et al: Surg Neurol 65:436, 2006. **B** and **E,** from Mori S et al: MRI atlas of human white matter, Amsterdam, 2005, Elsevier.*)

perforating branches of the anterior cerebral and anterior communicating arteries, particularly from a relatively large one called the **recurrent artery** (of **Heubner**) or **medial striate artery** (see Fig. 6-8). The anterior choroidal artery supplies inferior and posterior regions of the internal capsule. It overlaps the lenticulostriate arteries in supplying the posterior limb and provides most of the supply of the retrolenticular and sublenticular parts. Perforating branches of the posterior cerebral

artery also help supply the retrolenticular and sublenticular parts.

Small strokes in the internal capsule can obviously have major consequences. Hemorrhage of a lenticulostriate artery in the vicinity of the posterior limb can result in contralateral spastic paralysis and hemianesthesia. If the retrolenticular and sublenticular parts were also involved, visual deficits would be added to the symptoms. The auditory radiations would be damaged as well, but this

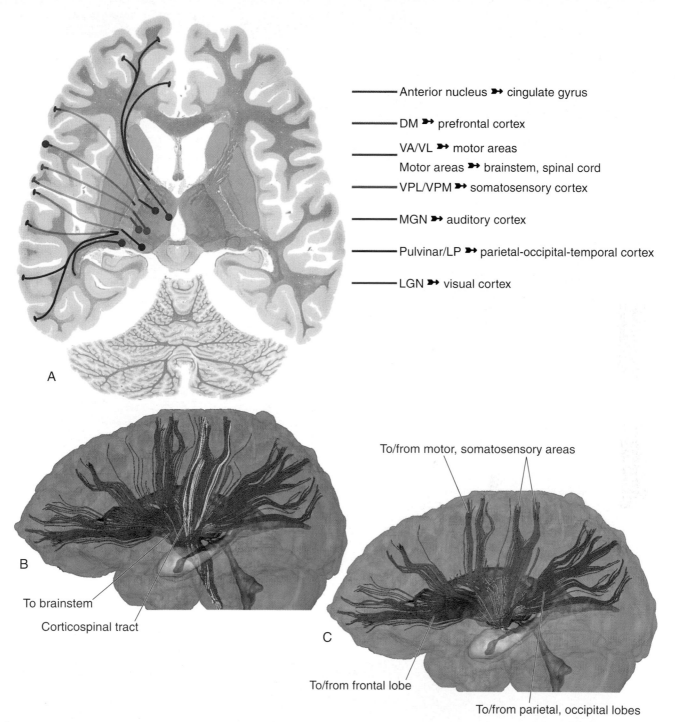

Anterior nucleus ➤ cingulate gyrus

DM ➤ prefrontal cortex

VA/VL ➤ motor areas

Motor areas ➤ brainstem, spinal cord

VPL/VPM ➤ somatosensory cortex

MGN ➤ auditory cortex

Pulvinar/LP ➤ parietal-occipital-temporal cortex

LGN ➤ visual cortex

A

B

To brainstem

Corticospinal tract

C

To/from motor, somatosensory areas

To/from frontal lobe

To/from parietal, occipital lobes

Figure 16-24 Principal components of the various parts of the internal capsule, as seen in an axial section (**A**) and in diffusion tensor images (**B** and **C**). **A,** The anterior nucleus and the pulvinar are not present in the plane of section shown, so no cell bodies are indicated. **B,** Fibers of different types overlap in some parts of the internal capsule. In this view, the corticospinal tract (white) and fibers on their way to the brainstem (corticopontine, corticobulbar; bright blue) obscure some other fibers. **C,** Once they are removed, additional components can be seen. DM, dorsomedial nucleus; LGN, lateral geniculate nucleus; LP, lateral posterior nucleus; MGN, medial geniculate nucleus; VA, ventral anterior nucleus; VL, ventral lateral nucleus; VPL, ventral posterolateral nucleus; VPM, ventral posteromedial nucleus. (**A,** modified from Nolte J, Angevine JB Jr: The human brain in photographs and diagrams, ed 3, St. Louis, 2007, Mosby. **B** and **C,** from Mori S et al: MRI atlas of human white matter, Amsterdam, 2005, Elsevier.)

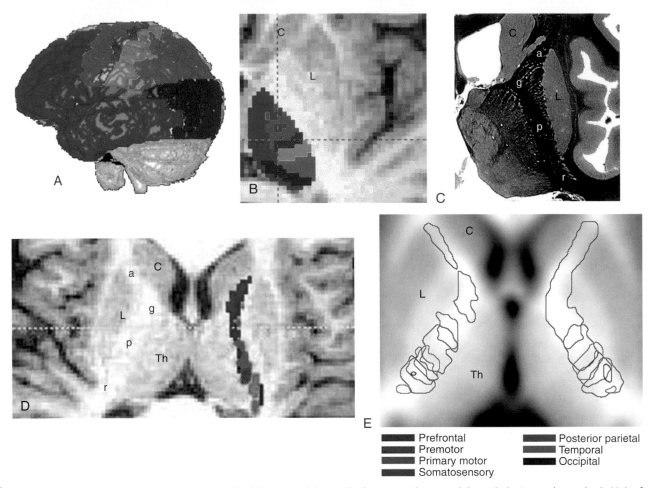

▬ Prefrontal		▬ Posterior parietal	
▬ Premotor		▬ Temporal	
▬ Primary motor		▬ Occipital	
▬ Somatosensory			

Figure 16-25 Mapping the connections between the thalamus and the cerebral cortex as they travel through the internal capsule. **A,** Major functional areas were laid out in the brain of a 33-year-old man, reconstructed in three dimensions from magnetic resonance images. **B,** A diffusion-weighted imaging protocol was used to infer the thalamic areas most strongly connected to each cortical functional area in the same subject (compare to Fig. 16-18). **C,** Axial section in approximately the same plane as in **B, D,** and **E. D,** The same protocol was used to infer the part of the internal capsule used by fibers going to and from each of the cortical areas in **A. E,** Composite data from 15 subjects, obtained using a protocol as in **B** and **D,** showing the average areas in the internal capsule occupied by fibers going to and from different cortical areas. Axons connected to prefrontal cortex account for half the area of the internal capsule, a reflection of the large extent of this cortex in human brains. a, g, p, and r, anterior limb, genu, posterior limb, and retrolenticular part of the internal capsule; C, caudate nucleus; L, lenticular nucleus; Th, thalamus. (*A, B, and D, from Behrens TEJ et al: Nat Neurosci 6:750, 2003. E, courtesy Dr. Mojtaba Zarei, University of Oxford. Based on Zarei M et al: J Magn Reson Imaging 25:48, 2007.*)

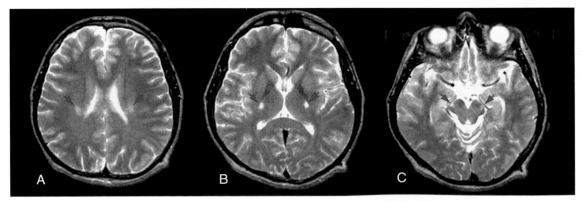

Figure 16-26 Dramatic demonstration of the location of the corticospinal tract in the corona radiata **(A)**, internal capsule **(B)**, and cerebral peduncle **(C)**. These T2-weighted magnetic resonance images are from a 34-year-old patient with a motor neuron disease (amyotrophic lateral sclerosis, or Lou Gehrig's disease) in which both upper and lower motor neurons degenerate. Increased signal intensity corresponding to the damaged corticospinal tracts is apparent at all three levels *(arrows)*. (*From Thorpe JW et al: J Neurol Neurosurg Psychiatry 61:314, 1996.*)

would produce relatively minor deficits because of the bilateral nature of the central auditory pathways.

SUGGESTED READINGS

Behrens TEJ, et al: Non-invasive mapping of connections between human thalamus and cortex using diffusion imaging. Nat Neurosci 6:750, 2003.

Boivie J: Central pain. In McMahon SB, Koltzenburg M, editors: Wall and Melzack's textbook of pain, ed 5, Edinburgh, 2005, Churchill Livingstone.

Carrera E, Bogousslavsky J: The thalamus and behavior: effects of anatomically distinct strokes. Neurology 66:1817, 2006.

Craig AD, et al: A thalamic nucleus specific for pain and temperature sensation. Nature 372:770, 1994.

Duvernoy HM: The human pineal gland: relationships with surrounding structures and blood supply. Neurol Res 22:747, 2000.
 Beautifully illustrated.

Erisir A, Van Horn SC, Sherman SM: Relative numbers of cortical and brainstem inputs to the lateral geniculate nucleus. Proc Natl Acad Sci U S A 94:1517, 1997.

Feig S, Harting JK: Corticocortical communication via the thalamus: ultrastructural studies of corticothalamic projections from area 17 to the lateral posterior nucleus of the cat and inferior pulvinar nucleus of the owl monkey. J Comp Neurol 395:281, 1998.

Giguere M, Goldman-Rakic PS: Mediodorsal nucleus: areal, laminar, and tangential distribution of afferents and efferents in the frontal lobe of rhesus monkeys. J Comp Neurol 277:195, 1988.

Gillilan LA: The arterial and venous blood supplies to the forebrain (including the internal capsule) of primates. Neurology 18:653, 1968.

Grieve KL, Acuña C, Cudeiro J: The primate pulvinar nuclei: vision and action. Trends Neurosci 23:35, 2000.

Groenewegen HJ, Berendse HW: The specificity of the "nonspecific" midline and intralaminar thalamic nuclei. Trends Neurosci 17:52, 1994.

Groothius DR, Duncan GW, Fisher CM: The human thalamocortical sensory path in the internal capsule: evidence from a small capsular hemorrhage causing a pure sensory stroke. Ann Neurol 2:328, 1977.

Guido W, Weyand T: Burst responses in the thalamic relay cells of the awake behaving cat. J Neurophysiol 74:1782, 1995.
 Elegant though technically demanding experiments demonstrating some of the factors that influence the response mode of lateral geniculate projection neurons during normal behavior.

Ilinsky IA, Kultas-Ilinsky K: Sagittal cytoarchitectonic maps of the Macaca mulatta thalamus with a revised nomenclature of the motor-related nuclei validated by observations on their connectivity. J Comp Neurol 262:331, 1987.

Jones EG: The thalamus, ed 2, New York, 2007, Cambridge University Press.

Jones EG, Leavitt RY: Retrograde axonal transport and the demonstration of non-specific projections to the cerebral cortex and striatum from thalamic intralaminar nuclei in the rat, cat, and monkey. J Comp Neurol 154:349, 1974.

Kawashima M, et al: Surgical approaches to the atrium of the lateral ventricle: microsurgical anatomy. Surg Neurol 65:436, 2006.

Kim JH, et al: Lesions limited to the human thalamic principal somatosensory nucleus (ventral caudal) are associated with loss of cold sensations and central pain. J Neurosci 27:4995, 2007.

Langworthy OR, Fox HM: Thalamic syndrome: syndrome of the posterior cerebral artery: a review. Arch Intern Med 60:203, 1937.

Lecourtier L, Kelly PH: A conductor hidden in the orchestra? Role of the habenular complex in monoamine transmission and cognition. Neurosci Biobehav Rev 31:658, 2007.

Lin C-S, et al: A major direct GABAergic pathway from zona incerta to neocortex. Science 248:1553, 1990.

Ludwig E, Klingler J: Atlas cerebri humani, Boston, 1956, Little, Brown.
 A collection of remarkable dissections of human brains.

Macchi MM, Bruce JN: Human pineal physiology and functional significance of melatonin. Front Neuroendocrinol 25:177, 2004.

Mitrofanis J: Some certainty for the "zone of uncertainty"? Exploring the function of the zona incerta. Neuroscience 130:1, 2005.

Montero UM: A quantitative study of synaptic contacts on interneurons and relay cells of the cat lateral geniculate nucleus. Exp Brain Res 86:257, 1991.

Mountcastle VB, Henneman E: The representation of tactile sensibility in the thalamus of the monkey. J Comp Neurol 97:409, 1952.
 An early physiological demonstration of the mapping of the body surface in VPL/VPM.

Pinault D: The thalamic reticular nucleus: structure, function and concept. Brain Res Rev 46:1, 2004.

Plets C, et al: The vascularization of the human thalamus. Acta Neurol Belg 70:687, 1970.
 Long and detailed.

Pritchard TC, et al: Projections of thalamic gustatory and lingual areas in the monkey, Macaca fascicularis. J Comp Neurol 244:213, 1986.

Romanski LM, et al: Topographic organization of medial pulvinar connections with the prefrontal cortex in the rhesus monkey. J Comp Neurol 379:313, 1997.

Ross ED: Localization of the pyramidal tract in the internal capsule by whole brain dissection. Neurology 30:59, 1980.

Rousseaux M, et al: Disorders of smell, taste, and food intake in a patient with a dorsomedial thalamic infarct. Stroke 27:2328, 1996.

Russchen FT, Amaral DG, Price JL: The afferent input to the magnocellular division of the mediodorsal thalamic nucleus in the monkey, Macaca fascicularis. J Comp Neurol 256:175, 1987.

Sadikot AF, Parent A, François C: The centre médian and parafascicular thalamic nuclei project respectively to the sensorimotor and associative-limbic territories in the squirrel monkey. Brain Res 510:161, 1990.

Sánchez-González MÁ, et al: The primate thalamus is a key target for brain dopamine. J Neurosci 25:6076, 2005.

Sandson TA, et al: Frontal lobe dysfunction following infarction of the left-sided medial thalamus. Arch Neurol 48:1300, 1991.

Saunders RC, Mishkin M, Aggleton JP: Projections from the entorhinal cortex, perirhinal cortex, presubiculum, and parasubiculum to the medial thalamus in macaque monkeys: identifying different pathways using disconnection techniques. Exp Brain Res 167:1, 2005.

Schmahmann JD: Vascular syndromes of the thalamus. Stroke 34:2264, 2003.

Sherman SM, Guillery RW: Exploring the thalamus and its role in cortical function, ed 2, Cambridge, 2006, MIT Press.
 An outstanding review of the circuitry, physiology, and probable modes of operation of thalamic relay and association nuclei.

Sugitani M: Electrophysiological and sensory properties of the thalamic reticular neurones related to somatic sensation in rats. J Physiol 290:79, 1979.

Ulrich DJ, Tamamaki N, Sherman SM: Brainstem control of response modes in neurons of the cat's lateral geniculate nucleus. Proc Natl Acad Sci U S A 87:2560, 1990.

Walker AE: The primate thalamus, Chicago, 1938, University of Chicago Press.

An early (and historically important) exposition of the thalamic terminology commonly used today.

Whitsel BL, et al: Thalamic projections to S-I in macaque monkey. J Comp Neurol 178:385, 1978.

The microarchitecture of the projection from VPL/VPM to the cortex, giving some idea of how remarkably detailed this projection is.

Wilkins RH, Brody IA: The thalamic syndrome. Arch Neurol 20:560, 1969.

A brief introduction to (and excerpted translation of) the original work: Dejerine J, Roussy G: Le syndrome thalamique, Rev Neurol 14:521, 1906.

Zarei M, et al: Two-dimensional population map of cortical connections in the human internal capsule. J Magn Reson Imaging 25:48, 2007.

Zhan XJ, et al: Current clamp and modeling studies of low-threshold calcium spikes in cells of the cat's lateral geniculate nucleus. J Neurophysiol 81:2360, 1999.

The Visual System

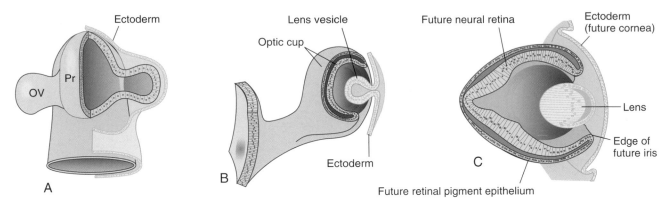

Figure 17-1 Embryological development of the eye. **A,** At about 4 weeks, the optic vesicle (OV) of each side has evaginated from the prosencephalon (Pr) in this head-on view. **B,** At about 5 weeks, the initially spherical optic vesicle has folded in on itself to form the two-layered optic cup; the optic cup partially envelops the lens vesicle, which is derived from surface ectoderm. **C,** At about 6 weeks, the lens vesicle has pinched off, and the remaining surface ectoderm has begun to form the epithelial covering of the cornea. The outer layer of the two-layered optic cup will go on to form the retinal pigment epithelium; the inner layer will form the neural retina. Anteriorly, both layers will grow around farther in front of the lens and participate in the formation of the ciliary body and iris. *(Redrawn from Hamilton WJ: Textbook of human anatomy, ed 2, St. Louis, 1976, Mosby.)*

It is clear from everyday experience that humans are a visually oriented species. Although it is arguable which of our senses is most important, loss of vision certainly has a greater impact on humans than loss of, for example, olfaction or taste. Partly because of its importance (and partly for anatomical and technical reasons discussed later), a great deal of research has been done on the visual system. Currently, more is known about the visual system than about any other sensory system, and it is likely that with further study we will understand in some detail how this portion of the central nervous system (CNS) actually works.

Some lizards, fish, and amphibians have a photosensitive pineal organ that constantly stares up at the sky as an unblinking third eye. In mammals, however, with very few exceptions, all photic information is transduced in the **rods** and **cones** of the **retina** and then conveyed to the brain by way of the axons of the output cells (called **ganglion cells**) of the retina. These axons, together with the axons of higher order cells on which they synapse, form a visual pathway that begins anteriorly in the eyes and ends posteriorly in the occipital lobes. Throughout most of this course a precise **retinotopic** arrangement of fibers is maintained, so that particular small regions of the retina are represented in particular small regions of more central parts of the pathway. Damage at many different locations within this system results in visual deficits, and knowledge of the anatomy involved makes it possible to understand these deficits. This in turn means that the same knowledge can be used to deduce the site of a lesion.

The Eye Has Three Concentric Tissue Layers and a Lens

Eyes and cameras both need to deal with similar sets of issues—maintaining a stable relationship between a focusing apparatus and a photosensitive surface, focusing on near and far objects, regulating the amount of light reaching the photosensitive surface, and recording the pattern of incoming light—so, not surprisingly, they have many analogous components. The retina is an outgrowth of the diencephalon (Fig. 17-1), and one result of this origin is numerous parallels between the eye and the brain and meninges. The eye can be thought of as formed from three roughly spherical, concentric tissue layers, with a lens suspended inside them (Fig. 17-2). Each layer contributes to different structures in different parts of the eye (Table 17-1).

The outermost tissue layer is continuous with the dura mater. Like the dura, it is a feltwork of collagenous connective tissue. Most of this layer forms the **sclera**, the "white of the eye." The dura acts as a sheath around the optic nerve, extending out around the eye and forming the sclera. Beginning at a circular transition zone called the **limbus**, the anterior sixth of this layer is the transparent **cornea**, which lets light into the eye.

The heavily vascularized middle layer, the **uvea,**[a] or **uveal tract**, is similar in some ways to the arachnoid and pia. This is the principal route through which blood vessels and nerves (other than the optic nerve) travel within the wall of the eye. Over most of its extent the uvea is sandwiched between the sclera and the retina as the densely pigmented **choroid.** Choroidal capillaries supply retinal photoreceptors, and choroidal pigment absorbs stray light (much like the flat black paint job inside a camera does). The uvea continues anteriorly to form the bulk of the **ciliary body** (containing the **ciliary muscle**) and the **stroma** of the **iris.**

The innermost layer is an outgrowth of the CNS and is itself a double-layered structure, reflecting its origin

---

[a]Uvea is Latin for "grape." This part of the eye apparently received its name for the aperture in its anterior portion that lets the rays in.

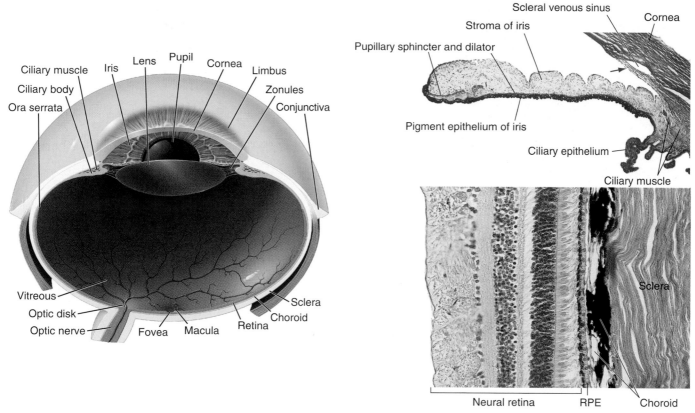

Figure 17-2 General structure of the eye as seen in a hemisection, with histological sections of the iris and ciliary body (upper inset) and the wall of the eye (lower inset). The arrow indicates the trabecular meshwork overlying the scleral venous sinus (see Fig. 17-3). The posterior chamber is a small chamber found between the ciliary body and the edge of the pupil, whereas the anterior chamber is the area between the iris and the cornea (see Fig. 17-3). RPE, retinal pigment epithelium. *(Inset from Rohen JW: Invest Ophthalmol 18:133, 1979.)*

Table 17-1	Derivatives of the Three Tissue Layers of the Eye		
Layer	**Posterior to Ora Serrata**	**Between Ora Serrata and Limbus**	**Anterior to Limbus**
Fibrous outer layer	Sclera	Sclera	Cornea
Vascular middle layer (uveal tract)	Choroid	Ciliary body (vascular core) Ciliary muscle	Iris (stroma)
Inner layer (neuroepithelial double layer)	Neural retina Retinal pigment epithelium	Ciliary body (double-layered ciliary epithelium)	Iris (posterior epithelial layers) Pupillary sphincter and dilator

from the two layers of infolded optic cup (see Fig. 17-1). Over most of its extent, this double layer comprises the retina, which lines the choroid. The outer portion of the **retina**, adjacent to the choroid, is the **retinal pigment epithelium**, whereas the inner portion, adjacent to the interior of the eye, is the **neural retina**. Under normal conditions no space exists between the pigment epithelium and the neural retina in adults. However, the mechanical connections between the two are not very strong, and under certain circumstances, this potential space opens and **retinal detachment** results (see Fig. 17-14E). Retinal receptors are metabolically dependent on pigment epithelial cells and on the adjacent

choroidal vasculature, so detached areas stop working. The photosensitive retina ends anteriorly at a serrated border (the **ora serrata**), but the same two layers continue as the double-layered **ciliary epithelium** covering the ciliary body and the double layer of pigmented epithelium covering the posterior surface of the iris.

Intraocular Pressure Maintains the Shape of the Eye

Cameras have rigid bodies, designed to keep the film in a stable position relative to the lens. In contrast, the shape of the eye (and position of the retina) is

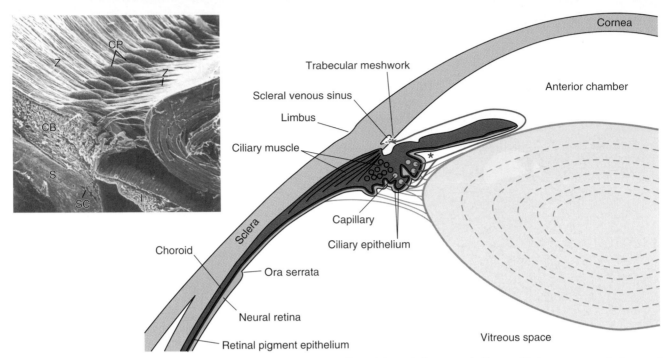

Figure 17-3 Production and circulation of aqueous humor. Components filtered through fenestrated ciliary capillaries are transported across the ciliary epithelium, enter the posterior chamber (*), move through the pupil into the anterior chamber, pass through the trabecular meshwork, and enter the scleral venous sinus. The inset is a scanning electron micrograph showing the zonular suspension of a monkey's lens; the view is as though you were in the vitreous space, looking diagonally outward toward the back of the lens. CB, ciliary body; CP, ciliary processes (the corrugated surface of the ciliary body, bulging between zonular fibers); I, iris; L, lens; S, sclera; SC, scleral venous sinus (Schlemm's canal); Z, zonules. *(Inset, from Rohen JW: Invest Ophthalmol 18:133, 1979.)*

maintained in much the same way as inflating a soccer ball maintains its shape. The collagenous sclera and cornea correspond to the wall of the soccer ball, and intraocular fluid pressure replaces air pressure. The pressure is generated by a now familiar process of fluid production, circulation, and reabsorption (Fig. 17-3). The ciliary body functions as a small outpost of choroid plexus, secreting **aqueous humor** across the ciliary epithelium and into the **posterior chamber**, the space between the iris and the lens. Pushed along by hydrostatic pressure, the aqueous humor passes through the pupil and into the **anterior chamber**, filters through the collagenous **trabecular meshwork** (analogous to arachnoid granulations) at the iridocorneal angle, and enters an endothelium-lined **scleral venous sinus** (the **canal of Schlemm**), which communicates directly with the venous drainage of the eye. The production rate (about 2 μL/min) is sufficient to completely replace the aqueous humor about 15 times a day. The space behind the lens, constituting most of the intraocular volume, is filled with gelatinous **vitreous** (Latin for "glassy") **humor**, so the resistance to aqueous outflow afforded by the trabecular meshwork and the wall of the scleral venous sinus causes a pressure of about 15 mm Hg that is transmitted throughout the eye, maintaining its shape.

In much the same way that blocking the circulation or reabsorption of cerebrospinal fluid causes increased intracranial pressure, headache, and neural damage, processes that interfere with the circulation or reabsorption of aqueous humor cause the painful condition of **glaucoma** and, ultimately, retinal damage (see Fig. 17-14F and G). Techniques to treat glaucoma include decreasing the production of aqueous humor from the ciliary body or increasing the outflow through the trabecular meshwork and into the canal of Schlemm.

The Cornea and Lens Focus Images on the Retina

Focusing an image requires refraction of light across one or more interfaces where there is a change in refractive index. The aqueous and vitreous humors have a refractive index only slightly lower than that of the lens, so the lens accounts for only about a third of the refractive power of the eye; its major role is adjusting the focus of the eye for near and far objects, as described later. Hence for nonaquatic vertebrates like humans, most of the refraction occurs at the air-water interface at the front surface of the cornea[b]; its curved shape, maintained by

---

[b]Fish and other aquatic animals obviously cannot use this mechanism. Instead, they have much larger, more spherical lenses, as well as adaptations to increase the difference in refractive index between the lens and the intraocular fluid.

intraocular pressure, accounts for humans' ability to see 90 degrees or more to the side (see Fig. 17-32).

One can imagine a variety of strategies for changing the focus of an optical device to **accommodate** to near objects—moving the photosensitive surface, moving the refractive elements, or changing the shape of the refractive elements. Different animals have adapted each of these strategies. Conventional cameras are adjusted for near or far objects by moving their lenses closer to or farther from the film; similarly, fish and most amphibians have intraocular muscles that move the lens back and forth. Arthropods cannot move or deform lenses that are part of the exoskeleton, but some have muscles that move the retina closer to or farther from the lens. Some animals have muscles attached to the cornea that can change its curvature. Terrestrial vertebrates use intraocular muscles to change the shape of the lens. The human lens is suspended by strands of connective tissue called **zonules** (see Fig. 17-3, inset), attached at one end to the lens and at the other end to the ciliary body. At rest, the tension of this zonular suspension keeps the lens slightly flattened and the eye focused on distant objects. The ciliary muscle has some fibers oriented circumferentially that act as a kind of sphincter; contraction of these fibers pulls the ciliary attachment points of the zonules toward the center of the pupil and relaxes some of the tension in the zonular suspension. Other ciliary muscle fibers are oriented parallel to the surface of the eye; contraction of these pulls the ciliary attachment points partly anteriorly and partly toward the center of the pupil, again relaxing some of the tension in the zonular suspension. Hence, somewhat counterintuitively, contraction of the ciliary muscle allows the lens to fatten as the eye accommodates to near objects: the posterior surface of the lens is embedded in the vitreous humor and does not move much, but the anterior surface bulges out slightly.

The Iris Affects the Brightness and Quality of the Image Focused on the Retina

The range of light intensities over which humans have useful vision, from starlight to bright sunlight, is an astonishing 10^{12} or so—a million million-fold. This is a much greater range of intensities than receptor potentials and frequencies of action potentials can encode directly, so there are mechanisms for adapting visual sensitivity to the ambient illumination. Most of these mechanisms depend on the physiology and wiring of retinal neurons, but in addition, the iris plays a role in regulating the amount of light reaching the retina. The two posterior epithelial layers are densely pigmented, and in brown-eyed individuals the stroma contains substantial additional pigment, so essentially all light reaching the retina must first pass through the **pupil**, the aperture in the middle of the iris.

The size of the pupil is controlled by two smooth muscles in the iris (see Fig. 17-2); both are highly unusual, in that they are derived from the same layers of neural ectoderm that give rise to the retina. The circumferentially arranged **pupillary sphincter** encircles the pupil at what was, embryologically, the edge of the optic cup.[c] The **pupillary dilator**, whose fibers are arranged like spokes radiating from the sphincter, is located at the interface between the pigment epithelial layers and the stroma. The sphincter is the stronger of the two, and reflex connections mediated by the optic and oculomotor nerves constrict the pupil in response to increased levels of illumination (see Fig. 17-39). The pupillary sphincter can contract by about 80%, much more than other muscles and enough to vary the diameter of the pupil from about 8 mm to 1.5 mm. However, this corresponds to only about a 30-fold change in area, consistent with the idea that retinal mechanisms play the major role in adjusting visual sensitivity.[d]

In addition to decreasing the amount of light reaching the retina, a smaller pupil improves the optical performance of the eye (just as, within limits, a smaller aperture improves the optical performance of a camera lens). This is particularly important when focusing on near objects (see Figs. 17-40 and 17-41).

A System of Barriers Partially Separates the Retina From the Rest of the Body

A further indication of the origin of the retina from the neural tube is a **blood-retina barrier** system, parallel to the three-part barrier system in and around the brain (see Fig. 6-27) that separates the neural retina from other parts of the body. The endothelial cells of **intraretinal capillaries**, like those of intracerebral capillaries, are joined by bands of tight junctions, forming a blood-retina barrier in the literal sense of the term. Capillaries in the ciliary body are leaky, but the **ciliary epithelium** prevents diffusion into the aqueous and vitreous humors, just as the choroid epithelium prevents diffusion into cerebrospinal fluid. Finally, substances in the sclera and choroid are unable to reach the retina because **retinal pigment epithelial** cells are also joined by tight junctions, forming a layer analogous to the arachnoid barrier; traffic between choroidal capillaries and photoreceptors is mediated by transport across the pigment epithelium.

---

[c]Signs of this optic cup origin are found in many species, including many fish and amphibians and even some mammals, whose pupillary sphincters contain visual pigment and contract autonomously in response to light.

[d]Continuing the camera analogy, the million million-fold range of light intensities over which humans have useful vision corresponds to about 40 f-stops. Pupillary constriction accounts for only about 4 f-stops.

The Retina Contains Five Major Neuronal Cell Types

One reason so much research has been done on the visual system is because of the overall anatomical simplicity of the neural retina relative to other parts of the nervous system. Although the neural retina contains hundreds of millions of neurons, there are only five basic types involved in the processing of visual information, and their patterns of interconnections are fundamentally the same throughout the retina.

The five cell types have their somata neatly arranged in three layers and make most of their synapses in two additional layers interposed between the layers of cell bodies. In each synaptic layer, one cell type brings visual information in, another type carries information out, and a third type serves as a laterally interconnecting element.

A simplified schematic illustration of these basic connection patterns is shown in Figure 17-4. Starting peripherally, photoreceptor cells stimulated by light project to the first layer of synapses, where they terminate on the aptly named **bipolar** and **horizontal cells.** Bipolar cells

then project to the next layer of synapses, whereas horizontal cells spread laterally and interconnect receptors, bipolar cells, and other horizontal cells. In the second layer of synapses, bipolar cells terminate on ganglion cells and **amacrine cells.**[e] Axons of ganglion cells leave the eye as the **optic nerve,** whereas processes of amacrine cells spread laterally and interconnect bipolar cells, ganglion cells, and other amacrine cells.

Retinal Neurons and Synapses Are Arranged in Layers

The entire retina is conventionally described as a 10-layered structure, beginning with the pigment epithelium (Fig. 17-5; see also Fig. 17-14); five of these layers are the layers of cell bodies and synapses just mentioned. In naming these layers, the term **nuclear** refers to cell bodies and the term **plexiform** to synaptic zones. **Inner** and **outer** refer to the number of synapses by which a structure is separated from the brain, so that, for

---

[e]Amacrine is Greek for "without a long process," referring to the fact that most amacrine cells do not have a conventional axon.

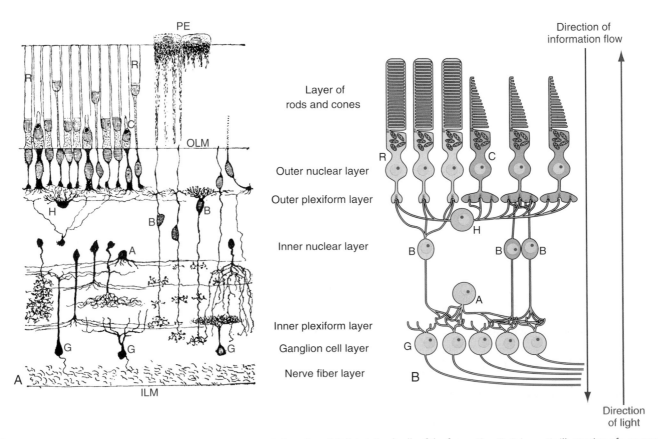

Figure 17-4 Cell types and their arrangement in the retina. **A,** Drawing of Golgi-stained cells of the frog retina. **B,** Schematic illustration of a generalized vertebrate retina showing retinal layers. A, amacrine cell; B, bipolar cell; C, cone; G, ganglion cell; H, horizontal cell; ILM, inner limiting membrane; OLM, outer limiting membrane; PE, pigment epithelium; R, rod. (**A,** *from Ramón y Cajal S: Histologie due système nerveux de l'homme et des vertébrés, vol 2, Paris, 1911, Maloine.*)

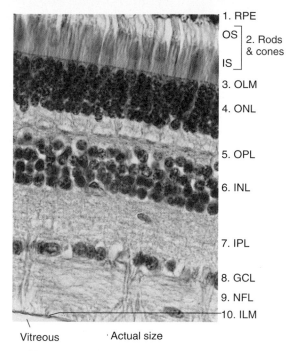

1. RPE
OS } 2. Rods & cones
IS
3. OLM
4. ONL
5. OPL
6. INL
7. IPL
8. GCL
9. NFL
10. ILM

Vitreous   Actual size

Figure 17-5 Light micrograph of human retina. The entire retina is only 200 to 300 μm thick; the tiny speck at the bottom of the photo shows the actual size of this piece of retina. GCL, ganglion cell layer; ILM, inner limiting membrane; INL, inner nuclear layer; IPL, inner plexiform layer; IS, inner segments; NFL, nerve fiber layer; OLM, outer limiting membrane; ONL, outer nuclear layer; OPL, outer plexiform layer; OS, outer segments; RPE, retinal pigment epithelium. *(Courtesy Dr. Allen L. Bell, University of New England College of Osteopathic Medicine.)*

example, photoreceptors are "outer" with respect to bipolar cells. From outside in, the 10 layers of the retina are as follows.

1. The **retinal pigment epithelium** is a single layer of polygonal, pigmented cells. One side of each cell adjoins the choroid, whose capillaries supply the avascular first two layers of the retina. The other side of each cell forms numerous fine processes that partially surround the outer portions of the receptor cells and obliterate the space that existed embryonically within the wall of the optic cup. Pigment epithelial cells are intimately involved metabolically with the receptors. They also play a role in absorbing light that has passed through the retina.

2. **Rods** and **cones** are the two different types of vertebrate photoreceptors. Each consists of several regions (Fig. 17-6): an **outer segment**, an **inner segment**, a cell body, and a synaptic terminal. (Strictly speaking, *rod* or *cone* refers to only the outer segment plus the inner segment of a photoreceptor cell, but these terms are commonly used to refer to entire receptors.)

The outer segment of a rod is relatively long and cylindrical, whereas that of a cone (except in the fovea) is shorter and tapered (Figs. 17-6 and 17-7). Each type of outer segment is filled with hundreds of flattened membranous sacs, or **disks.** In cones, the interior of most of these disks is continuous with

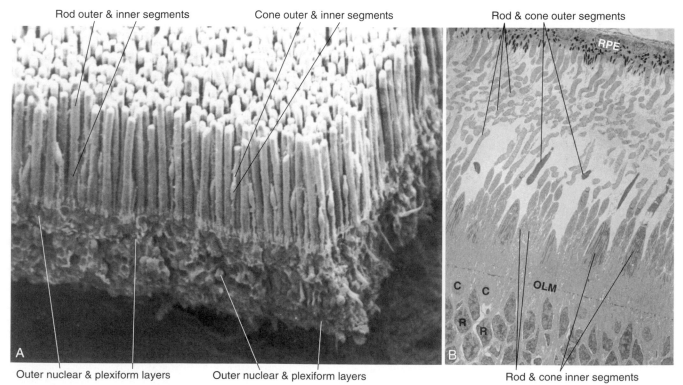

Figure 17-6 Electron micrographs of rods and cones. **A,** Scanning electron micrograph of the retina of a bullfrog. **B,** Electron micrograph of the photoreceptor layer of a rhesus monkey's retina. This section was taken from a region near the fovea but not in it, so both rods and cones are plentiful. The outer limiting membrane (OLM) is actually a row of intercellular junctions. The insertion of the tips of rod outer segments into the pigment epithelial layer is apparent. C, cone nucleus; R, rod nucleus; RPE, retinal pigment epithelium. (*A,* from Steinberg RH: Z Zellforsch 143:451, 1973. **B,** courtesy Dr. David Moran and Pamela Eller, University of Colorado Health Sciences Center.)

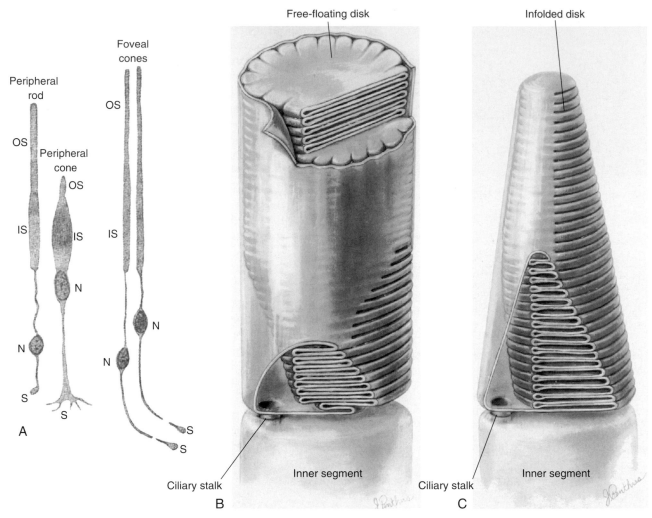

Figure 17-7 Ultrastructural differences between the outer segments of rods and cones. **A,** General shape of peripheral rods and cones and of foveal cones dissociated from a human retina. **B,** Rod outer segment (cut off near the top to be the same length as the cone outer segment in **C**); note that some disks toward the base of the outer segment are open to the outside world, but most disks are pinched off and completely surrounded by cytoplasm. **C,** Cone outer segment; note that this outer segment tapers toward its apex (hence its name) and that all its disks are infoldings of the plasma membrane, with their interiors still continuous with extracellular space. IS, inner segment; N, nucleus in cell body; OS, outer segment; S, synaptic ending. (**A,** from Ramón y Cajal S: Histologie due système nerveux de l'homme et des vertébrés, vol 2, Paris, 1911, Maloine. **B** and **C**, courtesy Dr. Richard W. Young, University of California at Los Angeles.)

extracellular space, but in rods, almost all the disks have pinched off from the external membrane and are wholly intracellular. The major protein constituent of the outer segment membranes of both rods and cones is the visual pigment, which is called **rhodopsin** in rods. (There is no universally accepted name for the visual pigments of cones, and they are often referred to simply as **cone pigments.**) Hence photons traversing the outer segment of a rod or cone must pass through hundreds or thousands of sheets of membrane, each full of visual pigment molecules. As one might expect from this localization of visual pigment, the outer segment is the site of visual transduction; photons absorbed here cause a receptor potential that then spreads to the rest of the cell. The photosensitive portion of the receptor

cells, oddly enough, is located in the part of the neural retina farthest removed from incoming light (i.e., the retina is inverted with respect to the path of light through it [see Figs. 17-2 and 17-4]). This curious situation is universally true among vertebrates. However, this does not detract substantially from visual sensitivity or acuity, because the retina is thin (see Fig. 17-5) and nearly transparent (Fig. 17-8), and because other anatomical modifications (discussed later) are found in the retinal area of greatest acuity.

Each outer segment is an elaborately specialized cilium that remains connected to its inner segment by a narrow ciliary stalk. The inner segments contain, among other organelles, a very prominent collection of mitochondria. These mitochondria supply the

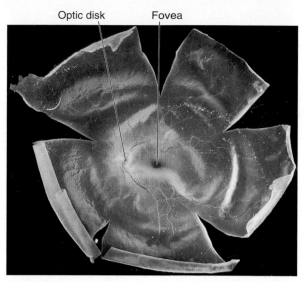

Optic disk   Fovea

Figure 17-8 An isolated human neural retina. *(Courtesy Dr. Dennis M. Dacey, University of Washington School of Medicine.)*

energy necessary for processes associated with transduction and for the synthesis of visual pigments. These pigments are continually renewed, being synthesized in the inner segment, transported through the ciliary stalk, and incorporated into disk membranes. "Old" disks at the apical ends of the outer segments of rods and cones are then phagocytosed by the pigment epithelium. (Certain types of retinal degeneration are caused by a defect in this renewal-phagocytosis process.)

As discussed later in this chapter, rods mediate low-acuity monochromatic vision in dim light, whereas cones mediate high-acuity color vision, but require more light to do so.

3. The **outer limiting membrane** was so named because it has the appearance of a distinct line when viewed with a light microscope. However, electron microscopy reveals it to be a row of intercellular junctions (see Fig. 17-6B). Elongated specialized glial cells called **Müller cells** span almost the entire retina, ending distally at the bases of the inner segments of the rods and cones. Here, adjacent Müller processes and inner segments are joined by junctional complexes, which collectively form the outer limiting membrane.

4. The **outer nuclear layer** consists of the cell bodies of the rods and cones.

5. The **outer plexiform layer** is the relatively thin synaptic zone in which receptors terminate on horizontal and bipolar cells and in which processes of horizontal cells spread laterally. The rods and cones synapse on separate subpopulations of bipolar cells and on different regions of some horizontal cells (see Figs. 17-24 and 17-25).

6. The **inner nuclear layer** contains the cell bodies of all the retinal interneurons as well as those of the Müller cells. The nuclei of horizontal cells are found near its distal edge, those of bipolar cells in the middle, and those of amacrine cells near its proximal edge. Bipolar cells conduct visual information through this layer, projecting to the second synaptic zone.

7. The **inner plexiform layer** is the relatively thick synaptic zone in which bipolar cells terminate on amacrine and ganglion cells, and processes of amacrine cells spread laterally. The actual pattern of interconnections is somewhat more complex than that shown in Figure 17-4. The amacrine cells provide one example of this added complexity: based on neurochemical and anatomical characteristics, more than 30 different types, each presumed to have a somewhat distinctive function, have been described.

8. The **ganglion cell layer** contains the cell bodies of the ganglion cells, whose dendrites ramify in the inner plexiform layer and whose axons leave the eye as the optic nerve. This cell layer is considerably thinner than either the outer or the inner nuclear layer in most retinal locations, reflecting the fact that there are about 5 million cones and about 100 million rods in a human retina, but only about 1 million ganglion cells. Clearly, a good deal of convergence is involved in retinal processing, but the convergence is not uniform across the retina. As discussed later, some regions are specialized for high spatial acuity and have little convergence, whereas other regions are specialized for high sensitivity and have a great deal of convergence.

Visual information travels in several parallel streams, just as somatosensory information travels rostrally through the spinal cord and brainstem in multiple parallel pathways. In the case of the visual system, the axons of several anatomically and functionally distinct classes of ganglion cells share the same optic nerve in their course toward the brain. In the primate visual system, approximately 80% of all ganglion cells form a single class of small cells that are particularly responsive to the colors of visual objects and to details of their shapes. Some general aspects of the distinctive connections of this and other ganglion cell classes are mentioned later in this chapter.

9. The **nerve fiber layer** is the collection of axons of ganglion cells that converge like spokes toward the **optic disk** or **optic papilla** (located posteriorly and slightly medial to the midline of the eye [see Fig. 17-2]), where they form the optic nerve. The central retinal artery, a branch of the ophthalmic artery, traverses the optic nerve and enters the eye at the optic disk. Hence the retina has a dual blood supply, with the outer two layers supplied by the choroidal

circulation (also fed by the ophthalmic artery) and the inner layers by the central retinal artery.

10. The **inner limiting membrane** is a thin basal lamina interposed between the vitreous and the proximal ends of the Müller cells.

The Retina Is Regionally Specialized

Cross sections through the retina do not have the same appearance at all locations. For example, no photoreceptors, interneurons, or ganglion cells are present at the optic disk, where the axons of ganglion cells leave the eye to form the optic nerve (Fig. 17-9). These axons originate near the vitreous, so they must turn posteriorly and traverse the retina before passing through the sclera. Because there are no photoreceptors at the optic disk, humans are blind to any object whose image falls on this part of the retina. Although the **blind spot** can be demonstrated easily (Fig. 17-10), we have no awareness as we walk around a blank spot in visual space. One might think this is because the left eye can see the part of the visual field that falls on the right eye's blind spot, and vice versa (see Fig. 17-32). This cannot be the explanation, though, because humans are unaware of the blind spot even with one eye closed. The real reason is that the

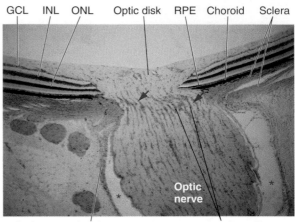

Figure 17-9 Light micrograph of a human optic disk, showing the absence of neuronal layers at this location. *Arrows* indicate bundles of optic nerve fibers passing through the lamina cribrosa, the perforated scleral zone at the optic disk. *, subarachnoid space surrounding the optic nerve; GCL, ganglion cell layer; INL, inner nuclear layer; ONL, outer nuclear layer; RPE, retinal pigment epithelium. *(Courtesy Dr. Allen L. Bell, University of New England College of Osteopathic Medicine.)*

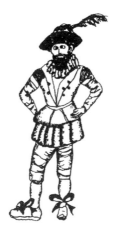

A

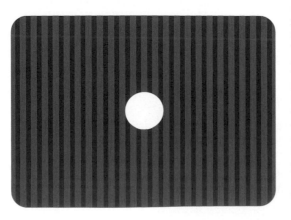

B

Figure 17-10 How to demonstrate your right eye's blind spot to yourself. **A,** Close your left eye, hold the book at arm's length, stare fixedly at the spot on the left side of the figure, and slowly move the book toward you. At some point about a foot from your face, the bearded gentleman's head will disappear. **B,** Demonstration of how the CNS "fills in" the blind spot. Again, close your left eye, stare at the black spot with your right eye, and move the book slowly toward you. When the image of the hole in the striped pattern falls on your blind spot, your brain will try to convince you that there are stripes where none exist. *(A, based on a technique of King Charles II, as recounted by Rushton WAH: Vision Res 19:255, 1979.)*

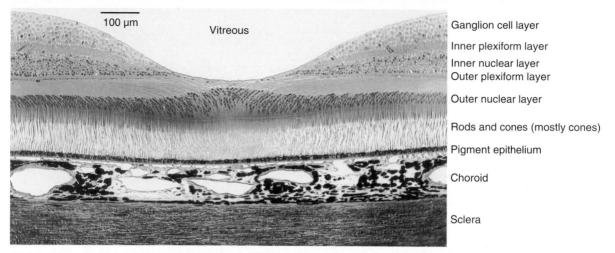

	Ganglion cell layer
	Inner plexiform layer
	Inner nuclear layer
	Outer plexiform layer
	Outer nuclear layer
	Rods and cones (mostly cones)
	Pigment epithelium
	Choroid
	Sclera

Vitreous

Figure 17-11 Fovea of a rhesus monkey. Note that all retinal elements (except the photoreceptors, which are all cones in the center of the fovea) are displaced to either side so that light needs to pass through only the outer nuclear layer before reaching the cones. The nerve fiber layer is scanty in this region because the axons of more laterally placed ganglion cells arc around the fovea on their way to the optic disk. *(From Fine BS, Yanoff M: Ocular histology, ed 2, New York, 1979, Harper & Row.)*

nervous system simply "fills it in." Humans are actually quite skillful at this, and patients with damage to their visual systems can become blind in surprisingly large areas of their visual fields without being aware of it.

Beginning near the lateral edge of the optic disk is a circular portion of the retina, about 5 mm in diameter, in which many of the cells contain a blue-absorbing pigment. This gives the area a yellowish color (see Fig. 17-8) when examined with appropriate illumination and has led to its being called the **macula lutea** (Latin for "yellow spot"), usually shortened to **macula.** In the center of the macula is a depression about 1.5 mm in diameter, called the **fovea,** which is particularly rich in cones. In the central part of the fovea is a pit, only about 350 μm across, which contains only elongated cones (no rods) and is directly in line with the visual axis (Fig. 17-11). The central fovea is specialized for vision of the highest acuity; all the neurons and capillaries that are present elsewhere (and that light would otherwise traverse before reaching the receptors) are collected around the edges of the fovea. Specialized interneurons called **midget bipolar cells** receive their inputs from individual foveal cones. These bipolars in turn contact individual **midget ganglion cells,** so that an anatomical basis for highly detailed foveal vision is maintained.[f]

---

[f]One might think it advantageous to continue the anatomical specializations of the fovea, such as small, tightly packed photoreceptors and no convergence, throughout the retina; this would give us highly detailed vision over our entire field of view. However, as Wässle and Boycott point out (Physiol Rev 71:447, 1991), foveal vision requires so much cerebral cortex (see Figs. 17-29 and 17-35) that using foveal specializations throughout the retina would necessitate 100 times as much cerebral cortex as we presently have available in the entire cerebrum. Instead, we use a very small fovea, together with precisely controlled eye movements that allow us to aim it at objects of interest (see Chapter 21).

The fovea is one extreme in a changing rod-cone distribution across the retina (Fig. 17-12). The packing density of cones decreases sharply outside the fovea, whereas that of rods increases, reaching a maximum just outside the macula. From here to the edge of the retina, the cone density remains at a low level, and the rod density slowly declines as well (Fig. 17-13). Given the properties of rods and cones, it follows from these distributions that the fovea is used for high-acuity color vision in reasonably bright light, whereas extrafoveal regions function at lower light levels.

Recently developed tomographic techniques allow retinal layers and regional specializations to be visualized in living, intact eyes (Box 17-1 and Fig. 17-14).

Retinal Neurons Translate Patterns of Light Into Patterns of Contrast

Analogies between eyes and cameras mostly cease at the level of the retina. Cameras and film are generally designed to produce accurate maps of patterns of illumination. The impression that the human visual system does the same is largely illusory. On the contrary, visual systems are specialized to recognize significant objects and features in visual scenes despite changes in angle of view, distance, and illumination. Receptor potentials in the array of retinal photoreceptors are the beginning of a neural process in which patterns of light are dissected into their components—areas of motion, boundaries between light and dark areas, boundaries between areas of different color, and other features—and the abstracted properties somehow reassembled into a unified perception. The brain, in effect, makes its "best guess" in interpreting patterns of light, and the results are sometimes inaccurate or go considerably beyond the information

Direction of view in *B* and *D*

Cone inner segments

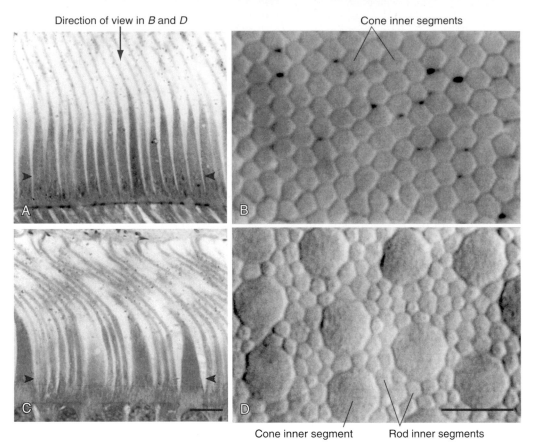

Cone inner segment   Rod inner segments

Figure 17-12 Differential distribution of rods and cones in the human retina. **A** and **C,** Standard histological sections parallel to the long axes of photoreceptor inner and outer segments in the fovea **(A)** and the midperipheral retina **(C). B** and **D,** The array of photoreceptors in comparable areas of another retina viewed end-on, using a special video microscopy technique (Nomarski differential interference contrast) that allows focusing on a particular cross-sectional plane of the sample. In this case, the plane of focus is one that cuts through the photoreceptor inner segments at the level indicated by the arrowheads in **A** and **C**. In the fovea **(B),** all the inner segments are of closely packed, slender cones, whereas in the midperipheral retina **(D),** the inner segments of fatter cones are interspersed among the rod inner segments. Scale marks in **C** (applies also to **A**) and **D** (applies also to **C**) = 10 μm. *(Modified from Curcio CA et al: J Comp Neurol 292:497, 1990.)*

received by the eye (Fig. 17-15; see also Figs. 17-22 and 17-23D). The blind spot hidden from our consciousness is one example; another is the feeling that we have sharp, clear, color vision throughout our visual fields, whereas this is true only for a small central region (see Fig. 17-18).

Photopigments Are G Protein–Coupled Receptors That Cause Hyperpolarizing Receptor Potentials

Rhodopsin and cone pigments are members of the same family of G protein–coupled receptors that mediate many postsynaptic effects and some other sensory transduction processes, such as olfaction. In the case of rods and cones, the ligand of the receptor protein **opsin,** rather than being a neurotransmitter or an odorant, is a vitamin A derivative **(11-*cis* retinal)** that enables the photopigments to absorb visible light. Slight differences among the opsins of rods and each of the three types of cones result in differences in the wavelengths absorbed preferentially by each photopigment (see Fig. 17-19A).

The only effect of light in the phototransduction process is to isomerize 11-*cis* retinal to all-*trans* retinal, which shortly thereafter dissociates from opsin. Isomerization of retinal causes a conformational change in the opsin to which it is bound, and opsin in its altered conformation activates nearby molecules of **transducin,** a G protein (Fig. 17-16). Each activated transducin in turn activates phosphodiesterase, an enzyme that hydrolyzes **cyclic guanosine monophosphate (cGMP).** This seemingly cumbersome process results in great amplification. Absorption of a single photon by one of the hundred million rhodopsins in a rod can activate dozens of transducins; each transducin-activated phosphodiesterase can hydrolyze about a thousand cGMP molecules per second.

The surface membranes of rod and cone outer segments contain cGMP-gated cation channels. In the dark, the cGMP concentration is relatively high, the cation channels are open most of the time, and a current carried mainly by Na^+ ions flows into the outer segment

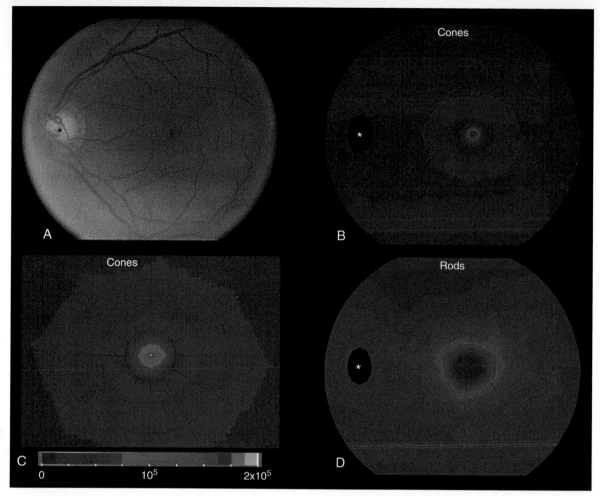

Figure 17-13 Differential distribution of rods and cones in the human retina. **A,** Funduscopic view of the left retina. Arteries and veins emerge from the optic disk (*) and arc around the fovea (F). **B** and **D,** Distributions of cones **(B)** and rods **(D)** in an area of retina comparable to that shown in **A.** Note the absence of photoreceptors in the optic disk (*), the foveal concentration of cones (shown enlarged in **C**), and the perifoveal concentration of rods. The scale at the lower left shows the number of cells per mm^2. (*A, courtesy Dr. Christine A. Curcio, University of Alabama at Birmingham. B to D, modified from Curcio CA et al: J Comp Neurol 292:497, 1990.*)

Optical Coherence Tomography: *Using Reflected Light to Visualize Cross Sections of Intraocular Structures*

The retina is much too thin for techniques such as magnetic resonance imaging to resolve its layers. For that reason, a new form of tomography, **optical coherence tomography (OCT)**, developed in the 1990s, has been a great advance in ophthalmology. The principle of OCT is simple. The retina is translucent (see Fig. 17-8), so a beam of light can penetrate it. As it does so, varying amounts are reflected back from different levels. For example, the nerve fiber layer is more reflective than the inner and outer nuclear layers. So by measuring the timing of changes in reflected light, one can make inferences about changes in tissue structure along the path of the beam; the reflection from the nerve fiber layer will arrive at the detector first, followed by the reflection from the ganglion cell layer, and so on. By repeating this process as the beam scans across the retina, two-dimensional pictures of the retina—cross sections, in effect—can be built up (see Figs. 17-14A to D).

Measuring the time delays of reflected signals is the basis of ultrasonography and radar, but light travels so quickly that its "echo" time cannot be measured in reflections from things as small as retinas. Instead, the delay times are measured indirectly, using an interfer-ometer. If the beam of light reflected from the retina is mixed with a reference beam reflected from a stationary surface, a time-varying interference pattern can be measured: at some points in time, the sample and reference beams will be in phase (constructive interference; large combined signal); shortly thereafter, the beams will be out of phase (destructive interference; small combined signal). The time between the peaks and troughs of the interference signal is a direct measure of changes in the distance traveled by the sample beam. The size difference between the peaks and the troughs is a measure of the amount of light reflected from that level of the retina; if there is not much reflection, there is not much interference.

OCT systems now make it possible to visualize a wide variety of retinal pathologies noninvasively, with a spatial resolution of less than 10 μm (see Fig. 17-14E). In addition, the infrared light used to make the scans is not scattered by cataracts, so it is possible to make images of retinas behind them. The infrared light also penetrates some other intraocular tissues well enough to make tomographic images of them possible (see Fig. 17-14F and G).

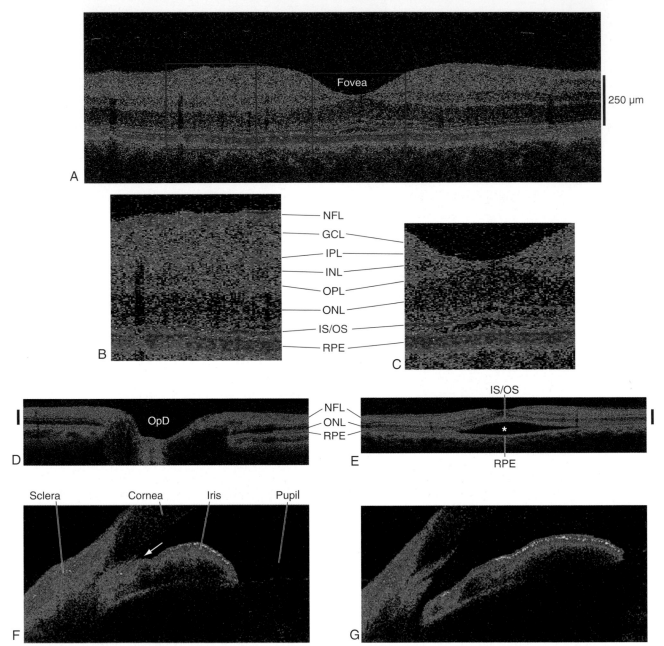

Figure 17-14 Use of optical coherence tomography (OCT) to visualize the retina and intraocular pathology. **A,** OCT image of the fovea and parafoveal retina. The outlined areas are enlarged in **B** and **C. D,** Normal optic disk (OpD) with a thick nerve fiber layer (NFL) converging on it from either side. Scale mark = 250 μm. **E,** A case of retinal detachment. The space (*) between the retinal pigment epithelium (RPE) and the photoreceptor layer (IS/OS) is apparent. The maintained reflectivity of the photoreceptor layer is a good prognostic sign, indicating probable recovery once the photoreceptors are reattached to the pigment epithelium. Scale mark = 250 μm. **F** and **G,** A case of acute angle-closure glaucoma in a 63-year-old woman who presented to the emergency department with a red, painful left eye and reduced vision. OCT revealed that her iris was edematous and bowed forward, presumably because of contact between the lens and the pupillary margin of the iris. The increased pressure in the posterior chamber pushed the iris forward, narrowing the angle (*arrow* in **F**) between the iris and cornea and obstructing the outflow of aqueous humor. A laser was used to perforate the peripheral iris, providing a direct route to the anterior chamber for aqueous trapped in the posterior chamber (much like using a shunt to treat hydrocephalus). Her left iris assumed a more normal configuration **(G),** and her symptoms resolved. GCL, ganglion cell layer; INL, inner nuclear layer; IPL, inner plexiform layer; IS/OS, photoreceptor inner and outer segments; ONL, outer nuclear layer; OPL, outer plexiform layer. (*A, B, D, and E, from Huang D et al: Optical coherence tomography. In Huang D et al, editors: Retinal imaging, Philadelphia, 2006, Mosby Elsevier. C, courtesy Dr. James G Fujimoto, Massachusetts Institute of Technology. F and G, from Kalev-Landoy M et al: Acta Ophthalmol Scand 85:427, 2007.*)

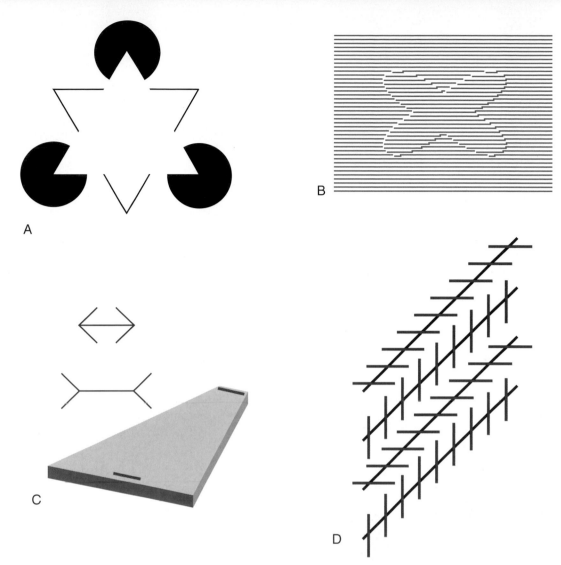

Figure 17-15 Some simple visual illusions. **A,** The Kanizsa triangle (named for Gaetano Kanizsa, who first described it in 1955), in which an illusory figure (here a white triangle) seems to be located in front of other objects, partially occluding them. In fact, nothing is there except black lines and notched disks. **B,** Slight displacement of some line segments causes the illusory appearance of a raised surface. **C,** Misperception of line length. In the Müller-Lyer illusion, the upper horizontal line appears shorter than the lower, even though both are the same length. The oppositely directed angles at the ends of these lines give false perspective cues. The two lines on the seemingly three-dimensional surface are also equal in length. **D,** The Zöllner illusion. All four black lines are actually parallel to one another.

(Fig. 17-17). As a result, rods and cones have a relatively depolarized resting potential of about −40 mV in the dark and release neurotransmitter (glutamate) at a steady rate onto processes of bipolar and horizontal cells. Light-induced hydrolysis of cGMP causes cation channels to close, the membrane hyperpolarizes toward the potassium equilibrium potential, and transmitter release declines.[g]

_____

[g]In a sense, therefore, our photoreceptors are really "darkness receptors," depolarizing and releasing more transmitter as the level of illumination decreases. Presumably because we evolved spending about half our time in light and half in darkness, this arrangement is not as metabolically inefficient as it sounds at first. There are even some fortuitous economies now that we spend more than half our time in the light.

Rods Function in Dim Light

Rods carry this amplification mechanism to an extreme, producing small but detectable electrical responses to single photons. Absorption of one photon by a dark-adapted rod causes transient closure of several hundred cation channels in the surface membrane, about a million ions are prevented from entering (see Fig. 17-17), and there is a small, brief decrease in the rate of transmitter release. This sensitivity comes at a price, however. Rods can respond only up to about moonlight levels of light intensity; they are saturated in room light and daylight. In addition, rod responses are slow (see Fig. 17-16A). Finally, the responses of multiple rods must be pooled to produce meaningful changes in the firing rate

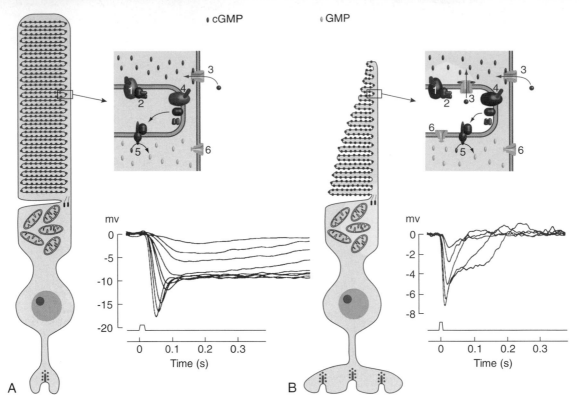

Figure 17-16 Phototransduction in rods **(A)** and cones **(B)**. In the dark, rhodopsin and cone pigments (1) bind 11-*cis* retinal, transducin is inactive (2), and cGMP-gated cation channels are open (3). Light isomerizes 11-*cis* retinal to all-*trans* retinal (4), activating transducin, which in turn activates an enzyme (phosphodiesterase) that hydrolyzes cGMP (5). Decreased availability of cGMP causes the cGMP-gated cation channels to close (6) and the photoreceptors to hyperpolarize. The voltage records show the responses of a monkey rod (left) and L (red-absorbing) cone (right) to 10-msec flashes of increasing intensity. The light intensity for the cone record was several thousand times greater than for the rod record, resulting in the absorption of about 40 times as many photons per flash by the cone. It can be seen that cones are less sensitive than rods, and their responses are faster and briefer. *(Voltage records, from Schneeweis DM, Schnapf JL: Science 268:1053, 1995.)*

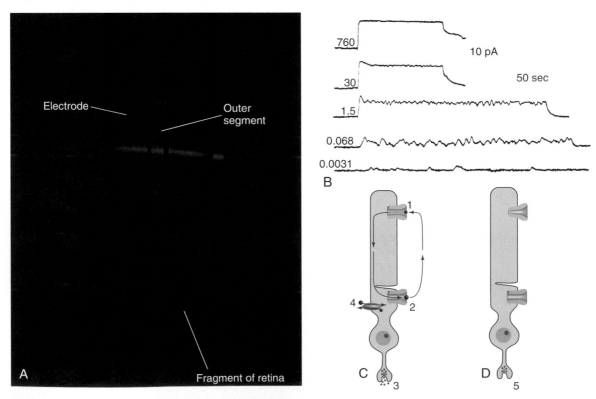

Figure 17-17 Current flow into retinal rods in the dark, and changes in this current flow in response to light. **A,** Drawing a single rod outer segment into a tightly fitting suction electrode allows all the current flowing into the outer segment to be recorded, both in the dark and in response to small slits of light. **B,** Reduction in current flow (upward deflections) in response to light of increasing intensity (given in photons/μm²/sec). The dimmest light causes transient reductions, reflecting channel closings in response to absorption of single photons; the brightest light completely terminates the current that flows in the dark. **C,** In the dark, current carried primarily by Na⁺ ions flows into the outer segment (1) through normally open cation channels and flows out of the inner segment (2) as K⁺ ions passing through normally open K⁺ channels. The resulting depolarization causes tonic release of glutamate from the receptor's synaptic terminal (3). Ionic concentration gradients are maintained by Na⁺/K⁺ pumps in the inner segment (4). **D,** In response to light, the outer segment cation channels close, the receptor hyperpolarizes, and glutamate release slows or ceases (5). *(A, courtesy Dr. Denis A. Baylor, Department of Neurobiology, Stanford University School of Medicine. B, from Baylor DA, Lamb TD, Yau K-Y: J Physiol 288:613, 1979.)*

of ganglion cells in response to dim light. Particularly in the peripheral retina, the outputs of thousands of rods converge on hundreds of bipolar cells before ultimately reaching single ganglion cells; hence spatial resolution in dim light is relatively poor.

All our retinal rods contain the same rhodopsin, making them incapable of discriminating color. Even though rhodopsin absorbs 500-nm light more effectively than light of other wavelengths (see Fig. 17-19A), every photon absorbed sets in motion the same G protein–coupled cascade. Hence a dim 500-nm stimulus causes the same receptor potential as a brighter 600-nm stimulus.

Populations of Cones Signal Spatial Detail and Color

Cones have smaller outer segments, less visual pigment, and smaller, briefer single-photon responses than rods. All this makes cones less sensitive (but faster) than rods (see Fig. 17-16B), and they require moonlight or greater levels of illumination to function effectively. Hence we use rods to see by starlight (**scotopic** vision), both rods and cones in moonlight (**mesopic** vision), and only cones for anything brighter than moonlight (**photopic** vision).

There is considerably less convergence in cone pathways than in rod pathways. This contributes further to the lower sensitivity of the cone system, because individual ganglion cells collect information from only a small number of cones. However, it also makes possible the resolution of fine spatial detail. Acuity is highest in the fovea (Fig. 17-18), where midget ganglion cells have receptive fields with centers the size of a single cone.

In contrast to the single class of retinal rods, cones come in more than one variety. Most mammals have two kinds: one that absorbs maximally in the blue or ultraviolet part of the spectrum, and another that absorbs at longer wavelengths. Humans and some other primates have three varieties, defined by the wavelength of light each absorbs most efficiently (Fig. 17-19A). Hence there are **long wavelength (L), middle wavelength (M),** and **short wavelength (S)** cones, also commonly referred to as **red**,[h] **green**, and **blue** cones. The absorption peak is determined by the kind of opsin a particular cone makes; each of the cone opsins binds the same 11-*cis* retinal as rhodopsin does. Multiple populations of cones are the starting point for color vision. Even though individual cones, like individual rods, can report only the number of photons absorbed and not their wavelength, the relative activity levels of multiple populations of cones provide information about wavelength (see Fig. 17-19B). The **trichromatic** nature of our color vision is indicated by the fact that any color in the spectrum can be matched

[h]Red cones are referred to as "red" because they are the most important for distinguishing colors at the red end of the spectrum, even though they absorb maximally in the yellow-green range.

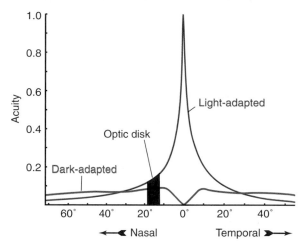

Figure 17-18 Spatial acuity of different retinal regions under different conditions of illumination. When using cones in bright light, acuity is highest in the fovea but falls off rapidly. When using rods in dim light, acuity is always less than with foveal cone vision, and it is zero in the fovea because no rods are present there. (*Redrawn from Ruch T, Patten HD, editors: Physiology and biophysics, ed 20, Philadelphia, 1979, WB Saunders.*)

by some combination of three primary colors (e.g., red, green, and blue) that stimulates the three populations of cones the same relative amounts as the test stimulus.

S cones account for only about 5% of the total cone population. L and M cones are more or less randomly intermingled, in a distribution that is surprisingly variable (Fig. 17-20). Among individuals with normal color vision, the ratio of L to M cones ranges from about 1:1 to more than 15:1. The genes for the red and green cone pigments are located next to each other on the X chromosome, and unequal crossing over during meiosis can cause one X chromosome to wind up with a missing or defective red or green gene. As a result, about 2% of the male population is red-green **color blind** (Fig. 17-21B and C) because of a lack of the red or green pigment (conditions called **protanopia** and **deuteranopia,** respectively). The incidence in females is much lower because they are likely to have at least one X chromosome with normal red and green genes. Lack of the blue cone pigment (**tritanopia;** see Fig. 17-21D) is rare and, because the blue gene is located on chromosome 7, is equally uncommon in males and females.

Ganglion Cells Have Center-Surround Receptive Fields

Once photons have been absorbed and receptor potentials produced, the rest of the work of the visual system is based on a series of synapses that begins in the outer plexiform layer and extends to and beyond the visual association areas of the occipital, temporal, and parietal lobes. At each level a certain amount of information processing takes place, so cortical neurons respond best to

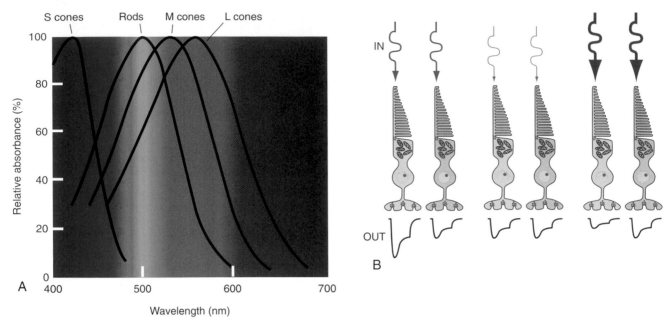

Figure 17-19 **A,** Absorption spectra of rod and cone visual pigments. **B,** Schematic indication of the necessity for multiple cone types to discriminate wavelengths. L cones produce receptor potentials of the same size in response to moderate green light, dim yellow light, or bright red light. M cones, however, produce receptor potentials of progressively decreasing size. Hence wavelength can be discriminated by comparing the outputs of different classes of cones. (For simplicity, light is indicated as reaching the cone outer segments directly; in reality, it would move in the opposite direction, traversing the cell bodies of the cones before reaching their outer segments.)

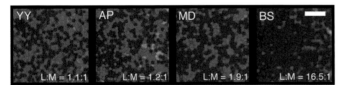

Figure 17-20 The distribution of S (blue), M (green), and L (red) cones just outside the center of the fovea in four males with normal color vision. These remarkable images were made with advanced optical techniques that allow individual cones to be seen and identified in intact eyes. *(From Hofer H, Singer B, Williams DR: J Vision 5:444, 2005.)*

stimuli that are quite different from those best able to stimulate individual rods and cones. A cell at any given level in the visual system, like a cell in the somatosensory system, can be characterized by its **receptive field,** which in this case refers to the retinal area in which changing conditions of illumination produce an alteration of the cell's activity. By extension, receptive fields of visual neurons can also be defined in terms of the particular part of the outside world whose image falls on this region of the retina. One initially surprising observation about the receptive fields of bipolar cells and more proximal neurons is that the intensity of illumination is relatively unimportant in determining the level of activity of most cells. Rather, the important parameter is the contrast between different areas of the receptive field. That is, the visual system is especially attuned to the detection of borders between light and dark areas, or between areas of different color. This is in large part responsible for the fairly constant appearance of objects

despite varying illumination. For example, the words on this page do not change their appearance when looked at in room light or sunlight, despite the fact that more light is reflected from the print in sunlight than from the white background in room light. Similarly, the colors of objects do not seem to change much, even though the spectral composition of the light we encounter changes drastically at different times of the day and in different locations. An orange in a bowl of fruit, for example, looks just about as orange when viewed at noon or at sunset, or in incandescent or fluorescent light, even though the proportions of various wavelengths it reflects are very different in these four conditions. Here again, the brain analyzes the patterns of light reaching the retina and makes its "best guess" about the reality they represent. Just as we can be fooled when assessing shapes and lines (see Fig. 17-15), our best guess about brightness and color can also be erroneous (Fig. 17-22).

Recordings from individual ganglion cells show that their receptive fields are composed of two concentric, roughly circular zones. Illumination of the central area (the **center**) causes either an increase or a decrease in the background firing rate (Fig. 17-23), whereas illumination of the peripheral area (the **surround**) has the opposite effect; hence there are **ON-center** and **OFF-center** receptive fields.

Simultaneous illumination of both center and surround causes relatively little change in firing rate because the antagonistic effects of the two areas roughly cancel each other. Cells of different functional classes vary in

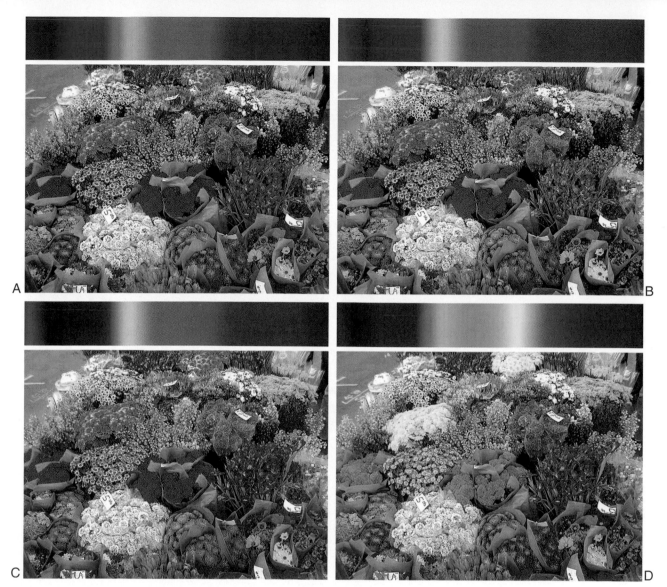

Figure 17-21 Simulations of how the spectrum and the array of flowers shown in **A** might appear to a protanope **(B)**, a deuteranope **(C)**, and a tritanope **(D)**. Although it is impossible to be sure that the subjective experience of someone with normal color vision viewing these simulations is the same as that of someone with one of these conditions, the difficulty in discriminating among various parts of the spectrum is apparent. Having only one cone population that absorbs in the green part of the spectrum **(B** and **C)**, for example, makes it difficult to discriminate among red, yellow, and green objects. *(Simulations produced using Colorfield Insight 1.0.1, Colorfield Digital Media, Inc.)*

the sizes of their receptive fields, their color sensitivity, and some temporal aspects of their responses, but usually not in their basic center-surround organization. Thus, even at the level of ganglion cells, the contrast between two different areas of the receptive field is of paramount importance.

Center-Surround Receptive Fields Are Formed in the Outer Plexiform Layer

The basic spatial organization of ganglion cell receptive fields develops in the outer plexiform layer. Bipolar cells do not make action potentials, but instead produce postsynaptic potentials in a center-surround pattern and pass this along to ganglion cells through excitatory

(glutamate) synapses (Fig. 17-24A). The properties of the centers of bipolar cell receptive fields reflect the "straight-through" receptor to bipolar cell path. All photoreceptors can do is increase or decrease their rate of glutamate release, so the fact that some bipolar cells depolarize and others hyperpolarize in response to illumination means that glutamate has opposite effects on these two populations of bipolar cells (a nice example of the idea that the effects of neurotransmitters are determined by the postsynaptic receptor). Briefly, the metabotropic glutamate receptor (mGluR6) a receptor that results in inhibitory activity when bound to glutamate, is found on the "ON" bipolar cells resulting in the inhibition of these "ON" bipolar cells in the dark when there is more glutamate.

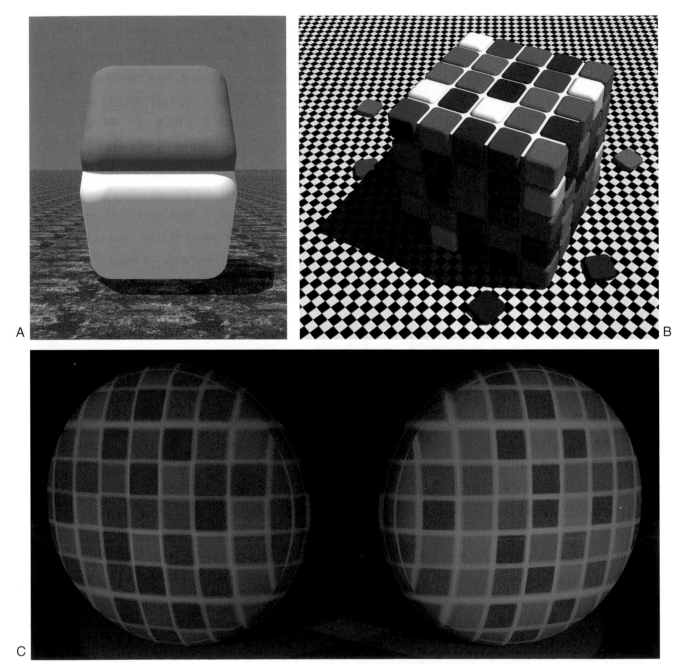

Figure 17-22 Three spectacular examples of how the brain can misjudge brightness or color. These illusions are so compelling that you will probably need to use the mask included at the back of this book to convince yourself of the brightness or color of some parts of the figures. In **A,** the upper gray panel looks much darker than the lower panel, but in fact they are the same. The adjoining dark and light gradients between the two panels make it look as though the upper panel is illuminated and the lower panel is in shadow. The brain apparently assumes that this amount of light reflected back from the illuminated (upper) surface signifies a relatively dark object, and that the same amount of light reflected back from the surface in shadow signifies a relatively light object. Similarly, in **B,** the upper face of the cube seems to be illuminated, and the front face seems to be in shadow. As a result, we interpret the central square in the upper face as brown and the central square in the front face as orange, even though they are identical. Finally, in **C,** the surface on the left seems to be illuminated by reddish light and that on the right by bluish light. As a result, we interpret the central squares of the two surfaces (each marked with a black dot) as differing in color, even though they are the same. *(Courtesy Drs. R. Beau Lotto and Dale Purves, Duke University Medical Center.)*

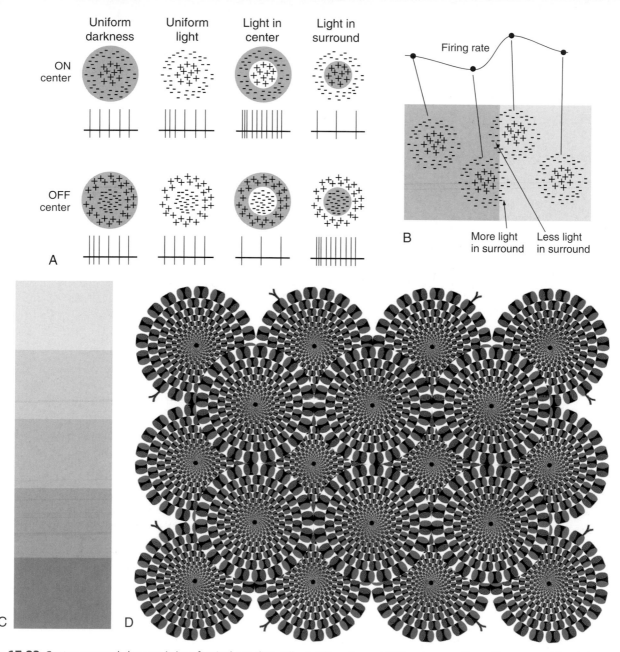

Figure 17-23 Center-surround characteristics of retinal ganglion cells. **A,** ON-center and OFF-center ganglion cells are named for their response to light in the center of the receptive field. Plus and minus signs indicate areas of the field where light causes increases or decreases in the firing rate. **B,** The antagonistic surround (in this case, using an ON-center cell as an example) results in an accentuation of the change in firing rate when an area of contrast moves across the receptive field. **C,** One result of this enhanced contrast sensitivity is the Chevreul illusion (one of a family of illusions usually called Mach bands). Each rectangle is a uniform shade of gray (you can verify this by covering up all but one square), but the darkness and lightness on either side of a transition appear exaggerated. **D,** Another probable result of this contrast sensitivity is the apparent motion seen in the Rotating Snakes illusion as your gaze moves across it. Some contrast jumps are processed faster than others, fooling motion-sensitive cells into thinking that parts of this stationary pattern are moving. (**D,** courtesy Dr. Akiyoshi Kitaoka, Ritsumeikan University.)

The "OFF" bipolar cells contain an inotropic glutamate receptor termed AMPA (α-amino-3-hydroxy-5-methyl-4-isoxazolepropionic acid receptor) that result in the influx of mainly Na cations resulting in the excitation of the "OFF" bipolar cells in the presence of glutamate. Hence, the bipolar cells begin to distinguish the photoreceptor message based on the amount of glutamate they receive.

Illumination of a given receptor causes it to hyperpolarize and release less glutamate. Illumination of its neighbors does just the opposite, causing it to release more glutamate; this is the basis of the surround in bipolar cell center-surround receptive fields. Although the mechanism of this effect is still unclear, it is mediated by horizontal cells (see Fig. 17-24B). Glutamate released by receptors depolarizes horizontal cells;

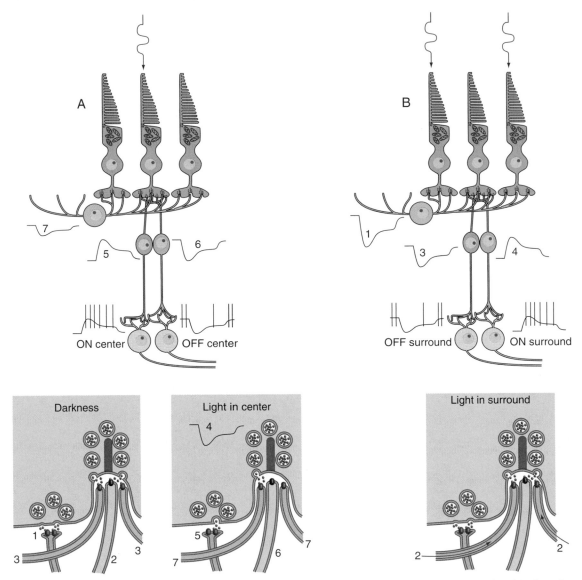

Figure 17-24 Formation of center-surround receptive fields at the level of bipolar cells, using foveal cones and midget bipolar cells as examples. **A,** Formation of receptive field centers. In the dark, photoreceptors are depolarized and release glutamate onto the superficial synapses made by OFF-center bipolar cells (1) and onto the invaginating processes of ON-center bipolar cells (2) and horizontal cells (3). Because of the nature of the postsynaptic receptor molecules, glutamate hyperpolarizes the processes of ON-center bipolar cells and depolarizes the other two kinds of processes. Hence in the dark, ON-center bipolar cells are relatively hyperpolarized, and horizontal cells and OFF-center bipolar cells are relatively depolarized. Light in the receptive field center hyperpolarizes the cone (4), decreases glutamate release, and reverses all these polarizations: ON-center bipolar cells (as their name implies) depolarize (5), and the ganglion cells to which they project fire more rapidly; OFF-center bipolar cells hyperpolarize (6); and horizontal cells also hyperpolarize (7), but only moderately, because glutamate is still being released onto their other processes. **B,** Role of horizontal cells in formation of the antagonistic surround. Light delivered to cones surrounding the central cone in **A** causes a large hyperpolarization of horizontal cells (1) because of diminished glutamate release on many of their processes. This hyperpolarization spreads to the synaptic terminal of the central cone (2), in turn causing increased release of glutamate (as though it just got darker in the center of the receptive field), hyperpolarization of the ON-center bipolar cell (3), and depolarization of the OFF-center bipolar cell (4). The mechanism of this increased glutamate release is still being investigated, but it probably involves the effects of altered pH in the synaptic cleft on voltage-gated Ca^{2+} channels in the photoreceptor synaptic terminal.

illumination removes this depolarization, causing them to hyperpolarize. The hyperpolarization spreads through horizontal cell processes to the synaptic terminals of nearby receptors, where it increases Ca^{2+} influx and glutamate release.

Further lateral interactions in the inner plexiform layer, mediated by amacrine cells, are thought to enhance the center-surround effect and to modify such things as the temporal characteristics of the ganglion cell response. For example, some ganglion cells respond only transiently to a change in illumination, whereas others show a maintained change in discharge rate. Many lower vertebrates have much more complex ganglion cell receptive fields, and there is a corresponding increase in the

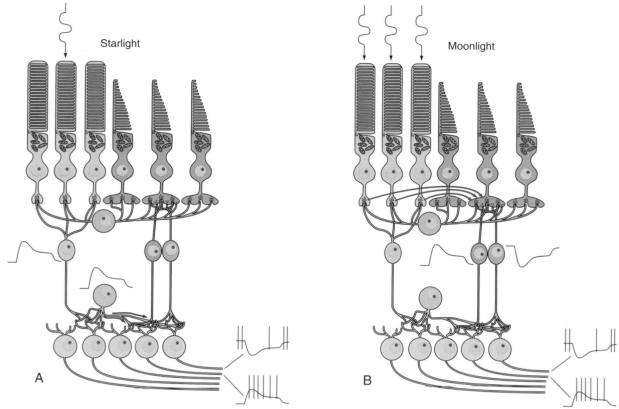

Figure 17-25 Rod signals reach ganglion cells through a remarkable system of special amacrine cells and modifiable gap junctions. At scotopic levels **(A)**, rod signals reach rod bipolar cells, which hyperpolarize in response to glutamate (so they depolarize in response to light). Rod bipolar cells terminate on processes of special amacrine cells, in turn depolarizing them. Gap junctions open between amacrine cell processes and the synaptic terminals of cone ON-center bipolar cells *(green arrow)*, allowing rod signals access to this branch of the cone circuitry. Other processes of the same amacrine cells make inhibitory (glycine) chemical synapses on the synaptic terminals of cone OFF-center bipolar cells *(red arrow)* and also on dendrites of OFF-center ganglion cells. At mesopic levels **(B)**, gap junctions between rod and cone terminals open *(green arrows)*, and rod receptor potentials gain access to the cone circuitry described in Figure 17-24.

thickness of the inner plexiform layer and a proliferation of amacrine cell synapses.

Every point in the visual field is represented by both ON-center and OFF-center ganglion cells. This means that in the fovea, for example, each cone synapses on two midget bipolar cells (as in Fig. 17-24), one of which depolarizes and one of which hyperpolarizes in response to increases in light intensity (and vice versa).[i] The two midget bipolar cells synapse on two midget ganglion cells, with the result that one of the ganglion cells fires faster whether light intensity increases or decreases. This presumably enhances the speed of visual processing: it takes much less time to determine that a cell's firing rate has increased than to determine that it has decreased.

---

[i]These midget bipolar cells are integral parts of the high-acuity pathway subserving foveal vision, but they are only part of the story. Each cone synapses on six other bipolar cells as well—three additional kinds of ON-center cells and three additional kinds of OFF-center cells. The functional significance of this distribution of cone information into eight different parallel pathways is still not understood.

Rod and Cone Signals Reach the Same Ganglion Cells

The entire range of light intensities, from scotopic threshold to bright sunlight, is signaled by the same population of ganglion cells. Cone signals reach ganglion cells by the circuitry just described. Rods use a more circuitous route that enables them to cleverly "hitch a ride" on parts of the cone circuitry (Fig. 17-25). At scotopic levels, rod signals reach special bipolar cells dedicated to rod function, which then transmit this information through amacrine cells to cone bipolar cells. At mesopic levels, gap junctions between rods and cones open, and rod receptor currents flow directly into the synaptic terminals of cones.

Half of the Visual Field of Each Eye Is Mapped Systematically in the Contralateral Cerebral Hemisphere

Ganglion cell axons travel in the optic nerve to the **optic chiasm,** where they undergo a partial decussation and enter one of the two **optic tracts.** Most of the fibers in each optic tract then terminate in the **lateral geniculate nucleus,** the thalamic relay nucleus for vision. Geniculate fibers travel through the internal capsule and corona radiata to primary visual cortex in the banks of the calcarine sulcus. In addition, a considerable number of optic tract fibers project directly to the midbrain and a few to the hypothalamus. Throughout the pathway from retina to cerebral cortex (and to the superior colliculus of the midbrain), the numbers of fibers and areas of representation for the macula are disproportionately large for the macula's actual size. This reflects the relatively small amount of convergence in the macula, which in turn reflects its specialization for high acuity.

Fibers From the Nasal Half of Each Retina Cross in the Optic Chiasm

The unmyelinated axons of ganglion cells collect at the optic disk, pierce the sclera in a region called the **lamina cribrosa** (see Fig. 17-9), acquire myelin sheaths, and form the optic nerve. Embryologically and in its adult anatomy, the optic nerve is actually a tract of the CNS and, as such, has meningeal coverings much like other areas. The sclera continues as its dural sheath, lined in turn by arachnoid and pia. The subarachnoid space around the optic nerve dead-ends at the back of the eye but communicates with the subarachnoid spaces around other parts of the brain. Increases in intracranial pressure are therefore transmitted to the optic nerve, compress it, and choke off both venous flow and axoplasmic transport. The resulting edema and engorgement of axons cause a characteristic swelling of the optic disk, called **papilledema,** which can be a valuable diagnostic sign of intracranial pressure often due to hydrocephalus.

Just anterior to the infundibular stalk, the two optic nerves partially decussate in the optic chiasm. All fibers from the nasal half of each retina cross to the contralateral optic tract; all fibers from the temporal half of each retina pass through the lateral portions of the chiasm without crossing and enter the ipsilateral optic tract. The result is that each optic tract contains the fibers arising in the temporal retina of the ipsilateral eye and the nasal retina of the contralateral eye. As indicated in Figure 17-26, this apparently curious partial decussation is exactly appropriate for delivering all the information from the contralateral visual field to each optic tract. Also, because much of the basis for depth perception involves a comparison of the slightly different views seen by our two eyes, it is necessary to bring together information from comparable areas of the two retinas, which the optic chiasm accomplishes.

From the optic tract to the visual cortex, cells and fibers representing corresponding areas of the two retinas (i.e., fibers carrying information about the same

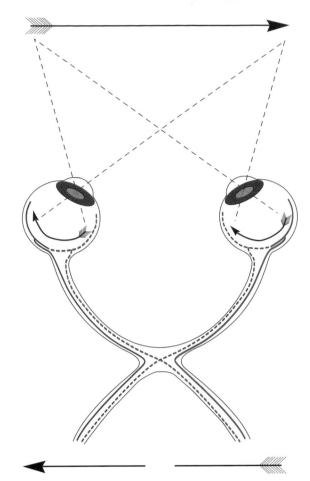

Figure 17-26 Schematic diagram illustrating the formation of the optic chiasm and tracts. All information from the temporal side of a vertical line passing through a given fovea enters the ipsilateral optic tract; all information from the nasal side crosses in the chiasm and enters the contralateral optic tract. The result, as indicated, is that each optic tract "looks at" the contralateral visual field.

area in the visual field) are located near each other, with the result that damage to the optic tract or more central parts of the pathway causes comparable (although not necessarily identical) visual deficits in both eyes.[j]

Most Fibers of the Optic Tract Terminate in the Lateral Geniculate Nucleus

The optic tract curves posteriorly around the cerebral peduncle, and most of its fibers terminate in the lateral geniculate nucleus (Fig. 17-27; see also Fig. 16-13). This is a six-layered, dome-shaped nucleus in which the optic tract fibers terminate in a precise retinotopic pattern.

---

[j]The retinotopic arrangement in the optic tract is only approximate because the fibers sort themselves not only by retinal origin but also by functional type. This is presumably the basis of clinical reports that partial optic tract damage, although uncommon, causes deficits mainly involving only selected aspects of visual function, such as color vision, or more extensive deficits in one eye than the other.

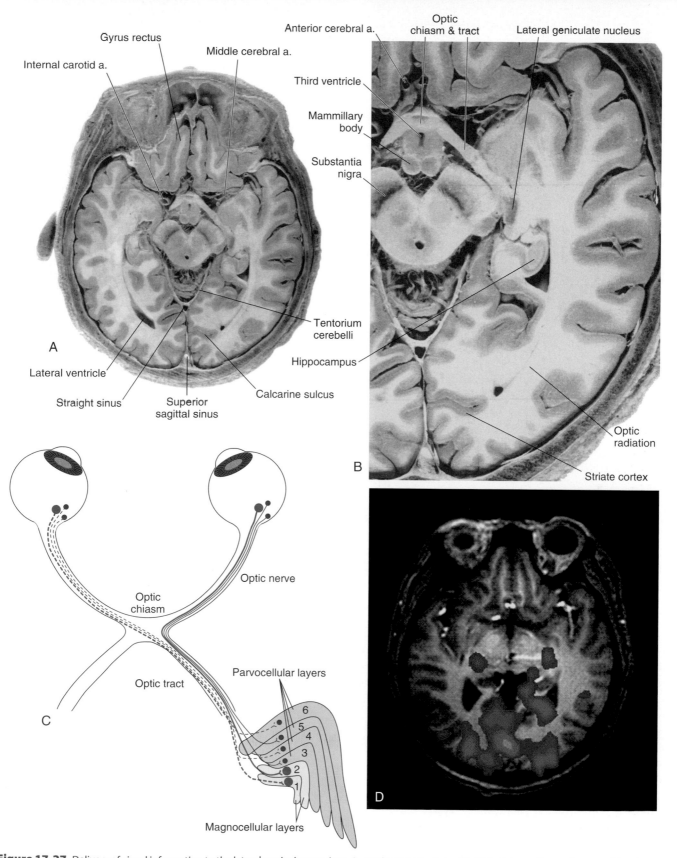

Figure 17-27 Delivery of visual information to the lateral geniculate nucleus. **A,** Axial section (enlarged in **B**) just above the confluence of the sinuses, showing most of the visual pathway. **C,** Projection from the retina to the lateral geniculate nucleus, indicating how information traveling in the magnocellular and parvocellular pathways, as well as information from the two eyes, remains segregated at the level of the lateral geniculate. Notice, however, that all information from a given point in the visual field ends up in a column that extends through all six geniculate layers. **D,** Functional magnetic resonance imaging data from a subject watching a red and black checkerboard in which the squares reversed color 8 to 10 times per second, superimposed on a T1-weighted axial slice at a level similar to that shown in **A.** The stimulus activates not only occipital cortex posteriorly but also the lateral geniculate nuclei (*). (**A** and **B,** courtesy Dr. John T. Willson, University of Colorado Health Sciences Center. **D,** from Chen W et al: Magn Reson Med 39:89, 1998.)

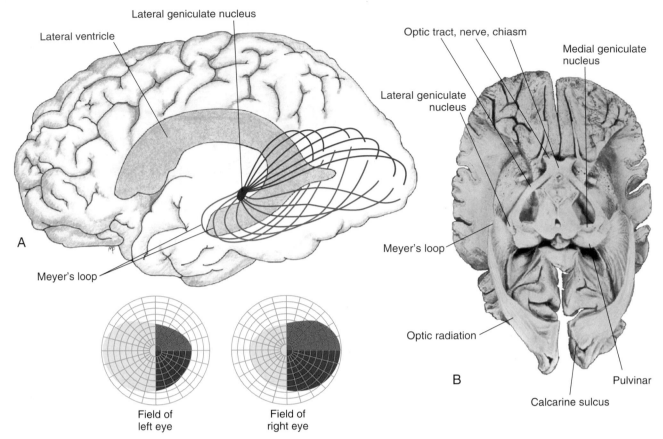

Lateral geniculate nucleus

Lateral ventricle

Optic tract, nerve, chiasm

Medial geniculate
nucleus

Lateral geniculate
nucleus

Meyer's loop

Meyer's loop

A

Optic radiation

B

Pulvinar

Calcarine sulcus

Field of
left eye

Field of
right eye

Figure 17-28 Two views of the optic radiation. **A,** Schematic illustration of the course of geniculocalcarine fibers as they loop over the lateral aspect of the lateral ventricle and then turn posteriorly to end in the banks of the calcarine sulcus on the medial surface of the hemisphere; note that the fibers representing inferior visual fields end in the upper bank, fibers representing superior visual fields end in the lower bank, and fibers representing the macula end most posteriorly. (See Fig. 17-32 for additional information about the mapping of visual fields.) **B,** Inferior aspect of a brain dissected to show the entire visual pathway, from optic nerve to striate cortex. (*B, from Ludwig E, Klingler J: Atlas cerebri humani, Boston, 1956, Little, Brown.*)

The pattern is about the same in each layer, so that a given point in the visual field is represented in a column of cells extending through all six layers. However, each layer receives input from only one eye: layers 1 (most inferior), 4, and 6 (most superior) from the contralateral eye, and layers 2, 3, and 5 from the ipsilateral eye (see Fig. 17-27C). Consistent with this anatomical arrangement, electrical recordings from the lateral geniculate nucleus reveal few cells that can be activated by both eyes.

Layers 3 to 6 contain small neurons that receive their inputs from the numerically dominant class of small ganglion cells sensitive to color and form. In view of their small neurons, these layers are referred to as the **parvocellular layers,** and this entire subdivision of the visual system is called the **parvocellular system.** Layers 1 and 2 contain larger neurons that receive their inputs from a separate class of larger ganglion cells that are more sensitive to movement and contrast. This subdivision, including the **magnocellular layers** (1 and 2) of the lateral geniculate nucleus, is referred to as the **magnocellular system.**

The Lateral Geniculate Nucleus Projects to Primary Visual Cortex

Fibers arising in the lateral geniculate nucleus project through the retrolenticular and sublenticular parts of the internal capsule, curve around the lateral wall of the lateral ventricle as the **optic radiation** (Fig. 17-28; see also Fig. 17-33), and terminate in the cortex adjacent to the calcarine sulcus. The optic radiation is sometimes called the **geniculocalcarine tract,** reflecting its origin and termination. Not all these fibers pass directly backward to the occipital lobe. Rather, they form a broad sheet covering much of the posterior and inferior horns of the ventricle. Fibers representing superior *visual field* quadrants (i.e., those representing inferior *retinal* quadrants) loop out into the temporal lobe **(Meyer's loop)** before turning posteriorly. As a result, temporal lobe damage can somewhat surprisingly produce a superior visual field deficit.

A retinotopic organization is maintained in the optic radiation. Fibers representing inferior visual fields are most superior, whereas those representing superior visual fields loop farthest out into the temporal lobe. Macular fibers occupy a broad middle area. The visual pathway is more dispersed in the optic radiation than elsewhere, and individual fibers still carry information from only one eye, so damage here often results in deficits that are overlapping but not identical in the two eyes.

The visual pathway ends retinotopically in the cortex above and below the calcarine sulcus (**area 17;** this numerical nomenclature, by which the cerebral cortex is divided into a series of areas called **Brodmann's areas,** is discussed in Chapter 22). Inferior visual fields project to the cortex above the calcarine sulcus, and superior fields project to the cortex below the sulcus. The macula is represented more posteriorly and peripheral fields more anteriorly (Figs. 17-29 and 17-30). Numerous myelinated fibers ramify within this cortex in a discrete layer that can be seen with the naked eye as a thin, white stripe (the **line of Gennari**) (Fig. 17-31; see also Fig. 17-27B). Hence primary visual cortex is also called **striate cortex.**

The striate cortex parallels the calcarine sulcus and extends for a short distance onto the posterior surface of the occipital lobe. It is surrounded by **area 18,** which in turn is surrounded by **area 19;** the two together make up most of the rest of the occipital lobe. Areas 18 and 19, together with related parts of the temporal and parietal lobes, are commonly referred to as **visual association cortex** or **extrastriate cortex** and are heavily interconnected with area 17. The parvocellular and magnocellular systems, as described later in this chapter, follow separate but interrelated routes through striate and extrastriate cortex.

Damage at Different Points in the Visual Pathway Results in Predictable Deficits

Visual fields are tested by moving a small object in from the periphery until the patient, with one eye covered, reports seeing it. By repeating this for many different directions of approach, a chart of the visual field can be made (Fig. 17-32). Each eye can normally see a surprising 90 degrees from the visual axis in a temporal direction (because of refraction by the cornea), but the field is less extensive in other directions because of obstruction by the nose, eyebrows, and cheeks. The area of overlap of the two visual fields is the area in which binocular vision is possible.

Deficits resulting from damage to various parts of the visual pathway are named according to certain conventions. Most importantly, visual defects are always named according to the visual field loss and not according to the area of the retina that is nonfunctional. Because the retinal image is inverted and reversed, damage to temporal areas of the retina causes nasal field losses, and damage to superior areas of the retina causes inferior

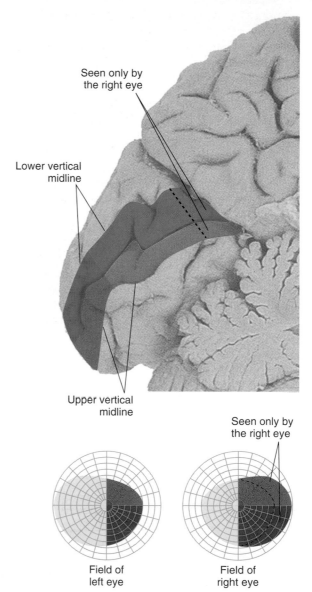

Figure 17-29 Map of the right visual field (of both eyes) in primary visual cortex of the left occipital lobe. The map is distorted so that the vertical midline lies above and below the calcarine sulcus, at the boundary between areas 17 and 18, and the horizontal meridian lies deep in the calcarine sulcus. The foveal representation extends a short distance beyond the medial surface of the occipital lobe, onto the occipital pole. There is considerably more primary visual cortex than it appears from this view; most is actually in the walls of the deep calcarine sulcus. *(Modified from Nolte J, Angevine JB Jr: The human brain in photographs and diagrams, ed 3, St. Louis, 2007, Mosby.)*

field losses. The combining form -*anopia* (or -*anopsia*) is used to denote loss of one or more quadrants of a visual field; **hemianopia** refers to loss of half a visual field, **quadrantanopia** to loss of one quarter of a visual field. Finally, the term **homonymous** denotes a condition in which the visual field losses are similar for both eyes, and **heteronymous** denotes a condition in which the two eyes have nonoverlapping field losses.

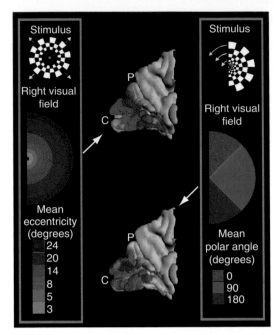

Figure 17-30 Retinotopic mapping of the right visual fields in the left occipital lobe, revealed by functional magnetic resonance imaging as a subject watched an expanding checkered annulus (upper image) or a rotating checkered stimulus (lower image). As indicated in Figure 17-29, the fovea is represented most posteriorly, and inferior visual fields most superiorly. Repeated colors farther from the calcarine sulcus (C) are the beginnings of additional retinotopic maps in extrastriate cortex. P, parietooccipital sulcus. *(From DeYoe EA et al: Proc Natl Acad Sci U S A 93:2382, 1996.)*

Homonymous losses may be **congruous** (essentially identical) or overlapping but **noncongruous.**

Using this terminology, it is possible to name the deficits resulting from damage at most locations in the visual pathway (Fig. 17-33); some of the names are real tongue-twisters. The overarching concept is that damage anterior to the optic chiasm affects only the ipsilateral eye, damage at the chiasm causes heteronymous deficits, and damage behind the chiasm causes homonymous deficits. A lesion of one optic nerve causes blindness of the ipsilateral eye. Damage in the central region of the optic chiasm, affecting the crossing fibers, causes a heteronymous hemianopia (in this case, **bitemporal hemianopia;** Fig. 17-34A). This most commonly results from midline pressure exerted by a tumor of the pituitary gland, which lies close to the chiasm (see Fig. 23-9). Lateral pressure on one side of the chiasm, affecting the noncrossing fibers on that side, causes **nasal hemianopia** of the ipsilateral eye. This occasionally results from an aneurysm at a branch point of the internal carotid artery, which lies adjacent to the chiasm (see Fig. 6-3). In the rare event of aneurysms of both internal carotid arteries, **binasal hemianopia** could result. Destruction of one optic tract interrupts all the fibers carrying information from the contralateral visual fields, causing contralateral **homonymous hemianopia.**

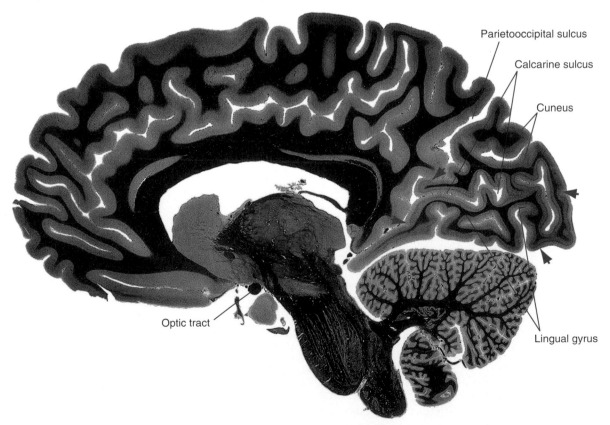

Figure 17-31 Parasagittal section, stained for myelin, showing the stripe of myelinated fibers that gave the striate cortex its name. The stripe ends abruptly *(arrows)* at the area 17–area 18 junction. Note that striate cortex extends a short distance beyond the medial surface of the occipital lobe, onto the occipital pole.

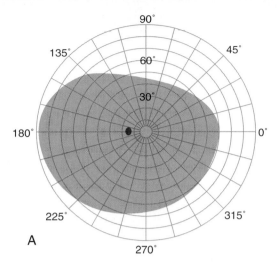

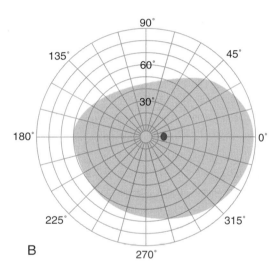

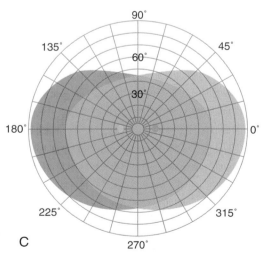

Figure 17-32 Normal visual field of the left eye **(A)**, the right eye **(B)**, and both eyes superimposed **(C)**. The blind spot of each eye is indicated in a darker color in **A** and **B**. The view is the patient's view of the charts on which the fields are being recorded.

Damage to the optic radiation can cause complete hemianopia (see Fig. 17-34B), but it is rarely this extensive; quadrant or sector deficits are more often the result. For example, a large destructive lesion of the left temporal lobe, interrupting the fibers of Meyer's loop (which represent inferior retinal quadrants), would produce **right homonymous superior quadrantanopia.** Lesions in either the optic radiation or visual cortex leave the pupillary light reflex undisturbed, as would be predicted from the anatomical pathways involved in this reflex (see Fig. 17-39).

In cases of massive damage to the visual cortex of one occipital lobe (e.g., after occlusion of one posterior cerebral artery near its origin from the basilar artery), contralateral homonymous hemianopia would be the expected result. In fact, it is frequently observed clinically that vision is preserved over much of the fovea. This phenomenon is called **macular** (or **foveal**) **sparing,** and its existence, extent, and basis have been a topic of debate for many years. Much or all of its origin probably lies in the disproportionately large representation of the fovea in the striate cortex; even very large cortical lesions may leave part of the foveal region undamaged, especially in cases of distal posterior cerebral artery occlusions that spare some of its branches. In addition, the distributions of the middle and posterior cerebral arteries overlap near the occipital pole (see Fig. 6-4). Therefore, even total occlusion of the posterior cerebral artery may allow for supply of part of the foveal region by the middle cerebral artery.

Some Fibers of the Optic Tract Terminate in the Superior Colliculus, Accessory Optic Nuclei, and Hypothalamus

The standard vertebrate plan of central visual connections includes not only a projection from the retina to the lateral geniculate nucleus (or its equivalent) but also a projection to the superior colliculus (or its equivalent). In lower vertebrates the collicular (or tectal) pathway is the more important, but in primates it is much less so. Nevertheless, the major inputs to the primate superior colliculus are still visual—one arising in the retina, and the second in the striate cortex. The retinal input consists of a substantial number of fibers in each optic tract that bypass the lateral geniculate nucleus, pass over the medial geniculate nucleus in a bundle called the **brachium of the superior colliculus** (or **superior brachium;** see Fig. 25-9), and terminate retinotopically in the superior colliculus and in the nearby **pretectal area** (described later) and other **accessory optic nuclei.** Some of these fibers are collaterals of axons that also terminate in the lateral geniculate nucleus, but most arise from separate subpopulations of ganglion cells. The cortical input consists of cells in area 17 that project to the superior colliculus (again via

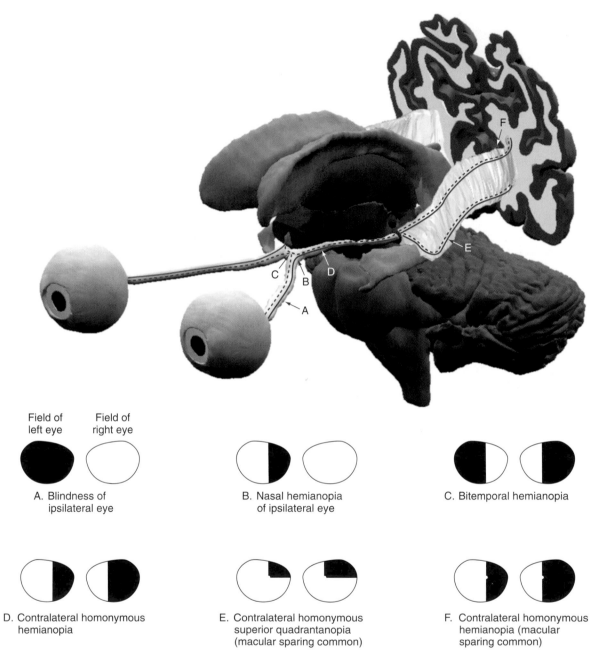

Figure 17-33 Visual field deficits caused by lesions at various points along the visual pathway. **A,** Destruction of one optic nerve causes blindness of the eye in which that nerve arises. **B,** Damage to one side of the optic chiasm destroys the noncrossing fibers from the ipsilateral eye; these fibers arise in the temporal retina, so nasal hemianopia of the ipsilateral eye results. **C,** Pressure on the middle of the optic chiasm, typically from a pituitary tumor, destroys the crossing fibers from both eyes, causing bitemporal hemianopia (one type of heteronymous hemianopia). **D,** Destruction of one optic tract causes contralateral homonymous hemianopia. **E,** Damage to one temporal lobe could destroy part of the optic radiation, specifically the fibers representing the contralateral superior quadrant of each visual field. Because the optic radiation is spread out near the lateral ventricle at this point, some fibers are likely to be spared; in this case, for example, the macular fibers remain intact. **F,** Massive damage to one occipital lobe (such as might be caused by occlusion of one posterior cerebral artery) causes contralateral homonymous hemianopia; the macular representation is very large, and some of it is likely to survive, resulting in macular sparing. (See Videos 17-1 and 17-2.)

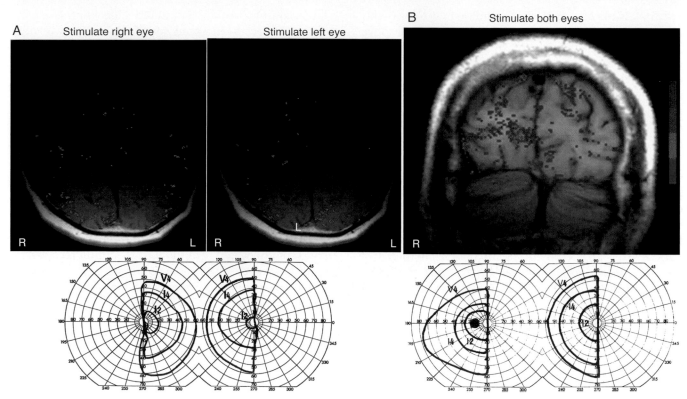

Figure 17-34 Visual field deficits demonstrated by functional magnetic resonance imaging and visual field mapping. In both cases, areas of intact vision were outlined three times, using progressively brighter or larger stimuli (V4 is 256 times larger than I4; I4 is 10 times brighter than I2). **A,** A 46-year-old man with a history of pulmonary tuberculosis developed a sellar tuberculoma that compressed his optic chiasm, resulting in bitemporal hemianopia. Monocular visual stimulation activated only the ipsilateral visual cortex because of damage to crossing fibers in the optic chiasm. **B,** A 58-year-old man had a stroke involving his left optic radiation, resulting in right homonymous hemianopia. Even though visual cortex appeared structurally normal bilaterally, visual stimulation of both eyes activated only his right visual cortex. (**A,** from Miki A et al: Am J Ophthalmol 122:404, 1996. **B,** from Miki A et al: Am J Ophthalmol 121:258, 1996.)

its brachium) and end in a pattern that coincides with the retinotopic map in the colliculus.

In addition to visual inputs, the superior colliculus receives (1) somatosensory inputs (sometimes referred to as the **spinotectal** or **spinomesencephalic tract**), many of them collaterals of fibers in somatosensory pathways ascending to the thalamus; (2) auditory inputs, chiefly by way of projections from the inferior colliculus; and (3) additional inputs from other areas of the cortex.

Efferent connections of the superior colliculus include projections to the reticular formation, the inferior colliculus, and the cervical spinal cord (the **tectospinal tract**). Of interest with respect to the visual system, the superior colliculus also projects to the posterior thalamus, notably to the lateral geniculate nucleus and the pulvinar. The pulvinar, in turn, projects to cortical areas 18 and 19, areas of visual association cortex.

The function of the human superior colliculus is not well understood. It is presumed to play a role in certain reflexes, such as orienting the head to visual (or other) stimuli, and in certain kinds of eye movements. However, no known clinical condition in humans can

be attributed specifically to damage to the superior colliculus. In contrast, after careful training, monkeys have been shown to have considerable visual capacity after extensive lesions of the striate cortex, particularly when dealing with moving stimuli. In a few rare cases of selective damage to the striate cortex, humans too have been found to have residual visual capacities that are strange and paradoxical: for example, despite having no conscious awareness of visual stimuli in the "blind" portions of their visual fields, they may be able to point to such stimuli quite accurately. There are a number of anatomical possibilities to account for this residual visual capacity; an example is the pathway to areas 18 and 19 via the superior colliculus and pulvinar. The relative importance of the various pathways is not known at present, just as the function of these pathways in the intact nervous system is not understood.

Photic input is involved in many neuroendocrine functions, so one might expect there to be a projection from the retina to the hypothalamus. This is in fact a standard feature of mammalian brains, originating from a small population of peculiar ganglion cells that are directly photosensitive[k] and ending in the **suprachiasmatic nucleus,** a small hypothalamic nucleus above the optic chiasm (see Fig. 23-4). Many of our physical functions wax and wane with a 24-hour rhythm (**circadian rhythm,** from the Latin words *circa* and *diem,* meaning "about a day"). For example, our body temperature rises and falls about a degree, being highest late in the afternoon and lowest early in the morning, when we are normally asleep. Many other circadian rhythms exist, involving such things as hormone secretion, eating, drinking, alertness, and excretion of various electrolytes. If no information about day length is available (as in the case of an animal living in constant light or constant darkness), the periods of these rhythms become a little longer than 24 hours. This implies that one or more "clocks" exist within our bodies and that, left to their own devices, these clocks are based on a period of slightly more than 24 hours; under normal circumstances, information about day length **entrains** these clocks to a period of 24 hours (see Fig. 23-5). The suprachiasmatic nucleus of the hypothalamus is the "master clock" for the timing of most (but not all) circadian rhythms; direct retinal input to the suprachiasmatic nucleus provides information for entraining these rhythms to a 24-hour cycle.

Primary Visual Cortex Sorts Visual Information and Distributes It to Other Cortical Areas

Receptive fields of cells in the lateral geniculate nucleus are generally similar to those of ganglion cells, as expected from the role of the thalamus as a gateway rather than a signal-processing center. The contrast detection mechanism is somewhat more efficient, so that uniform illumination causes less response than in the case of ganglion cells, but the basic center-surround organization is unchanged. Things do change, though, in striate cortex, where incoming visual information is dissected into its component elements (e.g., orientation, color, depth, motion) and distributed to a multitude of specialized extrastriate areas for further processing. This simultaneous, parallel processing in multiple cortical areas is a common strategy in the CNS and is thought to contribute to the speed of things such as visual perception, which is extraordinary. We can, for example, analyze a large, complex visual scene and decide whether it contains an object from some specified category in only 150 msec. This is much faster than would be expected if every element of the scene had to be analyzed sequentially by our relatively slow neurons.

Visual Cortex Has a Columnar Organization

Striate cortex is an array of repeated, modular collections of neurons occupying the cortex under each square millimeter of cortical surface. (Most or all neocortical areas, as described in Chapter 22, have a related modular organization.) Each module is an assembly of smaller columns in which most or all of the neurons have similar physiological properties (Fig. 17-35). For example, all the neurons in one column might respond best to stimuli received by the ipsilateral eye with similar contrast properties and in overlapping parts of the visual field. Neurons in an adjacent column might have the same properties except for a preference for stimuli received by the contralateral eye. Collectively, the columns making up one module analyze all aspects of the visual information arriving from discrete areas of the visual field. Modules in the foveal part of the retinotopic map analyze very small areas; modules in the peripheral part analyze areas hundreds of times larger. This means that many more modules are required for the foveal part of the field, largely accounting for its size in the retinotopic map (see Fig. 17-29).

The receptive fields of contrast-sensitive cortical neurons are more complicated than those of ganglion cells or lateral geniculate neurons, and names such as "simple," "complex," and "hypercomplex" have been coined to describe them. Simple cells respond best either to a dark bar on a light background or to a light bar on a dark background; uniform illumination has essentially no effect. In addition, the bar must be oriented at a particular angle. It has been hypothesized that the receptive fields of simple cells result from the convergence of a large number of geniculate axons onto a single cortical neuron; if the receptive fields of these axons fell along a straight line, a bar-shaped receptive field with flanking antagonistic areas could result. Complex and hypercomplex cells respond best to edges, bars, and corners with particular orientation and movement properties. Many of their properties, like those of the simple cells, can be explained by the convergence of simpler neurons onto a single cell.

Visual Information Is Distributed in Dorsal and Ventral Streams

This account of visual processing is obviously highly simplified. It is also selective, in that data dealing with color vision and binocular interactions have not been discussed. It is known, for example, that many cells in the primate visual system have wavelength-specific properties and that certain cortical neurons are sensitive

---

[k]These directly photosensitive ganglion cells use an unusual photopigment related to invertebrate pigments. Even though they can generate signals about light intensity all by themselves, they also receive inputs from rods and cones via bipolar and amacrine cells. The relative roles of the direct photosensitivity and the more usual retinal circuitry are not yet understood; the direct photosensitivity of these ganglion cells is activated only by bright light, and the rod-cone input may increase the range of intensities over which they operate. However, mutant mice with no rods or cones have essentially normal circadian rhythms.

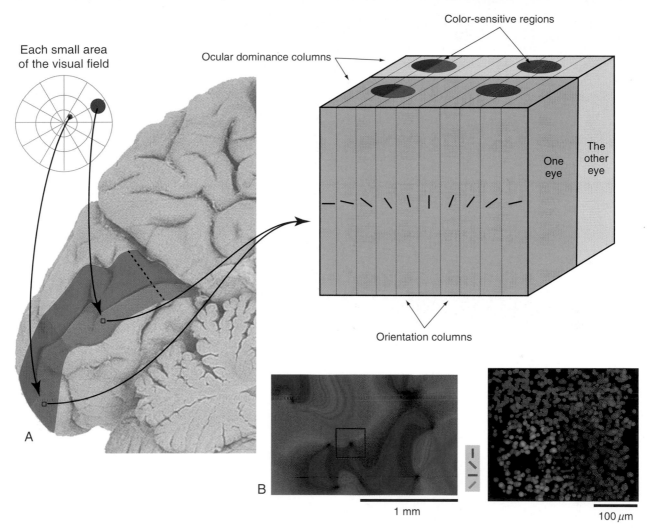

Figure 17-35 Organization of primary visual cortex. **A,** Area 17 is made up of a series of modules, each accounting for about 1 mm² of cortical surface area. Each module receives information from one area of the contralateral visual field—a very small area for foveal parts of the field, and a larger area for peripheral parts. As indicated in the schematic illustration on the right, modules are composed of small columns, portrayed here as slabs to keep things simple, in which the neurons throughout most of the depth of the cortex respond best to stimuli with a specific orientation and conveyed from one eye or the other. Collectively, the small slabs (orientation columns) cover all possible orientations. The half of the slabs in one module that prefer input from one eye constitute an ocular dominance column. Interspersed among the orientation columns are cylindrical assemblies of cells that are sensitive not to the orientation of a stimulus but rather to its spectral properties. **B,** Columns within a module are not actually oblong slabs. Orientation columns, shown here, are actually more like a pinwheel array of wedges. The image on the left is a view toward the surface of a cat's visual cortex. Optical imaging techniques were used to determine which small cortical areas were active in response to lines of different orientations, and active areas were color-coded according to the orientation key (e.g., neurons in green areas responded most to horizontal lines). The higher resolution image on the right shows how precise the arrangement is, extending all the way to the center of the pinwheel. In this study, the activity of individual neurons at multiple depths in the cortex was recorded using a Ca²⁺-sensitive fluorescent dye; each dot represents a single neuron, and the color coding is the same as in the image to the left. Other parts of the diagram in **A** were also simplified. For example, the color-sensitive regions do not extend through the entire thickness of the cortex. In addition, other properties such as motion and depth are mapped in a systematically distributed way in each module. **C** to **E,** Direct demonstration of ocular dominance columns in monkey visual cortex.

Continued

to the location of an object in three-dimensional space as well as to its size and shape. Aspects such as color and depth are processed in parallel with form and movement. These various qualities begin to be sorted out in the division of the lateral geniculate into parvocellular and magnocellular layers. The sorting continues as a partially separate, partially interconnected sequence of projections of the parvocellular and magnocellular systems through striate and extrastriate cortex. Although the details are incompletely understood, and the

independence of the two systems is far from total, the parvocellular system (color, detailed form) generally projects to more ventral portions of extrastriate cortex, and the magnocellular system (location, movement) projects to more dorsal portions (Fig. 17-36). One consequence is that damage to particular regions of extrastriate cortex can cause selective deficits in only some visual capabilities, such as the ability to distinguish colors, motion, or even something as specific as the identity of faces (Box 17-2; Figs. 17-37 and 17-38).

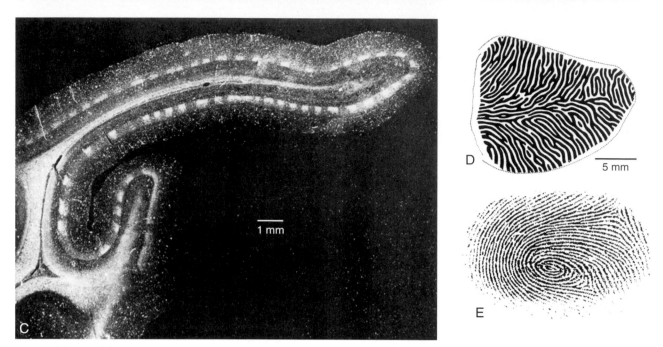

Figure 17-35, cont'd C, Autoradiograph of a section through the visual cortex of a monkey whose ipsilateral eye had been injected with a radioactive amino acid 2 weeks before sectioning. The amino acid was taken up by the ganglion cells of that eye, transported to the lateral geniculate nucleus (presumably after being incorporated into proteins), taken up by geniculate cells, and then transported to the visual cortex. Ocular dominance columns for the injected eye show up as light areas in layer IV (where the optic radiation terminates) in this autoradiograph seen with darkfield optics; the interspersed dark areas are ocular dominance columns for the contralateral eye. **D,** Reconstruction of the ocular dominance columns (seen as though one were looking down on the cortical surface) shows that the columns are really more or less parallel slabs. **E,** Fingerprint of a human index finger to the same scale as **D.** *(Diagram in **A,** based on Livingstone MS, Hubel DH: J Neurosci 4:309, 1984. **B,** adapted from Ohki K et al: Nature 442:925, 2006. **C** to **E,** from Hubel DH, Wiesel TN: Proc R Soc Lond B 198:1, 1977.)*

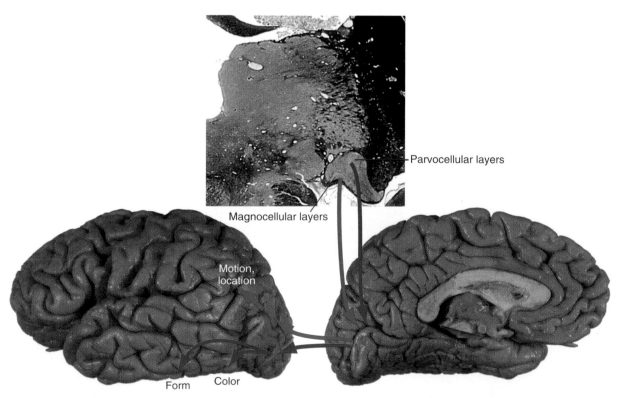

Figure 17-36 Schematic indication of the distribution of higher-order visual processing among different cortical areas. The actual distribution system is far more complex than illustrated here; for example, dozens of separate visual areas, related to one another by hundreds of sets of interconnections, have been described in primate cortex. However, in a very general sense, there is a dorsal stream of connections (dominated by the magnocellular system) concerned with the location and motion of objects and a ventral stream of connections (dominated by the parvocellular system) concerned with the form and color of objects.

BOX 17-2

Selective Loss of Some Visual Capabilities

Damage in posterior parts of the brain commonly affects either the optic radiation or striate cortex, affecting all function in parts of the visual field (see Fig. 17-33). In a few rare cases, however, patients have incurred bilateral damage to particular regions of extrastriate cortex, sparing primary visual cortex. Their visual fields were more or less intact, but they had selective visual deficits that illustrate strikingly the functional specialization of different parts of extrastriate cortex. Two such cases are reviewed here.

Motion Blindness

As a result of a superior sagittal sinus thrombosis, a 43-year-old woman suffered bilateral infarcts of lateral parts of the parietal, occipital, and posterior temporal lobes, including the area shown in Figure 17-37. Visual fields, color vision, depth perception, and reading were unaffected. Her ability to perceive moving sound sources or somatosensory stimuli moving across her skin was also unaffected, but she complained of a persisting deficit in perceiving visual motion:

She had difficulty, for example, in pouring tea or coffee into a cup because the fluid appeared to be frozen, like a glacier. In addition, she could not stop pouring at the right time since she was unable to perceive the movement in the cup (or a pot) when the fluid rose. Furthermore the patient complained of difficulties in following a dialogue because she could not see the movements of the face and, especially, the mouth of the speaker. In a room where more than two other people were walking she felt very insecure and unwell, and usually left the room immediately, because "people were suddenly here or there but I have not seen them moving." The patient experienced the same problem but to an even more marked extent in crowded streets or places, which she therefore avoided as much as possible. She could not cross the street because of her inability to judge the speed of a car, but she could identify the car itself without difficulty. "When I'm looking at the car first, it seems far away. But then, when I want to cross the road, suddenly the car is very near." She gradually learned to "estimate" the distance of moving vehicles by means of the sound becoming louder.*

Color Blindness and Prosopagnosia

A 51-year-old man experienced the abrupt onset of headache and confusion one evening. He did not lose consciousness but subsequently remembered nothing that occurred during the next 12 hours. He was taken home and helped to bed, and when he awoke the next morning he became aware of several visual deficits. He had bilateral loss of parts of his foveal visual fields above the horizontal meridian and an incomplete left superior homonymous quadrantanopia (see Fig. 17-38A). He also had some difficulty recognizing where he was if only using vision, but his most striking deficits were an inability to recognize colors (achromatopsia) or faces (prosopagnosia). The patient described these problems 6 months later:

Everything appears in various shades of grey. My shirts all look dirty and I can't tell one of them from the other. I have no idea which tie to wear. … I have difficulty in recognizing certain kinds of food on my plate, until I have tasted or smelled them. I can tell peas or bananas by their size and shape. An omelet, however, looks like a piece of meat and when I open a jar I never know if I'll find jam or pickles in it! … [When trying to identify faces] I can see the eyes, nose, and mouth quite clearly but they just don't add up. They all seem chalked in, like on a blackboard. I have to tell by the clothes or voice whether it is a man or woman, as the faces are all neutral. … The hair may help a lot, or if there is a moustache. … I cannot recognize people in photographs, not even myself. At the club I saw someone strange staring at me and asked the steward who it was. You'll laugh at me. I'd been looking at myself in a mirror. … I later went to London and visited several cinemas and theatres. I couldn't make head or tail of the plots. I never knew who was who.†

He also had trouble distinguishing different animals, especially in photographs, although not as much difficulty as he had with faces. He was nevertheless able to identify common objects with ease (as long as color was not a major factor), and his form, motion, and depth perception were preserved. An angiogram indicated partial occlusion of the right posterior cerebral artery. This presumably resulted in damage to visual cortex below the right calcarine sulcus, accounting for the deficits in the left visual fields. However, the smaller deficits in the right visual field imply damage to inferior parts of the left occipital lobe as well. Subsequent similar cases with computed tomography or magnetic resonance imaging verification of the lesion sites make it likely that this patient had bilateral damage in the lingual and occipitotemporal gyri, including the extrastriate areas indicated in Figure 17-38B.

*From Zihl J, von Cramon D, Mai N: Brain 106:313, 1983.
†From Pallis CA: J Neurol Neurosurg Psychiatry 18:218, 1955.

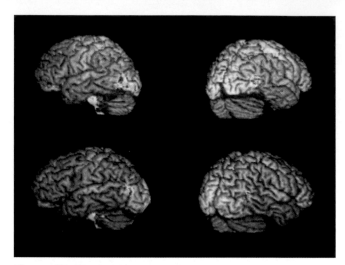

Figure 17-37 Combined positron emission tomography–magnetic resonance images demonstrating the cortical areas activated as subjects watched moving visual stimuli (versus stationary stimuli); each row of two images is from a different subject. *(From Watson JDG et al: Cereb Cortex 3:79, 1993.)*

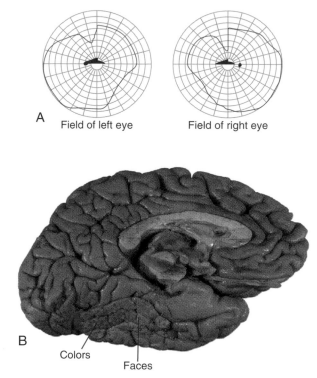

Figure 17-38 A case of achromatopsia and prosopagnosia. **A,** The patient's visual fields. Areas where vision was lost completely are black, and remaining intact parts of the visual fields are outlined. **B,** Cortical areas likely to have been damaged in this patient (in addition to inferior parts of striate cortex). *(**A,** redrawn from Pallis CA: J Neurol Neurosurg Psychiatry 18:218, 1955.)*

Early Experience Has Permanent Effects on the Visual System

The visual system provides a unique opportunity to study the extent to which connections within the CNS are genetically determined and unchangeable and the extent to which they can be influenced by the environment.

Recordings from neurons in the visual cortex of newborn cats and monkeys never previously exposed to light reveal that the basic properties of these neurons are similar to those of adults. This indicates that the wiring pattern of the visual system is, to a great extent, genetically determined and does not depend on visual input for its formation.

If, however, one eye of a newborn animal is covered for the first few months of its life, that eye will be permanently blind (in a perceptual sense) when uncovered (see Chapter 24). At the same time, cortical neurons respond only to stimulation of the eye that was not covered. This appears to be primarily the result of the replacement of "idle" synapses by connections that reflect activity in the noncovered eye.

This effect of covering an eye is specific to the first few months of life; no deficit results if it occurs later. Also, it is not simply a result of the eye not being exposed to light. If the eye is covered with translucent rather than opaque material so that the retina is exposed to light but not to patterns, the same functional blindness results. This is consistent with the fact that normal cortical neurons respond as poorly to diffuse illumination as they do to no illumination at all. This also corresponds to the finding that infantile cataracts (and even more

subtle defects) in humans can result in permanent blindness (called **amblyopia**), unless they are corrected at an early age.

Reflex Circuits Adjust the Size of the Pupil and the Focal Length of the Lens

Modern cameras have autoexposure and autofocus mechanisms; reflex connections beginning with the optic nerve take care of similar functions for the eye.

Illumination of Either Retina Causes Both Pupils to Constrict

Light directed into either eye causes both pupils to constrict. The response of the pupil of the illuminated eye is called the **direct pupillary light reflex,** whereas that of the other eye is called the **consensual pupillary light reflex.** The afferent limb of the reflex arc consists of optic tract axons, many of them from the same intrinsically photosensitive ganglion cells that project to the suprachiasmatic nucleus. These enter the brachium of the superior colliculus and terminate in the **pretectal area,** which is directly rostral to the superior colliculus at the junction between midbrain and diencephalon. Pretectal

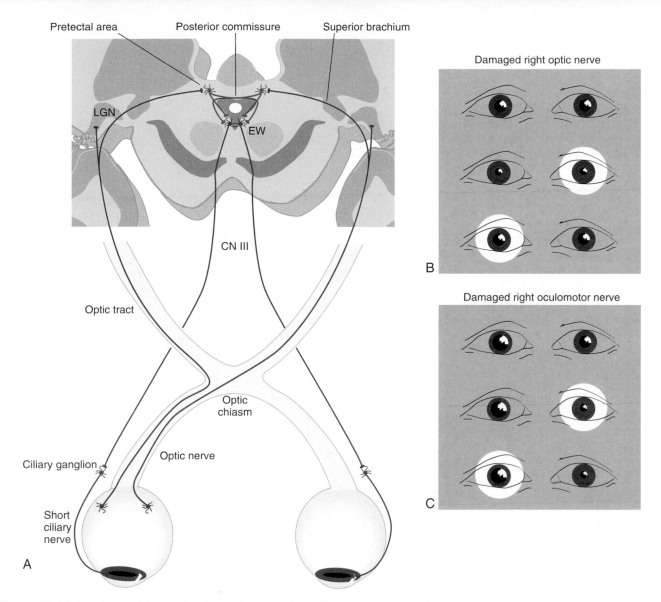

Figure 17-39 **A,** Pathway of the pupillary light reflex. **B** and **C,** Pupillary consequences of damage to one optic nerve or one oculomotor nerve, respectively. In each, the upper images show the relative sizes of pupils in the dark, and the middle and lower images show the expected responses to illumination of the left and right eyes, respectively. Note that when switching illumination from the left eye to the right eye in **B,** the right pupil dilates in a seemingly paradoxical fashion. This is the basis of the swinging flashlight test. (The right pupil in **C** is always dilated, and moving the illumination to the right eye causes no change.) CN III, oculomotor nerve; EW, Edinger-Westphal nucleus; LGN, lateral geniculate nucleus. *(**A,** modified from Nolte J: Elsevier's integrated neuroscience, Philadelphia, 2007, Mosby Elsevier.)*

neurons project bilaterally to the Edinger-Westphal nucleus, with fibers crossing through the posterior commissure (Fig. 17-39A). Preganglionic parasympathetic neurons in the Edinger-Westphal nucleus then project through the oculomotor nerve to the ciliary ganglion, where they synapse. Postganglionic fibers in the short ciliary nerves complete the reflex arc, synapsing on the smooth muscle cells of the pupillary sphincter.

Because one optic tract contains axons of ganglion cells in both eyes, and because each pretectal area projects bilaterally to the Edinger-Westphal nucleus, light directed into one eye causes the same amount of activity in the Edinger-Westphal nucleus on each side. This is the basis of the consensual light reflex. The result is that both pupils are ordinarily the same size, even if one eye is closed or only one eye is illuminated.

The pathways of the pupillary light reflex are utilized clinically in a procedure known as the **swinging flashlight test** for damage to one retina or optic nerve (see Fig. 17-39B). With the patient seated in a dimly lit room, a light source is quickly moved back and forth from one eye to the other while the examiner observes the behavior of each pupil in turn. For example, assume the right optic nerve is damaged. When the left eye is illuminated, both pupils will constrict. When the right eye is illuminated, the light reflex arc will be less effectively activated,

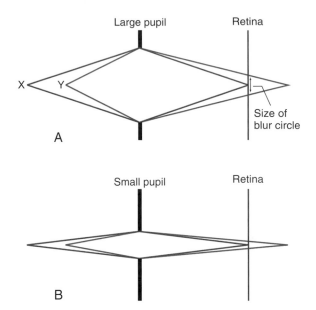

Figure 17-40 Effect of pupil size on depth of focus. **A,** When the eye is focused on objects at distance X and the pupil is large, the image of a point at distance Y will be out of focus and smeared out over a relatively large area. **B,** A smaller pupil results in a smaller blur circle for a point at distance Y; objects over a greater range of distances are now in acceptable focus.

and both pupils will dilate. Therefore, when the light is moved from the left eye to the right, the right pupil will dilate in a seemingly paradoxical fashion, indicating damage to the right retina or optic nerve.

Both Eyes Accommodate for Near Vision

When visual attention is directed to a nearby object, three things happen in a reflex manner: (1) **convergence** of the two eyes, so the image of the object falls on both foveae; (2) contraction of the ciliary muscle, a round muscle the encircles the lens, causing the lens to "round up" or thicken the lens (accommodation), so the image of the object is in focus on the retina; and (3) pupillary constriction, which improves the optical performance of the eye by reducing certain types of aberration and by increasing its depth of focus[1] (Fig. 17-40).

Unlike the pupillary light reflex, the **near reflex** or **accommodation reflex** requires the participation of cerebral cortex. The pathway involved is not completely understood, but at a minimum it includes the normal visual pathway to striate cortex, projections from there to visual association cortex, and from there to the superior colliculus or pretectal area or both (Fig. 17-41).

---

[1]Hence there are conflicting effects of pupillary constriction, which makes things more easily visible by improving the optical performance of the eye but less easily visible by reducing the amount of light reaching the retina. The CNS automatically figures out and implements the pupil size that is the best compromise for a given target distance and level of illumination.

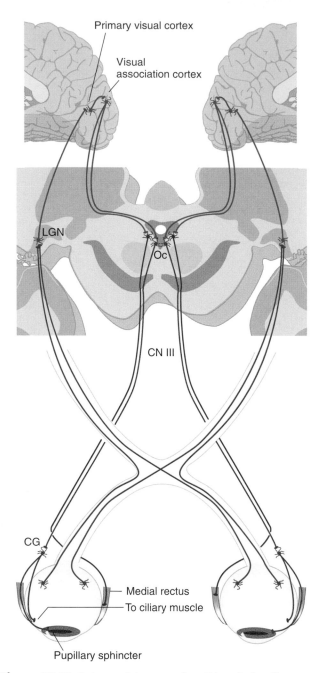

Figure 17-41 Pathway of the near reflex. Although the efferent projections from visual association cortex to the oculomotor nucleus are indicated as arising in the occipital lobe, the exact site of origin is not known with certainty. CG, ciliary ganglion; CN III, oculomotor nerve; LGN, lateral geniculate nucleus; Oc, oculomotor nucleus. *(Modified from Nolte J: Elsevier's integrated neuroscience, Philadelphia, 2007, Mosby Elsevier.)*

Impulses are then relayed to the oculomotor nucleus, stimulating medial rectus motor neurons and preganglionic parasympathetic neurons of the Edinger-Westphal nucleus. The cerebellum also plays a prominent role in the near reflex (see Chapter 21).

Although the same preganglionic parasympathetic fibers are thought to mediate the pupillary constriction of both the light reflex and the near reflex, these two types of constriction can nevertheless be dissociated in certain pathological conditions. An **Argyll Robertson pupil** refers to a condition (usually bilateral and a manifestation of neurosyphilis) in which the pupil constricts during the near reflex but not in response to light. The site of the lesion involved is not known with certainty, but it is often assumed to be in that portion of the pretectal area subserving the light reflex.

SUGGESTED READINGS

Albright TD, Desimone R, Gross CG: Columnar organization of directionally selective cells in visual area MT of the macaque. J Neurophysiol 51:16, 1984.

Bender MB, Bodis-Wollner I: Visual dysfunction in optic tract lesions. Ann Neurol 3:187, 1978.
  Clinical observations of nonidentical visual losses in the two eyes, or of selective deficits of only some visual functions, after optic tract damage.

Bouvier SE, Engel SA: Behavioral deficits and cortical damage loci in cerebral achromatopsia. Cereb Cortex 16:183, 2006.
  One example of the notion that the primary visual cortex and visual association cortex are not like a screen on which the retinal image is projected; rather, a number of different subareas deal selectively with different aspects of the visual world.

Büttner-Ennever JA, et al: Pretectal projections to the oculomotor complex of the monkey and their role in eye movements. J Comp Neurol 366:348, 1996.

Cadetti L, Thoreson WB: Feedback effects of horizontal cell membrane potential on cone calcium currents studied with simultaneous recordings. J Neurophysiol 95:1992, 2006.

Clarke S, Miklossy J: Occipital cortex in man: organization of callosal connections, related myelo- and cytoarchitecture, and putative boundaries of functional visual areas. J Comp Neurol 298:188, 1990.

Conway BR, et al: Neural basis for a powerful static motion illusion. J Neurosci 25:5651, 2005.
  A possible explanation for the Rotating Snakes illusion.

Curcio CA, et al: Human photoreceptor topography. J Comp Neurol 292:497, 1990.

Dougherty RF, et al: Visual field representations and locations of visual areas V1/2/3 in human visual cortex. J Vision 3:586, 2003.

Engles M, Wooten B, Hammond B: Macular pigment: a test of the acuity hypothesis. Invest Ophthalmol 48:2922, 2007.
  The standard hypothesis about the function of macular pigment is that it keeps blue light out of the fovea, reducing chromatic aberration. This may not be correct.

Franze K, et al: Müller cells are living optical fibers in the vertebrate retina. Proc Natl Acad Sci U S A 104:8287, 2007.
  A unique glial function that may partially compensate for our inverted retina.

Fu Y, Yau K-W: Phototransduction in mouse rods and cones. Pflugers Arch 454:805, 2007.

Gegenfurtner KR, Sharpe LT, editors: Color vision: from genes to perception, Cambridge, 1999, Cambridge University Press.

Gooley JJ, et al: Melanopsin in cells of origin of the retinohypothalamic tract. Nat Neurosci 4:1165, 2001.

Hankins MW, Peirson SN, Foster RG: Melanopsin: an exciting photopigment. Trends Neurosci 31:27, 2008.
  Melanopsin, the photopigment in a small percentage of retinal ganglion cells, is the basis of what is likely to be a fascinating evolutionary story.

Haxby JV, et al: Face encoding and recognition in the human brain. Proc Natl Acad Sci U S A 93:922, 1996.

Hofer H, Singer B, Williams DR: Different sensations from cones with the same photopigment. J Vision 5:444, 2005.

Holmes G: The organization of the visual cortex in man. Proc R Soc Lond B 132:348, 1945.

Horton JC, Hocking DR: An adult-like pattern of ocular dominance columns in striate cortex of newborn monkeys prior to visual experience. J Neurosci 16:1791, 1996.

Horton JC, Hoyt WF: The representation of the visual field in human striate cortex: a revision of the classic Holmes map. Arch Ophthalmol 109:816, 1991.

Hoyt WF, Luis O: The primate chiasm. Arch Ophthalmol 70:69, 1963.

Huang D, et al, editors: Retinal imaging, Philadelphia, 2006, Mosby Elsevier.

Hubel DH, Wiesel TN: Functional architecture of macaque monkey visual cortex. Proc R Soc Lond B 198:1, 1977.
  A detailed discussion of the elegant experiments on the primate visual system done by these two investigators over the previous 20 years.

Humphrey NK, Weiskrantz L: Vision in monkeys after removal of the striate cortex. Nature 215:595, 1967.

Ishikawa S, Sakiya H, Kondo Y: The center for controlling the near reflex in the midbrain of the monkey: a double labelling study. Brain Res 519:217, 1990.

Jampel RS: Representation of the near-response on the cerebral cortex of the macaque. Am J Ophthalmol 48:573, 1959.

Kalev-Landoy M, et al: Optical coherence tomography in anterior segment imaging. Acta Ophthalmol Scand 85:427, 2007.

Kanizsa G: Subjective contours. Sci Am 234:48, 1976.

Kedar S, et al: Congruency in homonymous hemianopia. Am J Ophthalmol 143:772, 2007.

Kupfer C: The projection of the macula in the lateral geniculate nucleus in man. Am J Ophthalmol 54:597, 1962.

Land MF, Nilsson D-E: Animal eyes, New York, 2002, Oxford University Press.
  A constantly fascinating account of all the different ways animals manage to see.

Leff A: A historical review of the representation of the visual field in primary visual cortex with special reference to the neural mechanisms underlying macular sparing. Brain Lang 88:268, 2004.

Livingstone M, Hubel D: Segregation of form, color, movement, and depth: anatomy, physiology, and perception. Science 240:740, 1988.
  An intriguing summary pointing out some striking correlations between the basic properties of visual system neurons and the way we perceive things visually.

Loewenfeld IE: The pupil: anatomy, physiology, and clinical applications, Boston, 1999, Butterworth-Heinemann.
  An encyclopedic review of the vast literature on pupils and irises.

Lotto RB, Purves D: The effects of color on brightness. Nat Neurosci 2:1010, 1999.
  An explanation of illusions like that shown in Fig. 17-22B.

Lotto RB, Purves D: An empirical explanation of color contrast. Proc Natl Acad Sci U S A 97:12834, 2000.
  An explanation of illusions like that shown in Fig. 17-22C.

Lucas RJ, Douglas RH, Foster RG: Characterization of an ocular photopigment capable of driving pupillary constriction in mice. Nat Neurosci 4:261, 2001.
  Mice with no rods or cones still have pupillary light reflexes.

Magoun HW, et al: The afferent path of the pupillary light reflex in the monkey. Brain 59:234, 1936.

Mills SL, Massey SC: Differential properties of two gap junctional pathways made by AII amacrine cells. Nature 377:734, 1995.
  A partial unraveling of the way rod signals piggyback on cone pathways at different light intensities.

Nordby K: Vision in a complete achromat: a personal account. In Hess RF, Sharpe LT, Nordby K, editors: Night vision: basic, clinical and applied aspects, Cambridge, 1990, Cambridge University Press.
  Rarely, someone is born with a complete absence of cones. As this personal description indicates, color blindness is only one of the consequences.

Ohki K, et al: Highly ordered arrangement of single neurons in orientation pinwheels. Nature 442:925, 2006.

Ott M: Visual accommodation in vertebrates: mechanisms, physiological response and stimuli. J Comp Physiol 192A:97, 2006.
Just about every conceivable mechanism is used by one animal or another.

Oyster CW: The human eye: structure and function, Sunderland, Mass, 1999, Sinauer Associates.
An extensive, well-written review of the retina, the rest of the eye, and its orbital surroundings.

Perry VH, Cowey A: Retinal ganglion cells that project to the superior colliculus and pretectum in the macaque monkey. Neuroscience 12:1125, 1984.

Pollack JG, Hickey TL: The distribution of retinocollicular axon terminals in rhesus monkey. J Comp Neurol 185:587, 1979.

Puce A, et al: Face-sensitive regions in human extrastriate cortex studied by functional MRI. J Neurophysiol 74:1192, 1995.

Purves D, Shimpi A, Lotto RB: An empirical explanation of the Cornsweet effect. J Neurosci 19:8542, 1999.
An explanation of illusions like that shown in Fig. 17-22A.

Ramachandran VS: Blind spots. Sci Am 266:86, 1992.
Games you can play with your blind spot.

Rao-Mirotznik R, et al: Mammalian rod terminal: architecture of a binary synapse. Neuron 14:561, 1995.
An interesting review of the synaptic specializations involved in passing along information about the absorption of single photons.

Reese BE, Cowey A: Fibre organization of the monkey optic tract. I. Segregation of functionally distinct optic axons. II. Noncongruent representation of the two half-retinae. J Comp Neurol 295:385 and 401, 1990.

Richter HO, et al: Functional neuroanatomy of the human near/far response to blur cues: eye-lens accommodation/vergence to point targets varying in depth. Eur J Neurosci 20:2722, 2004.

Rodieck RW, Watanabe M: Survey of the morphology of macaque retinal ganglion cells that project to the pretectum, superior colliculus, and parvicellular laminae of the lateral geniculate nucleus. J Comp Neurol 338:289, 1993.

Rohen JW: Scanning electron microscopic studies of the zonular apparatus in human and monkey eyes. Invest Ophthalmol 18:133, 1979.

Schiller PH, Sandell JH, Maunsell JHR: Functions of the ON and OFF channels of the visual system. Nature 322:824, 1986.

Schneider GE: Two visual systems. Science 163:895, 1969.
Differential effects of collicular and cortical damage on a hamster's visual capabilities.

Sherman SM, Koch C: The control of retinogeniculate transmission in the mammalian lateral geniculate nucleus. Exp Brain Res 63:1, 1986.
The lateral geniculate has an important role in regulating the access of visual information to the cerebral cortex.

Solomon SG, Lennie P: The machinery of colour vision. Nat Rev Neurosci 8:276, 2007.

Stein J, Walsh V: To see but not to read; the magnocellular theory of dyslexia. Trends Neurosci 20:147, 1997.
A review of the evidence that an abnormality in the visual channel specialized for the analysis of rapidly changing stimuli might underlie dyslexia.

Strauss O: The retinal pigment epithelium in visual function. Physiol Rev 85:845, 2005.

Tanaka K: Inferotemporal cortex and object vision. Annu Rev Neurosci 16:109, 1996.

Tassinari G, et al: Magno- and parvocellular pathways are segregated in the human optic tract. Neuroreport 5:1425, 1994.

Thorpe S, Fize D, Marlot C: Speed of processing in the human visual system. Nature 381:520, 1996.
Clever experiments showing how quickly we can extract significant features from complex visual scenes.

Tucker VA: The deep fovea, sideways vision and spiral flight paths in raptors. J Exp Biol 203:3745, 2000.
An intriguing look at the retinal and behavioral specializations used by hawks and eagles to spot prey from great distances and keep it in sight while diving after it.

Völgyi B, et al: Convergence and segregation of the multiple rod pathways in mammalian retina. J Neurosci 24:11182, 2004.

Walls GL: The vertebrate eye and its adaptive radiation, New York, 1967, Hafner Publishing Company.
A monumental, engrossing book describing the myriad variations in every part of the eye that adapt different species to their environments.

Wässle H, Boycott BB: Functional architecture of the mammalian retina. Physiol Rev 71:447, 1991.

Wässle H, et al: The rod pathway of the macaque monkey retina: identification of AII-amacrine cells with antibodies against calretinin. J Comp Neurol 361:537, 1995.

Weiskrantz L, et al: Visual capacity in the hemianopic field following a restricted cortical ablation. Brain 97:709, 1974.
Remarkable account of the visual capabilities remaining in one individual after known selective damage to his striate cortex.

Wilson JR: Circuitry of the dorsal lateral geniculate nucleus in the cat and monkey. Anat Embryol 147:1, 1993.

Wilson ME, Cragg BG: Projections from the lateral geniculate nucleus in the cat and monkey. J Anat 101:677, 1967.

Wong AMF, Sharpe JA: Representation of the visual field in the human occipital cortex: a magnetic resonance imaging and perimetric correlation. Arch Ophthalmol 117:208, 1999.

Wong KY, et al: Synaptic influences on rat ganglion-cell photoreceptors. J Physiol 582:279, 2007.

Wong-Riley MTT: Connections between the pulvinar nucleus and the prestriate cortex in the squirrel monkey as revealed by peroxidase histochemistry and autoradiography. Brain Res 134:249, 1977.

Zee PC, Manthena P: The brain's master circadian clock: implications and opportunities for therapy of sleep disorders. Sleep Med Rev 11:59, 2007.

Zeki S: A vision of the brain, London, 1993, Blackwell.
A well-written overview of central visual processing, with an emphasis on the history of ideas, clinical observations, and experiments regarding the localization of different aspects of visual function.

Zihl J, von Cramon D, Mai N: Selective disturbance of movement vision after bilateral brain damage. Brain 106:313, 1983.
Another example of the apparent parceling of visual cortical areas into regions dealing with particular aspects of a visual stimulus.

Overview of Motor Systems

Each of us has fewer than a million motor neurons with which to control muscles. Without them, we would be completely unable to interact with the outside world. With them, however, we are capable of an enormous range of complex activities, from automatic and semiautomatic movements such as postural adjustments to the characteristically human movements involved in speaking and writing. The way in which a wide variety of neural structures interact to make these activities possible is the topic of Chapters 18 to 20.

Each Lower Motor Neuron Innervates a Group of Muscle Fibers, Forming a Motor Unit

Lower motor neurons, the target of central nervous system (CNS) pathways and connections involved in motor control, are arranged in the spinal cord and brainstem in groups corresponding to individual muscles (see Fig. 10-10). The axons of lower motor neurons leave the CNS in anterior roots (or in motor roots of cranial nerves) and divide into terminal branches widely distributed in their target muscles. Each branch ends at the single neuromuscular junction of a muscle fiber (see Figs. 8-1 and 8-11). The combination of one motor neuron and all the muscle fibers it innervates is referred to as a **motor unit.** Motor units vary tremendously in size, in a way that makes functional sense: the size of the motor units in a given muscle is related to the degree of fine control involved in the use of that muscle. As examples, there may be only 2 or 3 muscle fibers in a motor unit in the stapedius, 10 in an extraocular muscle, 100 in a hand muscle, and 1000 in a large antigravity muscle such as the gastrocnemius (Fig. 18-1). Even within a single muscle, however, motor units vary in size and functional properties, as described shortly.

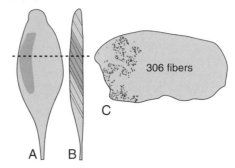

Figure 18-1 The muscle fibers of a single motor unit (type FR) in cat gastrocnemius. The general location of the group of fibers is indicated by shading on a drawing of the whole muscle **(A)** and a longitudinal section through the muscle **(B)**. On a cross section of the muscle **(C)**, each muscle fiber in the motor unit is indicated by a dot. *(Redrawn from Burke RE, Tsairis P: J Physiol 234:749, 1973.)*

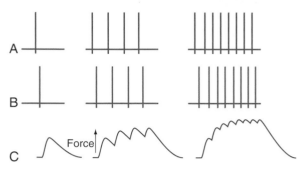

Figure 18-3 Relationships between action potentials in lower motor neurons **(A)**, action potentials in a postjunctional muscle fiber **(B)**, and force production by the muscle fiber **(C)**. *(Modified from Nolte J: Elsevier's integrated neuroscience, Philadelphia, 2007, Mosby Elsevier.)*

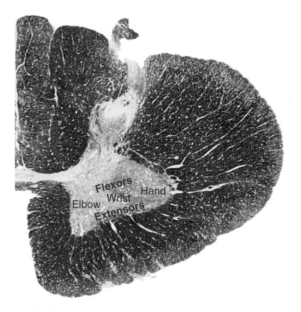

Figure 18-2 Somatotopic arrangement of motor neurons at C8. The large number of motor neurons for distal muscles accounts for the lateral expansion of the anterior horn at this level.

Lower Motor Neurons Are Arranged Systematically

Just as there are systematic maps in sensory pathways (see Fig. 10-22) and in cortical areas (see Figs. 3-30 and 17-29), so too is there a systematic arrangement of clusters of motor neurons. In the anterior horn of the spinal cord, for example, motor neurons for axial muscles are located medial to those for more distal muscles, and those for flexors are posterior to those for extensors (Fig. 18-2). This axial-distal mapping corresponds to the arrangement of descending pathways, some of which are important for postural adjustments of axial muscles, and others for the control of more distal musculature (see Fig. 18-8).

There Are Three Kinds of Muscle Fibers and Three Kinds of Motor Units

Invertebrates have both excitatory and inhibitory motor neurons, but in vertebrates, all lower motor neurons release acetylcholine onto nicotinic receptors of skeletal muscle. A single action potential in the axon of a lower motor neuron causes the release of acetylcholine at hundreds of active zones, resulting in a single action potential in the postjunctional muscle fiber (see Fig. 8-10). This in turn causes a twitch of the muscle fiber. Hence force production by vertebrate muscle fibers is related to the rate of firing of lower motor neurons: successive twitches sum temporally, much the way excitatory postsynaptic potentials do (Fig. 18-3).

Most muscles are called on to contract for different purposes. The gastrocnemius, for example, must contract weakly but for long periods when we stand upright, more strongly while running (which most of us cannot do for nearly as long as we can stand), and very strongly but very briefly during a jump. Corresponding to these requirements, there are three kinds of skeletal muscle fibers (Fig. 18-4), each populating one of three different types of motor unit (Fig. 18-5). **Red fibers (type I)** are thin, contain abundant mitochondria, and contract weakly and slowly but are able to sustain contractions for long periods. **White fibers (types IIa and IIb)** are larger, contain relatively few mitochondria, and contract in briefer, more powerful twitches. Type IIb fibers use glycolysis almost exclusively to fuel their contractions and fatigue very rapidly; type IIa fibers use a combination of oxidative metabolism and glycolysis and fatigue at intermediate rates. Most muscles contain all three fiber types randomly intermingled with one another, but in proportions that vary depending on the principal function of a given muscle.[a]

---

[a]In domestic fowl, for example, that do a lot of standing and running but little flying, dark meat is muscle with many red fibers, and white meat is muscle with many white fibers. The flight muscles of migratory birds, in contrast, are mostly dark meat.

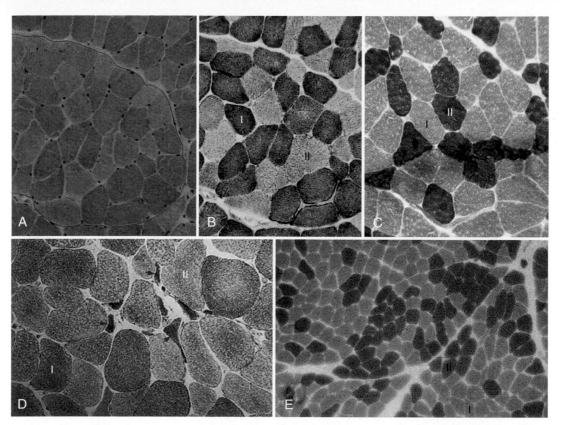

Figure 18-4 Demonstration of fiber types in cross sections of human skeletal muscle biopsies, and some characteristic changes that accompany neuropathology. **A,** Muscle fibers, each with nuclei (small red dots) at their periphery, are grouped into fascicles (Gomori trichrome stain); part of one fascicle is outlined. **B,** Staining for an oxidative enzyme (NADH dehydrogenase) found in mitochondria and the sarcoplasmic reticulum differentiates type I (I) and type II (II) fibers, which are more or less randomly interspersed with one another. **C,** Staining for myofibrillar ATPase (pH 9.4) also differentiates type I (I) and type II (II) fibers. **D,** Denervated muscle fibers atrophy, becoming small and angular in cross section *(arrows)*. **E,** Following partial loss of a muscle's lower motor neuron inputs, the remaining motor neurons sprout new endings that reinnervate nearby muscle fibers. Each reinnervated muscle fiber assumes the physiological properties of the other fibers in its newfound motor unit, with the result that fiber types become grouped rather than being interspersed. Here such fiber type grouping is shown at low magnification with an ATPase stain (pH 9.4). *(Courtesy Dr. Steven Ringel and Shelley Reed, University of Colorado Health Sciences Center.)*

All the muscle fibers in a motor unit are of a single type, with the result that there are three types of motor units (see Fig. 18-5). The smallest lower motor neurons innervate type I fibers, the largest innervate type IIb fibers, and motor neurons of intermediate size innervate type IIa fibers. The properties of each motor unit type can be predicted from the properties of the muscle fibers: type **S** (*slow-twitch*) motor units produce small amounts of force for prolonged periods, type **FF** (*fast-twitch, fatigable*) units produce large amounts of force for brief periods, and type **FR** (*fast-twitch, fatigue-resistant*) produce moderate amounts of force that can be sustained for moderate amounts of time (see Fig. 18-5).

Motor Units Are Recruited in Order of Size

The association of different muscle fiber types with motor neurons of different sizes is the basis of an elegantly simple mechanism for grading the force of muscle contraction. If two neurons have the same density of channels in their surface membranes, the smaller of the two neurons will have fewer total channels and a greater resistance to transmembrane current flow. Hence a given amount of synaptic current will cause a greater membrane potential change in the smaller neuron, making the smaller neuron more easily excitable. As the synaptic drive reaching the anterior horn increases, motor neurons reach threshold in order of increasing size (the **size principle**). S units are recruited first, and as they fire faster and faster, FR units are added. As the FR units increase their firing rate, FF units are added. This sequence is required to smoothly increase the force of muscle contraction, beginning with small increases from the background level of tone and ending with brief maximal contractions (Fig. 18-6). The elegant part is that it happens automatically, in all movements, simply by virtue of the increasing size of the motor neurons in the three types of motor unit.

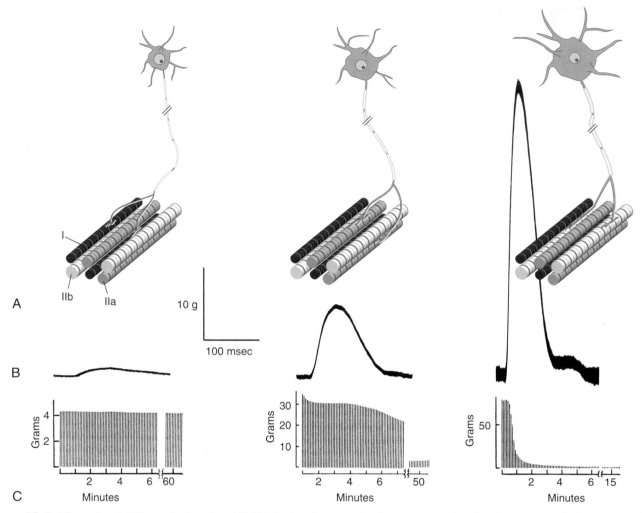

Figure 18-5 S (first column), FR (second column), and FF (third column) motor units of cat gastrocnemius, showing the anatomical components **(A)**, twitch response to a single stimulus **(B)**, and responses to intermittent bursts of action potentials **(C)** for each. The same time and force scale applies to all three twitches in **B**. (*B and C, modified from Burke RE et al: J Physiol 234:723, 1973.*)

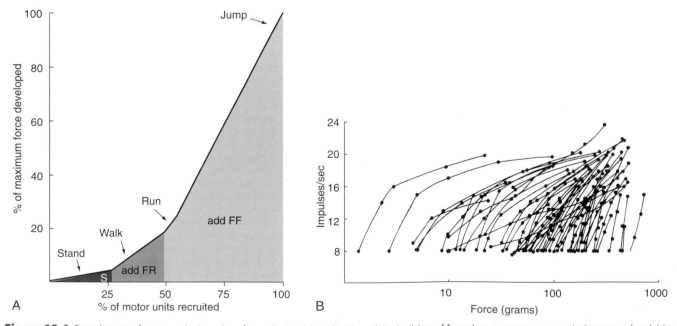

Figure 18-6 Recruitment of motor units in order of size. **A,** Graphic indication of the buildup of force in cat gastrocnemius during normal activities as motor units are recruited in order of size. **B,** Firing rates of 60 motor units in a human forearm muscle (extensor digitorum) during isometric contraction of increasing force; each line represents a single motor unit. Force production increases by individual units firing more rapidly and, simultaneously, by additional units being recruited. Note that the force scale is logarithmic, and later-recruited units provide greater increments of force. (*A, modified from Walmsley B, Hodgson JA, Burke RE: J Neurophysiol 41:1203, 1978. B, from Monster AW, Chan H: J Neurophysiol 40:1432, 1977.*)

Motor Control Systems Involve Both Hierarchical and Parallel Connections

The inputs that determine the level of activity of lower motor neurons can be divided very broadly into three overlapping classes (Fig. 18-7):

1. Built-in patterns of neural connections.
2. Descending pathways that modulate the activity of motor neurons; these effects may be either direct or indirect, by way of influences on built-in neural subsystems. Collectively, the neurons that give rise to these descending pathways are **upper motor neurons.**
3. Higher centers that influence the activity of descending pathways.

Damage to either upper or lower motor neurons (or muscle) causes weakness and a distinctive set of accompanying symptoms and signs. Damage to higher centers also causes distinctive movement abnormalities (e.g., involuntary movements, incoordination, difficulty initiating movement), but is not accompanied by substantial weakness.

Reflex and Motor Program Connections Provide Some of the Inputs to Lower Motor Neurons

The stretch reflex is an obvious and simple example of a built-in pattern of neural connections that controls, to some extent, the activity of motor neurons. Stretching a muscle stimulates its muscle spindles, whose afferent

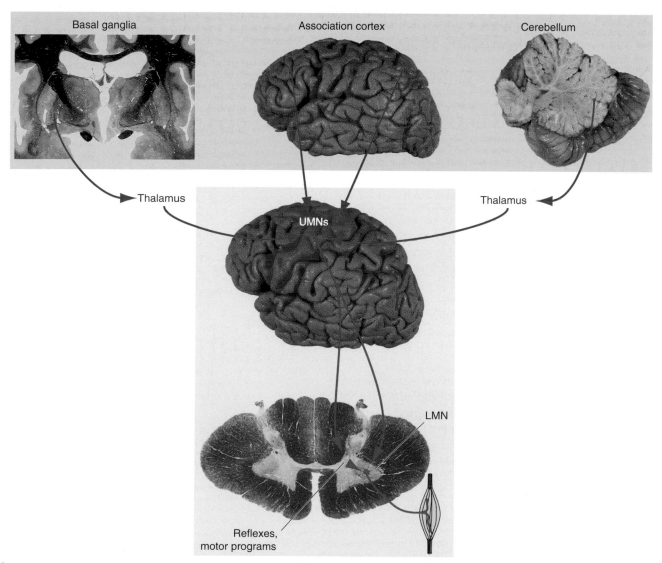

Figure 18-7 Major components and schematic connections involved in motor control. The cerebellum and basal ganglia participate in motor control primarily by influencing the output from cerebral cortex to the brainstem and spinal cord. (These connections are discussed in greater detail in Chapters 19 and 20.) Each also has additional outputs to brainstem nuclei (relatively minor for the basal nuclei, more substantial for the cerebellum). The association cortex, basal nuclei, and cerebellum play vital roles in the choice, design, and monitoring of movement but have no direct effect on lower motor neurons (LMN). For this reason, damage to structures in the lower box but not the upper box causes movement disorders in which weakness is prominent. (As indicated in Fig. 18-8, not all upper motor neurons [UMNs] live in the cerebral cortex.)

fibers end on motor neurons, which in turn causes the muscle to contract (see Fig. 10-11). Other reflexes, such as the flexor reflex (see Figs. 10-13 and 10-15), are more complex and involve a number of muscles and spinal segments. Finally, there are networks of interneurons in the brainstem and spinal cord that can act as pattern generators for rhythmic movements such as breathing and walking. Although some of the same interneurons involved in reflexes may also be part of the circuitry of these motor programs or **central pattern generators**, these programs are more than simply a stringing together of reflexes, each one triggering the next. One indication of this is the observation that the principal features of central pattern generators can persist in the absence of afferent input. As an extreme example, the spinal cord of a lamprey (a primitive, jawless fish) can be kept alive in a dish for several days. Such a spinal cord, completely isolated from the rest of the lamprey, can exhibit in its anterior roots oscillating bursts of action potentials that in an intact animal would produce rhythmic, coordinated swimming movements. Upper motor neurons and higher centers harness the basic elements of these central pattern generators and adapt them as necessary— for example, modifying a stepping cycle to avoid an obstacle.

Upper Motor Neurons Control Lower Motor Neurons Both Directly and Indirectly

Upper motor neurons, whose axons descend to the spinal cord (and to cranial nerve motor nuclei) to affect the activity of lower motor neurons, are located in both the cerebral cortex and the brainstem. The descending pathways involved, most of which have already been mentioned, are summarized in Figure 18-8. The **vestibulospinal tracts** (see Fig. 14-29) are important mediators of postural adjustments and head movements. The **corticospinal tract** (see Fig. 10-24) has traditionally been considered the principal mediator of voluntary movement, although, as discussed in this chapter, its real role is currently not entirely clear. The **reticulospinal tracts** (see Fig. 11-19) and, to a lesser extent, the **rubrospinal tract** are the principal alternative routes for the mediation of voluntary movement. The rubrospinal tract originates in the red nucleus, crosses to the other side of the midbrain, descends in the lateral part of the brainstem

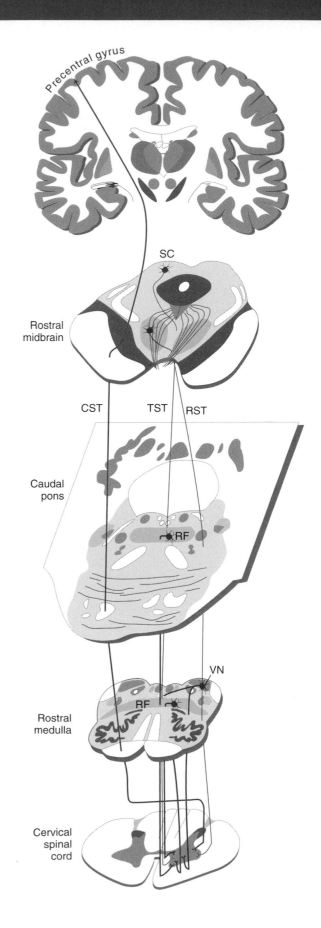

Figure 18-8 Principal locations and projections of upper motor neurons. Only one corticospinal fiber is indicated and is shown crossing the midline to join the lateral corticospinal tract. However, some corticospinal fibers, mostly headed for lower motor neurons for axial muscles, do not cross in the pyramidal decussation and join the anterior corticospinal tract. (See Video 18-1.) CST, corticospinal tract; RF, reticular formation; RST, rubrospinal tract; SC, superior colliculus; TST, tectospinal tract; VN, vestibular nuclei.

tegmentum, and travels through the lateral funiculus of the spinal cord along with the lateral corticospinal tract. The rubrospinal tract of humans is very small, and the reticulospinal tracts are the major alternative routes to the spinal cord. A **tectospinal tract** has also been described, descending from the superior colliculus through the contralateral anterior funiculus to cervical levels of the spinal cord. It likely has a role in reflexive turning of the head in response to visual stimuli; retrograde tracing studies indicate that such a reflex would be multisynaptic. The lateral corticospinal and rubrospinal tracts terminate primarily in lateral parts of the anterior horn, where they influence motor neurons for distal muscles. All the others terminate primarily in more medial parts of the anterior horn, where they influence the motor neurons for axial muscles important in postural adjustments.

Association Cortex, the Cerebellum, and the Basal Nuclei Modulate Motor Cortex

Even though corticospinal, rubrospinal, reticulospinal, and vestibulospinal fibers are able to influence lower motor neurons and their local connections, this still does not explain how a voluntary movement is made. There is activation of multiple areas of the frontal cortex, which occurs up to 2 seconds before a voluntary movement is made and that all such movement has an afferent component that initiates it. We can specify some of the structures and connections that must be involved, because damage to these structures and connections results in defective movements (see Fig. 18-7). In addition to the portions of the CNS already mentioned, these structures include the basal nuclei, the cerebellum, some areas of association cortex, and portions of the thalamus. The basal nuclei and the cerebellum are the subjects of Chapters 19 and 20, respectively, but the general way in which the various components of the motor system are interconnected is discussed here briefly. Cortical association areas are discussed in Chapter 22.

In one sense, the components of the motor system are organized hierarchically, as though association areas of cortex "decide" that a movement is called for; premotor areas of the cortex devise a plan for the movement and pass this information on to the motor cortex, which then issues commands to motor neurons either directly or indirectly, by way of nuclei and interneurons of the brainstem and spinal cord. In another sense, the components of the motor system are organized in parallel, much like the sensory pathways: messages are conveyed to the spinal cord not only from motor cortex but also from premotor areas themselves (see Fig. 18-11). The basal nuclei and cerebellum are involved in various aspects of planning and monitoring movements but have few or no outputs of their own to the spinal cord.

Rather, they act primarily by affecting motor and premotor cortex.

This is a very simplified overview of the central motor apparatus and omits a number of important details. Some of these details are mentioned in this and the next two chapters, whereas others are beyond the scope of this book. For example, no mention has been made of the role of sensory input to this system. Such input is clearly involved, because we can easily make appropriate modifications in the walking program to accommodate an increased load, such as a backpack, or modifications in the running program to accommodate the sight of an impending brick wall. A variety of pathological conditions reflect motor deficits resulting from sensory losses. One example already cited is the ataxia resulting from damage to the posterior columns. We can make simple movements involving single joints or basic rhythms fairly accurately without sensory feedback, but not more complex movements (Fig. 18-9) or corrections in response to perturbations.

The Corticospinal Tract Has Multiple Origins and Terminations

During the 19th century it was discovered that electrical stimulation of certain areas of the mammalian cerebral cortex causes movements of the contralateral side of the body. In humans the area with the lowest threshold for this effect lies in and near the anterior wall of the central

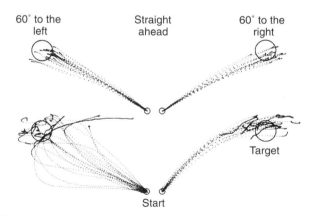

Figure 18-9 Ataxia caused by a somatosensory deficit. A normal subject (upper records) and a patient with a peripheral neuropathy that selectively affected large-diameter sensory fibers (lower records) used a computer mouse held in the right hand to move a cursor from a starting point to a target. The position of the mouse was digitized every 20 msec, producing a dotted-line record of hand movement. The subjects could see the position of the target and the cursor on the computer screen but not the mouse or the right hand holding it. The normal subject made the movements smoothly and accurately in either direction. The patient was inaccurate and somewhat irregular when moving to the right and had much more trouble when moving to the left, because this was a more complex movement of the right hand across the midline. *(From Gordon J, Ghilardi MF, Ghez C: J Neurophysiol 73:347, 1995.)*

sulcus (Fig. 18-10), so this area has come to be called the **primary motor cortex.** Subsequent work showed that there is a distorted mapping of the body in primary motor cortex (see Fig. 3-30), which shows up as stimulation of restricted cortical areas causing contraction of small groups of muscles or even single muscles. The **somatotopic** map is not as precise as Figure 3-30 seems to indicate—different body parts overlap and interdigitate with one another—but it is distorted in such a way that the parts of the body capable of intricate movements (such as the fingers and lips) have disproportionately large representations. The **motor homunculus** is similar in this way to the sensory homunculus in the somatosensory cortex of the postcentral gyrus, and this corresponds to (among other things) the notion that detailed sensory information is required for fine motor control.[b]

It was also known in the 19th century that the primary motor cortex contains giant pyramidal cells called **Betz cells,** whose axons descend to the spinal cord through the medullary pyramids; in addition, it was known that cerebral lesions that destroy motor cortex and adjoining areas or lesions that destroy the posterior limb of the internal capsule as the axons of Betz cells pass through it cause contralateral spastic paralysis. It therefore became accepted neurological thinking that the corticospinal tract (1) consists exclusively of large axons, (2) originates in the precentral gyrus, (3) proceeds exclusively to the anterior horn of the spinal cord, (4) is necessary for voluntary movement, and (5) is a tract whose destruction results in spastic paralysis. However, it gradually became apparent that this traditional description is incorrect in almost every way.

Corticospinal Axons Arise in Multiple Cortical Areas

The large (up to 22 µm) axons of Betz cells are included in the corticospinal tract, but they account for only about 3% of the tract's 1 million fibers. The vast majority of corticospinal fibers are much smaller, in the 1- to 4-µm range. In humans, up to 20% of the fibers that form the corticospinal tract synapse directly on motor neurons, and the majority of those are large-diameter fibers.

Betz cells are concentrated specifically in primary motor cortex, but only about half the corticospinal fibers originate in this cortical area. The remainder come from adjacent frontal motor areas and from the

[b]Other species have maps distorted in different but appropriate ways. For example, nearly two thirds of the fibers leaving an elephant's motor cortex are bound for its facial motor nucleus, reflecting an elephant's fine control over trunk movements; only one third of the fibers reach the spinal cord.

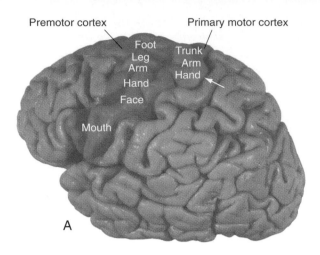

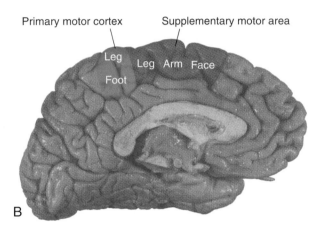

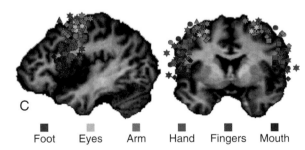

Figure 18-10 Location, extent, and somatotopic arrangement in motor areas of cerebral cortex; most of the primary motor cortex is hidden from view in the central sulcus. The indicated maps in premotor and supplementary motor areas are approximate at best; each of these includes multiple subareas, each with its own map, and not all are in register with one another. **A,** View of the lateral surface, seen from slightly above and behind. Although the detailed configuration of the central sulcus varies from one individual to another (see Fig. 3-6), the posteriorly directed bend *(arrow)* in its upper part is a reliable indicator of the level where the hand is represented. **B,** Medial surface. **C,** Compilation from multiple studies of the areas activated in premotor cortex as subjects used different body parts, imagined using them, or engaged in cognitive tasks that might ordinarily involve the use of those body parts. *(**C,** from Schubotz RI, von Cramon D Yves: Neuroimage 20:S120, 2003.)*

parietal lobe, particularly the somatosensory cortex of the postcentral gyrus. In view of this fact, the cortical complex on both sides of the central sulcus is sometimes referred to as the **sensorimotor cortex.** Hence primary motor cortex is neither the only source of corticospinal fibers nor the only cortical area involved in motor control. There are also maps of the body in the **premotor cortex** directly anterior to primary motor cortex and in the **supplementary motor area,** located on the medial surface of the hemisphere just anterior to the representation of the foot in primary motor cortex (see Fig. 18-10). (Much like the mosaic of visual association areas mentioned in Chapter 17, the premotor and supplementary motor areas are actually complexes of smaller areas. What used to be known as a single premotor area, for example, actually contains four separate and distinct motor areas; there are two separate areas in the supplementary motor area, and three more in the banks of the cingulate sulcus.) The premotor and supplementary motor areas provide another third of the corticospinal tract, and both also project to primary motor cortex (Fig. 18-11). All this corticospinal output passes through the posterior limb of the internal capsule, with fibers from primary motor cortex most posterior (Fig. 18-12), those from the supplementary motor area most anterior, and those from the premotor areas in between. The projection is somatotopically organized (Fig. 18-13) as far as the midbrain, but curiously, this organization is lost as the corticospinal tract traverses the pons.

Movements can be elicited by electrically stimulating the premotor and supplementary motor areas, but more current is required than in the case of primary motor cortex. In addition, the movements are more complex. Stimulating the premotor cortex may cause turning of the trunk to the opposite side or movement of the entire contralateral arm. Stimulating the supplementary motor area can cause bilateral movements, vocalizations, or the arrest of speech. Some of the movements elicited by stimulating premotor and supplementary motor cortex arise via direct connections and others via primary motor cortex. For example, hand movements can no longer be produced by stimulation of the supplementary motor area after primary motor cortex has been removed, whereas trunk movements are unaffected. However, these two cortical areas are much more than simply additional sources of motor command signals, as reflected in their projections to primary motor cortex. Both areas receive sets of inputs appropriate for planning movements, prominently including projections from prefrontal cortex (decision making) and parietal association cortex (information about the spatial relationships between body parts and the outside world). Both change their levels of activity before movements occur, and even if movements are only contemplated (see Fig. 18-14; also see Fig. 20-24). Although their

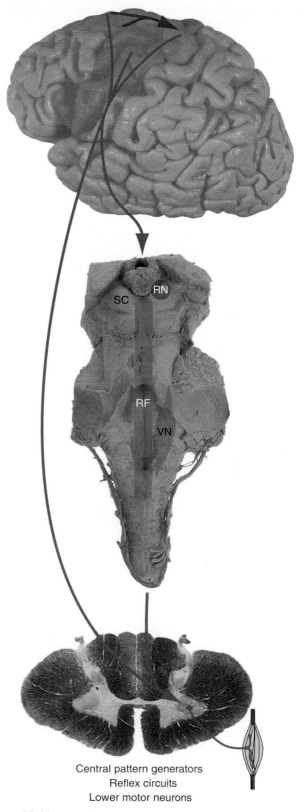

Figure 18-11 Projection of premotor and supplementary motor areas to primary motor cortex, and of all three motor areas to the brainstem and spinal cord. RF, reticular formation; RN, red nucleus; SC, superior colliculus; VN, vestibular nuclei.

Central pattern generators
Reflex circuits
Lower motor neurons

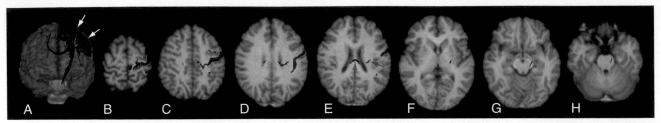

Figure 18-12 The path of axons leaving primary motor cortex, demonstrated with diffusion tensor imaging. **A,** In this anterior view, fibers can be seen leaving motor cortex *(white arrows)*. Some cross to the opposite hemisphere through the corpus callosum *(green arrow)*, but most enter the corticospinal tract *(blue arrow)*. **B** to **D,** Fibers leave motor cortex, enter the cerebral white matter, and travel through the centrum semiovale. **E,** Near the roof of the lateral ventricles, some cross through the corpus callosum *(green arrow)*, but most enter the corona radiata *(blue arrow)*. From there, the latter (corticospinal) fibers pass through the posterior limb of the internal capsule **(F)**, the middle of the cerebral peduncle **(G)**, and the basal pons **(H)**. *(Courtesy Dr. Mojtaba Zarei, University of Oxford.)*

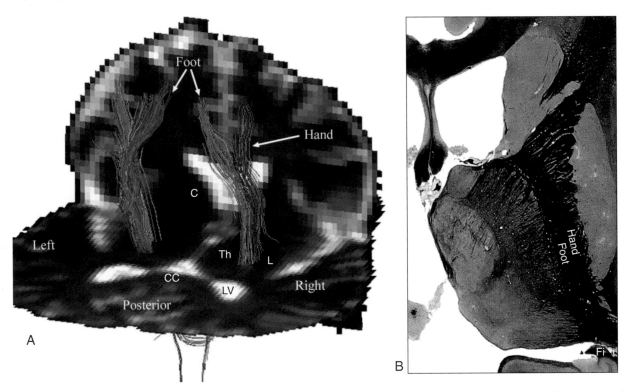

Figure 18-13 Typical somatotopic arrangement of corticospinal fibers in the posterior limb of the internal capsule. **A,** Diffusion tensor image showing the course of corticospinal fibers for the hand and foot. Foot fibers arise from the medial surface of the hemisphere and usually travel medial and slightly posterior to hand fibers, at least until they reach the brainstem. **B,** Relative positions of hand and foot fibers, about two thirds of the way back in the posterior limb of the internal capsule. C, caudate nucleus; CC, corpus callosum; L, lenticular nucleus; LV, lateral ventricle; Th, thalamus. *(**A,** adapted from Holodny AI et al: Radiology 234:649, 2005.)*

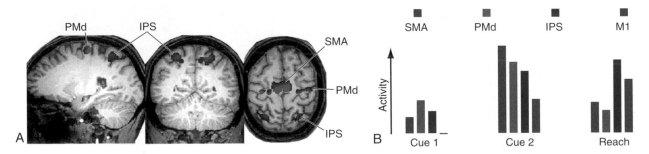

Figure 18-14 Participation of the supplementary motor area, premotor cortex, and parietal association cortex in planning movements. Subjects were given two sequential cues (which target to reach for, which hand to use) in random order, then reached for the target, all while functional magnetic resonance imaging measurements were being made. **A,** Areas that responded to both cues, but more to the second one (as though they were helping to assemble a plan for the reaching movement). **B,** Activity changes in four different cortical areas during the first and second cues and the reaching movement itself. The supplementary motor area, premotor cortex, and parietal association cortex all respond to the first cue, but they respond more to the second cue; parietal association cortex continues to respond during the movement because of the change in arm position. Primary motor cortex, in contrast, does not respond to the first cue and responds most vigorously during the movement. IPS, intraparietal sulcus (parietal association cortex); M1, primary motor cortex; PMd, dorsal premotor cortex; SMA, supplementary motor area. *(Adapted from Beurze SM et al: Integration of target and effector information in the human brain during reach planning. J Neurophysiol 97:188, 2007. Used with permission.)*

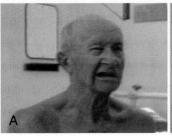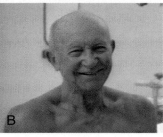

Figure 18-15 Selective weakness of lower facial muscles after cortical damage. This patient suffered a stroke that resulted in weakness of his left hand (not shown) and the left side of his face. When he tried to bare his teeth on request **(A),** weakness of the left lower facial muscles was apparent. However, when told a joke, he smiled almost symmetrically **(B).**

relative roles are not yet clear, premotor cortex may be more important for movements guided by external stimuli, such as reaching for a seen (or recently seen) object; the supplementary motor area may be more important in planning and learning complex, internally generated movements. The existence of multiple motor areas, each with its own access to lower motor neurons, is consistent with the observation that cortical damage sometimes causes the inability to move in some circumstances but not in others (Fig. 18-15).

Motor Cortex Projects to Both the Spinal Cord and the Brainstem

Corticospinal fibers, as their name implies, end in the spinal cord. However, in their course from cortex to cord, they give rise to large numbers of collaterals that end in a wide variety of locations, including the basal nuclei, the thalamus, the reticular formation, and various sensory nuclei such as the posterior column nuclei. Even within the spinal cord, some end in the posterior horn, others end in the intermediate gray matter, and a minority end directly on alpha and gamma motor neurons. Because of these numerous connections, it seems unlikely that the corticospinal tract has a single, easily specified function. The projections to sensory nuclei, for example, might serve to compensate somehow for the altered afferent activity caused by an impending movement. Projections to places such as the reticular formation work in the background, setting the stage for even the simplest movements. Most movements, particularly those involving the limbs, cause a shift in the body's center of mass and require a postural adjustment; these typically begin even before the limb movement is under way.

The corticospinal tract does, of course, have a major effect on motor neurons as well, both directly and indirectly by way of interneurons. In general, both alpha and gamma motor neurons are affected similarly. The utility

of this **alpha-gamma coactivation** can be seen in Figure 9-15. If only the alpha motor neurons were activated, during the resulting contraction the muscle spindles would be "destretched" and hence inactive. Stretch reflexes would thus be inoperative and unable to help compensate for sudden changes in load during the movement. Activating the gamma motor neurons as well serves to maintain spindle sensitivity throughout the movement.

Corticospinal Input Is Essential for Only Some Movements

Studies in which both medullary pyramids of monkeys were carefully and selectively severed have demonstrated that after an initial period of flaccid paralysis, surprisingly little chronic motor deficit results from a total loss of corticospinal function. In moving about their cages, these animals are virtually indistinguishable from normal monkeys. The only behaviorally obvious deficit is a permanent inability to use their fingers individually (e.g., to pick up a small object between thumb and forefinger). This corresponds to the evolution of corticospinal connections, which in most animals reach interneurons in the posterior horn and intermediate gray matter but not lower motor neurons. The lower motor neurons of primates capable of individual finger movements, in contrast, are contacted directly by corticospinal endings (Fig. 18-16). Loss of such finger movements is certainly serious for creatures who use their hands as much and as skillfully as many primates do, but it falls far short of being a generalized weakness or paralysis of voluntary movement.

If lesions of medial portions of the medullary reticular formation are added to the corticospinal lesion, a severe and permanent disability of the axial muscles results. Conversely, if lesions of the lateral portions of the medullary reticular formation are added to the corticospinal lesion, a severe and permanent disability of independent use of the arms (including, of course, the fingers) results. Evidently the reticulospinal or rubrospinal tract, or both, can compensate for the role normally played by the corticospinal tract in most aspects of voluntary movement.

Naturally occurring lesions in humans are seldom as neatly restricted as those in the monkeys just mentioned, and comparable cases of humans with selective damage to the pyramids are rare. However, there was once a neurosurgical procedure (whose rationale is explained in the next chapter) in which the corticospinal tract was cut in the cerebral peduncle. In these cases, the results were quite similar to those encountered with pyramid-sectioned monkeys, and relatively little chronic deficit resulted. Selective damage to the medullary pyramids of humans also causes less pronounced weakness and spasticity than does damage to motor areas of the cortex.

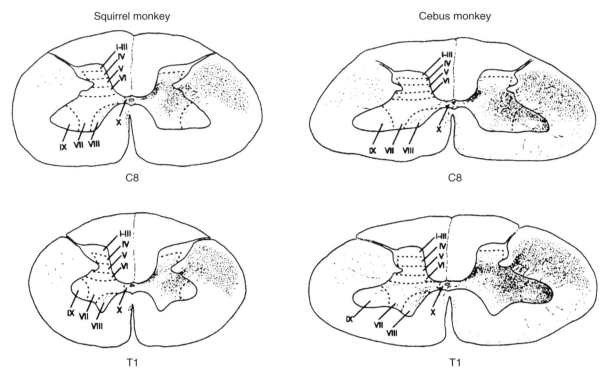

Squirrel monkey

Cebus monkey

C8

C8

T1

T1

Figure 18-16 Terminations of corticospinal axons (labeled by axoplasmic transport of a marker) in two species of monkey—one that does not use individual finger movements (squirrel monkey), and one that does (cebus monkey). In both species there is a broad band of corticospinal terminals in the intermediate gray, but only in the cebus monkey are there terminals in the lateral extension of the anterior horn, where finger motor neurons live. *(From Bortoff GA, Strick PL: J Neurosci 13:5105, 1993.)*

The reason for the apparent discrepancy can be seen in Figure 18-8. Damage to a medullary pyramid affects a select group of fibers—the final portions of corticospinal axons just before they reach the spinal cord. In contrast, damage to motor, premotor, or supplementary motor cortex or to the internal capsule affects not only corticospinal fibers but also projections from the cortex to the thalamus, basal nuclei, reticular formation, and other structures. Furthermore, even if it was possible to selectively damage only corticospinal fibers in the internal capsule, they would be affected before they gave off their many collaterals rather than after. Which part of this additional damage is responsible for the appearance of spasticity is not known with certainty, but the loss of projections from the premotor cortex to the reticular formation, and consequent reticulospinal dysfunction, is a likely cause.

Upper Motor Neuron Damage Causes a Distinctive Syndrome

The most common cause of upper motor neuron problems is a cerebrovascular accident involving the motor and premotor cortex or the posterior limb of the internal capsule. Immediately after the stroke, a period of flaccid paralysis ensues, analogous to spinal shock. After a period of days to weeks, tone and reflexes return and increase, and the situation resolves into **spastic hemi-** **plegia** or **hemiparesis.**[c] Tone is increased because stretch reflexes are increased in a velocity-dependent fashion (Fig. 18-17), so that when a muscle is stretched rapidly (such as when an examiner forcibly flexes a patient's leg), its resistance to further stretch increases greatly. (Slow stretch meets less resistance.) At some point this increased resistance suddenly melts away, and the limb collapses in flexion (or extension, if it was forcibly extended). This sudden collapse is called the **clasp-knife effect,** and it is often attributed to inhibition of motor neurons by reflex connections of Golgi tendon organs (see Fig. 10-12); inhibitory effects of other muscle receptors, however, are probably more important. Sudden stretch of a muscle may lead to **clonus,** a rapid series of rhythmic contractions maintained for the duration of the stretch. Increased tone is especially pronounced in the flexors of the arm and fingers and in the extensors of the leg, contributing to the typical hemiparetic stance and gait. This combination of hyperreflexia and

---

[c]Hemiplegia (from the Greek plegia, meaning "stroke"), strictly speaking, means total paralysis on one side. Because some voluntary movement returns after injury to the motor cortex or internal capsule, the condition is actually a hemiparesis (from the Greek paresis, meaning "slackening"), indicating weakness or partial paralysis.

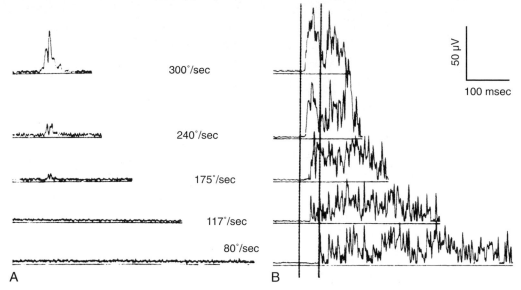

Figure 18-17 Biceps electromyograms from normal **(A)** and spastic **(B)** subjects in response to a 30-degree extension at the rates indicated. *(From Thilmann AF, Fellows SJ, Garms E: Brain 114:233, 1991.)*

hypertonia is spasticity. In addition, certain normal reflexes disappear, and some abnormal reflexes appear. The best known of the latter is Babinski's sign. Interestingly, Babinski's sign is normally seen in human infants before the corticospinal tract is fully myelinated and functional, and it is also seen after selective damage to the corticospinal tract in the cerebral peduncle or pyramid.

Some voluntary movement eventually returns, again in a characteristic pattern. Proximal muscles recover more than distal muscles, and movements of the fingers are the most severely and permanently affected. Skilled movements recover less than coarser movements of entire limbs do, suggesting that a major role of the corticospinal tract is to increase the speed and dexterity of movements whose basic characteristics can be generated by other descending pathways.

There Are Upper Motor Neurons for Cranial Nerve Motor Nuclei

Some corticospinal fibers, as we have seen, end directly on spinal motor neurons, whereas the rest end in the posterior horn, in the intermediate gray matter, or on interneurons of the anterior horn. Those not ending directly on motor neurons have a variety of effects, ranging from regulating the access of information to ascending pathways to affecting the activity of motor neurons via interneurons. In a similar manner, other fibers leave the cerebral cortex, descend through the internal capsule (immediately anterior to the corticospinal tract; see Fig. 18-19), and end in the brainstem on cells of sensory relay nuclei, the reticular formation, and

motor nuclei of some cranial nerves. Strictly speaking, this entire collection of fibers is the **corticobulbar tract.**[d] However, the term *corticobulbar tract* is commonly used to refer selectively to those fibers that affect the motor neurons of cranial nerves (Fig. 18-18). As in the spinal cord, some of these corticobulbar fibers end directly on motor neurons, particularly those for muscles over which we have the finest control (e.g., lip and tongue muscles). Most, however, act through interneurons of the reticular formation. The oculomotor, trochlear, and abducens nuclei receive no direct corticobulbar fibers; there are other peculiarities about the innervation of these nuclei, so they are treated separately in Chapter 21. Thus the following discussion pertains to the trigeminal, facial, and hypoglossal motor nuclei, nucleus ambiguus, and the spinal accessory nucleus.

In general, these nuclei receive a bilateral corticobulbar innervation, corresponding nicely to the way we often use muscles on both sides of the head and neck simultaneously (e.g., chewing, swallowing). The fibers originate from the face and mouth portion of motor cortex and from other areas of the frontal and parietal lobes as well. They accompany the corticospinal tract almost to the level of the nucleus they influence, where they part company with the corticospinal tract and end in the appropriate motor nucleus on both sides, or in the adjacent reticular formation. (Hence there is no single "corticobulbar decussation" analogous to the pyramidal decussation.) The major exception to this general pattern involves the facial motor nucleus. As mentioned in

---

[d]*Bulb* is an old term for the medulla or, by extension, for the entire brainstem.

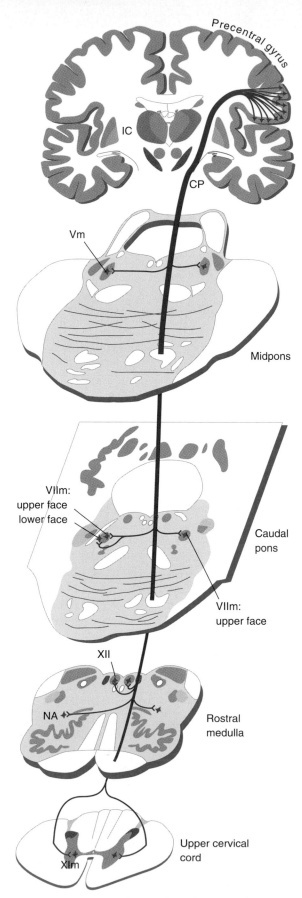

Figure 18-18 Corticobulbar pathway (except for cranial nerves III, IV, and VI). Three simplifications were used to keep the diagram manageable. First, corticobulbar fibers are shown ending directly on motor neurons, but most actually end on interneurons in the reticular formation. Second, corticobulbar fibers are shown with an equal bilateral distribution to the trigeminal, hypoglossal, and accessory nuclei. The trigeminal and hypoglossal nuclei and the trapezius motor neurons of the accessory nucleus often receive a preponderance of crossed fibers. Finally, all corticobulbar fibers are shown accompanying the corticospinal tract, whereas many actually leave this tract at various levels caudal to the cerebral peduncle and pursue a variety of aberrant courses through the brainstem. CP, cerebral peduncle; IC, internal capsule; NA, nucleus ambiguus; Vm, trigeminal motor nucleus; VIIm, facial motor nucleus; XII, hypoglossal nucleus; XIm, spinal accessory nucleus.

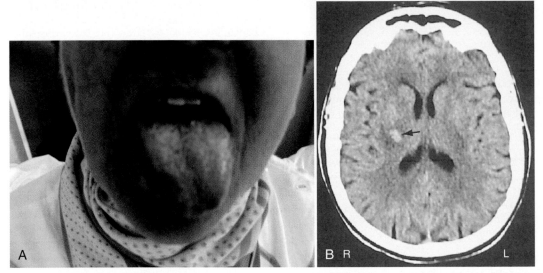

Figure 18-19 Tongue weakness caused by damage to corticobulbar fibers in the internal capsule. This 68-year-old hypertensive woman was referred to the neurology department after experiencing a sudden weakness in mastication and mild dysarthria. When she was asked to protrude her tongue, a left lingual paresis was evident **(A)**. Weakness of the left side of the tongue (and resulting deviation of the tongue to the left) is usually the result of damage to the left hypoglossal nerve or nucleus. In this case, however, the only abnormality revealed by computed tomography **(B)** was a small hemorrhage in the posterior limb of the right internal capsule *(arrow)*. *(From Gerace C, Fele RM, Pingi A: J Neurol Neurosurg Psychiatry 76:595, 2005.)*

Chapter 12, motor neurons to the lower facial muscles are innervated mainly by contralateral cortex (corresponding to the way we can contract muscles around the mouth asymmetrically), whereas those to upper facial muscles are innervated bilaterally. The result is that an individual with unilateral corticobulbar damage (e.g., a lesion of one cerebral peduncle) is unable to smile or bare the teeth symmetrically or puff out the contralateral cheek; however, the ability to blink and wrinkle the forehead on both sides remains (see Fig. 12-26). In addition, even though the hypoglossal and trigeminal motor nuclei and those neurons of the spinal accessory nucleus that innervate the trapezius[e] receive some input from the cortex of both hemispheres, the input from the contralateral side predominates (to a degree that varies from one individual to another). Hence, after damage to the motor cortex, internal capsule, or cerebral peduncle on one side, there may be slight (and typically transient) weakness of the contralateral trapezius and masseter and the contralateral side of the tongue (Fig. 18-19).

---

[e]Corticobulbar innervation of sternocleidomastoid motor neurons is still a matter of debate. It is observed clinically that motor cortex damage is frequently followed by weakness when turning the head toward the side contralateral to the lesion, implying that one cerebral hemisphere projects to motor neurons for the ipsilateral sternocleidomastoid. However, electrical studies indicate that corticobulbar fibers for this muscle are distributed bilaterally, with a contralateral preponderance. The apparent discrepancy may involve the role of other muscles, such as neck muscles and the platysma, in head turning.

SUGGESTED READINGS

Balagura S, Katz RG: Undecussated innervation to the sternocleidomastoid muscle: a reinstatement. Ann Neurol 7:84, 1980.

Beurze SM, et al: Integration of target and effector information in the human brain during reach planning. J Neurophysiol 97:188, 2007.

Brinkman J, Kuypers HGJM: Cerebral control of contralateral and ipsilateral arm, hand, and finger movements in the split-brain rhesus monkey. Brain 96:653, 1973.

Complex but interesting experiments whose results indicate that each cerebral hemisphere can exercise some control over the movements of both arms but not the fingers of both hands.

Brodal A: Self-observations and neuro-anatomical considerations after a stroke. Brain 96:675, 1973.

A fascinating account by an eminent neuroanatomist of a stroke he suffered and the pattern of his recovery. Such an individual can provide information about motor control and other cerebral functions that is probably impossible to obtain in any other way.

Bucy P, Keplinger JE, Siqueira EB: Destruction of the "pyramidal tract" in man. J Neurosurg 21:385, 1964.

Effects of cutting the corticospinal fibers in the cerebral peduncle.

Chainay H, et al: Foot, face and hand representation in the human supplementary motor area. Neuroreport 15:765, 2004.

Cruccu G, Fornarelli M, Manfredi M: Impairment of masticatory function in hemiplegia. Neurology 38:301, 1988.

Dietz V: Spinal cord pattern generators for locomotion. Clin Neurophysiol 114:137, 2003.

Gerace C, Fele RM, Pingi A: Capsular lingual paresis. J Neurol Neurosurg Psychiatry 76:595, 2005.

Gerloff C, et al: Stimulation over the human supplementary motor area interferes with the organization of future elements in complex motor sequences. Brain 120:1587, 1997.

Geyer S, et al: Functional neuroanatomy of the primate isocortical motor system. Anat Embryol 202:443, 2000.

Gilman S, Lieberman JS, Marco LA: Spinal mechanisms underlying the effects of unilateral ablation of areas 4 and 6 in monkeys. Brain 97:49, 1974.

How are motor and premotor cortex related to the mechanism of spasticity?

Gong S, et al: Cerebral cortical control of orbicularis oculi motoneurons. Brain Res 1047:177, 2005.
"Cortical control of OO motor activity is distributed bilaterally among multiple motor areas."

Grinevich V, Brecht M, Osten P: Monosynaptic pathway from rat vibrissa motor cortex to facial motor neurons revealed by lentivirus-based axonal tracing. J Neurosci 25:8250, 2005.
We have monosynaptic corticospinal inputs to motor neurons for finger muscles; rats have them for the muscles that move their whiskers.

Hallett M: Volitional control of movement: the physiology of free will. Clin Neurophysiol 118:1179, 2007.

Hallett M, Cruccu G: Corticobulbar tracts. Suppl Clin Neurophysiol 58:3, 2006.

Holodny AI, et al: Diffusion-tensor MR tractography of somatotopic organization of corticospinal tracts in the internal capsule: initial anatomic results in contradistinction to prior reports. Radiology 234:649, 2005.

Jürgens U, Alipour M: A comparative study on the cortico-hypoglossal connections in primates, using biotin dextranamine. Neurosci Lett 328:245, 2002.

Jürgens U, Ehrenreich L: The descending motorcortical pathway to the laryngeal motoneurons in the squirrel monkey. Brain Res 1148:90, 2007.

Kernell D: The motoneurone and its muscle fibres, Oxford, 2006, Oxford University Press.

Kiehn O: Locomotor circuits in the mammalian spinal cord. Annu Rev Neurosci 29:279, 2006.

Kleinschmidt A, Nitschke MF, Frahm J: Somatotopy in the human motor cortex hand area: a high-resolution functional MRI study. Eur J Neurosci 9:2178, 1997.

Kuypers HGJM: Corticobulbar connexions to the pons and lower brain-stem in man. Brain 81:364, 1958.

Lawrence DG, Kuypers HGJM: The functional organization of the motor system in the monkey. I. The effects of bilateral pyramidal lesions. II. The effects of lesions of the descending brain-stem pathways. Brain 91:1 and 15, 1968.
Two classic papers on the chronic effects of selective corticospinal lesions in primates, including information about which other descending pathways are able to compensate for loss of the corticospinal tract.

Libet B: Unconscious cerebral initiative and the role of conscious will in voluntary action. Behav Brain Sci 8:529, 1985.
Under certain conditions, electrical changes related to voluntary movement appear to start in the brain before a person is aware of having decided to move. This paper and the commentaries that follow it discuss these experiments, their validity, and their philosophical implications.

Matelli M, et al: Motor cortex. In Paxinos G, Mai JK, editors: The human nervous system, ed 2, San Diego, 2004, Elsevier Academic Press.

Morecraft RJ, et al: Cortical innervation of the facial nucleus in the non-human primate: a new interpretation of the effects of stroke and related subtotal brain trauma on the muscles of facial expression. Brain 124:176, 2001.

Nathan PW, Smith MC: The rubrospinal and central tegmental tracts in man. Brain 105:223, 1982.

Nathan PW, Smith MC, Deacon P: The corticospinal tracts in man: course and location of fibres at different segmental levels. Brain 113:303, 1990.

Newton JM, et al: Non-invasive mapping of corticofugal fibres from multiple motor areas—relevance to stroke recovery. Brain 129:1844, 2006.

Okano K, Tanji J: Neuronal activities in the primate motor fields of the agranular frontal cortex preceding visually triggered and self-paced movement. Exp Brain Res 66:155, 1987.
Description of a population of neurons in the supplementary motor area that change their firing rate many hundreds of milliseconds before a voluntary movement begins.

Pearce SL, et al: Responses of single motor units in human masseter to transcranial magnetic stimulation of either hemisphere. J Physiol 549:583, 2003.

Picard N, Strick PL: Imaging the premotor areas. Curr Opin Neurobiol 11:663, 2001.

Polit A, Bizzi E: Processes controlling arm movements in monkeys. Science 201:1235, 1978.
An article dealing with the motor abilities of a monkey receiving no afferent input from one arm.

Ralston DD, Ralston HJ, III: The terminations of corticospinal tract axons in the macaque monkey. J Comp Neurol 242:325, 1985.

Rathelot J-A, Strick PL: Muscle representation in the macaque motor cortex: an anatomical perspective. Proc Natl Acad Sci U S A 103:8257, 2006.

Schubotz RI, von Cramon DY: Functional-anatomical concepts of human premotor cortex: evidence from fMRI and PET studies. Neuroimage 20:S120, 2003.

Smithard DG, et al: The natural history of dysphagia following a stroke. Dysphagia 12:188, 1997.
Nucleus ambiguus may receive bilateral corticobulbar inputs, but losing half of them can still cause problems for a while.

Thaler D, et al: The functions of the medial premotor cortex. I. Simple learned movements. Exp Brain Res 102:445, 1995.

Thompson ML, Thickbroom GW, Mastaglia FL: Corticomotor representation of the sternocleidomastoid muscle. Brain 120:245, 1997.

Urban PP, et al: The course of cortico-hypoglossal projections in the human brainstem: functional testing using transcranial magnetic stimulation. Brain 119:1031, 1996.

Vytopil M, Jones HR, Jr: Mogul-clonus. Neurology 63:1130, 2004.
An unusual way for clonus to show up.

White LE, et al: Structure of the human sensorimotor system. I. Morphology and cytoarchitecture of the central sulcus. Cereb Cortex 7:18, 1997.

Yousry TA, et al: Localization of the motor hand area to a knob on the precentral gyrus: a new landmark. Brain 120:141, 1997.

Zilles K, et al: Mapping of human and macaque sensorimotor areas by integrating architectonic, transmitter receptor, MRI and PET data. J Anat 187:515, 1995.

Basal Nuclei

In 1817 James Parkinson, an English country physician, published a brief monograph entitled *An Essay on the Shaking Palsy,* in which he described the symptoms of several individuals who had the disease that now bears his name. Parkinsonian patients, as described in more detail later in this chapter, are characterized by tremor, generally increased muscle tone, and difficulty initiating voluntary movements, which are unusually small and slow once begun. This and related disorders, whose signs typically include some combination of slowed or dimin-ished movements, involuntary movements, and general-ized alterations in muscle tone, have come to be associated with damage to the basal nuclei. They were long referred to as **extrapyramidal disorders** to distinguish them from disorders involving the corticospinal (pyramidal) system. This terminology is no longer used because, as discussed later in this chapter, the two systems are ultimately inter-digitated; for example, many of the involuntary move-ments following basal nuclei damage are actually effected through the corticospinal tract.

The Basal Nuclei Include Five Major Nuclei

The term *basal nuclei* is slowly replacing the more traditional terminology—*basal ganglia;* both terms are appropriate and both are commonly used. The meaning of the term *basal nuclei* has evolved over time, but it is now used to refer to those structures whose damage causes the distinctive kinds of movement disorders (and other disorders) described in this chapter. These structures include some large subcortical nuclei of each cerebral hemisphere—the **putamen, caudate, nucleus accumbens,** and **globus pallidus**—together with the diencephalic **subthalamic nucleus** and the **substantia nigra** of the rostral midbrain (Figs. 19-1 and 19-2).

Various names are applied to different combinations of members of the basal nuclei (Fig. 19-3). The putamen,

caudate nucleus, and nucleus accumbens have a common embryological origin, identical histological appearances, and similar connections. One indication of this common origin is their physical continuity just above the orbital surface of the frontal lobe, where the head of the caudate merges with nucleus accumbens,[a] which in turn merges with the anterior part of the putamen. Another indication is the bridges of gray matter that cross the internal capsule between the putamen and the caudate nucleus, giving this region a

---

[a]Named historically for its physical location, its original name was nucleus accumbens septi—"nucleus leaning against the septum"—because the region of apparent fusion of the putamen and caudate nucleus seems to lean up against the base of the septum pellucidum (see Fig. 19-2A).

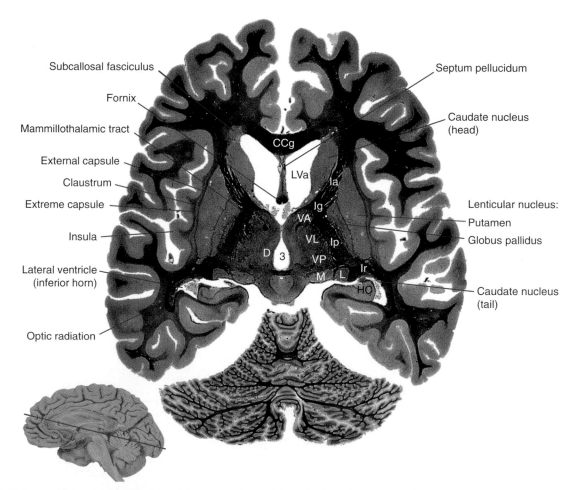

Figure 19-1 Basal nuclei and surrounding structures, as seen in an axial section. The claustrum is a plate of gray matter, suspected of playing a role in consciousness, that is layered between the putamen and the insular cortex. The external capsule, between the claustrum and the putamen, is a route through which many projections from the cerebral cortex reach the putamen; many cortical fibers reach the caudate nucleus through the subcallosal fasciculus. The extreme capsule houses association fibers that interconnect different cortical areas (see Chapter 22). 3, third ventricle; CCg, genu of the corpus callosum; D, dorsomedial nucleus; HC, hippocampus; Ia, Ig, Ip, and Ir, internal capsule—anterior limb, genu, posterior limb, and retrolenticular part; L, lateral geniculate nucleus; LVa, anterior horn of the lateral ventricle; M, medial geniculate nucleus; VA, VL, and VP, ventral anterior, ventral lateral, and ventral posterior nuclei. *(Adapted from Nolte J, Angevine JB Jr: The human brain in photographs and diagrams, ed 3, St. Louis, 2007, Mosby.)*

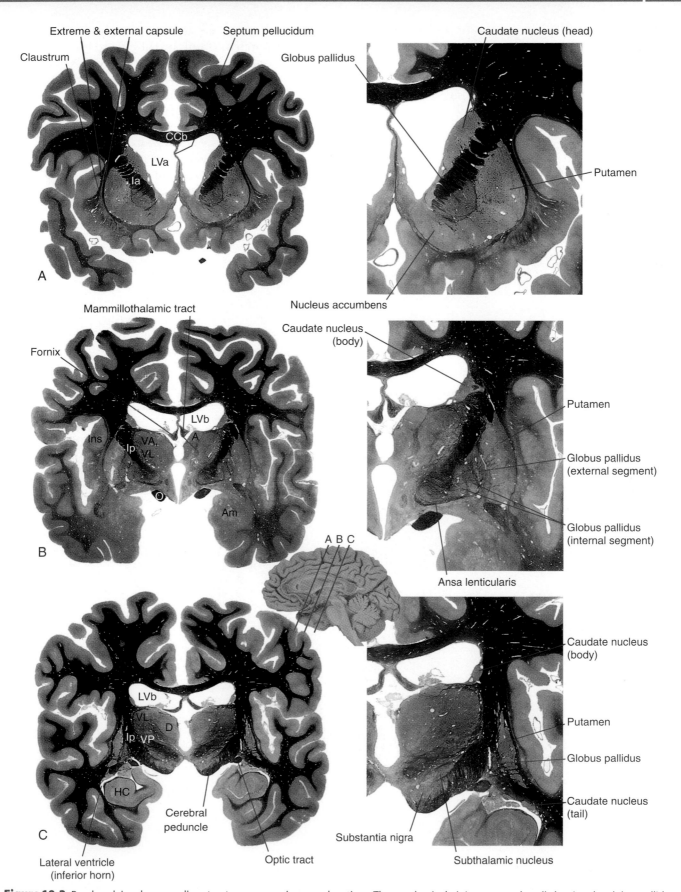

Figure 19-2 Basal nuclei and surrounding structures, as seen in coronal sections. The ansa lenticularis is an output bundle leaving the globus pallidus (see Fig. 19-15 and Video 19-1). A, anterior nucleus (of the thalamus); Am, amygdala; CCb, body of the corpus callosum; D, dorsomedial nucleus; HC, hippocampus; Ia and Ip, internal capsule—anterior limb and posterior limb; Ins, insula; LVa and LVb, anterior horn and body of the lateral ventricle; O, optic tract; VA, VL, and VP, ventral anterior, ventral lateral, and ventral posterior nuclei. *(Adapted from Nolte J, Angevine JB Jr: The human brain in photographs and diagrams, ed 3, St. Louis, 2007, Mosby.)*

striped appearance in many planes of section (Fig. 19-4). Because of this appearance, the putamen, caudate nucleus, and nucleus accumbens together are referred to as the **striatum.** The putamen and globus pallidus have different connections but are physically apposed,

BASAL GANGLIA

Striatum
    caudate nucleus
    nucleus accumbens
    putamen

Globus pallidus (pallidum)
    external segment (GPe)
    internal segment (GPi)

Lenticular nucleus

Subthalamic nucleus

Substantia nigra
    compact part (SNc)
    reticular part (SNr)

Figure 19-3 Terminology associated with the basal nuclei.

and together they are referred to as the **lenticular** or **lentiform nucleus** (from the Latin word for "lentil").

These assorted names give rise to prefixes and suffixes that are used to describe fibers coming from or going to different parts of the basal nuclei. *Strio-* and *-striate* are used for the striatum; thus *striopallidal* fibers go from, for example, the putamen to the globus pallidus, and *corticostriate* fibers go from the cerebral cortex to the putamen, caudate nucleus, or nucleus accumbens. The globus pallidus is also called the **pallidum,** so *pallidothalamic* fibers go from the globus pallidus to the thalamus. *Nigroreticular* fibers go from the substantia nigra to the reticular formation.

The Striatum and Globus Pallidus Are the Major Forebrain Components of the Basal Nuclei

The lenticular nucleus is shaped somewhat like a wedge cut from a sphere (see Figs. 19-1 and 19-2). The putamen (from the Latin for "husk"), which is approximately coextensive with the insula, forms the outermost portion of this wedge. It is separated from the more medial globus

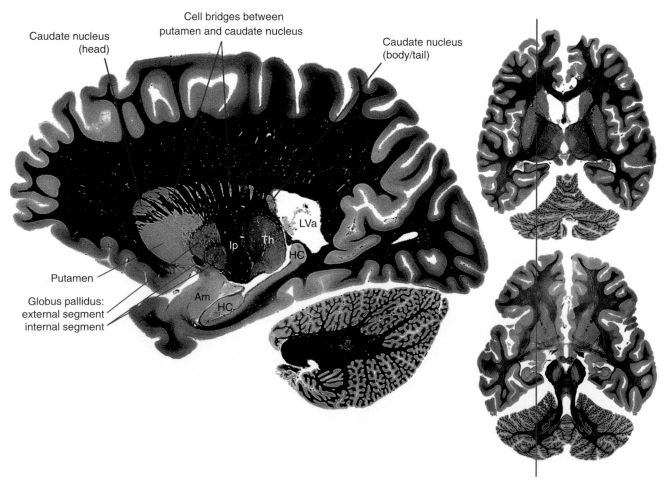

Figure 19-4 Parasagittal section showing how the striatum got its name. Am, amygdala; HC, hippocampus; Ip, posterior limb of the internal capsule; LVa, atrium of the lateral ventricle; Th, thalamus. *(Adapted from Nolte J, Angevine JB Jr: The human brain in photographs and diagrams, ed 3, St. Louis, 2007, Mosby.)*

pallidus by a thin **lateral medullary lamina** of myelinated fibers. The globus pallidus is itself divided into **internal** (medial) and **external** (lateral) portions by a **medial medullary lamina.** In unstained sections through the lenticular nucleus, the globus pallidus has a distinctively pale appearance as a result of the large number of myelinated fibers that originate from it or traverse it. (In myelin-stained sections such as those shown in Figs. 19-1 and 19-2, it is therefore relatively dark.)

The putamen is located where the diencephalon and telencephalon fuse during development (see Figs. 2-12 and 2-13). The caudate nucleus is found in the wall of the lateral ventricle and grows with it in a C-shaped course during development. The result is that the caudate nucleus (Latin for "nucleus with a tail") winds up with an enlarged **head** that bulges into the anterior horn, a **body** in the lateral wall of the body of the ventricle, and a slender **tail** that borders on the inferior horn (Fig. 19-5 and see Figs. 19-1 and 19-2). In the temporal lobe, the tail of the caudate nucleus is continuous with the amygdala, which in turn is continuous with the putamen (see Fig. 25-5).

The Subthalamic Nucleus and Substantia Nigra Are Interconnected With the Striatum and Globus Pallidus

The subthalamic nucleus, shaped like a biconvex lens enveloped in white matter, is located between the medial part of the cerebral peduncle and the thalamus (see Fig. 19-2C). Although relatively small, it has major interconnections with other parts of the basal nuclei (see Fig. 19-17).

The region referred to as the *substantia nigra* actually has two parts (Fig. 19-6)—a dorsal **compact part (SNc)** that contains closely packed, pigmented neurons, and a **reticular part (SNr)** nearer the cerebral peduncle that contains more loosely packed neurons, most of which are nonpigmented. These correspond to the two distinctly different ways in which the substantia nigra participates in the circuitry of the basal nuclei: the compact part provides widespread, modulatory, dopaminergic projections to other parts of the basal nuclei, whereas the reticular part is one of the basal nuclei output nuclei (Fig. 19-7 and see Fig. 19-9).

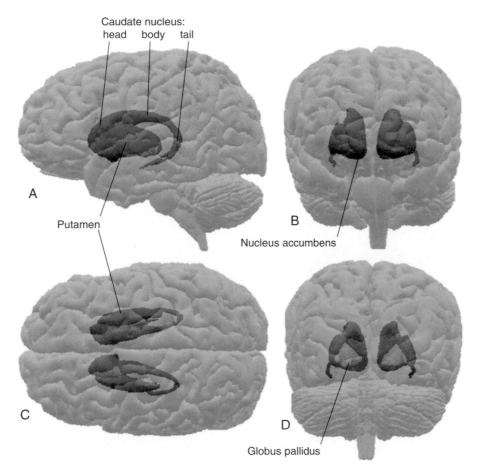

Figure 19-5 Three-dimensional reconstruction of the striatum and globus pallidus inside a translucent CNS, seen from the left **(A),** in front **(B),** above **(C),** and behind **(D).** (See Videos 19-2 and 19-3.)

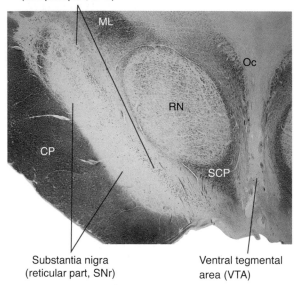

Substantia nigra
(compact part, SNc)

Figure 19-6 The compact (SNc) and reticular (SNr) parts of the substantia nigra. The dark dots that characterize SNc are individual dopaminergic neurons filled with neuromelanin. Nearby neurons in the ventral tegmental area (VTA) are also dopaminergic. CP, cerebral peduncle; ML, medial lemniscus; Oc, oculomotor nucleus; RN, red nucleus; SCP, cerebellar efferent fibers that ascend through the superior cerebellar peduncle.

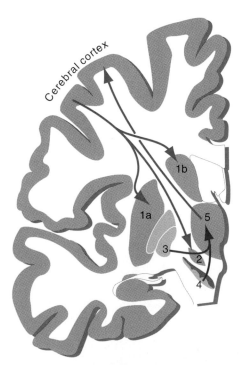

Figure 19-7 Principal inputs to and outputs from the basal nuclei. The major inputs come from cerebral cortex, reaching the putamen (1a), caudate nucleus (1b) (and nucleus accumbens, which is not present in this plane), and subthalamic nucleus (2). Outputs project from the internal segment of the globus pallidus (3) and the reticular part of the substantia nigra (4) to the thalamus (5), which in turn projects back to the cortex. These connections are mostly uncrossed, but there is some bilaterality (not shown). Excitatory connections are shown in *green*, inhibitory connections in *red*.

Basal Nuclei Circuitry Involves Multiple Parallel Loops That Modulate Cortical Output

Although the basal nuclei are best known for their role in motor control, mediated by their interactions with motor cortex and subcortical structures, it is now clear that they are more generally involved in many disparate cortical functions. The basis of this involvement is a series of loops, each starting with projections from an area of cerebral cortex to the basal nuclei and then returning, by way of the thalamus, to part of this cortical area. The cortical starting and ending points of each loop determine its function, with some related to movement, others to cognition, and still others to emotion and motivation. Interconnections within the basal nuclei determine the pattern of activity in each loop on a moment-to-moment basis.

Afferents From the Cortex Reach the Striatum and Subthalamic Nucleus; Efferents Leave From the Globus Pallidus and Substantia Nigra

Projections from the cerebral cortex reach the striatum and subthalamic nucleus (see Fig. 19-7), which in this sense are the principal input elements of the basal nuclei. Outputs leave from the internal segment of the globus pallidus (GPi) and the SNr. The links between these input and output structures are discussed a little later in this chapter. The corticostriate inputs and the projections back to the cortex from the thalamus all make excitatory (glutamate) connections, whereas the GPi-SNr outputs are all inhibitory (γ-aminobutyric acid [GABA]). There are multiple versions of this loop, all similar in principle but each utilizing different cortical areas and a distinctive portion of the striatum, globus pallidus, and other nuclei. Some loops begin and end in parietal or temporal association cortex, so interactions with the basal nuclei may characterize most cortical areas.

The major circuit through which the basal nuclei participate in the control of movement provides one example of such a loop. The striatum and globus pallidus form by far the largest part of the basal nuclei, yet they have no way to affect motor neurons directly (see Figs. 18-7 and 18-8). Thus the only way the basal nuclei can play a role in the control of movement is by influencing one or more of the descending pathways mentioned in the previous chapter. They do so primarily by affecting the activity of motor areas of the cerebral cortex (and, to a degree, through projections to the reticular formation). Somatosensory and motor areas project to a portion of the striatum (mostly putamen), which in turn projects by way of GPi to the ventral anterior and ventral lateral

(VA/VL) nuclei; the circuit is completed by projections from VA/VL back to motor areas of the cortex. Other basal nuclei loops use their own distinctive portions of the striatum, subthalamic nucleus, globus pallidus, substantia nigra, thalamus, and cerebral cortex. Collectively the loops roughly correspond to the putamen, caudate nucleus, and nucleus accumbens, which receive inputs from motor and somatosensory cortex, association cortex, and limbic areas, respectively (Fig. 19-8). The partitioning of connections among striatal subdivisions is not absolute. For example, limbic inputs reach not only nucleus accumbens but also adjoining parts of the putamen and caudate nucleus. For this reason, all these limbic-recipient regions are recognized as a separate striatal division called the **ventral striatum.**

Interconnections of the Basal Nuclei Determine the Pattern of Their Outputs

Most of the remaining connections of the basal nuclei fall into four categories: widespread dopaminergic projections from the compact part of the substantia nigra to other parts of the basal nuclei, especially the striatum; multiple inhibitory interconnections between different parts of the basal nuclei (see Fig. 19-13); excitatory projections from the subthalamic nucleus to the globus pallidus (see Fig. 19-17); and interconnections of thalamic intralaminar nuclei with the striatum and globus pallidus (Fig. 19-9 and see Fig. 19-14). A striking feature of these connections is the large proportion of inhibitory

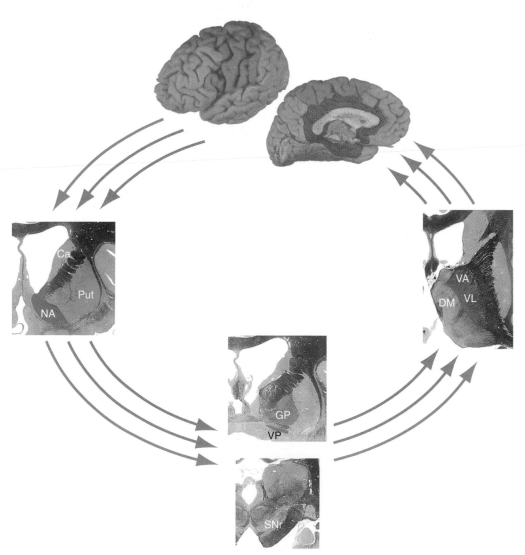

Figure 19-8 Parallel loops through the basal nuclei. In general, projections from association cortex emphasize the caudate nucleus, those from sensorimotor cortex emphasize the putamen, and those from limbic areas emphasize nucleus accumbens. However, the demarcations are not as absolute as this figure implies. For example, the frontal eye field (see Chapter 21) projects to the caudate nucleus, which is involved in eye movement control, and parietal association cortex projects to parts of the putamen as well as to parts of the caudate nucleus. Ca, caudate nucleus; DM, dorsomedial nucleus; GP, globus pallidus; NA, nucleus accumbens; Put, putamen; SNr, substantia nigra (reticular part); VA, ventral anterior nucleus; VL, ventral lateral nucleus; VP, ventral pallidum (a small extension of the globus pallidus under the anterior commissure).

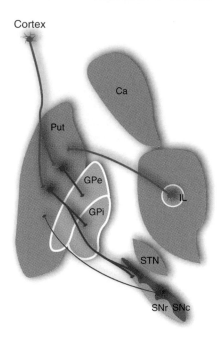

Figure 19-9 Major connections of the striatum. To keep things simple, only those of the putamen (Put) are shown, but the caudate nucleus (Ca) and nucleus accumbens (not shown in this plane) are wired in a similar fashion. Excitatory connections are shown in *green,* inhibitory connections in *red;* projections from the compact part of the substantia nigra (SNc) are shown in a third color, because dopamine is excitatory at some synapses and inhibitory at others. GPe and GPi, external and internal segments of the globus pallidus; IL, intralaminar nuclei of the thalamus; SNr, reticular part of the substantia nigra; STN, subthalamic nucleus.

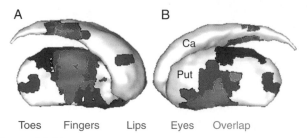

Toes Fingers Lips Eyes Overlap

Figure 19-10 Medial **(A)** and lateral **(B)** views of the left striatum, reconstructed from magnetic resonance imaging (MRI) scans, showing the somatotopic representation of body parts. Subjects repetitively flexed and extended their fingers or toes, contracted their lips, or looked from side to side while functional MRI measurements indicated the parts of the striatum where activity increased. Ca, caudate nucleus; Put, putamen. *(From Gerardin E et al: Cereb Cortex 13:162, 2003.)*

synapses. All the outputs from the striatum, globus pallidus, and reticular part of the substantia nigra are inhibitory, using GABA as a transmitter. The only prominent source of excitatory (glutamate) projections is the subthalamic nucleus.

In the account that follows, only the best documented connections of the basal nuclei are described. There are still many mysteries about the basal nuclei, and the precise function of most of these connections is unknown. However, there has been enough progress that some of the consequences of damage are beginning to make sense.

The Cerebral Cortex, Substantia Nigra, and Thalamus Project to the Striatum

The caudate nucleus, putamen, and ventral striatum receive inputs from the cerebral cortex, the substantia nigra (SNc) and nearby ventral tegmental area, and the intralaminar nuclei of the thalamus (see Fig. 19-9). The cortical input is by far the most massive of the three. These fibers originate in most areas of the cortex, pass through the internal and external capsules, and end in a roughly topographical pattern in the striatum. The putamen underlies the insula, at the base of the central sulcus, and receives most of the projections from the motor and somatosensory cortex; not surprisingly, body

parts are mapped out systematically in the putamen (Fig. 19-10). The caudate nucleus, as it curves around with the ventricular system, receives most of the projections from association areas; as the size and location of the head of the caudate might imply, the projection is particularly heavy from prefrontal cortex. Finally, the ventral striatum receives inputs not only from limbic cortex but also from the hippocampus and amygdala. Through these inputs, the basal nuclei are constantly informed about most aspects of cortical function. The compact part of the substantia nigra and the ventral tegmental area project systematically to all areas of the striatum (and to other parts of the basal nuclei) by way of very fine axons that use dopamine as their neurotransmitter. Destruction of this **nigrostriatal** pathway is the major factor causing Parkinson's disease (see Fig. 19-20). Finally, the intralaminar nuclei, especially the centromedian and parafascicular nuclei, project to the striatum. Many of these same fibers, as mentioned in Chapter 16, have collateral branches that end in the cerebral cortex. This **thalamostriate** pathway is particularly well developed in primates, but very little is known of its normal function. However, abnormal activity in this intralaminar nuclei→basal nuclei→intralaminar nuclei loop has been implicated in some basal nuclei disorders.

The cell types and their distributions are more or less uniform throughout the striatum, and it was once thought that it was functionally uniform as well. However, it is now known that the striatum is divided into discrete patches, or **striosomes,** embedded in a background **matrix,** with both compartments having distinctive types of connections and neurotransmitters (Fig. 19-11). It seems likely that the striosomes and matrix fit together in some as yet undefined modular way to form striatal functional units.

Different Parts of the Striatum Are Involved in Movement, Cognition, and Affect

The putamen, caudate nucleus, and ventral striatum, by virtue of their participation in different basal nuclei

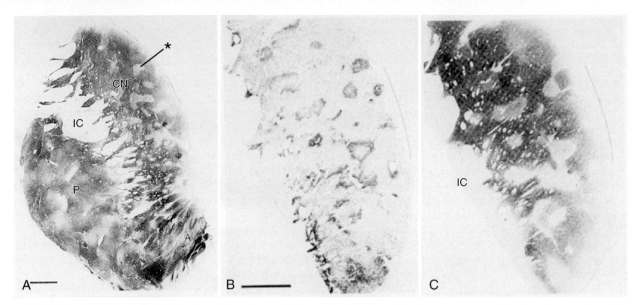

Figure 19-11 Chemical compartmentalization of the striatum. **A,** Coronal section through a human putamen (P) and caudate nucleus (CN), separated by the anterior limb of the internal capsule (IC), with the nucleus accumbens (A) forming the transition zone between the two. Histochemical staining for the enzyme acetylcholinesterase (AChE) was applied to the section, revealing that the striatum is made up of an AChE-rich background (matrix) with embedded AChE-poor regions (one indicated by an asterisk). The AChE-poor regions are about 300 to 600 μm wide and are often referred to as striosomes. Scale mark = 3 mm. Matrix and striosome regions have a number of other chemical differences. **B** and **C,** An example of these differences is shown in two adjacent coronal sections through the head of a human caudate nucleus. The section in **B** was stained immunocytochemically for enkephalin; the section in **C** was stained for AChE. High enkephalin levels are found precisely in the striosomes, especially around their peripheries. Scale mark = 3 mm. *(From Graybiel AM: Neurochemically specified subsystems in the basal nuclei. In Functions of the basal nuclei, Ciba Foundation Symposium 107, London, 1984, Pitman.)*

loops, have somewhat different functions. The putamen receives most of the inputs from motor and somatosensory areas of cortex and projects by way of the globus pallidus and thalamus to the motor, premotor, and supplementary motor areas. Corresponding to this, individual neurons in the putamen fire in conjunction with particular movements or positions (see Fig. 19-10). Thus the putamen is probably centrally involved in most of the motor functions of the basal nuclei. The caudate nucleus, in contrast, receives most of its inputs from association areas of cortex and projects by way of GPi-SNr and the thalamus mostly to prefrontal areas. Relatively few caudate neurons respond to movements or positions. Thus the caudate nucleus is likely more involved in cognitive functions and less directly in movement (Box 19-1). The limbic connections of the ventral striatum indicate its probable role in the initiation of drive-related behaviors (see Fig. 23-23).

The Striatum Projects to the Globus Pallidus and Substantia Nigra

Striatal efferents collect into numerous bundles of myelinated fibers that converge topographically (see Fig. 19-8) on the globus pallidus (see Fig. 19-9). Most of them are striopallidal fibers; some terminate in the internal segment of the globus pallidus, others in the external

segment. Still others pass through the globus pallidus and reach both parts of the substantia nigra.

The External Segment of the Globus Pallidus Distributes Inhibitory Signals Within the Basal Nuclei

The two segments of the globus pallidus have similar inputs but distinctly different sets of outputs. The external segment (GPe) receives inhibitory inputs from the striatum and excitatory inputs from the subthalamic nucleus. It then distributes widespread inhibitory (GABA) outputs to most other parts of the basal nuclei (Fig. 19-13). The functional map in the striatum continues into GPe, with different sectors dominated by inputs from the putamen, caudate nucleus, and ventral striatum. The functional significance of these far-flung inhibitory connections is still unknown, but inactivating specific subareas of GPe can mimic the movement, cognitive, and behavioral disturbances characteristic of different basal nuclei disorders.

The Internal Segment of the Globus Pallidus and the Reticular Part of the Substantia Nigra Provide the Output From the Basal Nuclei

GPi and SNr, like GPe, receive inhibitory inputs from the striatum and excitatory inputs from the subthalamic

BOX 19-1

A Case of Bilateral Damage to the Caudate Nucleus

Damage in the basal nuclei is usually associated with movement disorders, as in Parkinson's disease. However, the loop from association cortex, through the caudate nucleus, and ultimately back to prefrontal association cortex implies that caudate damage would result in findings related to those that occur after prefrontal damage (see Chapter 22). Several cases consistent with this idea have been reported, none more striking than that of a 25-year-old woman who incurred extensive bilateral damage to the head of the caudate nucleus (Fig. 19-12).

Before the onset of her illness she had been a high school honor student, was employed full-time, had been living independently, and was engaged to be married. From February to March of 1983 she suffered from daily headaches with occasional nausea and vomiting. In April she disappeared for 3 days. When found, she had undergone a dramatic personality change manifested by alterations in affect, motivation, cognition, and self-care. . . . Her abnormal behaviors included vulgarity, impulsiveness, easy frustration, violent outbursts, hypersomnia, enuresis, indifference, wandering, increased appetite, polydipsia, hypersexuality, minor criminal behavior including shoplifting and exposing herself, and poor hygiene. . . . [A year later] the patient had married and divorced, continued to be unemployed, and had little improvement in behavior. Two psychiatric hospitalizations and treatment with a variety of major tranquilizers were not beneficial.

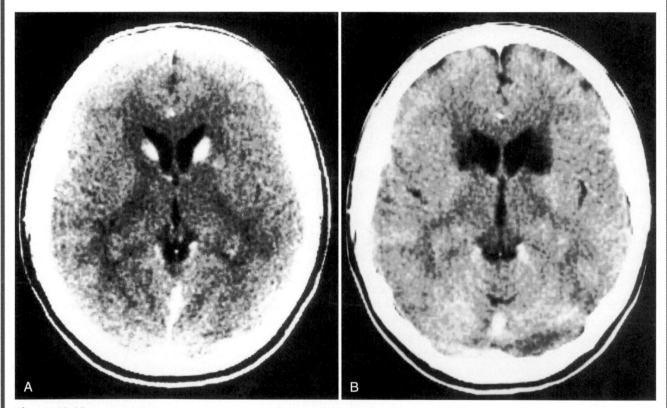

Figure 19-12 Contrast-enhanced computed tomography scans immediately after the 3-day disappearance of the patient described in Box 19-1 **(A)** and 8 months later **(B).** Contrast enhancement, indicative of pathology and blood-brain barrier breakdown, is seen in the head of the caudate nucleus bilaterally in the early scan. Eight months later, these areas are about the same density as cerebrospinal fluid, as though the heads of the caudate nuclei had degenerated. The cause of the pathology was never determined. *(From Richfield EK, Twyman R, Berent S: Ann Neurol 22:768, 1987.)*

From Richfield EK, Twyman R, Berent S: *Ann Neurol* 22:768, 1987.

nucleus (Fig. 19-14A). They also receive inputs from GPe, however, and their efferents are separate and distinct from those of GPe (see Fig. 19-14B). The internal pallidal segment projects mainly to the thalamus—an unusual example of seemingly specific inputs that use GABA—through two collections of fibers (Fig. 19-15). One collection, the **lenticular fasciculus,** runs directly through the internal capsule and then passes medially as a sheet of fibers between the subthalamic nucleus and the zona incerta. At the medial edge of the zona incerta,

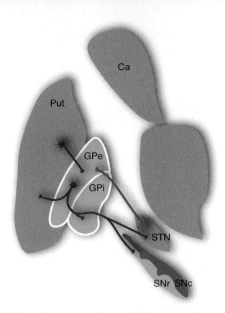

Figure 19-13 Major connections of the external segment of the globus pallidus (GPe); only striatal inputs from the putamen (Put) are shown, although the caudate nucleus (Ca) and ventral striatum are involved in similar ways. For simplicity, all the striatal projections to the internal segment of the globus pallidus (Gpi) and the reticular part of the substantia nigra (SNr) are shown as coming from the putamen. Most of those to SNr actually come from the caudate nucleus, and the ventral striatum projects to the ventral pallidum (see Fig. 23-22) and SNr. Excitatory connections are shown in *green,* inhibitory connections in *red.* SNc, compact part of the substantia nigra; STN, subthalamic nucleus.

the lenticular fasciculus makes a hairpin turn in a posterolateral direction and enters the thalamus. The second collection loops around the medial edge of the internal capsule as the **ansa lenticularis** (the Latin word *ansa* means "loop"); it joins the lenticular fasciculus and GABAergic fibers from SNr in the **thalamic fasciculus,**[b] which then enters the thalamus. The thalamic fasciculus terminates in a variety of thalamic nuclei. Fibers related to movement control end in VA/VL, those related to the caudate nucleus and prefrontal cortex end in the dorsomedial nucleus and in part of VA, and others end in the centromedian and parafascicular nuclei. VA/VL and the dorsomedial nucleus then project to frontal and other cortical areas, thus completing the principal circuit through the basal nuclei (see Figs. 19-7 and 19-8).

Most of these efferents from GPi-SNr to the thalamus also have a branch that descends to an area of the midbrain reticular formation adjacent to the decussation of the superior cerebellar peduncles (the **pedunculopontine nucleus**). Finally, a smaller number of GPi-SNr efferents reach the superior colliculus and the habenula. Those to the superior colliculus play a role in the control

of eye movements (see Chapter 21); the function of the connections with the habenula is unknown.

The Subthalamic Nucleus Is Part of Additional Pathways Through the Basal Nuclei

As Figure 19-16 shows, the subthalamic nucleus is located right across the internal capsule from the globus pallidus. The small bundles of fibers that cross the internal capsule and interconnect these two nuclei are collectively called the **subthalamic fasciculus.** The subthalamic nucleus provides a powerful excitatory input to GPi-SNr neurons and is thereby thought to have important effects on the pattern of inhibitory output from the basal nuclei, but it does more than this. Major inputs to the subthalamic nucleus (Fig. 19-17) arise not just in GPe but also in the cerebral cortex (especially motor areas). These cortical inputs provide the most rapid access to basal nuclei output nuclei (cortex→subthalamic nucleus→GPi) and are thought by some to play a central role in basal nuclei functions. Just as in the case of the striatum and GPe, different sectors of the subthalamic nucleus deal with motor, cognitive, and affective functions.

Part of the Substantia Nigra Modulates the Output of the Striatum and Other Parts of the Basal Nuclei

As mentioned earlier, the substantia nigra is actually two structures, with two distinctly different functions.

The reticular part of the substantia nigra resembles in many respects a displaced portion of the internal segment of the globus pallidus. Like GPi, the SNr receives inputs from the striatum, GPe, and subthalamic nucleus and projects to VA/VL and the dorsomedial nucleus of the thalamus (see Fig. 19-14). In addition, there are projections from SNr to the superior colliculus and the reticular formation (pedunculopontine nucleus). The connection with the superior colliculus is one route through which the basal nuclei participate in the control of eye movements (see Chapter 21).

The pigmented neurons of SNc and the medially adjacent ventral tegmental area (VTA), which use dopamine as their neurotransmitter, blanket the basal nuclei with modulatory inputs. A massive, topographically organized projection to the striatum is the best known, but most other parts of the basal nuclei also receive these inputs. These dopaminergic endings ultimately modulate the output from GPi-SNr (see Fig. 19-21D). Defects in this influence can result in movement disorders (putamen connections) and presumably in cognitive deficits as well (caudate connections). Comparable dopaminergic projections to the ventral striatum arise mainly in the VTA and have been implicated in such limbic functions as responses to novel or rewarding stimuli. SNr and VTA receive important inputs from the striatum and globus

[b]This complex bundle also includes cerebellar output fibers described in the next chapter.

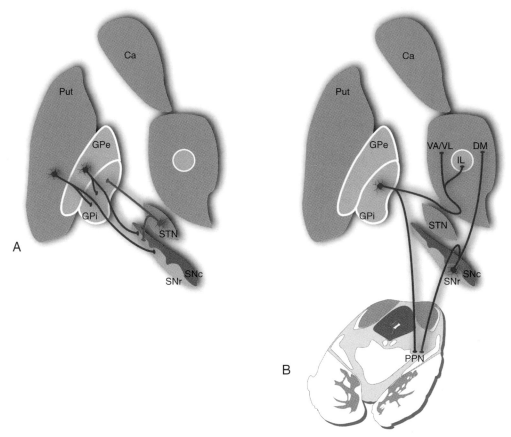

Figure 19-14 Major afferents to **(A)** and efferents from **(B)** the internal segment of the globus pallidus (GPi) and the reticular part of the substantia nigra (SNr). Excitatory connections are shown in *green*, inhibitory connections in *red*. Ca, caudate nucleus; DM, dorsomedial nucleus; GPe, external segment of the globus pallidus; IL, intralaminar nuclei; PPN, pedunculopontine nucleus; Put, putamen; SNc, compact part of the substantia nigra; STN, subthalamic nucleus; VA/VL, ventral anterior and ventral lateral nuclei.

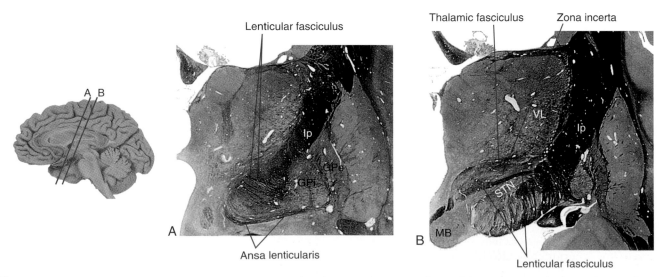

Figure 19-15 Efferents from the globus pallidus, seen in coronal sections. **A,** Enlargement of part of the section in Figure 19-2B, showing fibers of the lenticular fasciculus passing through the posterior limb of the internal capsule (Ip) and the ansa lenticularis hooking around it. **B,** Part of a coronal section through the mammillary bodies (MB) and ventral lateral nucleus (VL). Once they have crossed the internal capsule (Ip), fibers of the lenticular fasciculus move medially between the subthalamic nucleus (STN) and the zona incerta. They hook around the medial edge of the zona incerta and join with the ansa lenticularis and ascending cerebellar fibers to form the thalamic fasciculus. Planes of section are indicated in the inset to the left.

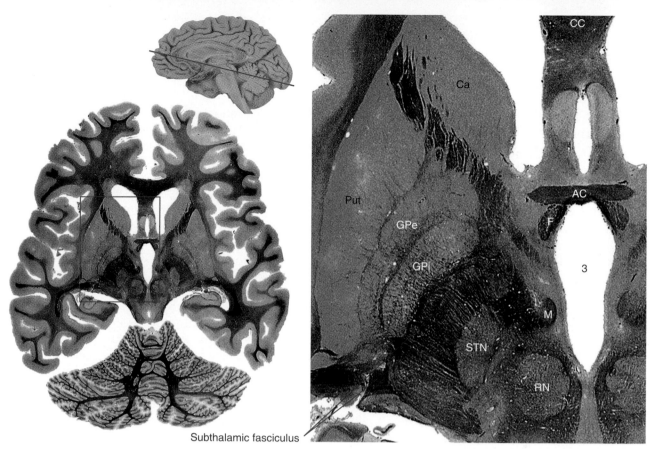

Subthalamic fasciculus

Figure 19-16 Subthalamic fasciculus as seen in an axial section. Subthalamic fasciculus is a collective term for the small bundles of fibers that pass through the internal capsule, interconnecting the subthalamic nucleus (STN) and the external (GPe) and internal (GPi) segments of the globus pallidus. 3, third ventricle; AC, anterior commissure; Ca, head of the caudate nucleus; CC, genu of the corpus callosum; F, fornix; M, mammillothalamic tract; Put, putamen; RN, red nucleus.

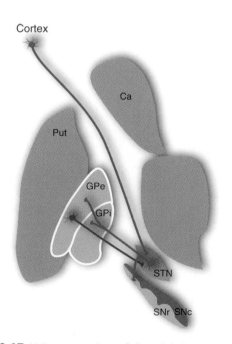

Figure 19-17 Major connections of the subthalamic nucleus (STN). Excitatory connections are shown in *green,* inhibitory connections in *red.* Ca, caudate nucleus; GPe and GPi, external and internal segments of the globus pallidus; Put, putamen; SNc and SNr, compact and reticular parts of the substantia nigra.

pallidus, so in some way, the basal nuclei are able to control their own supply of dopamine.

Perforating Branches From the Cerebral Arterial Circle (of Willis) Supply the Basal Nuclei

Like other deep structures located superior to the cerebral arterial circle, the basal nuclei receive their blood supply from small ganglionic or perforating branches of arteries in and adjacent to the circle. One would therefore expect the substantia nigra and subthalamic nucleus, located just below the posterior thalamus (see Fig. 19-2C), to be supplied by branches from posterior portions of the arterial circle. The striatum and globus pallidus are mostly anterior to this level (see Fig. 19-1), so their supply should come from more anterior portions of the circle. Hence the substantia nigra and subthalamic nucleus are supplied mainly by perforating branches of the posterior cerebral and posterior communicating arteries, the striatum by perforating branches of the middle cerebral artery (also referred to as **lenticulostriate** or **lateral striate arteries**), and the globus pallidus by the anterior choroidal artery (see Fig. 6-22).

Branches of the anterior cerebral artery help supply the striatum in the vicinity of nucleus accumbens and the head of the caudate nucleus; one of these is a particularly large branch referred to as the **medial striate artery** (of Heubner; see Fig. 6-8).

Many Basal Nuclei Disorders Result in Abnormalities of Movement

Involuntary movements, problems initiating movements, and disturbances of muscle tone figure prominently in the best known disorders involving the basal nuclei. The involuntary movements of **hyperkinetic disorders** are customarily subdivided into tremors and states of **chorea, athetosis,** and **ballismus.** Disturbances of tone may be such that tone is increased in flexors and extensors generally (as in the rigidity of Parkinson's disease) or only in some muscles, so that the patient's body is bent or twisted into an abnormal, relatively fixed posture. The latter condition is called **dystonia.** In still other cases, tone may be decreased.

Patients with chorea (from the Greek word for "dance") exhibit a series of nearly continuous, rapid movements of the face, tongue, or limbs (usually the distal portions of the limbs). The movements often resemble fragments of normal voluntary movements. **Huntington's disease** (**chorea**) is a hereditary disorder characterized by neuronal degeneration that is particularly severe in the striatum, especially in the caudate nucleus (Fig. 19-18), and affects neurons in the cerebral cortex and elsewhere to a lesser extent. Typically, symptoms first appear between the ages of 30 and 50 years as some combination of involuntary choreiform movements and alterations of mood or cognitive function. The movements slowly become more pronounced, and this symptom is followed or accompanied by gradually worsening dementia and personality changes. The chorea is presumably caused by striatal degeneration, and the dementia by some combination of caudate and cortical degeneration. This is a particularly nasty disease because it is inherited in an autosomal dominant pattern, but usually does not appear until after individuals are old enough to have started families. The defective gene has been localized to the short arm of chromosome 4, and tests are now available to determine whether an individual is indeed a carrier and will develop the disease. Hence it is also possible to determine whether half the children of an individual at risk are likely to be affected.

Athetosis (from a Greek word meaning "without position") is characterized by slow, writhing movements, most pronounced in the hands and fingers, so that a patient may be unable to keep the affected limb in a fixed position. The responsible lesion seems to be in the striatum. All intermediate forms between chorea and athetosis are seen, and questionable cases are often referred to as **choreoathetosis**. No one knows why a particular lesion in the striatum induces one state rather than the other.

Hemiballismus (*ballismus* comes from a Greek word meaning "jumping about") is one of the most dramatic disorders of the basal nuclei. Its most prominent characteristic is wild flailing movements of one arm and leg. The responsible lesion is usually in the contralateral

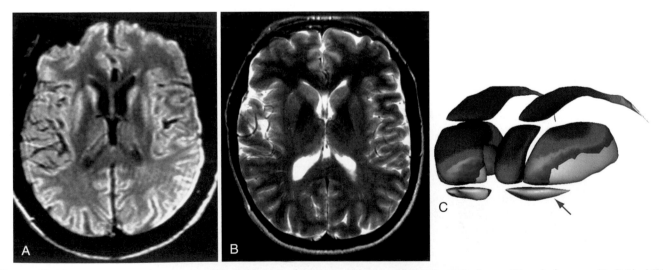

Figure 19-18 Axial magnetic resonance imaging (MRI) scans of a 29-year-old man with Huntington's disease (**A**) and of a normal individual (**B**). Notice how much smaller the caudate nucleus and putamen are in **A,** and how the anterior horn of the lateral ventricle has expanded to take up the volume vacated by the caudate nucleus. **C,** MRI reconstructions of various parts of the striatum of 20 patients with early Huntington's disease reveals that there is a dorsal-ventral gradient in the pattern of degeneration. Areas in *red* show the most degeneration, areas in *blue* the least. In early stages, the ventral striatum (*arrow*) is affected little. (**A,** *courtesy Dr. Erwin B. Montgomery Jr., University of Wisconsin Medical School.* **B,** *courtesy Dr. Roger Bird, St. Joseph's Hospital, Phoenix.* **C,** *from Douaud G et al: Neuroimage 32:1562, 2006.*)

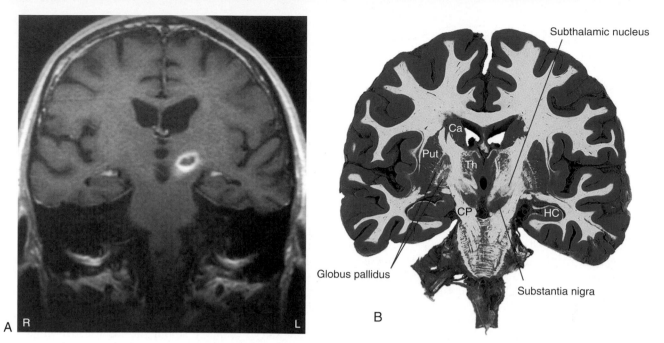

A R L

B

Subthalamic nucleus

Globus pallidus

Substantia nigra

Figure 19-19 Hemiballismus. **A,** A 65-year-old HIV-positive man developed, over the course of several months, "unintentional, forceful flinging movements of his right arm and leg." Contrast-enhanced coronal magnetic resonance imaging revealed a rim-enhancing mass (an appearance characteristic of an abscess) in the location of the subthalamic nucleus (compare to **B**). The involuntary movements resolved after several weeks of anti-toxoplasmosis treatment. **B,** Longitudinal slice of a normal brain in approximately the same plane as **A**. Ca, caudate nucleus; CP, cerebral peduncle; HC, hippocampus; Put, putamen; Th, thalamus. (**A**, *from Provenzale JM, Schwarzschild MA: AJNR Am J Neuroradiol 15:1377, 1994.* **B,** *prepared by Pamela Eller, University of Colorado Health Sciences Center.*)

subthalamic nucleus (Fig. 19-19). Hemiballismus is most often seen in older people, caused by a stroke involving a small ganglionic branch of the posterior cerebral artery. The reason movements are seen contralateral to the lesion is apparent from Figures 19-7 and 19-17: each subthalamic nucleus is related by way of GPi-SNr and VA/VL primarily to the ipsilateral motor cortex, which in turn is concerned with movements of the contralateral side of the body.

Parkinson's disease, the most prominent of the **hypokinetic disorders,** is the most common and best known disease involving the basal nuclei (Fig. 19-20). The symptoms are variable in severity and onset, but they usually include rigidity, slow and reduced movements, a stooped posture, and tremor. The **rigidity** is caused by increased tone in all muscles, although strength is nearly normal and reflexes are not particularly affected. The rigidity may be uniform throughout the range of movements imposed by an examiner (called **plastic** or **lead-pipe rigidity**), or it may be interrupted by a series of brief relaxations (called **cog-wheel rigidity**). Thus parkinsonian rigidity is quite distinct from spasticity; in spastic patients, muscle tone is increased selectively in the extensors of the leg and the flexors of the arm and can be overcome in the clasp-knife reaction, and stretch reflexes are hyperactive. The difficulty in moving (**bradykinesia,** or slow movements; **hypokinesia,** or few movements) is shown by such things as decreased blinking,

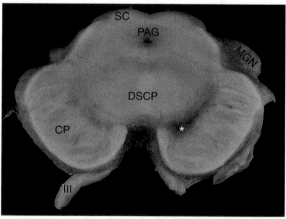

Figure 19-20 The midbrain of a patient with Parkinson's disease, showing loss of pigmentation in the compact part of the substantia nigra (*), more pronounced on the left side. CP, cerebral peduncle; DSCP, decussation of the superior cerebellar peduncles; III, oculomotor nerve; MGN, medial geniculate nucleus; PAG, periaqueductal gray; SC, superior colliculus. (*Courtesy Dr. Naomi Rance, University of Arizona College of Medicine.*)

an expressionless face, and the absence of the arm movements normally associated with walking. Bradykinesia and hypokinesia are fundamental deficits; they are not simply the result of rigidity, because patients whose rigidity is not pronounced can nevertheless have great difficulty moving. Finally, the tremor is a **resting tremor**

BOX 19-2

A Model for Movement Control by the Basal Nuclei

Each small portion of the internal segment of the globus pallidus makes inhibitory synapses in the restricted portion of the thalamus to which it projects. Thalamocortical projections are excitatory. Hence changes in the activity of a small portion of GPi would be expected to cause inverse changes in the activity of a corresponding small cortical area. This is the basis of a prominent model of basal nuclei function that suggests that a direct pathway from cortex→striatum→GPi-SNr→thalamus→cortex may facilitate selected cortical activity (Fig. 19-21A), while activity in an indirect pathway involving the subthalamic nucleus suppresses other cortical activity (Fig. 19-21B). A further implication is that decreased activity of neurons in the subthalamic nucleus should cause disorders that include many involuntary movements (hyperkinetic disorders), whereas increased activity of subthalamic neurons should cause hypokinetic disorders. Many of the clinical observations in basal nuclei disorders are consistent with this model. The involuntary movements of hemiballismus result from direct damage to the contralateral subthalamic

nucleus, which the model predicts would decrease the firing rate of GPi-SNr neurons (Fig. 19-21C). Conversely, the model also predicts that removal of the dopaminergic input to the striatum would result in increased subthalamic activity, increased Gpi-SNr activity (Fig. 19-21D and E), and hypokinesia, such as that seen in Parkinson's disease.

As successful as the direct-indirect pathway model has been in making sense of some of the symptoms and therapeutic interventions described elsewhere in this chapter, there is more to the story. There are many additional basal nuclei connections that are not included; for example, about half the synapses on GPi neurons come not from the striatum or the subthalamic nucleus but from GPe. In addition, a simple decrease or increase in GPi firing rate apparently does not underlie hyperkinetic and hypokinetic movement disorders, because the VA/VL action potential frequency is about the same in Huntington's and Parkinson's patients. It now appears that changes in the *pattern* of firing in various parts of the basal nuclei are responsible for the symptoms in such disorders.

---

characteristically involving the hands in a "pill-rolling" movement; it diminishes during voluntary movement and increases during emotional stress.

The parts of the basal nuclei not involved primarily in movement have been implicated in analogous disorders that include involuntary activation of other parts of the central nervous system (CNS), such as the stereotyped behaviors of Tourette's syndrome and the repetitive, intrusive thoughts of obsessive-compulsive disorder (OCD). Consistent with this, some of the same treatment strategies (described shortly) effective in dealing with basal nuclei movement disorders have been used successfully to treat severe cases of Tourette's and OCD.

Anatomical and Neurochemical Properties of the Basal Nuclei Suggest Effective Treatments for Disorders

Many disorders of the basal nuclei include striking **positive signs** (e.g., chorea, ballistic movements, rigidity, tremor) in which motor neurons are made to fire when they should not; they may also include **negative signs** (e.g., hypokinesia), in which motor neurons cannot easily be made to fire. Subsets of the basal nuclei connections described in this chapter have been used to try to explain these clinical observations (Box 19-2).

Postmortem examination of the brains of patients with Parkinson's disease indicated that damage is most consistently evident in the substantia nigra (Fig. 19-20), reflecting degeneration of the pigmented nigral cells

that normally manufacture dopamine and transport it to the striatum. It was therefore reasoned that if the dopamine could somehow be replaced, the symptoms might be ameliorated. Dopamine does not cross the blood-brain barrier, but administration of L-dopa (levodopa), a precursor of dopamine that does cross the barrier, reverses some of the functional abnormalities seen in Parkinson's disease (Fig. 19-22). Although this form of therapy has been a great help for many patients, it also has a number of shortcomings. After several years of L-dopa treatment, for example, many patients develop rapidly fluctuating responses to treatment, or L-dopa–induced involuntary movements. Therefore the search has continued for other therapeutic approaches.

In his original description, Parkinson remarked on a patient whose tremors disappeared on one side after suffering a stroke. This seems consistent with the idea that altered activity in the cortex→basal nuclei→cortex loop underlies these movement disorders, and it was reasoned some time ago that surgical intervention in part of the loop might alleviate some symptoms. Because the globus pallidus affects motor areas of the cortex by way of the VA/VL complex, logical sites for surgical destruction might seem to be GPi or VA/VL. Somewhat astoundingly, this turns out to be partially effective. Stereotactic lesions in the VA/VL region (**thalamotomy;** VL is the principal target) or, more commonly, in the internal segment of the globus pallidus or its output pathways (**pallidotomy**) are reasonably successful in relieving the tremor and rigidity of parkinsonism, the

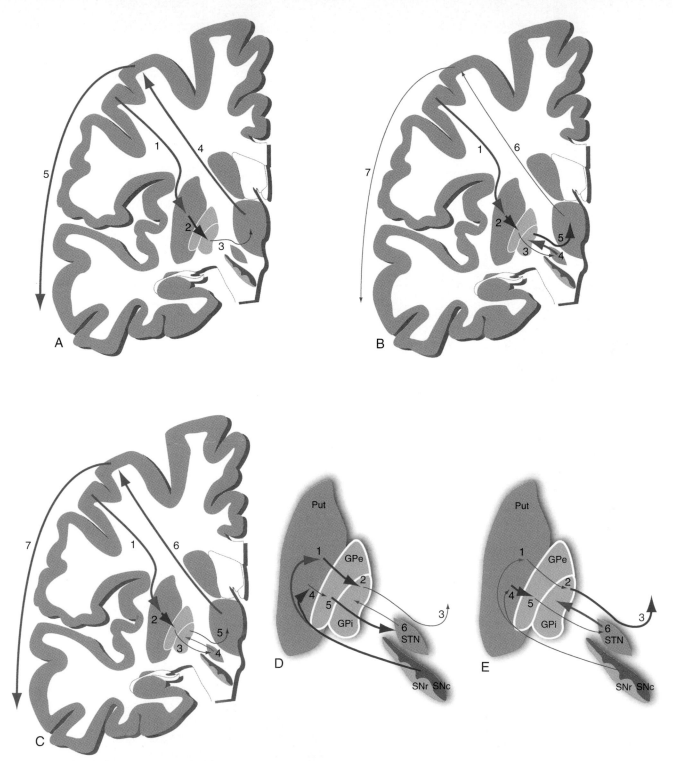

Figure 19-21 One model that uses some of the excitatory *(green)* and inhibitory *(red)* interactions in the basal nuclei to explain how they might function together to affect cortical output in health and disease. This is by no means a complete depiction of all such interactions in the basal nuclei, but it does illustrate how the alteration of a single element can unbalance the entire system. The level of activity in each pathway is roughly indicated by the thickness of a line. **A,** Proposed effect of the direct pathway through the basal nuclei in a normal individual. Excitatory corticostriatal fibers (1) activate inhibitory neurons in the striatum (2). The striatum inhibits the internal segment of the globus pallidus (GPi; 3) and the reticular part of the substantia nigra (SNr; not shown), thus disinhibiting the thalamus (4). This allows the thalamus to facilitate certain cortical outputs (5). **B,** Effect of the indirect pathway, utilizing the subthalamic nucleus (STN), in a normal individual. In this case, cortical input and striatal output (1, 2) diminish output from the external segment of the globus pallidus (GPe; 3), leading indirectly to increased inhibition of the thalamus (4, 5) and diminished cortical output (6, 7). Acting in parallel, the direct and indirect pathways (**A** and **B**) could facilitate activity in some cortical areas while inhibiting activity in others. **C,** Loss of excitatory subthalamic projections (4) disinhibits the thalamus (5), leading to a failure to suppress some cortical outputs (6, 7), which could manifest as involuntary movements (e.g., hemiballismus). **D,** The striatal neurons projecting into the direct and indirect pathways have different dopamine receptors: dopamine excites the former (1) and inhibits the latter (4). Hence dopamine facilitates movement, suppressing GPi output (3) through both the direct (1, 2) and indirect (4, 5, 6) pathways. **E,** In Parkinson's disease, the model predicts that loss of dopaminergic neurons from the compact part of the substantia nigra (SNc) will cause decreased activity in the direct pathway (1, 2) and increased activity in the indirect pathway (4, 5, 6), both of which enhance the output of GPi and SNr (3). The resulting inhibition of the thalamus causes a diminished cortical output, which could underlie bradykinesia and hypokinesia. Put, putamen.

flailing movements of hemiballismus, and some other involuntary movements and abnormalities of tone. Carefully placed lesions can even improve negative signs such as hypokinesia (Fig. 19-23). In the case of hemiballismus, the excessive activity of the basal nuclei is apparently expressed primarily through the corticospinal tract. This tract has been sectioned in the cerebral peduncle in a few humans (on the side contralateral to the ballistic movements) for the relief of hemiballismus. The involuntary movements were permanently abolished, and a transient, flaccid paralysis ensued on the

side contralateral to the surgery; however, as noted in the previous chapter, there were rather limited long-term deficits.

Considering the proximity of VA/VL and GPi to structures such as the internal capsule, this type of surgery has always been a last resort, and other forms of treatment have long been sought. A more recent surgical approach involves implanting electrodes in the globus pallidus or subthalamic nucleus and providing chronic stimulation with high-frequency bursts (**deep brain stimulation**); this has the effect of replacing the abnormal activity in these nuclei with regular trains of action potentials—in effect, removing the abnormal activity. This has now become a widespread treatment for advanced Parkinson's disease. The subthalamic nucleus and internal segment of the globus pallidus are favored targets, there is also evidence that stimulation of the pedunculopontine nucleus and the centromedian/ parafascicular thalamic nuclei may be effective in treating motor abnormalities.

Another initially promising area of research involved attempts to replace degenerated nigral cells. Because the CNS is largely isolated from the immune system, rejection of implanted tissue is not as great a concern as in other organs, and dopaminergic cells from human fetal midbrains (and even the midbrains of other mammals) have been successfully implanted into the striatum of a small number of patients with Parkinson's disease. The implantation of stem cells has thus far produced disappointing results.

Additional avenues of research in basal nuclei disorders were opened by the development of a primate model of Parkinson's disease. In the early 1980s several

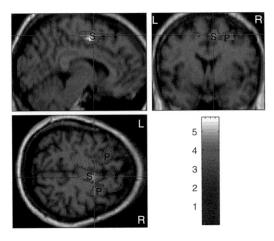

Figure 19-22 Increased blood flow in the supplementary motor area (S) and premotor cortex (P) of Parkinson's disease patients during movement following treatment with L-dopa. Blood flow was measured by functional magnetic resonance imaging (fMRI) as patients moved a joystick in response to hearing a tone. Areas where blood flow increased more following L-dopa treatment are shown superimposed on T1-weighted MRI scans. *(From Haslinger B et al: Brain 124:558, 2001.)*

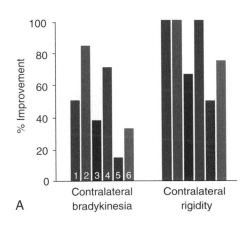

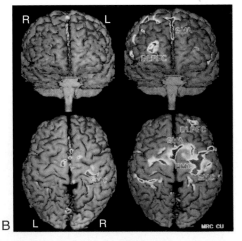

Figure 19-23 Improvement in motor system function of Parkinson's disease patients following unilateral pallidotomy. **A,** Improvements in clinical measures of bradykinesia and rigidity in six different patients 3 to 4 months after surgery. **B,** Cerebral blood flow increases during left-handed joystick movements before *(left)* and 18 weeks after *(right)* a right-sided pallidotomy. Both sets of positron emission tomography scans were obtained 12 hours after the 64-year-old patient's last dose of medication, and the results were superimposed on a reconstruction of the patient's brain derived from magnetic resonance images. Blood flow increased in the supplementary motor area (SMA), premotor cortex (PMC), and dorsolateral prefrontal cortex (DLPFC), primarily ipsilateral to the side of the pallidotomy. SMC, sensorimotor cortex adjacent to the central sulcus. *(A, plotted from data in Samuel M et al: Brain 120:1301, 1997. B, from Ceballos-Baumann AO et al: Lancet 344:814, 1994.)*

young individuals with what appeared to be severe Parkinson's disease were found to have injected themselves with a "synthetic heroin" that turned out to be meperidine contaminated with a compound called MPTP (1-methyl-4-phenyl-1,2,3,6-tetrahydropyridine). It was quickly found that MPTP is selectively toxic to dopaminergic neurons of the primate substantia nigra. This made certain types of controlled experiments more feasible and also lent credence to the idea that some as yet unidentified environmental agents (possibly pesticides) play an important role in most cases of Parkinson's disease.

The basal nuclei have proved to be a treasure trove of chemically coded neural subsystems. The dopaminergic projection from the substantia nigra to the striatum is one example, but there are many others. The many common features of the various syndromes caused by damage to diverse parts of the basal nuclei give rise to the concept that these neural structures form a finely tuned system in which malfunction of any part can throw the whole system out of balance. Thus a decrease in dopamine levels in the striatum causes parkinsonian symptoms. This can occur naturally (in Parkinson's disease) or as a side effect of drugs that act as dopamine antagonists (e.g., phenothiazines used for psychiatric disorders). In contrast, increased levels of dopamine in the striatum, as in parkinsonian patients who receive too much L-dopa, can cause choreiform and athetoid movements, as though the system were now tilted in the opposite direction. The study of these neurochemical balancing mechanisms is an active area of research.

SUGGESTED READINGS

Afonso F, et al: Treatment of motor and non-motor features of Parkinson's disease with deep brain stimulation. Lancet 11:429–442, 2012.

Albin RL, Mink JW: Recent advances in Tourette syndrome research. Trends Neurosci 29:175, 2006.

Alexander GE, DeLong MR, Strick PL: Parallel organization of functionally segregated circuits linking basal ganglia and cortex. Annu Rev Neurosci 9:357, 1986.

Alexander L: The vascular supply of the striopallidum. Res Publ Assoc Res Nerv Ment Dis 21:77, 1942.

Aouizerate B, et al: Deep brain stimulation of the ventral caudate nucleus in the treatment of obsessive-compulsive disorder and major depression. J Neurosurg 101:682, 2004.

Bergman H, Wichmann T, DeLong MR: Reversal of experimental parkinsonism by lesions of the subthalamic nucleus. Science 249:1436, 1990.
   Work emphasizing the critical role of the subthalamic nucleus in the movement abnormalities seen in multiple basal ganglia disorders, including Parkinson's disease.

Carpenter MB: Athetosis and the basal ganglia: review of the literature and study of forty-two cases. Arch Neurol Psychiatry 63:875, 1950.

Cory-Slechta DA, et al: Developmental pesticide models of the Parkinson disease prototype. Environ Health Prospect 113:1263–1270, 2005.

Crick FC, Koch C: What is the function of the claustrum? Phil Trans R Soc B 360:1271–1279, 2005.

Dauer W, Przedborski S: Parkinson's disease: mechanisms and models. Neuron 39:889, 2003.

Deng YP, et al: Differential loss of striatal projection systems in Huntington's disease: a quantitative immunohistochemical study. J Chem Neuroanat 27:143, 2004.

Denian JM, Menetrey A, Charpier S: The lamellar organization of the rat substantia nigra pars reticulata: segregated patterns of striatal afferents and relationship to the topography of corticostriatal projections. Neuroscience 73:761, 1996.

Detante O, et al: Globus pallidus internus stimulation in primary generalized dystonia: a $H_2^{15}O$ PET study. Brain 127:1899, 2004.

Dick JPR, et al: Simple and complex movements in a patient with infarction of the supplementary motor area. Mov Disord 1:255, 1986.
   Clinical evidence bearing on the relationship between the putamen and the supplementary motor area.

Dishman PS: Paradoxical aspects of parkinsonian tremor. Mov Disord 23:168, 2008.

Douaud G, et al: Distribution of grey matter atrophy in Huntington's disease patients: a combined ROI-based and voxel-based morphometric study. Neuroimage 32:1562, 2006.

Emre M: Dementia associated with Parkinson's disease. Lancet Neurol 2:229, 2003.

Feekes JA, Cassell MD: The vascular supply of the functional compartments of the human striatum. Brain 129:2, 2006.

Fine J, et al: Long-term follow-up of unilateral pallidotomy in advanced Parkinson's disease. N Engl J Med 342:1708, 2000.

François C, et al: Behavioural disorders induced by external globus pallidus dysfunction in primates. II. Anatomical study. Brain 127:2055, 2004.

Freed CR, et al: Transplantation of embryonic dopamine neurons for severe Parkinson's disease. N Engl J Med 344:710, 2001.

Gerardin E, et al: Foot, hand, face and eye representation in the human striatum. Cereb Cortex 13:162, 2003.

Goldman PS, Nauta WJH: An intricately patterned prefrontocaudate projection in the rhesus monkey. J Comp Neurol 171:369, 1977.
   Early results indicating that the traditional view of the striatum as a uniformly organized structure is an oversimplification.

Grabli D, et al: Behavioural disorders induced by external globus pallidus dysfunction in primates. I. Behavioural study. Brain 127:2039, 2004.

Graybiel AM, Ragsdale CW, Jr: Histochemically distinct compartments in the striatum of human, monkey, and cat demonstrated by acetylthiocholinesterase staining. Proc Natl Acad Sci U S A 75:5723, 1978.
   Additional results, complementary to those of Goldman and Nauta, indicating that the striatum is a jigsaw puzzle in terms of both connections and neurotransmitters.

Guehl D, et al: Tremor-related activity of neurons in the "motor" thalamus: changes in firing rate and pattern in the MPTP vervet model of parkinsonism. Eur J Neurosci 17:2388, 2003.

Guridi J, Lozano AM: A brief history of pallidotomy. Neurosurgery 41:1169, 1997.

Haber SN, Gdowski MJ: Basal ganglia. In Paxinos G, Mai JK, editors: The human nervous system, ed 2, San Diego, 2004, Elsevier Academic Press.

Hamani C, et al: The subthalamic nucleus in the context of movement disorders. Brain 127:4, 2004.

Holt DJ, Graybiel AM, Saper CB: Neurochemical architecture of the human striatum. J Comp Neurol 384:1, 1997.

Hopkins DA, Niesser LW: Substantia nigra projections to the reticular formation, superior colliculus and central gray in the rat, cat and monkey. Neurosci Lett 2:253, 1976.

Hore J, Meyer-Lohmann J, Brooks VB: Basal ganglia cooling disables learned arm movements of monkeys in the absence of visual guidance. Science 195:584, 1977.

Karachi C, et al: The pallidosubthalamic projection: an anatomical substrate for nonmotor functions of the subthalamic nucleus in primates. Mov Disord 20:172, 2005.

Kemp JM, Powell TPS: The connexions of the striatum and globus pallidus: synthesis and speculation. Philos Trans R Soc Lond B 262:441, 1971.

An early hypothesis of basal ganglia connectivity, before the multiple parallel loops were found.

Langston JW, et al: Chronic parkinsonism in humans due to a product of meperidine-analog synthesis. Science 219:979, 1983.

One of the original descriptions of MPTP-induced parkinsonism.

Lévesque M, Parent A: The striatofugal fiber system in primates: a reevaluation of its organization based on single-axon tracing studies. Proc Natl Acad Sci U S A 102:11888, 2005.

Many individual axons leaving the striatum terminate in GPe, GPi, and SNr.

Lindvall O, et al: Grafts of fetal dopamine neurons survive and improve motor function in Parkinson's disease. Science 247:574, 1990.

Marsden CD, Obeso JA: The functions of the basal ganglia and the paradox of stereotaxic surgery in Parkinson's disease. Brain 117:877, 1994.

The paradox lies in trying to explain why damage to the globus pallidus or VA/VL does not impair movement further.

Martin JP: The basal ganglia and posture, Tunbridge Wells, UK, 1967, Pitman Medical Publishing.

Menzies L, et al: Integrating evidence from neuroimaging and neuropsychological studies of obsessive-compulsive disorder: the orbitofronto-striatal model revisited. Neurosci Biobehav Rev 32:525, 2008.

Middleton FA, Strick PL: Basal ganglia and cerebellar loops: motor and cognitive circuits. Brain Res Rev 31:236, 2000.

Misgeld U: Innervation of the substantia nigra. Cell Tissue Res 318:107, 2004.

Morizane A, Li J-Y, Brundin P: From bench to bed: the potential of stem cells for the treatment of Parkinson's disease. Cell Tissue Res 331:323, 2008.

Nambu A, Tokuno H, Takada M: Functional significance of the cortico-subthalamo-pallidal "hyperdirect" pathway. Neurosci Res 43:111, 2002.

Obeso JA, Benabid AL, Koller WC, editors: Deep brain stimulation for Parkinson's disease and tremor. Neurology 55(Suppl 6), 2000.

Olanow CW, et al: A double-blind controlled trial of bilateral fetal nigral transplantation in Parkinson's disease. Ann Neurol 54:403–414, 2003.

Pahapill PA, Lozano AM: The pedunculopontine nucleus and Parkinson's disease. Brain 123:1767, 2000.

Perlmutter JS, Mink JW: Deep brain stimulation. Annu Rev Neurosci 29:229, 2006.

Pessiglione M, et al: Thalamic neuronal activity in dopamine-depleted primates: evidence for a loss of functional segregation within basal ganglia circuits. J Neurosci 25:1523, 2005.

Provenzale JM, Schwarzschild MA: Hemiballismus. AJNR Am J Neuroradiol 15:1377, 1994.

Redmond DE, Jr, et al: Behavioral improvement in a primate Parkinson's model is associated with multiple homeostatic effects of human neural stem cells. Proc Natl Acad Sci U S A 104:12175, 2007.

Rodriguez-Oroz MC, et al: Bilateral deep brain stimulation in Parkinson's disease: a multicentre study with 4 years follow-up. Brain 128:2240, 2005.

Romanelli P, et al: Somatotopy in the basal ganglia: experimental and clinical evidence for segregated sensorimotor channels. Brain Res Rev 48:112, 2005.

Sadikot AF, Parent A, François C: The centre median and parafascicular thalamic nuclei project respectively to the sensorimotor and associative-limbic striatal territories in the squirrel monkey. Brain Res 510:161, 1990.

Singer HS: Tourette's syndrome: from behaviour to biology. Lancet Neurol 4:149, 2005.

Smith Y, Parent A: Differential connections of caudate nucleus and putamen in the squirrel monkey (Saimiri sciureus). Neuroscience 18:347, 1986.

Soares J, et al: Role of external pallidal segment in primate parkinsonism: comparison of the effects of 1-methyl-4-phenyl-1,2,3,6-tetrahydropyridine-induced parkinsonism and lesions of the external pallidal segment. J Neurosci 24:6417, 2004.

Simply increasing the firing rate of GPi neurons does not necessarily cause a hypokinetic disorder.

Stefani A, et al: Bilateral deep brain stimulation of the pedunculopontine and subthalamic nuclei in severe Parkinson's disease. Brain 130:1596, 2007.

Tang JKH, et al: Firing rates of pallidal neurons are similar in Huntington's and Parkinson's disease patients. Exp Brain Res 166:230, 2005.

But the firing patterns are different.

van Domburg PHMF, ten Donkelaar HJ: The human substantia nigra and ventral tegmental area: a neuroanatomical study with notes on aging and aging diseases. Adv Anat Embryol Cell Biol 121:1, 1991.

Walker FO: Huntington's disease. Lancet 369:218, 2007.

Whittier JR: Ballism and the subthalamic nucleus (nucleus hypothalamicus; corpus Luysi): review of the literature and study of thirty cases. Arch Neurol Psychiatry 58:672, 1947.

Cerebellum

20

Chapter Outline

Cerebellum means "little brain," and in a real sense, it is: it accounts for only about 10% of the mass of the brain, but the cerebellum contains as many neurons as all the rest of the central nervous system (CNS) combined. This semidetached mass of neural tissue covers most of the posterior surface of the brainstem, tethered there by three pairs of fiber bundles called **cerebellar peduncles.** Sensory inputs of virtually every description find their way to the uniquely structured cortex of the cerebellum, which in turn projects (via a set of **deep cerebellar nuclei**) to various sites in the brainstem and thalamus. Although the cerebellum is extensively concerned with the processing of sensory information, and although it has few ways to influence motor neurons directly, it is considered part of the motor system because cerebellar damage results in abnormalities of equilibrium, postural control, and coordination of voluntary movements.

The Cerebellum Can Be Divided Into Both Transverse and Longitudinal Zones

The outside of the cerebellum has a banded appearance, as though its surface were folded like an accordion (Figs. 20-1 and 20-2). This folding is a successful way to increase surface area; by some estimates, if the cortex could be unfolded into a flat sheet, it would be more than 1 meter long (Fig. 20-3). Deep **fissures,** most easily seen in sagittal sections (see Fig. 20-2E), indent the cerebellar surface. Smaller creases indent the walls of these deep fissures, with the result that the entire cerebellar surface is made up of cortical ridges called **folia,**[a] most of which are transversely oriented; prominent fissures are the basis of common systems of dividing the cerebellum into **lobes** and **lobules.** Beneath the cortex is a mass of white matter, the **medullary center** of the cerebellum, which is composed of fibers going to or coming from the cerebellar cortex.

Transverse Fissures Divide the Cerebellum Into Lobes

The first fissure to appear during development is the **posterolateral fissure,** which separates the **flocculonodular lobe** from the **body of the cerebellum (corpus cerebelli).** In humans, the body of the cerebellum is by far the larger of the two parts, and the posterolateral fissure is so deep that the **flocculus** of each side is almost pinched off from the rest of the cerebellum (see Figs.

[a]Because the white matter of the cerebellum has a treelike appearance in sagittal sections (see Fig. 20-2E), it was named arbor vitae ("tree of life") by early anatomists. In a continuation of the tree analogy, each of the cortical folds on the surface of the arbor vitae is called a folium (Latin for "leaf," as in foliage).

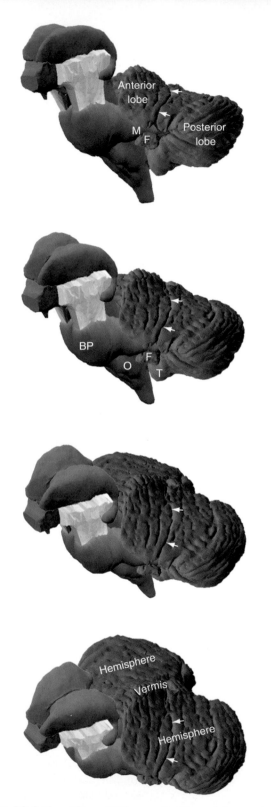

Figure 20-1 Three-dimensional reconstructions of the cerebellum, brainstem, and diencephalon. The primary fissure *(arrows)* subdivides most of the cerebellum into an anterior and posterior lobe, each straddling the midline and including part of a midline zone (the vermis) and part of each hemisphere. (See Videos 20-1 and 20-2.) BP, basal pons; F, flocculus (an additional part of each hemisphere); M, middle cerebellar peduncle; O, olive; T, tonsil (part of the posterior lobe).

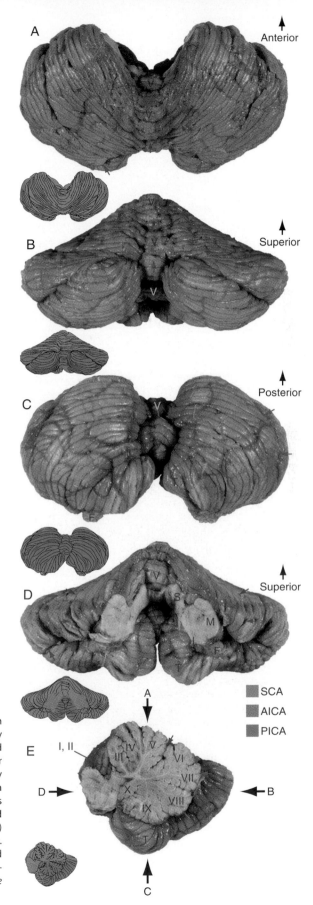

Figure 20-2 Gross anatomy and blood supply of the cerebellum, seen from above **(A)**, behind **(B)**, below **(C)**, in front **(D)**, and hemisected **(E)**. The primary fissure, marking the division between the anterior and posterior lobes, is indicated by *blue arrows*. The horizontal fissure, which prominently subdivides the posterior lobe, is indicated by *green arrows*. In the hemisected view **(E)**, the depth of many of the cerebellar fissures is apparent; these are used to divide the vermis into a number of lobules, commonly referred to by roman numerals. The same fissures continue laterally and divide up the cerebellar hemispheres (see also Fig. 20-4 and Table 20-1). Vermal lobules I and II are thin plates of cerebellar tissue (the lingula) that cover the roof of the rostral fourth ventricle; vermal lobule X is the nodulus. AICA, anterior inferior cerebellar artery; F, flocculus; I, M, and S, inferior, middle, and superior cerebellar peduncles; PICA, posterior inferior cerebellar artery; SCA, superior cerebellar artery; T, tonsil; V, vermis. *(Modified from Nolte J, Angevine JB Jr: The human brain in photographs and diagrams, ed 3, St. Louis, 2007, Mosby.)*

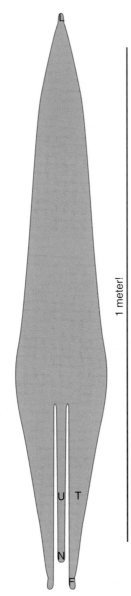

Figure 20-3 What the human cerebellar cortex would look like if it could be peeled off the surface of the cerebellum and laid out as a flat sheet. The deep notches at the bottom indicate that some of the transverse bands of cerebellar cortex (e.g., the flocculus and nodulus; see Fig. 2-11D) lose their continuity during development. F, flocculus; L, lingula; N, nodulus; T, tonsil; U, uvula. *(Redrawn from Braitenberg V, Atwood RP: J Comp Neurol 109:1, 1958.)*

20-1 and 20-2D). The **primary fissure,** a prominent landmark in midsagittal sections of the cerebellum, subdivides the body of the cerebellum into **anterior** and **posterior lobes.**

Functional Connections Divide the Cerebellum Into Longitudinal Zones

The cerebellum can also be divided into longitudinal zones, perpendicular to the fissures, which cut across the anterior, posterior, and flocculonodular lobes (Fig.

20-4). The most medial zone, straddling the midline, is the **vermis** (Latin for "worm"). On either side of the vermis is a large **cerebellar hemisphere.** Each hemisphere is subdivided into a **medial zone,** a longitudinal strip adjacent to the vermis (sometimes called the intermediate or paravermal zone), and a larger **lateral zone.** The vermis is fairly clearly set off from the hemispheres on the inferior surface of the cerebellum[b] (see Fig. 20-2C), but other longitudinal lines of separation are not as obvious from the outside (see Fig. 20-2A). The demarcation into longitudinal zones is based primarily on patterns of connections and on functional differences, as described shortly; cerebellar cortex has the same structure everywhere and is smoothly continuous from one hemisphere across the midline to the other.

The fissures that carve the cerebellum into lobules and folia are continuous across the midline during development, so each transverse wedge of cerebellum has a vermal portion and a more lateral portion. For example, the **nodulus** is the vermal portion of the flocculonodular lobe and continues laterally into the flocculus. The **tonsils** are the hemispheral portions just across the posterolateral fissure from the flocculi; appropriately enough, their vermal continuation is the **uvula.** An assortment of exotic names is applied to the lobules and the vermal areas of the corpus cerebelli (Table 20-1; see Fig. 20-4), and a roman numeral system is commonly used as well; for the most part, however, these names and numbers are of limited utility in clinical settings. (One exception is the tonsil. Because this is the part of the cerebellum adjacent to the foramen magnum, expanding masses in the posterior fossa can cause tonsillar herniation and compression of the medulla [see Fig. 4-19D].)

Three Peduncles Convey the Inputs and Outputs of Each Half of the Cerebellum

The cerebellum is attached to the brainstem by three peduncles on each side (Figs. 20-5 and 20-6). The **inferior cerebellar peduncle,** composed mainly of afferents to the cerebellum from the spinal cord and brainstem, has two parts. Most of it is the **restiform** ("ropelike") **body,** which ascends through the rostral medulla, growing larger as it accumulates cerebellar afferents. At the pontomedullary junction it turns posteriorly toward the cerebellum, and additional fibers travel over its medial surface as the **juxtarestiform body** (see Fig. 15-6)

---

[b]Vermis originally referred to the midline zone of the inferior surface of the cerebellum, which has a sinuous, wormlike appearance and is clearly set off from the hemispheres (see Fig. 20-2C). It is now used to refer to the midline strip throughout the cerebellum, even though its borders are harder to distinguish on the superior surface.

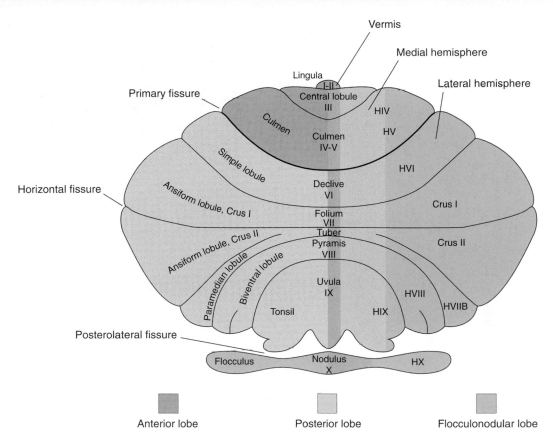

Figure 20-4 Cerebellar terminology on a schematic cerebellum, projected as though it were flattened out with its vermis in one plane (compare with Fig. 20-2). The general division into transversely oriented lobes is indicated on the left side of the diagram, and the division into longitudinal zones is indicated on the right. Also included is terminology for the various subdivisions of the vermis and lobules of the hemispheres. On the left side of the diagram are terms classically used for human cerebellar hemispheres. In the middle, both classic names and roman numerals are indicated for the vermis. On the right side is the roman numeral–based system more commonly used today for the hemispheres. This consists mostly of a series of lateral extensions of the vermal numbers, with an H added to signify hemisphere. The exceptions are crus I and crus II; these are parts of lobule HVII that are greatly expanded in the human cerebellum. *(Drawing modified from Larsell O: Anatomy of the nervous system, ed 2, New York, 1951, Appleton-Century-Crofts. Terminology based on Schmahmann JD et al: Neuroimage 10:233, 1999.)*

Table 20-1	Terminology for Parts of the Cerebellum

Vermis	Other Names	Hemisphere	Other Names
I	Lingula*		
II	Lingula*	HII	Lingula*
III	Central lobule	HIII	Central lobule
IV, V	Culmen	HIV, HV	Culmen anterior quadrangular lobule
VI	Declive	HVI	Simple lobule
			Posterior quadrangular lobule
VII	Upper part: folium	Crus 1	HVIIA, crus I
	Lower part: tuber		Ansiform lobule, crus I
			Superior semilunar lobule
		Crus II	HVIIA, crus II
			Ansiform lobule, crus II
			Inferior semilunar lobule
		HVIIB	Paramedian lobule
			Gracile lobule
VIII	Pyramis	HVIII	Biventral
IX	Uvula	HIX	Tonsil
X	Nodulus	HX	Flocculus

*Lobule I is a speck of vermal cortex in the roof of the rostral fourth ventricle. Lobule II extends a short distance into the hemisphere.

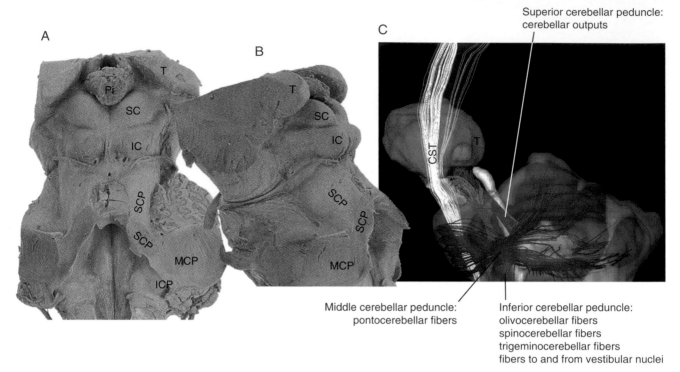

Figure 20-5 Posterior (**A**) and lateral (**B**) views of the severed cerebellar peduncles. **C,** Diffusion tensor image of a lateral view of the brainstem, showing the courses and an overview of the contents of the cerebellar peduncles (for more details, see Table 20-3). CST, corticospinal tract; IC, inferior colliculus; ICP, inferior cerebellar peduncle; MCP, middle cerebellar peduncle; Pi, pineal gland; SC, superior colliculus; SCP, superior cerebellar peduncle; T, thalamus. (**C,** from Mori S et al: MRI atlas of human white matter, Amsterdam, 2005, Elsevier.)

interconnecting the cerebellum and vestibular nuclei. The **middle cerebellar peduncle** (or **brachium pontis**—the "arm of the pons"), the largest of the three, emerges laterally from the basal pons. It is composed of afferents to the cerebellum from the pontine nuclei of the contralateral side. The **superior cerebellar peduncle** (or **brachium conjunctivum**[c]—the "joined-together arm," named for its decussation; see Figs. 11-11, 11-13, 11-14, 11-16, 11-17, and 20-22) contains the major efferent pathways from the cerebellum to the red nucleus and thalamus.

Deep Nuclei Are Embedded in the Cerebellar White Matter

A series of **deep cerebellar nuclei** is buried in the medullary center of each side of the cerebellum (Fig. 20-7). The

most lateral is the **dentate nucleus,** a crumpled sheet of cells that resembles the inferior olivary nucleus. Most of the fibers in the superior cerebellar peduncle originate from the dentate nucleus and emerge from its medially facing mouth, or **hilus** (see Fig. 20-6C). Medial to the dentate nucleus is the **interposed nucleus,** which in humans has two distinct subdivisions—an anterior and lateral **emboliform nucleus,** and a posterior and medial **globose nucleus.** (Because of their positions, the emboliform and globose nuclei are sometimes referred to as the anterior and posterior interposed nuclei, respectively.) Finally, the most medial of the deep cerebellar nuclei is the **fastigial nucleus.**

Inputs Reach the Cerebellar Cortex as Mossy and Climbing Fibers

The cortex of the cerebellum has a uniform three-layered structure (Fig. 20-8). The most superficial layer is the **molecular layer,** consisting mainly of the axons and dendrites of various cerebellar neurons. Deep to the molecular layer is the Purkinje layer, consisting of large neurons called **Purkinje cells.** Finally, adjacent to the medullary center is the **granular layer,** composed mainly of small **granule cells** arranged in a stratum many cells thick. The molecular and granular layers also contain

---

[c]There is a bit of a logical inconsistency in using the terms superior cerebellar peduncle and brachium conjunctivum synonymously. Brachium conjunctivum refers specifically to the large mass of cerebellar efferents bound mostly for the red nucleus and the thalamus (see Fig. 20-21), whereas the total superior cerebellar peduncle also includes a few cerebellar afferents, such as those of the anterior spinocerebellar tract, and many fibers that turn caudally and head for the inferior olivary nucleus.

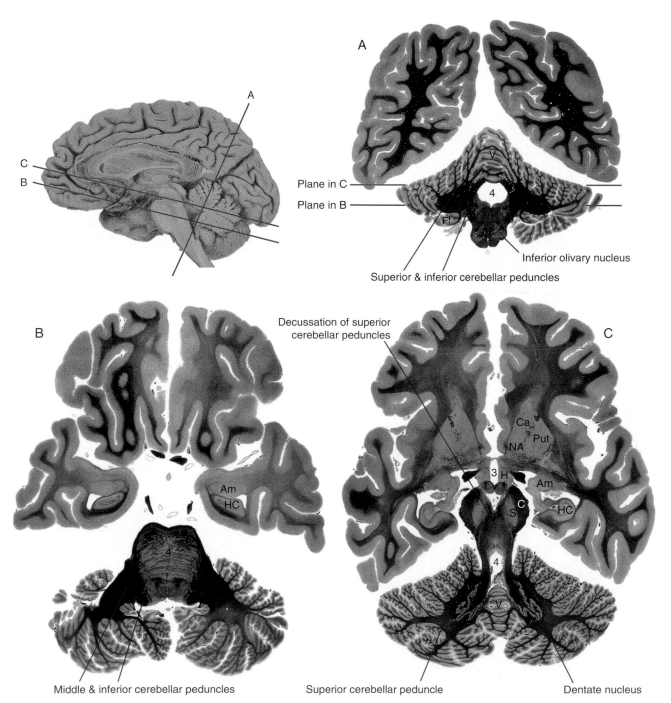

Plane in C

Plane in B

Inferior olivary nucleus

Superior & inferior cerebellar peduncles

Decussation of superior
cerebellar peduncles

Am
HC

Ca
Put
NA
3 H
Am
C
S
HC
4
V

Middle & inferior cerebellar peduncles

Superior cerebellar peduncle

Dentate nucleus

Figure 20-6 Cerebellar peduncles as seen in coronal and axial sections. **A,** Coronal section that passes tangentially through the inferior cerebellar peduncle as it turns posteriorly and enters the cerebellum. **B,** Axial section showing the middle cerebellar peduncle connecting the cerebellum and basal pons. The inferior cerebellar peduncle is cut in cross section just below the level at which it enters the cerebellum. **C,** Axial section slightly superior to **B,** showing the superior cerebellar peduncles leaving the cerebellum, entering the brainstem, and decussating in the midbrain. 3, third ventricle; 4, fourth ventricle; Am, amygdala; C, cerebral peduncle; Ca, caudate nucleus; Fl, flocculus; H, hypothalamus; HC, hippocampus; NA, nucleus accumbens; Put, putamen; S, substantia nigra; V, vermis. *(Modified from Nolte J, Angevine JB Jr: The human brain in photographs and diagrams, ed 3, St. Louis, 2007, Mosby.)*

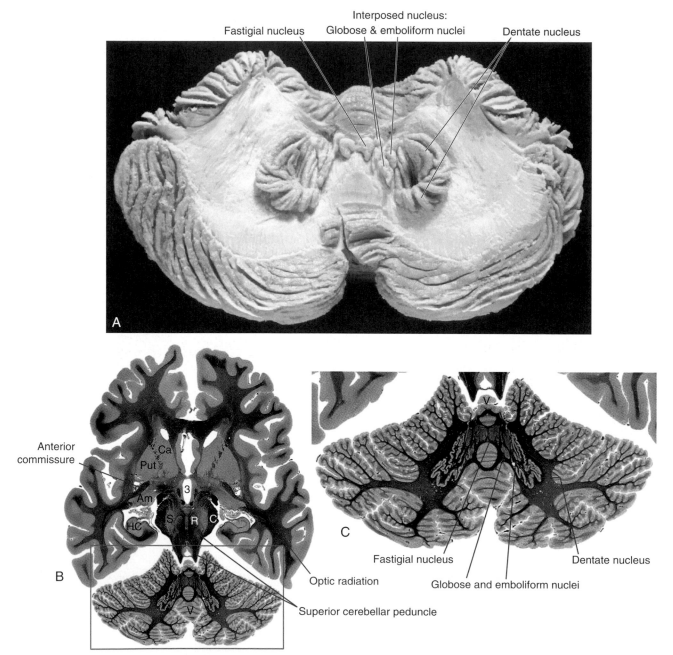

Interposed nucleus:
Fastigial nucleus   Globose & emboliform nuclei   Dentate nucleus

Anterior
commissure

Ca
Put

3

Am

HC   S   R   C

Optic radiation

V

Superior cerebellar peduncle

Fastigial nucleus   Dentate nucleus

Globose and emboliform nuclei

Figure 20-7 Deep cerebellar nuclei. **A,** Dissection demonstrating the deep nuclei of the human cerebellum. **B,** The deep nuclei as seen in an axial section slightly superior to that shown in Figure 20-6C (enlarged in **C**). (See Video 20-3.) 3, third ventricle; Am, amygdala; C, cerebral peduncle; Ca, caudate nucleus; HC, hippocampus; Put, putamen; R, red nucleus; S, substantia nigra; V, vermis. (**A,** *from Gluhbegovic N: J Anat 137:396, 1983.*)

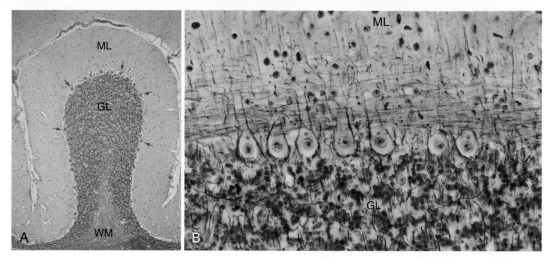

Figure 20-8 Light micrographs of cerebellar cortex. **A,** Cross section of a single folium from a human cerebellum (stained with hematoxylin and eosin). The molecular layer (ML) adjacent to the pial surface of the cerebellum contains relatively few neurons and is the main site of synaptic interactions between cerebellar interneurons and Purkinje cells. The granular layer (GL), adjacent to the central white matter (WM) of the cerebellum, contains the tightly packed cell bodies of tiny granule cells (see Fig. 20-11). Between the molecular and granular layers is a single layer of large Purkinje cells (*arrows*). **B,** Higher-magnification view of the Purkinje cell layer of monkey cerebellar cortex (Bodian silver stain), showing the large cell bodies of these neurons (some indicated by *) surrounded by silver-stained processes of cerebellar interneurons. Purkinje cell dendrites project into the molecular layer, where they are contacted by parallel fibers whose parent axons arise in the granular layer. *(Courtesy Dr. Nathaniel T. McMullen, University of Arizona College of Medicine.)*

characteristic types of interneurons (Fig. 20-9 and see Fig. 20-14B), but the fundamental circuitry of the cerebellar cortex can be described in terms of Purkinje cells, granule cells, and the afferents to the cortex (see Fig. 20-14A).

Purkinje cells are the only neurons whose axons leave the cerebellar cortex. They are, in addition, among the most anatomically distinctive neurons found in the nervous system. Each Purkinje cell has an intricate, extensive dendritic tree (see Fig. 1-4A) that is flattened out in a plane perpendicular to the long axis of the folium in which it resides (Fig. 20-10). Each granule cell (see Fig. 20-10) sends its axon into the molecular layer, where it bifurcates to form a fine, unmyelinated **parallel fiber** (Fig. 20-11) that extends for about 5 mm along the long axis of the folium. During its course, each parallel fiber passes through and synapses on the dendritic trees of Purkinje cells (as many as 500 of them). Each of us is estimated to have an incredible 10^{11} granule cells—half the neurons in the CNS—and each of our 25 million Purkinje cells receives synapses from perhaps 10^5 of them.

The cerebellum receives modulatory inputs from places such as the locus ceruleus and the raphe nuclei (see Figs. 11-24 and 11-27). There are also two distinctive sets of afferent fibers to the cerebellar cortex: **climbing fibers** and **mossy fibers.** A single climbing fiber ends directly on each Purkinje cell, winding around its dendrites like ivy climbing a trellis (Fig. 20-12); in the process, it makes tens of thousands of excitatory synapses, and collectively, these form the most powerful excitatory input in the nervous system. All of these climbing fibers arise in the contralateral inferior olivary nucleus. All of the rest of the afferents to the cerebellar cortex are mossy fibers. Mossy fibers end on the dendrites of granule cells, so this is a less direct route to the Purkinje cells (mossy fiber→granule cell→parallel fiber→Purkinje cell).

Purkinje Cells of the Cerebellar Cortex Project to the Deep Nuclei

Although Purkinje cell axons are the only route out of the cerebellar cortex, few of them leave the cerebellum itself. Rather, they project to the deep nuclei, which in turn give rise to the cerebellar output (Fig. 20-13). However, the deep nuclei are not just simple relay stations (Fig. 20-14C). For example, climbing fibers and many mossy fibers send collateral branches to the deep nuclei. It has been suggested that these inputs provide a tonic excitatory drive to neurons of the deep nuclei, and that inhibitory projections from Purkinje cells then modulate the firing rates of these neurons. In addition to giving rise to axons that leave the cerebellum, the deep nuclei project back to the same areas of cerebellar cortex from which they receive Purkinje axons. The functional implications of these additional connections are not fully understood, but they make it less surprising that the consequences of cerebellar damage are much more severe and long lasting when the deep nuclei are included in the lesion.

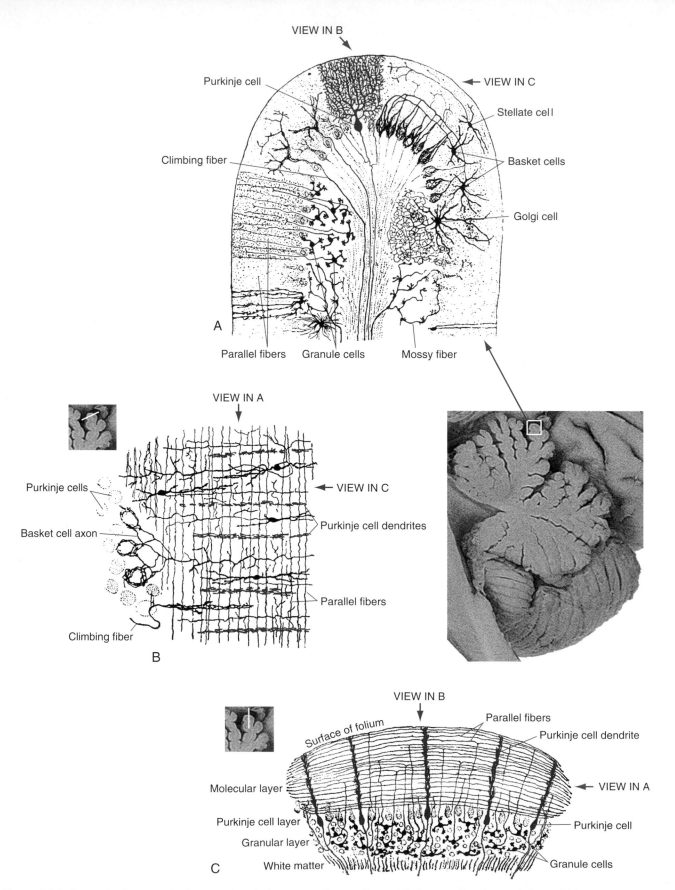

Figure 20-9 Composite drawings of Golgi-stained cerebellar neurons, from sections cut in three nearly orthogonal planes. **A,** Transverse section cut perpendicular to the long axis of a folium, showing mossy fibers, climbing fibers, and the major neuronal cell types of the cerebellar cortex. The elements of the principal circuit through the cerebellar cortex (see Fig. 20-14A) can be seen clearly. Other cell types in the cerebellar cortex: **basket cells,** whose dendrites spread out in the molecular layer and whose axons branch to enclose the cell bodies of a series of Purkinje cells; **stellate cells,** whose axons and dendrites all ramify in the molecular layer; and **Golgi cells,** whose dendrites spread out in the molecular layer and whose axons end on granule cell dendrites. **B,** A section parallel to the long axis of a folium, cut at an oblique angle so that it passes through the molecular layer on the right and the Purkinje cell layer on the left. This view demonstrates how the parallel fibers and the flattened dendritic trees of Purkinje cells are oriented perpendicular to each other. **C,** Another section parallel to the long axis of a folium, this time perpendicular to its surface, to demonstrate the layers of the cerebellar cortex. *(Modified from Ramón y Cajal S: Histologie du système nerveux de l'homme et des vertébrés, Paris, 1909, 1911, Maloine.)*

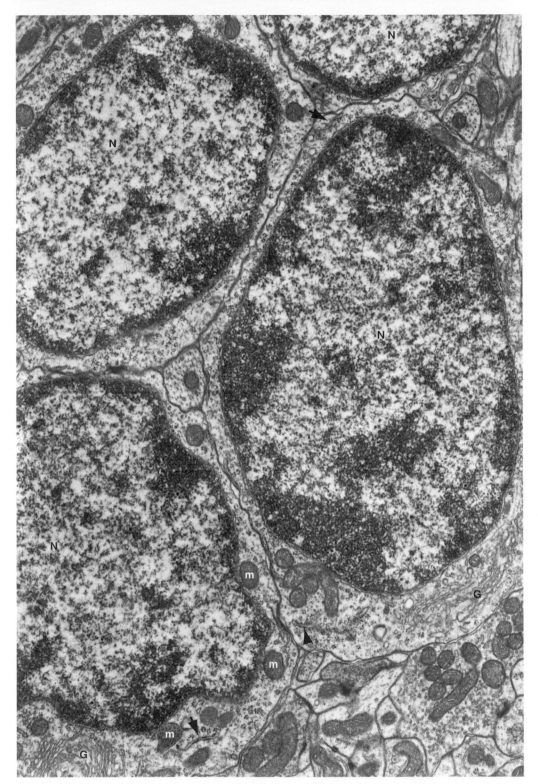

Figure 20-10 Granule cells of rat cerebellar cortex. These neurons are so small that each cell body is occupied almost entirely by the nucleus (N). However, the scanty cytoplasm contains typical organelles such as mitochondria (m), Golgi cisternae (G), and tiny Nissl bodies *(arrows)*. Each neuron is only about 5 μm in diameter, meaning that a row of 5000 of them would be only an inch long. *(From Pannese E: Neurocytology: fine structure of neurons, nerve processes, and neuroglial cells, New York, 1994, Thieme Medical Publishers.)*

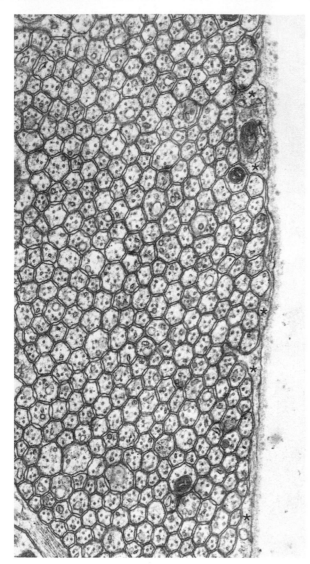

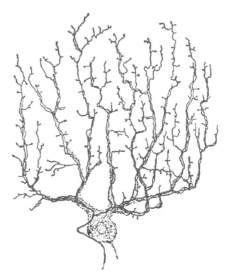

Figure 20-12 Drawing of a Golgi-stained climbing fiber *(green)*, demonstrating the origin of its name as it climbs up the dendritic tree of a Purkinje cell *(red)*. *(Modified from Ramón y Cajal S: Histologie du système nerveux de l'homme et des vertébrés, Paris, 1909, 1911, Maloine.)*

Figure 20-11 Regular array of parallel fibers in the molecular layer of rat cerebellar cortex (same plane as in Fig. 20-10). Only a thin glial covering (*) separates some parallel fibers from the surface of the cerebellum. Despite the tiny size of these unmyelinated axons (about 0.2 μm in diameter), each contains the usual microtubules and neurofilaments. *(From Pannese E: Neurocytology: fine structure of neurons, nerve processes, and neuroglial cells, New York, 1994, Thieme Medical Publishers.)*

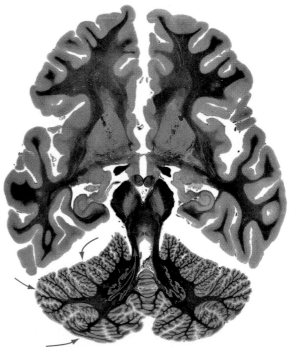

Inputs to cortex

Figure 20-13 Fundamental organization of the cerebellum: inputs→cerebellar cortex→deep nuclei→output targets. Most of the inputs to the cortex and outputs from the deep nuclei are excitatory *(green)*. The projections from the cortex to the deep nuclei, in contrast, are all inhibitory *(red)* axons of Purkinje cells.

Each Side of the Cerebellum Affects the Ipsilateral Side of the Body

There are many crossings of the midline in the various circuits interconnecting the cerebellum and other parts of the CNS, ultimately forming the basis for the fact that one cerebral hemisphere controls skeletal muscle of the contralateral limbs, but one half of the cerebellum influences movements of the ipsilateral limbs (see Figs. 3-33 and 20-23). For example, pontine nuclei receive inputs from the ipsilateral cerebral cortex and project to the contralateral half of the cerebellum (see Fig. 20-16), and one half of the cerebellum projects to the contralateral thalamus (see Fig. 20-20).

Details of Connections Differ Among Zones

The cerebellum is involved in equilibrium, in the control of muscle tone and posture, and in the coordination of voluntary movements; thus it would seem reasonable for it to receive vestibular, spinal, and cerebral cortical

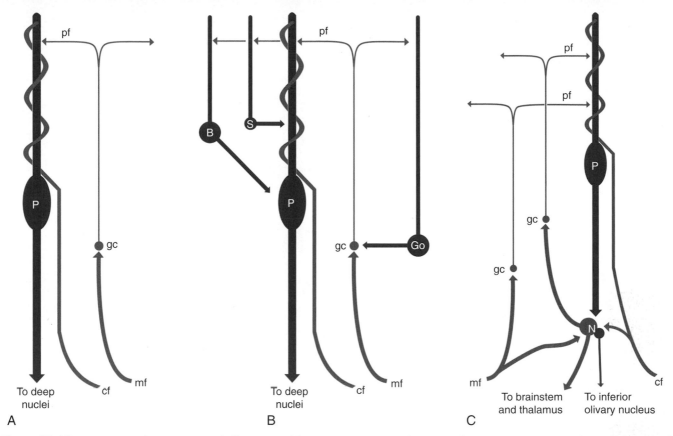

Figure 20-14 Connections of neurons in cerebellar cortex. Inhibitory connections are shown in *red,* excitatory in *green.* **A,** Schematic diagram of the principal circuit through the cerebellar cortex. Climbing fibers (cf) reach Purkinje cells (P) directly, and information from mossy fibers (mf) reaches them indirectly by way of granule cells (gc) and parallel fibers (pf). **B,** Additional interconnections in cerebellar cortex. One striking thing about the cerebellar cortex is the large amount of inhibition used in processing there: the mossy fiber–granule cell inputs and the climbing fiber inputs are excitatory, but everything else is inhibitory. Golgi cells (Go) make inhibitory feedback connections onto granule cells. Basket cells (B) and stellate cells (S) make inhibitory synapses on the cell bodies and dendrites, respectively, of Purkinje cells. Finally, synapses of Purkinje cells are all inhibitory. **C,** Schematic diagram of the general interconnections of cerebellar cortex and deep cerebellar nuclei. Climbing fibers and many mossy fibers send collaterals to cells of deep nuclei (N) before continuing to cerebellar cortex, where climbing fibers end directly on Purkinje cells and mossy fibers influence Purkinje cells indirectly through the granule cell→parallel fiber pathway. Purkinje cells, in turn, end on cells of deep nuclei. The deep nuclei contain two populations of neurons. One sends mossy fibers to cerebellar cortex as well as massive numbers of fibers to extracerebellar sites in the brainstem and thalamus. The other is a collection of small neurons that send inhibitory (GABA) projections to the contralateral inferior olivary nucleus. *(Modified from Thach WT: Brain Res 40:89, 1972.)*

inputs. This is indeed the case, and even though cerebellar cortex has the same anatomical appearance everywhere, different areas are concerned with particular functions. The flocculonodular lobe and part of the uvula receive vestibular inputs, so this area is referred to as the **vestibulocerebellum.** Most of the vermis and medial hemispheres (except for the nodulus and uvula) receive spinal inputs and so are called the **spinocerebellum.** Projections from the cerebral cortex (via relays in the pontine nuclei) form the major input to lateral parts of the cerebellar hemispheres, so the lateral hemispheres are sometimes referred to as the **cerebrocerebellum** or the **neocerebellum.** There is a certain amount of overlap of these functional divisions in terms of connections. For example, the spinocerebellum receives afferents from pontine nuclei, and parts of it also receive vestibular afferents.

Different areas of the cerebellar cortex are preferentially related not only to particular inputs but also to particular deep nuclei. The dentate nucleus receives projections mainly from the lateral parts of the cerebellar hemispheres, the interposed nucleus from the medial hemispheres, and the fastigial nucleus from the vermis (Fig. 20-15 and Table 20-2).

Cerebellar Cortex Receives Multiple Inputs

The cerebellar cortex receives some of its complement of mossy fibers from the deep cerebellar nuclei; the remaining mossy fibers carry information from four principal extracerebellar sources (Fig. 20-16): the vestibular nerve and nuclei, the spinal cord, the reticular formation, and the cerebral cortex (via pontine nuclei).

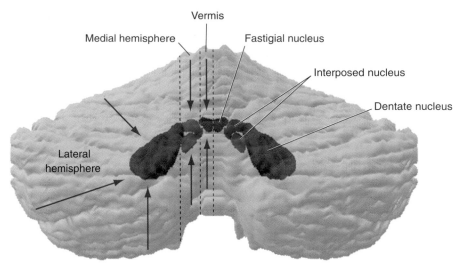

Figure 20-15 Projections from cerebellar cortex to deep cerebellar nuclei. The cortex is generally divided into three longitudinal zones that project in a medial-to-lateral sequence to the fastigial, interposed, and dentate nuclei. In addition, there is a projection (not shown) from the vermis and flocculonodular lobe directly to the vestibular nuclei. (See Video 20-4.)

Table 20-2	Divisions of the Cerebellum		
Anatomical Division	**Phylogenetic Division**	**Functional Division**	**Nucleus**
Anterior lobe	Paleocerebellum	Spinal cerebellum	Interposed
	Primary Fissure		
Posterior lobe	Neocerebellum	Cerebral cerebellum	Dentate
	Posterolateral Fissure		
Flocculonodular lobe	Archicerebellum	Vestibulocerebellum	Fastigial

Projections from different parts of the reticular formation largely parallel those from vestibular and spinal sites. The climbing fiber input to the cerebellar cortex, as mentioned previously, arises in the inferior olivary nucleus.

Vestibular Inputs Reach the Flocculus and Vermis

Some primary vestibular afferents enter the cerebellum through the juxtarestiform body (see Fig. 15-6) and end as mossy fibers in the nodulus and uvula. A larger number of second- and higher-order fibers, arising in the vestibular nuclei and reticular formation, follow the same course to the flocculonodular lobe and most of the vermis, bilaterally.

The Spinal Cord Projects to the Vermis and Medial Hemisphere

A great deal of somatosensory information (principally from various mechanoreceptors of the skin, muscles, and joints) reaches the vermis and medial hemisphere. Some of it reaches the cerebellum directly via the spinocerebellar tracts and the cuneocerebellar tract (see Fig. 10-23). Some arrives indirectly by way of the reticular formation. Not surprisingly, similar information from the head also reaches the cerebellum from the trigeminal system. All the trigeminal nuclei participate in this projection to some extent, but the bulk of it arises in the rostral two thirds of the spinal nucleus (interpolar and oral nuclei). The anterior spinocerebellar tract travels in the superior cerebellar peduncle, but all the rest of the somatosensory input from both body and head traverses the inferior cerebellar peduncle (Table 20-3).

Cerebral Cortex Projects to the Cerebellum by Way of Pontine Nuclei

The area of white matter in each cerebral peduncle is considerably larger than a medullary pyramid (Fig. 20-17), reflecting the fact that each cerebral peduncle contains about 21 million fibers, only about 1 million of which continue into the ipsilateral pyramid. Some of the remaining 20 million fibers are bound for the reticular formation or for the motor nuclei of cranial nerves, but the vast majority end in ipsilateral pontine nuclei. The pontine nuclei of one side contain about 12 million neurons that project through the middle cerebellar peduncle to virtually all parts of the cerebellar cortex.[d]

_____

[d]Pontocerebellar input to the flocculonodular lobe is sparse, and the nodulus may receive none at all.

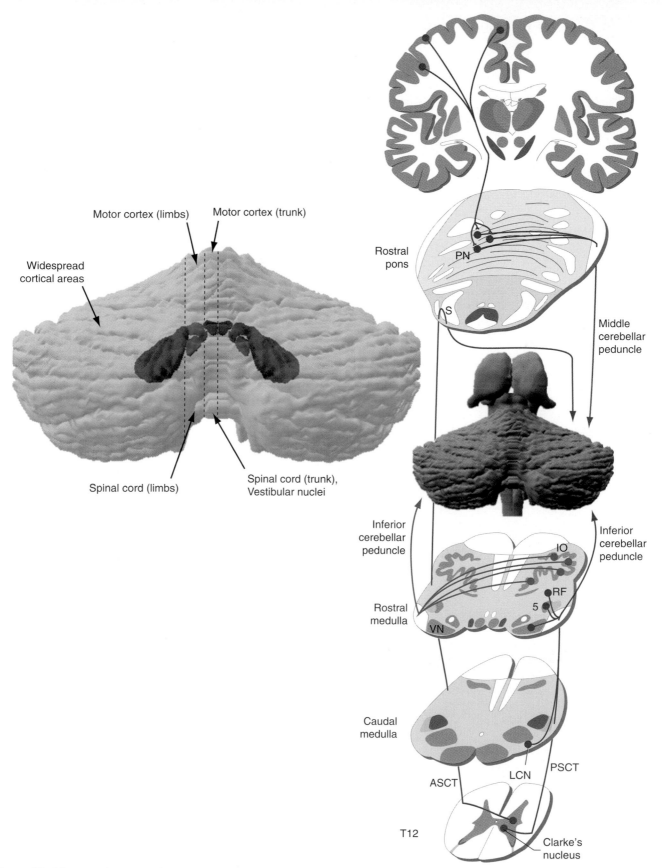

Figure 20-16 Principal inputs to the cerebellar cortex. As explained further in the text, spinocerebellar, cuneocerebellar, and trigeminocerebellar fibers end in the vermis and medial hemisphere; fibers from the vestibular nerve and nuclei end mainly in the flocculonodular lobe (not shown) and vermis; pontocerebellar fibers, conveying information from the cerebral cortex, end throughout the cerebellar cortex, as do olivocerebellar fibers. 5, spinal trigeminal nucleus; ASCT, anterior spinocerebellar tract; IO, inferior olivary nucleus; LCN, lateral cuneate nucleus; PN, pontine nuclei; PSCT, posterior spinocerebellar tract; RF, reticular formation; S, superior cerebellar peduncle; VN, vestibular nuclei.

Table 20-3	Inputs to Cerebellar Cortex*

Tract	Origin	Termination	Peduncle
Anterior spinocerebellar	Contralateral spinal cord	Vermis and intermediate zone, mostly ipsilateral to origin (recrosses in cerebellum)	Superior
Posterior spinocerebellar	Clarke's posterior thoracic nucleus	Vermis and intermediate zone, mostly ipsilateral	Inferior
Cuneocerebellar	Lateral cuneate nucleus	Vermis and intermediate zone, mostly ipsilateral	Inferior
Vestibulocerebellar[†]	Vestibular ganglion	Ipsilateral nodulus and uvula	Inferior[‡]
Vestibulocerebellar[§]	Vestibular nuclei	Flocculus, nodulus, and vermis, bilaterally	Inferior[‡]
Reticulocerebellar	Lateral, paramedian, reticular tegmental nuclei	Mainly vermis and intermediate zone, mostly ipsilateral	Inferior and middle[‖]
Trigeminocerebellar	Spinal and main sensory nuclei (V)	Vermis and intermediate zone, mostly ipsilateral	Inferior
Olivocerebellar	Inferior olivary, accessory olivary nuclei	All contralateral areas	Inferior
Pontocerebellar	Pontine nuclei	Contralateral anterior and posterior lobes, some to ipsilateral vermis	Middle

*Not including inputs from the deep cerebellar nuclei or modulatory inputs from places such as the raphe nuclei and locus ceruleus.
[†]Primary afferents.
[‡]Juxtarestiform body.
[§]Second-order fibers.
[‖]The reticular tegmental nucleus projects through the middle cerebellar peduncle.

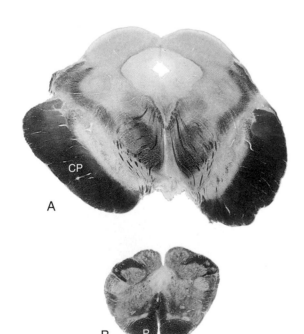

Figure 20-17 Cross sections of the rostral midbrain **(A)** and the caudal medulla **(B)** at the same magnification, showing the relative sizes of the cerebral peduncle (CP) and pyramid (P).

Almost all these fibers cross the midline in the basal pons and reach the contralateral half of the cerebellum; indeed, the pathway is usually treated as entirely crossed. However, some fibers (particularly some of those destined for the vermis) enter the ipsilateral middle cerebellar peduncle or have multiple branches that end bilaterally.

The corticopontocerebellar pathway is therefore a mammoth one, dwarfing the corticospinal tract by comparison. Several areas of the cerebral cortex project to the pontine nuclei (Fig. 20-18), but in most species contributions from the vicinity of the central sulcus predominate (i.e., from the motor and premotor cortex and from somatosensory cortex and adjacent parts of the parietal lobe). There are also projections from other parts of the cortex, such as visual, limbic, and association areas. In most animals these are not as heavy as the others just mentioned, but in humans they have added prominence (see Fig. 20-26). The vermis and medial hemispheres preferentially receive their cortical input from the motor cortex of the precentral gyrus, and the pathway is somatotopically organized so that the pontocerebellar fibers end in the same pattern as those carrying information from the spinal cord. The lateral parts of the cerebellar hemispheres, in contrast, receive most of their cortical input from premotor, somatosensory, and association areas of the cerebral cortex.

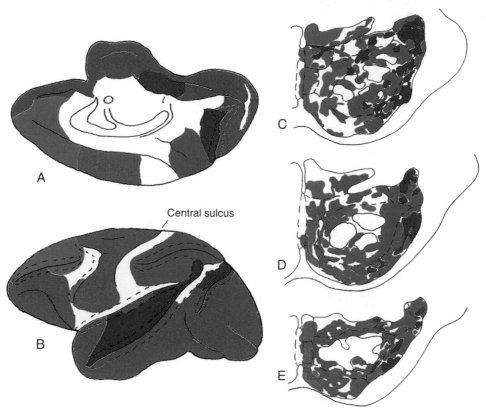

Central sulcus

Figure 20-18 Diagram of the basal pons of a rhesus monkey, illustrating the distribution of projections derived from association cortices in the prefrontal *(purple),* posterior parietal *(blue),* temporal *(red),* and parastriate and parahippocampal regions *(orange)* and from motor, premotor, and supplementary motor areas *(green).* The medial **(A)** and lateral **(B)** surfaces of the cerebral hemisphere are shown at the left, and sections through the basal pons in the rostral pons **(C),** midpons **(D),** and caudal pons **(E)** are shown on the right. Areas in white depict cortical regions that project to the pons, but details regarding the terminations are incomplete; note that this includes limbic areas such as the cingulate gyrus. Cortical areas shown in yellow are not currently thought to have pontine projections. There is a complex mosaic of terminations in the pons, with each cerebral region having preferential sites of pontine terminations. There is considerable interdigitation of the terminations but almost no overlap. *(Modified from the cover figure accompanying Schmahmann JD: Hum Brain Mapping 4:174, 1996.)*

Climbing Fibers Arise in the Contralateral Inferior Olivary Nucleus

The inferior olivary nucleus (actually a complex of a **principal** and two **accessory** olivary nuclei) is unique among structures providing afferents to the cerebellum. All olivary efferents emerge medially, enter the contralateral inferior cerebellar peduncle, and divide into 5 to 10 branches in the cerebellar white matter. All the branches of a given axon end in a narrow parasagittal strip as the single climbing fibers of 5 to 10 Purkinje cells (Fig. 20-19). Collectively, the efferents from one inferior olivary nucleus blanket the entire contralateral cerebellar cortex with climbing fibers, with particular small olivary areas systematically mapped onto particular small areas of cerebellar cortex.

The information these climbing fibers convey comes from diverse sources, including the spinal cord, the red nucleus, the cerebral cortex, and the cerebellum itself. Fibers from the ipsilateral red nucleus, forming the bulk of the central tegmental tract, are numerically the most important olivary input in primates. Somatosensory

inputs, all crossed, reach the inferior olivary complex both directly (via **spinoolivary** fibers) and indirectly (through relays in the posterior column nuclei); comparable inputs also arise from the trigeminal sensory nuclei. A few fibers from the cerebral cortex of both sides, mostly from motor cortex, also reach the olive. Finally, there is a topographically highly organized projection from the small γ-aminobutyric acid (GABA)ergic neurons in the contralateral dentate and interposed nuclei to the inferior olivary complex (Fig. 20-20). These form part of a large series of parallel loops reminiscent of those seen in the basal ganglia, in which small areas of cerebellar cortex, through small parts of the deep nuclei, project to the same parts of the inferior olive from which they receive climbing fibers. Such loops, together with their connections to the pontine nuclei, red nucleus, thalamus, and other sites, may be the basic functional units in cerebellar circuitry.

The inferior olivary nuclear complex's widespread connections make it key in cerebellar function. Selective destruction of the inferior olive in experimental animals has acute effects similar to those of destruction of the

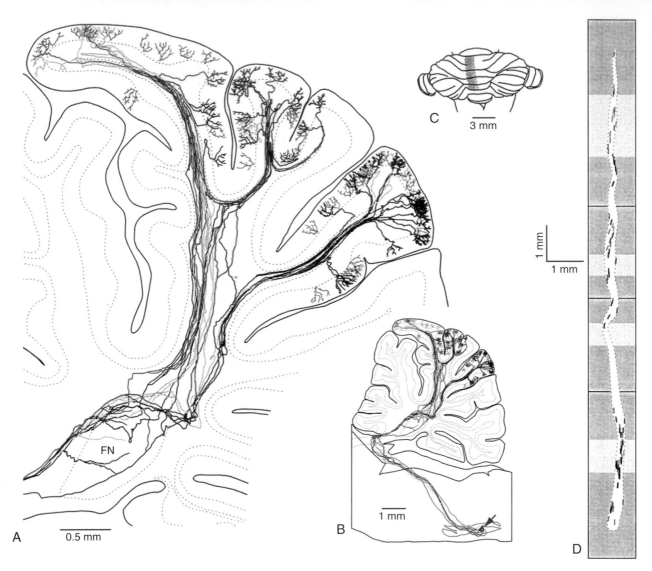

Figure 20-19 Reconstruction of single olivary efferents on their way to ending as climbing fibers in the cerebellar cortex of a rat. **A,** Six olivocerebellar axons (indicated by six different colors) enter the cerebellum and divide into 42 branches, each of which ends as a climbing fiber. Along the way they give off additional branches to the fastigial nucleus (FN). **B,** Lower magnification view with the site of the tracer injection in the contralateral inferior olivary nucleus indicated *(arrow)*. **C,** All the climbing fibers from this small olivary area end in the shaded parasagittal strip in the contralateral half of the vermis. **D,** Higher magnification of a flattened-out view of the parasagittal strip in **C.** Pale gray areas indicate what were formerly the crests of folia, dark gray areas indicate the walls of fissures, and individual climbing fibers are indicated with the same colors as in **A.** All the climbing fibers from a given olivary neuron end in a parasagittal strip 200 to 300 μm wide. *(From Sugihara I, Wu H-S, Shinoda Y: J Neurosci 21:7715, 2001.)*

entire contralateral half of the cerebellum (described later). After recovery from these acute effects, there is a persistent deficit in the motor learning functions of the cerebellum (described later).

Visual and Auditory Information Reaches the Cerebellum

The cerebellum utilizes not just somatosensory and vestibular information but also visual and auditory and even olfactory and visceral inputs. Visual information arrives from a subset of pontine nuclei (in the posterolateral part of the basal pons), which in turn receive it

from visual cortical areas and the superior colliculus. The reticular tegmental nucleus also projects visual information to the flocculus, where it is used in the control of eye movements (see Chapter 21). Auditory information probably reaches pontine nuclei from auditory cortical areas and the inferior colliculus.

Multiple cerebellar areas become active in response to sensory stimulation, depending on the task at hand. Simple detection of visual and auditory stimuli activates the vermis approximately midway along its length (i.e., in the same general area that receives somatosensory information from the head), probably reflecting participation in movement toward the stimulus. More complex tasks, such as discriminating among different stimuli, activate lateral parts of the posterior lobe (even if no movement is involved).

Each Longitudinal Zone Has a Distinctive Output

The entire output of the cerebellar cortex is provided by axons of Purkinje cells. Some of these, arising in the flocculonodular lobe and in parts of the vermis of both anterior and posterior lobes, leave the cerebellum via the juxtarestiform body and end in the vestibular nuclei. This provides the only direct access the cerebellar cortex has to motor neurons of the spinal cord (via the vestibulospinal tracts); all other Purkinje axons end in the deep cerebellar nuclei. They do so in an orderly medial-to-lateral way: the vermis projects to the fastigial nucleus, the medial hemisphere projects to the interposed nucleus, and the lateral hemisphere projects to the dentate nucleus (see Fig. 20-15).

Most neurons of the deep nuclei use glutamate as a neurotransmitter and make excitatory synapses on neurons they contact (as noted earlier, the projection from the deep nuclei to the inferior olivary nucleus arises from a separate population of inhibitory neurons that use GABA as their neurotransmitter). The output connections of the fastigial nucleus are distinctive, whereas those of the dentate and interposed nuclei are similar to each other. In addition to the connections described in the next two sections, all the deep nuclei project back to the cerebellar cortex.

The Vermis Projects to the Fastigial Nucleus

Fastigial nucleus output is directed primarily to the brainstem, ending in the vestibular nuclei of both sides and in the reticular formation, mainly contralaterally (see Fig. 20-20). Fibers that end ipsilaterally go right out through the juxtarestiform body. Those bound for contralateral targets cross the midline within the cerebellum, loop over the superior cerebellar peduncle as the **uncinate fasciculus** (or **hook bundle**), and descend through the contralateral juxtarestiform body. A few fibers also project to the contralateral ventral lateral/ventral anterior (VL/VA) nuclei of the thalamus and to the contralateral cervical spinal cord.

The Medial and Lateral Parts of Each Hemisphere Project to the Interposed and Dentate Nuclei

The major output from the cerebellum is the brachium conjunctivum, which arises in the dentate and interposed nuclei and leaves the cerebellum as the bulk of the superior cerebellar peduncle. This peduncle joins the brainstem in the rostral pons (see Fig. 11-14); at this

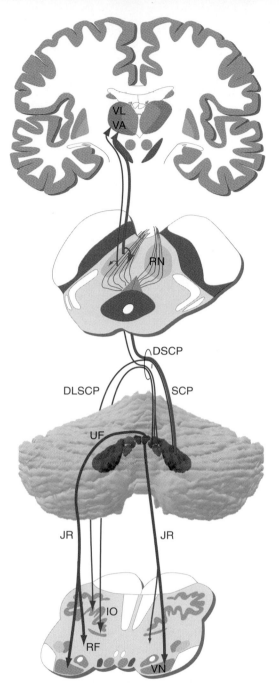

Figure 20-20 Principal efferent connections of the deep cerebellar nuclei. The fastigial nucleus projects bilaterally to the vestibular nuclei (VN) and the reticular formation (RF); a few fibers (not shown) reach the contralateral ventral lateral (VL) and ventral anterior (VA) nuclei of the thalamus. The interposed nucleus (globose + emboliform) projects to the magnocellular red nucleus (RN) and to the VL/VA nuclei; the dentate nucleus projects to the parvocellular red nucleus and to VL/VA. Both the interposed and dentate nuclei also send inhibitory fibers to the contralateral inferior olivary complex (whether the fastigial nucleus does so is uncertain). (See Video 20-5.) DLSCP, descending limb of the superior cerebellar peduncle; DSCP, decussation of the superior cerebellar peduncle; IO, inferior olivary nucleus; JR, juxtarestiform body; SCP, superior cerebellar peduncle; UF, uncinate fasciculus.

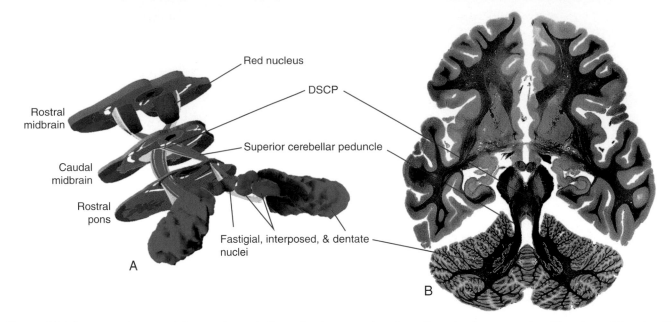

Figure 20-21 Origin and course of the superior cerebellar peduncle, as seen in a three-dimensional reconstruction **(A)** and an axial section **(B).** DSCP, decussation of the superior cerebellar peduncles. *(B, modified from Nolte J, Angevine JB Jr: The human brain in photographs and diagrams, ed 3, St. Louis, 2007, Mosby.)*

level, some fibers turn caudally as the **descending limb of the superior cerebellar peduncle** (see Fig. 20-20). Many of these are the inhibitory fibers on their way to the inferior olivary nucleus; others end in the reticular formation. Most of the fibers, however, continue rostrally, decussate in the midbrain (Fig. 20-21; see also Figs. 11-16 and 11-17), and reach the red nucleus, where some of them terminate. The red nucleus, like the substantia nigra, is actually two nuclei with different connections juxtaposed to each other—in this case, a caudal, large-celled (**magnocellular**) nucleus and a rostral, small-celled (**parvocellular**) nucleus. Neurons of the magnocellular red nucleus give rise to the rubrospinal tract, whereas those of the parvocellular nucleus project to the inferior olivary nucleus. In most mammals the magnocellular red nucleus is the larger of the two, but in apes and especially humans, the situation is reversed: the human magnocellular nucleus (and rubrospinal tract) is very small, and nearly all of what appears as the red nucleus in sections of the human brainstem is the parvocellular nucleus. Fibers from the dentate nucleus preferentially terminate in the parvocellular part of the red nucleus, and those from the interposed nucleus preferentially terminate in the magnocellular part (Fig. 20-22). The function of the dentate nucleus→ parvocellular red nucleus→inferior olivary nucleus→ cerebellar cortex→dentate nucleus loop, which is particularly well developed in humans, is still a mystery. It may be involved in the motor learning functions of the cerebellum (described later in this chapter).

The remaining majority of the fibers of the brachium conjunctivum pass through or around the red nucleus, join the thalamic fasciculus, and end in the VL/VA complex of the thalamus. The dentate and interposed nuclei project to separate but interdigitated groups of cells in the thalamus. From these thalamic cells, dentate information is conveyed to motor and premotor cortex, whereas information from the interposed nucleus is conveyed selectively to the limb areas of motor cortex (see Fig. 20-22).

The Lateral Hemispheres Are Involved in Planning and Skilled Movements

The lateral hemispheres form the largest part of the human cerebellum. The major neural circuit in which they are involved is the great loop from several areas of cerebral cortex to the cerebellum and back to motor and premotor cortex (see Fig. 20-22A). This circuitry suggests that the cerebellar hemispheres may be involved in the planning of movements, acting by influencing the output of motor cortex. Consistent with this notion, most neurons in the dentate nucleus change their firing rates before voluntary movements occur, and indeed, many of them change firing rates even before activity in motor cortex changes. (This is not to say that voluntary movements are *initiated* in the cerebellum, because in anticipation of a movement, various areas of cerebral association cortex become active even before the dentate nucleus does.) Currently, the most prevalent hypothesis about the function of the lateral hemisphere–dentate nucleus portion of the cerebellum is that it participates in the planning and programming of voluntary movements, particularly learned, skillful movements that

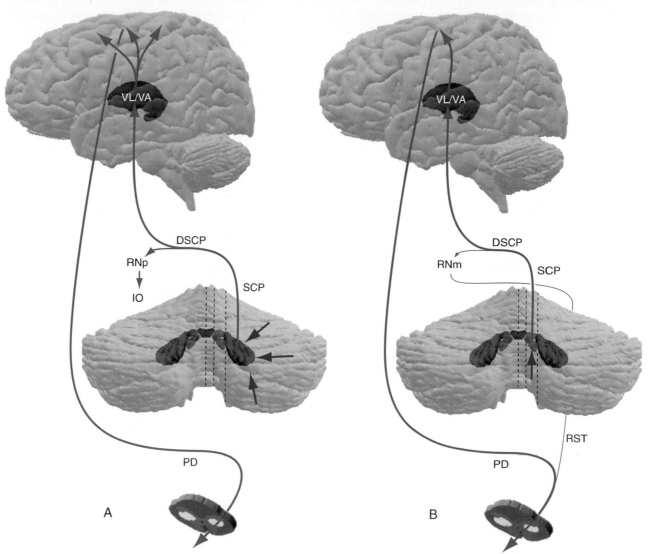

Figure 20-22 The principal output circuits through which the lateral and medial hemispheres of the cerebellum influence movement. Excitatory connections are indicated in *green,* inhibitory connections in *red.* **A,** The lateral hemispheres receive input via the pontine nuclei from widespread areas of cerebral cortex (not shown); then, via the dentate nucleus, superior cerebellar peduncle (SCP), and ventral lateral and ventral anterior (VL/VA) nuclei, they influence the output of motor and premotor cortex. Note that this cerebellar output crosses the midline in the decussation of the superior cerebellar peduncles (DSCP) and that the output from motor and premotor cortex recrosses the midline in the pyramidal decussation (PD). The result is that one lateral cerebellar hemisphere affects the ipsilateral side of the spinal cord and brainstem. (The projection from the dentate nucleus to the parvocellular red nucleus [RNp] and from there to the inferior olive [IO] is also indicated, although its role in influencing movement is not known.) **B,** Output connections of the medial hemisphere are similar in many respects to lateral hemisphere circuitry, but in this case the limb areas of primary motor cortex are the main targets; premotor cortex is less involved. However, the magnocellular red nucleus (RNm) and rubrospinal tract (RST) also have a minor role. Here again, there are compensating decussations: cerebellar output fibers cross in the decussation of the superior cerebellar peduncles, and rubrospinal fibers cross on their way to the spinal cord. The few fastigial fibers that reach the VL/VA nuclei behave in a similar manner, but their information is relayed to the trunk area of motor cortex.

become more rapid, precise, and automatic with practice. This is consistent with the clinical observation that although a great deal of compensation may take place after cerebellar injury, deficits in learned, skillful movements (e.g., piano playing) may be permanent. Note that the connections between cerebral and cerebellar hemispheres are crossed (see Fig. 20-22A). This means that, for example, the left side of the cerebellum is related to motor cortex on the right. Because the right motor cortex controls the left side of the body, the symptoms resulting

from unilateral cerebellar damage would be expected (and are found) on the ipsilateral side of the body.

The Medial Hemispheres Are Involved in Adjusting Limb Movements

The major inputs to the medial hemispheres (paravermal cortex) are superimposed, somatotopically arranged projections from the motor cortex and spinal cord (see Fig. 20-16). The major output of this part of the

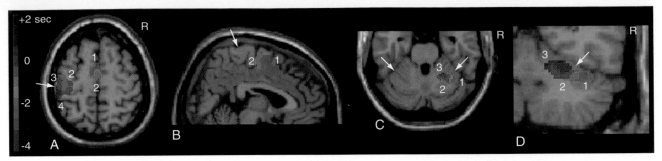

Figure 20-23 A series of axial (**A** and **C**), sagittal (**B**), and coronal (**D**) fMRI images showing the coordinated timing of maximal changes in cerebral and cerebellar blood flow before, during, and after voluntary movements. A subject was asked to press a button with his or her right thumb at any self-selected time during the 14 seconds after a cue. Blood flow began to increase 3 to 4 seconds before the movement in cingulate motor and anterior supplementary motor areas (**A1, B1**); then the increase moved into left premotor and posterior supplementary motor areas over about the next 2 seconds (**A2, B2**). Blood flow increased in primary motor cortex at about the time the movement began (**A3**), then increased in somatosensory cortex as information from the moving thumb arrived (**A4**). A parallel sequence was observed in the cerebellum. Shortly after the first cerebral changes, blood flow increased in the right lateral cerebellar hemisphere (**C1, D1**); this was still about 2 seconds before the movement began, consistent with the lateral hemisphere's role in planning it. As the movement began (**C2, D2**) and progressed (**C3, D3**), blood flow increased in the right medial hemisphere, consistent with a role in adjusting the movement. *Arrows* in **A** and **B** indicate the central sulcus; arrows in **C** and **D** indicate the primary fissure. (*Adapted from Hülsmann E, Erb M, Grodd W: Neuroimage 20:1485, 2003.*)

cerebellum is via the interposed nucleus back to motor cortex (through VL/VA; see Fig. 20-22B) and to the magnocellular red nucleus. Thus the medial hemispheres can influence spinal cord motor neurons through the corticospinal tract and also, to a minor extent, through the rubrospinal pathway. This led to the hypothesis that the intermediate zone of the cerebellum compares the commands emanating from motor cortex (it receives this information via pontine nuclei) with the actual position and velocity of the moving part (it receives this information via spinocerebellar and similar tracts) and then, by way of the interposed nucleus, issues correcting signals. This is consistent with the observation that most neurons of the interposed nucleus have firing rates related to voluntary movements, but unlike those of dentate neurons, their rates tend to change *during* rather than *before* movement (Fig. 20-23). Note that here again, a given side of the cerebellum winds up affecting ipsilateral motor neurons (e.g., left side of cerebellum→right thalamus→right motor cortex→left side of spinal cord).

The Vermis Is Involved in Postural Adjustments

The vermis includes the representation of the trunk conveyed by the spinocerebellar tracts. Its major outputs reach the vestibular nuclei and the reticular formation, both through the fastigial nucleus and through direct projections to the vestibular nuclei. The vestibulospinal and reticulospinal tracts then influence spinal motor neurons. Because this part of the cerebellum has so little effect on more rostral levels of the CNS, it seems reasonable that it should be most concerned with the regulation of posture and of stereotyped movements that are programmed in the brainstem and spinal cord. For example, the cerebellum-vestibulospinal pathway is partly responsible for rhythmic modulation of the basic pattern of walking movements generated in the spinal cord.

The Flocculus and Vermis Are Involved in Eye Movements

The principal connections of the flocculonodular lobe are with the vestibular nerve and nuclei, implying that it should have something to do with the maintenance of equilibrium. As discussed in the next section, this is indeed the case, and damage to this part of the cerebellum causes a general disequilibrium and vertigo, as though some controls had been removed from the vestibular nuclei. In addition, the flocculus has a special role in the coordination of slow eye movements (see Chapter 21), which is not surprising in view of the involvement of the vestibular nuclei in eye movements. Deciding how to track a moving target visually is not as easy as it sounds, because a target's image moves across the retina if the target, the eyes, or the head moves. Some Purkinje cells in the flocculus receive all three kinds of information, make the appropriate computations, and reflect true target velocity in their output.

The Cerebellum Is Involved in Motor Learning

We usually think of learning in terms of facts and concepts, although we also learn in terms of becoming more skilled in various kinds of movements. A common example is agility of the hands and feet in playing a piano; another is the skillful handball shots that can be developed over time. Evidence is accumulating that the cerebellum plays a special role in at least some forms of motor learning (Fig. 20-24). Two well-studied examples

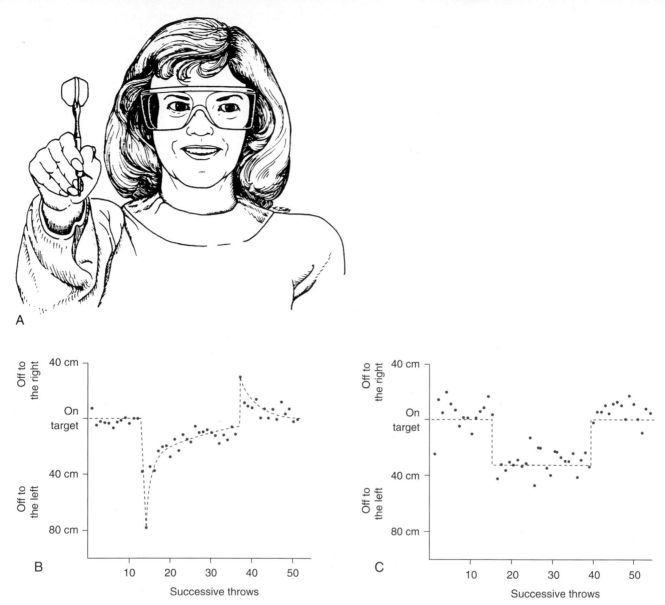

Figure 20-24 Example of the involvement of the cerebellum in motor learning—in this case, learning to alter one's dart-throwing technique while wearing prisms that displace images to one side. **A,** The experimental arrangement. The subject is wearing spectacles containing prisms that bend the path of light 15 degrees to the right. The effect of the prisms can be seen by the apparent displacement of the part of her face behind the spectacles and by the deviation of her eyes 15 degrees to her left; she is actually looking directly at you but must deviate her eyes to compensate for the prisms. **B,** The effect of prism spectacles on the dart-throwing ability of a normal subject. When the spectacles are first put on, the subject's throws become wide to the left. After a little practice, the throws become reasonably accurate again. At this point, the thrower would look like the subject in **A,** with her gaze deviated to one side but the dart aimed straight ahead. When the spectacles are removed, throws deviate to the right but then quickly become accurate again. **C,** The effect of prism spectacles on the dart-throwing ability of a patient with degenerative disease of the inferior olivary nuclei. In this case there is no compensation for the prism spectacles, and throws are wide to the left for as long as the spectacles are worn. *(Redrawn from Thach WT, Goodkin HP, Keating JG: Annu Rev Neurosci 15:403, 1992.)*

are described in this section, and the physiological basis is discussed in Chapter 24.

The vestibuloocular reflex was mentioned briefly in Chapter 14 (see Fig. 14-31). This reflex occurs during head movement, moving the eyes the same amount as the head but in the opposite direction. That is, the gain of the reflex is one: every degree of head movement elicits a degree of compensating eye movement. The result is that the direction of gaze stays constant, and the

visual world remains stable. The basic circuitry of the reflex is a simple three-neuron chain (see Fig. 14-32). The afferent limb is formed by vestibular primary afferents. These synapse on cells of the vestibular nuclei, which in turn project to the motor neurons of extraocular muscles. If the optics of the eye were to change (e.g., if someone started to wear glasses), a reflex gain of one might no longer be appropriate, and in fact, the vestibuloocular reflex arc is remarkably adaptable to changes in visual input. As an extreme example, if an experimental animal or a human subject wears reversing prisms, so that eye or head movement in one direction causes apparent movement in the opposite direction, an unaltered vestibuloocular reflex would be counterproductive. However, if the prisms are worn continuously as the subject moves about, the gain of the reflex will slowly change until, by the end of a day or so, it actually reverses direction. When the prisms are removed, the gain of the reflex slowly reverts to its usual state. Removal of the flocculus, or removal of a particular area of the inferior olivary nucleus, prevents these adaptive changes in the gain of the vestibuloocular reflex.

Some forms of conditioned responses also depend on the cerebellum. The best-studied example is a conditioned blink response. A puff of air directed at a rabbit's cornea elicits a reflex blink. If the puff of air is regularly preceded by a sound, after a while the sound itself elicits the same blink. Removal of a particular small area of the interposed nucleus abolishes the conditioned response of the ipsilateral eye, even though both the reflex response to the air puff and the conditioned response of the contralateral eye are unaffected. Lesions of the inferior olivary nucleus prevent acquisition of the conditioned response by the contralateral eye of an unconditioned animal. If the response was acquired before the olivary lesion, it slowly fades after the lesion, as though the inferior olivary nucleus is required to establish and sustain the conditioned response.

The exact locations of the modifiable synapses underlying these long-term changes are not yet known with certainty. However, it seems possible that similar changes may underlie the acquisition of skilled, voluntary movements in general.

The Cerebellum Is Also Involved in Cognitive Functions

Despite the fact that most corticopontine neurons reside in motor or somatosensory cortex, there are also many in limbic and association areas (see Fig. 20-18). The parts of the cerebellar cortex that deal with inputs from association cortex—the lateral hemispheres—are greatly expanded in humans (Fig. 20-25), as is the contingent of corticopontine fibers from association cortex (especially prefrontal cortex; Fig. 20-26). The human dentate nucleus has two parts see Fig. 20-25D)—a dorsal part that projects (through VL/VA) to motor cortex, and a larger ventral part that projects (through VL/VA and the dorsomedial nucleus) to prefrontal cortex; the ventral part is selectively enlarged in humans. All this is consistent with clinical reports that cerebellar damage or malformation can be associated with a variety of cognitive or behavioral disturbances, and with positron emission tomography (PET) and functional magnetic resonance

imaging (fMRI) studies indicating increased blood flow in different parts of the cerebellum during purely cognitive tasks. Just as the basal nuclei were traditionally associated primarily with movement but are now thought to have broader functions, the apparent role of the cerebellum in nonmotor functions is receiving increasing attention. It has been suggested that connections between the lateral hemispheres of the posterior lobe and association cortex are involved in cognition and that connections between more medial parts of the cerebellum and limbic cortex (as well as cerebellum-hypothalamus interconnections) play a role in affective and autonomic functions.

Clinical Syndromes Correspond to Functional Zones

Despite the fact that the cerebellum is functionally divided into longitudinal vermis–medial hemisphere–lateral hemisphere zones, syndromes referable to individual zones are rarely seen clinically. For example, for a lesion to destroy only the medial hemisphere on one side, it would need to extend from the superior surface of the cerebellum near the midbrain to the inferior surface of the cerebellum overlying the medulla. The lesion would also need to extend into the depths of the cerebellar fissures. It is extremely unlikely that this could happen without damaging other parts of the cerebellum and possibly parts of the brainstem. As a result, what is typically seen clinically are problems referable to the vermis, to one or both sides of the body of the cerebellum as a whole, or to the flocculonodular lobe.

Midline Damage Causes Postural Instability

The malnutrition that often accompanies chronic alcoholism causes degeneration of the cerebellar cortex that typically starts at the anterior end of the anterior lobe and spreads posteriorly. A great deal of the anterior lobe is occupied by vermis and medial hemisphere (see Fig. 20-4), and the legs are represented most anteriorly (Fig. 20-27). The result is a syndrome (called the **anterior lobe syndrome**) in which the legs are primarily affected; the most prominent symptom is a broad-based, staggering gait, similar in many ways to that seen after damage to the flocculonodular lobe. In the anterior lobe syndrome, however, there is a general incoordination, or **ataxia** (Greek for "lack of order"), of leg movements, even when the trunk is supported.

Lateral Damage Causes Limb Ataxia

Most of the cerebellum is made up of the lateral hemispheres, and with a few exceptions (e.g., the anterior lobe syndrome just mentioned), this is the region most

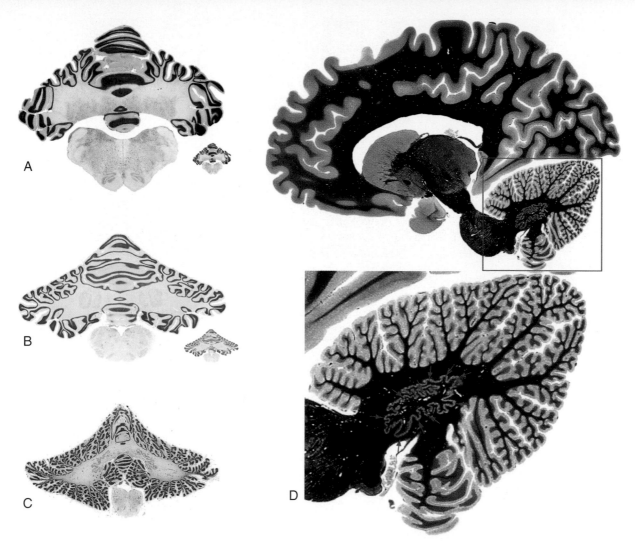

Figure 20-25 Evolutionary changes in the cerebellum. **A** to **C,** Nissl-stained coronal sections through the cerebella of a cat, rhesus monkey, and human, respectively, all enlarged to the same size; **C** and the smaller images in **A** and **B** are shown at about half actual size. The vermis occupies proportionally less of the cerebellum in humans, the cortex of the posterior lobe is more intricately convoluted, and the total area of cerebellar cortex is greatly increased. **D,** The dentate nucleus has two parts, a dorsal part *(blue arrows)* and, in humans, an expanded ventral part *(orange arrows)*. *(**A** to **C,** from www.brainmuseum.org, courtesy Dr. Wally Welker; supported by NSF grant 0131028. **D,** courtesy Dr. Jay B. Angevine Jr., University of Arizona College of Medicine.)*

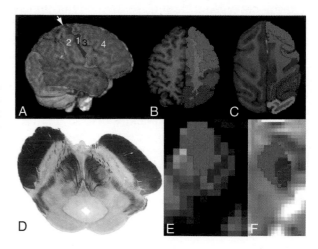

Figure 20-26 Evolutionary changes in prefrontal contributions to corticopontine fibers. **A,** Major functional areas were laid out on a brain reconstructed in three dimensions from MRI scans, including primary motor and somatosensory cortex (1, 2), premotor cortex (3), and prefrontal cortex (4, possibly including some posterior premotor areas). The top of the central sulcus is indicated by an arrow. **B** and **C,** Axial MRI scans of a human and macaque monkey brain, respectively, with the same cortical areas indicated. A diffusion-weighted imaging protocol was used to infer the projection of each cortical functional area through the cerebral peduncle of a human (**D** and **E**) and a macaque monkey (**F**). Twice as much of the human cerebral peduncle is occupied by fibers that arise in prefrontal cortex compared with the monkey. *(**A** to **C, E,** and **F,** adapted from Ramnani N et al: Cereb Cortex 16:811, 2006.)*

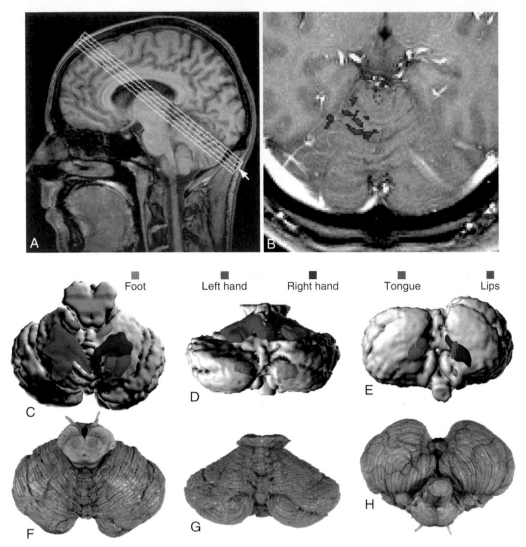

Figure 20-27 Demonstration of somatotopy in the human cerebellum using fMRI. **A** and **B,** Somatotopy in the anterior lobe of a single subject. The planes of section used in **A** were parallel to the peak of the tentorium cerebelli and the superior surface of the anterior lobe; the plane of section in **B** is indicated by an *arrow* in **A. B,** Areas of increased blood flow during repeated flexion and extension of the ipsilateral hand *(red, orange)* or foot *(blue).* Hand movement activated multiple small areas, all of them separate from the area activated by foot movements. **C** to **E,** The average areas of maximum activation in 46 subjects as they moved various body parts, seen from above **(C),** behind **(D),** and below **(E). F** to **H,** Views of a human cerebellum in approximately the same orientations as in **C** to **E.** *(A and B, from Nitschke MF et al: Brain 119:1023, 1996. C to E, from Grodd W et al: Hum Brain Mapping 13:55, 2001. F to H, from Nolte J, Angevine JB Jr: The human brain in photographs and diagrams, ed 3, St. Louis, 2007, Mosby.)*

heavily damaged in lesions of the body of the cerebellum. The result is called the **neocerebellar syndrome,** which is characterized by a variable combination of changes in muscle tone, reflexes, and the coordination of voluntary movements, all ipsilateral to the side of the lesion.

Widespread decreases in muscle tone (**hypotonia**) may occur acutely with small lesions, so that the limbs offer little resistance to passive movement and the muscles feel abnormally soft and flaccid. Stretch reflexes are often reduced (**hyporeflexia**), and as a result of the hypotonia, a limb may swing back and forth after a reflex contraction (**pendular reflexes**).

Most prominent, however, is a lack of coordination of voluntary movements. This is caused by a fundamental deficit in the timing of movements and the regulation of their rates. As shown in Figure 20-28, voluntary movements take longer than usual to initiate, and there are problems in stopping them or changing their direction. This manifests in a number of different ways: patients are likely to overshoot or undershoot targets (**dysmetria**); corrective movements as patients near a target have the appearance of a tremor (**intention tremor**); and rapid alternating movements, such as repeatedly pronating and supinating the forearm, may be especially difficult (**dysdiadochokinesia**). Note that the intention tremor of cerebellar disease is quite different from the resting tremor seen in Parkinson's disease, partly because it is seen *during* voluntary movements and partly because it is not as rhythmic or regular. When

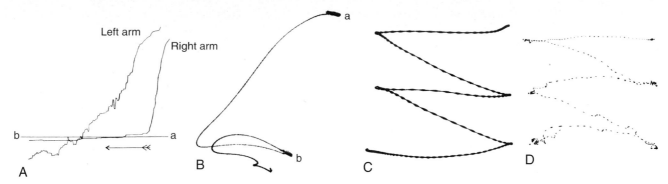

Figure 20-28 Movements made by patients with cerebellar lesions (all involving one or both hemispheres), recorded by the simple but ingenious technique of photographing a light bulb attached to the patient's finger (**B, C,** and **D**) or by recording the movement on a revolving drum (**A**). **A,** A patient with left-sided cerebellar damage attempts to stretch two similar springs and then keep them stretched to the level of the line ab; time progresses from right to left in this record. The normal right arm moves promptly and accurately, but the left arm starts slowly, moves slowly, makes many small corrective movements, overshoots the line, and is then unable to maintain a constant stretch. **B,** A patient attempts to touch his nose (at b) with the tip of his finger, starting from point a above his head; the movement has two distinct parts instead of being a smooth, continuous sweep (decomposition of movement), and the patient misjudges the range (dysmetria), striking his nose and then making irregular corrective movements. **C** and **D,** A patient with right-sided cerebellar damage moves each hand back and forth between a series of small targets; the light attached to his fingertip was flashing at a constant rate, so the separation between spots is a measure of finger velocity. The left hand (**C**) performs smoothly and accurately, but the right hand (**D**) moves at varying speeds and has particular difficulty stopping and changing direction. *(From Holmes G: Brain 62:1, 1939.)*

complex movements involving more than one joint are performed, the timing of different parts may be defective in different ways, leading to **decomposition of movement** (see Fig. 20-28B). Hence damage to the lateral hemispheres causes ataxia because of defective planning of movements, and damage to the medial hemispheres (in the anterior lobe syndrome) causes ataxia because of defective adjustments of movements in progress. The complex movements used in speaking may also be affected in this way; the normal flow and rhythm of speech are disrupted, and successive syllables may emerge slowly and separated from each other (**scanning speech**).

Although the cerebellar hemispheres use large amounts of sensory information to help in the programming of skilled voluntary movements, it is important to note again that the neocerebellar syndrome is not accompanied by any sensory deficits. Gordon Holmes (a famous British neurologist) described a patient who had incurred damage to his right cerebellar hemisphere. "The movements of my left arm," the patient noted, "are done subconsciously, but I have to think out each movement of the right arm. I come to a dead stop in turning and have to think before I start again."

Damage to the Flocculus Affects Eye Movements

The nodulus sits on the roof of the caudal part of the fourth ventricle. Tumors called *medulloblastomas* occasionally arise in the roof of the ventricle, usually in young children; they are the most common cause of damage to the flocculonodular lobe. Affected individuals have a general loss of equilibrium—they sway from side to side when standing, walk with a staggering, wide-based gait,

and tend to fall over. The basic mechanisms used in moving the limbs are unaffected, so that when the trunk is supported (e.g., when lying in bed), movements of the arms and legs are normal. In contrast to the findings after damage to the cerebellar hemispheres, there is no tremor, and both reflexes and muscle tone remain normal. A variety of problems with eye movement are also seen, such as difficulty with pursuit eye movements, with maintaining eccentric gaze, or with making accurate voluntary eye movements (see Chapter 21). However, eye movement disorders may be found after damage to other cerebellar regions as well. As a further consequence of these tumors, the lateral and median apertures of the fourth ventricle may be squeezed shut, with ensuing noncommunicating hydrocephalus.

SUGGESTED READINGS

Aas J-E: Subcortical projections to the pontine nuclei in the cat. J Comp Neurol 282:331, 1989.

Altman J, Bayer SA: Development of the cerebellar system: in relation to its evolution, structure, and functions, Boca Raton, Fla, 1997, CRC Press.

Andersen BB, Gundersen HJG, Pakkenberg B: Aging of the human cerebellum: a stereological study. J Comp Neurol 466:356, 2003.

Angevine JB, Jr, Mancall EL, Yakovlev PI: The human cerebellum: an atlas of gross topography in serial sections, Boston, 1961, Little, Brown.
A review of various systems of cerebellar nomenclature and terminology together with a collection of beautiful sections cut in several different planes.

Asanuma C, Thach WT, Jones EG: Distribution of cerebellar terminations and their relation to other afferent terminations in the ventral lateral thalamic region of the monkey. Brain Res Rev 5:237, 1983.

Burman K, Darian-Smith C, Darian-Smith I: Macaque red nucleus: origins of spinal and olivary projections and terminations of cortical inputs. J Comp Neurol 423:179, 2000.

Carpenter MB, Batton RR, III: Connections of the fastigial nucleus in the cat and monkey. Exp Brain Res Suppl 6:250, 1982.

Claeys KG, et al: Involvement of multiple functionally distinct cerebellar regions in visual discrimination: a human functional imaging study. Neuroimage 20:840, 2003.

Desmond JE, et al: Lobular patterns of cerebellar activation in verbal working-memory and finger-tapping tasks as revealed by functional MRI. J Neurosci 17:9675, 1997.

Fiez JA, et al: Impaired non-motor learning and error detection associated with cerebellar damage: a single case study. Brain 115:155, 1992.
A particularly well-studied case of cognitive changes after cerebellar damage.

Flumerfelt BA, Otabe S, Courville J: Distinct projections to the red nucleus from the dentate and interposed nuclei in the monkey. Brain Res 50:408, 1973.

Gerwig M, Kolb FP, Timman D: The involvement of the human cerebellum in eyeblink conditioning. Cerebellum 6:38, 2007.

Glickstein M: Cerebellar agenesis. Brain 117:1209, 1994.
It is sometimes claimed that individuals with congenital absence of the cerebellum have normal or near-normal motor functions. This paper argues that published studies indicate "cerebellar agenesis is always associated with profound motor deficits."

Glickstein M, Yeo C: The cerebellum and motor learning. J Cogn Neurosci 2:69, 1990.
A brief but enjoyable review of the history of theories about cerebellar function and of evidence that it is important for motor learning.

Gottwald B, et al: Evidence for distinct cognitive deficits after focal cerebellar lesions. J Neurol Neurosurg Psychiatry 75:1524, 2004.

Gould BB, Graybiel AM: Afferents to the cerebellar cortex in the cat: evidence for an intrinsic pathway leading from the deep nuclei to the cortex. Brain Res 110:601, 1976.

Grant G, Xu Q: Routes of entry into the cerebellum of spinocerebellar axons from the lower part of the spinal cord: an experimental study in the cat. Exp Brain Res 72:543, 1988.

Grodd W, et al: Sensorimotor mapping of the human cerebellum: fMRI evidence of somatotopic organization. Hum Brain Mapp 13:55, 2001.

Habas C, Cabanis EA: Cortical projections to the human red nucleus: a diffusion tensor tractography study with a 1.5-T MRI machine. Neuroradiology 48:755, 2006.

Herrup K, Kuermerle B: The compartmentalization of the cerebellum. Ann Rev Neurosci 20:61, 1997.
The beginnings of a molecular basis for the medial-lateral and anterior-posterior subdivisions of the cerebellum.

Holmes G: The cerebellum of man. Brain 62:1, 1939.
Still the all-time great description of the neocerebellar syndrome in humans and the source of the striking illustrations in Figure 20-28.

Hülsmann E, Erb M, Grodd W: From will to action: sequential cerebellar contributions to voluntary movement. Neuroimage 20:1485, 2003.

Ikeda M: Projections from the spinal and the principal sensory nuclei of the trigeminal nerve to the cerebellar cortex in the cat, as studied by retrograde transport of horseradish peroxidase. J Comp Neurol 184:57, 1979.

Kalil K: Projections of the cerebellar and dorsal column nuclei upon the inferior olive in the rhesus monkey: an autoradiographic study. J Comp Neurol 188:43, 1979.

Kelly RM, Strick PL: Cerebellar loops with motor cortex and prefrontal cortex of a nonhuman primate. J Neurosci 23:8432, 2003.

Langer T, et al: Afferents to the flocculus of the cerebellum in the rhesus macaque as revealed by retrograde transport of horseradish peroxidase. J Comp Neurol 235:1, 1985.

Langer T, et al: Floccular efferents in the rhesus macaque as revealed by autoradiography and horseradish peroxidase. J Comp Neurol 235:26, 1985.

Larsell O, Jansen J: The comparative anatomy and histology of the cerebellum: the human cerebellum, cerebellar connections, and the cerebellar cortex, Minneapolis, 1972, University of Minnesota Press.

Mainland JD, et al: Olfactory impairments in patients with unilateral cerebellar lesions are selective to inputs from the contralesional nostril. J Neurosci 25:6362, 2005.

Manni A, Petrosini L: A century of cerebellar somatotopy: a debated representation. Nat Rev Neurosci 5:241, 2004.

Marinković S, et al: The anatomical basis for the cerebellar infarcts. Surg Neurol 44:450, 1995.
A nice review of the blood supply of the cerebellum.

Martin TA, et al: Throwing while looking through prisms. I. Focal olivocerebellar lesions impair adaptation. II. Specificity and storage of multiple gaze-throw calibrations. Brain 119:1183 and 1199, 1996.

Marx JJ, et al: Topodiagnostic implications of hemiataxia: an MRI-based brainstem mapping analysis. Neuroimage 39:1625, 2008.

Matano S: Brief communication: proportions of the ventral half of the cerebellar dentate nucleus in humans and great apes. Am J Phys Anthropol 114:163, 2001.

McCormick DA, Steinmetz JE, Thompson RF: Lesions of the inferior olivary complex cause extinction of the classically conditioned eyeblink response. Brain Res 359:120, 1985.

Meyer-Lohmann J, Hore J, Brooks VB: Cerebellar participation in generation of prompt arm movements. J Neurophysiol 40:1038, 1977.
What happens to voluntary movements when one dentate nucleus is temporarily disabled?

Middleton FA, Strick PL: Basal ganglia and cerebellar loops: motor and cognitive circuits. Brain Res Rev 31:236, 2000.

Mihailoff GA: Cerebellar nuclear projections from the basilar pontine nuclei and nucleus reticularis tegmenti pontis as demonstrated with PHA-L tracing in the rat. J Comp Neurol 330:130, 1993.

Mulholland PJ: Susceptibility of the cerebellum to thiamine deficiency. Cerebellum 5:55, 2006.

Murphy MG, O'Leary JL: Neurological deficit in cats with lesions of the olivocerebellar system. Arch Neurol 24:145, 1971.

Orlovsky GN: Activity of vestibulospinal neurons during locomotion. Brain Res 46:85, 1972.
The activity is rhythmically modulated, and the modulation disappears after cerebellar lesions.

Palay SL, Chan-Palay V: Cerebellar cortex: cytology and organization, New York, 1974, Springer-Verlag.
A beautiful book, full of Golgi-stained cells and electron micrographs.

Papka M, Ivry RB, Woodruff-Pak DS: Selective disruption of eyeblink classical conditioning by concurrent tapping. Neuroreport 6:1493, 1995.
Clever experiments suggesting that you can use multiple memory systems simultaneously, but only for one task each.

Payne JN: The cerebellar nucleo-cortical projection in the rat studied by the retrograde fluorescent double-labelling method. Brain Res 271:141, 1983.

Pijpers A, et al: Precise spatial relationships between mossy fibers and climbing fibers in rat cerebellar cortical zones. J Neurosci 26:12067, 2006.

Ramnani N, et al: The evolution of prefrontal inputs to the cortico-pontine system: diffusion imaging evidence from macaque monkeys and humans. Cereb Cortex 16:811, 2006.

Sanes JN, Dimitrov B, Hallet M: Motor learning in patients with cerebellar dysfunction. Brain 113:103, 1990.

Schmahmann JD, Ko R, MacMore J: The human basis pontis: motor syndromes and topographic organization. Brain 127:1269, 2004.

Schmahmann JD, Sherman JC: The cerebellar cognitive affective syndrome. Brain 121:561, 1998.

Schmahmann JD, et al: Three-dimensional MRI atlas of the human cerebellum in proportional stereotaxic space. Neuroimage 10:233, 1999.

The methodology and a subset of the pictures from the Schmahmann et al (2000) atlas.

Schmahmann JD, et al: MRI atlas of the human cerebellum, San Diego, 2000, Academic Press.

A superb depiction of cerebellar anatomy in coronal, axial, and sagittal planes.

Schoch B, et al: Functional localization in the human cerebellum based on voxelwise statistical analysis: a study of 90 patients. Neuroimage 30:36, 2006.

Schwarz C, Schmitz Y: Projection from the cerebellar lateral nucleus to precerebellar nuclei in the mossy fiber pathway is glutamatergic: a study combining anterograde tracing with immunogold labeling in the rat. J Comp Neurol 381:320, 1997.

Schweighofer N, Doya K, Kuroda S: Cerebellar aminergic neuromodulation: towards a functional understanding. Brain Res Rev 44:103, 2004.

Snider RS: Recent contributions to the anatomy and physiology of the cerebellum. Arch Neurol Psychiatry 64:196, 1950.

A summary of the electrophysiologically determined mapping of the cerebral cortex and the body surface onto the cerebellar cortex.

Sugihara I, Wu H-S, Shinoda Y: The entire trajectories of single olivocerebellar axons in the cerebellar cortex and their contribution to cerebellar compartmentalization. J Neurosci 21:7715, 2001.

Sultan F, Braitenberg V: Shapes and sizes of different mammalian cerebella. A study in quantitative comparative neuroanatomy. J Hirnforsch 34:79, 1993.

Tavano A, et al: Disorders of cognitive and affective development in cerebellar malformations. Brain 130:2646, 2007.

Thach WT: Timing of activity in cerebellar dentate nucleus and cerebral motor cortex during prompt volitional movement. Brain Res 88:233, 1975.

Thompson RF: The neurobiology of learning and memory. Science 233:941, 1986.

A review by one of the principal investigators of the role of the cerebellum in classical conditioning.

Tolbert DL, Bantli H, Bloedel JR: Organizational features of the cat and monkey cerebellar nucleocortical projection. J Comp Neurol 182:39, 1978.

Van Essen DC: Surface-based atlases of cerebellar cortex in the human, macaque, and mouse. Ann N Y Acad Sci 978:468, 2002.

The findings: 0.8 cm^2 of cerebellar cortex for a mouse, 60 cm^2 for a macaque, 600 cm^2 for a human.

Victor M, Adams RD, Mancall EL: A restricted form of cerebellar cortical degeneration occurring in alcoholic patients. Arch Neurol 1:578, 1959.

Voogd J: Cerebellum and precerebellar nuclei. In Paxinos G, Mai JK, editors: The human nervous system, ed 2, San Diego, 2004, Elsevier Academic Press.

Wu H-S, Sugihara I, Shinoda Y: Projection patterns of single mossy fibers originating from the lateral reticular nucleus in the rat cerebellar cortex and nuclei. J Comp Neurol 411:97, 1999.

Zhu J-N, et al: The cerebellar-hypothalamic circuits: potential pathways underlying cerebellar involvement in somatic-visceral integration. Brain Res Rev 52:93, 2006.

Eye Movements

Photoreceptors are sensitive but slow, and all animals with image-forming eyes have mechanisms to prevent images of interest from moving across the retina too quickly to be analyzed. (Using the camera analogy from Chapter 17, our eyes behave in many respects like cameras with a shutter speed of about $\frac{1}{10}$ of a second.) A widespread strategy is to use some combination of eye movements and head or body movements to keep the direction of gaze constant, except for brief periods during which gaze shifts (Fig. 21-1). Additional complications are added by having a fovea, which results in good spatial acuity for only a small area of central vision (see Fig. 17-18). Finally, effective binocular vision requires precise alignment of the two eyes. All this necessitates a highly accurate system for controlling eye position and movement.

Our eyes do a fairly remarkable job of tracking (or moving to look at) various objects as we and the objects move about in three-dimensional space. Throughout this process the two eyes stay appropriately aligned with each other. Two general types of movement are involved: (1) **conjugate movements,** in which the two eyes move the same amount in the same direction, as when visually tracking an object moving about at a fixed distance from us, and (2) **vergence movements,** in which the two eyes move in opposite directions, as in the **convergence** that occurs when looking at a nearby object. Normally, conjugate and vergence movements are smoothly integrated so that images of the outside world fall on the two retinas in proper registration. The central nervous system (CNS) circuits that control eye movements for these various purposes have many properties in common with those described in the last three chapters for the control of other skeletal muscles—upper and lower motor neurons, central pattern generators, and interactions with the basal ganglia and cerebellum.

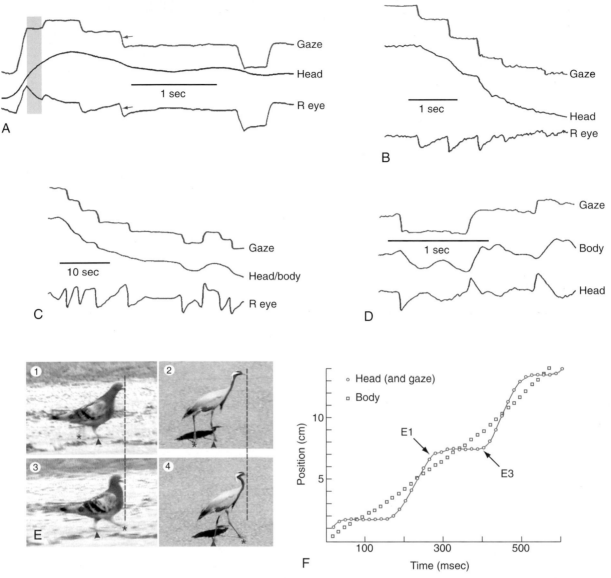

Figure 21-1 Gaze-holding by several different animal species, interrupted by quick movements that redirect gaze. **A-D** are seen from above as they go about various activities, **E** and **F** from the side. **A,** Movements of the right eye and head of a human standing at a sink and filling a kettle, getting ready to prepare a cup of tea. Most of the time his head and eyes move in exactly opposite directions, so that the direction of gaze (the sum of eye and head movement) does not change; one such period is indicated by *shading.* Every few hundred milliseconds his eyes move rapidly *(blue arrow),* shifting his gaze *(green arrow;* in this case, from the right faucet-handle to the stream of water flowing into the kettle). **B,** The orientation of the head, right eye, and gaze of a goldfish, as it turns while swimming in a tank of water. **C,** A rock crab *(Pachygrapsus marmoratus)* uses the same strategy as it walks around. The head obviously cannot move independently, but the eyestalks move to counteract body/head movements; periodic faster movements of the eyestalks redirect gaze. **D,** The eyes of flies are fixed in their heads and cannot move independently, but this blowfly *(Calliphora erythrocephala)* uses slow and fast head movements to compensate for body movements and to redirect gaze. **E,** Many species of birds appear to bob their heads back and forth as they walk, but this is illusory. What they really do is take advantage of their long necks to thrust their heads forward, then hold their heads stationary until the body catches up. These successive frames from a videocamera show a pigeon (E1, E3) and a crane (E2, E4) walking from left to right. E1 and E2 are just after a head thrust has been completed, E3 and E4 are just before another one starts. During each step, the beak stays stationary, one foot *(arrowhead)* stays planted, and the other foot *(asterisk)* and the body move forward. **F,** Relative positions of the body and head (and gaze) of a pigeon as it walks, showing periods of stable gaze in between head thrusts. *(A-D, modified from Land MF: J Comp Physiol A185:341, 1999. B, redrawn from Easter SS Jr, Johns PR, Heckenslively D: J Comp Physiol 92:23, 1974. C, redrawn from Paul H, Nalbach H-O, Varjú D: J Exp Biol 154:81, 1990. D, redrawn from Land MF: Nature 243:299, 1973. E, from Necker R: J Comp Physiol A193:1177, 2007. F, redrawn from Frost BJ: J Exp Biol 74:187, 1978.)*

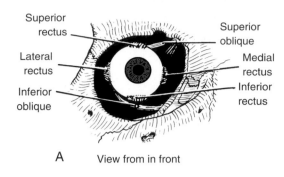

A   View from in front

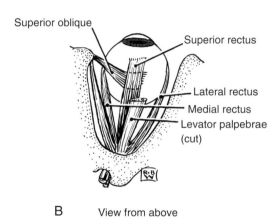

B   View from above

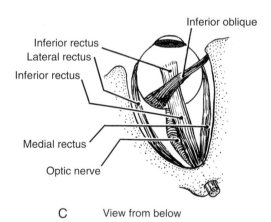

C   View from below

Figure 21-2 Anterior **(A),** superior **(B),** and inferior **(C)** views of the extraocular muscles of the right eye. *(Modified from von Noorden GK: Atlas of strabismus, ed 4, St. Louis, 1983, Mosby.)*

Six Extraocular Muscles Move the Eye in the Orbit

Six small **extraocular muscles** (Fig. 21-2) rotate each eye in its orbit, like a ball in a socket. Four **rectus** ("straight") muscles (**medial, lateral, superior,** and **inferior**) originate from a common tendinous ring (the annulus of Zinn) in the back of the orbit and insert *anteriorly* in the sclera, 5 to 8 mm from the limbus. Two **oblique** muscles,

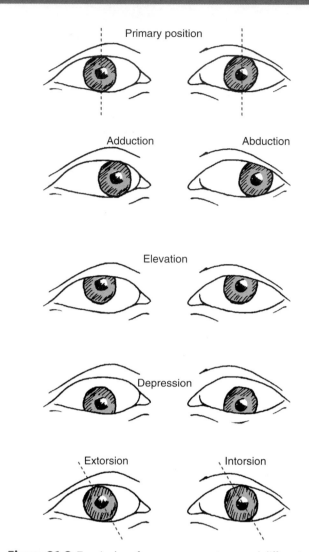

Figure 21-3 Terminology for eye movements around different axes.

as the name implies, pass obliquely over the surface of the eye and insert in the sclera of its *posterior* half. The **superior oblique** originates near the common tendinous ring, from the sphenoid bone at the back of the orbit, but it takes an unusual course in reaching the eye. Near the front of the orbit, the superior oblique tendon passes through a fibrous loop (the **trochlea**[a]) attached to the frontal bone, turns laterally and posteriorly, and inserts in the sclera of the posterior half of the eye. The **inferior oblique** originates anteriorly and medially from the floor of the orbit, passes across the inferior surface of the eye, and inserts posteriorly.

Different patterns of contraction of the six extraocular muscles rotate the eye horizontally (**adduction** = toward midline, **abduction** = away from midline), vertically (**elevation** = up, **depression** = down), or around its anterior-posterior axis (**extorsion** = rotate out, **intorsion** = rotate in) (Fig. 21-3). As you recall from Chapter 12, these muscles are innervated by three sets of cranial nerves.

---

[a]Trochlea, from which the fourth cranial nerve derives its name, is Greek for "pulley."

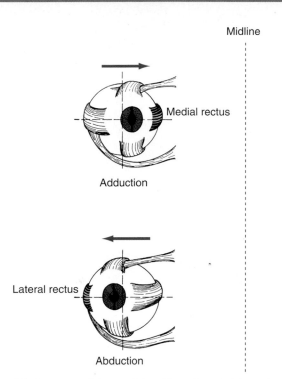

Figure 21-4 Actions of the medial and lateral recti of the right eye. *(Modified from Moses RA, editor: Adler's physiology of the eye, ed 5, St. Louis, 1970, Mosby.)*

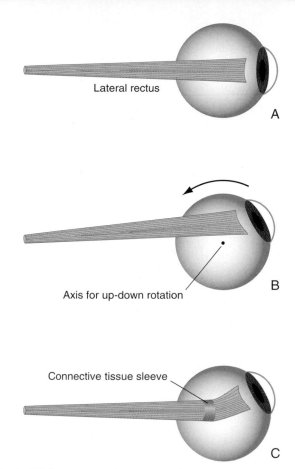

Figure 21-5 Limitation of the action of the lateral rectus by its connective tissue suspension within the orbit. **A,** With the eyes in primary position, the lateral rectus extends along the equator of the eye and abducts it by rotating it around a vertical axis. **B,** If the lateral rectus was attached only at its origin at the common tendinous ring and its insertion in the sclera, intermediate parts of it would be free to slide over the surface of the eye during eye movements. If the eye was elevated, for example, the insertion point would move above the center of rotation of the eye, and lateral rectus contraction would elevate the eye further in addition to abducting it. **C,** The functional insertion of the lateral rectus is the point at which it emerges from its connective tissue sleeve, so even if the eye is elevated, contraction mainly causes abduction.

Cranial nerve III (oculomotor) innervates the majority of the muscles, including the superior, medial, and inferior rectus as well as the inferior oblique. The lateral rectus is innervated by cranial nerve VI (abducens), and the superior oblique is innervated by cranial nerve IV (trochlear).

The Medial and Lateral Recti Adduct and Abduct the Eye

The medial and lateral recti are situated in a horizontal plane, so contractions of these muscles rotate the eye around a vertical axis. This makes their actions straightforward (Fig. 21-4)—the medial rectus adducts and the lateral rectus abducts the eye. Both muscles pass through sleeves of connective tissue (referred to as **pulleys**) as they travel from the common tendinous ring toward the eye, emerging a little posterior to their insertion points on the sclera. The pulleys, in turn, have connective tissue attachments to the walls of the orbit, so the positions of the muscles are constrained within the orbit as the eye moves. As a result, adduction and abduction continue to be the principal effects of the medial and lateral recti, even if the eye starts out in an elevated or depressed position (Fig. 21-5). The superior and inferior recti and the inferior oblique have similar pulleys (in this sense, the superior oblique is not as different from the other extraocular muscles as it seems to be). The pulleys form important parts of an elaborate mechanical suspension system that helps control rotations of the eye; half the fibers of the recti and inferior oblique actually attach to the pulleys rather than the sclera, adjusting pulley positions as the eye moves.

The Superior and Inferior Recti and the Obliques Have More Complex Actions

The actions of the superior and inferior recti and the obliques are not quite so straightforward, because the anatomical axis of the orbit is deviated about 23 degrees laterally from the visual axis of the eye (Fig. 21-6). The result, as indicated for the superior rectus and superior oblique in Figure 21-7 but equally true for the inferior rectus and inferior oblique, is that when one of these muscles contracts, it looks as though the eye should rotate around an axis that is neither vertical nor transverse nor anterior-posterior. Consequently, each of these four muscles has one principal action and weaker additional actions (Fig. 21-8). However, the pulley system constrains their directions of pull, and these secondary actions come into play only in eccentric gaze. Starting

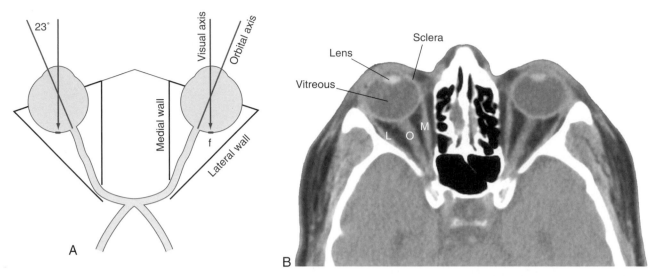

Figure 21-6 Relative orientations of the eyes and orbits. **A,** The eye, when focused for far vision, points more or less straight ahead so that images land on the fovea (f). Because the lateral wall of each orbit is oriented about 45 degrees from the sagittal plane, the axis of the orbit, along which the superior and inferior recti appear to pull, is oriented about 23 degrees from the visual axis. **B,** Computed tomography scan of a 68-year-old man showing the relationship between the eyes and the medial and lateral walls of the orbits. L, lateral rectus; M, medial rectus; O, optic nerve. (**B,** *courtesy Dr. Raymond F. Carmody, University of Arizona College of Medicine.*)

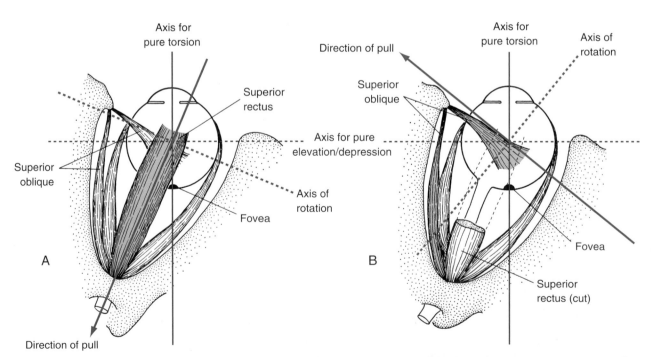

Figure 21-7 Apparent directions of pull and axes of rotation of the right superior rectus **(A)** and superior oblique **(B),** relative to the axes of rotation for pure torsion or pure elevation or depression. In reality, connective tissue suspensions make the superior rectus more of a pure elevator and the superior oblique more of a pure intorter than these diagrams indicate. (*Modified from Moses RA, editor: Adler's physiology of the eye, ed 5, St. Louis, 1970, Mosby.*)

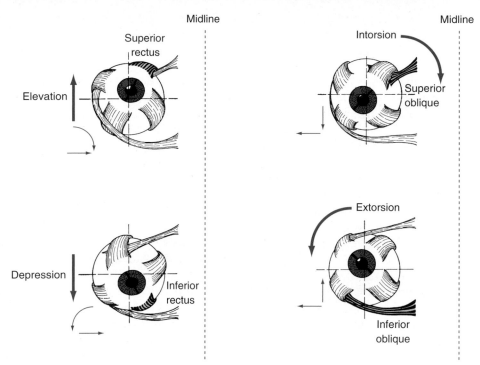

Figure 21-8 Actions of the right superior and inferior recti and obliques. Each has a primary action *(large arrows)* and two secondary actions *(small arrows)* when starting from the primary position. The actions are determined both by the direction of insertion of a muscle's tendon and by the position of the insertion. For example, the superior rectus and superior oblique both insert on the superior surface of the globe. However, the superior rectus inserts anteriorly and pulls posteriorly, so it elevates the eye. In contrast, the superior oblique inserts posteriorly and pulls in part anteriorly (see Fig. 21-7), so part of its action is depression. The extent of the secondary actions of the superior and inferior recti is somewhat exaggerated in this figure; connective tissue pulleys constrain their actions to nearly pure elevation and depression, respectively, in straight-ahead gaze. *(Modified from Moses RA, editor: Adler's physiology of the eye, ed 5, St. Louis, 1970, Mosby.)*

from straight-ahead gaze, the superior and inferior recti largely take care of elevation and depression, respectively; similarly, the superior and inferior obliques cause intorsion and extorsion, respectively.

To keep things reasonably simple in this chapter, torsional movements are not discussed,[b] and adduction, abduction, elevation, and depression are treated as the result of contraction of just one of the rectus muscles. However, eye movements actually involve coordinated changes in the activity of all six extraocular muscles (Table 21-1), some contracting and some relaxing in response to changing levels of input from the oculomotor, trochlear, and abducens nuclei (see Figs. 12-4 to 12-6). For example, adduction involves simultaneous contraction of the medial, superior, and inferior recti and relaxation of the lateral rectus and the superior and inferior obliques; the intorsion and extorsion of the superior and inferior recti cancel each other.

---

[b]We tend not to think much about torsional movements, but if you tilt your head to one side, both of your eyes counterrotate in partial compensation. Such tilting does not disturb images on the fovea too much, so torsional movements are less important for us than for more lateral-eyed animals.

Table 21-1	Extraocular Muscles Contributing to Movements Around Different Axes

Movement	Principal Muscle	Other Muscles Contributing
Adduction	Medial rectus	Superior rectus Inferior rectus
Abduction	Lateral rectus	Superior oblique Inferior oblique
Elevation	Superior rectus	Inferior oblique
Depression	Inferior rectus	Superior oblique
Extorsion	Inferior oblique	Inferior rectus
Intorsion	Superior oblique	Superior rectus

There Are Fast and Slow Conjugate Eye Movements

Conjugate movements serve one of two general purposes—to move an object's image onto the fovea or to keep it there (see Fig. 21-1). We use fast, steplike eye movements called **saccades** (from a French word meaning "a pull on the reins") to redirect gaze so a different image falls on the fovea. The same neural machinery comes into play whenever these brief, rapid movements are called for—to move our eyes voluntarily in any given direction, to glance over at something in the periphery, and in the fast phase of nystagmus. We use multiple kinds of smooth, slower eye movements to keep an image on the fovea, corresponding to the fact that an image can move on the retina if we move or if the object moves. The **vestibuloocular reflex (VOR)** (see Figs. 14-31 and 14-32) compensates for head movements, supplemented in this function by **optokinetic** movements (see Fig. 14-33A); for large head movements, these smooth eye movements become the slow phase of nystagmus. **Smooth pursuit movements** are used to track a visual stimulus that is itself moving. Without special training, we are unable to move our eyes smoothly unless an image starts to leave the fovea (Box 21-1).

A network of neural structures distributed through the brainstem, cerebellum, and cerebral hemispheres is involved in the initiation and coordination of conjugate eye movements (Fig. 21-10). Basically it involves reflex

connections and central pattern generators for these eye movements, located in the brainstem, together with cerebral and cerebellar centers that are able to trigger or modulate these brainstem mechanisms. The brainstem centers differ for different kinds of movement, but the cerebral and cerebellar centers overlap. No corticobulbar fibers reach the abducens, trochlear, or oculomotor nuclei directly (see Figs. 21-13 and 21-16).

Fast, Ballistic Eye Movements Get Images Onto the Fovea

Saccades and the fast phases of nystagmus are extremely rapid, reaching velocities of 700 degrees/second (Fig. 21-11). This is too fast for the visual system to provide useful feedback under most circumstances,[c] and fast eye movements generally behave as though the CNS computes the size of the required movement in advance (which takes about 200 msec), initiates the movement, and makes no corrections during its course. These preprogrammed movements are referred to as *ballistic*. One of the few ways in which saccades are altered once they begin is through the superimposition of the VOR, which compensates for head movements during a saccade (as in the period indicated by blue and green arrows in Fig. 21-1A).

Motor Programs for Saccades Are Located in the Pons and Midbrain

Moving an eye at 700 degrees/second to a target requires a brief, strong contraction of one or more extraocular

---

[c]We do not have a sensation of blurred vision during these fast eye movements (even though images move across the retina very rapidly) because the CNS suppresses or ignores visual input during these brief periods.

BOX 21-1

Smooth Eye Movements Usually Require Either a Vestibular Stimulus or a Target Moving Across the Retina

It generally comes as a surprise that, with the head stationary, we cannot voluntarily move our eyes smoothly unless we are tracking a slowly moving object (Fig. 21-9A). This is easily demonstrated, however. Watch someone's eyes as he or she tries to move them slowly and smoothly while there is nothing to track, or concentrate on your own eyes while you try to do the same thing. In either case the result will be the same: a series of rapid, jerky movements (saccades; see Fig. 21-9B). Some individuals can learn to have voluntary control of smooth tracking movements, but under normal circumstances and for most people, this is impossible. Interestingly, real moving stimuli in other sensory modalities provide, to varying degrees, an adequate stimulus for some smooth movements. For example, many people can use smooth eye movements to track their own index fingers moving back and forth in the dark (see Fig. 21-9C), even though they are unable to use such eye movements to track imaginary moving fingers. Similarly, smooth eye movements can be used to track a moving sound source in the dark (although less successfully than when using a somatosensory stimulus).

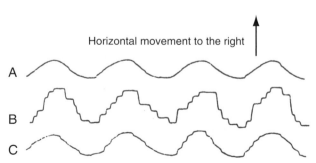

Figure 21-9 Recordings of the horizontal eye movements of a normal subject in an otherwise dark room as he tracked an LED moving back and forth **(A)**, tried to imagine an LED moving back and forth and track it with his eyes **(B)**, and tried to follow the position of his finger as he moved his arm back and forth in the dark **(C)**; upward deflections indicate movement to the right. Movements with a somatosensory assist are much smoother than those with only an imaginary target. You can approximate this experiment by closing your eyes and concentrating on how they move as you try to track an imaginary target or your own moving finger. *(From Hashiba M et al: Acta Otolaryngol Suppl 525:158, 1996.)*

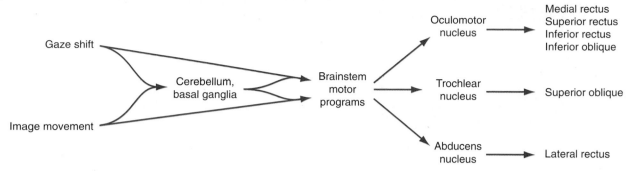

Figure 21-10 Schematic overview of eye movement control systems. Central pattern generators in the brainstem project through lower motor neurons to extraocular muscles, as indicated. Interconnections between the cerebellum, basal ganglia, and cerebral centers that initiate eye movements are described further in the text; this schematic overview is not meant to indicate, for example, that the basal ganglia project directly to the central pattern generators.

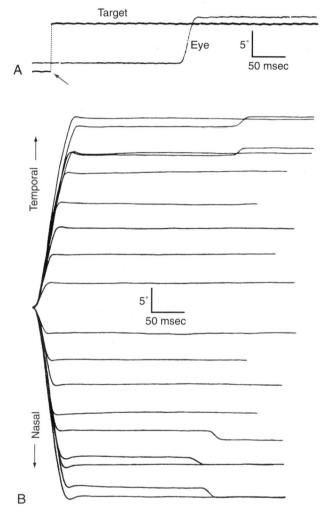

Figure 21-11 Time course of saccades, shown in recordings of the horizontal eye movements of a monkey trained to make gaze shifts (with head stationary) to follow a target that makes occasional jumps in position; upward deflections indicate movement to the right. **A,** After a target jump *(arrow),* the monkey makes a rapid (about 580 degrees/sec) saccade to its new position after a latency of about 200 msec. **B,** Larger and larger target jumps elicit saccades of increasing duration and peak velocity. Saccades in response to the largest target jumps are often a little too small and are followed by a corrective saccade after an additional 200- to 250-msec latency. *(From Fuchs AF: J Physiol 191:609, 1967.)*

muscles, followed by a weaker, sustained contraction to keep the eye in its new position. This is accomplished by central pattern generators whose circuitry resides in the brainstem: appropriate patterns of excitation are provided to motor neurons in the abducens, trochlear, or oculomotor nuclei by specialized areas of the pontine and mesencephalic reticular formation.

The neural machinery for generating rapid horizontal movements is located in the medial reticular formation of the pons near the abducens nucleus, a region commonly referred to by the logical but cumbersome name **paramedian pontine reticular formation (PPRF)**. Signals from this region project to the abducens nucleus and the nucleus of the medial longitudinal fasciculus (MLF) for connection to the contralateral CN III lower motor neurons of the medial rectus, with each PPRF directing movements to the ipsilateral side (see Fig. 21-13).

The machinery for rapid vertical movements is located in the reticular formation just dorsomedial to the red nucleus at the midbrain-diencephalon junction (in a region called the **rostral interstitial nucleus of the medial longitudinal fasciculus,** or **riMLF**). The riMLF on each side has a peculiar pattern of connections: it projects bilaterally to the motor neurons for all the elevator muscles of both eyes and to the motor neurons for the ipsilateral inferior rectus and the contralateral superior oblique. Hence unilateral damage here causes little or no deficit of upward gaze (because the other side can compensate), but there is some weakness of downward gaze (because one depressor of each eye cannot be activated). However, some of the connections required for upward saccades apparently involve more dorsal parts of the midbrain as well, because one of the common early effects of pineal tumors is selective paralysis of upward gaze (together with disturbances of convergence).

The Frontal Eye Field and Superior Colliculus Trigger Saccades to the Contralateral Side

Saccades are the eye movements we routinely use to explore the world visually during activities as varied as

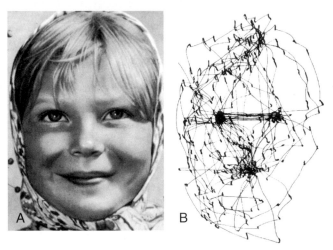

Figure 21-12 Using saccades to scan visual scenes. **A,** A photograph called "Girl from Volga," which a subject was asked to look at for 2 minutes. **B,** Recordings of eye position during this 2-minute period. Thin lines represent saccades between points of fixation, which center around parts of the face of greatest visual interest. The subject has no conscious sensation of making these saccades or of having brief periods of blurred vision. Rather, the CNS ignores inputs during the saccades and combines the visual inputs during the periods of fixation into a single, unified visual perception. *(From Yarbus AL: Eye movements and vision, New York, 1967, Plenum Press.)*

filling a teakettle (see Fig. 21-1A), scanning scenes and pictures (Fig. 21-12), and reading. Cortical control of saccades parallels that of other voluntary movements, with an equivalent of primary motor cortex, contributions from other cortical areas, and interactions with the basal nuclei and cerebellum.

The **frontal eye field** is located just in front of the representation of the face in the precentral gyrus, in the posterior portion of the middle frontal gyrus and the banks of the precentral sulcus (Fig. 21-13); it is prominently involved in the initiation of saccades. Stimulation here causes horizontal or oblique conjugate movements to the contralateral side, mediated in part by direct projections to the PPRF and in part by projections to the superior colliculus, which in turn projects to the PPRF. Part of the supplementary motor area (the **supplementary eye field**) and part of the parietal lobe (the **parietal eye field**) also participate in the initiation of saccades. Just as in the case of outputs from motor-related areas to the spinal cord (see Fig. 18-11), they do so through both connections with the frontal eye field and direct projections to the brainstem. Stimulation of these areas also elicits saccades, and, as in the case of other voluntary movements, it is assumed that each of these cortical areas has a distinctive role. The parietal eye field may be especially involved in more automatic saccades to things that appear in the periphery, and the supplementary eye field may be involved in sequences of multiple saccades.

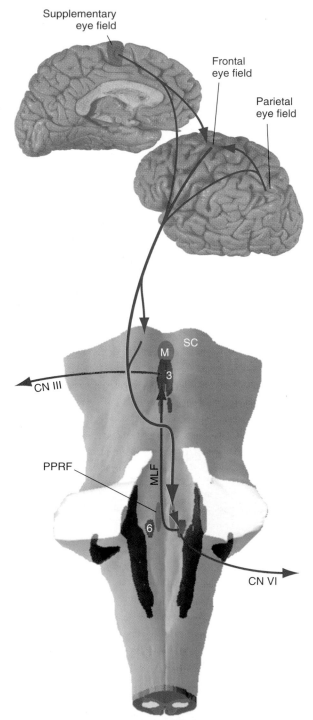

Figure 21-13 Cortical areas and brainstem circuitry involved in generating saccades to the right. 3, oculomotor nucleus; 6, abducens nucleus; M, midbrain reticular formation; MLF, medial longitudinal fasciculus; PPRF, paramedian pontine reticular formation; SC, superior colliculus.

Damage to the frontal eye field of one hemisphere causes the inability to look voluntarily to the contralateral side. It can easily be shown, however, that the appropriate muscles are not paralyzed, because other movements, such as those of the VOR, remain intact.

Vertical eye movements are not impaired after a unilateral lesion, and even the deficit in horizontal movements is only temporary, with recovery usually occurring in a matter of days. The relative roles of increased activity of the superior colliculus, other cortical areas, and the contralateral frontal eye field in this recovery of function are unclear. However, combined damage to the frontal eye fields and superior colliculi causes a severe and long-lasting deficit in the ability to generate saccades.

Slow, Guided Eye Movements Keep Images on the Fovea

The eye movements used to keep images from moving off the fovea are slower than saccades—typically up to only about 100 degrees/second—slow enough to utilize continuous feedback from the vestibular and visual systems to regulate their speed and duration. As noted earlier, images move on the retina if you or some part of the outside world moves. These things often happen simultaneously (think about playing any sport that involves a ball), and we have smoothly integrated mechanisms, all funneling through the vestibular nuclei, to deal with both.

Vestibuloocular and Optokinetic Movements Compensate for Head Movement

One of the greatest threats to the stability of images on the retina is the constant head movement that occurs as creatures walk, run, fly, or swim through their environments, and all jawed vertebrates use essentially similar mechanisms to deal with this. Head movement not only stimulates the semicircular canals and otolithic organs but also causes the image of the outside world to begin sweeping across the retina; both sets of sensory signals are used to generate compensatory eye movements.

The semicircular canals developed in parallel with the extraocular muscles (Box 21-2) and form the afferent limb of the VOR (see Figs. 14-31 and 14-32). As described in Chapter 14, this is a three-neuron reflex arc[d] that generates compensatory eye movements in the opposite

---

[d]Except in the case of reflex contraction of the medial rectus, which requires an additional interneuron whose cell body is in the abducens nucleus.

direction from head movements. Primary afferents have cell bodies in the vestibular ganglion, interneurons in the vestibular nuclei, and motor neurons in the abducens, trochlear, and oculomotor nuclei. The VOR, with a latency of only about 15 msec, is the fastest mechanism available for generating compensatory eye movements and is particularly effective at dealing with the

---

BOX 21-2

Using the Same Vestibuloocular Reflex for Eyes With Different Orientations

The vestibuloocular system appeared early in vertebrate phylogeny and has not changed much in its essentials. Each semicircular canal is nearly parallel to the plane in which two extraocular muscles of each eye pull, and increased activity of the semicircular canal selectively excites one of those muscles in each eye and inhibits its antagonist (Table 21-2). This creates some interesting challenges for the VOR because, although the orientations of the semicircular canals are more or less the same in all jawed vertebrates, not all animals' eyes are situated in their heads the same way. Consider the example of rotating a lateral-eyed rabbit and a frontal-eyed human about an anterior-posterior axis (i.e., an axis passing through the bridge of the nose and the occiput). For a rotation that moves the left ear downward, the appropriate compensatory eye movements for a rabbit would be elevation of the left eye and depression of the right eye; for a human, the appropriate movements would be torsional—intorsion of the left eye and extorsion of the right. Yet in both, the rotation causes depolarization of hair cells in the left anterior and posterior canals and contraction of the left superior rectus and superior oblique. The remarkable resolution of this apparent conflict lies in the fact that as orbits evolved into different positions, so did the origins, insertions, and paths of extraocular muscles (Fig. 21-14). The result is that contraction of a rabbit's left superior oblique and superior rectus produces elevation of the left eye; contraction of the same two muscles in a human produces intorsion.

Table 21-2	Effects of Increased Activity of Individual Semicircular Canals on Extraocular Muscles			
Canal	Excitation (Ipsilateral)	Inhibition (Ipsilateral)	Excitation (Contralateral)	Inhibition (Contralateral)
Anterior	Superior rectus	Inferior rectus	Inferior oblique	Superior oblique
Posterior	Superior oblique	Inferior oblique	Inferior rectus	Superior rectus
Horizontal	Medial rectus	Lateral rectus	Lateral rectus	Medial rectus

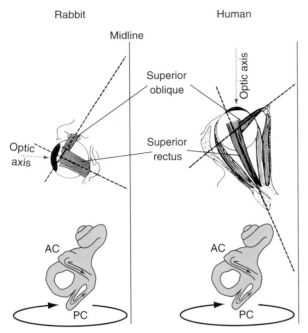

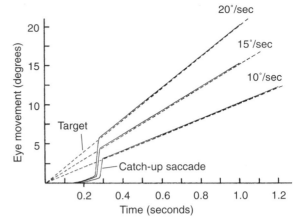

Figure 21-15 Time course of smooth pursuit movements, shown in recordings of the horizontal eye movements of a monkey trained to track (with head stationary) a target moving to the right. Smooth pursuit starts sooner than a saccade could, about 150 msec after target movement begins, but by then, the target's image has moved off the fovea. The CNS "knows" this will happen, however, and generates a saccade at about 250 msec that places the target's image back on the fovea. *(From Fuchs AF: J Physiol 191:609, 1967.)*

Figure 21-14 Effects of the same rotation (rolling to the left) on the left eye of a rabbit and a human; the view is as if you were looking down from above on both subjects. The insertion of the rabbit's superior oblique is anterior, so both the superior oblique and the superior rectus elevate the eye; the torsions of the two muscles cancel each other. The insertion of the human superior oblique is posterior, so it is a depressor that, in this movement, cancels the elevation of the superior rectus; both muscles combine to intort the eye. AC, anterior semicircular canal; PC, posterior semicircular canal. *(Modified from Simpson JI, Graf W: Ann N Y Acad Sci 374:20, 1981.)*

high-frequency components of head movements during locomotion. Interactions between the flocculus and the brainstem can cancel part or all of the VOR, allowing combined use of head and eye movements to shift gaze or follow targets (e.g., canceling the VOR if you decide to move your head to look at something else).

The VOR is not so effective with prolonged or low-frequency components of movement, which call into play a complementary system of compensatory optokinetic movements. Motion-sensitive ganglion cells project not only to the lateral geniculate nucleus and superior colliculus but also to a series of small **accessory optic nuclei** in the rostral midbrain. These in turn project to the vestibular nuclei, stimulating the same neurons that drive the VOR and producing eye movements that oppose image movement on the retina. This brainstem optokinetic system is present but rudimentary in humans, having been largely supplanted by cortically driven smooth pursuit movements (which also utilize the vestibular nuclei; see the next section).

Smooth Pursuit Movements Compensate for Target Movement

The development of a fovea adds a requirement for another kind of eye movement, one designed to keep the

images of small but interesting objects on the fovea even if an object is moving relative to the background.[e] This is accomplished by smooth pursuit movements (Fig. 21-15; see also Fig. 21-9), which use visual feedback to keep images of moving targets on the fovea. For objects that move too fast to track or that change speed or direction unpredictably, a combination of saccades and smooth pursuit is used (see Fig. 21-15).

We typically decide whether something is interesting enough to track, implying that cerebral cortex takes the lead in initiating pursuit movements. The arrangement is similar to that for saccades (see Fig. 21-13), but in this case, motion-sensitive extrastriate areas work in concert with the frontal and supplementary eye fields (Fig. 21-16). The rest of the circuitry suggests a probable evolutionary relationship between smooth pursuit movements and VOR cancellation. Both utilize the cerebellum (especially the flocculus) and vestibular nuclei, which makes smooth pursuit the only kind of movement known that requires the cerebellum for its generation. The cerebellar connection, in place since the days when its main function was VOR cancellation, may account for the seemingly peculiar observation that unilateral damage to the cortical areas in Figure 21-16 causes pursuit deficits in both directions, but a greater

---

[e]"Lateral-eyed afoveate animals are happy prisoners of their VORs. Foveate animals in hot pursuit of a dodging prey could not afford this." (From Robinson DA: The biology of eye movements. In Albert DM, Jakobiec FA, editors: Principles and practice of ophthalmology, Philadelphia, 1994, WB Saunders.)

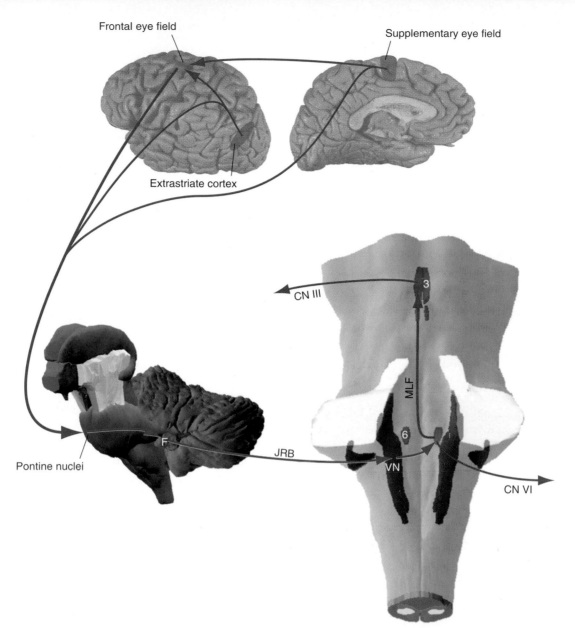

Figure 21-16 Cortical areas and other neural circuitry involved in smooth pursuit movements. 3, oculomotor nucleus; 6, abducens nucleus; F, flocculus; JRB, juxtarestiform body; MLF, medial longitudinal fasciculus; VN, vestibular nuclei.

deficit when tracking toward the side *ipsilateral* to the damage.

Changes in Object Distance Require Vergence Movements

Images of objects moving in any direction in a frontal plane move the same distance across both retinas, providing a signal that can be used to guide conjugate movements. Movements toward or away from the eyes, however, cause images to fall on increasingly disparate parts of the two retinas (Fig. 21-17). In addition, because the eye is well focused on only a particular range of

depths for any accommodative state of the lens, the same movements may cause image blurring. Both retinal disparity and accommodation signals are used to guide vergence eye movements.

The central pattern generator for vergence is located in the reticular formation of the rostral midbrain, near the oculomotor nuclei—just where it needs to be to implement the components of the near reflex (see Fig. 17-41). Vergence movements are initiated by a network of cortical areas similar to those involved in saccades and pursuit. Extrastriate areas involved in depth perception participate, along with the frontal and supplementary eye fields and possibly the parietal eye field. Consistent with this are observations that damage to the

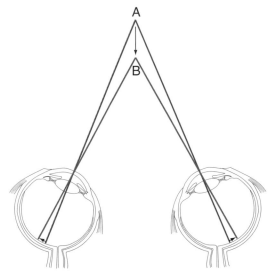

Figure 21-17 Retinal disparity created by images at different depths. With the eyes converged so that the image of an object at A falls on both foveae, images of objects at other depths, such as B, fall on disparate points on the two retinas. This disparity information is used by the CNS to figure out how to change convergence when looking from A to B.

midbrain and occasionally to the occipital lobes interferes with convergence, whereas damage to more caudal portions of the brainstem (including the MLF) does not.

The Basal Nuclei and Cerebellum Participate in Eye Movement Control

One of the multiple, parallel loops through which the basal nuclei affect cortical output (see Chapter 19) directly influences the production of saccades and pursuit movements (Fig. 21-18). The input side of the loop originates in the frontal and supplementary eye fields and other cortical areas and projects to the body of the caudate nucleus (see Fig. 19-10). The output side involves modulation of the frontal and supplementary eye fields and the superior colliculus by varying levels of inhibition emerging from the substantia nigra (reticular part). Consistent with this pattern of connections, patients with basal nuclei disorders such as Parkinson's and Huntington's diseases exhibit a variety of eye movement abnormalities reminiscent of the abnormalities of other movements. These include involuntary saccades during attempted steady gaze, small saccades, diminished numbers of spontaneous saccades, and slowed smooth pursuit.

The cerebellum plays a critical role in eye movements of all types. Although there is considerable overlap, the vermis is related more to fast movements and vergence, and the flocculus and nodulus to slow movements. In addition, functional imaging studies indicate that the lateral hemispheres are active during the planning of eye

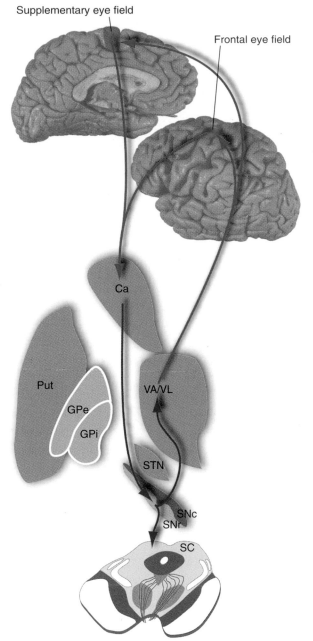

Figure 21-18 Basal ganglia connections affecting eye movements; other areas, such as the parietal eye field, probably feed into the same loop, but the connections of the frontal and supplementary eye fields are the best known. Excitatory connections are in green, inhibitory connections in red. See Chapter 19 for additional details. Ca, caudate nucleus; GPe and GPi, external and internal segments of the globus pallidus; Put, putamen; SC, superior colliculus; SNc and SNr, compact and reticular parts of the substantia nigra; STN, subthalamic nucleus; VA/VL, ventral anterior and ventral lateral nuclei.

movements. Some of these roles are comparable to cerebellar involvement in other movements, but others are unique:

1. Vermal areas in the upper part of the posterior lobe (referred to as the **oculomotor vermis;** Fig. 21-19A) help regulate the timing of muscle contractions

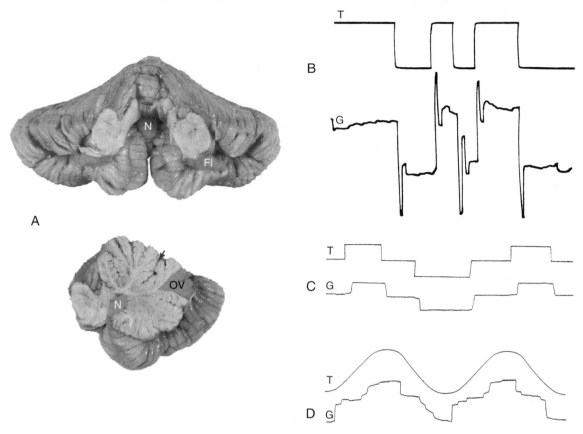

Figure 21-19 Cerebellum and eye movements. **A,** Cerebellar areas prominently involved in the production or coordination of eye movements. Arrow, primary fissure; Fl, flocculus; N nodulus; OV, oculomotor vermis. **B** to **D,** Eye movement abnormalities following damage to the cerebellum or its connections. **B,** Horizontal saccades of the right eye of a patient 1 month after surgical removal of a midline cerebellar tumor (medulloblastoma). When the patient tries to shift gaze in response to target steps, saccades are dysmetric and overshoot the target. **C,** Horizontal eye movements of a 73-year-old woman with an infarct in the right basal pons, including the pontine nuclei, which are known to convey visual motion signals to the cerebellum for use in pursuit movements. Saccades were normal **(C),** but smooth pursuit movements **(D)** were nearly absent, mostly replaced by saccades. G, direction of gaze; T, target position. *(**B,** from Selhorst JB et al: Brain 99:497, 1976. **C** and **D,** from Gaymard B et al: J Neurol Neurosurg Psychiatry 56:799, 1993.)*

during saccades. Damage here causes dysmetric saccades (see Fig. 21-19B) comparable to the dysmetric limb movements seen after damage to other parts of the cerebellum (see Fig. 20-28).

2. The role of the cerebellum in at least some forms of motor learning was mentioned in Chapter 20. The flocculus is essential for changing the gain of the VOR in response to changes affecting the optics of the eye. Similarly, the flocculus, sometimes in conjunction with the vermis, underlies plasticity of other eye movements such as saccades. This allows a degree of compensation for such things as changes in the strength of an extraocular muscle.

3. As noted earlier in this chapter, pursuit movements are unique in requiring the cerebellum for their very production. Damage to the flocculus causes substantial slowing of pursuit movements, and extensive cerebellar damage results in their total abolition (see Fig. 21-19C and D).

4. The cerebellum is also involved in, but not essential for, vergence movements. This may be related not just to the coordination of vergence but also to the need to adjust VOR gain on a moment-to-moment basis, depending on how far away objects are (Fig. 21-20), which happens automatically as part of the near reflex.

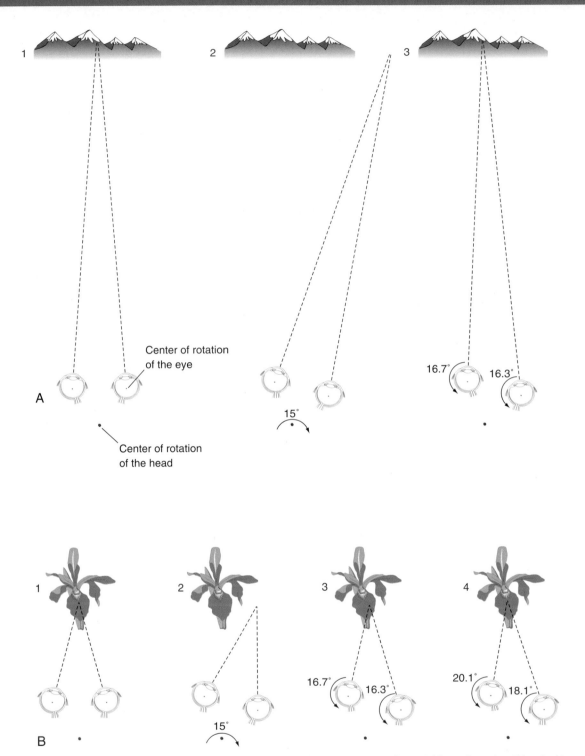

Figure 21-20 Different VOR gains are required to keep the image of a distant object or a near object stable on the retina. When looking at a distant object **(A1)**, the centers of rotation of the head and the eyes are close to each other, relative to the distance to the object. As a result, a VOR gain of 1 is appropriate: turning the head 15 degrees to the right **(A2)** can be compensated for by turning each eye about 15 degrees to the left **(A3)**. (A little more than 15 degrees is required in this example, because the eyes and the mountains are much closer to each other than they would be in reality.) When looking at a near object **(B1)** the centers of rotation of the head and the eyes are significantly different, relative to the distance to the object. As a result, turning the head 15 degrees to the right **(B2)** can no longer be compensated for by turning each eye about 15 degrees to the left **(B3)**, and a VOR gain greater than 1 is required **(B4).**

SUGGESTED READINGS

Bahill AT, LaRitz T: Why can't batters keep their eye on the ball? Am Sci 72:249, 1984.

Because the relatively slow speed of pursuit eye movements makes it impossible.

Basso MA, Pokorny JJ, Liu P: Activity of substantia nigra pars reticulata neurons during smooth pursuit eye movements in monkeys. Eur J Neurosci 22:448, 2005.

Baumann O, et al: Differences in cortical activation during smooth pursuit and saccadic eye movements following cerebellar lesions. Exp Brain Res 181:237, 2007.

Recent work on the role of the lateral hemispheres of the cerebellum in eye movements.

Bender MB: The oculomotor decussation. Am J Ophthalmol 54:591, 1962.

Evidence about the level at which corticobulbar fibers to the PPRF cross the midline.

Berryhill ME, Chiu T, Hughes HC: Smooth pursuit of nonvisual motion. J Neurophysiol 96:461, 2006.

Bogousslavsky J, Meienberg O: Eye-movement disorders in brainstem and cerebellar stroke. Arch Neurol 44:141, 1987.

Burr DC, Morrone MC, Ross J: Selective suppression of the magnocellular visual pathway during saccadic eye movements. Nature 371:511, 1994.

Carpenter RHS: Movements of the eyes, ed 2, London, 1988, Pion Limited.

Cui D-M, Yan Y-J, Lynch JC: Pursuit subregion of the frontal eye field projects to the caudate nucleus in monkeys. J Neurophysiol 89:2678, 2003.

Demer JL: Pivotal role of orbital connective tissues in binocular alignment and strabismus: the Friedenwald Lecture. Invest Ophthalmol 45:729, 2004.

Erkelen CJ, Steinman RM, Collewijn H: Ocular vergence under natural conditions. II. Gaze shifts between real targets differing in distance and direction. Proc R Soc Lond B 236:441, 1989.

Estanol B, Romero R, Corvera J: Effects of cerebellectomy on eye movements in man. Arch Neurol 36:281, 1979.

Frost BJ: The optokinetic basis of head-bobbing in the pigeon. J Exp Biol 74:187, 1978.

Gamlin PD: Neural mechanisms for the control of vergence eye movements. Ann N Y Acad Sci 956:264, 2002.

Gaymard B, et al: Smooth pursuit eye movement deficits after pontine nuclei lesions in humans. J Neurol Neurosurg Psychiatry 56:799, 1993.

Gottlieb JP, Bruce CJ, MacAvoy MG: Smooth eye movements elicited by microstimulation in the primate frontal eye field. J Neurophysiol 69:786, 1993.

Graf W, Baker R: The vestibuloocular reflex of the adult flatfish. I. Oculomotor organization. II. Vestibulooculomotor connectivity. J Neurophysiol 54:887 and 900, 1985.

Flatfish (e.g., flounder) start out like any other fish, then wind up with both eyes on one side of their body, but their semicircular canals don't change. This is the story of CNS changes that compensate for the mismatch.

Green JP, Newman NJ, Winterkorn JS: Paralysis of downgaze in two patients with clinical-radiologic correlation. Arch Ophthalmol 111:219, 1993.

Grossbras M-H, et al: An anatomical landmark for the supplementary eye fields in human revealed with functional magnetic resonance imaging. Cereb Cortex 9:705, 1999.

Heide W, Kurzidim K, Kömpf D: Deficits of smooth pursuit eye movements after frontal and parietal lesions. Brain 119:1951, 1996.

Hikosaka O, Takikawa Y, Kawagoe R: Role of the basal ganglia in the control of purposive saccadic eye movements. Physiol Rev 80:953, 2000.

Horn AKE, Büttner-Ennever JA: Premotor neurons for vertical eye movements in the rostral mesencephalon of monkey and human: histologic identification by parvalbumin immunostaining. J Comp Neurol 392:413, 1998.

Krauzlis RJ: The control of voluntary eye movements: new perspectives. Neuroscientist 11:124, 2005.

Land MF: Motion and vision: why animals move their eyes. J Comp Physiol [A] 185:341, 1999.

Leigh RJ, Zee DS: The neurology of eye movements, ed 4, New York, 2006, Oxford University Press.

The best reference work currently available.

Lim KH, Poukens V, Demer JL: Fascicular specialization in human and monkey rectus muscles: evidence for anatomic independence of global and orbital layers. Invest Ophthalmol 48:3089, 2007.

The global layer inserts into the sclera, and the orbital layer inserts into that muscle's connective tissue pulley.

Lynch JC, Hoover JE, Strick PL: Input to the primate frontal eye field from the substantia nigra, superior colliculus, and dentate nucleus demonstrated by transneuronal transport. Exp Brain Res 100:181, 1994.

Müri RM, et al: Location of the human posterior eye field with functional magnetic resonance imaging. J Neurol Neurosurg Psychiatry 60:445, 1996.

Necker R: Head-bobbing of walking birds. J Comp Physiol A193:1177, 2007.

Optican LM, Zee DS, Chu FC: Adaptive response to ocular muscle weakness in human pursuit and saccadic eye movements. J Neurophysiol 54:110, 1985.

Oyster CW: The extraocular muscles. In Oyster CW, editor: The human eye: structure and function, Sunderland, Mass, 1999, Sinauer Associates.

Peltsch A, et al: Saccadis impairments in Huntington's disease. Exp Brain Res 186:457, 2008.

Pierrot-Deseilligny C, et al: Saccade deficits after a unilateral lesion affecting the superior colliculus. J Neurol Neurosurg Psychiatry 54:1106, 1991.

Pierrot-Deseilligny CH, et al: Effects of cortical lesions on saccadic eye movements in humans. Ann N Y Acad Sci 956:216, 2002.

Rambold H, et al: Palsy of "fast" and "slow" vergence by pontine lesions. Neurology 64:338, 2005.

Robinson DA: The biology of eye movements. In Albert DM, Jakobiec FA, editors: Principles and practice of ophthalmology, Philadelphia, 1994, WB Saunders.

An excellent account by one of the pioneers in figuring out the actions of the extraocular muscles.

Rosano C, et al: Pursuit and saccadic eye movement subregions in human frontal eye field: a high-resolution fMRI investigation. Cereb Cortex 12:107, 2002.

Rosano C, et al: The human precentral sulcus: chemoarchitecture of a region corresponding to the frontal eye fields. Brain Res 972:16, 2003.

Schiller PH, True SD, Conway JL: Deficits in eye movements following frontal eye-field and superior colliculus ablations. J Neurophysiol 44:1175, 1980.

Selhorst JB, et al: Disorders in cerebellar ocular motor control. I. Saccadic overshoot dysmetria: an oculographic, control system and clinico-anatomical analysis. Brain 99:497, 1976.

Tian J-R, Lynch JC: Slow and saccadic eye movements evoked by microstimulation in the supplementary eye field of the cebus monkey. J Neurophysiol 74:2204, 1995.

Tucker VA: The deep fovea, sideways vision and spiral flight paths in raptors. J Exp Biol 203:3745, 2000.

Hawks and eagles have foveae that point 45 degrees away from the midline, allowing them to scan wide areas from high up in the air with great acuity. But there would be too much air resistance if they dove straight down with their heads cocked at 45 degrees, keeping a fovea pointed at something. Read how they get around this problem.

Ugolini G, et al: Horizontal eye movement networks in primates as revealed by retrograde transneuronal transfer of rabies virus: differences in monosynaptic input to "slow" and "fast" abducens motoneurons. J Comp Neurol 498:762, 2006.

There may be different sets of abducens motor neurons for different kinds of movements.

Vahedi K, et al: Horizontal eye movement disorders after posterior vermis infarctions. J Neurol Neurosurg Psychiatry 58:91, 1995.

Wardak C, et al: Contribution of the monkey frontal eye field to covert visual attention. J Neurosci 26:4228, 2006.

The frontal eye fields may do more than change the direction in which the eyes point.

Wurtz RH: Vision for the control of movement. Invest Ophthalmol 37:2131, 1996.

The role of the superior colliculus in the generation of saccades.

Cerebral Cortex

The cerebral cortex is a sheet of neurons and their interconnections; about 1800 cm^2 (2 ft^2) in surface area, cover the corrugated surface of the cerebral hemispheres in a layer just a few millimeters thick. This thin layer of gray matter accounts for nearly half the weight of the brain and is estimated to contain about 25 billion neurons, interconnected by more than 100,000 km of axons receiving an incredible 10^{14} synapses. The corrugation into gyri and sulci, a mechanism for increasing the area of cortex, is reasonably constant in its major features (Fig. 22-1).

One of the more striking changes that has occurred in the course of the evolution of vertebrate brains is the tremendous increase in the relative size of the cerebral

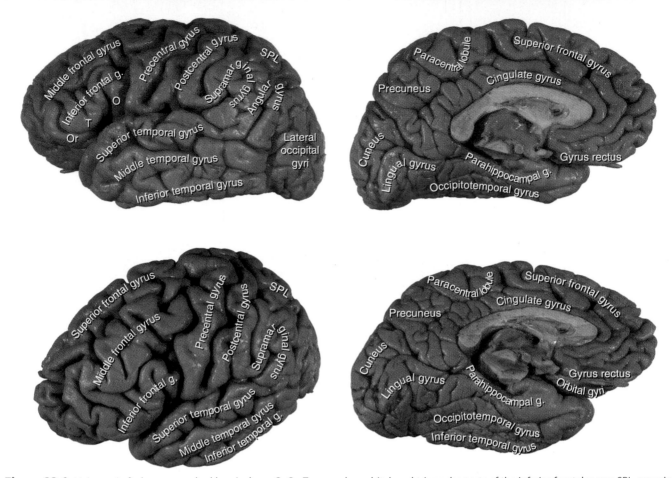

Figure 22-1 Major gyri of a human cerebral hemisphere. O, Or, T, opercular, orbital, and triangular parts of the inferior frontal gyrus; SPL, superior parietal lobule.

hemispheres and the even greater increase in the area of cerebral cortex on their surfaces. One inference drawn from this fact (and supported by abundant clinical and functional imaging evidence) is that the cerebral cortex has a critical role in the abilities and activities that reach their highest level of development in humans (or, in some cases, are unique in humans). Obvious examples are language and abstract thinking. These are, of course, not the only functions of the cerebral cortex; basic aspects of perception, movement, and adaptive response to the outside world also depend on it.

Most Cerebral Cortex Is Neocortex

Cerebral cortex does not have the same structure everywhere. Almost all the cortex that can be seen on the outside of the brain is of a type called **neocortex,** *neo* referring to the idea that it appeared fairly late in vertebrate evolution. Reptiles have cerebral cortex, but all of it consists of three-layered types that continue in humans as **paleocortex** (*paleo* = "old") and **archicortex** (*archi* = "beginning"), named in reference to their supposedly

more ancient origins.[a] Paleocortex covers some restricted parts of the base of the telencephalon (Fig. 22-2), and most of the hippocampus is archicortex. Neocortex has a different structure, described shortly, and develops interposed between the paleocortex and archicortex, separated from them by cortical transition zones with intermediate structures. Some mammals have relatively little neocortex, but it expands greatly in primates, accounting for about 95% of the total cortical area in humans. This expansion causes the apparent rotation of the cerebral hemispheres into their characteristic C shape, with paleocortex and archicortex at the two ends of the C (see Fig. 2-13).

All neocortical areas go through a period during development in which they have a six-layered structure. This layered appearance is altered in some areas of the adult brain, but in view of its uniform early

---

[a]Although the pattern of evolution of cerebral cortex continues to be debated, the earliest vertebrates probably had telencephalic regions that, although not cortical in structure, were the forerunners of paleocortex, archicortex, and neocortex. In that sense, one is not "newer" than the others.

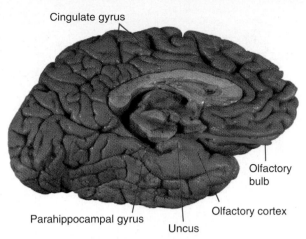

Cingulate gyrus

Olfactory bulb

Olfactory cortex

Parahippocampal gyrus

Uncus

Figure 22-2 Nonneocortical areas visible on the surface of the brain. There are also transition zones (not indicated) at the edges of the cingulate and parahippocampal gyri, interposed between olfactory cortex and neocortex and between the hippocampus and neocortex.

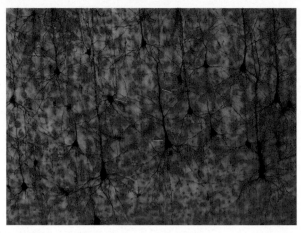

Figure 22-3 Golgi-stained cerebral cortex. The cell body *(red arrowhead)* and apical and basal dendrites *(red arrows)* of a pyramidal cell, and the cell body of a nonpyramidal cell *(orange arrow)* are indicated. *(Courtesy Dr. Nathaniel T. McMullen, University of Arizona College of Medicine.)*

development, neocortex is also referred to as **homogenetic cortex** or **isocortex**. In contrast, paleocortex and archicortex never go through such a six-layered stage and are referred to collectively as **heterogenetic cortex** or **allocortex** (from the Greek word *allo,* meaning "other"). The hippocampus is a component of the limbic system (see Chapter 23), and paleocortex, which develops in conjunction with the olfactory system (see Chapter 13), is closely interconnected with limbic structures; the remainder of this chapter deals with neocortex.

Pyramidal Cells Are the Most Numerous Neocortical Neurons

Pyramidal cells, the most numerous neurons of the neocortex, are named for their shape (Fig. 22-3). These cells have a conical cell body from which a series of spine-studded dendrites emerge—a long **apical dendrite** that leaves the "top" of each cell and ascends vertically toward the cortical surface, and a series of **basal dendrites** that emerge from around the base of the cell and spread out horizontally. Pyramidal cells range in size from less than 10 µm in diameter all the way up to the giant pyramidal cells (**Betz cells**) of the motor cortex, which are among the largest neurons in the central nervous system (CNS), some measuring more than 100 µm from their base to the beginning of the apical dendrite. Most or all pyramidal cells have long axons that leave the cortex to reach other cortical areas or various subcortical sites, where they make excitatory (glutamate) synapses. The remaining cortical neurons are spoken of collectively as **nonpyramidal cells.** Many are small (often less than 10 µm), multipolar **stellate** (or **granule**) **cells,** but a variety of other types and sizes have been described (Fig. 22-4). With few exceptions, nonpyramidal cells have short axons that remain within the cortex. One kind of nonpyr-

amidal cell has spine-covered dendrites, receives inputs from the thalamus, and makes excitatory (glutamate) synapses on nearby neurons; most or all of the others make inhibitory (γ-aminobutyric acid) synapses on their targets. Hence pyramidal cells are the principal output neurons of the neocortex, and nonpyramidal cells are the principal interneurons.

The **dendritic spines** of pyramidal cells (see Fig. 1-4E) are preferential sites of excitatory synaptic contacts and have been the source of considerable interest. They are not merely devices for increasing dendritic surface area, since the area of dendrites located between spines is sparsely populated with synaptic contacts. It has been suggested that dendritic spines may be the sites of synapses that are selectively modified as a result of learning, because small changes in the geometry of a spine can cause relatively large changes in its electrical or diffusional properties and therefore in the efficacy of that synapse. Certain cases of mental retardation are accompanied by faulty development of dendritic spines, including misshapen spines and/or an overabundance of spines, but which is cause and which is effect (if either) is not known. Certainly, however, the most remarkable change that occurs in the cortex after birth is the tremendous expansion of the dendritic trees of its neurons and a parallel increase in the number of dendritic spines. It should be noted that spines are not unique to cortical pyramidal cells; they are also found on the dendrites of some other neurons, such as Purkinje cells (see Fig. 8-16) and many striatal neurons.

Neocortex Has Six Layers

The cells of the neocortex are arranged in a series of six layers, more apparent in some areas than in others. Just as in the case of cerebellar cortex (see Figs. 20-9 and 20-10), the most superficial layer is a cell-poor **molecular**

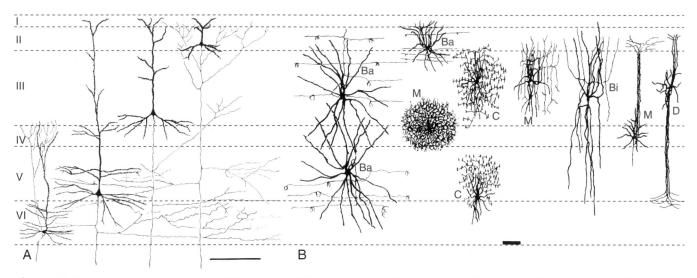

Figure 22-4 Neocortical neurons. **A,** Pyramidal neurons in different layers have characteristically different soma sizes and patterns of distribution of axon collaterals. **B,** Nonpyramidal neurons come in a variety of sizes and shapes; many have names attributable to their shapes. Basket cells (Ba) are usually large and make basket-shaped endings that partially surround the cell bodies of pyramidal cells. Other kinds of smaller multipolar cells (M) may have elaborate dendritic and axonal arborizations. Chandelier cells (C) have vertically oriented synaptic "candles" that end on the initial segments of pyramidal cell axons. Bipolar cells (Bi) have dendrites that both ascend and descend, and double bouquet cells (D) have axons that both ascend and descend. *(A, from Jones EG: Identification and classification of intrinsic circuit elements in the neocortex. In Edelman GM, Gall WE, Cowan WM, editors: Dynamic aspects of neocortical function, New York, 1984, John Wiley & Sons. B, from Hendry SHC, Jones EG: J Neurosci 1:390, 1981.)*

layer. The deepest neocortical layer is the **polymorphic** (or **multiform**) **layer,** which is populated largely by fusiform-shaped modified pyramidal cells. In between the molecular and polymorphic layers are four layers alternately populated mostly by small cells or mostly by large pyramidal cells. The layers are commonly designated by roman numerals and by names, as indicated in Figure 22-5. Myelin staining reveals vertically oriented bundles of cortical afferents and efferents, as well as horizontal bands through which these fibers and intracortical axons spread. Two particularly prominent horizontal bands are contained in layers IV and V and are called, respectively, the **outer** and **inner bands of Baillarger.**

Neocortex does not have the same striking regularity as cerebellar cortex; its six cell layers are not equally prominent everywhere. Areas that give rise to many long axons (e.g., the motor cortex) would be expected to have numerous large pyramidal cells, and this is indeed the case (Fig. 22-6A). In these areas, nonpyramidal cells appear minor by comparison, and layers II through V are dominated by large pyramidal cells to the extent that individual layers are no longer obvious. Because of the apparent lack of stellate (granule) cells, such cortex is called **agranular.** In contrast, primary sensory areas project mainly to adjacent cortical areas and do not give rise to many long axons. They have a corresponding dearth of large pyramidal cells; here too, layers II through V look like one continuous layer, but in this case they are dominated by small cells (both pyramidal and nonpyramidal; see Fig. 22-6A). Such cortex is therefore called **granular cortex** or **koniocortex** (from the Greek word

konia, meaning "dust," referring to the numerous tiny cells). There is a continuum of structural types ranging from thick (up to 4.5 mm) agranular cortex to thin (as little as 1.5 mm) granular cortex (Fig. 22-7). The intermediate kinds, in which the six neocortical layers are relatively distinct, are called **homotypical** cortices (rather than granular and agranular cortices, which are collectively called **heterotypical;** see Fig. 22-6B).

The differences among cortical areas are to some extent more apparent than real. Beneath a square millimeter of any area of mammalian cortex, whether from a hamster or a human, lie approximately the same number of neurons (roughly 100,000). The major exception is the binocular portion of the primary visual cortex of primates, where the neurons are packed more densely. About 80% of the neurons in all cortical areas are pyramidal cells. Hence 80% of the neurons in granular cortex are very small pyramidal cells. Different cortical areas have different appearances and functions because of the relative sizes of the cell types, the complexities of their dendritic trees, and the patterns of their connections. This fundamental similarity of all cortical areas is one aspect of the notion, discussed a little later in this chapter, that the cerebral cortex may be a large array of small, repeated functional units.

Different Neocortical Layers Have Distinctive Connections

Afferents to the cortex come from two general places: other cortical areas and subcortical sites. Afferents from other cortical sites, by far the majority, may arise in the

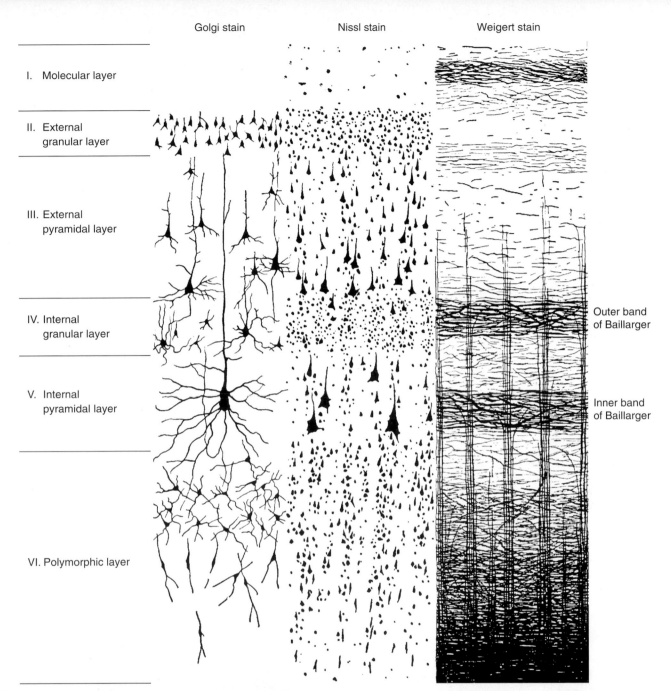

Golgi stain   Nissl stain   Weigert stain

I. Molecular layer

II. External
granular layer

III. External
pyramidal layer

IV. Internal
granular layer

Outer band
of Baillarger

V. Internal
pyramidal layer

Inner band
of Baillarger

VI. Polymorphic layer

Figure 22-5 Cross section of neocortex stained by three different methods; the six cortical layers are indicated. The Golgi stain reveals the shapes of the arborizations of cortical neurons by completely staining a small percentage of them. The Nissl method stains the cell bodies of all neurons, showing their shapes and packing densities. The Weigert method stains myelin, revealing the horizontally oriented bands of Baillarger and the vertically oriented collections of cortical afferents and efferents. *(From Brodmann K: Vergleichende Lokalisation lehre der Grosshirnrinde in ihren Prinzipien dargestellt auf Grund des Zellenbaues, Leipzig, 1909, JA Barth.)*

same hemisphere (**association fibers**) or in the contralateral hemisphere (**commissural fibers**). The predominant subcortical source of afferents is the thalamus, and its pattern of projections is described in Chapter 16. Other subcortical sites, such as the locus ceruleus and other chemically coded nuclei, also provide modulatory afferents to the cortex (see Chapter 11 and later in this chapter).

These various types of incoming fibers ramify within the cortex in different patterns (Fig. 22-8). For example, afferents from thalamic relay nuclei end primarily in the middle layers, as in the dense arborizations in layer IV

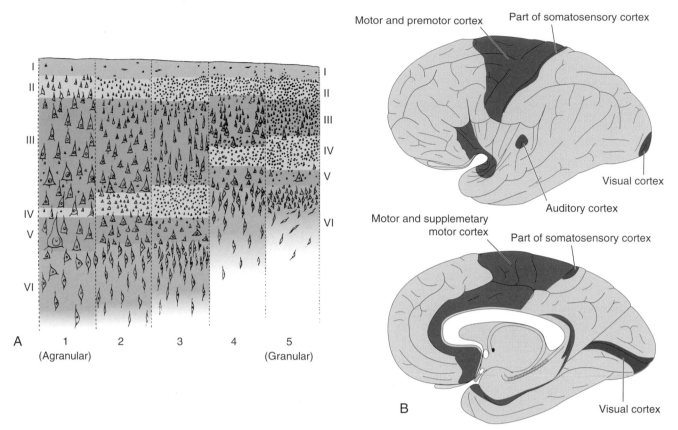

Figure 22-6 **A,** Different types of neocortex. At the two extremes are the heterotypical cortices: agranular cortex (1) dominated by large pyramidal cells, and granular cortex (5, koniocortex) dominated by small cells. Areas with intermediate structures in which six layers can be discerned more clearly are homotypical and were divided into three types by von Economo: 2, frontal type; 3, parietal type; 4, polar type. **B,** Distribution of heterotypical cortex. The lateral view, above, is drawn as though the lateral sulcus had been pried open, exposing the insula. Agranular cortex *(green)* is found primarily in motor areas, granular cortex *(blue)* primarily in sensory areas (compare with Fig. 22-13). *(Modified from von Economo C: The cytoarchitectonics of the human cerebral cortex, Oxford, 1929, Oxford University Press.)*

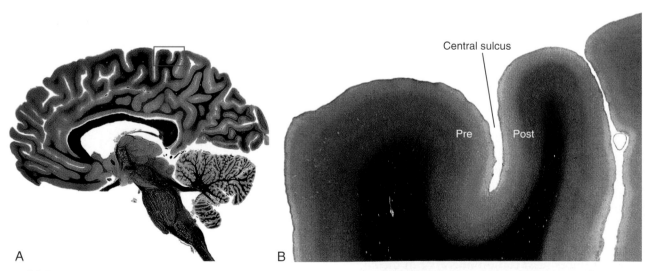

Figure 22-7 Agranular (motor) cortex of the precentral gyrus (Pre) and granular (somatosensory) cortex of the postcentral gyrus (Post), seen in a parasagittal section. The area outlined in **A** is enlarged in **B**. The differing cortical thickness on opposite sides of the central sulcus is apparent. *(A, from Nolte J, Angevine JB Jr: The human brain in photographs and diagrams, ed 3, St. Louis, 2007, Mosby.)*

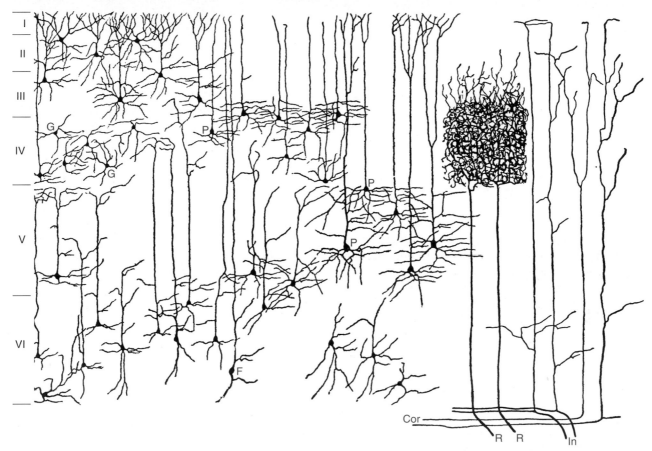

Figure 22-8 Types of cortical neurons seen in Golgi-stained cerebral cortex from a mouse; the main types of cortical afferents are shown on the right. Cells: F, fusiform-shaped modified pyramidal cells; G, granule (stellate) cells; P, pyramidal cells. Afferents: Cor, association fibers from other cortical areas; In, fibers from intralaminar thalamic nuclei; R, fibers from thalamic relay nuclei. Note the strongly vertical orientation of many cortical elements. *(From Lorente de Nó R: Cerebral cortex: architecture, intracortical connections, motor projections. In Fulton JF: Physiology of the nervous system, ed 3, Oxford, 1949, Oxford University Press.)*

of fibers from sensory relay nuclei[b]; fibers from other thalamic nuclei and from other cortical areas ascend vertically and terminate diffusely along their course in distinctive patterns (e.g., those from intralaminar nuclei mostly in layer VI, and those from other cortical areas mostly in layers II and III).

Efferents from the cortex, like afferents to it, must be connected either with other cortical areas or with subcortical sites. Efferents to subcortical sites, mentioned in various places throughout this book, mostly descend through the internal capsule. The longest ones continue through the cerebral peduncle, the basal pons, and the medullary pyramids, finally extending all the way to the spinal cord. Others reach an assortment of additional subcortical sites, including the caudate nucleus and putamen, the thalamus, the superior colliculus, the red nucleus, the reticular formation, pontine nuclei, motor neurons of cranial and spinal nerves, and various sensory nuclei of the brainstem and spinal cord. Some corticostriate fibers travel through the external capsule. Just as afferents to the cortex have a distinctive laminar pattern of termination, efferents from the cortex have a laminar pattern of origin. Although there is substantial overlap, layer III is the major source of corticocortical fibers, layer V of corticostriate fibers, fibers to the brainstem and spinal cord, and layer VI of regulatory projections back to the thalamus.

The Corpus Callosum and Anterior Commissure Interconnect the Two Cerebral Hemispheres

Most efferents to the cortex of the contralateral hemisphere pass through the **corpus callosum,** as described later in this chapter (see Fig. 22-28). Those interconnecting parts of the temporal lobes (particularly inferior

[b]Because the line of Gennari in striate cortex (see Fig. 17-31) represents a particularly large outer band of Baillarger and is located in layer IV, it is often assumed that it represents the massive projection from the lateral geniculate nucleus to the striate cortex. However, cutting all the afferents to the striate cortex does not cause the line of Gennari to degenerate. It is known that it exists in both sighted and blind individuals. It is thought to be a collection of intracortical axons, although the details of its structure and function are still unknown.

parts) traverse the **anterior commissure,** along with crossing fibers from the anterior olfactory nucleus (see Figs. 13-17 and 13-18).

Association Bundles Interconnect Areas Within Each Cerebral Hemisphere

Efferents to ipsilateral cortical areas come in all lengths, from very short ones that never leave the cortex, to U-shaped fibers that dip under one sulcus to reach the next gyrus, to longer association fibers that travel to a different lobe; collectively, they account for a large majority of the axons in the white matter of each hemisphere. The longer fibers collect into reasonably well-defined bundles that can be found by dissection (Fig. 22-9A) and now by diffusion tensor imaging (Fig. 22-9B to D). The most prominent of these association bundles are the **superior longitudinal fasciculus,** the **superior** and **inferior occipitofrontal fasciculi,** and the **cingulum.** The superior longitudinal fasciculus (also called the **arcuate fasciculus**) sweeps along in a great arc above the insula between the frontal lobe and posterior portions of the hemisphere, where it fans out among the parietal, occipital, and temporal lobes. The superior occipitofrontal fasciculus, as its name implies, runs between the frontal lobe and superior parts of the parietal and occipital lobes. It travels parallel to the corpus callosum and, for much of its course, is located between the corpus callosum and the caudate nucleus. Here it lies adjacent to the **subcallosal fasciculus,** a pale-staining bundle of fibers on their way from several cortical areas to the caudate nucleus (see Fig. 19-1). The inferior occipitofrontal fasciculus passes below the insula between the frontal and occipital lobes, traversing the temporal lobe along the way. Its fibers fan out at both ends of the fasciculus, and those at its anterior end lie adjacent to the **uncinate fasciculus** (from the Latin *uncus,* meaning "hook"), an association bundle that hooks around the margin of the lateral sulcus to interconnect the orbital cortex and anterior temporal cortex. Finally, the cingulum courses within the cingulate gyrus and continues around within the parahippocampal gyrus to nearly complete a circle. None of these association bundles is a discrete, point-to-point pathway from one place to another; rather, fibers travel in both directions and enter

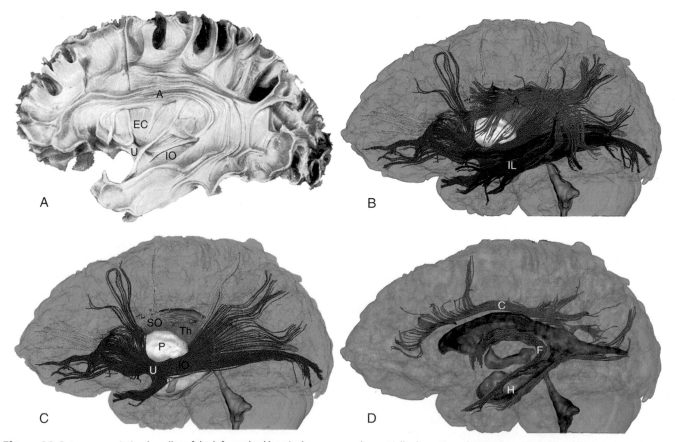

Figure 22-9 Long association bundles of the left cerebral hemisphere, as seen by partially dissecting a hemisphere (**A**) and in diffusion tensor images (**B** to **D**). A, arcuate (superior longitudinal) fasciculus; C, cingulum; EC, extreme capsule; F, fornix and stria terminalis (see Chapter 23); H, hippocampus; IL, inferior longitudinal fasciculus; IO, inferior occipitofrontal fasciculus; P, putamen; SO, superior occipitofrontal fasciculus (combined with the subcallosal fasciculus adjacent to it); Th, thalamus; U, uncinate fasciculus. (**A,** *from Ludwig E, Klingler J: Atlas cerebri humani, Boston, 1956, Little, Brown.* ***B*** *to* ***D,*** *from Mori S et al: MRI atlas of human white matter, Amsterdam, 2005, Elsevier.*)

and leave each pathway all along its course. The inferior occipitofrontal fasciculus provides a good example of this. Few of its fibers actually extend all the way between the occipital and frontal lobes. Rather, those in the posterior part of this fasciculus interconnect occipital and temporal areas and are often considered separately as the **inferior longitudinal fasciculus;** anterior fibers travel through inferior parts of the **extreme capsule** to interconnect the superior temporal gyrus, the insula, and orbital and prefrontal cortex.

Neocortex Also Has a Columnar Organization

Even though the cortex is horizontally laminated, there is also a vertical organization ("vertical" meaning perpendicular to the surface). Apical dendrites of pyramidal cells have vertical courses, as do afferents to the cortex and the axons of some intracortical cells (see Fig. 22-8); even the cell bodies of cortical neurons often look as though they are arranged in vertical columns (see Fig. 22-5). Both physiological and anatomical studies have shown that this is not just an illusion. If an electrode is slowly advanced through somatosensory cortex along a path perpendicular to the cortical surface, all the cells encountered respond with about the same latency to the same type of stimulus delivered to about the same region of the body. Similarly, all the cells along a vertical path through visual cortex respond best to bars or edges with the same orientation in about the same part of the visual field (see Fig. 17-35A); if the electrode is moved 50 μm or so across the surface of the cortex, cells with a different preferred stimulus orientation are encountered. Furthermore, most cells along such a vertical path respond better to stimulation of one eye than to stimulation of the other eye; cells in a nearby vertical region may have not only a different preferred stimulus orientation but also a different preferred eye. The picture that has emerged is one in which the cortex is organized into vertical slabs or columns, each 50 to 500 μm wide, in which some parameter (e.g., stimulus orientation) is constant for all cells.

This kind of columnar organization most likely reflects a general strategy used in the construction of neocortex. Anatomical tracing techniques make it possible to visualize the columns (see Fig. 17-35C), and there are indications that columnar organization is widespread. For example, in at least some cortical areas, afferents from the thalamus, from other ipsilateral cortical areas, and from contralateral cortical areas end in vertical slabs separated by slabs that do not receive that particular kind of input. Throughout the neocortex, the basic building blocks appear to be "minicolumns" about 50 μm in diameter containing about 100 neurons; dozens of minicolumns, linked by horizontal intracortical connections, make up larger functional modules such as the hypercolumns in visual cortex (see Fig. 17-35A).

Neocortical Areas Are Specialized for Different Functions

Consider the "simple" visual examination of an object. This involves analysis of its size, shape, color, movement, and position in space; correlation of that object with objects seen in the past; cross-correlation of the appearance of the object with its sound, smell, and other properties; and decision making about, for instance, whether to run away or to grab it. Not surprisingly, large expanses of cortex are involved in even simple activities such as this, and the performance of complex tasks can be impaired by damage to widely separated cortical areas. Nevertheless, many years of clinical experience have shown that reasonably predictable deficits are found after damage at various cerebral sites. This means that a given function is actually localized in a particular area, that the area performs one crucial step in the function, or that the area facilitates the activity of one or more other structures. Whichever is the case, the consistent association of some deficits with certain areas of damage provides a useful diagnostic tool, and we often speak as though functions are localized to specific cortical areas.

Different Neocortical Areas Have Subtly Different Structures

Seeing that various cortical areas are structurally distinct from one another in fairly obvious ways (e.g., granular vs. agranular cortex; [see Fig. 22-6A] or striate vs. extrastriate cortex [see Fig. 17-31]), a number of anatomists have sought to map the cortex in terms of these differences and often of considerably more subtle differences. One mapping system whose terminology has come into widespread use is that devised by Korbinian Brodmann, who divided the neocortex of each hemisphere into 44 areas (Fig. 22-10). The boundaries between many of these areas are not precise, as they often grade into each other by degrees. In addition, as noted previously, the correlation of functions with specific anatomical areas is not nearly as precise as was once hoped. Nevertheless, many of the areas described by Brodmann correspond remarkably well to areas defined by other measures of connection or function, and many of the numbers proposed by him are still commonly used for reference purposes (Table 22-1).

Although each of us has roughly the same total amount of cerebral cortex, there are surprisingly large variations in the sizes of particular areas. The areas of visual, somatosensory, and motor cortex may vary by a factor of 2 to 3 among typical individuals. Because the total neocortical area is much more constant than this, someone with a larger than average visual cortex presumably has other areas that are smaller than average. Whether these differences in area are correlated with

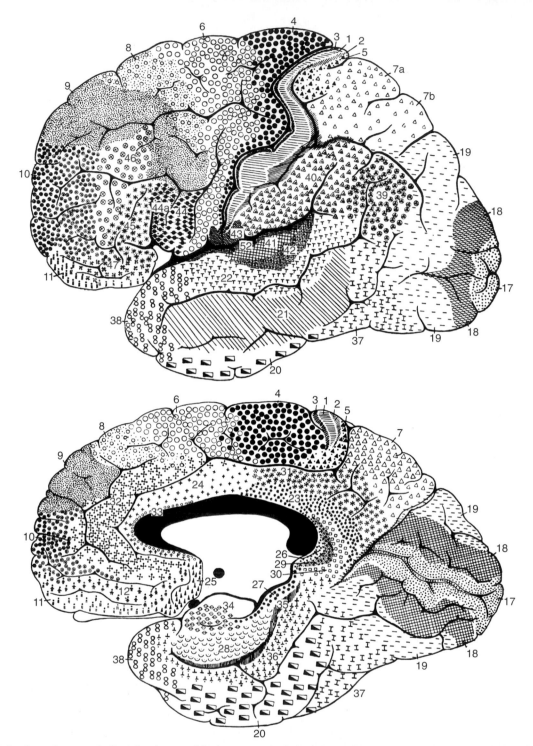

Figure 22-10 Brodmann's anatomically defined areas of the human cerebral cortex (see Table 22-1). *(From Brodmann K: Vergleichende Lokalisation lehre der Grosshirnrinde in ihren Prinzipien dargestellt auf Grund des Zellenbaues, Leipzig, 1909, JA Barth.)*

Table 22-1		Selected Brodmann's Areas	
Lobe	Number	Location	Other Names
Frontal	4	Precentral gyrus, anterior paracentral lobule	Primary motor area; M1
	6	Superior and middle frontal gyri, precentral gyrus	Premotor area, supplementary motor area
	44, 45	Inferior frontal gyrus (opercular and triangular parts)	Broca's area (on the left)
Parietal	3, 1, 2	Postcentral gyrus, posterior paracentral lobule	Primary somatosensory area; S1
	5, 7	Superior parietal lobule	Somatosensory association area
	39	Inferior parietal lobule	Angular gyrus
	40	Inferior parietal lobule	Supramarginal gyrus
Occipital	17	Banks of calcarine sulcus	Primary visual area; V1
	18, 19	Surrounding 17	Visual association areas; V2, V3, V4, V5
Temporal	41	Transverse temporal gyri	Primary auditory area; A1
	42	Transverse temporal gyri	Auditory association area; A2
	22	Superior temporal gyrus	Auditory association area; posterior portion (on the left) = Wernicke's area

differences among individuals in various skills and functional capacities is not known.[c]

There Are Sensory, Motor, Association, and Limbic Areas

The neocortex of each cerebral hemisphere is usually considered to be made up of **primary sensory areas** (receiving inputs from thalamic sensory relay nuclei), a **primary motor area** (giving rise to much of the corticospinal tract), **association areas,** and **limbic areas.** Somatosensory cortex occupies the postcentral gyrus, visual cortex the banks of the calcarine sulcus, auditory cortex the transverse temporal gyri, and motor cortex part of the precentral gyrus. These areas are characterized by a topographical organization in which the bodies' surface, the range of audible frequencies, or the outside world is mapped onto the cortical surface (see Figs. 3-30, 14-19, and 17-29). These maps are distorted (Box 22-1; Fig. 22-11), so that highly discriminating or finely controlled parts of the nervous system or body have disproportionately large representations (e.g., the fovea in visual cortex, the fingers in motor and somatosensory cortex).

These primary areas are the cortical zones most directly related to the outside world, and they account for most of the cortex in many mammals. Primates, especially humans, have vast repertoires of ways to use and respond to sensory inputs; this is thought to result

[c]Mark Twain apparently alluded to this possibility: "I never could keep a promise. I do not blame myself for this weakness, because the fault must lie in my physical organization. It is likely that such a liberal amount of space was given to the organ which enables me to make promises that the organ which should enable me to keep them was crowded out." (From Twain M: The innocents abroad, New York, 1869, Charles L Webster. Recounted in Harvey PH, Krebs JR: Science 249:140, 1990.)

BOX 22-1

Star-Nosed Moles, Revisited

Star-nosed moles (see Box 9-1) have an elaborate array of 11 appendages, or rays, surrounding each nostril that are used for somatosensory exploration of their environment. Corresponding to the behavioral importance of these rays, more than 50% of the mole's somatosensory cortex is used to process information from them (see Fig. 22-11). Further details of the somatosensory map, though not apparent in Figure 22-11, also make functional sense. The moles move their noses around as they travel through their tunnels, contacting objects more or less at random with the rays. If contact is made by one of the first 10 rays, the animal reorients its nose so that the object can be explored in more detail by ray 11, a small, ventrally directed ray just above the mouth. If the object feels like it might be good to eat, it gets gobbled up. Interestingly, ray 11 has fewer Eimer's organs (see Fig. 9-11) than almost any other ray, but each of these ray-11 organs has four times more cortical space devoted to it than do the organs from the other rays. This behavior pattern and cortical organization have been likened to the way we detect a visual target in the periphery and then point our foveae at it.

from a progressive increase in the amount of association cortex over the course of mammalian evolution (Fig. 22-12). Association cortex is commonly divided into two broad types. Some of the areas adjacent to a primary area are **unimodal association areas** (Fig. 22-13), devoted to an elaboration of the business of that primary area. Thus areas 18 and 19, which surround the primary visual cortex, are part of the **visual association cortex.** Similarly, parts of the superior parietal lobule, much of

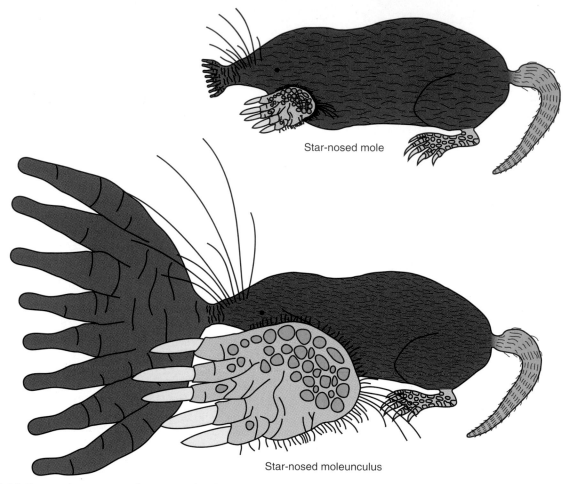

Figure 22-11 The actual proportions of a star-nosed mole compared with the proportions of the map of its body surface in somatosensory cortex. *(Courtesy Dr. Kenneth C. Catania, Vanderbilt University.)*

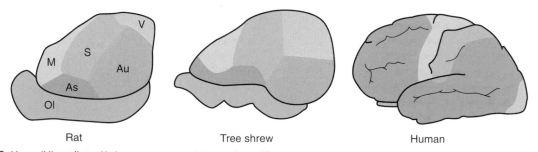

Figure 22-12 Motor (M), auditory (Au), somatosensory (S), visual (V), olfactory (Ol), and association (As) areas of the cerebral hemispheres of three different mammalian species. All three brains are drawn the same size, even though the human brain is far larger than the other two; the relative and absolute increase in the amount of association cortex is apparent. *(Modified from Penfield W: Speech, perception and the cortex. In Eccles JC, editor: Brain and conscious experience, New York, 1966, Springer-Verlag.)*

the superior temporal gyrus, and premotor and supplementary motor cortex are involved in somatosensory, auditory, and motor functions, respectively. This still leaves the inferior parietal lobule and large portions of the frontal and temporal lobes. Neurons in these areas typically respond to multiple sensory modalities and may change their response properties under different circumstances. For example, a neuron in the inferior parietal lobule might respond to a visual stimulus, but *only* if it is something interesting, such as a cue or a piece of food. These **multimodal** or **heteromodal association areas** are therefore thought to be concerned with high-level intellectual functions.

Although there is a great deal of validity to this broad view of cortical organization, it is also a considerable oversimplification. For one thing, the distinction between primary areas and association areas is not nearly as clear as the traditional formulation implies.

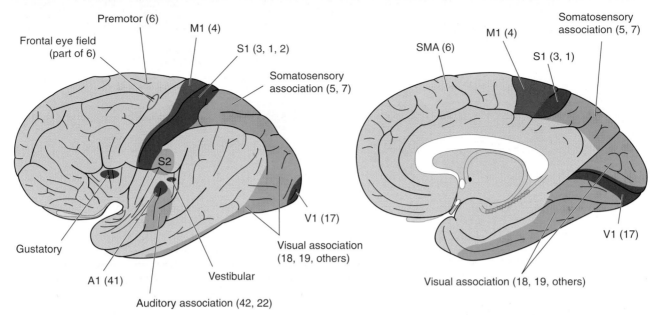

Figure 22-13 Summary diagram of primary and unimodal association areas. The lateral view, as in Figure 22-6, is drawn as though the lateral sulcus had been pried open, exposing the insula. Visual association cortex is particularly extensive in primate brains, occupying not only most of the occipital lobe but also much of the temporal lobe. Many of these various functional areas are associated with one or more of Brodmann's anatomically defined areas, although sometimes the correspondence is only approximate; commonly used Brodmann numbers are indicated in parentheses (area 2 usually does not extend onto the medial surface of the hemisphere). A1, M1, S1, V1, primary auditory, motor, somatosensory, and visual cortex; S2, second somatosensory area; SMA, supplementary motor area. *(Modified from von Economo C: The cytoarchitectonics of the human cerebral cortex, Oxford, 1929, Oxford University Press.)*

One example given in an earlier chapter is the finding that the corticospinal tract originates not just from the classical primary motor cortex but also from other areas, including somatosensory cortex. As another example, there are types of cortex intermediate between primary and association (see Fig. 22-15), just as there are transitional areas between isocortex and allocortex. In addition, the concepts that primary sensory areas receive all the input (which is then acted on in a more complex fashion by the association cortex) and that motor activity is formulated in association areas and funnels down to the primary motor area for expression are certainly not completely correct. Monkeys (and humans as well) with extensive damage to the precentral or postcentral gyrus are not rendered unable to move or to perceive tactile stimuli. They are impaired in these capacities, but the fact that they suffer only a partial disability indicates that other cortical areas also play a role and that these other areas can function independently of the primary areas, at least to some extent[d] (Fig. 22-14). The details of how different areas of the cortex and other parts of the CNS cooperate to produce a simple voluntary move-

ment or simple visual perception are still largely mysterious, but progressively more is becoming understood.

Primary Somatosensory Cortex Is in the Parietal Lobe

Somatosensory information traveling rostrally in the medial lemniscus and the spinothalamic tract relays in the ventral posterolateral (VPL) and ventral posteromedial (VPM) nuclei and projects through the posterior limb of the internal capsule mainly to areas 3, 1, and 2. These are three long, parallel strips of cortex that together occupy almost the entire postcentral gyrus; most of area 3 is in the posterior wall of the central sulcus, and most of area 2 is in the anterior wall of the postcentral sulcus. These areas not only are structurally distinct from one another, but they also differ in their connections and properties; the body surface is mapped separately in each area, but when going from area 3 to 1 to 2, the characteristics change from primary somatosensory cortex to the beginnings of somatosensory association cortex (Fig. 22-15). Cells in area 3 receive most of the thalamocortical projections from VPL and VPM; cells in areas 1 and 2 receive progressively less input from the thalamus and progressively more from other cortical areas. Cells in area 3 have receptive fields that reflect activity in particular kinds of receptors, whereas those in areas 1 and 2 have more complex receptive fields that respond to things such as limb position or the shape of an object touching the skin. In the strict sense of the term, area 3 is primary somatosensory cortex, but

[d]The extent to which this is true varies in different association areas and in different species. In primates, for example, some portions of visual and somatosensory association cortex absolutely depend on the primary areas for their continued function, whereas other portions do not.

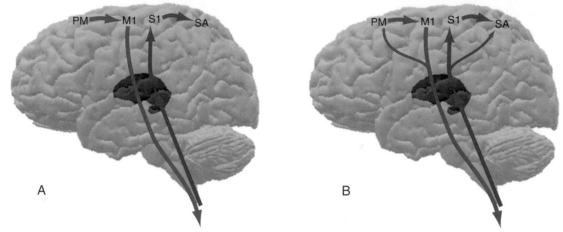

Figure 22-14 Cortical connections in sensory and motor systems. The somatosensory system is used as an example in this illustration, but the same principles apply to other sensory systems. **A,** Traditional serial processing. In this view, all sensory inflow from the thalamus ends in the primary sensory cortex (S1, primary somatosensory cortex), which then processes the information and passes it on to association areas (SA, somatosensory association cortex). Similarly, all motor outflow originates in the primary motor cortex (M1), which receives its inputs from motor association areas such as premotor cortex (PM). **B,** Combination of serial and parallel processing. In this view, sensory inflow from the thalamus is distributed to both primary and association areas. Similarly, motor outflow originates in both primary motor and motor association areas. In both cases, the primary area is of major importance, but association areas have some connections in parallel.

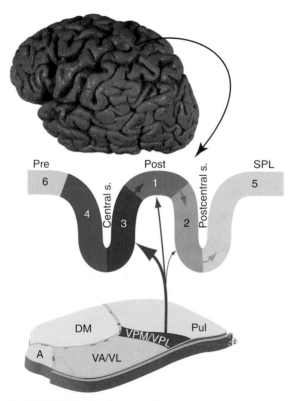

Figure 22-15 Pattern of connections of somatosensory cortex, as seen in a section through the precentral (Pre) and postcentral (Post) gyri and the superior parietal lobule (SPL). Numbers refer to Brodmann's areas (see Fig. 22-10 and Table 22-1). Moving from area 3 to 1 to 2, each successive area receives less input from the thalamus and more from other somatosensory cortical areas. A, anterior nucleus; DM, dorsomedial nucleus; Pul, pulvinar; VA/VL, ventral anterior and ventral lateral nuclei; VPM/VPL, ventral posteromedial and ventral posterolateral nuclei.

because the postcentral gyrus as a whole is the most prominent area concerned with somatic sensation, it is usually referred to as the **primary (first) somatosensory area** (or **S1**).

Another somatosensory association area called the **second somatosensory area (S2)** has also been described; it receives inputs not only from S1 but also, to a lesser extent, directly from VPL and VPM. It occupies part of the parietal operculum, and much of it is buried in the lateral sulcus, possibly extending onto the insula. S2 is also somatotopically organized, but its order is the reverse of that in S1; that is, the face areas of both maps are adjacent to each other, and the rest of the S2 map extends into the lateral sulcus. The cells in S2 often have bilateral receptive fields, so that touching either of two symmetrically placed sites activates them.

Stimulation of the postcentral gyrus in conscious humans produces sensations usually described as tingling or numbness in a contralateral part of the body whose location is related in an orderly way to the site stimulated (see Fig. 3-30). The sensations generally do not resemble those caused by natural stimuli such as bending a hair or touching the skin, presumably because electrical stimulation of the cortex is a poor imitation of the pattern of activity set up by natural stimuli. Interestingly, sensations of pain can rarely be elicited from the postcentral gyrus, rather the concept of a pain matrix, whereby disparate regions of cerebral cortex form a network that is at least partially dedicated to pain perception, is emerging. Large lesions affecting the entire postcentral gyrus cause considerable impairment of the finer aspects of somatic sensation (e.g., judging the exact location or intensity of a stimulus) and a serious deficit in the sense of position and movement of the affected parts, but such damage does not abolish tactile sensation or the sensation of pain. Indeed, on the few occasions when removal of the postcentral cortex was tried as a treatment for intractable pain, the patient's pain was usually relieved only partially and briefly, and this was often followed by a hyperpathic state reminiscent of thalamic pain. In contrast, small lesions affecting only the part of the postcentral gyrus adjacent to the central sulcus cause not a loss of pain and temperature sensation but rather difficulty localizing painful stimuli in the somatotopically appropriate part of the body on the contralateral side. Corresponding to this clinical observation, neurons specifically responsive to painful stimuli have been found in the somatosensory cortex of monkeys at about the junction between areas 3 and 1. However, processing of pain information is not the exclusive province of S1. Pain-sensitive neurons have also been found in S2 and other areas, and functional imaging studies have demonstrated increased blood flow in S1, S2, part of the insula, and anterior cingulate cortex in response to painful stimuli. S1 is now thought to be important for localizing painful stimuli, and the other areas (especially the insula and cingulate gyrus) are thought to be responsible for the unpleasantness of pain.

Primary Visual Cortex Is in the Occipital Lobe

The retinotopic projection from the lateral geniculate nucleus to the banks of the calcarine sulcus, conveying information about the contralateral visual field, is described in Chapter 17. This primary visual cortex (**V1,** also called **striate cortex;** see Fig. 17-31) corresponds to area 17 of Brodmann's map. Peripheral parts of the visual field are represented anteriorly, the fovea has a disproportionately large representation located posteriorly, and the vertical meridian is represented along the upper and lower borders of area 17 (see Fig. 17-29). Although area 17 looks fairly small on maps such as those in Figures 22-10 and 22-13, it really occupies a substantial amount of the cortical surface and appears small only because most of it forms the walls of the deep calcarine sulcus.

A two-part visual association cortex occupies the rest of the occipital lobe. Area 18 surrounds area 17 and is itself surrounded by area 19. This association cortex receives its visual information both from area 17 and via the superior colliculus–pulvinar pathway. Areas 18 and 19 are themselves complex mosaics of smaller, retinotopically organized areas—one interested in the movements of objects, another in the colors of objects, and still others in other properties. Additional visual association areas occupy much of the temporal lobe (see Fig. 22-13), reflecting the importance of vision for primates.

The relative roles of primary visual cortex and visual association cortex in human vision are not completely understood. However, it is safe to say that the primary area is extremely important, because its destruction results in a total or near-total loss of conscious awareness of visual stimuli. A simplified view of its function, then, is that the primary visual cortex does some initial processing of inputs from the lateral geniculate nucleus (e.g., combining inputs from the two eyes and beginning to analyze depth), then distributes this information to the various subareas of visual association cortex where motion, color, and other parameters are analyzed more elaborately (see Fig. 17-36). If this is true, bilateral lesions of visual association cortex could conceivably disrupt single aspects of visual function. (Such cases would also be extremely rare, because they would have to involve symmetrically placed areas and spare the optic radiations.) A few cases have in fact been reported (see Box 17-2) in which bilateral damage to the inferior surfaces of the occipital lobes caused color blindness or in which more lateral damage near the occipital-temporal junction caused motion blindness.

Primary Auditory Cortex Is in the Temporal Lobe

The superior surface of the temporal lobe forms one wall of the lateral sulcus. One or two **transverse temporal gyri** (of Heschl; see Fig. 14-18) cross the posterior part of this surface and form Brodmann's areas 41 and 42. Area 41 is granular cortex (like areas 3 and 17) and receives most of the auditory radiation from the medial geniculate nucleus via the sublenticular part of the internal capsule; thus it serves as **primary auditory cortex,** or **A1** (Fig. 22-16). Just as the body is mapped onto the postcentral gyrus (**somatotopy**) and the retina is mapped onto striate cortex (**retinotopy**), the spectrum of audible frequencies is mapped onto area 41 (**tonotopy;** see Fig. 14-19). Area 42 is adjacent to area 41 and receives auditory information from both area 41 and the medial geniculate nucleus. This is analogous to the arrangement found in the second somatosensory area (S2), so area 42 is often referred to as **A2.** Area 42 is itself flanked by area 22, which forms much of the superior temporal gyrus and is called the **auditory association cortex.**

At levels rostral to the cochlear nuclei, both ears are represented in the auditory pathway of each side of the brain, although the contralateral ear predominates (see Chapter 14). As a result, even total destruction of auditory cortex on one side has relatively little effect on hearing. An individual with such damage may have some difficulty localizing sounds on the contralateral side and may have some subtle hearing loss that is greater for the contralateral ear, but the deficits are not nearly comparable in magnitude to those that follow unilateral damage to somatosensory or visual cortex. If the auditory association cortex of area 22 is damaged in the dominant hemisphere, severe language problems ensue, as discussed later in this chapter.

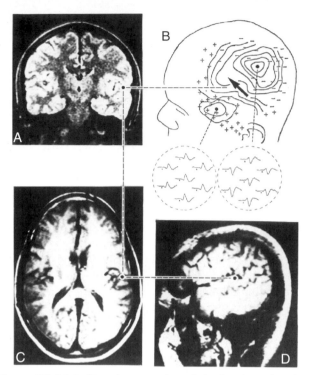

Figure 22-16 Striking demonstration of the location of auditory cortex on the superior surface of the temporal lobe in a living human. The current flows associated with nerve impulses are accompanied by fluctuating external magnetic fields. The fields and their fluctuations are tiny, but the changes can be measured using extremely sensitive recording instruments based on special detectors called superconducting quantum interference devices (SQUIDs). Magnetic field changes can then be mapped using a technique called magnetoencephalography. In the study shown here, 1-kHz tone bursts 400 msec in duration were presented to the right ear, and the resulting magnetic field changes were mapped over the left hemisphere **(B)**; some of the actual magnetic field change recordings are shown in the circular insets. The calculated source of these field changes was then mapped as a dot onto coronal, horizontal, and sagittal magnetic resonance images of the same individual **(A, C,** and **D,** respectively). *(From Yamamoto T et al: Proc Natl Acad Sci U S A 85:8732, 1988.)*

There Are Primary Vestibular, Gustatory, and Olfactory Areas

Gustatory information, relayed from VPM through the posterior limb of the internal capsule, reaches the frontal operculum and part of the anterior insula. These seem like logical places for gustatory cortex, because part is near both the representation of the tongue in somatosensory cortex and orbital olfactory cortex (see Chapter 13); however, these probable gustatory areas are rarely exposed during surgical procedures, so little direct information is available. A few cases have been reported in which stimulation of the frontal operculum or nearby insula caused sensations of taste or in which seizures originating in this vicinity were preceded by an aura that included sensations of taste.

The vestibular area was long thought to be located in the superior temporal gyrus and posterior insula near auditory cortex (see Fig. 22-13), because stimulation of

this region sometimes produces a sensation of movement or dizziness. Although this is the most important vestibular cortical area (see Fig. 14-30), there are also cortical projections from the vestibular system to the parietal lobe near the representation of the head in primary somatosensory cortex. All these vestibular areas are somewhat different from other primary sensory areas in that they respond to somatosensory and visual stimuli as well, consistent with the way all three of these systems contribute to the sense of position and movement.

The olfactory system is unique in that it does not relay in the thalamus before reaching its primary sensory area, and the primary olfactory cortex is paleocortical rather than neocortical (see Fig. 13-17). Primary olfactory cortex projects both directly and by way of the dorsomedial nucleus to olfactory association cortex on the orbital surface of the frontal lobe (see Fig. 13-19).

Most Motor Areas Are in the Frontal Lobe

Just as the somatosensory, visual, and auditory systems have multiple representations in the cortex, there are several areas from which movements can be elicited. **Primary motor cortex** corresponds to Brodmann's area 4, occupying a tapering strip in the precentral gyrus, mostly in the anterior wall of the central sulcus. Area 4 is agranular, the thickest cortex in the brain, and contains a preponderance of large pyramidal cells, including giant pyramidal cells (Betz cells). In the mid-19th century, before motor cortex had been explored electrically, the British neurologist Hughlings Jackson predicted the pattern in which movements are mapped on the precentral gyrus, based on his careful observation of patients with epileptic foci in this area. He noted that such patients typically had seizures that started as twitching in one part of the body and then spread to other regions on the same side in a sequence that was similar from one patient to another. This sequence corresponds to the now-familiar homunculus for the motor cortex, which is generally parallel to the homunculus found in the somatosensory cortex (Fig. 22-17). As might be expected from the distortions of the motor homunculus, Jackson also observed that these seizures were more likely to begin as twitching of the fingers or lips. Such attacks are still referred to as **jacksonian seizures** and the spread of motor activity as a **jacksonian march.** Stimulation of area 4 in conscious humans causes discrete movements involving one muscle or a small group of muscles (e.g., flexion of a single finger joint) that the patient is unable to prevent.[e] The movements are always contralateral to the side stimulated, except in movements of the palate, the pharynx, the masseter, and often the tongue (but not the lower face), where the

_____

[e]However, the patient has no sensation of willing the movement.

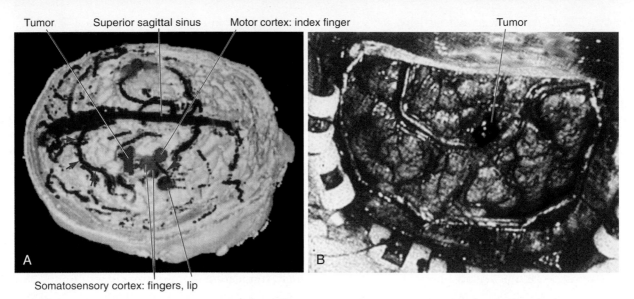

Tumor   Superior sagittal sinus   Motor cortex: index finger   Tumor

A

B

Somatosensory cortex: fingers, lip

Figure 22-17 Use of functional imaging to map cortical areas before neurosurgery. A 56-year-old woman with a history of metastatic breast cancer began to experience tingling and numbness of her left hand and forearm. MRI was combined with magnetic resonance angiography and magneto-encephalography during finger movements or touching of her fingers or lower lip, yielding a detailed map of functional areas, the cortical surface, and cerebral veins **(A)**. At surgery **(B),** this map's correspondence with the actual anatomy was apparent. *(From Gallen GC, Bucholz R, Sobel DF: Surg Neurol 42:523, 1994.)*

movements are bilateral; this corresponds nicely to the partly crossed–partly uncrossed corticobulbar (cortico-nuclear) projection (see Fig. 18-18).

Several cortical areas in addition to area 4 give rise to corticospinal fibers and to other cortical efferents that participate in motor control (see Fig. 18-11). Among them is area 6, which is agranular cortex similar to area 4, except that it lacks Betz cells. Movements can be elicited by stimulating area 6 on the lateral surface of the hemisphere (**premotor cortex**), but the threshold is slightly higher than in area 4, the movements are slower, and they are more likely to involve larger groups of muscles. Corticospinal fibers also arise in the somato-sensory cortex of the postcentral gyrus, and movements can be elicited from this region too, according to a pattern identical to the somatosensory homunculus. Finally, the **supplementary motor area** is located on the medial surface of the hemisphere, anterior to the representation of the foot in primary motor cortex, in the medial extension of area 6 (see Fig. 22-13). Stimulation of the supplementary motor area causes movements that are usually described as the assumption of postures and may involve muscles on both sides of the body. For example, there might be a turning of the head and trunk to the contralateral side, accompanied by a raising of the contralateral arm.

The multiple representations of movement in the cerebral cortex, with a primary area and several other nearby areas, are similar to the situation in sensory systems. In this case, too, the primary motor area seems to be the most important in terms of the deficits that follow its destruction. Lesions of area 4 cause an initial contralateral flaccid paralysis, which resolves fairly quickly into hemiparesis accompanied by mild spasticity. The paresis is worse for more distal muscles, and its effects are most evident when fine, skilled movements (e.g., individual finger movements) are attempted. There is disagreement about the degree of spasticity (or whether there is any at all) after damage restricted to area 4, but the spasticity is certainly slight compared with that seen in cases of more widespread cortical damage or lesions of the internal capsule. Selective damage to area 6 or to the supplementary motor area does not produce paralysis or reflex changes, but if such damage accompanies destruction of the primary motor area, full-blown spastic hemiparesis results.

The Right and Left Cerebral Hemispheres Are Specialized for Different Functions

All the functions discussed thus far have been related equally to both cerebral hemispheres, so the hemisphere in which a lesion occurs makes a difference only insofar as determining the side of the body on which a deficit is found. In contrast, it has long been known that language deficits are far more likely to occur after damage to the left hemisphere than to the right. Thus it appears that language tends to be lateralized in the human brain, and the hemisphere that is more important for the comprehension and production of language is now commonly called the **dominant hemisphere.** The "other" hemisphere is known as the **nondominant hemisphere,** although this is rather chauvinistic terminology because (as will be seen) the so-called nondominant hemisphere is quite superior in some things.

Nearly all right-handed people (at least 95%) have dominant left hemispheres. The majority of left-handed people are also left-dominant, although left-handers are more likely than right-handers to have dominant right hemispheres or to have some language representation in each hemisphere. Thus the side that is dominant is correlated to some extent with handedness, but regardless of whether an individual is left-handed or right-handed, the left hemisphere is more likely to be dominant.

On casual inspection, brains look bilaterally symmetrical, but searches for an anatomical basis for the lateralization of language have revealed that a variety of asymmetries actually exist. As discussed in the next section, certain cortical areas abutting the lateral sulcus are important for linguistic functions, so the consistent asymmetries found in the vicinity of the lateral sulcus are of great interest in this regard. The part of the superior surface of the superior temporal gyrus located posterior to primary auditory cortex is called the **planum temporale** (or **temporal plane**) and is, on average, considerably larger on the left than on the right. Because the lateral border of the planum temporale forms part of the lower bank of the lateral sulcus, it stands to reason that the lateral sulcus should extend farther posteriorly on the left than on the right. This too has been found to be the case (Fig. 22-18). These asymmetries are present

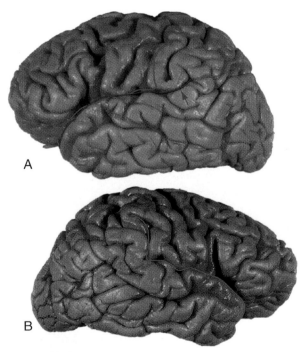

Figure 22-18 Typical asymmetry of the two lateral sulci. The lateral sulci of the left **(A)** and right **(B)** hemispheres of a single brain were traced, and the right lateral sulcus was then reversed and overlaid on the left. The left lateral sulcus extends farther posteriorly than the right does *(arrow)*, corresponding to the fact that the planum temporale is usually larger on the left. *(Adapted from Nolte J, Angevine JB Jr: The human brain in photographs and diagrams, ed 3, St. Louis, 2007, Mosby. Based on the method in Rubens AB, Mahowald MW, Hutton JT: Neurology 26:620, 1976.)*

before birth, which seems to indicate that left hemisphere dominance for language is, at least in part, genetically determined.

Language Areas Border on the Lateral Sulcus, Usually on the Left Hemisphere

Stimulation of the part of motor cortex where the mouth is represented causes an inability to speak and at the same time produces involuntary grunts, cries, or other forms of vocalization. This is similar to what happens when any other part of motor cortex is stimulated: there is a discrete movement during which the patient is powerless to use those muscles for anything else. However, there are other areas whose stimulation on the dominant side causes the patient to cease speaking but not to do something else with the vocal muscles; more strikingly, stimulation of these areas can cause the patient to make linguistic errors or be unable to find appropriate words. The two best known are **Broca's area,** in the opercular and triangular parts of the inferior frontal gyrus, and **Wernicke's area,** in the posterior part of the superior temporal gyrus (continuing in a functional sense into the planum temporale and the inferior parietal lobule). Because these areas largely surround the lateral fissure (of Sylvius), they are commonly referred to as the **perisylvian language zone.**

Inability to use language (i.e., loss of the use of or access to the set of symbols that humans use to represent concepts) is called **aphasia.** (This is not necessarily the same thing as loss of the ability to communicate. If you were in a foreign country where a different language was spoken, for example, you would still be able to communicate and understand to some extent through things such as intonation, mimicry, and gestures.) Broca's and Wernicke's areas form the basis of the traditional framework that accounts for the two broad categories of aphasia—**nonfluent** and **fluent,** depending on the ease with which words can be produced (Box 22-2; Figs. 22-19 and 22-20). Broca's aphasics produce few words, either written or spoken, and often use stock phrases repeatedly when responding to questions or requests (e.g., "OK," "Oh boy!"); other words are produced only with great difficulty. They tend to leave out all but the most meaningful words in a sentence and to speak or write in a telegraphic manner. In contrast to their difficulties in producing language, Broca's aphasics have relatively less difficulty comprehending it. Wernicke's aphasics, in contrast, are able to produce written and spoken words, but the words or the sequences in which they are used are defective in their linguistic content. There may be substitutions of one letter or word for another (**paraphasia**), insertion of new and meaningless words (**neologisms**), or stringing together of words and phrases in an order that conveys little or no meaning (**jargon aphasia**). This suggests that such patients have difficulty comprehending whether their own speech makes sense, and indeed,

Nonfluent and Fluent Aphasia

The difference between nonfluent and fluent language production can be illustrated by transcriptions of the speech of two patients as they tried to describe a drawing of a picnic scene*
(see Fig. 22-19).

Patient MN was a right-handed, 62-year-old man who had a stroke in the anterior distribution of the left middle cerebral artery (see Fig. 22-20A). When tested at 2 years after the stroke, his language profile was consistent with moderately severe Broca's aphasia. His spoken language was characterized by single-word utterances that contained articulation errors but was largely intelligible. His utterances were lacking grammatical structure, consisting primarily of nouns and a few verbs. When asked to describe the picnic scene, he said:

"picnic ... flying kite ... swimming ... house ... tree ... pouring water ... boat ... trees ... okay ... car."

Patient JS was a right-handed, 65-year-old man who had a stroke in the posterior distribution of the left middle cerebral artery (see Fig. 22-20B). His initial diagnosis was conduction aphasia. At 3½ years after the stroke, his speech was fluent, with a relatively normal sentence structure, but word-finding difficulties were evident. When describing the picnic scene, he said: "In the pier, somebody is fishing. Somebody is playing into the water. The man with the kite has the jeans with the pocket deal." His word-finding difficulties were more noticeable when he was asked to perform a naming task. For example, when trying to name a paper clip he said, "safety pin, no, the little clip."

*Cases courtesy Dr. Pelagie M. Beeson, University of Arizona.

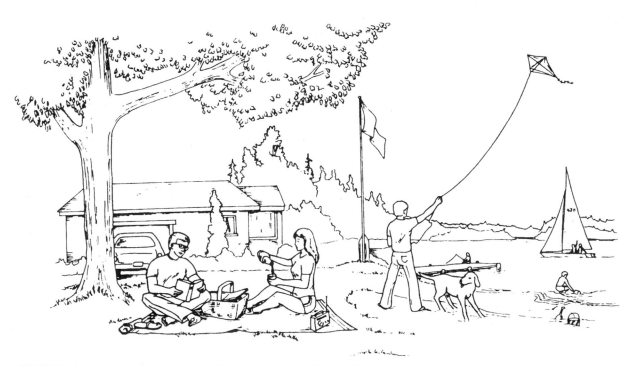

Figure 22-19 Picnic scene that the two patients from Box 22-2 were asked to describe. *(From Kertesz A: Western aphasia battery, copyright © 1982 by Harcourt Assessment, Inc. Reproduced with permission. All rights reserved.)*

Wernicke's aphasics are relatively more deficient in the comprehension of language generally.

These two broad types of aphasia have traditionally been interpreted in terms of Broca's area containing motor programs for the generation of language and Wernicke's area containing mechanisms for the formulation of language. Destruction of Broca's area would thus deprive the motor cortex of the instructions needed to generate language, but the muscles involved would be normal in other activities; comprehension of language would be relatively unaffected. Destruction of Wernicke's area would leave Broca's area unchecked, so that words could be produced without regard for their meaning. These core perisylvian language areas, interconnected through the arcuate (superior longitudinal) fasciculus (see Fig. 22-9), would then be sufficient to allow someone

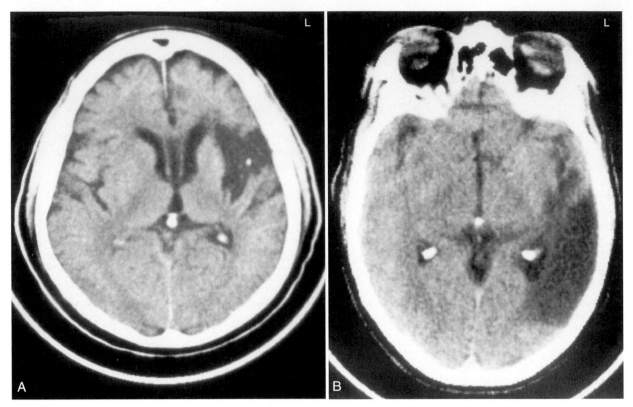

Figure 22-20 Computed tomography scans of the two patients in Box 22-2 near the time of testing. **A,** Patient MN. Note that the infarct includes not only part of the left inferior frontal gyrus but also the left insula. **B,** Patient JS, showing damage more posteriorly in the left temporal-parietal region.

to hear spoken language (using Wernicke's area) and repeat it (using Broca's area), and damage within the perisylvian zone would cause impaired repetition. For example, it would be predicted that selective destruction of the arcuate fasciculus would leave Broca's area unchecked and would result in a form of fluent aphasia. Cases have been reported (with lesions near the predicted site) in which the patient speaks like a Wernicke's aphasic but has relatively intact comprehension, because Wernicke's area itself is undamaged. This syndrome is called **conduction aphasia.** Additional aphasic syndromes have been accounted for by disruption of other inputs to Broca's or Wernicke's area (Table 22-2). Hence **transcortical aphasias** are caused by damage outside the perisylvian language zone. They have features of Broca's or Wernicke's aphasia because the respective areas have been deprived of important inputs, but repetition is relatively spared.

This traditional model is appealingly simple and often successful in explaining a variety of aphasic disorders, but it is certainly an oversimplification. Functional imaging studies have shown increased blood flow in extensive networks of multiple cortical areas during most language tasks. In addition, not all aphasic patients have damage in the expected location. For example, damage restricted to Broca's area causes only a mild, temporary deficit in fluency; patients with severe, per-

sistent Broca's aphasia have more extensive damage that involves the insula and possibly the head of the caudate nucleus (Box 22-3; Fig. 22-21). Similarly, patients with persistent Wernicke's aphasia typically have extensive lesions that include not just the superior temporal gyrus but also parts of the middle temporal gyrus and inferior parietal lobule. Finally, damage that includes the supramarginal gyrus is thought to be the basis for conduction aphasia; a lesion of the arcuate fasciculus alone is insufficient. Despite these complications, however, it is consistently found that within the cortical areas important for language, more anterior lesions result in greater deficits in the production of language, and more posterior lesions result in greater deficits in comprehension (Fig. 22-22).

Communication by language involves more than just selecting words and then assembling them according to grammatical rules. Most of the emotional content, and part of the linguistic content as well, is conveyed by varying emphases. This is true of language generally, but especially of spoken language. For example, depending on how they are said, the words "Jack is here" could be a statement of fact or a question; they could convey a feeling of happiness or dread. The rhythmic and more or less musical aspects of speech are called **prosody.** The right hemisphere plays a special role in producing and comprehending the affective aspects of the prosody of

Table 22-2 Major Aphasia Syndromes

Aphasia Type	Fluency	Repetition	Comprehension	Typical Lesion Location*
Broca's	↓	↓	±	
Transcortical motor	↓	±	±	
Global	↓	↓	↓	
Wernicke's	±	↓	↓	
Transcortical sensory	±	±	↓	
Conduction	±	↓	±	

±, Relatively intact (although rarely normal); ↓, conspicuously impaired.
*Often involves deep structures as well.

BOX 22-3

Broca's Original Patient

The idea that particular mental functions are associated with specific cortical areas has not always been accepted. Following the decline of phrenology in the early 19th century, the prevailing view was that cognitive functions such as language were the result of the cerebral cortex working as an undivided structure. Even so, some investigators began to provide evidence that localized cortical damage could cause predictable deficits. The most famous and influential of these was the demonstration in 1861 by Paul Broca, a French physician, of an association between damage to the "third frontal convolution" (the inferior frontal gyrus) and the loss of language production.

In April 1861, Broca encountered a patient named Leborgne who had a 20-year history of inability to produce meaningful words. He had been nicknamed "Tan" because "he could no longer produce but a single syllable, which he usually repeated twice in succession; regardless of the question asked him, he always responded: *tan, tan,* combined with varied expressive gestures. This is why, throughout the hospital, he is known only by the name *Tan*."* Leborgne died a week later and at autopsy was found to have long-standing damage to his left inferior frontal gyrus (see Fig. 22-21A). Although attention was focused on the cortical area that came to bear Broca's name, the damage was clearly more extensive, affecting additional cortical areas (including the insula) and parts of the basal nuclei (see Fig. 22-21C and D).

Over the next 2 years, Broca investigated seven more cases of loss of spoken language. As in the case of Leborgne, all seven had left hemisphere damage. In an 1865 paper, Broca was one of the first to describe the idea of hemispheric dominance for language.

*From Broca P: Bulletins de la Société d'anatomie (Paris), 2e serie 6:330, 1861. Translated in Dronkers NF et al: Brain 130:1532, 2007.

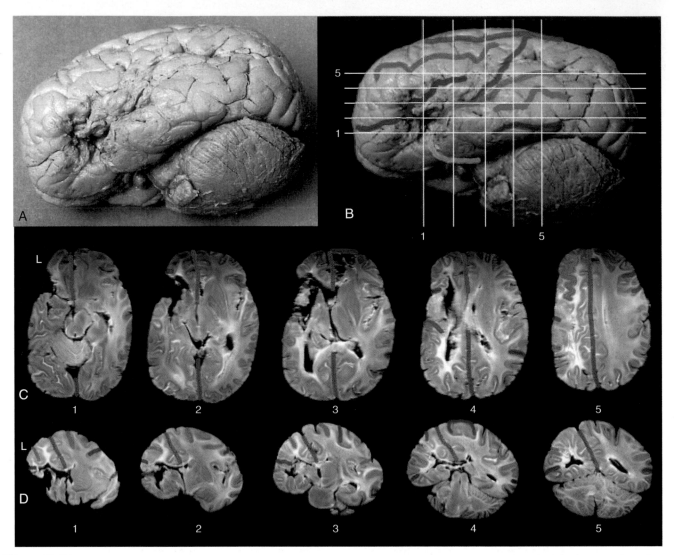

Figure 22-21 The brain of Leborgne (Box 22-3), which was preserved in alcohol at autopsy in 1861. **A,** View from the left, showing a large lesion centered in the inferior frontal gyrus but extending farther into the frontal, anterior temporal, and even parietal lobes; the right hemisphere appears to be normal. **B,** The same view as in **A,** with planes of the magnetic resonance images in **C** and **D** indicated. Prominent sulci were colored, including the central and lateral sulci (*dark blue* and *light blue*) and the inferior frontal sulcus *(red)*. **C** and **D,** Axial and coronal MRI scans. Damage in the left inferior frontal gyrus is apparent **(C2, D1),** but there is also extensive damage on the left to the insula **(C2-3, D2-3);** basal nuclei **(C2-3, D1-2);** deep white matter, including the arcuate fasciculus **(C4-5, D2-5);** and other sites. *(Adapted from Dronkers NF et al: Brain 130:1532, 2007.)*

speech. The system for generating and comprehending prosody is apparently organized in a fashion analogous to the left hemisphere system for producing and comprehending language. That is, the right inferior frontal gyrus is involved in *producing* prosody, and the right posterior temporoparietal region in *comprehending* it. One of the first patients described with a deficit related to prosody was a schoolteacher with right frontal damage who began to have difficulty controlling her students because she was unable to convey anger or authority by voice or gesture (even though the feelings were there). She had **motor aprosodia.** Patients with more posterior lesions on the right may have **sensory aprosodia** and have difficulty comprehending the emotional content of the speech or gestures of others.

Parietal Association Cortex Mediates Spatial Orientation

The **posterior parietal cortex,** the part of the parietal lobe posterior to S1, is filled with association areas. Some of these are unimodal, grading into the visual association areas of the occipital and temporal lobes, the auditory association areas of the temporal lobe, and somatosensory cortex in the postcentral gyrus. Damage to these areas can cause sensory-specific **agnosias.** *Agnosia* (from the Greek word for "lack of knowledge") means the inability to recognize the identity or some other property of objects when using a given sense, even though that sense is basically intact. Visual agnosias, for example, may entail an inability to recognize faces or to perceive the movement of visual objects (see Box 17-2),

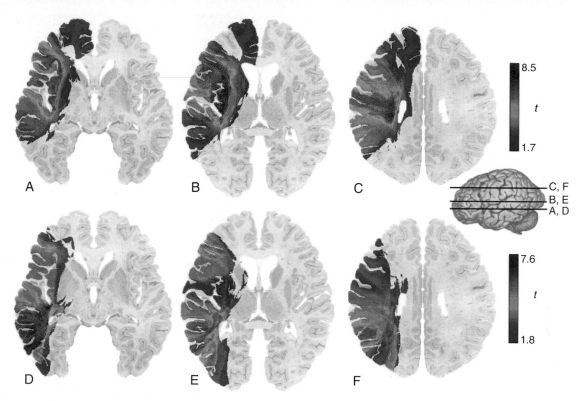

Figure 22-22 Associations between sites of damage and aphasia symptoms in 101 aphasic stroke patients. The likelihood that a patient with impaired fluency had damage at different sites in three axial levels is indicated in **A** to **C**; *red* and *blue* indicate high and low probabilities, respectively. The likelihood that a patient with impaired auditory comprehension had damage at different sites in the same three axial levels is indicated in **D** to **F.** Impaired fluency is associated with damage extending beyond Broca's area, commonly affecting the insula **(B)** and deep white matter **(C).** Impaired comprehension is associated with damage extending beyond Wernicke's area, commonly affecting the middle temporal gyrus **(D)** and inferior parietal lobule **(F).** Nevertheless, impaired fluency is clearly associated with more anterior infarcts than impaired comprehension is. *(From Bates E et al: Nat Neurosci 6:448, 2003. Brain slices and brain inset adapted from DeArmond SJ, Fusco MM, Dewey MM: Structure of the human brain: a photographic atlas, ed 3, New York, 1989, Oxford University Press.)*

even using intact parts of the visual fields; the sensory specificity shows up as a retained ability to do similar tasks using other senses, such as recognizing people by their voices or perceiving the movement of something across the skin. Tactile and auditory (and even gustatory and olfactory) agnosias, though less common, have also been reported. There even appear to be the equivalents of dorsal and ventral streams (see Fig. 17-36) in the somatosensory and auditory systems. Someone with a normal audiogram, for example, might be selectively unable to recognize the identity of environmental sounds or to perceive the location or movement of a sound source.

The rest of the posterior parietal cortex is a series of interrelated multimodal areas, centered on the intraparietal sulcus (Fig. 22-23). Collectively, they keep track of the shifting relationships between body parts and things in the outside world, factoring in motivation, attention, and the relevance of different objects. The parietal eye field (see Fig. 21-13) is one such area, monitoring the relationship between eye position and not just visual objects but also sound sources and body parts. Analogous areas in or near the intraparietal sulcus are tuned

to arms and hands and participate in reaching for objects or grasping them. Each of these parietal multimodal areas is tightly coupled to a premotor area, and the resulting frontoparietal circuits swing into action whenever we shift attention to different parts of the environment. Removal of the posterior parietal cortex from a monkey causes neglect of the contralateral half of the body; even though the tactile threshold is unchanged, the limbs on that side are used little, and reaching with them is inaccurate. The consequences of large lesions of the right parietal lobe in humans are similar, but more complex.[f] Such a patient has difficulty with spatial orientation to everything on the left and may completely ignore the halves of objects to the left (Fig. 22-24) and even the left half of his or her own body. The most common cause is a stroke in the territory of the middle

---

[f]In this discussion of parietal lobe syndromes, some types of symptoms are related to right-sided damage and others to left-sided damage. It is assumed (but generally not proved) that these sides correspond in a given patient to the sides nondominant and dominant for language, respectively. Certainly this is true in a large majority of patients.

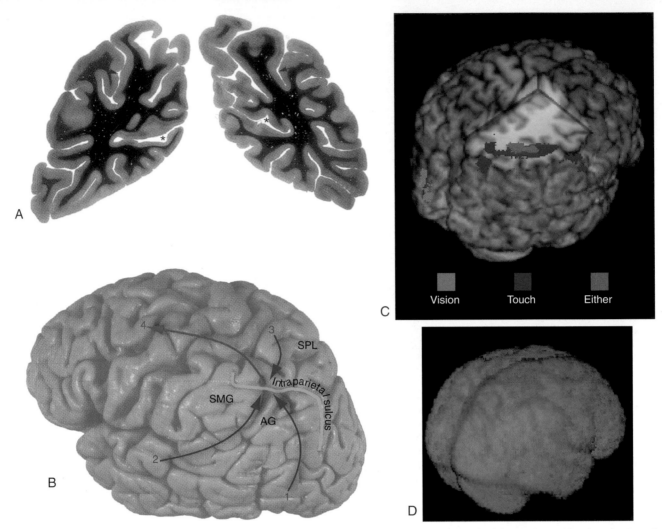

Figure 22-23 Parietal association cortex. **A,** Coronal section showing the intraparietal sulcus *(arrows)* in both hemispheres. Like the calcarine sulcus (*), the intraparietal sulcus is deep and has a lot of cortex in its walls. **B,** General pattern of connections of parietal multimodal areas in and near the intraparietal sulcus. Each receives converging inputs from visual (1), auditory (2), and somatosensory (3) association cortex and projects to a selected premotor area (4). AG, angular gyrus; SMG, supramarginal gyrus; SPL, superior parietal lobule. **C,** Functional MRI study showing areas of increased blood flow as subjects tried to judge the orientation of a grating that they looked at or touched. Each task activated unimodal areas in the occipital and parietal lobes, respectively, but both activated a multimodal area in the right intraparietal sulcus. **D,** Combined PET and MRI study of increased blood flow during tasks that required increasing amounts of mental rotation of objects. When humans are asked to look at an object, such as a number or a letter, that has been rotated and quickly decide whether the object started out in its proper orientation or was mirror-reversed, they solve the problem by imagining the object rotating back to its original orientation and then using their "mind's eye" to examine it. As subjects performed increasingly more demanding tasks of this type, blood flow selectively increased in the region of the right intraparietal sulcus, shown by superimposing the PET data on a three-dimensional MRI reconstruction. **(C,** from Kitada R et al: J Neurosci 26:7491, 2006. **D,** from Harris IM et al: Brain 123:65, 2000.)

cerebral artery (see Fig. 6-4); such a lesion is rarely confined to the parietal lobe and is often accompanied by hemiparesis and a hemisensory loss. The patient may deny that anything is wrong with the affected limbs and may even maintain that they are someone else's limbs. In some cases of **contralateral neglect,** there is a general deficit in spatial orientation that shows up as difficulty following maps or finding locations, even in familiar surroundings. Functional imaging has revealed that humans use parietal association cortex, especially that of the right hemisphere, when simply thinking during tasks that require the mental manipulation of objects (see Fig. 22-23D).

Contralateral neglect less frequently follows left parietal damage, and when it does, it is usually transient. This is because the right hemisphere is dominant for spatial attention. After left hemisphere damage, the right hemisphere can direct attention to both the contralateral and ipsilateral sides, but after right hemisphere damage, the left hemisphere can only manage to attend to the contralateral side, so the left side of the world is neglected.

Contralateral neglect has traditionally been attributed to damage in the right inferior parietal lobule, but damage to the frontal areas with which it is connected can also cause neglect. In addition, just as studies have

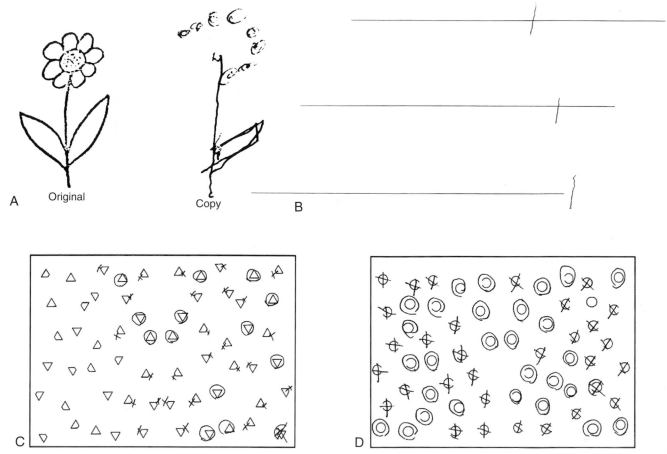

Figure 22-24 Left hemineglect, typically occurring after right parietal damage. **A,** A patient was asked to copy a drawing and omitted multiple parts of the left side. **B,** A 77-year-old man with a right frontoparietal stroke was asked to bisect lines on a piece of paper. All the bisections were off to the right. As the lines moved farther to the left, the errors grew greater, until he finally missed the line entirely. **C** and **D,** Two different patients with right middle cerebral artery strokes were asked to circle complete figures and cross out incomplete figures. **C,** A 55-year-old man with damage to the parietal, temporal, and frontal lobes, the insula, and the caudate nucleus and putamen neglected most of the figures on the left side of the page. However, he marked the figures on the right side of the page correctly. **D,** A 70-year-old man with damage mostly confined to the parietal and temporal lobes marked figures on both sides of the page. However, if a circle located anywhere on the page had a gap on the left, the gap was usually missed. (**A,** from Heilman KM, Valenstein E, editors: Clinical neuropsychology, ed 2, New York, 1985, Oxford University Press. **B,** courtesy Dr. Sarah Orjada, Brandeis University. **C** and **D,** from Ota H et al: Neurology 57:2064, 2001.)

shown that aphasia syndromes involve lesions more extensive than or sometimes outside the "classical" language areas, damage outside these frontoparietal circuits (especially in the right superior temporal gyrus) has been implicated in neglect syndromes. These multiple sites may reflect the possibility that neglect is not a single syndrome. Some patients, for example, neglect everything to their left (see Fig. 22-24C), whereas others neglect the left sides of all objects, wherever they are (see Fig. 22-24D).

Although right parietal association areas are more important for spatial attention, comparable areas on the left are more important for assembling the bits of sensory information needed to plan movements accurately. Damage here can cause peculiar disabilities called **apraxias** (from the Greek word for "lack of action"), in which a patient is unable to perform some actions, even though the muscles required are perfectly sound and

able to perform the same action in a different context. An apraxic patient might be unable to touch her nose with her index finger when asked to imitate the examiner's movement but be quite capable of doing so spontaneously if her nose itched. There are several subcategories of apraxias and numerous theories about whether some types are based on language deficits, spatial disorientation, or other more basic problems. As in the case of neglect, damage outside the left parietal lobe, especially left frontal damage, can cause forms of apraxia. Apraxia of mouth and face movements, for example, often accompanies left frontal lesions and is a prominent part of Broca's aphasia.

Prefrontal Cortex Mediates Working Memory and Decision Making

The part of each frontal lobe anterior to areas 4 and 6 is referred to as **prefrontal cortex,** and it has a different role from that of the other cortical areas considered in this chapter. Prefrontal cortex does not cause movements when stimulated, and it does not contain any primary sensory areas. Instead, it is centrally involved in controlling the activities of other cortical areas—to such an extent that it is seen as underlying the **executive functions** of the brain: planning, insight, foresight, and many of the most basic aspects of personality. Consistent with this, prefrontal cortex expanded dramatically during mammalian evolution (see Fig. 22-12) and now occupies the inside of the distinctively large forehead of humans.

Different prefrontal areas share extensive interconnections with the dorsomedial nucleus of the thalamus. These play an important role in the workings of this cortical area, as shown by the observation that lesions of the dorsomedial nucleus have effects that are in some ways similar to those of prefrontal damage. In a functional sense, and in terms of patterns of connections with other parts of the forebrain, there are two broad sets of prefrontal areas (Fig. 22-25). The parts exposed on the lateral convexity (**dorsolateral prefrontal cortex**) have massive interconnections with parietal multimodal cortex and somatosensory, visual, and auditory association areas (via the long association bundles mentioned earlier; see Fig. 22-9). Many neurons in analogous regions of monkey prefrontal cortex respond to various kinds of stimuli, but they respond especially vigorously when the stimulus is gone and the monkey's task is to remember it briefly to receive a reward. This is consistent with the idea that dorsolateral prefrontal cortex plays a critical role in **working memory,** the ability to keep "in mind" recent events or the moment-to-moment

results of mental processing. (A common example of working memory is remembering a telephone number until you have finished keying it in.) Patients with damage in this prefrontal area have problems with planning, solving problems, and maintaining attention.

In contrast, **ventromedial prefrontal cortex** (extending into orbitofrontal and anterior cingulate areas) is interconnected more with limbic structures such as the amygdala, as described further in Chapter 23. Patients with damage here are impulsive and have trouble suppressing inappropriate responses and emotional reactions; some psychopathic conditions are thought to be a reflection of orbitofrontal dysfunction. An early clue to the role of this area in human behavior was provided by an unfortunate accident in the 19th century. In 1848, Phineas Gage, the foreman of a railroad construction crew, was setting a charge of explosives in a hole in rock, using a 13-pound, $3\frac{1}{2}$-foot iron tamping rod. The charge exploded and blew the tamping iron through the front of his head (Fig. 22-26), destroying a good deal of his ventromedial prefrontal cortex. Remarkably, he survived the accident and regained his physical health in a few weeks. However, his personality changed dramatically. Before the accident he had been hardworking, responsible, clever, and thoroughly respectable. After the accident he seemed to lose most of his industriousness and his awareness of social responsibilities.[g] He wandered aimlessly from job to job, exhibiting himself and his tamping iron in various carnivals. He was tactless and impulsive in his behavior, not particularly concerned about his future or the consequences of his actions.

We routinely combine cognitive strategies and emotional reactions to situations when making decisions and plans, reflecting constant collaboration between dorsolateral and ventromedial areas (Box 22-4; Fig. 22-27).

Various means of separating the prefrontal cortex from the rest of the brain (procedures called **prefrontal lobotomy** or **leukotomy**) were used in the first half of the 20th century as a treatment for certain severe psychoses and other conditions, but these operations were largely abandoned decades ago in favor of drug therapy. The procedures were done bilaterally, but similar (though

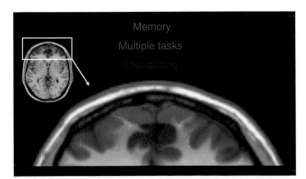

Figure 22-25 Functional specialization of different prefrontal areas near the frontal pole. Data from 104 different functional imaging studies published from 1995 to 2005 were combined to produce a map indicating where blood flow was most likely to increase during three different kinds of tasks. Memory refers to studies in which subjects recalled events from their past; multiple tasks to studies in which subjects used multiple mental efforts (e.g., task switching, predicting future events); and mentalizing to studies in which subjects inferred the mental or emotional states of themselves or others (e.g., judging emotional states by looking at pictures of facial expressions). The map was made to be bilaterally symmetrical because, for these tasks, there was little asymmetry near the frontal pole; other prefrontal activities are more lateralized (see Fig. 22-27). *(From Gilbert SJ et al: J Cog Neurosci 18:932, 2006.)*

---

[g]"The equilibrium or balance, so to speak, between his intellectual faculties and animal propensities, seems to have been destroyed. He is fitful, irreverent, indulging at times in the grossest profanity (which was not previously his custom), manifesting but little deference for his fellows, impatient of restraint or advice when it conflicts with his desires, at times pertinaciously obstinate, yet capricious and vacillating, devising many plans of future operation, which are no sooner arranged than they are abandoned. … In this regard his mind was radically changed, so decidedly that his friends and acquaintances said that he was 'no longer Gage.'" (Harlow HM: Recovery from the passage of an iron bar through the head, Mass Med Soc Publ 2:327, 1868.)

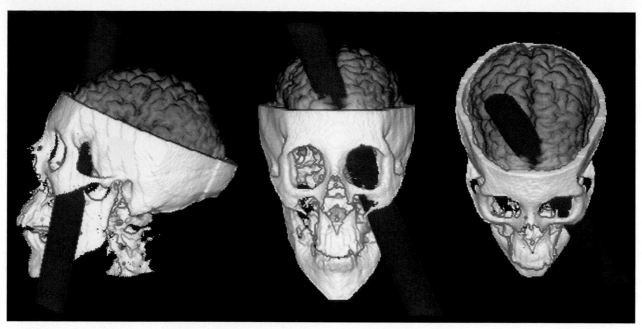

Figure 22-26 The probable relationship between Phineas Gage's brain and the tamping iron, based on a modern reexamination of his skull and the entry and exit wounds. Ventrolateral prefrontal areas were heavily damaged, but motor cortex, Broca's area, and most dorsolateral prefrontal areas were probably spared. *(From the cover illustration accompanying Damasio H et al: Science 264:1102, 1994.)*

Reason and Emotion in the Ultimatum Game

One of the ways humans differ markedly from other species is that humans defer or even give up personal rewards in favor of fairness to other members of society. Fairness has a value of its own for humans and gets factored into decision making. This generates constant conflict, as in the mixed feelings engendered by paying taxes. Resolving such conflict involves a constant interplay between prefrontal cortex and other areas more concerned with emotion and motivation.

This interplay is illustrated dramatically in the Ultimatum Game, a simple economic game with two moves. One player proposes a way to divide a known sum of money with another player. The second player responds by accepting or rejecting the offer. If the offer is accepted, the proposer and responder get the amounts of money specified in the offer; if the offer is rejected, no one gets anything. Easy, right? The only rational response seems to be to accept all offers, because some money is better than none. In fact, however, that is not how people behave. Players instead accept all offers of 50% or more of the money; when offered progressively less than 50%, they are more and more likely to perceive the offer as unfair and reject it (see Fig. 22-27A), even if that means forgoing significant amounts of money. Wrestling with the decision is associated with activation of the insula and anterior cingulate gyrus (limbic-related areas; see Chapter 23) and of the right dorsolateral prefrontal cortex (see Fig. 22-27B).

The role of dorsolateral prefrontal cortex in controlling behavior in the Ultimatum Game (and in everyday activities) is hinted at by looking at changes in blood flow, but it is demonstrated more directly by inactivating it. Current passed through a coil placed on the scalp induces a localized magnetic field that passes through the skull and brain. The magnetic field in turn causes current flow in the brain, changing the activity of nearby neurons. Single pulses of **transcranial magnetic stimulation (TMS)** typically make cortical neurons under the coil fire a brief burst of action potentials, whereas repetitive pulses can disrupt the activity of a small region of cortex, creating a "temporary lesion." Inactivating dorsolateral prefrontal cortex in this way on the right (but not the left) makes responders in the Ultimatum Game more likely to accept unfair offers, even though they still perceive them to be unfair (see Fig. 22-27C).

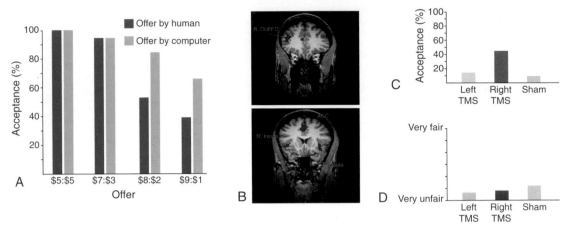

Figure 22-27 The Ultimatum Game and cortical activity (Box 22-4). **A,** Typical results of a series of games in which $10 was available to be divided. As offers began to dip below $5, they were progressively less likely to be accepted. Offers made by a computer were less likely to be rejected, indicating that responders are more willing to punish humans who make unfair offers, even if both the proposer and the responder lose in the process. **B,** Areas where blood flow (assessed by fMRI) increased more when pondering unfair offers than when pondering fair offers. **C,** Rates of acceptance of unfair offers (20% of available money) tripled when right (but not left) dorsolateral prefrontal cortex activity was disrupted. **D,** Despite the increased rate of acceptance in **C,** the offers were still perceived as very unfair. ACC, anterior cingulate cortex; DLPFC, dorsolateral prefrontal cortex, TMS, transcranial magnetic stimulation. (**A** and **B,** from Sanfey AG et al: Science 300:1755, 2003. **C,** from Knoch D et al: Science 314:829, 2006.)

less pronounced) effects were seen after unilateral operations. There was considerable variation from one patient to another, but individuals so treated typically became carefree and often apparently euphoric, which was the beneficial effect sought; someone suffering from intractable pain, for example, would admit that there was no decrease in the pain after a prefrontal leukotomy but would no longer be bothered by it. Unfortunately, though not surprisingly in view of current knowledge of prefrontal connections and functions, many also became more reckless in their behavior; powers of concentration, attention span, initiative, spontaneity, and abstract reasoning all suffered.

The Corpus Callosum Unites the Two Cerebral Hemispheres

The corpus callosum, which interconnects the two cerebral hemispheres, is by far the largest fiber bundle in the human brain. It contains somewhere around 250 million axons; most of them interconnect roughly mirror-image sites, but a substantial number end in areas different from, but related to, those in which they arise. Area 17 of one hemisphere, for example, projects to areas 18 and 19 of the contralateral hemisphere. Nearly all cortical areas receive commissural fibers (Fig. 22-28), with a few notable exceptions such as the hand area of somatosensory and motor cortex and all of area 17 not representing areas adjacent to the vertical midline. The commissural fibers to and from much of the temporal lobe, particularly its inferior parts, pass through the anterior commissure.

We all know from common experience that something initially seen in one visual field can be identified if presented later in the contralateral visual field (e.g., we can recognize the elements of a picture after it has been reversed left to right). The same is true for other sensory modalities such as touch[h]; similar transfers from one hemisphere to the other can be demonstrated easily in experimental animals. The importance of the corpus callosum for these transfers can be shown dramatically in experiments involving bisection of the optic chiasm of experimental animals. This destroys all fibers crossing from each eye to the contralateral lateral geniculate nucleus, so anything presented to one eye reaches only the ipsilateral cerebral hemisphere. Such animals, despite having bitemporal visual field deficits, continue to show normal transfer of learning from one side to the other. However, if the corpus callosum is also sectioned, the animals no longer show this transfer. It is even possible to train them to give two completely different responses to the same stimulus, depending on which eye sees the stimulus.

Section of the corpus callosum has been used as a treatment of last resort for some human patients suffering from intractable epilepsy, to prevent seizures from spreading from one hemisphere to the other. The procedure generally ameliorates the epilepsy, and otherwise, the patients seem more or less unchanged; however,

---

[h]Even though parts of the somatosensory and visual cortices receive no commissural fibers, all areas of the parietal and occipital association cortices do, so each hemisphere has access to data from the contralateral half of the body and the outside world.

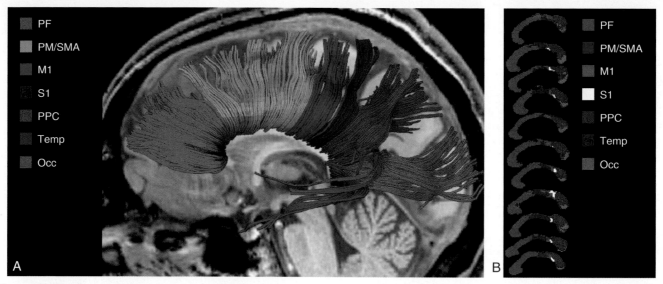

Figure 22-28 Topography of the human corpus callosum, demonstrated with diffusion tensor imaging. A very large proportion interconnects cortex anterior to the precentral gyrus, reflecting the size of this area in human brains. **A,** Callosal fibers of a single male subject, superimposed on a sagittal MRI scan. **B,** The origins or destinations of fibers at different locations in the corpus callosum of 11 different individuals (7 male, 4 female); anterior is to the left. M1, primary motor cortex; Occ, occipital lobe; PF, prefrontal cortex; PM, premotor cortex; PPC, posterior parietal cortex; S1, primary somatosensory cortex; SMA, supplementary motor area; Temp, temporal lobe. (**A,** *from Hofer S, Frahm J: Neuroimage 32:989, 2006.* **B,** *from Zarei M et al: J Anat 209:311, 2006.*)

careful testing reveals some remarkable alterations. Words flashed in the right visual field can be read normally, but words flashed in the left field cannot be read, and the patient denies having seen them. As far as spoken or written responses to visual stimuli are concerned, these "split-brain" patients behave as though they have a left homonymous hemianopia. This is thoroughly consistent with the notion of dominance of the left hemisphere for language, which can organize and execute a spoken or written response; visual stimuli in the left field reach the right hemisphere, which no longer has access to the language areas. However, it is easy to show that the right hemisphere is still quite functional. For example, a picture of an object can be flashed in the left visual field, and the patient asked to pick out that object manually from an assortment on a table; this can be done (usually with the left hand), even though the patient denies having seen anything. This is a clear indication that the right hemisphere has some capacity for the comprehension of language and the organization of nonverbal responses.

Continued testing of such patients has yielded some general concepts of hemisphere function that, by and large, confirm and extend the conclusions drawn from studies of patients with unilateral brain damage. The left hemisphere in most people is dominant not only for language (Fig. 22-29A) but also for mathematical ability and the ability to solve problems in a sequential, logical fashion. The right hemisphere is superior in some aspects of musical skills, in recognition of faces, and in tasks requiring comprehension of spatial relationships

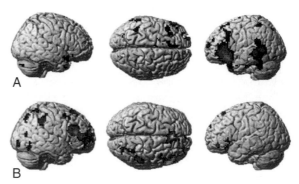

Figure 22-29 Hemispheric lateralization in a typical subject, demonstrated by fMRI. **A,** Areas with increased blood flow during all three language tasks utilized (generating multiple words that begin with a given letter, judging whether two words are synonyms, naming pictures). **B,** Areas with increased blood flow as the same subject judged whether a series of lines had been bisected accurately. (*From Jansen A et al: Neuroimage 33:204, 2006.*)

(see Fig. 22-29B); after callosal section, a right-handed patient is likely to be able to draw and copy better with the left hand than with the right hand. Problems are solved in a more comprehensive, holistic fashion by the right hemisphere. As noted previously, the right hemisphere also has some capacity for comprehension of language. The corpus callosum ordinarily welds the two hemispheres together into a unitary consciousness. After section of the corpus callosum, individuals develop close cooperation between their two hemispheres and subtle methods of cross-cueing, but each hemisphere still appears to have separate conscious experiences, creating a knotty philosophical problem.[i]

These same studies of split-brain patients also indicate that there is probably somewhat more bilaterality in the connections of somatic sensory and motor pathways than is commonly acknowledged. With time and practice, each hemisphere acquires not only a great deal of control over ipsilateral proximal muscles but also considerable awareness of stimuli applied to the ipsilateral side of the body.

Disconnection Syndromes Can Result From White Matter Damage

It stands to reason that we could not reach out for a seen object unless visual information could somehow influence the activity of motor cortex. This has been corroborated experimentally in monkeys: cuts in the parietal lobe that destroy the long association bundles connecting the frontal and occipital lobes interfere with the ability to carry out movements guided by vision in the contralateral visual field. **Disconnection syndromes** that are similar in principle have been proposed (and in some cases shown fairly convincingly) to account for some of the complex disorders that follow cerebral damage in humans.

The classic example of a disconnection syndrome is **pure word blindness,** or **alexia without agraphia.** Patients with this rare condition are able to write (thus no agraphia) but are unable to read (alexia)—even words they have just finished writing; they almost always have a right homonymous hemianopia as well. Alexia without agraphia occasionally follows a stroke that involves the left posterior cerebral artery, if it causes destruction of the left visual cortex (hence the hemianopia) and the splenium of the corpus callosum (Fig. 22-30). As a result, the language areas of the left hemisphere are cut off from all visual input; the destroyed left visual cortex can supply no input, and the intact right visual cortex can supply none because the route through the corpus callosum is blocked. Because the language areas themselves are undamaged and still connected to motor cortex, comprehension of verbal language and produc-

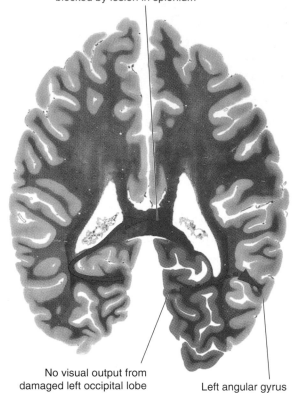

Visual output from right occipital cortex blocked by lesion in splenium

No visual output from damaged left occipital lobe

Left angular gyrus

Figure 22-30 Diagram of a lesion that would cause pure word blindness (alexia without agraphia). Destruction of the left visual cortex prevents information from the right visual field from reaching language areas of the left hemisphere, such as the left angular gyrus. Destruction of the splenium of the corpus callosum prevents information from the left visual fields from reaching the language areas because the route from the right visual cortex to the left hemisphere is blocked. The language areas themselves are undamaged, so the production of language and the comprehension of speech are intact.

tion of both verbal and written language are relatively unaffected.

Several other disconnection syndromes have been proposed or demonstrated, and the concept is valuable in terms of understanding some disorders of higher cerebral function. Callosal section represents an ultimate example. Conduction aphasia, in which Broca's and Wernicke's areas seem disconnected from each other, was once thought to be another example (although it now seems that damage to cortex, and not just to the arcuate fasciculus, is required to produce this syndrome). Disconnections of language areas from different sensory areas or from motor cortex have been invoked to explain some cases of agnosia or apraxia.

Consciousness and Sleep Are Active Processes

The various perceptual and cognitive processes described so far in this chapter generally operate on a

---

[i]"Everything we have seen so far indicates that the surgery has left these people with two separate minds, that is, two separate spheres of consciousness. What is experienced in the right hemisphere seems to be entirely outside the realm of awareness of the left hemisphere. This mental division has been demonstrated in regard to perception, cognition, volition, learning, and memory. One of the hemispheres, the left, dominant or major hemisphere, has speech and is normally talkative and conversant. The other, the minor hemisphere, however, is mute or dumb, being able to express itself only through nonverbal reactions." (Sperry RW: In Eccles JC, editor: Brain and conscious experience, New York, 1966, Springer-Verlag.) Not everyone agrees with Sperry's conclusion.

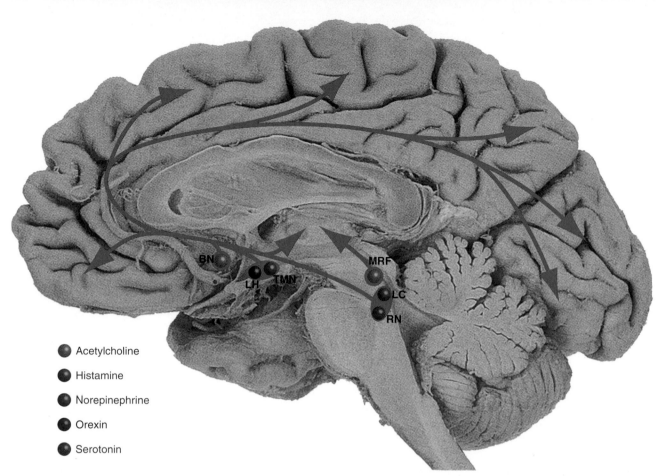

Figure 22-31 Major components of the subcortical modulatory network that, together with the cerebral cortex, maintains consciousness and regulates its level. Cholinergic innervation of the thalamus comes mostly from the midbrain reticular formation (MRF), and that of the cortex comes mostly from the basal nucleus (of Meynert; BN); other parts of the network typically project to both thalamus and cortex. LC, locus ceruleus; LH, lateral hypothalamus; RN, raphe nuclei; TMN, tuberomammillary nucleus (so named because it sits between the tuberal hypothalamus and the mammillary body; see Chapter 23).

background of **consciousness.** Although no universally accepted definition of consciousness exists, we all have an intuitive understanding of what it means—roughly, a state of self-awareness in which it is possible to direct attention and manipulate abstract ideas. Consciousness has both a **content** and a **level.** The content varies from moment to moment, reflecting the activity and interactions of different cortical areas. The level of consciousness also varies from moment to moment (e.g., alert, drowsy), but consciousness itself does not "reside" as a single entity in any particular part of the brain. Rather, it arises somehow from interactions among many neural structures. Remarkably large cortical areas can be destroyed without abolishing consciousness, and no single cortical area is crucial for maintaining it. Not even a fully intact cerebral cortex, all by itself, is conscious. Maintenance of normal cortical function depends on modulatory inputs from a network of subcortical nuclei (Fig. 22-31). These include the brainstem reticular activating system (see Chapter 11; cholinergic and other projections from the reticular formation,

noradrenergic projections from the locus ceruleus, and serotonergic projections from the raphe nuclei), cholinergic projections from the basal nucleus, and some unique projections from the hypothalamus. The last include histaminergic neurons near the mammillary body and neurons in the lateral hypothalamus that secrete two closely related neuropeptides called **orexins** (hypocretins).[j] Some parts of this network depolarize thalamic neurons, shifting them toward a tonic mode (see Fig. 16-15) in which they are able to transmit information accurately to the cerebral cortex. Others project directly to widespread cortical areas; most do both.

---

[j]In 1998 two different groups of investigators described the same pair of neuropeptides. One group (Cell 92:573, 1998) named them *orexins,* from the Greek word for "appetite," because they are found in a region of the hypothalamus related to feeding behavior. The second group (Proc Natl Acad Sci U S A 95:322, 1998) named them *hypocretins,* because they are produced by hypothalamic neurons and have a structural resemblance to the gut hormone secretin. Both terms are still in use.

(This does not imply that consciousness resides in this subcortical network either; your car will not run without a battery, but when it is running, the battery is not the source of power.)

Pathological loss of consciousness requires bilateral damage, either to extensive areas of cortex or white matter or to extensive parts of the modulatory network. Because major parts of the modulatory network either originate in or traverse the midbrain reticular formation, bilateral destruction of this area causes **coma,** a state of unconsciousness from which a patient cannot be aroused. Similarly, bilateral diencephalic damage can cause coma, as can extensive bilateral cerebral damage (e.g., from toxicity or metabolic derangements). Unilateral damage, no matter how extensive, does not cause coma. Coma generally has a poor prognosis that varies with the age of the patient and the cause of the coma, but it rarely lasts more than a week or two. In that period it may evolve to a **vegetative state,** in which brainstem functions are more or less intact, some aspects of sleep-wake cycles (see later) return, but the patient shows no signs of meaningful interaction with the environment. Vegetative states can persist for years with medical support and are fraught with ethical dilemmas.

Sleep, in contrast, is a normally occurring state of unconsciousness from which we can be aroused. Mammals, birds, and reptiles all spend regular parts of the day or night asleep, and most other species have regular periods of reduced activity that may be comparable to sleep. Despite this near universality, the overall, one main function of sleep is still largely unknown. It looks like a restful state, but the amount of energy saved during a night's sleep is minimal. Sleep plays some role in learning and memory, but seemingly not enough to justify the large amount of valuable time we spend at it. It was once thought that sleep is a passive process reflecting a decreased level of excitation of the subcortical modulatory network and a consequent "shutting down" of the cerebral cortex. However, it is now apparent that active mechanisms play a major role and that specific neural structures periodically induce sleep by systematically inhibiting parts of the network.

There Are Two Forms of Sleep

Our sleep is of two different kinds (Fig. 22-32). The first, called **non-REM** sleep, includes several stages in which the electroencephalogram (EEG) gets progressively slower and more synchronized. Non-REM sleep culminates in periods of **slow-wave sleep,** so named because the EEG is dominated by synchronous waves at various low frequencies, principally less than 4 Hz (**delta waves**). The slow waves arise as a result of interactions between cortical neurons and rhythmically bursting thalamic neurons (see Fig. 16-15). During slow-wave sleep, muscle tone is somewhat reduced, heart rate and breathing are

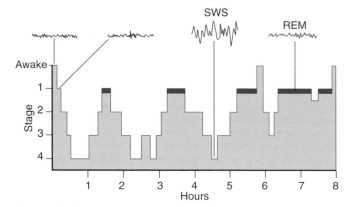

Figure 22-32 Typical sequence of sleep stages and EEG changes in a young adult. SWS, slow-wave sleep. *(Adapted from Nolte J: Elsevier's integrated neuroscience, Philadelphia, 2007, Mosby Elsevier.)*

Table 22-3	Major Characteristics of Non-REM and REM Sleep	
	Non-REM Sleep	**REM Sleep**
Other names	Synchronized Slow-wave (deeper stages)	Desynchronized Paradoxical
EEG	Large, slow, desynchronized (deeper stages)	Small, fast, synchronized
Muscle tone	Decreased	Almost abolished
Arousal threshold	Progressively higher	Highest
Mental activity	Vague dreams	Detailed, visual, emotional dreams
Autonomic activity	Increased parasympathetic Slow, regular pulse and respiration	Increased sympathetic Irregular pulse and respiration

slowed but steady, cerebral blood flow is somewhat reduced relative to wakefulness (Fig. 22-33A), and subjects awakened from this state seldom report long, elaborate dreams. Roughly every 90 to 120 minutes we shift into the second type of sleep, called **desynchronized sleep,** in which thalamic neurons are back in the tonic mode and the EEG is dominated by low-voltage, high-frequency activity that is not organized into obvious waves and is remarkably similar to the activity seen in the waking state. Despite the fact that the EEG looks like that of wakefulness, an individual is harder to awake from this stage than from slow-wave sleep; as a result, desynchronized sleep is also called **paradoxical sleep.** Desynchronized sleep is a very peculiar state, substantially different from non-REM sleep (Table 22-3), with several distinctive properties: there is a nearly complete abolition of muscle tone, and the transmission of impulses over at least some sensory pathways is greatly

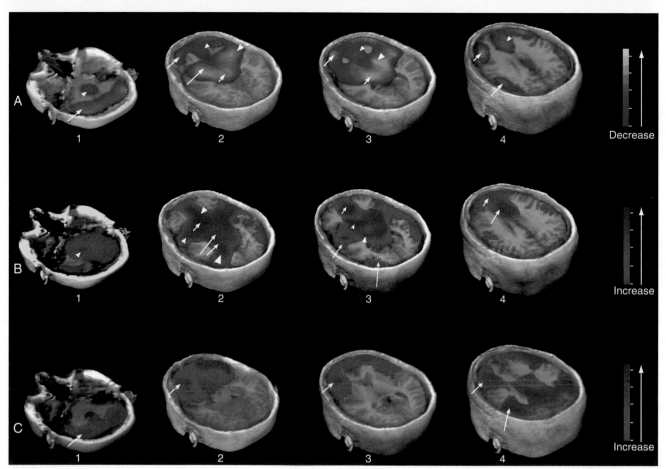

Figure 22-33 An amazing PET study in which changes in cerebral blood flow were followed in 37 healthy young men as they slept; sleep stages were monitored simultaneously. Data from all 37 subjects were averaged to produce a composite figure showing the regional differences in blood flow between wakefulness and slow-wave sleep **(A)**, slow-wave sleep and REM sleep **(B)**, and REM sleep and wakefulness **(C)**. **A,** Slow-wave sleep (vs. wakefulness) entails decreased blood flow in the reticular formation of the pons and midbrain (**1,** *arrowhead;* **2,** *short arrow*), thalamus (**3,** *short arrow*), limbic cortex in the insula (**2,** *large arrowhead*), orbital (**2,** *medium arrow* and *small arrowhead*) and cingulate (**3** and **4,** *small arrowheads*) gyri, dorsolateral prefrontal cortex (**3,** *medium arrow;* **4,** *short arrow*), and parietal multimodal cortex (**4,** *medium arrow*). Blood flow also decreases in the cerebellum (**1,** *arrow*) and basal ganglia (**2,** *long arrow;* **3,** *large arrowhead*). **B,** Moving from slow-wave sleep into REM sleep entails blood flow increases in the reticular formation of the pons and midbrain (**1,** *arrowhead;* **2,** *long arrow*), thalamus (**3,** *medium arrowhead*), limbic cortex in the insula (**2,** *small arrowhead*), and medial orbital (**2,** *medium arrowhead*), cingulate (**3,** *short arrow;* **4,** *medium arrow*), and parahippocampal (**2,** *medium arrow*) gyri. Blood flow also increases in visual (**2,** *large arrowhead;* **3,** *long arrow*) and auditory (**3,** *medium arrow*) association cortex, medial prefrontal cortex (**4,** *short arrow*), and basal nuclei (**2,** *short arrow;* **3,** *small arrowhead*). Notably, blood flow stays depressed in dorsolateral prefrontal and parietal multimodal cortex. **C,** Blood flow in many areas is at near waking levels during REM sleep. Wakefulness finally restores blood flow to dorsolateral prefrontal cortex (**3,** *arrow;* **4,** *medium arrow*), parietal multimodal cortex (**4,** *long arrow*), lateral orbital cortex (**2,** *arrow*), and the cerebellum (**1,** *arrow*). *(From Braun AR et al: Brain 120:1173, 1997.)*

decreased; blood pressure rises a little, and heart rate and breathing become erratic; we become reptile-like, in the sense that hypothalamic regulation of body temperature ceases. Superimposed on this background are coincident phasic events. There are bursts of inhibition of motor mechanisms, so the last vestige of tone in most muscles is eliminated for brief periods. Some twitching movements manage to break through the inhibition, most prominently bursts of rapid eye movements (REMs). The latter phenomenon gives rise to the most common name for desynchronized sleep, which is **REM sleep.** Subjects awakened from REM sleep are likely to report that they were having visually detailed, often emotionally charged dreams. By most measures, large

areas of the cerebral cortex are in an awake state during REM sleep, but because of the blockade of sensory pathways, their activity is generated internally; blood flow to multimodal areas remains reduced (Fig. 22-33B), lending credibility to dream events that would seem bizarre during wakefulness.

Both Brainstem and Forebrain Mechanisms Regulate Sleep-Wake Transitions

Most aspects of the anatomical substrates of sleep and wakefulness were first worked out in experimental animals, and lesions in the reticular formation at different longitudinal levels figured prominently in these early investigations. Damage to the reticular formation of the rostral midbrain results in a continuously synchronized EEG similar to that of slow-wave sleep, at least in the acute stages after the operation. This fits with the scheme in Figure 22-31, because it destroys some parts of the reticular activating system and disconnects the remainder from the cerebrum. Not surprisingly, damage below the rostral medulla has little effect on sleep-wake cycles, because the reticular activating system remains intact and connected. An initially surprising observation was that after midpontine damage an animal shows signs of constant wakefulness rostral to the lesion, at least during the acute stages after the operation. This indicates not only that the parts of the reticular activating system crucial for wakefulness are contained in the midbrain and rostral pons but also that parts of the medullary and caudal pontine reticular formation have a role in periodically turning the reticular activating system off and on.

There is more to the story, however. The role of hypothalamic parts of the modulatory network were first described during World War I, when von Economo noted that encephalitic damage to the posterior hypothalamus was associated with the hypersomnia of sleeping sickness (encephalitis lethargica), as though the posterior hypothalamus is a wakefulness-promoting region. He also noted that less common encephalitic damage to the anterior hypothalamus was associated with insomnia. More recent work has established the locations of the neurons responsible, their chemical identities, and an initial understanding of how the hypothalamic and brainstem parts of the network are coordinated. Orexin neurons have excitatory connections with all the other parts of the wakefulness-promoting network and may be particularly important in coordinating network activity during wakefulness. The widespread excitatory projections of histaminergic neurons are also important (hence the drowsiness caused by many antihistamines). Finally, the cholinergic projections from the basal nucleus to the cerebral cortex also promote arousal and wakefulness. Conversely, neurons in the most anterior part of the hypothalamus (the **preoptic area**; see Chapter 23) send inhibitory projections to most or all parts of the wakefulness-promoting network (Fig. 22-34). How these projections interact with those from the caudal brainstem is not fully known, but the preoptic projections probably play the major role in intact nervous systems. Continued activity of the hypothalamic centers is probably responsible in some cases for the evolution of coma into a vegetative state: about 10 to 15 days after damage to the mesencephalic reticular formation in experimental animals, the forebrain once again begins to cycle through the synchronized and desynchronized EEGs of sleep and wakefulness.

Sleep is a periodic process, influenced by both the time of day and recent sleep history. Humans sleep at night for about 7 to 8 hours, but we sleep sooner and

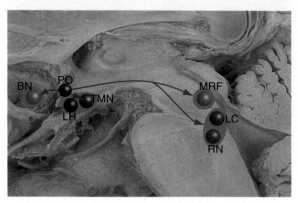

Figure 22-34 Inhibition of the wakefulness-promoting network by projections from the preoptic area (PO). Projections from the medullary reticular formation (not shown) also inhibit parts of the network. BN, basal nucleus (of Meynert); LC, locus ceruleus; LH, lateral hypothalamus; MRF, midbrain reticular formation; RN, raphe nuclei; TMN, tuberomammillary nucleus.

longer after losing sleep the night before. The basic periodicity comes from a biological clock in the hypothalamus (see Fig. 23-5). The need to make up for lost sleep arises in part from the accumulation of various substances in the brain during wakefulness. Adenosine is a prominent example, building up in CNS extracellular spaces as the day wears on and inhibiting parts of the modulatory network (particularly the cholinergic parts). Caffeine, used around the world in various forms to combat sleepiness, works in part by blocking adenosine receptors at these sites. Likewise, melatonin secreted from the pineal gland as a hormone builds up toward the evening and acts at melatonin receptors on the superchiasmatic nucleus of the hypothalamus, resulting in an overall decrease in "awake machinery" of the hypothalamus.

Control Circuits for REM Sleep Are Located in the Brainstem

The basic anatomical control mechanisms for REM sleep are more localized than those for slow-wave sleep and are entirely contained in the brainstem. Once non-REM sleep has begun, neurons in the pontine reticular formation become active periodically, causing neurons in the locus ceruleus and raphe nuclei to cease firing entirely and midbrain cholinergic neurons to fire faster (Table 22-4). The cholinergic neurons in turn project to the thalamus and other parts of the brainstem, initiating an episode of REM sleep (Fig. 22-35). Thalamic neurons return to tonic mode, and the EEG becomes desynchronized. Various parts of the brainstem are responsible for other components; reticular neurons near the locus ceruleus, for example, cause inhibition of lower motor neurons and the loss of muscle tone. Cats with bilateral damage just ventral to the locus ceruleus have REM sleep without atonia and appear to "act out" their dreams.

Table 22-4	Firing Patterns of Modulatory Neurons During Non-REM and REM Sleep				
Nucleus	**Transmitter**	**Wakefulness**	**Non-REM Sleep**	**REM Sleep**
Preoptic area	GABA	−	++	++
Lateral hypothalamus	Orexin	++	+	−*
Tuberomammillary nucleus†	Histamine	++	+	−
Raphe nuclei	Serotonin	++	+	−*
Locus ceruleus	Norepinephrine	++	+	−*
Midbrain reticular formation	Acetylcholine	++	−	++

GABA. γ-aminobutyric acid.
*These neurons resume firing shortly before the end of each REM sleep episode and are thought to have a role in terminating the episode.
†See Chapter 23.

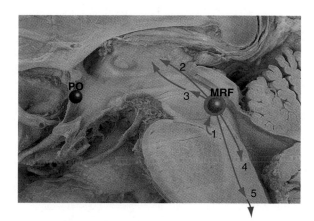

Figure 22-35 Control circuitry for REM sleep. Excitatory (probably glutamate) projections from the pontine reticular formation (1) activate cholinergic neurons in the midbrain reticular formation (MRF). These in turn depolarize thalamic neurons either directly (2) or indirectly (3) and also project to eye movement control centers (4) and inhibitory reticulospinal neurons (5). PO, preoptic area of the hypothalamus.

Activity of noradrenergic and serotonergic neurons helps keep the REM machinery suppressed during wakefulness. Multiple mechanisms contribute to turning it on and off periodically once sleep has begun, and in some conditions, components of REM sleep may either appear at inappropriate times or not appear when they should. **Narcolepsy** is a disorder characterized by intrusions of elements of REM sleep into periods of wakefulness. Patients have irresistible urges to sleep for brief periods during the day and almost immediately enter into REM sleep. Even when awake and alert, they may have sudden, brief losses of muscle tone (**cataplexy**), particularly during emotionally charged situations. As they fall asleep at night, narcoleptic patients may have episodes of paralysis or hallucinations while still awake. Conversely, patients (usually older men) with **REM sleep behavioral disorder** flail about in a coordinated way during REM sleep, in a manner consistent with the activities in their dreams. A large majority of narcoleptic patients have drastically depleted populations of orexin neurons, providing an indication that the hypothalamus plays an important role in the control of REM episodes.

SUGGESTED READINGS

Aboitiz F, et al: Fiber composition of the human corpus callosum. Brain Res 598:143, 1992.

Adamantidis AR, et al: Neural substrates of awakening probed with optogenetic control of hypocretin neurons. Nature 450:420, 2007.
Unbelievably cool experiments in which mice were genetically engineered to express a bacterial rhodopsin in their orexin neurons. Light delivered to the hypothalamus while they slept made them wake up.

Aglioti SM, et al: Taste laterality in the split brain. Eur J Neurosci 13:195, 2001.

Ahern GL, et al: Right hemisphere advantage for evaluating emotional facial expressions. Cortex 27:193, 1991.

Alvarez VA, Sabatini BL: Anatomical and physiological plasticity of dendritic spines. Annu Rev Neurosci 30:79, 2007.

Basheer R, et al: Adenosine and sleep-wake regulation. Prog Neurobiol 73:379, 2004.

Bates E, et al: Voxel-based lesion-symptom mapping. Nat Neurosci 6:448, 2003.

Bechara A, et al: Dissociation of working memory from decision making within the human prefrontal cortex. J Neurosci 18:428, 1998.
Differing effects of dorsolateral and ventromedial prefrontal damage.

Bernat JL: Chronic disorders of consciousness. Lancet 367:1181, 2006.

Bogousslavsky J: Frontal stroke syndromes. Eur Neurol 34:306, 1994.

Braun AR, et al: Regional cerebral blood flow throughout the sleep-wake cycle: an H₂¹⁵O PET study. Brain 120:1173, 1997.

Brodmann K: Brodmann's: localisation in the cerebral cortex, trans. Garey LJ, New York, 2006, Springer.
An annotated translation of the original work.

Catani M, Ffyttche DH: The rises and falls of disconnection syndromes. Brain 128:2224, 2005.

Catani M, et al: Occipito-temporal connections in the human brain. Brain 126:2093, 2003.

Catania KC, Kaas JH: Somatosensory fovea in the star-nosed mole: behavioral use of the star in relation to innervation patterns and cortical representation. J Comp Neurol 387:215, 1997.

Clarke S, et al: Auditory agnosia and auditory spatial deficits following left hemispheric lesions: evidence for distinct processing pathways. Neuropsychologia 38:797, 2000.

Creutzfeldt OD: Cortex cerebri: performance, structural and functional organization of the cortex, New York, 1995, Oxford University Press.

Critchley M: The parietal lobes, London, 1953, Edward Arnold, Ltd.
The classic clinical work on the various syndromes resulting from parietal lesions.

Damasio H, et al: The return of Phineas Gage: clues about the brain from the skull of a famous patient. Science 264:1102, 1994.

Datta S, MacLean RS: Neurobiological mechanisms for the regulation of mammalian sleep-wake behavior: reinterpretation of historical evidence and inclusion of contemporary cellular and molecular evidence. Neurosci Biobehav Rev 31:775, 2007.

Di Virgilio G, et al: Cortical regions contributing to the anterior commissure in man. Exp Brain Res 124:1, 1999.

Dougherty RF, et al: Visual field representations and locations of visual areas V1/2/3 in human visual cortex. J Vision 3:586, 2003.
Use of modern imaging techniques to study the variability in the sizes of visual areas.

Douglas R, Markram H, Martin K: Neocortex. In Shepherd GM, editor: The synaptic organization of the brain, ed 5, New York, 2004, Oxford University Press.

Downar J, et al: A multimodal cortical network for the detection of changes in the sensory environment. Nat Neurosci 3:277, 2000.
The right hemisphere is better at noticing changes in any modality.

Dronkers NF, et al: Paul Broca's historic cases: high resolution MR imaging of the brains of Leborgne and Lelong. Brain 130:1532, 2007.

Feinberg TE, Farah MJ, editors: Behavioral neurology and neuropsychology, ed 2, New York, 2003, McGraw-Hill.

Finger S: Paul Broca: cortical localization and cerebral dominance. In Minds behind the brain, New York, 2000, Oxford University Press.

Fletcher PC, Henson RNA: Frontal lobes and human memory: insights from functional imaging. Brain 124:849, 2001.

Foote SL, Morrison JH: Extrathalamic modulation of cortical function. Annu Rev Neurosci 10:67, 1987.

Frackowiak RSJ, et al: Human brain function, ed 2, San Diego, 2003, Academic Press.
A review of methods and findings from the ongoing revolution in functional brain imaging.

Galaburda AM, et al: Right-left asymmetries in the brain. Science 199:852, 1978.

Gazzaniga MS, editor: The cognitive neurosciences III, ed 3, Cambridge, Mass, 2004, MIT Press.

Geschwind N: Disconnexion syndromes in animals and man. I and II. Brain 88(237):585, 1965.
Scholarly and influential papers arguing forcefully for the concept of complex syndromes caused by disconnections of various cerebral areas from one another.

Gilbert SJ, et al: Functional specialization within rostral prefrontal cortex (area 10): a meta-analysis. J Cog Neurosci 18:932, 2006.

Gironell A, de la Calzada MD, Sagales T: Absence of REM sleep and unaltered non-REM sleep caused by a haematoma in the pontine tegmentum. J Neurol Neurosurg Psychiatry 59:195, 1995.

Goldman PS, Nauta WJH: Columnar distribution of corticocortical fibers in the frontal association, limbic, and motor cortex of the developing rhesus monkey. Brain Res 122:393, 1977.

Gordon HW, Bogen JE: Hemispheric lateralization of singing after intracarotid sodium amylobarbitone. J Neurol Neurosurg Psychiatry 37:727, 1974.

Graff-Radford NR, Welsh K, Godersky J: Callosal apraxia. Neurology 37:100, 1987.

Grefkes C, Fink GR: The functional organization of the intraparietal sulcus in humans and monkeys. J Anat 207:3, 2005.

Gücer G: The effect of sleep upon the transmission of afferent activity in the somatic afferent system. Exp Brain Res 34:287, 1979.

Haaxma R, Kuypers HGJM: Intrahemispheric cortical connexions and visual guidance of hand and finger movements in the rhesus monkey. Brain 98:239, 1975.
Direct experimental demonstration of a type of disconnection syndrome.

Hallett M: Transcranial magnetic stimulation and the human brain. Nature 406:147, 2000.

Harris IM, et al: Selective right parietal lobe activation during mental rotation: a parametric PET study. Brain 123:65, 2000.

Hendry SHC, Jones EG: Sizes and distributions of intrinsic neurons incorporating tritiated GABA in monkey sensory-motor cortex. J Neurosci 1:390, 1981.

Herkenham M: Laminar organization of thalamic projections to the rat neocortex. Science 207:532, 1980.

Hillis AE: Aphasia: progress in the last quarter of a century. Neurology 69:200, 2007.

Hillis AE, et al: Anatomy of spatial attention: insights from perfusion imaging and hemispatial neglect in acute stroke. J Neurosci 24:3161, 2005.

Hofer S, Frahm J: Topography of the human corpus callosum revisited—comprehensive fiber tractography using diffusion tensor magnetic resonance imaging. Neuroimage 32:989, 2006.

Iannetti GD, Mouraux A: From the neuromatrix to the pain matrix (and back). Exp Brain Res 205:1–12, 2010.

Irwin SA, et al: Dendritic spine structural anomalies in fragile-x mental retardation syndrome. Cerebral Cortex 10:1038–1044, 2000.

Jansen A, et al: The assessment of hemispheric lateralization in functional MRI—robustness and reproducibility. Neuroimage 33:204, 2006.

Jensen K, Call J, Tomasello M: Chimpanzees are rational maximizers in an ultimatum game. Science 318:107, 2007.
In contrast to humans, chimps seem to take what they can get.

Jones EG, Coulter JD, Wise SP: Commissural columns in the sensory-motor cortex of monkeys. J Comp Neurol 188:113, 1979.

Jones EG, Powell TPS: An anatomical study of converging sensory pathways within the cerebral cortex of the monkey. Brain 93:793, 1970.
A study of the stepwise radiations of auditory, visual, and somatosensory information from the primary receiving areas to parts of the association cortex—done by the straightforward but clever technique of lesioning a primary area, tracing the degenerating fibers, and making lesions where the degeneration terminates.

Jouandet ML, Gazzaniga MS: Cortical field of origin of the anterior commissure of the rhesus monkey. Exp Neurol 66:381, 1979.

Kaas JH: The organization of callosal connections in primates. In Reeves AG, Roberts DW, editors: Epilepsy and the corpus callosum II, New York, 1995, Plenum Press.

Karnath H-O, Ferber S, Himmelbach M: Spatial awareness is a function of the temporal not the posterior parietal lobe. Nature 411:950, 2001.
Computed tomography studies of a series of patients indicating that, contrary to a century of neurological dogma, the critical area damaged in at least some patients with left-sided neglect may be the right superior temporal gyrus and not the right inferior parietal lobule.

Kell CA, et al: The sensory cortical representation of the human penis: revisiting somatotopy in the male homunculus. J Neurosci 25:5984, 2005.
The location of the genitals in the classic homunculus (Fig. 3-30) always seemed odd. This functional imaging study used electric toothbrushes and fMRI to demonstrate a more logical location.

Kenshalo DR, Jr, Isensee O: Responses of primate SI cortical neurons to noxious stimuli. J Neurophysiol 50:1479, 1983.

Kitada R, et al: Multisensory activation of the intraparietal area when classifying grating orientation: a functional magnetic resonance imaging study. J Neurosci 26:7491, 2006.

Kleinman JT, et al: Right hemispatial neglect: frequency and characterization following acute left hemisphere stroke. Brain Cog 64:50, 2007.

Knoch D, et al: Diminishing reciprocal fairness by disrupting the right prefrontal cortex. Science 314:829, 2006.

Kryger MH, Roth T, Dement WC, editors: Principles and practice of sleep medicine, ed 4, Philadelphia, 2005, WB Saunders.

Land EH, et al: Colour-generating interactions across the corpus callosum. Nature 303:616, 1983.

Clever experiments showing that if the contrast comparisons needed to make decisions about color involve areas that span the vertical midline, the corpus callosum gets into the act.

LaPierre D, Braun CMJ, Hodgkins S: Ventral frontal deficits in psychopathy: neuropsychological test findings. Neuropsychology 33:139, 1995.

Lau HC, Passingham RE: Unconscious activation of the cognitive control system in the human prefrontal cortex. J Neurosci 27:5805, 2007.

"These results suggest that the cognitive control system in the prefrontal cortex is not exclusively driven by conscious information, as has been believed previously.".

LeDoux JE, Wilson DH, Gazzaniga MS: A divided mind: observations on the conscious properties of the separated hemispheres. Ann Neurol 2:417, 1977.

An individual with some bilateral language representation may not give the same responses with each hemisphere after section of the corpus callosum.

Lhermitte F: Human autonomy and the frontal lobes. II. Patient behavior in complex and social situations: the "environmental dependency syndrome. Ann Neurol 19:335, 1986.

Quantitative measurement of the effects of prefrontal damage is difficult, but simple observation provides fascinating insights.

Libet B, et al: Subjective referral of the timing for a conscious sensory experience: a functional role for the somatosensory specific projection system in man. Brain 102:193, 1979.

How do we decide when a tactile stimulus occurs? Is it at the instant of physical contact, when the first electrical activity reaches the postcentral gyrus, or after this activity has rattled around the cortex for a while? A fascinating and provocative paper that addresses this question experimentally.

Mahowald MW, Schenck CH: Dissociated states of wakefulness and sleep. Neurology 42(Suppl 6):44, 1992.

An early description of syndromes in which fragments of sleep or wakefulness intrude on each other.

Makris N, et al: The occipitofrontal fascicle in humans: a quantitative, in vivo, DT-MRI study. Neuroimage 37:1100, 2007.

McCormick DA, Bal T: Sleep and arousal: thalamocortical mechanisms. Annu Rev Neurosci 20:185, 1997.

Mesulam M-M: Cholinergic pathways and the ascending reticular activating system of the human brain. Ann N Y Acad Sci 757:169, 1995.

Mesulam M-M, editor: Principles of behavioral and cognitive neurology, ed 2, New York, 2000, Oxford University Press.

Miller BL, Cummings JL, editors: The human frontal lobes: functions and disorders, ed 2, New York, 2007, Guilford Press.

Mori S, et al: MRI atlas of human white matter, Amsterdam, 2005, Elsevier.

Mountcastle VB: The columnar organization of the neocortex. Brain 120:701, 1997.

Mukhametov LM: Sleep in marine mammals. Exp Brain Res Suppl 8:227, 1984.

Porpoises have evolved the novel technique of sleeping with one hemisphere at a time.

Nauta WJH: The problem of the frontal lobe: a reinterpretation. J Psychiatr Res 8:167, 1971.

Nieuwenhuys R: The neocortex: an overview of its evolutionary development, structural organization and synaptology. Anat Embryol 190:307, 1994.

Northcutt RG, Kaas JH: The emergence and evolution of mammalian neocortex. Trends Neurosci 18:373, 1995.

Ohno K, Sakurai T: Orexin neuronal circuitry: role in the regulation of sleep and wakefulness. Front Neuroendocrinol 29:70, 2008.

Ota H, et al: Dissociation of body-centered and stimulus-centered representations in unilateral neglect. Neurology 57:2064, 2001.

Owen AM, et al: Using functional magnetic resonance imaging to detect covert awareness in the vegetative state. Arch Neurol 64:1098, 2007.

The title well describes the scary prospects.

Pakkenberg B, Gundersen HJG: Neocortical neuron number in humans: effect of sex and age. J Comp Neurol 384:312, 1997.

Paul LK: Agenesis of the corpus callosum: genetic, developmental and functional aspects of connectivity. Nat Rev Neurosci 8:287, 2007.

Once thought to be very rare, this surprisingly common malformation offers insights into how the left and right hemispheres normally work together.

Penfield W, Rasmussen T: The cerebral cortex of man, New York, 1950, Macmillan.

A review of the results of cortical stimulation in a large series of patients and the results of localized cortical excisions from these patients.

Penfield W, Roberts L: Speech and brain-mechanisms, Princeton, NJ, 1959, Princeton University Press.

Posner JB, et al: Plum and Posner's diagnosis of stupor and coma, ed 4, New York, 2007, Oxford University Press.

An authoritative new edition of the classic reference in the field.

Powell TPS: Certain aspects of the intrinsic organization of the cerebral cortex. In Pompeiano O, Ajmone Marsan C, editors: Brain mechanisms and perceptual awareness, IBRO Monograph Series, vol 8, New York, 1981, Raven Press.

A nice review of the evidence concerning the uniform organization of cerebral cortex. Although some of the details may be inaccurate, the general concept appears to be correct.

Price BH, et al: The compartmental learning disabilities of early frontal lobe damage. Brain 113:1383, 1990.

An important paper about two patients who suffered extensive prefrontal damage at an early age, indicating that, "in comparison with other types of brain damage which disrupt cognitive development, frontal damage acquired early in life appears to provide the neurological substrate for a special type of learning disability in the realms of insight, foresight, social judgment, empathy, and complex reasoning.".

Price CJ: The anatomy of language: contributions from functional imaging. J Anat 197:335, 2000.

Purpura DP: Dendritic spine "dysgenesis" and mental retardation. Science 186:1126, 1974.

Rechtschaffen A, et al: Physiological correlates of prolonged sleep deprivation in rats. Science 221:182, 1983.

Reed CL, Caselli RJ, Farah MJ: Tactile agnosia: underlying impairment and implications for normal tactile object recognition. Brain 119:875, 1996.

Rolls ET, et al: Emotion-related learning in patients with social and emotional changes associated with frontal lobe damage. J Neurol Neurosurg Psychiatry 57:1518, 1994.

"Patients often reported verbally that the contingencies had changed, but were unable to alter their behaviour appropriately. These impairments occurred independently of IQ or verbal memory impairments.".

Ross ED, Monnot M: Neurology of affective prosody and its functional-anatomic organization in right hemisphere. Brain Lang 104:51, 2008.

Russell IS, Ochs S: Localization of a memory trace in one cortical hemisphere and transfer to the other hemisphere. Brain 86:37, 1963.

We know that inputs spread to both hemispheres under normal circumstances via the corpus callosum. This interesting paper describes what happens if one hemisphere is temporarily inactivated during the acquisition of a memory.

Sallanon M, et al: Long-lasting insomnia induced by preoptic neuron lesions and its transient reversal by muscimol injection into the posterior hypothalamus in the cat. Neuroscience 32:669, 1989.

Sanfey AG, et al: The neural basis of economic decision-making in the Ultimatum Game. Science 300:1755, 2003.

Saper CB, Scammell TE, Lu J: Hypothalamic regulation of sleep and circadian rhythms. Nature 437:1257, 2005.

Sauerland EK, Harper RM: The human tongue during sleep: electromyographic activity of the genioglossus muscle. Exp Neurol 51:160, 1976.

> If the muscles of your tongue follow the general pattern and become flaccid during REM sleep, why don't you get into trouble by inhaling it? Read this article and find out.

Scalaidhe SPÓ, Wilson FAW, Goldman-Rakic PS: Areal segregation of face-processing neurons in prefrontal cortex. Science 278:1135, 1997.

> Different prefrontal areas for different working memories.

Schmahmann JD, Pandya DN: Fiber pathways of the brain, New York, 2006, Oxford University Press.

> A beautifully illustrated, painstaking account of the cerebral white matter of primates.

Scott TR, et al: Gustatory responses in the frontal opercular cortex of the alert cynomolgus monkey. J Neurophysiol 56:876, 1986.

Shapiro CM, et al: Slow-wave sleep: a recovery period after exercise. Science 214:1253, 1981.

> An old hypothesis about sleep is that we do it as some sort of "restorative" process. Our sleep patterns do not change much after ordinary exercise, but they do after running a marathon.

Sherin JE, et al: Activation of ventrolateral preoptic neurons during sleep. Science 271:216, 1996.

Small DM, et al: Gustatory agnosia. Neurology 64:311, 2005.

Sperry RW: Lateral specialization in the surgically separated hemispheres. In Schmitt FO, Worden FG, editors: The neurosciences: third study program, Cambridge, Mass, 1974, MIT Press.

> A general review of results from humans with a sectioned corpus callosum by the principal figure in this type of research.

Steriade M, McCarley RW: Brain control of wakefulness and sleep, ed 2, New York, 2005, Springer.

Stewart L, et al: Music and the brain: disorders of musical listening. Brain 129:2533, 2006.

Sweet RA, Dorph-Petersen K-A, Lewis DA: Mapping auditory core, lateral belt, and parabelt cortices in the human superior temporal gyrus. J Comp Neurol 491:270, 2005.

Szentagothai J: The neuron network of the cerebral cortex: a functional interpretation. Proc R Soc Lond B 201:219, 1978.

Talbot JD, et al: Multiple representations of pain in human cerebral cortex. Science 251:1355, 1991.

> PET scanning studies indicating that the perception of pain is accompanied by increased blood flow at least in the contralateral S1, S2, and cingulate gyrus.

Tang Y, Nyengaard JR: A stereological method for estimating the total length and size of myelin fibers in human brain white matter. J Neurosci Methods 73:193, 1997.

Teuber HL: The brain and human behavior. In Held R, Leibowitz HW, Teuber HL, editors: Handbook of sensory physiology, vol 8, Perception, New York, 1978, Springer-Verlag.

> An interesting, scholarly, wide-ranging correlation of deficits and brain damage in humans and experimental animals.

Thomson AM, Bannister AP: Interlaminar connections in the neocortex. Cereb Cortex 13:5, 2003.

Trampe R, et al: Do the congenitally blind have a stria of Gennari? First intracortical insights in vivo. Cerebral Cortex 21:2075–2081, 2011.

Treede R-D, et al: Cortical representation of pain: functional characterization of nociceptive areas near the lateral sulcus. Pain 87:113, 2000.

Triarhou LC: The percipient observations of Constantin von Economo on encephalitis lethargica and sleep disruption and their lasting impact on contemporary sleep research. Brain Res Bull 69:244, 2006.

Van den Pol AN: Narcolepsy: a neurodegenerative disease of the hypocretin system? Neuron 27:415, 2000.

Villablanca J: Behavioral and polygraphic study of "sleep" and "wakefulness" in chronic decerebrate cats. Electroencephalogr Clin Neurophysiol 21:562, 1966.

> In the chronic state after a rostral mesencephalic transection, the portions of the CNS both rostral and caudal to the transection are capable of some manifestations of sleep and wakefulness; amazingly enough, they do so with completely independent rhythms.

Wada J, Rasmussen T: Intracarotid injection of sodium Amytal for the lateralization of cerebral speech dominance: experimental and clinical observations. J Neurosurg 17:266, 1960.

Wada JA, Davis AE: Fundamental nature of human infant's brain asymmetry. Can J Neurol Sci 4:203, 1977.

> We are born not only with built-in anatomical asymmetries but also, apparently, with built-in physiological asymmetries.

Watanabe M: Reward expectancy in primate prefrontal neurons. Nature 382:629, 1996.

Watson RT, et al: Normal tactile threshold in monkeys with neglect. Neurology 34:917, 1984.

Weyand TG, Boudreaux M, Guido W: Burst and tonic modes in thalamic neurons during sleep and wakefulness. J Neurophysiol 85:1107, 2001.

Woolsey TA, van der Loos H: The structural organization of layer IV in the somatosensory region (SI) of mouse cerebral cortex: the description of a cortical field composed of discrete cytoarchitectonic units. Brain Res 17:205, 1970.

> A special kind of columnar organization described in a delightful paper.

Yamadori A, et al: Preservation of singing in Broca's aphasia. J Neurol Neurosurg Psychiatry 40:221, 1977.

Zarei M, et al: Functional anatomy of interhemispheric cortical connections in the human brain. J Anat 209:311, 2006.

Zhang HQ, et al: Parallel processing in cerebral cortex of the marmoset monkey: effect of reversible SI inactivation on tactile responses. J Neurophysiol 76:3633, 1996.

Drives and Emotions: The Hypothalamus and Limbic System

We seldom perceive things in a completely neutral fashion. Various sights and sounds make us happy, sad, or angry; some tastes and smells are extremely gratifying, others disgusting. Such feelings engendered by sensory inputs are ultimately the result of brains wired to promote survival and reproduction, and they are variable depending on current physiological needs and the social situation. Food, for example, becomes more attractive when one is hungry and less attractive when it is overpriced. Hence, any anatomical substrate for feelings and emotions needs to include at least some neocortical areas as the basis for conscious awareness of them. The same system would also need to be heavily interconnected with the hypothalamus, because sensory inputs that arouse an emotion also initiate autonomic responses such as salivating and gearing up the alimentary tract, or pumping adrenaline and diverting blood to skeletal muscles.

The **limbic system** is the name given to the portions of the brain primarily concerned with such responses and behaviors. As discussed in some detail later in this chapter and in the next one, it includes the **cingulate** and **parahippocampal gyri** (see Fig. 3-13), the **amygdala,** and the **hippocampus.** In view of the preceding

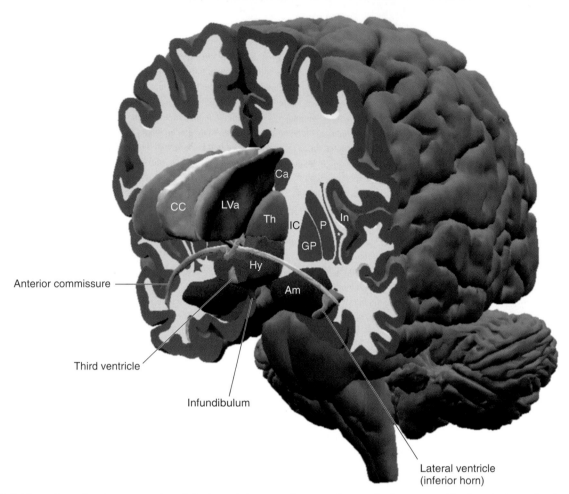

Figure 23-1 Three-dimensional reconstruction of the hypothalamus and surrounding cerebral structures. The hypothalamus has been rendered with a flat anterior surface because the preoptic area (see Fig. 23-4), which envelops the anterior end of the third ventricle but is in front of the plane sometimes used to separate the diencephalon and telencephalon, was not included. *, claustrum; Am, amygdala; Ca, caudate nucleus; CC, corpus callosum; GP, globus pallidus; Hy, hypothalamus; IC, internal capsule; In, insula; LVa, anterior horn of the lateral ventricle; P, putamen; Th, thalamus.

discussion, it is not surprising that the components of the limbic system appeared early in vertebrate phylogeny and that, in terms of its connections, the limbic system is interposed between the hypothalamus and the neocortex. That is, limbic structures serve as bridges between autonomic and voluntary responses to changes in the environment. Our response to a chilly room provides a simple example. There are autonomic responses to the chill, coordinated by the hypothalamus, such as cutaneous vasoconstriction and shivering. We also become consciously aware of the chill and may choose to put on more clothes or throw another log on the fire.

The Hypothalamus Coordinates Drive-Related Behaviors

The hypothalamus (Fig. 23-1) is a small portion of the diencephalon (weighing only about 4 g), but it is important as a nodal point in pathways concerned with autonomic, endocrine, emotional, and somatic functions

(Fig. 23-2)[a] that are generally designed to maintain our internal environment in a physiological range (i.e., to promote homeostasis). For example, stimulation of appropriate hypothalamic areas in experimental animals can cause vasodilation, feeding behavior, or alterations of pituitary function. Its functions extend beyond this, however, into more complex interactions involved in drives and emotional behaviors; stimulation of overlapping hypothalamic areas can elicit responses such as rage, sleep, or sexual behavior. Participation in these multiple functions is based on a widespread set of

---

[a]Although it often appears in diagrams such as Figure 23-2 that the hypothalamus-autonomic-pituitary system works in a realm separate and distinct from that controlling skeletal muscle, this is not the case. We have only one nervous system, and its parts work in a coordinated way to achieve desired outcomes. A simple set of examples is provided by the great variety of afferent and efferent limbs in reflexes that include autonomic fibers: light causes parasympathetic pupillary responses, a sudden loud noise is likely to cause sympathetic responses, cold causes shivering, and so on.

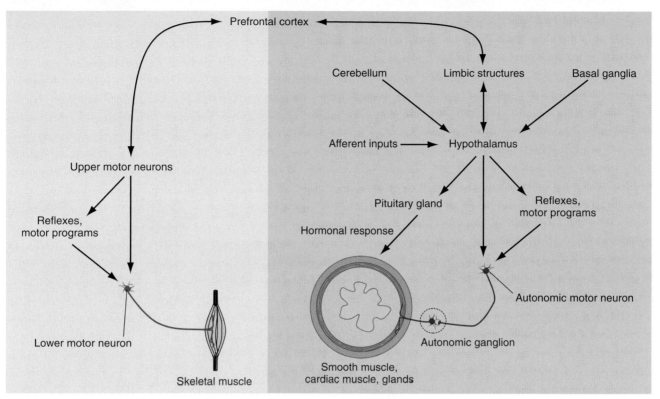

Figure 23-2 Overview of the pivotal role of the hypothalamus in drive-related activities. The hypothalamus can affect autonomic motor neurons both directly and through visceral motor programs in the brainstem and spinal cord, and it can influence visceral structures through its control over the pituitary gland (see Fig. 23-10). It can also stimulate somatic responses through connections with limbic structures that interconnect the hypothalamus and neocortex. The latter are two-way connections, providing us with a degree of voluntary control over responses that may be physiologically desirable but do not fit the current circumstances in some other way (e.g., "grin and bear it"). The cerebellum and basal ganglia also have connections with the hypothalamus, but their roles in the planning and coordination of drive-related activities are still poorly understood and are not discussed in this chapter.

connections that fall into three principal categories: (1) interconnections with various components of the limbic system, (2) outputs that influence the pituitary gland, and (3) interconnections with various visceral and somatic nuclei, both motor and sensory, of the brainstem and spinal cord. The hypothalamus is divided into a number of nuclei and areas, as described shortly. Each of these different nuclei and areas has more or less distinctive connections, but for the sake of simplicity, most of these connections are discussed here as though the hypothalamus were by and large a uniform structure.

The Hypothalamus Can Be Subdivided in Both Longitudinal and Medial-Lateral Directions

The inferior surface of the hypothalamus (see Figs. 3-16 and 3-17), exposed directly to subarachnoid space, is bounded by the optic chiasm, the optic tracts, and the posterior edge of the mammillary bodies. This area, exclusive of the mammillary bodies, is called the **tuber cinereum** (Latin for "gray swelling"; Fig. 23-3A). The **median eminence** protrudes ventrally from the surface of the tuber cinereum and is continuous with the

infundibular stalk, which in turn is continuous with the **posterior lobe of the pituitary.** The infundibular stalk and posterior lobe together constitute the **neurohypophysis.**

The medial surface of the hypothalamus (see Fig. 23-3B) extends anteriorly to the lamina terminalis, superiorly to the hypothalamic sulcus, and posteriorly to the caudal edge of the diencephalon. As in the case of the brainstem, transverse planes are sometimes used to define the anterior and posterior boundaries—in this case, a plane passing through the posterior commissure and the posterior edge of the mammillary bodies, and another passing through the anterior edge of the optic chiasm and the posterior edge of the anterior commissure. Also as in the case of the brainstem, however, functionally related neural tissue continues through both these planes. For example, the neural tissue immediately in front of the anterior plane is structurally and functionally continuous with the hypothalamus (see Fig. 23-3B and C). Therefore this region, the **preoptic area,** is treated instead as part of the anterior hypothalamus.

The hypothalamus can be subdivided from front to back into **anterior, tuberal,** and **posterior** regions. The

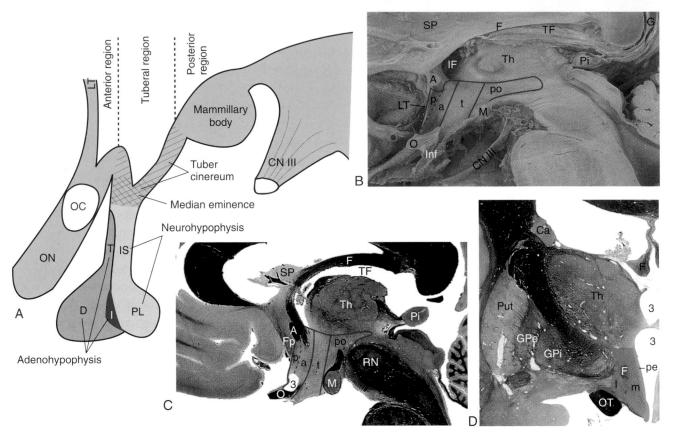

Figure 23-3 **A,** Regions of the hypothalamus and pituitary in midsagittal view. The entire area filled with diagonal lines is the tuber cinereum. The crosshatched portion of the tuber cinereum is the median eminence. **B,** The medial surface of the hypothalamus. **C,** Myelin-stained parasagittal section of the diencephalon, near the midline. **D,** Myelin-stained coronal section of the diencephalon and basal ganglia, showing the medial-lateral subdivision of the hypothalamus. The dashed red lines in **B** and **C** indicate the transverse plane sometimes used as the diencephalon-telencephalon boundary; the area between this plane and the lamina terminalis (the preoptic area) is considered here to be part of the hypothalamus. 3, third ventricle (optic recess in **C**); A, anterior commissure; a, p, po, and t, anterior, preoptic, posterior, and tuberal regions of the hypothalamus; Ca, caudate nucleus; D, distal part of the adenohypophysis; F, fornix; Fp, precommissural part of the fornix (see Fig. 24-17); G, great cerebral vein (of Galen); GPe, external segment of the globus pallidus; GPi, internal segment of the globus pallidus; I, intermediate part of the adenohypophysis; IF, interventricular foramen; Inf, infundibulum; IS, infundibular stalk; l, m, and pe, lateral, medial, and periventricular regions of the hypothalamus; LT, lamina terminalis; M, mammillary body (part of the posterior hypothalamus); O or OC, optic chiasm; ON, optic nerve; OT, optic tract; Pi, pineal gland; PL, posterior lobe of the pituitary; Put, putamen; RN, red nucleus; SP, septum pellucidum; T, tuberal part of the adenohypophysis; TF, transverse fissure; Th, thalamus.

anterior region is the part above the optic chiasm, the tuberal region is the part above and including the tuber cinereum, and the posterior region is the part above and including the mammillary bodies. In addition, the entire hypothalamus of each side is divided into three longitudinal zones (see Fig. 23-3D). The thin **periventricular zone,** in the wall of the third ventricle, is a rostral continuation of the periaqueductal gray. The **lateral zone,** lateral to the fornix as this fiber bundle traverses the hypothalamus, is a rostral continuation of the reticular formation. The periventricular and lateral zones include collections of neurons and are also avenues through which ascending and descending axons enter, leave, or traverse the hypothalamus; the **medial zone** between them is populated by a series of hypothalamic nuclei (Fig. 23-4; Table 23-1).

The periventricular zone is traversed by the **dorsal longitudinal fasciculus,** a bundle of hypothalamic afferents and efferents (see Fig. 23-6B and C). It also contains a small **suprachiasmatic nucleus** and a larger **arcuate nucleus.** The suprachiasmatic nucleus is tiny—less than 1 mm³ and fewer than 10,000 neurons on each side—but it is the "master clock" for our circadian rhythms (Fig. 23-5A). The free-running period of cells in the suprachiasmatic nucleus is typically about 25 hours (see Fig. 23-5B), but it receives direct projections from the retina that entrain it to the actual day length. Its neurons also contain numerous melatonin receptors, and the nighttime rise in pineal melatonin secretion is thought to provide an additional signal that helps "set" the circadian clock. The arcuate nucleus, as described later in this chapter, is critically involved in feeding behavior.

The lateral zone consists mainly of scattered cells interspersed among the longitudinally running fibers of the **medial forebrain bundle.** Anteriorly, it is continuous

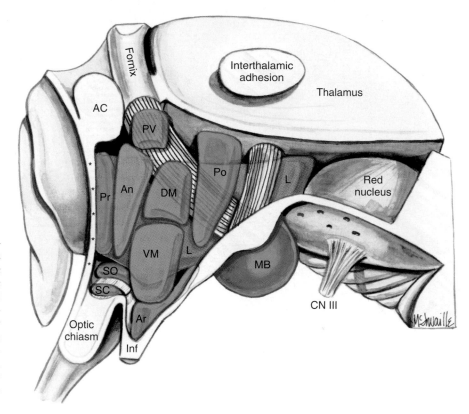

Figure 23-4 Principal nuclei of the hypothalamus (most of the periventricular zone has been removed for clarity). *, lateral terminalis; AC, anterior commissure; An, anterior nucleus; Ar, arcuate (infundibular) nucleus; CN, cranial nerve; DM, dorsomedial nucleus; Inf, infundibular stalk; L, lateral nucleus; MB, mammillary body; Po, posterior nucleus; Pr, medial preoptic nucleus; PV, paraventricular nucleus; SC, suprachiasmatic nucleus; SO, supraoptic nucleus; VM, ventromedial nucleus. (*Modified from Nauta WJH, Haymaker W: The hypothalamus, Springfield, Ill, 1969, Charles C Thomas.*)

Table 23-1	Hypothalamic Nuclei		
Region	**Periventricular Zone**	**Medial Zone**	**Lateral Zone**
Anterior	Suprachiasmatic nucleus	Medial preoptic nucleus	Lateral preoptic nucleus
		Anterior nucleus	Lateral nucleus
		Paraventricular nucleus	
		Supraoptic nucleus	
Tuberal	Arcuate nucleus	Dorsomedial nucleus	Lateral tuberal nuclei
		Ventromedial nucleus	Tuberomammillary nucleus
			Lateral nucleus
Posterior		Mammillary body	Lateral nucleus
		Posterior nucleus	

with the lateral preoptic nucleus, an important sleep-promoting area (see Fig. 22-34); caudally, it is continuous with the midbrain reticular formation. Part of the supraoptic nucleus intrudes into it, as do clumps of cells called **lateral tuberal nuclei.** It also contains the small **tuberomammillary nucleus,** the source of histaminergic fibers that project widely to the cerebral cortex and thalamus and participate in the sleep-wake cycle (see Fig. 22-31). Otherwise it is undivided.

The medial zone contains a number of nuclei (see Table 23-1). Anteriorly, these include two distinctive nuclei containing large neurosecretory cells: the **supraoptic** and **paraventricular nuclei.** The supraoptic

nucleus sits astride the optic tract, extending into the lateral hypothalamic zone; the paraventricular nucleus is higher up in the wall of the third ventricle, near the anterior commissure. Most cells of the supraoptic nucleus and many cells of the paraventricular nucleus secrete hormones that travel down the axons of these cells and are released in the neurohypophysis. The hormones involved and the pathway traversed by them are discussed later in this chapter (see Fig. 23-10). The medial tuberal region is subdivided into dorsal and ventral portions called the **dorsomedial** and **ventromedial nuclei,** respectively. In addition, clusters of orexin-containing neurons near the fornix, extending into the

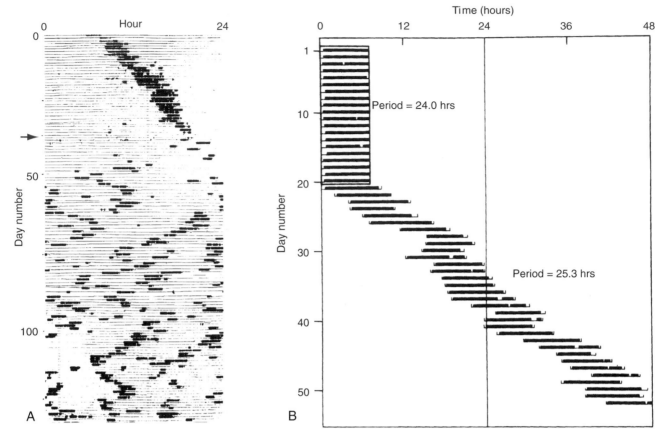

Figure 23-5 Dependence of circadian rhythms on the suprachiasmatic nucleus. **A,** Wheel-running behavior of a hamster over a period of several months while living in constant light. Each horizontal line represents a single day, and each thickening represents a period of wheel running. Wheel running starts out clearly rhythmic, with a prominent episode approximately every 25 hours. On day 37 *(arrow)* the suprachiasmatic nucleus was destroyed bilaterally, and the wheel running subsequently became almost random. **B,** Entrainment of circadian rhythms by environmental cues. These are the sleep records of a 22-year-old man living in a laboratory situation with no cues about the time of day. Thick bars represent time asleep, and thin lines indicate time in bed but awake. For the first 20 days, the subject was awakened every 24 hours and chose to go to bed at about the same time every day (without knowing what time it was). After day 20 he self-selected his own sleep time (i.e., his circadian rhythms were allowed to run freely with no entraining cues). As a result, he went to bed about an hour later on each successive day; the free-running period was 25.3 hours. *(**A,** from Turek FW: Nature 292:289, 1981. **B,** from Czeisler CA et al: Sleep 4:1, 1981.)*

lateral and posterior hypothalamus, are the source of a second set of widespread wakefulness-promoting projections (see Fig. 22-31). The medial mammillary region contains the **mammillary body** (actually a complex of several nuclei) and the **posterior hypothalamic nucleus,** part of which is continuous with the periaqueductal gray matter of the midbrain.

Hypothalamic Inputs Arise in Widespread Neural Sites

Neural inputs to the hypothalamus arise in two general areas (Fig. 23-6): (1) various parts of the forebrain, particularly components of the limbic system, and (2) the brainstem and spinal cord. Afferents from the brainstem and spinal cord convey visceral and somatic sensory information, whereas those from limbic structures convey information relevant to the role of the hypothalamus in mediating many of the autonomic and somatic aspects of affective states. The connections of limbic

components with one another and with the hypothalamus are discussed later in this chapter and are mentioned only briefly here.

Most Inputs From the Forebrain Arise in Limbic Structures

Major forebrain afferents to the hypothalamus arise in the (1) **septal nuclei** and nearby parts of the basal forebrain, including the ventral striatum; (2) hippocampus; (3) amygdala; (4) insula, orbitofrontal cortex, and a few other related cortical areas; and (5) retina.

The septal nuclei (see Fig. 25-2), prominent components of the limbic system located adjacent to the septum pellucidum, project fibers to the hypothalamus through the medial forebrain bundle. The medial forebrain bundle is built like a frayed rope, with fibers entering and leaving it at many levels as it traverses the lateral hypothalamic zone and extends into the brainstem tegmentum. This is a bidirectional bundle that also contains afferents from the brainstem to the hypothalamus,

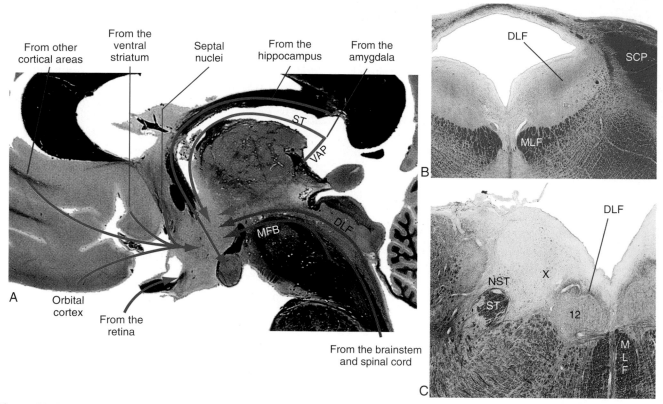

Figure 23-6 A, Major inputs to the hypothalamus. DLF, dorsal longitudinal fasciculus; MFB, medial forebrain bundle; ST, stria terminalis; VAP, ventral amygdalofugal pathway (see Fig. 23-20). **B** and **C,** Location of the dorsal longitudinal fasciculus (DLF) in the rostral pons and rostral medulla. 12, hypoglossal nucleus; MLF, medial longitudinal fasciculus; NST, nucleus of the solitary tract; SCP, superior cerebellar peduncle; ST, solitary tract; X, dorsal motor nucleus of the vagus.

hypothalamic efferents passing both rostrally and caudally, fibers interconnecting different hypothalamic levels, and fibers passing through the hypothalamus on their way to someplace else.

The major output from the hippocampus is contained in the fornix. This fiber bundle arches around under the corpus callosum and through the hypothalamus, where many of its fibers reach the mammillary body (see Fig. 24-17).

The amygdala projects fibers to the hypothalamus by two different routes. Some travel through the **stria terminalis,** a long, curved fiber bundle that accompanies the caudate nucleus. Others take a shorter course and pass under the lenticular nucleus directly to the hypothalamus (see Fig. 23-20).

There are direct projections from the cerebral cortex to the hypothalamus. These arise mainly in the orbital and medial prefrontal cortex of the frontal lobe and in the insula and join the medial forebrain bundle. There are also contributions from the cingulate gyrus and some other cortical areas.

Finally, the projections from photosensitive retinal ganglion cells to the suprachiasmatic nucleus play a key role in entraining circadian rhythms.

Inputs From the Brainstem and Spinal Cord Traverse the Medial Forebrain Bundle and Dorsal Longitudinal Fasciculus

An assortment of sensory inputs (in addition to those from the retina) reaches the hypothalamus by several routes. Some involve synapses in various portions of the reticular formation and periaqueductal gray; others arrive directly from sites such as the solitary and parabrachial nuclei. Some of these afferents travel in the medial forebrain bundle; others are contained in the dorsal longitudinal fasciculus (see Fig. 23-6B and C), a collection of thinly myelinated fibers that pass through the periventricular and periaqueductal gray of the brainstem and then fan out in the hypothalamic wall of the third ventricle. Still other afferents enter the hypothalamus as collaterals of fibers in other pathways such as the spinothalamic tract.

Ascending axons from brainstem monoamine-containing neuronal groups—locus ceruleus, raphe nuclei, and the ventral tegmental area—also traverse the medial forebrain bundle on their way to innervate the cerebral cortex (see Figs. 11-24, 11-26, and 11-27). Along the way, some terminate in the hypothalamus.

The Hypothalamus Contains Intrinsic Sensory Neurons

In addition to receiving various types of visceral and somatic information through the brainstem pathways just mentioned, the hypothalamus contains neurons that are directly responsive to physical stimuli. Some of these cells are sensitive to the temperature of the hypothalamus itself, whereas the activity of others is sensitive to such things as blood osmolality (Fig. 23-7) or the concentration of glucose or certain hormones in blood passing through the hypothalamus.

Hypothalamic Outputs Largely Reciprocate Inputs

Some efferent pathways from the hypothalamus reciprocate the afferent pathways (Fig. 23-8). Thus the hypothalamus projects to the septal nuclei, hippocampus, amygdala, and the brainstem and spinal cord by way of

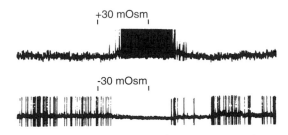

+30 mOsm

-30 mOsm

Figure 23-7 Patch-clamp recordings from a rat supraoptic neuron as it was exposed to hypertonic and hypotonic solutions. Hypertonic solutions cause the neuron to shrink, mechanosensitive ion channels to open, and a burst of action potentials. Hypotonic solutions cause the reverse. *(From Oliet SHR, Bourque CW: Nature 364:341, 1993.)*

the same fiber bundles that carry afferents to the hypothalamus. Efferents to the cerebral cortex, rather than focusing on limbic areas, blanket the cortex with widespread projections in a manner similar to that of the monoamine-containing fibers from the brainstem; the two most prominent examples are histaminergic fibers from the tuberomammillary nucleus and orexinergic fibers from the tuberal and posterior hypothalamus. A few pathways are totally or predominantly efferent in nature. The prominent **mammillothalamic tract,** for example, passes from the mammillary body to the anterior nucleus of the thalamus. Shortly after leaving the mammillary body, many of these same axons send branches to the midbrain reticular formation through the **mammillotegmental tract.**

The Hypothalamus Controls Both Lobes of the Pituitary Gland

The final efferent pathways from the hypothalamus are of great functional importance because they control the **pituitary gland** (or **hypophysis**). The pituitary is a two-part gland (Fig. 23-9), with a posterior lobe that develops as a downward outgrowth from the diencephalon and an **anterior lobe** that develops from the roof of the mouth; the anterior lobe, together with its upward extension around the infundibular stalk, constitutes the **adenohypophysis.** The hypothalamus has a separate control system for each lobe: a neural projection to the neurohypophysis and a vascular link with the adenohypophysis.

The supraoptic and paraventricular nuclei, as mentioned previously, contain large neurosecretory cells.

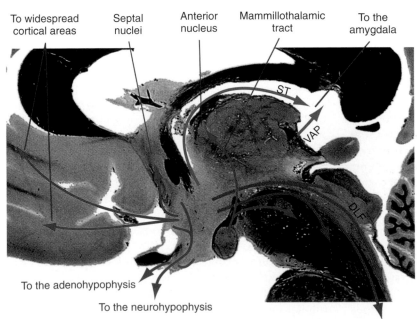

To widespread cortical areas

Septal nuclei

Anterior nucleus

Mammillothalamic tract

To the amygdala

ST

VAP

DLF

To the adenohypophysis

To the neurohypophysis

To the brainstem and spinal cord

Figure 23-8 Major outputs from the hypothalamus. *DLF,* dorsal longitudinal fasciculus; *ST,* stria terminalis; *VAP,* ventral amygdalofugal pathway (see Fig. 23-20).

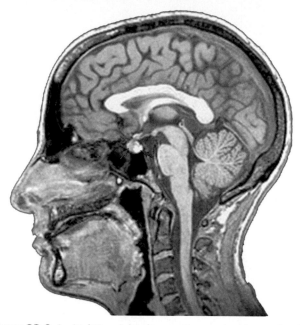

Figure 23-9 Sagittal T1-weighted magnetic resonance image showing the anterior *(green arrow)* and posterior *(blue arrow)* lobes of the pituitary gland. *(Courtesy Dr. Elena M. Plante, University of Arizona.)*

(The paraventricular nucleus also contains numerous smaller cells, many of which project as hypothalamic efferents to the dorsal motor nucleus of the vagus nerve, the intermediolateral cell column of the spinal cord, and other sites.) The large neurosecretory cells of the supraoptic and paraventricular nuclei produce two peptide hormones, each nine amino acids in length; a given cell produces only one of the two hormones. The first is **antidiuretic hormone** (**ADH,** or **vasopressin**), whose principal physiological function as a hormone[b] is to increase the reabsorption of water in the kidney and thereby decrease the production of urine. The second is **oxytocin** (from Greek words meaning "rapid birth"), a similar peptide that causes contraction of uterine and mammary smooth muscle and is important in parturition and milk ejection. Both hormones travel down the axons of their parent cell bodies by axoplasmic flow, bound to a carrier protein (**neurophysin**). These neurosecretory cells are electrically excitable, and the passage of action potentials down their axons causes release of their hormones from bulbous endings adjacent to capillaries in the median eminence, infundibular stalk, and posterior lobe of the pituitary (Fig. 23-10A). Most of the axons arise in the supraoptic nucleus, so this pathway is called the **supraopticohypophyseal tract.**

The adenohypophysis secretes a multitude of hormones whose discussion is beyond the scope of this book. It has long been known that electrical stimulation of certain areas of the hypothalamus can modulate the rates of secretion of these hormones, but there are no neural connections that can explain this modulation. This drew attention to the **hypophyseal portal system** as a vascular connection between the hypothalamus and the adenohypophysis (see Fig. 23-10B). The **superior hypophyseal artery,** a branch of the internal carotid, breaks up into a capillary bed in the median eminence and proximal part of the infundibular stalk. Blood in these capillaries then re-collects into **hypophyseal portal vessels,** which travel down the infundibular stalk and break up into a second capillary bed in the adenohypophysis. Small peptides,[c] called **hypothalamic releasing hormones** and **inhibiting hormones,** are secreted by cells of the arcuate nucleus and nearby sites in the wall of the third ventricle,[d] travel down the axons of these cells, and are released into the bloodstream in the first capillary bed. (The median eminence is one of the circumventricular organs [see Fig. 6-29], and its capillaries are fenestrated [see Fig. 6-30].) From there the releasing and inhibiting hormones travel down the hypophyseal portal vessels to the adenohypophysis, where they act. As their names imply, releasing hormones promote the release of particular hormones, whereas inhibiting hormones prevent this release. The entire collection of axons carrying these releasing and inhibiting factors is called the **tuberoinfundibular** or **tuberohypophysial tract.**

The relatively small cells that secrete releasing and inhibiting factors are commonly referred to as the **parvocellular neurosecretory system,** as distinguished from the **magnocellular neurosecretory system** of larger neurons in the supraoptic and paraventricular nuclei that secrete oxytocin and vasopressin.

The same small hypothalamic peptides are also found in other neurons in widespread areas of the central nervous system (CNS) and in other cells of the body as well. This is reminiscent of the situation with enkephalins and endorphins, briefly discussed in Chapter 11. A slowly emerging picture is that, in some respects, the brain is a much more "distributed" organ than it is normally considered to be—that is, it may use the same chemical both as a neurotransmitter acting locally on a postsynaptic neuron and as a hormone acting at a distance, both actions working toward the same physiological goal.

---

[b]Both vasopressin and oxytocin, like the hypothalamic releasing and inhibiting hormones discussed shortly, also serve as neurotransmitters or neuromodulators, so their total physiological roles extend beyond their functions as hormones.

---

[c]The major exception is dopamine, which inhibits the release of prolactin.

[d]Some of these are located in the paraventricular nucleus, which therefore contains three distinct cell types—large neurons that secrete oxytocin or vasopressin, smaller neurons that secrete releasing or inhibiting hormones, and neurons that project to the brainstem and spinal cord.

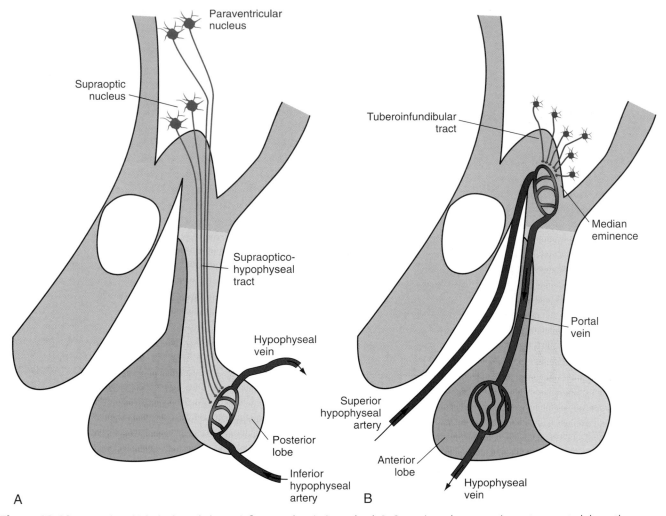

Figure 23-10 Routes by which the hypothalamus influences the pituitary gland. **A,** Oxytocin and vasopressin are transported down the axons of magnocellular neurons of the supraoptic and paraventricular nuclei, reaching capillaries of the posterior lobe. **B,** Parvocellular neurons in the arcuate nucleus and nearby regions of the walls of the third ventricle secrete releasing and inhibiting hormones in the median eminence, where they gain access to the hypophyseal portal system and, through it, reach the anterior lobe. The inferior hypophyseal artery (not shown) also participates in the hypophyseal portal system, giving rise to capillary sinusoids in the lower part of the infundibulum.

Perforating Branches From the Circle of Willis Supply the Hypothalamus

The infundibular stalk is located just about in the middle of the circle of Willis (see Fig. 6-3), and the inferior surface of the entire hypothalamus is more or less surrounded by the circle. The arterial supply of the hypothalamus is derived from a series of small perforating or ganglionic arteries arising from arteries in and adjacent to the circle of Willis (see Fig. 6-22). Specifically, small branches of the anterior cerebral and anterior communicating arteries supply the preoptic and supraoptic regions; paramedian branches arising from the posterior communicating arteries and the proximal portions of the posterior cerebral arteries supply the tuberal and mammillary regions; lenticulostriate branches from proximal portions of the middle cerebral arteries, together with anterior choroidal branches, help supply the lateral hypothalamus.

The Hypothalamus Collaborates With a Network of Brainstem and Spinal Cord Neurons

The connections of the hypothalamus with the limbic system, pituitary gland, and brainstem put it in a good position to control various visceral functions and activities involved in drives and emotional states. Consistent with this, many hypothalamic "centers" have been described and implicated in feeding and drinking behavior, temperature regulation, gut motility, sexual activity, and numerous other such functions. Few of these responses are actually organized in the hypothalamus, however. Instead, much like the motor control system (see Fig. 18-7), the hypothalamus is in some ways like a collection of upper motor neurons, projecting in part directly to (preganglionic) autonomic motor neurons and in part to central pattern generators (see Fig. 23-2). Consistent with this, fragments of most behavior patterns elicited by stimulating a hypothalamic location

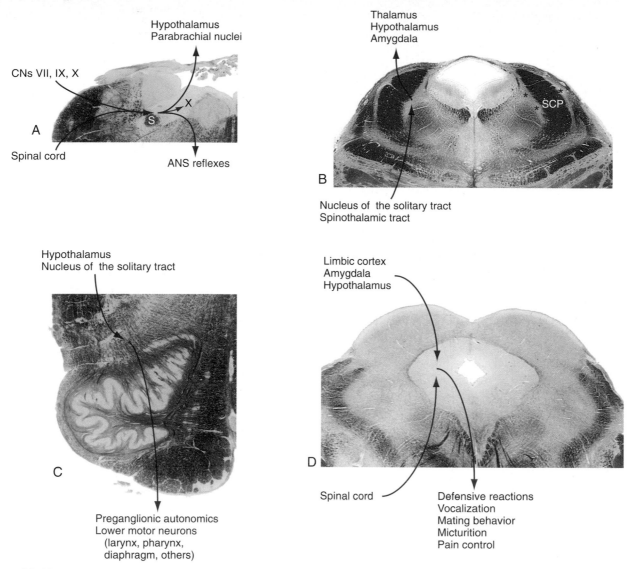

Figure 23-11 Major patterns of connections of parts of the brainstem interconnected with the hypothalamus. **A,** The nucleus of the solitary tract receives visceral afferents from cranial nerves (through the solitary tract [S]) and the spinal cord, and projects to autonomic motor neurons in the dorsal motor nucleus of the vagus (X) and elsewhere and to central pattern generators. Its outputs reach the hypothalamus and limbic system in part directly and in part through other nuclei such as the parabrachial nuclei. **B,** The parabrachial nuclei (*) convey visceral, pain, and temperature information to the hypothalamus, thalamus (and from there to the insula), and amygdala. **C,** Central pattern generators for coordinated autonomic and somatic responses to physiological challenges are located in the reticular formation. Those in the ventrolateral rostral medulla are important for cardiovascular and respiratory responses. **D,** The periaqueductal gray orchestrates complex responses, especially to threatening situations, guided by inputs from the cerebrum. ANS, autonomic nervous system; SCP, superior cerebellar peduncle.

can be elicited by stimulating appropriate sites in the brainstem.

A network of heavily interconnected brainstem areas works together with the hypothalamus to implement many aspects of drive-related behavior. Four prominent components of this network (Fig. 23-11) are the nucleus of the solitary tract, the **parabrachial nuclei,** the ventrolateral reticular formation of the rostral medulla, and the periaqueductal gray. Although these are all interconnected with one another and with other parts of the brainstem and diencephalon, each has a distinctive major function.

The nucleus of the solitary tract is the principal visceral sensory nucleus located in the brainstem. Primary afferents in cranial nerves VII, IX, and X conveying information about taste (see Figs. 13-4 and 13-6) and about conditions in internal organs all terminate there. In addition, second-order fibers convey visceral information that reached the spinal cord through sympathetic nerves. The nucleus of the solitary tract in turn projects into visceral reflex arcs (e.g., to the dorsal motor nucleus of the vagus) and to more rostral levels of the CNS.

The parabrachial nuclei (so named for their proximity to the superior cerebellar peduncle, or brachium conjunctivum) also deal with visceral sensory information, but they have a more general role in conveying information that is the basis of a subjective sense of well-being (or not-so-well-being). They receive inputs from the nucleus of the solitary tract dealing with bodily functions, as well as spinothalamic inputs dealing with pain and temperature. They then forward this to forebrain structures involved in drives and emotions, especially the hypothalamus, amygdala, and thalamus.

A series of central pattern generators for responses to physiological challenges is distributed through the reticular formation. Those in the ventrolateral reticular formation of the rostral medulla are particularly important for cardiovascular and respiratory functions, but there are others (e.g., the pontine micturition center; see Fig. 23-13). Although some of these pattern generators affect autonomic outputs almost exclusively (e.g., cardiovascular responses), others, such as those involved in respiration, swallowing, micturition, defecation, and sexual function, provide nice examples of the coordinated use of autonomic motor neurons and lower motor neurons.

The periaqueductal gray is best known as the origin of a descending pain-control pathway (see Fig. 11-21), but this is only part of what it does. Columns of neurons in the periaqueductal gray orchestrate complex behavioral responses, especially to threatening stimuli, by projecting to central pattern generators in other parts of the brainstem. Signals emanating from the periaqueductal gray of a frightened cat, for example, initiate tachycardia, piloerection, arching of the back, hissing, and, in some situations, analgesia.

Normal Micturition Involves a Central Pattern Generator in the Pons

Control of micturition (urination)[e] epitomizes the way both smooth muscle and skeletal muscle participate in numerous routine activities; analogous sets of connections, not detailed here, underlie respiration, ingestion and defecation, sexual functions, and other activities.

The urinary bladder is essentially a muscular container that switches back and forth between two states: long periods in a **storage mode,** alternating with brief periods in an **elimination mode.** Being **continent** means having conscious control of the switch. Peristaltic waves in the ureters push urine from the kidneys into the bladder. If the pressure in the bladder (the **intravesical**[f] pressure) becomes greater than the outflow resistance, urine gets eliminated. The pressure in the bladder is controlled by the **detrusor** (the layer of smooth muscle in the bladder wall) and by the mechanical properties of the bladder wall. Outflow resistance is controlled by

[e]Micturition is derived from a Latin word, urination from a Greek word. Both mean the same thing.

[f]From the Latin word *vesica,* meaning "bladder" or "blister." So a synaptic vesicle is a "small bladder."

smooth muscle in the neck of the bladder (forming an internal urethral sphincter), by the elasticity of the urethra, and by the **external urethral sphincter,** a band of striated muscle surrounding the proximal urethra.

The bladder spends most of its time in storage mode, maintained in that state by sympathetic inputs and the lack of parasympathetic activity (Fig. 23-12, left side). Preganglionic sympathetic neurons from T11 to L2 project to the inferior mesenteric ganglion (one of the prevertebral ganglia). Postganglionic sympathetic neurons then promote relaxation of the detrusor by releasing norepinephrine on postganglionic parasympathetic ganglion cells in and near the bladder wall and on the detrusor itself (the latter has a relatively minor effect). At the same time, outflow resistance is maintained by tonic contraction of the external sphincter, innervated not by autonomic neurons but rather by

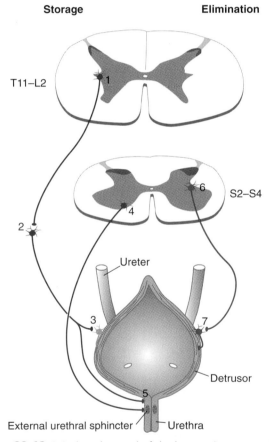

Figure 23-12 Spinal cord control of the lower urinary tract. As the bladder fills (left side of figure), intravesical pressure is minimized by T11-L2 preganglionic sympathetic neurons (1) that synapse on postganglionic neurons (2) in the inferior mesenteric ganglion; these in turn inhibit postganglionic parasympathetic neurons in the bladder wall (3). Outflow resistance is high because lower motor neurons in Onuf's nucleus (4) activate the external sphincter, and sympathetics activate smooth muscle in the bladder neck (5). During elimination mode (right side of figure), all this is reversed. Sympathetics and sphincter motor neurons slow down or fall silent, reducing outflow resistance. Sacral preganglionic parasympathetic neurons (6) synapse on postganglionic neurons (7) in the bladder wall; these in turn activate the detrusor, increasing intravesical pressure.

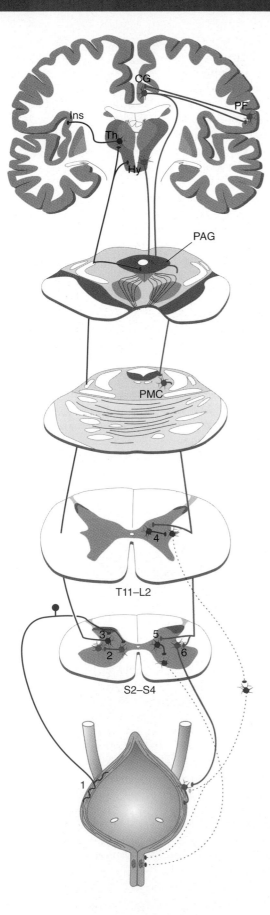

Figure 23-13 Neural connections involved in normal micturition. To simplify the diagram, ascending connections are shown on the left and descending connections on the right; in reality, both are bilateral. Tension receptors in the bladder wall (1) project to interneurons subserving the vesicovesical reflex (2), which has little effect in normal adults. The same primary afferents also synapse on tract cells (3) that convey information about bladder fullness to the periaqueductal gray (PAG), hypothalamus (Hy), and thalamus (Th) and from there to visceral sensory cortex in the insula (Ins). The periaqueductal gray integrates sensory inputs, inputs from the hypothalamus, and cortical inputs representing activity in prefrontal (PF) and limbic (cingulate gyrus; CG) areas. Periodically, the periaqueductal gray activates the pontine micturition center (PMC), which in turn inhibits sympathetic (4) and lower motor neurons (5) to the bladder and activates parasympathetics (6) to the detrusor.

lower motor neurons from a small cluster in S2 called **Onuf's nucleus** (which also innervates the external anal sphincter). The intrinsic elasticity of the ureter and some sympathetically innervated smooth muscle in the neck of the bladder also contribute to outflow resistance. As a result, the bladder fills with relatively little rise in intravesical pressure (because the detrusor is relaxed).

The bladder periodically switches to elimination mode (see Fig. 23-12, right side), in which the parasympathetics take over and storage conditions are reversed. Lower motor neurons in Onuf's nucleus are inhibited, reducing outflow resistance. Shortly thereafter, T11-L2 sympathetics are inhibited, S2-S4 parasympathetics are activated, the detrusor contracts, and intravesical pressure increases.

In infants, the switch from storage to elimination mode is mediated by spinal cord circuitry, in the form of a **vesicovesical reflex** through which stretch of the bladder wall causes detrusor contraction (Fig. 23-13, left side). In adults, the vesicovesical reflex is suppressed (in much the same way as Babinski's sign and other spinal cord circuitry is suppressed), and brainstem components come into play. The same information about tension in the bladder wall that feeds into the vesicovesical reflex also ascends bilaterally through the middle of the lateral funiculus to the periaqueductal gray, hypothalamus, and thalamus (ventral posteromedial [VPM] nucleus). VPM in turn relays it to visceral sensory cortex in the insula, leading to conscious awareness of the state of the bladder. The periaqueductal gray collects information about the status of the bladder and also about things such as the current social situation (see Fig. 23-13, right side; Fig. 23-14). When the time is right, it sends a signal to a pattern generator in the rostral pons called the **pontine micturition center,** which turns on the elimination mode and coordinates normal micturition.

Lesions in various parts of this micturition circuitry cause changes reminiscent of those that follow damage to lower and upper motor neurons and their connections. Lesions of the conus medullaris or cauda equina are comparable to lower motor neuron damage. The detrusor can no longer contract, and the only two

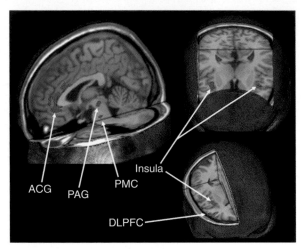

Figure 23-14 Compilation of data from five functional imaging studies, showing areas activated when subjects perceived their bladders to be full (vs. empty). ACG, anterior cingulate gyrus; DLPFC, dorsolateral prefrontal cortex; PAG, periaqueductal gray; PMC, pontine micturition center. *(Adapted from Kavia RBC, DasGupta R, Fowler CJ: J Comp Neurol 493:27, 2005. Prepared using MRIcro software; Rorden C, Brett M: Behav Neurol 12:191, 2000.)*

sources of pressure in the lower urinary tract are the propulsion of urine through the ureters and the intrinsic elasticity of the bladder neck and urethra. As a result, the bladder fills beyond its normal size, even though the pressure stays low (because the detrusor cannot contract); bladder pressure eventually exceeds urethral pressure, and overflow incontinence results. In the absence of catheterization or some other treatment, a lot of urine remains in the bladder constantly, inviting urinary tract infections. Damage between the sacral cord and the pons causes the same pattern of bladder inactivity during the period of spinal shock. The vesicovesical reflex then becomes hyperactive, just as stretch reflexes become hyperactive. This creates a situation in which the bladder automatically tries to empty itself, even at lower than normal volumes. However, the external sphincter never gets the signal that would normally descend from the pontine micturition center telling it to relax, so bladder pressure builds up until it overcomes the sphincter. This can have serious consequences, because the high pressure is transmitted retrogradely to the kidneys and can damage them. Lesions above the pons do not affect the basic micturition reflex, but because the pontine micturition center factors in more than just bladder status before sending signals to the spinal cord, other abnormalities can result, such as difficulty suppressing urination or diminished social awareness.

The Hypothalamus and Associated Central Pattern Generators Keep Physiological Variables Within Narrow Limits

A whole host of internal parameters—temperature, pH, water and glucose concentrations, and many others—need to be maintained within narrow limits for bodies to function optimally. Changes in any of them typically cause autonomic and endocrine responses as well as behavioral drives, all acting in a coordinated way to counteract the change. The maintained value is usually referred to as a **set point,** much like the setting of a thermostat; deviation of some variable from the set point creates an error signal, which in turn activates mechanisms that decrease the error signal (in the case of the thermostat example, by turning on the furnace or air conditioner). Set points may not always be reference values stored someplace in the CNS, but the concept provides a useful way to think about homeostatic processes.

Temperature regulation, through which we maintain a body temperature of about 37°C, is a well-known example. About 20% of the neurons in the medial preoptic nucleus are directly warm-sensitive, firing faster as their temperature increases. The same neurons receive information about skin temperature and the temperature of internal organs, either through branches of spinothalamic fibers or through projections from the parabrachial nuclei. Directly or indirectly, these warm-sensitive neurons excite central pattern generators for heat-dissipation mechanisms and inhibit pattern generators for heat-retention and heat-production mechanisms. Different pattern generators have different thresholds, so they can be recruited systematically. We remain comfortable in a range of environmental temperatures, for example, because small temperature changes can be counteracted by sympathetically mediated cutaneous vasoconstriction (conserving heat) or vasodilation (dissipating heat). Larger temperature changes bring more powerful mechanisms into play—sweating, shivering, metabolic production of heat. As mentioned earlier, they also make us feel uncomfortable, leading to behavioral responses such as shedding or adding clothes or seeking out a cooler or warmer room.

Body water is also closely regulated, and another group of medial preoptic neurons collects data from several sources for this purpose. Decreased water volume causes a decrease in blood volume and an increase in its osmolality. The decreased blood volume (and pressure) stimulates receptors *(baroreceptors)* in and near the heart; this is transmitted via the glossopharyngeal and vagus nerves to the nucleus of the solitary tract. The increased osmolality is detected by osmoreceptive neurons in the vascular organ of the lamina terminalis (one of the circumventricular organs; see Fig. 6-29). Finally, decreased blood flow to the kidney leads to elevated blood levels of angiotensin II, a peptide hormone, which is detected by neurons in the subfornical organ (another circumventricular organ). All three sets of neurons project to the medial preoptic nucleus, which in turn projects to the ADH-secreting neurons of the supraoptic and paraventricular nuclei, leading to increased reabsorption of water by the kidneys. At the same time, signals about decreased water volume reach the cerebral cortex, leading to feelings of thirst and a search for water.

Regulation of food intake and energy balance is much more complicated, but the same themes of multiple feedback signals about nutrient levels and stores, together with coordinated endocrine, autonomic, and behavioral responses, are seen here as well. Early studies found that bilateral lesions in the ventral part of the medial tuberal hypothalamus produce animals that overeat and get fat, leading to the notion that this part of the hypothalamus contains a "satiety center." Conversely, destruction of the lateral hypothalamus in the tuberal region ("feeding center") produces animals that do not eat and may actually starve to death unless force-fed postoperatively. Much as medial preoptic neurons combine sources of information about temperature or water balance, neurons in the arcuate nucleus combine signals relevant to feeding behavior. Arcuate neurons receive projections from the nucleus of the solitary tract dealing with stomach distention and the contents of the stomach and intestines, are directly sensitive to glucose and other nutrients, and have receptors for several peptide hormones whose levels fluctuate in proportion to nutrient levels. Two important examples of the latter are **ghrelin** and **leptin.** Ghrelin is secreted by the stomach at rates that increase with time since the last meal; it binds to arcuate neurons and stimulates feeding behavior and energy storage. Leptin is produced by adipocytes and has the opposite effect. Changes or abnormalities in ghrelin or especially leptin signaling are now thought to underlie many cases of obesity. Arcuate neurons in turn project to parvocellular neurosecretory neurons (affecting pituitary production of thyrotropin and other hormones), to autonomic pattern generators in the brainstem and spinal cord, and to neurons in the lateral hypothalamus (many of them the same orexin neurons that are active in promoting wakefulness) that stimulate feeding behavior.

Because so many things are packed together in the hypothalamus, discrete lesions often do not cause single changes such as hypothermia or obesity. Bilateral lesions of the medial tuberal region provide an instructive example of both the multiple effects from discrete lesions and the involvement of the hypothalamus in emotional

behavior. Cats with bilateral ventromedial lesions overeat and get fat and are also extremely nasty.[g] They respond with full-blown hissing rages to innocuous stimuli. Similar rage responses can be elicited by stimulation of the adjacent lateral tuberal hypothalamus of an intact cat. The attacks are coordinated and well directed but cease the moment the stimulus does. The ways in which such emotional responses are related, under normal circumstances, to activity in the limbic system are discussed later in this chapter.

Limbic Structures Are Interposed Between the Hypothalamus and Neocortex

In 1878 Paul Broca pointed out that a general feature of mammalian brains is a great horseshoe-shaped rim of cortex surrounding the junction between the diencephalon and each cerebral hemisphere (see Fig. 3-13). The ends of the arc are joined by olfactory areas at the base of the brain so that a complete loop is formed, with the olfactory tract and bulb extending anteriorly like the handle of a tennis racket. He referred to this ring of cortex at the margin of the hemisphere as the limbic lobe (from the Latin *limbus,* meaning "border") and suggested that the entire lobe might be concerned with the sense of smell. However, the limbic lobe includes the cingulate and parahippocampal gyri and is associated with the nearby amygdala and hippocampus, and it soon became apparent that olfaction is not the primary responsibility of these areas. For example, although some dolphins have no olfactory bulbs and are thought to be completely anosmatic, they nevertheless have an amygdala, a hippocampus, and a well-developed limbic lobe. Cases have been reported of humans with congenital absence of the olfactory bulb and tracts but with apparently normal limbic lobes. Finally, subsequent anatomical and physiological experiments showed that, aside from the already mentioned olfactory areas at the base of the brain, the limbic lobe does not receive a particularly large amount of olfactory input.

In 1937 James Papez proposed that the limbic lobe instead was organized as an anatomical substrate for drive-related and emotional behavior. He noted that the hippocampus is interposed between the cingulate gyrus and the hypothalamus (see Fig. 24-20) and suggested that the cingulate gyrus and its widespread neocortical connections are the basis for experiencing emotions, whereas the hypothalamus and its connections are responsible for some of the outward manifestations of emotions. The basic reasoning was correct, but it is now clear that the amygdala and its connections are more centrally involved in emotional experiences and responses, and the hippocampus has a primary role in some forms of learning and memory (see Chapter 24). The conglomerate of the limbic lobe, its connections,

---

[g]"One of my own most striking memories is of huge, fat, and extremely hostile cats with ventromedial hypothalamic lesions. When they observed laboratory visitors through the bars, thankfully strong bars, of their cages, they appeared to have a singular interest in attack. They gave every sign of dedication to the goal of destroying the visitor. Their great size made the threat something not to be taken lightly." (From Isaacson RL: The limbic system, New York, 1974, Plenum Press, p. 85.)

and a few additional structures has come to be referred to as the limbic system. There is no universal agreement on the total list of structures that should be included in the term *limbic system,* but all authors would include the cingulate and parahippocampal gyri, some adjoining areas of cortex (see Fig. 23-16), the hippocampus, the amygdala, and the septal nuclei; most would include the hypothalamus, parts of the midbrain reticular formation, and the olfactory areas. Beyond that, the boundaries get fuzzy; some authors include various thalamic and neocortical regions interconnected with undisputed limbic components, whereas others do not.

The Hippocampus and Amygdala Are the Central Components of the Two Major Limbic Subsystems

Limbic cortical areas and other limbic components serve as bridges between multimodal association areas (especially in the frontal lobe) and the hypothalamus. The two major limbic subsystems are centered around the amygdala and the hippocampus (Fig. 23-15) and include cortical areas that extend beyond the cingulate and parahippocampal gyri (Fig. 23-16); structurally similar cortex extends over the uncus and across the insula and orbital cortex, so the limbic lobe as it is

currently envisioned forms a complete ring of cortex. The amygdala subsystem utilizes ventromedial prefrontal, anterior temporal, and insular cortex as its liaison with the neocortex generally, and it has a close relationship with the dorsomedial nucleus of the thalamus. The output end (in terms of programming or triggering behavioral outputs) is a continuous core of neural tissue extending from the septal area through the hypothalamus and into the midbrain reticular formation. The medial forebrain bundle is its principal longitudinal fiber pathway. The hippocampal subsystem, as described further in Chapter 24, utilizes posterior cingulate and parahippocampal cortex as its liaison with the neocortex generally, and it has a close relationship with the anterior thalamic nucleus and the mammillary body.

The Amygdala Is Centrally Involved in Emotional Responses

The amygdala is a collection of about a dozen nuclei lying beneath the uncus of the limbic lobe, at the anterior end of the hippocampus and the inferior horn of the lateral ventricle (Fig. 23-17; see also Fig. 23-20). It merges with the periamygdaloid cortex, which forms part of the surface of the uncus, and with the parahippocampal

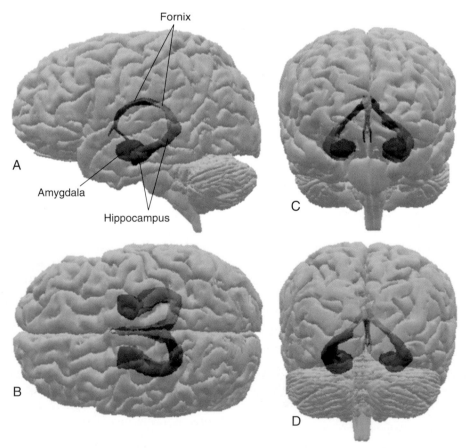

Figure 23-15 Three-dimensional reconstruction of the hippocampus, fornix, and amygdala inside a translucent CNS, seen from the left **(A)**, in front **(B)**, above **(C)**, and behind **(D)**.

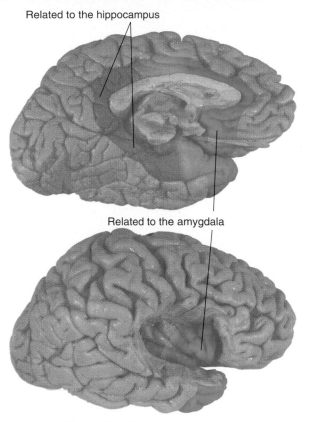

Related to the hippocampus

Related to the amygdala

Figure 23-16 Limbic areas of cortex.

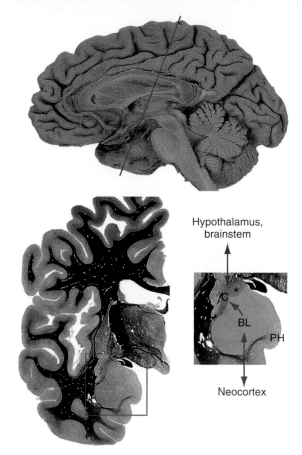

Hypothalamus,
brainstem

Neocortex

Figure 23-17 Subdivision of the amygdala into basolateral (BL), central (C), and medial (*) nuclei. The basic pattern of connections of the basolateral and central nuclei is indicated. PH, parahippocampal gyrus.

gyrus. The nuclei are subdivided into a **medial, central, and basolateral group,** each of which plays a different role in amygdalar function. The medial nuclei abut the periamygdaloid cortex, are interconnected with the olfactory system, and are relatively small in humans. The central nuclei are also small, but their interconnections with the hypothalamus and related brainstem nuclei (e.g., periaqueductal gray) underlie one aspect of the amygdala's involvement in emotional responses. The basolateral nuclei, by far the largest part of the human amygdala, are in some ways like a cortex without layers; they contain pyramidal neurons, are continuous with parahippocampal cortex, and are extensively interconnected with other cortical areas (Fig. 23-18; see also 23-21). Projections from the basolateral nuclei to the central nuclei provide a key link between the experience of emotions and their expression. The amygdala receives its blood supply from branches of the anterior choroidal artery.

The Amygdala Receives a Wide Variety of Sensory Inputs

The amygdala receives a great deal of sensory input, of two general types (see Fig. 23-18). Much of it is the familiar type about sights, sounds, touches, smells, and tastes. Olfactory information arrives at the medial nuclei, both directly from the olfactory bulb and from olfactory

cortex. The rest reaches the basolateral nuclei from the thalamus and from unimodal visual, auditory, somatosensory, and gustatory association areas. A second kind of sensory input, dealing in a more general sense with levels of physical and emotional comfort and discomfort, also reaches the basolateral nuclei from orbital and anterior cingulate cortex and especially the insula (Box 23-1; Fig. 23-19). Finally, visceral sensory inputs reach the central nuclei from the hypothalamus and from brainstem sites such as the periaqueductal gray and parabrachial nuclei.

These inputs arrive via four routes (Fig. 23-20): (1) from the hypothalamus and septal nuclei through the stria terminalis, a long, curved bundle that travels in the wall of the lateral ventricle beside the caudate nucleus and the thalamostriate (or terminal) vein; (2) from the thalamus and hypothalamus, and from orbital and anterior cingulate cortex, through the **ventral amygdalofugal pathway** (not the best name for this pathway, because it contains both afferents and efferents); (3) from the olfactory bulb and olfactory cortex through the lateral olfactory tract; and (4) directly from temporal lobe structures such as neocortical areas and the hippocampus.

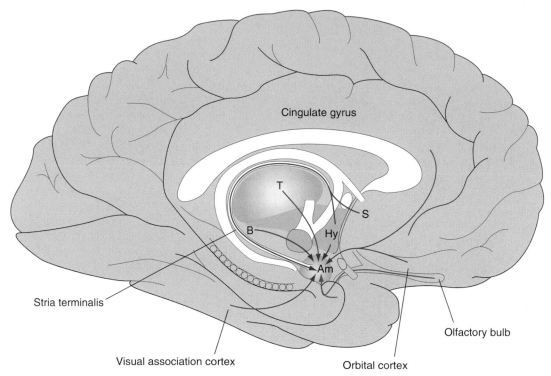

Figure 23-18 Major inputs to the basolateral *(blue)*, central *(red)*, and medial *(green)* nuclei of the amygdala (Am). Only inputs from visual association cortex to the basolateral nuclei are shown, although there are similar projections from most or all unimodal sensory areas. The inputs from limbic cortex to the basolateral nuclei also include a major projection from the insula, which is not present in this view. B, brainstem (periaqueductal gray, parabrachial nuclei, other nuclei); Hy, hypothalamus; S, septal nuclei; T, thalamus (multiple nuclei). *(Modified from Warwick R, Williams PL: Gray's anatomy, Br ed 35, Philadelphia, 1973, WB Saunders.)*

BOX 23-1

The Pleasure of Gentle Touch*

Tactile sensation is usually thought of in terms of large-diameter afferents and the dorsal column–medial lemniscus pathway, with small-diameter fibers relegated to roles in pain, temperature, and visceral sensations. However, many of the unmyelinated afferents (C fibers) that innervate hairy skin respond not to harmful stimuli or temperature changes, but rather to soft, gentle stroking; they are lacking in glabrous skin. Such receptors seem poorly suited for discriminative tactile sensation because of the slow conduction velocity of C fibers, and their role was mysterious for a long time. Ordinarily they cannot be stimulated selectively, because stroking the skin also stimulates receptors with large-diameter axons. A rare patient has now provided insight into their function.

At the age of 31, GL developed an autoimmune syndrome that resulted in degeneration of all the large-diameter sensory fibers in her spinal nerves; her cranial nerves remained mostly intact. When studied 23 years later, "she denied having any touch sensibility below the nose," although she reported that "her perceptions of temperature, pain and itch are intact." Testing revealed that she was unable to detect vibration on her arm or the palm of her hand (see Fig. 23-19A), consistent with a loss of large-diameter fibers. Nor could she detect

gentle stroking with a soft watercolor brush when it was applied to the palm of her hand (where there are no C-touch receptors). When the same stroking was applied to her forearm, however, "she reported that, if she really concentrated, she was able to perceive a faint and diffuse touch sensation, which she described as 'a pressure.'" The forearm stimuli seemed less intense to her than to control subjects, but just as pleasant (see Fig. 23-19B).

Functional magnetic resonance imaging (fMRI) revealed that stroking GL's forearm (see Fig. 23-19C and E) activated the contralateral insula and premotor cortex, but neither primary somatosensory cortex nor the second somatosensory area. In contrast, the same stimulus applied to control subjects activated not only the contralateral insula and premotor cortex but also primary somatosensory cortex on the contralateral side and the second somatosensory area bilaterally (see Fig. 23-19D and F).

Other work has shown that a similar or overlapping area of the insula is activated in all of us in response to a wide variety of stimuli that make us feel comfortable or uncomfortable—pain, temperature changes, fatigue, even looking at picture of a loved one or a picture of someone else who is seemingly in pain (see Fig. 23-25).

*Based on Olausson H et al: Nat Neurosci 5:900, 2002.

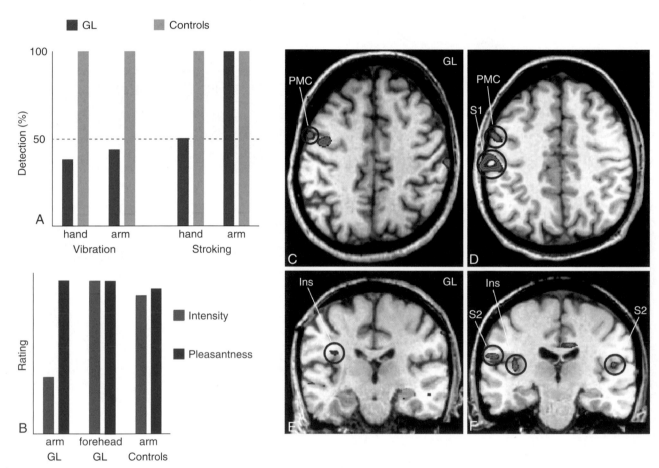

Figure 23-19 Psychophysical testing and functional imaging during stimulation of C-touch receptors. **A,** Detection of various stimuli by patient GL (see Box 23-1) and control subjects; the *dashed line* indicates a chance level of detection. **B,** Rating of the intensity and pleasantness of gentle brushing by GL and control subjects. GL rated both intensity and pleasantness the same as controls did when the stimulus was applied to her forehead (where innervation was still normal). The same stimulus was perceived as equally pleasant but less intense when applied to her forearm. **C to F,** Functional MRI demonstration of areas activated in GL (**C** and **E**) and control subjects (**D** and **F**) during gentle brushing of the forearm. Ins, insula; PMC, premotor cortex; S1, primary somatosensory cortex; S2, second somatosensory area. *(From Olausson H et al: Nat Neurosci 5:900, 2002.)*

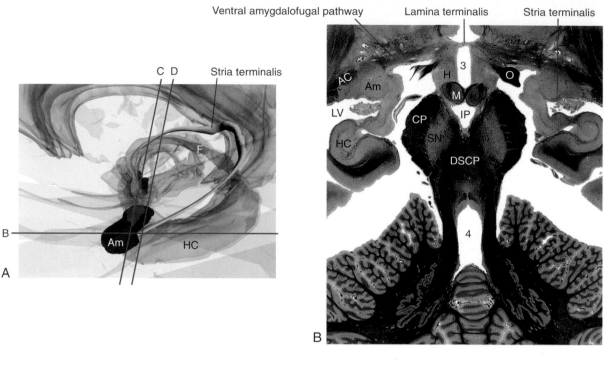

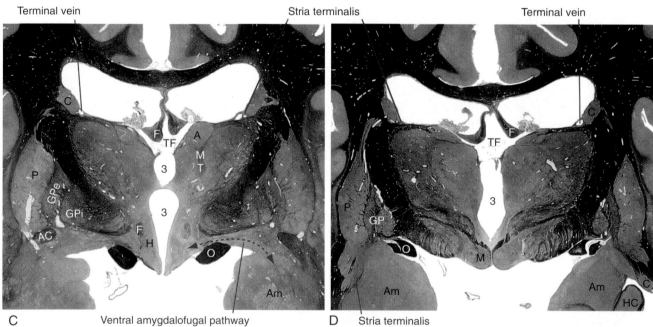

Figure 23-20 Location of the amygdala and related fiber bundles. **A,** Three-dimensional reconstruction with the planes of section shown in **B, C,** and **D** indicated. 3, third ventricle; 4, fourth ventricle; A, anterior thalamic nucleus; AC, anterior commissure; Am, amygdala; C, caudate nucleus; CP, cerebral peduncle; DSCP, decussation of the superior cerebellar peduncles; F, fornix; GP, globus pallidus; GPe, external segment of globus pallidus; GPi, internal segment of globus pallidus; H, tuberal hypothalamus; HC, hippocampus; IP, interpeduncular cistern; LV, lateral ventricle (inferior horn); M, mammillary body; MT, mammillothalamic tract; O, optic tract; P, putamen; SN, substantia nigra; TF, transverse fissure. (**A,** prepared by Cheryl Cotman. **A** to **D,** modified from Nolte J, Angevine JB Jr: The human brain in photographs and diagrams, ed 3, St. Louis, 2007, Mosby.)

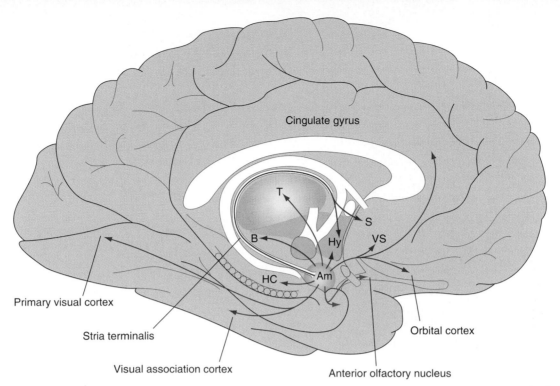

Figure 23-21 Major outputs from the basolateral *(blue)*, central *(red)*, and medial *(green)* nuclei of the amygdala (Am). These take three routes: (1) the stria terminalis, which reaches the septal nuclei (S) and hypothalamus (Hy); (2) the ventral amygdalofugal pathway (see Fig. 23-20B and C) to the hypothalamus (Hy), thalamus (T; mainly the dorsomedial nucleus), widespread areas of ventromedial prefrontal and insular cortex, ventral striatum (VS), olfactory structures, and various brainstem sites (B); and (3) direct projections to the hippocampus (HC) and temporal and other neocortical areas. Only visual cortical areas are shown, although there are similar projections to most or all primary and unimodal sensory areas. *(Modified from Warwick R, Williams PL: Gray's anatomy, Br ed 35, Philadelphia, 1973, WB Saunders.)*

The Amygdala Projects to the Cerebral Cortex and Hypothalamus

Fibers also leave the amygdala through the stria terminalis and the ventral amygdalofugal pathway to reach many of the same areas that send afferents to it (Fig. 23-21). Fibers in the ventral pathway pass underneath the lenticular nucleus and spread out to blanket the base of the brain, ending in the septal nuclei and the hypothalamus, olfactory regions such as the anterior olfactory nucleus, the anterior perforated substance and piriform cortex, and the orbital and anterior cingulate cortices. Some reach the **ventral striatum,** which includes the area of fusion of the putamen and the head of the caudate nucleus (the nucleus accumbens [see Figs. 19-2 and 19-5]), together with adjacent portions of the striatum. The ventral striatum in turn projects to an extension of the globus pallidus, the **ventral pallidum,** beneath the anterior commissure (Fig. 23-22). The ventral striatum and pallidum are links in a basal ganglia circuit similar to that involved in motor functions. In this case, however, the inputs to the basal ganglia are from limbic structures such as the amygdala and hippocampus; the outputs relay in the dorsomedial nucleus of the thalamus rather than the ventral anterior–ventral lateral nuclear complex and influence prefrontal and orbital frontal cortex. This limbic connection with the basal ganglia is presumably a route through which drive-related information can influence decisions about movement, and it apparently functions more generally in the neural circuitry that makes associations between stimuli and rewards (Fig. 23-23); virtually anything that is expected to be pleasurable causes increased release of dopamine in the ventral striatum by way of projections from the ventral tegmental area (see Fig. 11-26). Many ventral amygdalofugal fibers turn dorsally in the diencephalon and reach the dorsomedial nucleus of the thalamus. Finally, some amygdalar efferents enter neither the stria terminalis nor the ventral pathway but rather pass directly to extensive cortical areas in the temporal lobe and beyond. Some reach the hippocampus and related cortical areas. Others extend all the way to primary sensory areas.

The Amygdala Is Involved in Emotion-Related Aspects of Learning

The connections of the amygdala suit it perfectly for linking the perception of objects and situations with appropriate emotional responses, particularly but not solely in times of danger. Inputs from unimodal areas and the thalamus inform it of the nature of things in the

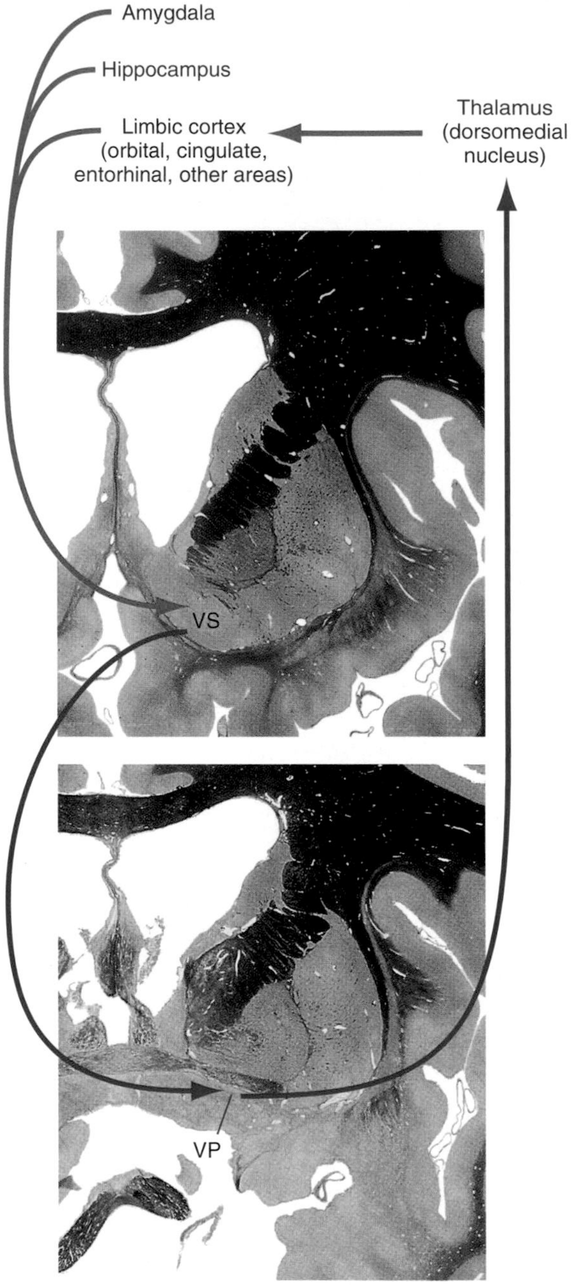

Amygdala

Hippocampus

Limbic cortex
(orbital, cingulate,
entorhinal, other areas)

Thalamus
(dorsomedial
nucleus)

VS

VP

Figure 23-22 Overview of the limbic loop through the basal ganglia. Only major connections are indicated, although others are known. For example, there are direct projections from the ventral striatum to the hypothalamus and amygdala. Excitatory connections are shown in green, inhibitory connections in red. VP, ventral pallidum; VS, ventral striatum.

outside world, and inputs from places such as limbic cortex and the hypothalamus inform it about the current physiological and emotional state (Box 23-2; Fig. 23-24). Outputs to the ventral striatum, hypothalamus, and brainstem initiate emotional responses; those to limbic cortex contribute to emotional experience; and those to sensory cortical areas heighten awareness when that would be advantageous.

Recognition of Emotion Without Awareness*

Everyone has probably had the experience of feeling uncomfortable without knowing why, hinting that maybe the pathways leading to conscious awareness are partially independent of the pathways leading to emotional responses. Some patients with prosopagnosia (see Box 17-2), for example, have measurable autonomic responses to some familiar faces, despite no conscious recognition of them.

The role of the amygdala in these emotional responses was demonstrated in the case of an unfortunate 52-year-old physician who had a stroke affecting the left occipital lobe and parts of the left parietal and temporal lobes (see Fig. 23-24). Initially he had signs of right-sided weakness and fluent aphasia, which soon resolved, but he was left with right homonymous hemianopia (see Fig. 17-33). Thirty-six days later he had a second stroke, this one affecting the right occipital lobe. When tested several months later, "he could not detect movement or colors, or even the presence of a strong light source. He was unable to identify any geometric shapes or objects—large or small—in the visual modality alone, and had to rely on hearing and touch in his everyday activities." Despite being cortically blind, when asked to "guess," he was often able to distinguish the emotional expressions in pictures of faces (angry, sad, or frightened vs. happy), even though he was unable to distinguish between other kinds of pictures. While he looked at pictures of angry, sad, or frightened faces (but not happy faces), blood flow, measured by fMRI, increased in his right amygdala (see Fig. 23-24).

*Based on Pegna AJ et al: Nat Neurosci 8:24, 2005.

The role of the amygdala in subjective feelings (presumably involving interactions with both ventromedial prefrontal cortex and the hypothalamus) has been demonstrated in numerous studies. When an animal's amygdala is stimulated, it most often stops whatever it was doing and becomes very attentive. This may be followed by responses of defense, raging aggression, or fleeing. Amygdalar stimulation in humans can cause a variety of emotions, but the most common is fear, accompanied by all its normal autonomic manifestations (e.g., dilation of the pupils, release of adrenaline, increased heart rate). Conversely, bilateral destruction of the amygdala causes a great decrease in aggression, and as a result, such animals are tame and placid. This is part of a distinctive kind of memory deficit, one that impairs the ability to learn or remember the appropriate emotional and autonomic responses to stimuli. Our brains are genetically programmed to find some things pleasurable (e.g., sweet

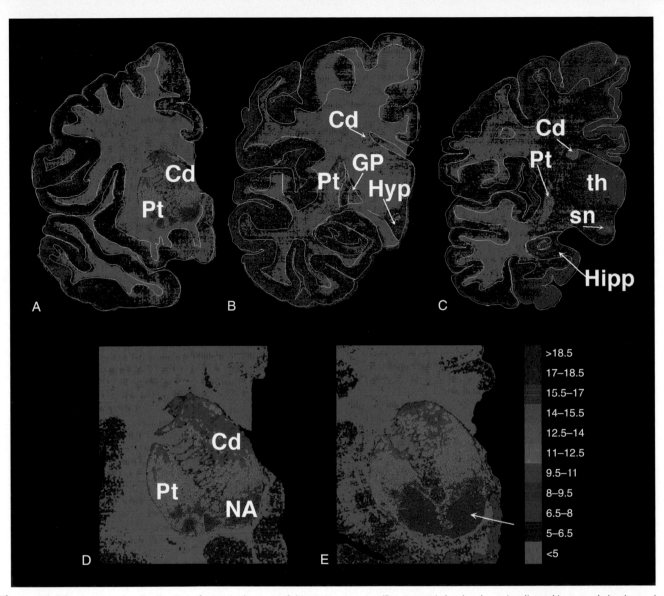

Figure 23-23 Mapping the distribution of a particular type of dopamine receptor (D_3 receptor) that has been implicated in reward circuitry, using a radioactive ligand. In coronal sections of normal brain (**A** to **D**) the receptor is preferentially localized in the ventral striatum, particularly the nucleus accumbens (NA). In the brain of a chronic cocaine user who died of a cocaine overdose **(E)**, this preferential distribution is even more pronounced. The color bar at the lower right shows the color coding of receptor density, measured as radioligand binding (fmol/mg). Cd, caudate nucleus; GP, globus pallidus; Hipp, hippocampus; Hyp, hypothalamus; Pt, putamen; sn, substantia nigra; th, thalamus. *(From Staley JK, Mash DC: J Neurosci 16:6100, 1996.)*

tastes, gentle stroking), but throughout life we all learn to associate other things with pleasure or pain, with good or bad outcomes. (Here in the Southwest, for example, the sight of a scorpion or a snake causes automatic sympathetic responses.) Amygdalar damage prevents the acquisition of these response patterns. Similar emotional responses are a part of social interactions. We ordinarily feel bad when we watch or even think about the suffering of others, for example, and some of the same circuitry involved in subjective pain has been implicated in this reaction (Fig. 23-25). The interplay between cognition and emotions plays an important role in decision making (see Box 22-4), and this is a

two-way street: interactions between dorsolateral and ventromedial prefrontal cortex are involved in the conscious control of emotions (Fig. 23-26).

Finally, there is obvious survival value in remembering the circumstances of pleasurable and painful events, and the amygdala plays a role in this as well. The hippocampus is centrally involved in the formation of memories of facts and events (see Chapter 24), and projections from the basolateral amygdala to the hippocampus (see Fig. 23-21) help determine *which* facts and events will be committed to memory. It is a common experience that facts or events associated with strong emotions are more likely to be remembered. (For

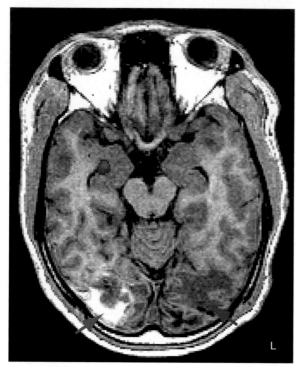

Figure 23-24 Axial MRI scan of the 52-year-old physician described in Box 23-2, showing damaged areas in the left *(red arrow)* and right *(green arrow)* occipital lobes and increased blood flow in the right amygdala as he looked at pictures of angry, sad, or frightened faces. *(From Pegna AJ et al: Nat Neurosci 8:24, 2005.)*

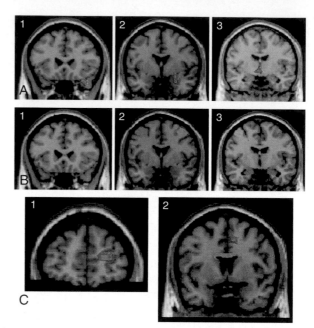

Figure 23-26 Regulation of emotions by conscious effort involves both dorsolateral and ventromedial prefrontal cortex. Ten young male subjects (average age 23.5 years) watched erotic films in two different conditions. In one **(A)** they were instructed to relax and react normally, and in the other **(B)** they were instructed to suppress any sexual feelings. Subjects in the first condition reported sexual arousal, and fMRI demonstrated increased blood flow in the right temporal pole **(A1)**, right amygdala **(A2)**, and hypothalamus **(A3)**. Subjects in the second condition reported much lower levels of sexual arousal, and fMRI demonstrated no increased blood flow in any of these areas **(B1-3)**. However, in the second condition, blood flow did increase in the right dorsolateral prefrontal **(C1)** and anterior cingulate **(C2)** cortex. *(From Beauregard M, Lévesque J, Bourgouin P: J Neurosci 21:RC165, 2001.)*

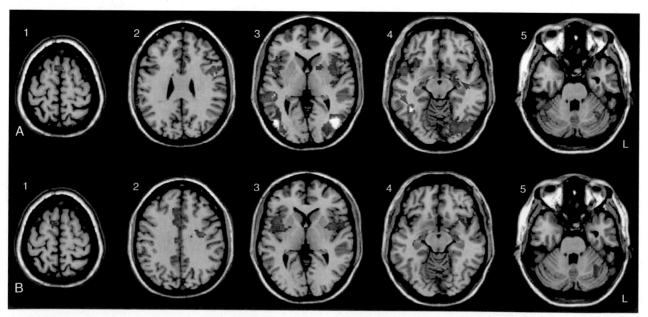

Figure 23-25 Areas of increased blood flow, measured by fMRI, in subjects watching videotapes of the faces of patients in pain **(A)** and themselves receiving a painfully hot stimulus **(B)**. In both conditions, there was activation of medial prefrontal cortex **(A1-2, B1-2)** and the insula **(A3, B3)**. Only when watching the faces of others in pain was there activation of the face-recognition area in the right occipitotemporal gyrus **(A4,** *green arrow)* and the left amygdala **(A4,** *red arrow)*. The lateral cerebellum was also activated in both conditions **(A5, B5)**, consistent with this structure's role in more than just movement (see Chapter 20). *(From Botvinick M et al: Neuroimage 25:312, 2005.)*

example, most Americans who were old enough at the time can easily recall where they were and what they were doing when John F. Kennedy was assassinated or when the space shuttle *Challenger* exploded or when the twin towers in New York City fell.)

Bilateral Temporal Lobe Damage Causes a Complex, Devastating Syndrome

One classic technique for studying the function of a structure is to remove it or destroy it and then see what happens. Removing the temporal lobe back to the level of primary auditory cortex should certainly incapacitate the limbic system to a great extent, because the amygdala and most of the hippocampus and parahippocampal gyrus would be lost. When this is done to animals bilaterally, the following constellation of deficits results (called the **Klüver-Bucy syndrome** for the investigators who first described it).

1. The animals are fearless and placid, showing an absence of emotional reactions. They do not respond to threats, to social gestures by other animals, or to objects they would normally flee from or attack.
2. Male animals become hypersexual and are impressively indiscriminate in their choice of sex partners. They are likely to mount other animals of the same gender, animals of whatever species may be available, or inanimate objects.
3. They show an inordinate degree of attention to all sensory stimuli, as though ceaselessly curious. They respond to every object within sight or reach by sniffing it and examining it orally. If the object can in any sense be considered edible, they eat it. Partly because of this, they eat much more than normal animals.
4. Although they incessantly examine all objects in sight, these animals recognize nothing and may pick up the same thing over and over. This was called "psychic blindness" by Klüver and Bucy and would now be called *visual agnosia*.

The Klüver-Bucy syndrome has been fractionated to some extent: the placidity and hypersexuality result from destruction of the amygdala, and the visual agnosia from damage to visual association areas on the inferior surface of the temporal lobe. The composite syndrome is tremendously detrimental.[h] Leaving aside the visual agnosia, it is as though all the behavior patterns central to satisfying basic drives are intact, but the animal can no longer tell when and in what context to use them.

---

[h]"A monkey which approaches every enemy to examine it orally will conceivably not survive longer than a few hours if turned loose in a region with a plentiful supply of enemies. We doubt that a monkey would be seriously hampered under natural conditions, in the wild, by a loss of its prefrontal region, its parietal lobes or its occipital lobes, as long as small portions of the striate cortex remained intact." (Klüver H, Bucy PC: Arch Neurol Psychiatry 42:979, 1939.)

SUGGESTED READINGS

Adams JH, Daniel PM, Prichard MML: Observations on the portal circulation of the pituitary gland. Neuroendocrinology 1:193, 1965–66.

Allen LS, et al: Two sexually dimorphic cell groups in the human brain. J Neurosci 9:497, 1989.
  Both are contained in the preoptic anterior hypothalamus, a region known to be involved in the production of gonadotropin-releasing factor.

Andy OJ, Stephan H: The septum in the human brain. J Comp Neurol 133:383, 1968.
  There is a tendency to think of the septal area as small and rudimentary in humans, but this paper argues that in fact it reaches its highest development in us.

Antunes-Rodrigues J, et al: Neuroendocrine control of body fluid metabolism. Physiol Rev 84:169, 2004.

Beauregard M, Lévesque J, Bourgouin P: Neural correlates of conscious self-regulation of emotion. J Neurosci 21:RC165, 2001.

Benarroch EE: Thermoregulation: recent concepts and remaining questions. Neurology 69:1293, 2007.

Bergland RM, Page RB: Pituitary-brain vascular relations: a new paradigm. Science 204:18, 1979.
  Results that indicate that the pituitary portal system may not be so straightforward; for example, it may at times function in reverse, transporting adenohypophyseal hormones to the brain.

Blessing WW: Lower brain stem regulation of visceral, cardiovascular, and respiratory function. In Paxinos G, Mai JK, editors: The human nervous system, ed 2, San Diego, 2004, Elsevier Academic Press.

Botvinick M, et al: Viewing facial expressions of pain engages cortical areas involved in the direct experience of pain. Neuroimage 25:312, 2005.

Braak H, Braak E: The hypothalamus of the human adult: chiasmatic region. Anat Embryol 175:315, 1987.

Carrive P, Morgan MM: Periaqueductal gray. In Paxinos G, Mai JK, editors: The human nervous system, ed 2, San Diego, 2004, Elsevier Academic Press.

Craig AD: How do you feel? Interoception: the sense of the physiological condition of the body. Nat Rev Neurosci 3:655, 2002.

DeGroat WC: Integrative control of the lower urinary tract: preclinical perspective. Br J Pharmacol 147(Suppl2):S25, 2006.

Dierickx K: Immunocytochemical localization of the vertebrate cyclic nonapeptide neurohypophyseal hormones and neurophysins. Int Rev Cytol 62:120, 1980.

Duvernoy HM: The human hippocampus: functional anatomy, vascularization and serial sections with MRI, ed 3, Berlin, 2005, Springer-Verlag.
  A meticulously detailed and beautifully illustrated book.

Fry M, Ferguson AV: The sensory circumventricular organs: brain targets for circulating signals controlling ingestive behavior. Physiol Behav 91:413, 2007.

Gaffan D, Murray EA: Amygdalar interaction with the mediodorsal nucleus of the thalamus and the ventromedial prefrontal cortex in stimulus-reward associative learning in the monkey. J Neurosci 10:3479, 1990.

Gao Q, Horvath TL: Neurobiology of feeding and energy expenditure. Annu Rev Neurosci 30:367, 2007.

Guillemin R: Peptides in the brain: the new endocrinology of the neuron. Science 202:390, 1978.

Hamann SB, et al: Amygdala activity related to enhanced memory for pleasant and aversive stimuli. Nat Neurosci 2:289, 1999.

Hardy JD, Hellon RF, Sutherland K: Temperature-sensitive neurones in the dog's hypothalamus. J Physiol 175:242, 1964.

Heimer L, Van Hoesen GW: The limbic lobe and its output channels: implications for emotional functions and adaptive behavior. Neurosci Biobehav Rev 30:126, 2006.
  A beautifully illustrated recent review.

Hofman MA, Zhou J-N, Swaab DF: Suprachiasmatic nucleus of the human brain: immunocytochemical and morphometric analysis. Anat Rec 244:552, 1996.

Holstege G: Micturition and the soul. J Comp Neurol 493:15, 2005.

Holstege G, Mouton LJ, Gerrits NM: Emotional motor system. In Paxinos G, Mai JK, editors: The human nervous system, ed 2, San Diego, 2004, Elsevier Academic Press.

Jänig W: The integrative action of the autonomic nervous system: neurobiology of homeostasis, Cambridge, 2006, Cambridge University Press.

Katter JT, Burstein R, Giesler GJ, Jr: The cells of origin of the spino-hypothalamic tract in cats. J Comp Neurol 303:101, 1991.

Kavia RBC, DasGupta R, Fowler CJ: Functional imaging and the central control of the bladder. J Comp Neurol 493:27, 2005.

Klüver H, Bucy PC: Preliminary analysis of functions of the temporal lobes in monkeys. Arch Neurol Psychiatry 42:979, 1939.
  Still interesting reading.

Kosfield M, et al: Oxytocin increases trust in humans. Nature 435: 673, 2005.
  A fascinating look at the participation of neuropeptide pathways in social interactions.

Koutcherov Y, et al: Organization of the human paraventricular hypothalamic nucleus. J Comp Neurol 423:299, 2000.

Kringelbach ML, Rolls ET: The functional neuroanatomy of the human orbitofrontal cortex: evidence from neuroimaging and neuropsychology. Prog Neurobiol 72:341, 2004.

LeDoux JE, Romanski L, Xagoraris A: Indelibility of subcortical emotional memories. J Cog Neurosci 1:238, 1989.
  Work on the role of the amygdala in learning the emotional significance of stimuli.

Levin BE: Why some of us get fat and what we can do about it. J Physiol 583:425, 2007.

Lilly R, et al: The human Klüver-Bucy syndrome. Neurology 33: 1141, 1983.

Machne X, Segundo JP: Unitary responses to afferent volleys in amygdaloid complex. J Neurophysiol 19:232, 1956.
  Single cells that respond equally well to a brief shock to the sciatic nerve and to a whiff of something.

Malamud N: Psychiatric disorder with intracranial tumors of limbic system. Arch Neurol 17:113, 1967.

Middleton JW, Keast JR: Artificial autonomic reflexes: using functional electrical stimulation to mimic bladder reflexes after injury or disease. Autonom Neurosci 113:3, 2004.
  Using anatomical details to devise ways to improve bladder function after spinal cord injury.

Mosko SS, Moore RY: Neonatal suprachiasmatic nucleus lesions: effects on the development of circadian rhythms in the rat. Brain Res 164:17, 1979.

Nagashima K, et al: Neuronal circuitries involved in thermoregulation. Autonom Neurosci 85:18, 2000.

Nakamura K, Morrison SF: A thermosensory pathway that controls body temperature. Nature Neurosci 11:62, 2008.

Nathan PW, Smith MC: The location of descending fibres to sympathetic neurons supplying the eye and sudomotor neurons supplying the head and neck. J Neurol Neurosurg Psychiatry 49:187, 1986.

Olausson H, et al: Unmyelinated tactile afferents signal touch and project to insular cortex. Nat Neurosci 5:900, 2002.

Papez JW: A proposed mechanism of emotion. Arch Neurol Psychiatry 38:725, 1937.
  The evidence was not very strong by today's standards, but the idea has been extremely influential anyway.

Pegna AJ, et al: Discriminating emotional faces without primary visual cortices involves the right amygdala. Nat Neurosci 8:24, 2005.

Reeves AG, Plum F: Hyperphagia, rage, and dementia accompanying a ventromedial hypothalamic neoplasm. Arch Neurol 20:616, 1969.

Reiman EM, et al: Neuroanatomical correlates of anticipatory anxiety. Science 243:1071, 1989.
  Positron emission tomography studies implicating the anterior ends of the temporal lobes in the neural circuitry underlying feelings of fear and anxiety.

Ressler KJ, Mayberg HS: Targeting abnormal neural circuits in mood and anxiety disorders: from the laboratory to the clinic. Nat Neurosci 10:1116, 2007.
  Emerging uses of deep brain stimulation, transcranial magnetic stimulation, and related techniques to treat psychiatric disorders.

Rolls ET: The brain and emotion, New York, 2000, Oxford University Press.

Rosene DL, van Hoesen GW: Hippocampal efferents reach widespread areas of cerebral cortex and amygdala in the rhesus monkey. Science 198:315, 1977.

Sack RL, et al: Entrainment of free-running circadian rhythms by melatonin in blind people. N Engl J Med 343:1070, 2000.

Salloway S, Malloy P, Cummings JL, editors: The neuropsychiatry of limbic and subcortical disorders, Washington, DC, 1997, American Psychiatric Press.

Saper CB: The central autonomic nervous system: conscious visceral perception and autonomic pattern generation. Annu Rev Neurosci 25:433, 2002.

Saper CB: Hypothalamus. In Paxinos G, Mai JK, editors: The human nervous system, ed 2, San Diego, 2004, Elsevier Academic Press.

Schoenbaum G, et al, editors: Linking affect to action: critical contributions of the orbitofrontal cortex. Ann NY Acad Sci 1121:2007.

Sims KS, Williams RS: The human amygdaloid complex: a cytologic and histochemical atlas using Nissl, myelin, acetylcholinesterase and nicotinamide adenine dinucleotide phosphate diaphorase staining. Neuroscience 36:449, 1990.

Swaab DF, et al: Functional neuroanatomy and neuropathology of the human hypothalamus. Anat Embryol 187:317, 1993.

van Esseveldt LKE, Lehman MN, Boer GJ: The suprachiasmatic nucleus and the circadian time-keeping system revisited. Brain Res Rev 33:34, 2000.

Wasman M, Flynn JP: Directed attack elicited from hypothalamus. Arch Neurol 6:220, 1962.

Young JK, Stanton GB: A three-dimensional reconstruction of the human hypothalamus. Brain Res Bull 35:323, 1994.

Zald DH: The human amygdala and the emotional evaluation of sensory stimuli. Brain Res Rev 41:88, 2003.

Zhu J-N, et al: The cerebellar-hypothalamic circuits: potential pathways underlying cerebellar involvement in somatic-visceral integration. Brain Res Rev 52:93, 2006.

Formation, Modification, and Repair of Neuronal Connections

Previous chapters may have made it sound as if the parts of the nervous system are interconnected in rigid, immutable ways, but this is far from accurate. The details of the nervous system are much too complex to be completely laid out genetically. Instead, only the general layout of the nervous system is specified genetically; later stages of development are a time of great **plasticity,** in which neurons and their connections are adjusted extensively to match the nervous system to the body and the world in which it lives. The peril of this high level of developmental plasticity is the potential production of permanent neural abnormalities if something is wrong with the environment.

Once the matching process is complete, plasticity is reduced but not abolished; ongoing adjustments of connections and synaptic strength underlie processes such as learning and memory. This relative stability of the mature nervous system carries a complementary peril: a limited ability to repair itself after disease or injury. However, experimental methods of enhancing

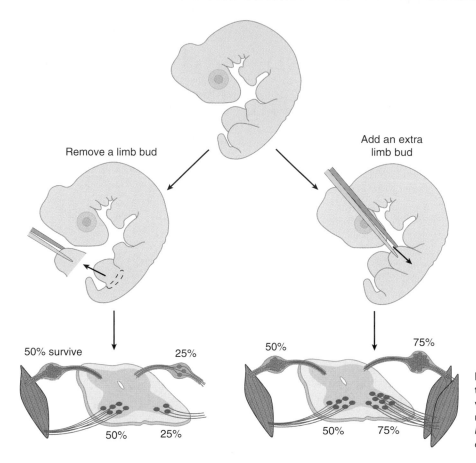

Remove a limb bud

Add an extra limb bud

50% survive   25%

50%   25%

50%   75%

50%   75%

Figure 24-1 Effect of removing or adding target tissue during development on the survival of dorsal root ganglion cells and lower motor neurons. *(Redrawn from Sanes DH, Reh TA, Harris WA: Development of the nervous system, ed 2, San Diego, 2005, Academic Press.)*

the remaining plasticity, or of reactivating the processes at work during development, are beginning to offer promising approaches to treatment.

Both Neurons and Connections Are Produced in Excess During Development

The central nervous system (CNS) develops from the neural tube as a series of modules, each supplying the neurons and connections needed for particular functions. The result is most apparent in the spinal cord, where individual segments contain the motor neurons, interneurons, and primary afferent connections for specific regions of the body (see Figs. 10-1 and 10-4). Comparable modules come into play in other parts of the CNS, including brainstem segments with particular sets of cranial nerve nuclei and forebrain zones that provide particular sets of neurons.

The final number of neurons, and the number and pattern of connections of these neurons, varies from one module to another. Again, this is most apparent in the spinal cord, where different segments wind up with, for example, different numbers of lower motor neurons or different populations of autonomic motor neurons (see Fig. 10-8). The initially surprising mechanism accounting for these level-to-level differences is that each

module produces an excess of neurons, and each of these neurons makes more widespread connections than are necessary. The matching process is one of winnowing the surplus neurons and retracting inappropriate connections.

Neurotrophic Factors Ensure That Adequate Numbers of Neurons Survive

Early experiments with chicks showed that the number of embryonically produced dorsal root ganglion cells, lower motor neurons, and autonomic ganglion cells that survive into adulthood depends on the amount of target tissue with which these neurons interact during development (Fig. 24-1). The basis of this effect is **neurotrophic factors**[a] that are produced in limited quantities by target tissues, taken up by peripheral nerve endings, and transported retrogradely to neuronal cell bodies. Neurons compete for these factors during development, and those that acquire sufficient quantities survive. One

---

[a]*Trophic* comes from a Greek word meaning "nourishment," reflecting initial assumptions that neurotrophic factors had growth-promoting functions. They actually work by preventing the activation of programmed cell death (apoptosis), in which specific degradative enzymes are synthesized and proceed to disassemble affected neurons.

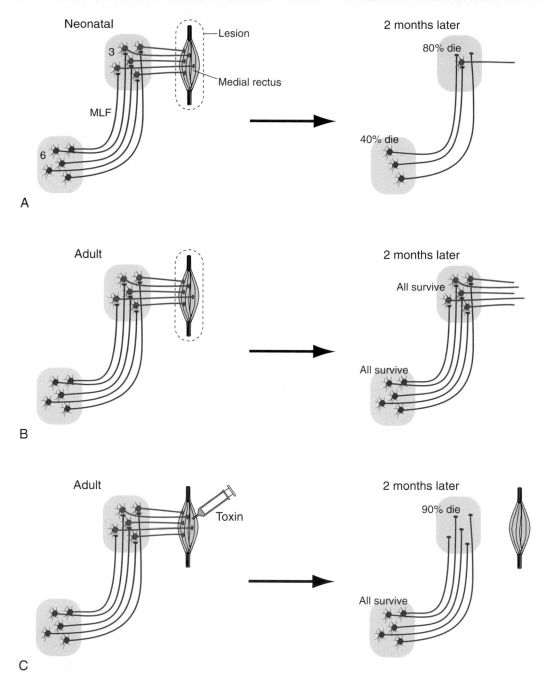

Figure 24-2 The precise and nearly exclusive projection of internuclear neurons in the abducens nucleus (6) to medial rectus motor neurons in the oculomotor nucleus (3; see Fig. 12-9) provides a convenient means to test the dependence of these internuclear neurons on their postsynaptic targets. **A,** Unilateral removal of the medial rectus (together with the terminals of medial rectus motor neurons) from a neonatal rat results in death of most medial rectus motor neurons. This in turn reduces the supply of neurotrophic factors to internuclear neurons, and many of them die. **B,** Adult neurons are less dependent on trophic factors for their survival, so the same medial rectus removal from an adult rat does not result in the death of any motor neurons (although they go through a period of metabolic changes in the weeks following the lesion; see Fig. 24-27). Internuclear neurons also survive, but this could be due to survival of motor neurons or to decreased dependence on trophic factors. **C,** Injection of an adult medial rectus with a cytotoxic lectin (ricin) results in death of almost all medial rectus motor neurons. Internuclear neurons still survive, consistent with decreased dependence on trophic factors. MLF, medial longitudinal fasciculus. *(Based on Morcuende S et al: Exp Neurol 195:244, 2005.)*

result of normal development is that thoracic spinal segments, with less tissue to innervate and a smaller supply of trophic factors, lose more motor neurons and other neurons than do cervical segments. Trophic interactions are not limited to neurons with processes in peripheral nerves (Fig. 24-2A), and throughout the nervous system, roughly half of all newborn neurons die.

A host of neurotrophic factors have now been characterized. **Nerve growth factor (NGF),** the first discovered and most famous, is part of a family of small proteins called **neurotrophins.** Other members include **brain-derived neurotrophic factor (BDNF), neurotrophic factor-3 (NT-3),** and **neurotrophic factor-4/5 (NT-4/5).** The neurotrophins act primarily on neurons, but many other neurotrophic factors are active in both the nervous system and other parts of the body. For example, the glial cell line derived trophic factors (GDNF) play important roles in glial and neuronal development and survival, with recent studies demonstrating the importance of GDNF and the survival of dopamine neurons in models of Parkinson's disease. Different types of peripheral nervous system (PNS) neurons depend on particular neurotrophins or combinations of neurotrophins for their early survival. For example, sympathetic ganglion cells and dorsal root ganglion cells with free nerve endings are especially sensitive to NGF, vestibular ganglion neurons to BDNF, and spiral ganglion neurons to NT-3. Most CNS neurons are less selective and respond to multiple neurotrophic factors, although there are exceptions (e.g., the cholinergic neurons of the basal nucleus [see Fig. 11-28] are especially sensitive to NGF).

Axonal Branches Are Pruned to Match Functional Requirements

Later in development, neurotrophic factors cease to be essential for the survival of many neurons (see Fig. 24-2B and C) but continue to have a major role in determining which dendrites and axon branches flourish while determining which wither and retract. Immature neurons are considerably more promiscuous in both receiving and making synaptic connections than are adult neurons. Some are as seemingly peculiar as neurons in the occipital lobe that project to the spinal cord, or other cortical neurons with one branch that traverses the corpus callosum and another that enters the internal capsule. In a series of activity-dependent processes that mostly begin after the period of cell death and extend well beyond birth, connections that contribute less effectively to function are withdrawn; for the most part, connections at which there is correlated presynaptic and postsynaptic activity are retained, and others are pruned away. (This is not to say that the total number of *synapses* decreases. The surviving connections become more complex and elaborate, and the total number of synapses increases.)

One well-studied example is the innervation of skeletal muscle fibers by motor neurons (Fig. 24-3). The neuromuscular junction of each skeletal muscle fiber is initially innervated during fetal life by terminal branches of two or more motor neurons. Starting at about midgestation (after the period of naturally occurring motor neuron death is over), some of these terminal branches begin to withdraw, and the remaining branches expand to take over the vacated territory. Near the time of birth,

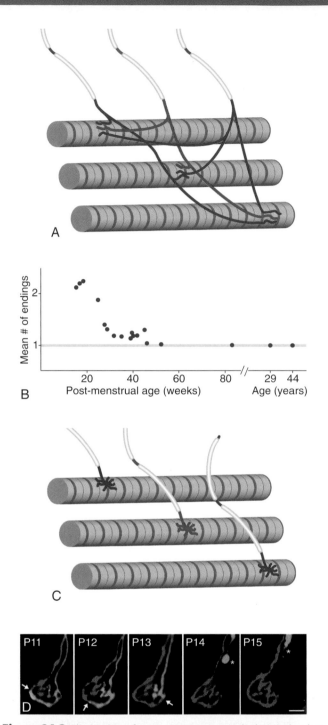

Figure 24-3 Elimination of motor neuron terminals during development. **A,** Through midgestation, most muscle fibers are innervated by terminals of multiple motor neurons. **B,** The average number of axon terminals innervating each human psoas muscle fiber at different perinatal ages (normal term is about 40 postmenstrual weeks), compared with two adults. **C,** The final adult configuration, achieved by a few weeks after birth. **D,** Direct demonstration of one motor axon displacing another over the course of 4 days, beginning 11 days postnatally (P11). Mice were genetically engineered to express two different fluorescent proteins in the axons of different motor neurons, and the same sternocleidomastoid neuromuscular junction was examined repeatedly. Red fluorescence indicates acetylcholine receptors in the postjunctional membrane underlying the axon terminals. The green axon takes over the territory of the blue axon for a couple of days *(arrows),* then the blue axon retreats (*). (**B,** redrawn from Gramsbergen A et al: Early Hum Dev 49:49, 1997. **D,** from Walsh MK, Lichtman JW: Neuron 37:67, 2003.)

each muscle fiber is left with a singly innervated neuromuscular junction.

Similar elimination of axonal branches is widespread in the CNS. Two thirds of the axons in the corpus callosum of a newborn monkey, for example, die off during the first few months of life; those that survive acquire myelin sheaths and permanent connections. Something comparable undoubtedly happens in the human corpus callosum, although it probably extends over several years. Likewise, there is an excess of corticospinal axons at birth, including large numbers of uncrossed projections that retract over a period of years (Fig. 24-4); most of these are probably branches of neurons whose functionally most important connections lie elsewhere, as in the temporary occipital corticospinal projections referred to earlier. The process leading to innervation of individual cerebellar Purkinje cells in adults by single climbing fibers (see Figs. 20-13, 20-14, and 20-20) provides another example (Fig. 24-5), this one analogous to the development of singly innervated neuromuscular junctions. Each immature Purkinje cell receives limited synaptic inputs from multiple climbing fibers; all but one retract, and the remaining climbing fiber extends over the proximal dendrites and forms a much more powerful distributed synapse.

Pruning of Neuronal Connections Occurs During Critical Periods

The time available for matching CNS connections to the environment is normally limited to a series of **critical periods** during which plasticity is maximal; the wiring patterns achieved during these periods are more or less permanent. This has been studied most extensively in primary visual cortex, where changes in the systematic organization of hypercolumns (see Fig. 17-35) can be examined in detail. Lateral geniculate neurons receive input from just one eye (see Fig. 17-27C) and pass it along to neurons in layer IV of the primary occipital cortex (see Fig. 17-35C). Outputs from layer IV then converge on neurons in other layers, with the result that most of these neurons respond, at least to some extent, to inputs from both eyes (Fig. 24-6A); this is the beginning of binocular vision and depth perception. Covering one eye of an adult cat for long periods causes no change in these properties of cortical neurons. In striking contrast, however, covering one eye for the first 2 to 3 months of life results in nearly all cells being responsive only to the eye that had not been covered (see Fig. 24-6B). This is a permanent effect associated specifically with early deprivation; leaving the previously deprived eye uncovered does not restore its ability to activate cortical neurons. Clear functional deficits accompany these physiological changes. Although the pupillary light reflex is normal, the animal behaves as though blind when using the previously covered eye. Segregated monocular inputs to layer IV are present at birth in humans and

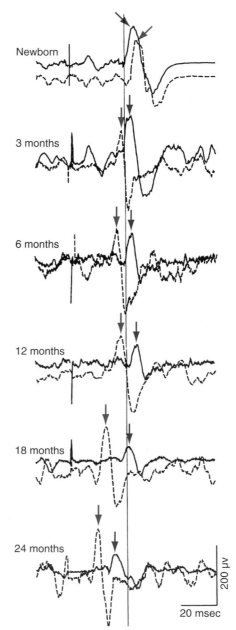

Figure 24-4 Mass electrical activity (electromyogram) of the right *(dashed traces, green arrows)* and left *(solid traces, blue arrows)* biceps in response to transcranial magnetic stimulation (see Box 22-4) of left motor cortex. All recordings were made from the same subject at different ages. The response of the biceps ipsilateral to the stimulated cortex slowly becomes smaller over a period of years, while the response of the contralateral biceps becomes larger and faster. *(From Eyre JA et al: Neurology 57:1543, 2001.)*

monkeys, and these compete with each other for synaptic sites (much like the competition for space at neuromuscular junctions). If one eye is occluded, as by an infantile cataract, inputs from the other eye expand in layer IV to take over its territory; the result is **amblyopia** (Greek for "dim vision"), in which vision is poor in that eye despite a normal retina.

Competition between the two eyes is also revealed if the two eyes are not normally aligned early in life (see

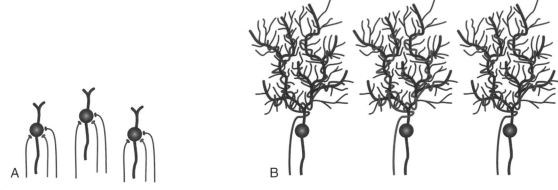

Figure 24-5 **A,** Purkinje cells initially receive simple synapses on their cell bodies from multiple olivary axons that will later become climbing fibers. **B,** As the elaborate Purkinje cell dendritic tree develops, all but one olivary axon branch withdraws from each. The remaining branch forms that Purkinje cell's single climbing fiber.

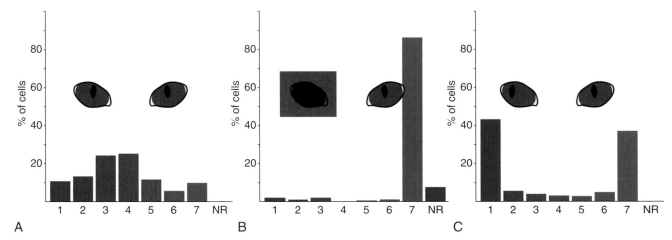

Figure 24-6 Critical period for binocular interactions in primary visual cortex. **A,** Normal binocular sensitivity of neurons in the primary visual cortex of adult cats. The neurons were divided into seven groups, depending on how exclusively they responded to one eye or the other. Neurons in groups 1 and 7 responded only to light in the contralateral or ipsilateral eye, respectively; group 4 responded equally well to light in either eye. Few or no neurons were unresponsive to light (NR). **B,** After opening an eye that had been covered for the first 2 to 3 months of life, almost no cortical neurons responded to it. **C,** After strabismus during the critical period (caused by cutting the medial rectus in one eye), nearly all cortical neurons responded to one eye or the other, but not both. (**A,** *replotted from Wiesel TN, Hubel DH: J Neurophysiol 26:1003, 1963.* **B,** *replotted from Wiesel TN, Hubel DH: J Neurophysiol 28:1029, 1965.* **C,** *replotted from Hubel DH, Wiesel TN: J Neurophysiol 28:1041, 1965.*)

Fig. 24-6C), thus disrupting the correlated visual information that ordinarily reaches cortical neurons from the two eyes. The input from one eye or the other then takes over at almost all cortical neurons; binocular vision and depth perception are impaired permanently.

Experience-dependent plasticity during critical periods is also found in the auditory and somatosensory systems. Similarly, prevention of limb use during early life (presumably analogous to covering an eye) leads to abnormal development of corticospinal terminals in the spinal cord (Fig. 24-7). Normal terminals fail to develop later in life, and fine movement control continues to be impaired.

Critical periods extend to the acquisition of more complex skills as well. For example, children learn languages much more easily and successfully than adults do. This is a complicated process that starts early in life and extends into the teenage years. Very young infants

are able to discriminate among the speech sounds of all human languages. Starting at about 6 months of age, they get better at detecting different sounds heard from caregivers in their native language and start to lose the ability to discriminate among speech sounds they have not heard, that is, some sounds of nonnative languages (Fig. 24-8A). Much of this process is complete by 1 year of age and presumably corresponds to the refinement of synaptic connections someplace in auditory association cortex. Acquisition of more subtle aspects of language continues for years after this but does not go on indefinitely; learning a new language fluently is considerably more difficult after about age 16 (see Fig. 24-8B). Comparable phenomena are found with other complex skills. Six-month-old infants, for example, can distinguish equally well between a familiar face and a novel face, whether it belongs to a human or a monkey. Nine-month-old infants, like adults, are much better at

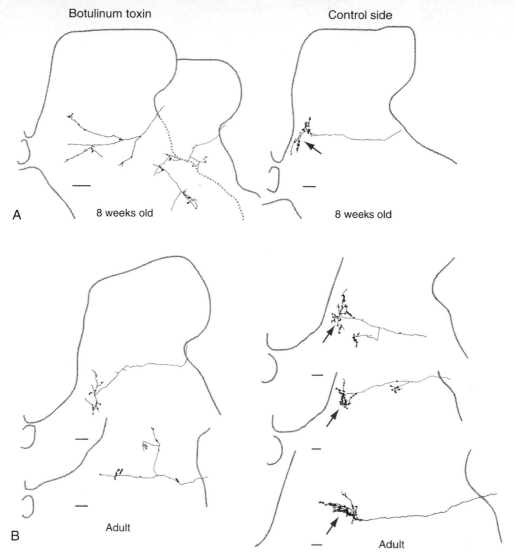

Figure 24-7 Critical period for the development of fine motor control. Use of one forelimb was prevented during weeks 3 to 7 of a kitten's life—the time when some corticospinal branches are retracted and others become much more elaborate—by injecting botulinum toxin (see Box 8-1) into the elbow flexors and extensors and the wrist flexors. Single corticospinal axons were then examined in the C8 segment. **A,** At 8 weeks, a week after the botulinum toxin had worn off, corticospinal axons on the previously paralyzed side had failed to develop the elaborate sprays of synaptic endings *(arrow)* seen on the normal side. **B,** The immature corticospinal endings persisted into adulthood. Scale bars = 100 μm. *(From Martin JH et al: J Neurosci 24:2122, 2004.)*

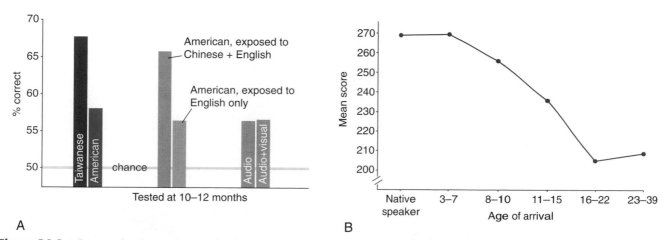

Figure 24-8 Influence of early exposure on the development of language skills. **A,** Ability of 10- to 12-month-old infants to distinguish Chinese speech sounds, as measured by a head-turning test. By this age, American infants exposed only to English are less able to distinguish such sounds than are Taiwanese infants exposed only to Chinese (left bars). Middle bars, It does not take a lot of experience to preserve the ability to distinguish sounds in any language. Exposing American infants to Chinese speakers 12 times for 25 minutes/session while they were 9 months old prevents this decline in ability to distinguish Chinese speech sounds. Right bars, Preserving speech-discrimination ability appears to require not just sound exposure but also social interaction. Listening to recordings of the same Chinese speakers, or watching movies of them with sound, fails to prevent the decline in ability. **B,** Scores on an English grammar test by 46 native Korean or Chinese speakers who had arrived in the United States at various ages from 3 to 39 years. Scores declined as the age of arrival increased, until leveling off in the late teenage years. *(A, replotted from Kuhl PK, Tsao F-M, Liu H-M: Proc Natl Acad Sci U S A 100:9096, 2003. B, replotted from Johnson JS, Newport EL: Cog Psychol 21:60, 1989.)*

distinguishing between human faces than monkey faces. There are at least hints of critical-period effects on virtually every human cognitive ability.

Critical periods draw to a close at different times in different parts of the brain (Fig. 24-9), in part due to the onset of processes that restrict the ability of the adult CNS to respond effectively to damage; these are described later in the chapter. Not surprisingly, the refinement of synapses in multimodal areas, which depend on inputs from unimodal areas, takes longest.

Synaptic Connections Are Adjusted Throughout Life

Developmental processes, including those that occur during critical periods, complete the basic wiring of the nervous system. However, synaptic connections continue to be adjusted, albeit on a smaller scale, throughout life. Some of the changes are short-term consequences of activity at most or all synapses, lasting milliseconds to minutes; others last years and are the basis for long-term processes such as learning and memory. Changes in presynaptic or postsynaptic Ca^{2+} concentrations play a key role in many of the mechanisms of synaptic modification.

There Are Short-Term and Long-Term Adjustments of Synaptic Strength

The voltage-gated Ca^{2+} channels essential for chemical synaptic transmission (see Fig. 8-6) permit the influx of Ca^{2+} faster than it can be sequestered. The result is a brief increase in presynaptic Ca^{2+} concentrations, of a

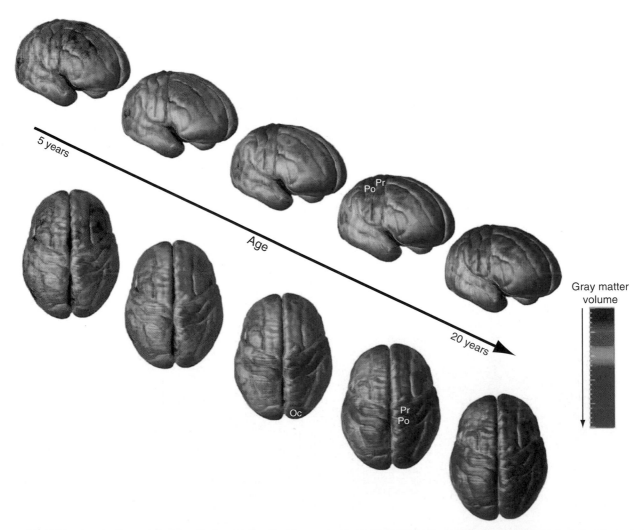

Figure 24-9 Mapping the time course of cortical maturation by using magnetic resonance imaging to measure the decrease in regional gray matter as an indicator of synaptic pruning. Each of 13 subjects was scanned four times at intervals of approximately 2 years, and the results were combined to follow changes over time. Primary areas such as motor, somatosensory, and visual cortex in the precentral (Pr) and postcentral (Po) gyri and the occipital lobe (Oc) mature first, and multimodal association areas in the parietal, frontal, and temporal lobes mature last. *(From Lenroot RK, Giedd JN: Neurosci Biobehav Rev 30:718, 2006.)*

size dictated by the frequency of invading action potentials. This in turn facilitates transmitter release and causes **potentiation** of transmission at that synapse—an increase in transmitter release in response to subsequent action potentials that abates within a few minutes. Other changes accompanying routine synaptic transmission can cause complementary short-term **depression,** also lasting minutes or less, through both presynaptic and postsynaptic mechanisms (Fig. 24-10A). High-frequency stimulation can cause depletion of vesicles and smaller subsequent releases; transmitter can bind to presynaptic **autoreceptors,** usually decreasing transmission; continued binding of transmitter generally makes postsynaptic receptors less sensitive for a little while (much as sensory receptors adapt to continued stimulation); and retrograde signals such as nitric oxide act briefly at many synapses.

More prolonged effects on synaptic strength, collectively called **long-term potentiation (LTP)** and **long-term depression (LTD),** can act through almost any part of a synapse (see Fig. 24-10B and C); these are the basis of the lasting changes that occur during critical periods and in learning and memory. The best known examples of each occur at the postsynaptic membranes of glutamate synapses on pyramidal and many other neurons,

where two different kinds of ionotropic receptors usually coexist. **AMPA receptors**[b] are typical ligand-gated channels that cause depolarization by allowing nonselective passage of Na^+ and K^+ ions. **NMDA receptors** are also ligand gated but have the additional property of being voltage sensitive (see Fig. 8-20); they open only if they bind glutamate *and* the membrane is already depolarized. In addition, NMDA receptors allow passage of not just Na^+ and K^+ but also Ca^{2+}. Collectively, these properties make NMDA receptors eminently suited to initiate activity-dependent changes in synaptic strength. In the presence of background depolarization—caused, for example, by high-frequency inputs, correlated activity at nearby synapses, or changes in modulatory inputs during increased attention—glutamate release results in not only further depolarization but also Ca^{2+} influx. Ca^{2+} influx in turn sets in motion intracellular signaling pathways that result in the phosphorylation of the AMPA channel that can modulate Na+ conductance but also

---

[b]Like NMDA receptors, AMPA receptors are named for a glutamate analog that they bind selectively. AMPA receptors bind α-amino-3-hydroxyl-5-methyl-4-isoxazole-propionate; NMDA receptors bind N-methyl-D-aspartate.

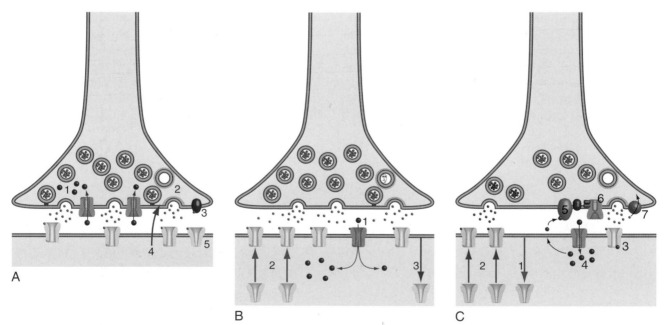

Figure 24-10 A sampling of the mechanisms involved in synaptic plasticity. **A,** Short-term enhancement is mediated by Ca^{2+} effects in presynaptic endings, such as residual Ca^{2+} increasing the likelihood of vesicle fusion (1). Short-term depression can be mediated presynaptically or postsynaptically by mechanisms including depletion of the supply of vesicles (2), binding of transmitter by presynaptic autoreceptors (3), retrograde signaling (4), and desensitization of postsynaptic receptors (5). **B,** Long-term potentiation (LTP) and long-term depression (LTD) at many glutamate synapses is initiated by Ca^{2+} entering through postsynaptic NMDA channels (1). Large amounts of Ca^{2+} entry cause more AMPA receptors to be inserted in the postsynaptic membrane (2), causing LTP; smaller amounts result in LTD by causing internalization of AMPA receptors (3). **C,** Several other mechanisms of long-term adjustments of synaptic strength—some Ca^{2+} dependent and others not—have been described. These include removal (1) and insertion (2) of GABA receptors, enzymatic modification of postsynaptic receptors (3), and retrograde signaling with longer-lasting effects. One prominent example of the last is endocannabinoid signaling, in which postsynaptic Ca^{2+} entry (4) causes the release of endocannabinoids that bind to presynaptic CB1 receptors (5), which in turn affects Ca^{2+} channels (6) and other parts of the presynaptic apparatus. Finally, at some synapses, alterations in the activity of transmitter reuptake pumps (7) can change the duration of action of neurotransmitters.

the insertion or removal of AMPA receptors at that synapse. More AMPA receptors make the synapse more sensitive to subsequent glutamate release (LTP); fewer receptors make it less sensitive (LTD). Early stages of LTP and LTD, lasting hours, are based on the insertion or removal of AMPA receptors already present in the presynaptic ending. The changes can be stabilized and persist for years through later stages that involve communication with the nucleus and protein synthesis.

Multiple Memory Systems Depend on Adjustments of Synaptic Strength

Although we tend to think of memory as a unitary function and to associate it with remembering facts and events, there are in fact multiple kinds of memory, each depending on different sets of CNS structures (Fig. 24-11). Memory of events and facts—remembering what you had for dinner last night (**episodic** memory), or remembering that Yankee Stadium is in the Bronx or the meaning of a word (**semantic** memory)—is called **declarative** (or **explicit**) memory, indicating that these items are accessible to consciousness and can be *declared* as remembered events or facts. Memory that manifests more as subconsciously generated responses to events or stimuli is called **nondeclarative** (or **implicit**) memory. Nondeclarative memory is more varied and includes memories of skills and procedures—how to play handball or pinochle—as well as conditioned reflexes and seemingly automatic emotional reactions to certain situations. Just as we normally combine the activities of multiple eye movement control systems in real-life situations, we combine different kinds of memory in most learning tasks. The knowledge of how

to get to school or work, for example, is a mixture of learned habits and procedures and remembered facts.

Most forms of memory, especially declarative memory, have multiple steps. Some form of information is first encoded and enters **working memory,** basically the small amount of information that we can keep "in mind" at one time. Some fraction of the things that enter working memory then goes through a **consolidation** phase, becoming **long-term** memories stored in parts of the CNS.

Cortical Maps Are Adjusted Throughout Life

The cerebral cortex is the site of long-term storage of several forms of memory, both declarative and nondeclarative. These take the form of networks of neurons, interconnected by strengthened (or sometimes new) synapses. One way in which expanded synaptic connections among cortical neurons are manifest is in the reorganization of cortical maps. These maps were traditionally considered stable in adults, but it is now clear that parts of them can expand or shrink substantially (Fig. 24-12). Extended, skilled use of a body part causes its representation in motor and somatosensory cortex to expand at the expense of neighboring areas; the changes start within hours, so they probably depend on preexisting, previously inactive connections. Conversely, in cases of immobilization or amputation, surrounding areas take over the territory of the affected part. If damage occurs early in life, before plasticity has declined to its adult level, the changes can be extensive (see Fig. 24-12D and E). An extreme example is the conversion of visual cortex to other functions in the congenitally blind (Box 24-1; Figs. 24-13 and 24-14).

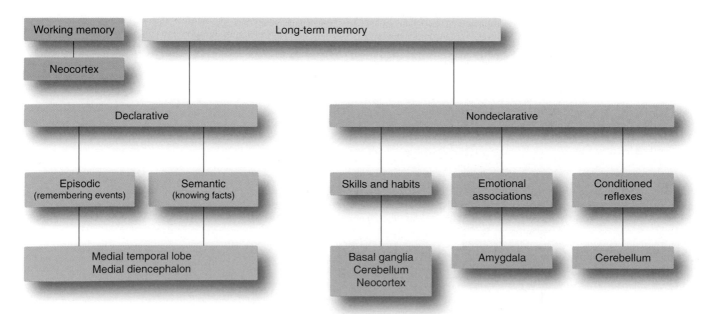

Figure 24-11 Major categories of learning and memory, and the principal parts of the CNS associated with each.

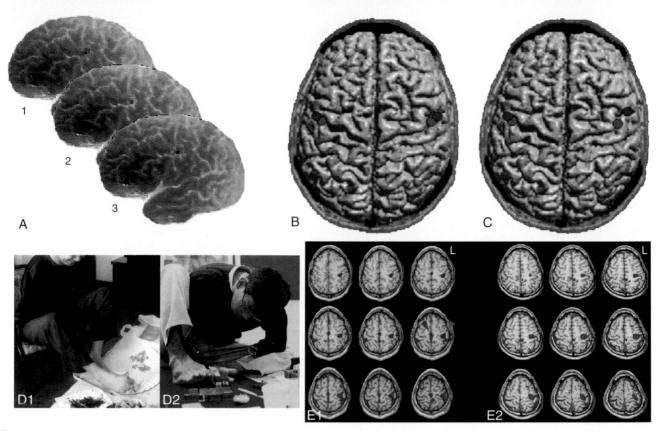

Figure 24-12 Plasticity in cortical maps. **A,** Short-term plasticity in motor cortex. The subject was a 54-year-old woman who had been blind all her life and worked as a Braille proofreader. The area of left motor cortex devoted to her right first dorsal interosseous muscle was mapped using transcranial magnetic stimulation on a Friday after she had been reading Braille all week (1), at the end of a 10-day vacation during which she read little Braille (2), and at the end of the next week of work (3). Activity-dependent changes in the amount of motor cortex devoted to this muscle used in Braille reading can be seen easily. Consistent with these changes, she reported difficulty reading Braille at normal speeds for a period of time after her vacation. **B** and **C,** Use-dependent changes in somatosensory cortex in professional musicians. **B,** Average source of evoked potentials after electrically stimulating the contralateral median *(red)* and ulnar *(blue)* nerves in 35 nonmusicians, providing a measure of the size of the hand representation in somatosensory cortex. **C,** Average source of evoked potentials after electrically stimulating the contralateral median *(red)* and ulnar *(blue)* nerves in 15 right-handed violin players. By this measure, the representation of the left hand in somatosensory cortex is enlarged substantially. **D** and **E,** Much more extensive changes in motor cortex in two individuals who lost both upper extremities early in life and subsequently learned to perform very skilled movements with their feet. **D1,** A 30-year-old man who had bilateral amputations at the shoulder at age 4 following a high-voltage accident went on to become a professional painter and sculptor. **D2,** A 33-year-old man who had amputations at age 8 above the left elbow and below the right shoulder, also following a high-voltage accident. He too went on to become a sculptor and is shown carving a stone seal. **E1** and **E2,** Functional magnetic resonance imaging of both men as they performed a flexion-extension task with their right toes reveals activation in the paracentral lobule *(blue arrow),* where the foot is represented (see Fig. 3-30), and also laterally in the precentral gyrus *(green arrow)* at a level where the hand would ordinarily be represented. *(A, from Pascual-Leone A et al: Ann Neurol 38:910, 1995. **B** and **C,** from Schwenkreis P et al: Eur J Neurosci 26:3291, 2007. **D** and **E,** from Yu X et al: Magn Reson Imaging 24:45, 2006.)*

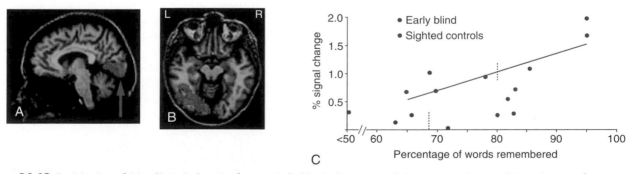

Figure 24-13 Participation of "visual" cortical areas of congenitally blind subjects in verbal memory tasks. **A** and **B,** Activation of primary visual cortex **(A)** and left visual association areas **(B)** as one subject tried to recall words from a recently learned list. **C,** The amount of activation measured in studies such as those shown in **A** and **B** is highly correlated with the number of words remembered 6 months later. Note that the average memory score for the blind subjects is superior to that for the sighted controls *(vertical dashed lines)* and that there is little or no occipital activation in sighted controls during the verbal memory task. *(A and B, from Pascual-Leone A et al: Annu Rev Neurosci 28:377, 2005. **C,** redrawn from Amedi A et al: Nat Neurosci 6:758, 2003.)*

BOX 24-1

Changing the Function of Visual Cortex

What happens to a cortical area deprived of its principal functional input? Remarkably, it gets involved in other functions, to a degree that depends on the age at which the deprivation began. After 5 days of continuous blindfolding, the occipital cortex of normal humans is activated during tasks in which they identify objects by touch (but not while simply touching things); within hours of removing the blindfold, the occipital activation disappears. These changes are much too rapid to be accounted for by the growth of new long-distance connections (which does not happen much in adult brains; see later sections of this chapter). Rather, they are probably based on already present corticocortical connections that are ordinarily inactive or used in other ways.

Permanent loss of vision leads to greater, sustained use of visual areas for other functions. Blind humans reading Braille, for example, have increased blood flow in both primary visual and visual association areas. Those who became blind early in life have much greater occipital activation and become more proficient in Braille reading. This is not just a transfer of tactile functions to visual areas, however; it is more an involvement of formerly visual areas in language and cognitive functions. The same occipital areas are activated in such individuals by verbal language tasks and by learning lists of words (see Fig. 24-13), accounting at least in part for the superior ability of blind humans to perform some nonvisual tasks.

The essential role that the occipital lobes can play in Braille reading was demonstrated in a recent unfortunate case. A 63-year-old woman who had been blind from birth and was a proficient Braille reader collapsed at work and was taken to a hospital. T2-weighted magnetic resonance imaging revealed bilateral infarction in the territory of the posterior cerebral artery (see Fig. 24-14), which resulted in loss of the ability to read Braille.

On the second day, when she tried to read a Braille card sent to her, she was unable to do so. She stated that the Braille dots "felt flat" to her, though she described being able to concentrate and determine whether or not there was a raised dot in a given position in an isolated cell of Braille. Nonetheless, when attempting to read Braille normally, she found that she could not extract enough information to determine what letters, and especially what words, were written. She likened her impairment to "having the fingers covered by thick gloves." Despite her profound inability to read, she was struck by the fact that she did not notice any similar impairment in touch discrimination when trying to identify the roughness of a surface or locate items on a board. She was able to identify her house-key by touch in order to ask a friend to check on her cat at home, and she was similarly able to identify different coins tactually without any difficulty. … Twelve months after her stroke she continued to be unable to read Braille and had resorted to the use of a computer with voice recognition software, otherwise she remained active and continued to work.*

*From Hamilton R et al: Neuroreport 11:237, 2000.

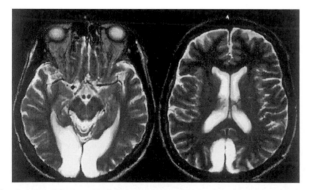

Figure 24-14 T2-weighted axial magnetic resonance images showing the extent of bilateral occipital damage in the patient described in Box 24-1. *(From Hamilton R et al: Neuroreport 11:237, 2000.)*

The Hippocampus and Nearby Cortical Regions Are Critical for Declarative Memory

Neurosurgeons discovered (by accident) in the early 1950s that after bilateral removal of the medial parts of the temporal lobe[c] (or after unilateral removal from patients with preexisting damage on the other side), humans have a striking memory deficit (Box 24-2; Fig. 24-15). After such surgery, patients have severe **anterograde amnesia**—they are unable to form new episodic or semantic memories. There is typically some **retrograde amnesia** for events that occurred before the surgery, often worse for episodic than for semantic memories, but beyond some point in the past, early memories are intact. A new item such as a list of numbers or a dictated phrase can be retained in working memory for a little while if the patient has nothing else to do but concentrate on it, but it disappears at the first distraction. Intelligence is more or less undisturbed, but this is still an enormously debilitating problem. Imagine being perpetually unable to remember new acquaintances,

_____

[c]Even though the hippocampus underlies cortical areas that are usually described as parts of the limbic lobe, this area is also commonly referred to as the medial temporal lobe because of its continuity with the temporal lobe of gross anatomy.

BOX 24-2

A Famous Case of Amnesia

A particularly famous case of amnesia, one of the first described as a result of surgical intervention, is a man referred to by the initials HM. HM began to have minor seizures in 1936, when he was 10 years old. The cause has never been clear—there was a family history of epilepsy, and he sustained a head injury with loss of consciousness when he was 9. The seizures became generalized when he was 16, got progressively worse, and could not be controlled by the anticonvulsants available at the time. In 1953, when he was 27, an experimental operation was performed in the hope of alleviating his seizures. The anterior 5 to 6 cm of his medial temporal lobe was removed bilaterally (see Fig. 24-15), including the amygdala and most of the hippocampus and parahippocampal gyrus.

Following the surgery, HM's seizures were much improved (though not eliminated), but there was an additional dramatic, unexpected result. Although his IQ actually increased (probably because of the lower doses of anticonvulsant that became possible), HM had a profound anterograde amnesia that never improved. He was unable to add new words to his vocabulary, remember people he met after 1953, or recall events that happened after his surgery.

HM's memory deficit has been studied extensively and described in detail. He has a degree of retrograde amnesia, apparently more severe for episodic than semantic memories. Other deficits can be attributed to damage outside the hippocampus and parahippocampal gyrus. He has a normal olfactory threshold, but, consistent with damage to olfactory cortical areas (see Figs. 13-17 and 13-8), he is unable to discriminate among different odors or identify anything by smell. He is impaired in keeping track of his internal states, presumably because of the removal of both amygdalae. For example, his feelings of hunger or thirst do not change after eating or drinking, and he has difficulty discriminating between things that are warm and painfully hot.

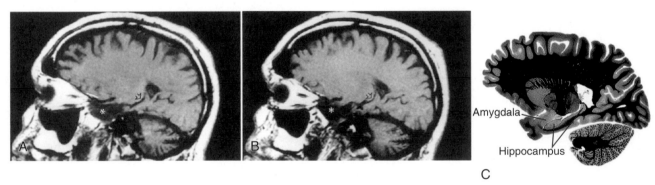

Figure 24-15 T1-weighted parasagittal magnetic resonance images of the left (**A**) and right (**B**) sides of HM's brain, made when he was 66 years old (almost 40 years after his surgery). The areas from which anterior parts of his medial temporal lobes had been removed are indicated by asterisks, and the preserved posterior parts of his hippocampi by open arrows. **C,** Parasagittal section of an unoperated brain, showing the anterior temporal structures missing in **A** and **B**. HM's cerebellar atrophy (compare **A** and **B** to **C**) is attributed to his longtime treatment with phenytoin for seizure control. (**A** and **B,** from Corkin S et al: J Neurosci 17:3964, 1997.)

unable to keep track of events in the lives of relatives and old friends, unable to complete simple tasks because of inability to remember why they were begun, and unable to read a story because there is no memory of sentences preceding the current one.

Interestingly, the amnesia that occurs after bilateral hippocampal damage applies only to declarative memories and not to the learning of new skills and procedures. Such a patient could, for example, learn in repeated attempts how to assemble a jigsaw puzzle more and more skillfully at the same rate as a normal individual, despite having no memory of ever seeing the puzzle before (see Fig. 24-23).

Because the hippocampus is a major part of the medial temporal lobe, and because a declarative memory deficit occurs when there appears to be little damage other than to the two hippocampi, the function of laying down or consolidating new memories has been attributed to this portion of the limbic system. (Memories themselves must reside elsewhere in the CNS—presumably as distributed sets of connections in neocortical association areas—because old memories can still be retrieved after medial temporal damage.)

The Hippocampus Is a Cortical Structure That Borders the Inferior Horn of the Lateral Ventricle

Paleocortex and archicortex occupy most of the surface of each cerebral hemisphere in lower vertebrates. As the area devoted to neocortex expands through phylogeny, archicortex moves dorsally and then rolls around

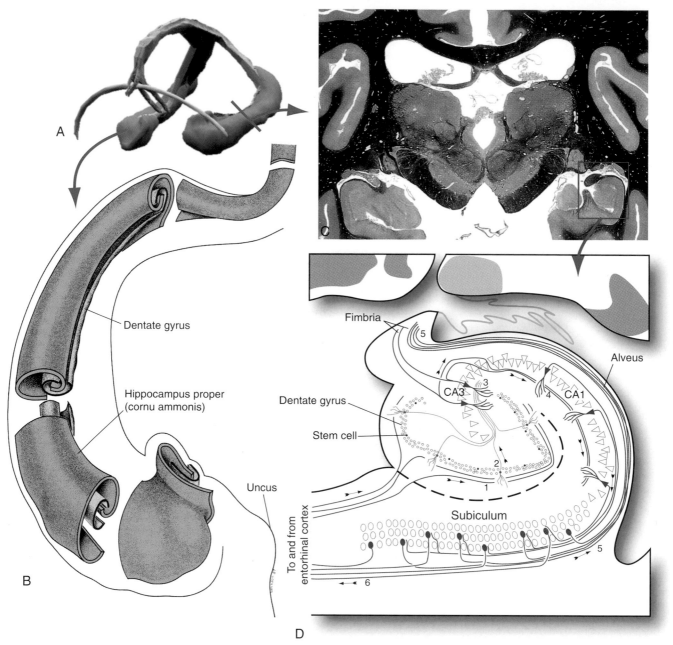

Figure 24-16 Structure of the hippocampus. **A,** Three-dimensional reconstruction of the hippocampi and fornix. **B,** Arrangement of the dentate gyrus and hippocampus proper (cornu ammonis) as two interlocking C-shaped (in cross section) cortical structures. **C,** Coronal section through the dentate gyrus, hippocampus proper, and subiculum. **D,** Schematic diagram showing the general arrangement of cells and fibers in the hippocampus. A few hippocampal efferents arise from pyramidal cells of the hippocampus proper (CA), but most, as indicated, arise from the subiculum. Note that the major route of information flow through the hippocampus is a one-way circuit, starting with inputs from entorhinal cortex (1) and then passing successively through the dentate gyrus (2), two sectors of hippocampal pyramidal cells (3, 4), and the subiculum. Finally, subicular neurons project either through the fornix (5) or directly back to entorhinal cortex (6). As discussed later in this chapter, a small population of neural stem cells is located in deep parts of the dentate gyrus. (See Videos 24-1 and 24-2.) (**B,** modified from Duvernoy HM: The human hippocampus: functional anatomy, vascularization and serial sections with MRI, ed 3, Berlin, 2005, Springer-Verlag. **C,** modified from Nolte J, Angevine JB Jr: The human brain in photographs and diagrams, ed 3, St. Louis, 2007, Mosby.)

in a C-shaped pattern onto the medial surface of the hemisphere, whereas the paleocortex moves ventrally onto the base of the brain. With the continued expansion of the hemisphere in primates, the hippocampus becomes one more structure that is carried around in a great arc (see Fig. 2-13)—in this case ending up in the temporal lobe as the floor of the inferior horn of the lateral ventricle (Fig. 24-16). Traces of its heritage are revealed by a thin, rudimentary strand of gray matter (the **hippocampal rudiment,** or **indusium griseum**), continuous with the hippocampus, that is left behind on the dorsal surface of the corpus callosum and by the long, curved course of the **fornix,** the most prominent hippocampal output pathway (Fig. 24-17).

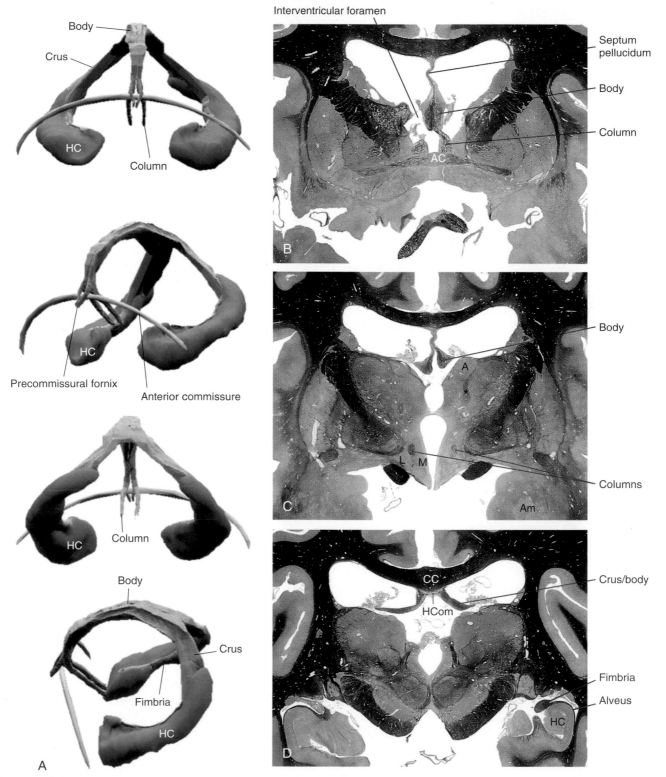

Figure 24-17 Origin and course of the fornix. This bundle, mostly efferents from the hippocampus (HC), begins as fibers that collect on the ventricular surface of the hippocampus proper as the alveus. The fibers move medially to form the fimbria of the hippocampus and then part company with the hippocampus near the splenium of the corpus callosum to become the crus of the fornix. The two crura converge on the midline, forming the body of the fornix; as they do so, a few fibers are exchanged between the two crura in the hippocampal commissure (HCom). The body of the fornix diverges again near the anterior commissure (AC) and interventricular foramen into the columns of the fornix. Most of these fibers continue on through the hypothalamus as the postcommissural fornix, ending primarily in the mammillary bodies. Nearly half, however, split off in front of the anterior commissure as the precommissural fornix, ending primarily in the septal nuclei and ventral striatum. **A** shows three-dimensional reconstructions of this course. **B, C,** and **D** are coronal sections at the levels of the anterior commissure, anterior thalamus, and posterior thalamus, respectively. (See Video 24-3.) *, mammillothalamic tract; A, anterior nucleus of the thalamus; Am, amygdala; CC, corpus callosum; L, M, lateral and medial zones of the tuberal hypothalamus. (**B** to **D**, modified from Nolte J, Angevine JB Jr: The human brain in photographs and diagrams, ed 3, St. Louis, 2007, Mosby.)

The hippocampus is a curved and recurved sheet of cortex folded into the medial surface of the temporal lobe. Transverse sections (see Fig. 24-16) reveal that it has three distinct zones: the **dentate gyrus,** the **hippocampus proper,**[d] and the **subiculum.** In such sections, the dentate gyrus and the hippocampus proper have the form of two interlocking Cs. The subiculum is a transitional zone, continuous with the hippocampus proper at one of its edges and with the cortex of the parahippocampal gyrus at the other edge. The entire hippocampus has a length of about 5 cm in the parahippocampal gyrus from its anterior end at the amygdala to its tapering, posterior end near the splenium of the corpus callosum. Along this course numerous small blood vessels enter the hippocampus from the adjacent subarachnoid space by penetrating the dentate gyrus, thus giving this gyrus the beaded or toothed appearance for which it was named.

The Fornix Is a Prominent Output Pathway From the Hippocampus

The hippocampus proper and the dentate gyrus are three-layered structures, with a superficial **molecular layer** and a deep **polymorphic layer,** both similar to the layers of the same name in the neocortex. The intermediate stratum is a **granule cell layer** in the dentate gyrus and a **pyramidal cell layer** in the hippocampus proper. The molecular layer of the hippocampus proper faces the dentate gyrus, and the hippocampal equivalent of subcortical white matter is a layer of fibers called the **alveus** that lies just beneath the ependymal lining of the ventricle (see Fig. 24-16). The molecular layer of the dentate gyrus faces the subarachnoid space, and its output fibers, which do not leave the hippocampus, project directly into the hippocampus proper. The subiculum, as mentioned previously, is the zone of transition from the hippocampus proper to the parahippocampal gyrus and changes gradually from three-layered to six-layered cortex.

The alveus contains both afferents to and efferents from the hippocampus (primarily the latter). These fibers collect into a bundle called the **fimbria** (Latin for "fringe") **of the hippocampus** at the edge of the choroid fissure (see Fig. 24-16). As the hippocampus ends near the splenium of the corpus callosum, the fimbria becomes a detached bundle called the **crus** ("leg") **of the fornix.** The two crura converge and join in the midline to form the **body of the fornix,** which travels forward at the inferior edge of the septum pellucidum (see Fig. 24-17). At the interventricular foramen, the fornix turns inferiorly and posteriorly, diverging through the middle of the hypothalamus toward the mammillary bodies, termed the **columns of the fornix** (see Figs. 23-4 and 24-17C).

The connections of the hippocampus have been mapped in ruthless detail and in three dimensions. Proceeding around its C shape (as seen in transverse sections), the hippocampus proper has been divided into several zones,[e] all of whose connections differ somewhat from one another and from those of the subiculum and dentate gyrus. Along the course of the hippocampus through the temporal lobe, its connections change. Finally, afferents from different sources end at different levels on the apical dendrites of hippocampal pyramidal cells. The high degree of order has made the hippocampus very attractive for anatomical and physiological research, particularly in studies of neural plasticity and regeneration. However, to keep matters manageable, the following account treats the hippocampus, by and large, as a uniform structure.

Entorhinal Cortex Is the Principal Source of Inputs to the Hippocampus

By far the most prominent source of afferents to the hippocampus is the adjacent entorhinal cortex (Fig. 24-18). Entorhinal cortex receives relatively minor olfactory inputs, but it also receives massive projections from widespread areas of association cortex, including the posterior cingulate gyrus (via the cingulum), orbital cortex (via the uncinate fasciculus), and multimodal areas of the frontal, parietal, and temporal lobes. These additional connections provide the hippocampus with a vast repertoire of information that is potentially available for declarative memories. In addition, modulatory cholinergic inputs from the septal nuclei that reach the hippocampus through the fornix, as well as inputs that reach it directly from the amygdala, affect the probability that any given bit of information will be retained. Finally, a few fibers arrive from the contralateral hippocampus by passing from one crus of the fornix to the other beneath the splenium of the corpus callosum in the **hippocampal commissure,** a small commissure near the site where the two crura join to form the body of the fornix; this connection is rudimentary in humans.

---

[d]Also called *Ammon's horn* (or cornu ammonis, after an Egyptian deity with ram's horns) because of the way the hippocampi curve downward and outward from the hippocampal rudiment into the temporal lobes. Hippocampal nomenclature has a long, colorful, and not entirely logical history, as discussed by F. T. Lewis in "The Significance of the Term Hippocampus" (J Comp Neurol 35:213, 1923-1924). In this book, the terms *hippocampus* and *hippocampal formation* are used interchangeably to refer to the combination of dentate gyrus, hippocampus proper, and subiculum.

[e]These zones, each a narrow longitudinal strip of the hippocampus proper, are commonly referred to as *CA fields* (CA being an abbreviation for cornu ammonis). Hence neurons of the dentate gyrus project primarily to CA3 pyramidal cells, whose axon collaterals project to CA2 and CA1 pyramidal cells. CA1 in turn projects to the subiculum, where most of the output from the hippocampus arises (see Fig. 24-16).

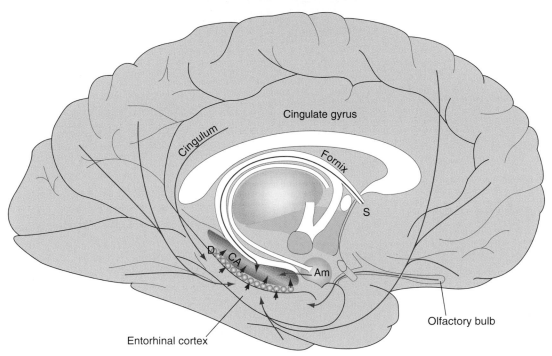

Figure 24-18 Afferents to the hippocampus. The major source is the entorhinal cortex, which in turn collects inputs from widespread association areas and from the olfactory bulb. Entorhinal cortex projects to the dentate gyrus (D), which projects to the hippocampus proper (CA). Other hippocampal inputs arrive directly from the amygdala (Am) and via the fornix from the septal nuclei (S) and contralateral hippocampus (not shown). Other modulatory inputs, such as those from the locus ceruleus, are not indicated. For simplicity, all neocortical inputs are shown projecting only to entorhinal cortex, although some reach parts of the hippocampus directly. Similarly, all inputs from the amygdala are shown projecting only to the hippocampus proper, although some reach entorhinal cortex and other nearby areas. *(Modified from an illustration in Warwick R, Williams PL: Gray's anatomy, Br ed 35, Philadelphia, 1973, WB Saunders.)*

Hippocampal Outputs Reach Entorhinal Cortex, the Mammillary Body, and the Septal Nuclei

Hippocampal outputs arise mainly in the subiculum, with some contribution from the hippocampus proper. Although most fibers project directly back to the entorhinal cortex as well as to other cortical areas, the most prominent output pathway anatomically is the fornix (Fig. 24-19). Fornix fibers arch forward under the corpus callosum along the path depicted in Figure 24-17 (except for the few that cross in the hippocampal commissure). At the level of the interventricular foramen, many fibers split off in front of the anterior commissure as the **precommissural fornix** (see Fig. 24-17A). Most of these end nearby in the septal and preoptic nuclei and ventral striatum, but some continue on to reach orbital and anterior cingulate cortex. The remaining fibers of the fornix (the **postcommissural fornix**) do one of two things: some turn sharply posteriorly and end in the anterior thalamic nucleus, whereas the rest travel through the hypothalamus in the column of the fornix and end mainly in the mammillary body (although many end in other hypothalamic areas or in the midbrain reticular formation). Because the mammillothalamic tract ends in the anterior nucleus (Fig. 24-17C), the hippocampus can influence this part of the thalamus both directly and indirectly.

The anterior thalamic nucleus projects to the cingulate gyrus, thus completing a great loop through the diencephalon and telencephalon (Fig. 24-20). Beginning in the hippocampus, the pathway proceeds through the fornix to the mammillary body and from there, in sequence, to the anterior thalamic nucleus, the cingulate gyrus and part of the parahippocampal gyrus (the entorhinal cortex), and finally back to the hippocampus. James Papez pointed out in 1937 that this loop provided for interactions among the neocortex, limbic structures, and hypothalamus, and proposed that it might be the anatomical substrate of emotional experience. Though undoubtedly a great oversimplification (for one thing, hippocampal connections are considerably more complex than this loop indicates), this idea provided the impetus for a great deal of research into the structure and function of the limbic system; the loop is still known as the **Papez circuit.**

Bilateral Damage to the Hippocampus or Medial Diencephalon Impairs Declarative Memory

A variety of changes in autonomic and endocrine function have been described as resulting from hippocampal stimulation or damage in experimental animals, consistent with the connections between the hippocampus and the septal nuclei and hypothalamus; a number of

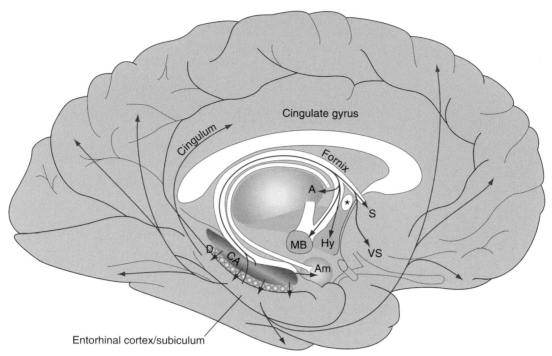

Figure 24-19 Efferents from the hippocampus. One major efferent pathway is the fornix, through which fibers reach an assortment of anteriorly situated forebrain structures, including the anterior nucleus of the thalamus (A), the mammillary body (MB) and other parts of the hypothalamus (Hy), the septal nuclei (S), and the ventral striatum (VS). Some fibers of the precommissural fornix spread beyond the septal nuclei and ventral striatum and reach orbital and anterior cingulate cortices. In addition, many fibers pass directly from the subiculum to the entorhinal cortex, to the amygdala (Am), or backward along the cingulum to the posterior cingulate gyrus. For simplicity, the entorhinal cortex and subiculum are lumped together, although they have distinctive but overlapping connections (e.g., the subiculum projects mostly to entorhinal cortex but also has some outputs to other cortical areas). *, anterior commissure; CA, hippocampus proper; D, dentate gyrus. *(Modified from an illustration in Warwick R, Williams PL: Gray's anatomy, Br ed 35, Philadelphia, 1973, WB Saunders.)*

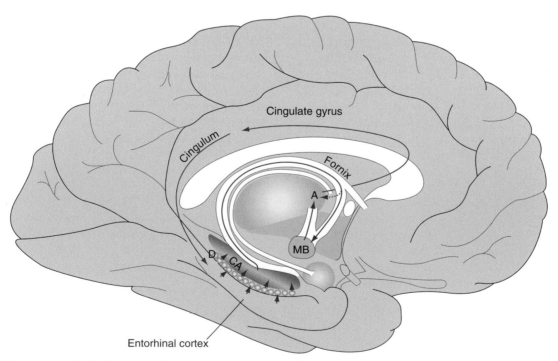

Figure 24-20 The Papez circuit. The shortcut from the hippocampus directly to the anterior thalamic nucleus, not part of the circuit as originally proposed, is indicated by a dashed line. A, anterior thalamic nucleus; CA, hippocampus proper; D, dentate gyrus; MB, mammillary body. *(Modified from an illustration in Warwick R, Williams PL: Gray's anatomy, Br ed 35, Philadelphia, 1973, WB Saunders.)*

behavioral changes have been described as well. The most prominent role of the hippocampus, however, is in the consolidation of declarative memories. This role extends to the connections of the hippocampus with other parts of the CNS.

Damage to the mammillary bodies (which occurs over the course of widespread damage to the periaqueductal and periventricular gray matter as a result of chronic alcoholism) is also correlated with anterograde amnesia. The condition is called **Korsakoff's psychosis.** Patients so afflicted may have relatively intact intelligence but an inability to form new declarative memories. They typically make up answers as they go along, concealing to some extent the memory loss (hence a wonderful alternative name for Korsakoff's psychosis is the **amnestic confabulatory syndrome**). This led to the appealing notion that the entire Papez circuit is involved in learning and memory. Unfortunately, things are rarely as simple as they seem, and understanding of the hippocampal role in memory has developed slowly. For example, bilateral destruction of the cingulum causes no particular memory loss,[f] and destruction of the fornix does not cause a memory deficit comparable in magnitude to that seen after medial temporal damage. In addition, there have been cases in which reported destruction of the mammillary bodies was not accompanied by memory loss, yet several cases in which the mammilothalamic tract has resulted in memory impairment. Some investigators claim that the only common factor in all cases of Korsakoff's psychosis is bilateral damage to the medial thalamus (i.e., the dorsomedial nuclei) that tends to include the dorsomedial and anterior nuclei.

Explanations for these apparent discrepancies have come from the realization that there are multiple kinds of memory systems working in parallel with one another (see Fig. 24-11), as well as from increased knowledge of hippocampal anatomy. As mentioned previously, humans with amnesia can still learn new motor skills, indicating that this form of learning does not require an intact hippocampus. In general, varieties of learning and memory not built around the conscious recall of specific items, such as pattern recognition, habits, conditioned autonomic reactions to stimuli, and motor skills, are now known not to depend on the hippocampus. Rather, the hippocampus and nearby cortical areas (such as entorhinal cortex) play a crucial role, one that slowly diminishes over years, in consolidating explicit memories of facts and events. Because the hippocampus has

major outputs that do not travel through the fornix (see Fig. 24-19), damage to the fornix does not cause a profound impairment of memory. Similarly, damage restricted to the hippocampus and sparing entorhinal and nearby cortices causes only partial amnesia. The critical structure whose damage causes Korsakoff's psychosis has still not been determined with certainty.

The Amygdala Is Centrally Involved in Emotional Memories

One prominent category of nondeclarative memory is emotional associations, in which the amygdala plays a central role. Throughout life we develop associations between stimuli that are intrinsically neutral (e.g., a soft buzzing sound) and good or bad outcomes (e.g., a mosquito bite). These emotional "tags" develop as patterns of strengthened synapses in the basolateral amygdala, in turn initiating autonomic and behavioral responses through the central nuclei of the amygdala (Fig. 24-21). Information about sights, sounds, and other stimuli reaches the basolateral amygdala rapidly through the thalamus and more slowly from cortical association areas (see Fig. 23-18). Information about painful and rewarding stimuli reaches the same neurons. An intrinsically pleasant or unpleasant stimulus (an **unconditioned stimulus**) by itself causes an emotional response. Pairing of such stimuli with neutral stimuli causes activation of NMDA receptors, followed by LTP, in basolateral neurons. A subsequent phase of protein synthesis consolidates this pairing in the amygdala, so that later exposure to the same formerly neutral stimulus (now a **conditioned stimulus**) causes an emotional response. Conditioned responses to simple stimuli can be mediated rapidly by the pathway through the thalamus, then modified appropriately by the slower pathway through the cortex (e.g., "False alarm!" or "Worse than I thought!"). Bilateral damage to the amygdala blocks the acquisition of such conditioned emotional responses without affecting declarative memory for the conditioning trials themselves; damage to the medial temporal lobes that spares the amygdala does just the opposite (Fig. 24-22).

We are also more likely to remember situations in which something good or bad happened, an effect mediated largely by projections from the amygdala to the hippocampus (see Fig. 24-18). The resulting declarative memories (sometimes called "flash-bulb" memories) may not be more accurate than other declarative memories, but seem unusually vivid.

The Basal Ganglia Are Important for Some Forms of Nondeclarative Memory

Much of what we learn in life is based on gradually acquired experience rather than explicitly stated rules. An example is choosing a route to drive to work based

---

[f]Interestingly, bilateral section of the cingulum causes emotional changes similar to those seen after prefrontal leukotomy, a type of change that might be expected after damage to the limbic system. This operation has been used on an experimental basis as a treatment for intractable pain and for certain psychiatric disorders.

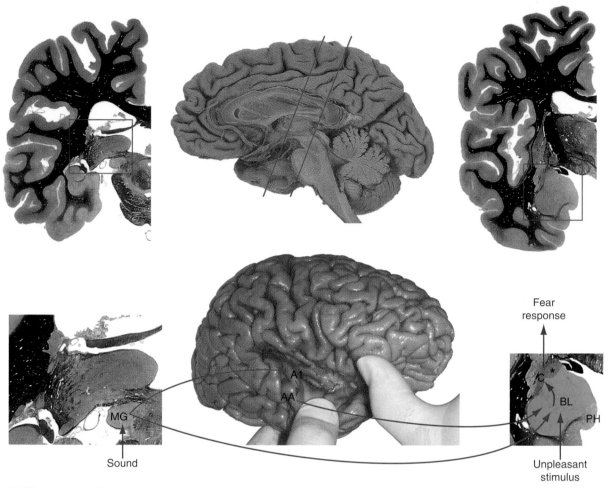

Figure 24-21 Conditioned fear in response to sounds is a well-studied example of emotional learning. Inputs from the medial geniculate nucleus (MG), auditory association cortex (AA), and places such as the parabrachial nuclei (conveying inputs about well-being or its opposite) all converge on neurons in the basolateral amygdala (BL). Paired activation of the parabrachial and other inputs potentiates the response to the latter, allowing innocuous sounds to trigger emotional responses via the central nuclei (C) of the amygdala. *, medial nuclei of the amygdala; A1, primary auditory cortex; PH, parahippocampal gyrus.

on the weather, the time of day, and other factors that we combine in a probabilistic way. The basal ganglia, through their interactions with the frontal lobes and other cortical areas (see Fig. 19-8), are particularly important for such nondeclarative learning of habits, procedures, and patterns of behavior. We ordinarily combine declarative memories of particular events (e.g., remembering a particularly difficult commute on a rainy day) with the subconscious learning of patterns and probabilities, but the two can be dissociated. Patients with Parkinson's disease, for example, have small and slow movements but are also impaired in this type of implicit learning (Fig. 24-23).

The Cerebellum Is Important for Some Forms of Nondeclarative Memory

Even though no one understands quite how it does it, the cerebellum is a learning machine involved in mul-

tiple forms of nondeclarative memory. Plasticity in the elaborately crisscrossing network of cortical synapses (see Fig. 20-10) adds learning to the basic functions of the anatomically laid out longitudinal cerebellar zones (see Fig. 20-16). Plasticity is accomplished through the use, with some cerebellar idiosyncrasies, of a full complement of the plasticity mechanisms illustrated in Figure 24-10. LTD is prominent in the cerebellar cortex, especially at the enormous number of parallel fiber–Purkinje cell synapses. Purkinje cells are unusual in having no NMDA receptors, but they use an alternative system of Ca^{2+} signaling to regulate the AMPA receptors at parallel fiber–Purkinje cell synapses. The powerful excitatory input provided by climbing fibers elicits a brief opening of voltage-gated Ca^{2+} channels with each spike. Any parallel fiber input that is active during the resulting transient elevation of Ca^{2+} concentration sets in motion a complementary process that results in the removal of AMPA receptors at that synapse (i.e., LTD). At

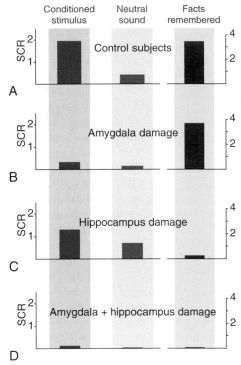

Figure 24-22 Differential effects of damage to the amygdala and hippocampus on emotional and declarative learning, as shown in four control subjects and three patients with neurological damage. A startling sound (a boat horn at 100 dB) was used to elicit sympathetic responses, as measured by a skin conductance response (SCR). All subjects had a comparable SCR (not shown) to the boat horn and only a small response to a neutral tone. **A,** Control subjects had an SCR to neutral sounds that were paired with the boat horn (i.e., conditioned stimuli), and they were able to remember factual details of the conditioning session (declarative memory). **B,** A patient with a rare disorder that caused bilateral degeneration of the amygdala showed no conditioned responses but was able to remember factual details of the conditioning session. **C,** In contrast, a patient with bilateral lesions of the hippocampus (as a result of cardiac arrest and hypoxic damage) had nearly normal conditioning but remembered no details of the conditioning session. **D,** Despite having a normal SCR to the boat horn, a patient with extensive bilateral medial temporal damage, including the amygdala (from herpes simplex encephalitis), showed neither conditioning nor declarative memory of the conditioning session. *(Replotted from Bechara A et al: Science 269:1115, 1995.)*

the same time, Purkinje cells initiate retrograde endocannabinoid signaling at sites where climbing fibers and parallel fibers are simultaneously active, suppressing glutamate release by the parallel fibers for tens of seconds. Climbing fibers seem to be the key elements in cerebellar learning, delivering "teaching" or "error" signals during the activity of selected parallel fibers.

These and other mechanisms of synaptic weakening and strengthening occur throughout the cerebellar cortex (and deep nuclei); the connections of particular areas dictate the functions affected. Hence plastic changes in the flocculus adjust the gain of the vestibulo-ocular reflex, and changes in a particular part of the vermis can adjust the parameters of saccades (see Fig. 21-19). The medial hemispheres and other parts of the

vermis are involved in adjusting additional reflexes involving skeletal muscles; one example described in Chapter 20 is conditioned eye blinks (also see Fig. 20-25). Finally, consistent with their connections with widespread neocortical areas (see Fig. 20-19), the lateral hemispheres are involved in learning more complex motor and sensory skills, especially in the early stages of learning (Fig. 24-24).

PNS Repair Is More Effective Than CNS Repair

The adult nervous system does not repair itself as well as some other parts of the body do (see Fig. 24-28). Once the developmental period of abundant plasticity is completed, neurons downregulate the activity of growth-related genes and turn to maintenance activities. In addition, the adult CNS actively discourages the processes that earlier led to wholesale rearrangement of connections. As a result, possibilities for regrowth become more limited.

Adult neurons that die because of injury, stroke, or disease are rarely replaced (but see the later section on new neurons). The consequences of less serious injury depend on whether it happens in the PNS or CNS.

Peripheral Nerve Fibers Can Regrow After Injury

Transection of an axon in the PNS is followed by a characteristic set of events (Fig. 24-25). Over a period of a week or two, the severed axon segment and its myelin (when present) are removed in a process of **Wallerian degeneration.** Schwann cells jettison their myelin, which fragments and gets gobbled up by Schwann cells and macrophages. Schwann cells proliferate and secrete trophic factors, which signal the affected neuron to downregulate genes for things like synapse-related proteins and upregulate growth-related genes (e.g., those for cytoskeletal components). This shows up cytologically as **chromatolysis** ("loss of color")—the euchromatic nucleus moves off to one side, the neuronal cell body swells, and ribosomes disperse, resulting in a seeming loss of Nissl substance (total RNA actually increases). As the neuron attends to regrowing an axon, normal interactions between it and its presynaptic and postsynaptic partners are disrupted, causing **retrograde transneuronal** changes such as retraction of synapses and **anterograde transneuronal** changes such as atrophy of skeletal muscle fibers (see Fig. 18-4D).

In favorable cases, a new axon reaches the previously denervated target, and everything returns to normal. This can happen in crush injuries, in which basal laminae and connective tissue elements remain continuous and can guide regrowing axons. Following transection, however, recovery is rarely complete because, without

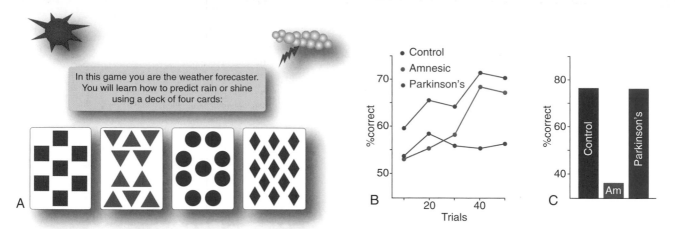

Figure 24-23 Differential effects of damage to the basal ganglia and hippocampus on a probabilistic learning task and on declarative learning. **A,** The probabilistic learning task. Subjects were shown various combinations of four cards that had different probabilities of predicting rain or shine. They were not told the probabilities; they were told only whether they were correct or incorrect after each trial. It was impossible to memorize the solution, and subjects felt like they were guessing. **B,** Control subjects started out performing at about a chance level (50%) on this task but improved over 50 trials. A group of 12 amnesic subjects with bilateral damage to the hippocampus or medial diencephalon improved to the same degree, but a group of 20 patients with Parkinson's disease continued to perform at chance levels. **C,** Nevertheless, the Parkinson's patients remembered details of the testing session as well as controls did, but the amnesic subjects (Am) did not. *(Redrawn and replotted from Knowlton BJ, Mangels JA, Squire LR: Science 273:1399, 1996.)*

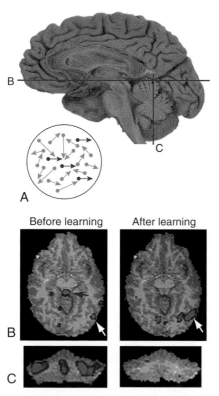

Figure 24-24 Cerebellar participation in perceptual learning. **A,** The learning task. Subjects watched successive frames in which dots jumped about in a seemingly random pattern (examples of distances and directions are indicated by the arrows attached to each dot). However, about 20% of the dots actually moved the same distance in the same direction (colored blue in this example, but not in the actual experiment). The subjects were asked whether there was a general sense of motion in one direction or another (in this example, to the left or to the right). During the first few trials (before learning) their performance was at chance levels, but with repeated exposure it climbed to nearly 100% in a few minutes (after learning). **B,** As learning progressed, activity in cortical areas responsive to visual motion (see Fig. 17-37) expanded *(white arrows)*. Activity in the superior colliculus *(blue arrow)* declined, probably reflecting this structure's role in visual attention. **C,** As learning began, the cerebellum, especially the lateral hemispheres, was highly active. This activity almost disappeared as the task was learned and the cerebral cortex took over. *(From Vaina LM et al: Proc Natl Acad Sci U S A 95:12657, 1998.)*

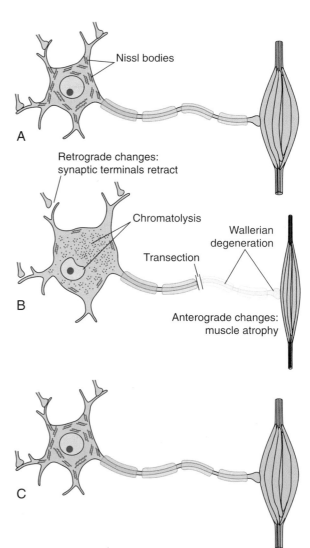

Figure 24-25 Wallerian degeneration in the PNS. **A,** A lower motor neuron is used as an example, although similar phenomena follow transection of autonomic and sensory fibers in peripheral nerves. **B,** Wallerian degeneration and chromatolysis following axonal transection, together with retrograde and anterograde changes that typically accompany them. **C,** With luck, accurate reinnervation is achieved, and everything returns to normal. *(Adapted from Nolte J: Elsevier's integrated neuroscience, Philadelphia, 2007, Mosby Elsevier.)*

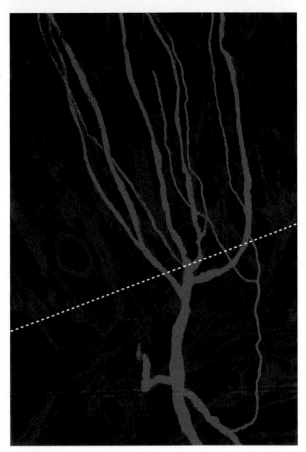

Figure 24-26 A single fluorescent axon in a transgenic mouse divides into multiple branches as it regenerates from proximal *(bottom)* to distal across a transection in a sciatic nerve. The plane at which the distal nerve stump begins is indicated by a dashed line. Laminin *(red fluorescence)* in the distal stump is arranged longitudinally, parallel to the regenerating axonal branches. *(From Witzel C, Rohde C, Brushart TM: J Comp Neurol 485:183, 2005.)*

this guidance, regrowing axons are not very selective (Fig. 24-26), and aberrant reinnervation commonly results. One well-known example ("crocodile tears" syndrome) occurs after facial nerve injury when the lacrimal gland is innervated by some fibers that should go to salivary glands, resulting in tearing while eating.

CNS Glial Cells Impede Repair After Injury

Wallerian degeneration also follows transection of CNS axons, but it is much slower—lasting months or even years—and usually has a very different outcome (Figs. 24-27 and 24-28). Astrocytes and oligodendrocytes do not provide trophic factors to spur regrowth, and in fact, they actively impede the attempts of affected neurons to regenerate. As a result, chromatolysis is usually briefer and less pronounced than after PNS damage, transected axons grow local sprouts near the site of injury but do not reestablish connections, and their parent cell bodies atrophy. If the transection is near a neuron's cell body, it

may even die. There can be permanent anterograde and retrograde transneuronal effects in neurons extensively interconnected with a damaged neuron.

Astrocytes hypertrophy and wall off an injured area, preventing the spread of inflammation into neighboring, undamaged parts of the CNS. In the process, however, they form a dense glial scar that blocks regrowing axons (Fig. 24-29). This is not simply a physical barrier; hypertrophic (**reactive**) astrocytes increase their production of extracellular matrix molecules, especially **chondroitin sulfate proteoglycans** (CSPGs), that inhibit the growth of neural processes. Interestingly, the deposition of CSPGs increases at the end of critical periods, suggesting that one of their roles in healthy nervous systems is to prevent the growth of new connections once things are wired appropriately.

Following white matter damage, oligodendrocytes also jettison their myelin, but in this case, they do not help clean up the debris. Instead, this is accomplished slowly, mainly by microglia, so myelin fragments persist for a long time following CNS damage. Because myelin and oligodendrocytes contain several other growth-inhibiting molecules, this further impedes regrowth. Myelination, in parallel with CSPG deposition, coincides with the end of critical periods.

CNS neurons are not inherently unable to grow new axons. For example, axons in a severed tract can regrow through a peripheral nerve graft. Hence, some combination of enhancing the regenerative responses of injured neurons and blocking inhibitory glial responses offers real hope of improved recovery after CNS damage.

Limited Numbers of New Neurons Are Added to the CNS Throughout Life

It was long thought that all neurons were produced during development and that neurons lost to damage or disease could not be replaced. The existence of mammalian **neural stem cells**—cells that can produce new CNS neurons—was not generally accepted until the 1990s. Stem cells have now been found in the walls of all the ventricles, but most of them sit there in a latent state throughout life. There are only two regions where stem cells give rise to new neurons throughout life. A population in the **subgranular zone** of the dentate gyrus (see Fig. 24-16D) produces new granule cells. A population in the **subventricular zone** of the lateral ventricle, overlying the head of the caudate nucleus, produces new inhibitory interneurons that migrate to the olfactory bulb (Fig. 24-30). The normal role of these newborn neurons is still not known with certainty, although there is evidence that some of the new granule cells are integrated into hippocampal circuitry and are involved in learning. However, devising ways to control the activity of the stem cells offers the potential of neuronal replacement therapies.

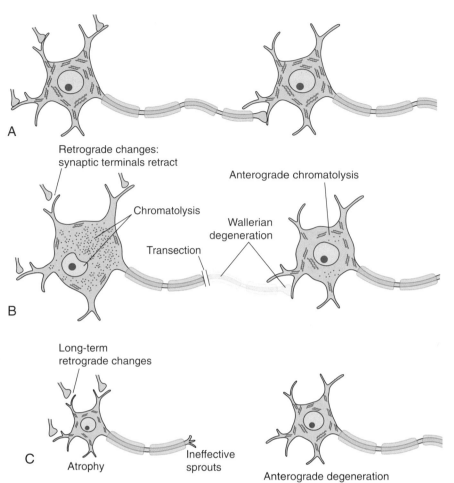

A

Retrograde changes:
synaptic terminals retract

Anterograde chromatolysis

Chromatolysis

Wallerian
degeneration

Transection

B

Long-term
retrograde changes

Atrophy

Ineffective
sprouts

Anterograde degeneration

C

Figure 24-27 Wallerian degeneration in the CNS. **A,** Normal connection between one neuron and another. **B,** Wallerian degeneration and chromatolysis following axonal transection, together with retrograde and anterograde changes that typically accompany them. **C,** CNS axons form sprouts near the site of injury, but these rarely travel far or make synapses. Anterograde and retrograde changes persist, and the neuron often atrophies. *(Adapted from Nolte J: Elsevier's integrated neuroscience, Philadelphia, 2007, Mosby Elsevier.)*

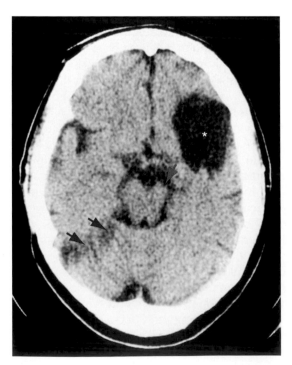

Figure 24-28 Computed tomography scan of a patient who had suffered a stroke in part of the territory of the left middle cerebral artery years earlier. The cortex and part of the basal ganglia in that area died and have been removed, leaving a cavity filled with cerebrospinal fluid (*). Wallerian degeneration can be seen in the form of a shrunken left cerebral peduncle *(green arrow; also see Fig. 16-26)*. Transneuronal atrophy can be seen in the right half of the cerebellum *(red arrows)*. *(Courtesy Dr. Raymond F. Carmody, University of Arizona College of Medicine.)*

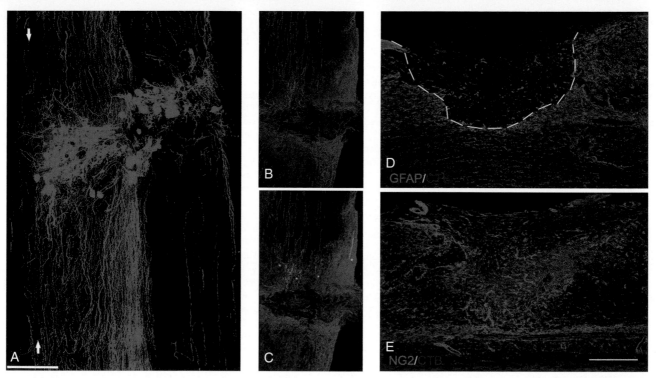

Figure 24-29 Block of axon growth by chondroitin sulfate proteoglycans (CSPGs). **A,** Sagittal section of the cervical spinal cord of a rat, showing an implant of dorsal root ganglion cells with processes growing rostrally (upward) and caudally from these cells through the posterior columns. The dorsal root ganglion cells were taken from a transgenic mouse that expressed green fluorescent protein in these cells. The arrows indicate the border between fasciculus cuneatus and the dorsal horn; scale mark, 200 μm. **B,** Similar processes stop growing when they reach a wound that transected the right posterior column. The red fluorescence indicates glial fibrillary acidic protein (GFAP), an intermediate filament protein produced by astrocytes, and shows the glial scar around the edges of the wound. **C,** The same view as in **B,** but stained to show CSPGs produced by astrocytes in the scar. **D,** Another sagittal section of rat spinal cord, showing axons in fasciculus gracilis stopping at the glial scar surrounding a wound that transected the posterior columns; caudal is to the right. The axons had been labeled with a fluorescent marker, cholera toxin B (CTB), transported from the sciatic nerve. **E,** Treatment with an antibody to NT-2 (a CSPG prominent in glial scars) allowed axons to grow past the scar surrounding a similar wound. (**A** to **C,** from Davies SJA et al: J Neurosci 19:5810, 1999. **D** and **E,** from Tan AM et al: J Neurosci 26:4729, 2006.)

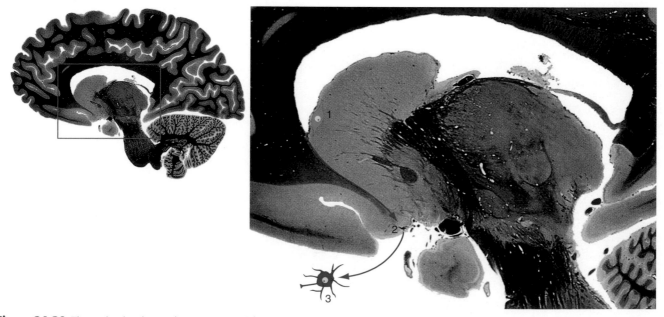

Figure 24-30 The path taken by newborn neurons (1) from the subventricular zone to the lateral olfactory tract (2) and from there into the olfactory bulb, maturing into an inhibitory interneuron (3) once it gets there.

SUGGESTED READINGS

Altman J: Are new neurons formed in the brains of adult mammals? Science 135:1127, 1962.
Long ignored but eventually verified.

Amedi A, et al: Early "visual" cortex activation correlates with superior verbal memory performance in the blind. Nat Neurosci 6:758, 2003.

Andersen P, et al, editors: The hippocampus book, New York, 2007, Oxford University Press.

Bechara A, et al: Double dissociation of conditioning and declarative knowledge relative to the amygdala and hippocampus in humans. Science 269:1115, 1995.

Berardi N, et al: Molecular basis of plasticity in the visual cortex. Trends Neurosci 26:369, 2003.

Bharwadj RD, et al: Neocortical neurogenesis in humans is restricted to development. Proc Natl Acad Sci U S A 103:12564, 2006.
Ingenious experiments using fallout from Cold War nuclear testing to show that humans do not produce significant numbers of neocortical neurons postnatally.

Bibel M, Barde Y-A: Neurotrophins: key regulators of cell fate and cell shape in the vertebrate nervous system. Genes Dev 23:2919, 2000.

Bliss TVP, Lømo T: Long-lasting potentiation of synaptic transmission in the dentate area of the anaesthetized rabbit following stimulation of the perforant path. J Physiol 232:331, 1973.
The original description of long-term potentiation.

Brenowitz SD, Regehr WD: Associative short-term synaptic plasticity mediated by endocannabinoids. Neuron 45:419, 2005.

Busch SA, Silver J: The role of extracellular matrix in CNS regeneration. Curr Opin Neurobiol 17:120, 2007.

Chauvet N, Prieto M, Alonso G: Tanycytes present in the adult rat mediobasal hypothalamus support the regeneration of monoaminergic axons. Exp Neurol 151:1, 1998.
Axons can regrow through those rare parts of the CNS that lack astrocytes.

Chevaleyre V, Takahashi KA, Castillo PE: Endocannabinoid-mediated synaptic plasticity in the CNS. Annu Rev Neurosci 29:37, 2006.

Corkin S, et al: H. M.'s medial temporal lobe lesion: findings from magnetic resonance imaging. J Neurosci 17:3964, 1997.

Curtis MA, et al: Human neuroblasts migrate to the olfactory bulb via a lateral ventricular extension. Science 315:1243, 2007.

Dancause N, et al: Extensive cortical rewiring after brain injury. J Neurosci 25:10167, 2005.
For some cortical areas, maybe much more than expected.

David S, Aguayo AJ: Axonal elongation into peripheral nervous system "bridges" after central nervous system injury in adult rats. Science 214:931, 1981.

Davies SJA, et al: Robust regeneration of adult sensory axons in degenerating white matter of the adult rat spinal cord. J Neurosci 19:5810, 1999.

Doyon J, Penhune V, Ungerleider LG: Distinct contribution of the cortico-striatal and cortico-cerebellar systems to motor skill learning. Neuropsychology 41:252, 2003.

Duvernoy HM: The human hippocampus: functional anatomy, vascularization and serial sections with MRI, ed 3, Berlin, 2005, Springer-Verlag.
A meticulously detailed and beautifully illustrated book.

Egan DA, Flumerfelt BA, Gwyn DG: Axon reaction in the red nucleus of the rat: perikaryal volume changes and the time course of chromatolysis following cervical and thoracic lesions. Acta Neuropathol 37:13, 1977.

Emsley JG, et al: Adult neurogenesis and repair of the adult CNS with neural progenitors, precursors, and stem cells. Prog Neurobiol 75:321, 2005.

Eriksson PS, et al: Neurogenesis in the adult human hippocampus. Nat Med 4:1313, 1998.

Eyre JA, et al: Evidence of activity-dependent withdrawal of corticospinal projections during human development. Neurology 57:1543, 2001.

Faulkner JR, et al: Reactive astrocytes protect tissue and preserve function after spinal cord injury. J Neurosci 24:2143, 2004.

Finney EM, Fine I, Dobkins KR: Visual stimuli activate auditory cortex in the deaf. Nat Neurosci 4:1171, 2001.

Galea MP, Darian-Smith I: Postnatal maturation of the direct corticospinal projections in the macaque monkey. Cereb Cortex 5:518, 1995.

Garcez PP, et al: Axons of callosal neurons bifurcate transiently at the white matter before consolidating an interhemispheric projection. Eur J Neurosci 25:1384, 2007.

Gramsbergen A, et al: Regression of polyneural innervation in the human psoas muscle. Early Hum Dev 49:49, 1997.

Gross CG: Neurogenesis in the adult brain: death of a dogma. Nat Rev Neurosci 1:67, 2000.

Hamburger V: Regression versus peripheral control of differentiation in motor hypoplasia. Am J Anat 102:365, 1958.

Hamilton R, et al: Alexia for Braille following bilateral occipital stroke in an early blind woman. Neuroreport 11:237, 2000.

Harrison RV, Gordon KA, Mount RJ: Is there a critical period for cochlear implantation in congenitally deaf children? Analyses of hearing and speech perception performance after implantation. Dev Psychobiol 46:252, 2005.

Hashimoto K, Kano M: Postnatal development and synapse elimination of climbing fiber to Purkinje cell projection in the cerebellum. Neurosci Res 53:221, 2005.

Hebben N, et al: Diminished ability to interpret and report internal states after bilateral medial temporal lobe resection: Case HM. Behav Neurosci 99:1031, 1985.

Hensh TK: Critical period regulation. Annu Rev Neurosci 27:549, 2004.

Hubel DH, Wiesel TN: Binocular interaction in striate cortex of kittens reared with artificial squint. J Neurophysiol 28:1041, 1965.

Johnson JS, Newport EL: Critical period effects in second language learning: the influence of maturational state on the acquisition of English as a second language. Cog Psychol 21:60, 1989.

Kishimoto Y, Kano M: Endogenous cannabinoid signaling through the CB_1 receptor is essential for cerebellum-dependent discrete motor learning. J Neurosci 26:8829, 2006.

Knowlton BJ, Mangels JA, Squire LR: A neostriatal habit learning system in humans. Science 273:1399, 1996.

Kuhl PK, Tsao F-M, Liu H-M: Foreign-language experience in infancy: effects of short-term exposure and social interaction on phonetic learning. Proc Natl Acad Sci U S A 100:9096, 2003.

LaMantia AS, Rakic P: Axon overproduction and elimination in the corpus callosum of the developing rhesus monkey. J Neurosci 10:2156, 1990.

LeDoux JE, Romanski L, Xagoraris A: Indelibility of subcortical emotional memories. J Cog Neurosci 1:238, 1989.
Work on the role of the amygdala in learning the emotional significance of stimuli.

Lenroot RK, Giedd JN: Brain development in children and adolescents: insights from anatomical magnetic resonance imaging. Neurosci Biobehav Rev 30:718, 2006.

Martin JH, et al: Corticospinal system development depends on motor experience. J Neurosci 24:2122, 2004.

Martin JH, et al: Activity- and use-dependent plasticity of the developing corticospinal system. Neurosci Biobehav Rev 31:1125, 2007.

Massey JM, et al: Increased chondroitin sulfate proteoglycan expression in denervated brainstem targets following spinal cord injury creates a barrier to axonal regeneration overcome by chondroitinase ABC and neurotrophin-3. Exp Neurol 209:426, 2008.

Merabet LB, Amedi A, Pascual-Leone A: Activation of the visual cortex by Braille reading in blind subjects. In Lomber SG, Eggermont JJ, editors: Reprogramming the cerebral cortex: plasticity following central and peripheral lesions, Oxford, 2006, Oxford University Press.

Moran LB, Graeber MB: The facial nerve axotomy model. Brain Res Rev 44:154, 2004.

Morcuende S, et al: Abducens internuclear neurons depend on their target motoneurons for survival during early postnatal development. Exp Neurol 195:244, 2005.

Morris RGM, et al: Selective impairment of learning and blockade of long-term potentiation by an N-methyl-D-aspartate receptor antagonist, AP5. Nature 319:774, 1986.

Navarro X, Vivó M, Valero-Cabré A: Neural plasticity after peripheral nerve injury and regeneration. Prog Neurobiol 82:163, 2007.

Nelson CA, III, et al: Cognitive recovery in socially deprived young children: the Bucharest Early Intervention Project. Science 318:2007, 1937.

Packard MG, Knowlton BJ: Learning and memory functions of the basal ganglia. Annu Rev Neurosci 25:563, 2002.

Papez JW: A proposed mechanism of emotion. Arch Neurol Psychiatry 38:725, 1937.
  The evidence was not very strong by today's standards, but the idea has been extremely influential anyway.

Pascalis O, de Haan M, Nelso CA: Is face processing species-specific during the first year of life? Science 296:1321, 2002.

Pascual-Leone A, et al: The role of reading activity on the modulation of motor cortical outputs to the reading hand in Braille readers. Ann Neurol 38:910, 1995.

Pascual-Leone A, et al: The plastic human brain cortex. Annu Rev Neurosci 28:377, 2005.

Phelps EA: Human emotion and memory: interactions of the amygdala and hippocampal complex. Curr Opin Neurobiol 14:198, 2004.

Richardson PM, Issa VMK: Peripheral injury enhances central regeneration of primary sensory neurones. Nature 309:791, 1984.
  Somewhat paradoxically, cutting the peripheral process of a dorsal root ganglion cell jump-starts its growth responses and makes it better able to deal with subsequent section of its central branch.

Rosene DL, van Hoesen GW: Hippocampal efferents reach widespread areas of cerebral cortex and amygdala in the rhesus monkey. Science 198:315, 1977.

Sadato N, et al: Activation of the primary visual cortex by Braille reading in blind subjects. Nature 380:526, 1996.

Savio T, Schwab ME: Lesioned corticospinal tract axons regenerate in myelin-free rat spinal cord. Proc Natl Acad Sci U S A 87:4130, 1990.

Schwenkreis P, et al: Assessment of sensorimotor cortical representation asymmetries and motor skills in violin players. Eur J Neurosci 26:3291, 2007.

Scoville WB, Milner B: Loss of recent memory after bilateral hippocampal lesions. J Neurol Neurosurg Psychiatry 20:11, 1957.
  The original description of patient HM.

Shen Y, Linden DJ: Long-term potentiation of neuronal glutamate transporters. Neuron 46:715, 2005.

Shimony JS, et al: Diffusion tensor imaging reveals white matter reorganization in early blind humans. Cereb Cortex 16:2006, 1653.

Snyder JS, et al: A role for adult neurogenesis in spatial long-term memory. Neuroscience 130:843, 2005.

Stanfield BB, O'Leary DDM: The transient corticospinal projection from the occipital cortex during the postnatal development of the rat. J Comp Neurol 238:236, 1982.

Szpunar KK, Watson JM, McDermott KB: Neural substrates of envisioning the future. Proc Natl Acad Sci U S A 104:642, 2007.
  "Episodic memory may, at its heart, be the ability to vividly represent oneself in time, in both the past and the future … individuals, be they depressive patients, young children, or amnesics, who are unable to vividly recollect their past, also seem to be unable to form specific mental images of the future."

Tan AM, et al: Antibodies against the NG2 proteoglycan promote the regeneration of sensory axons within the dorsal columns of the spinal cord. J Neurosci 26:4729, 2006.

Vaina LM, et al: Neural systems underlying learning and representation of global motion. Proc Natl Acad Sci U S A 95:12657, 1998.

Vargas ME, Barres BA: Why is Wallerian degeneration in the CNS so slow? Annu Rev Neurosci 30:153, 2007.

Weiss S, et al: Multipotent CNS stem cells are present in the adult mammalian spinal cord and ventricular neuroaxis. J Neurosci 16:7599, 1996.

Wiesel TN, Hubel DH: Single-cell responses in striate cortex of kittens deprived of vision in one eye. J Neurophysiol 26:1003, 1963.

Wiesel TN, Hubel DH: Comparison of the effects of unilateral and bilateral eye closure on cortical unit responses in kittens. J Neurophysiol 28:1029, 1965.

Witzel C, Rohde C, Brushart TM: Pathway sampling by regenerating peripheral axons. J Comp Neurol 485:183, 2005.

Xie F, Zheng B: White matter inhibitors in CNS axon regeneration failure. Exp Neurol 209:302, 2008.

Xu J, Wall JT: Rapid changes in brainstem maps of adult primates after peripheral injury. Brain Res 774:211, 1997.

Yu X, et al: The activation of the cortical hand area by toe tapping in two bilateral upper-extremities amputees with extraordinary foot movement skill. Magn Reson Imaging 24:45, 2006.

Zucker RS, Regehr WG: Short-term synaptic plasticity. Annu Rev Physiol 64:355, 2002.

Zweifel LS, Kuruvilla R, Ginty DD: Functions and mechanisms of retrograde neurotrophin signalling. Nat Rev Neurosci 6:615, 2005.

Atlas of the Human Forebrain[a]

25

When the nervous system is discussed in terms of functional subsystems, as in the preceding chapters, it is sometimes difficult to envision how the various parts are related to the whole. Therefore an abbreviated atlas is provided here using the same philosophy as in Chapter 15, with a wide variety of forebrain structures and a few brainstem structures labeled.

Only major structures that are mentioned prominently in this book are indicated. In addition, to keep the number of labels manageable, cerebral sulci and gyri are generally left unlabeled, and a number of structures that appear repeatedly are not labeled every time they appear. Very abbreviated descriptions of labeled structures are provided; additional details can be found elsewhere in the text and in the glossary.

---

[a]All figures modified from Nolte J, Angevine JB Jr: The human brain in photographs and diagrams, ed 3, St Louis, 2007, Mosby.

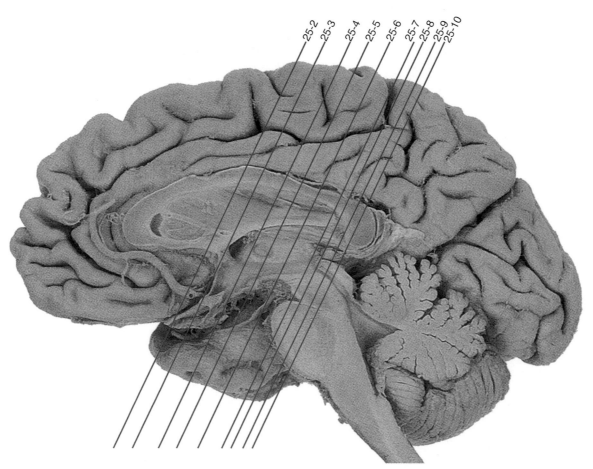

25-2
25-3
25-4
25-5
25-6
25-7
25-8
25-9
25-10

Figure 25-1 Planes of the sections shown in Figures 25-2 to 25-10.

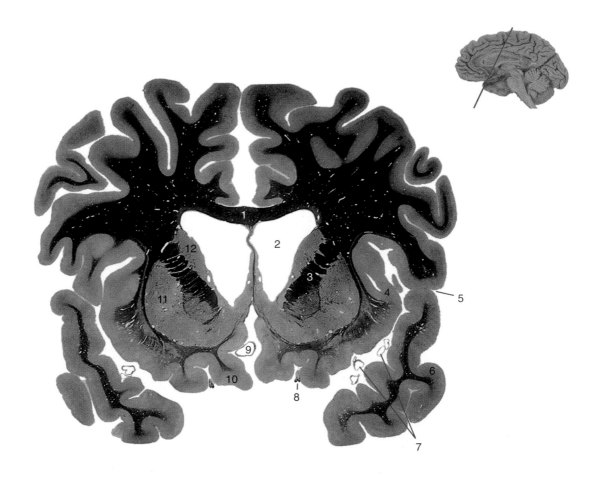

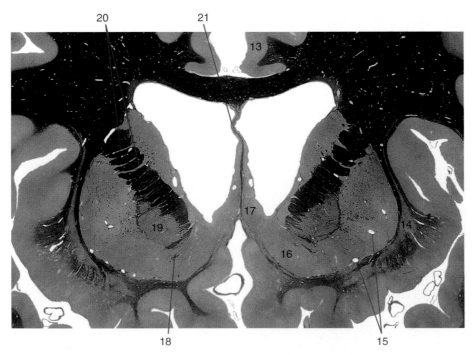

Figure 25-2 Anterior horn of the lateral ventricle.

1. Corpus callosum (body). Commissural fibers interconnecting most cortical areas.
2. Anterior horn of the lateral ventricle.
3. Anterior limb of the internal capsule. Contains projections to and from prefrontal and anterior cingulate cortex, including those from the dorsomedial and anterior nuclei of the thalamus.
4. Insula. Includes gustatory and visceral cortex.
5. Lateral sulcus (Sylvian fissure).
6. Anterior end of the temporal lobe (temporal pole). Limbic cortex.
7. Branches of the middle cerebral artery. Will emerge from the lateral sulcus and supply the lateral surface of the cerebral hemisphere.
8. Olfactory tract. Projections from the olfactory bulb to the piriform cortex and amygdala.
9. Anterior cerebral artery. Branches parallel the corpus callosum and supply the medial surface of the frontal and parietal lobes.
10. Gyrus rectus. Part of orbital frontal cortex; extensive limbic connections, particularly in circuits involving the amygdala.
11. Putamen. The part of the striatum with predominantly motor connections.
12. Caudate nucleus (head). The part of the striatum predominantly connected with association cortex.
13. Cingulate gyrus. Extensive limbic connections: anteriorly in circuits involving the amygdala, and posteriorly in circuits involving the hippocampus.
14. Claustrum. Reciprocal connections with cerebral cortex, poorly understood function.
15. Lenticulostriate arteries. Small perforating branches of the middle cerebral artery.
16. Nucleus accumbens. The part of the striatum with predominantly limbic connections.
17. Septal nuclei. Reciprocally connected with the amygdala, hippocampus, hypothalamus, and other limbic structures.
18. Projections from the anterior olfactory nucleus on their way to the anterior commissure.
19. Globus pallidus (external segment). Afferents from the striatum, efferents to the subthalamic nucleus and other parts of the basal ganglia.
20. Gray bridges between the putamen and caudate nucleus; part of the reason the striatum got its name.
21. Septum pellucidum. Paired membrane separating the two lateral ventricles.

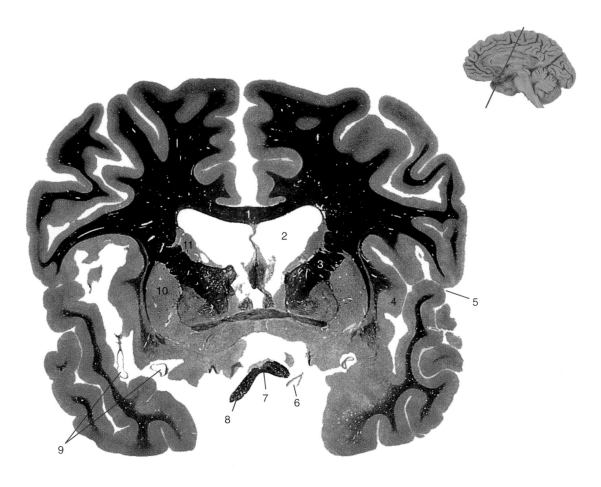

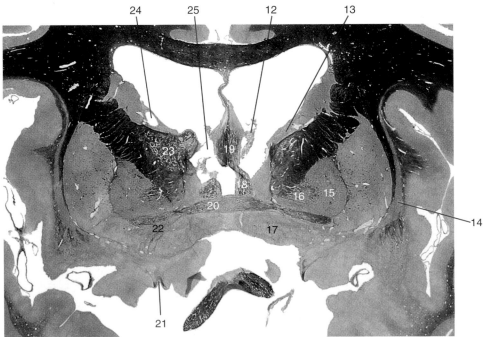

Figure 25-3 Anterior commissure.

1. Corpus callosum (body). Commissural fibers interconnecting most cortical areas.
2. Junction between the anterior horn and body of the lateral ventricle.
3. Genu of the internal capsule. Contains projections to and from frontal cortex.
4. Insula. Includes gustatory and visceral cortex.
5. Lateral sulcus (Sylvian fissure).
6. Internal carotid artery, just before it bifurcates into the anterior and middle cerebral arteries.
7. Optic chiasm, where optic nerve fibers from the nasal half of each retina decussate.
8. Optic nerve. Axons of retinal ganglion cells on their way to the lateral geniculate nucleus, superior colliculus, and a few other sites.
9. Branches of the middle cerebral artery. Will emerge from the lateral sulcus and supply the lateral surface of the cerebral hemisphere.
10. Putamen. The part of the striatum with predominantly motor connections.
11. Caudate nucleus (junction between the head and body). The part of the striatum predominantly connected with association cortex.
12. Choroid plexus adjacent to the interventricular foramen.
13. Stria terminalis. Efferents from the amygdala to the septal nuclei, basal forebrain, and hypothalamus.
14. Claustrum. Reciprocal connections with cerebral cortex, poorly understood function.
15. Globus pallidus (external segment). Afferents from the striatum, efferents to the subthalamic nucleus and other parts of the basal ganglia.
16. Globus pallidus (internal segment). Afferents from the striatum and subthalamic nucleus, efferents to the thalamus and midbrain reticular formation.
17. Basal forebrain. Includes the basal nucleus (of Meynert), groups of large cholinergic neurons that innervate most forebrain areas.
18. Column of the fornix. Efferents from the hippocampus to the septal nuclei, basal forebrain, and mammillary body.
19. Body of the fornix. Efferents from the hippocampus to the septal nuclei, basal forebrain, and mammillary body.
20. Anterior commissure. Commissural fibers interconnecting the temporal lobes, together with a few crossing olfactory fibers.
21. Olfactory tract. Projections from the olfactory bulb to the piriform cortex and amygdala.
22. Ventral pallidum. Limbic extension of the globus pallidus, with inputs from nucleus accumbens.
23. Reticular nucleus, covering the anterior (and lateral) surface of the thalamus. Afferents from the thalamus and cerebral cortex, GABAergic efferents to the thalamus.
24. Terminal (thalamostriate) vein, adjacent to the stria terminalis.
25. Interventricular foramen.

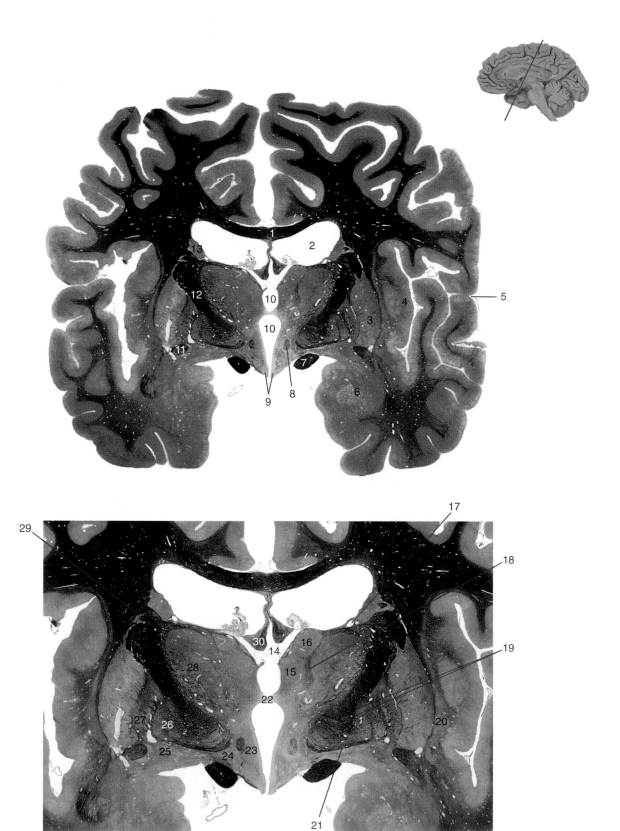

Figure 25-4 Anterior thalamus.

1. Corpus callosum (body). Commissural fibers interconnecting most cortical areas.
2. Body of the lateral ventricle.
3. Putamen. The part of the striatum with predominantly motor connections.
4. Insula. Includes gustatory and visceral cortex.
5. Lateral sulcus (Sylvian fissure).
6. Amygdala. A collection of nuclei forming the core of one of the two major limbic circuits.
7. Optic tract. Axons of ganglion cells from half of each retina, on their way to the lateral geniculate nucleus, superior colliculus, and a few other sites.
8. Column of the fornix. Efferents from the hippocampus to the mammillary bodies.
9. Median eminence of the hypothalamus. Former attachment point of the infundibular stalk.
10. Third ventricle. The two portions indicated are separated by the interthalamic adhesion (massa intermedia).
11. Fibers that will cross in the anterior commissure, interconnecting the temporal lobes.
12. Posterior limb of the internal capsule. Contains projections to and from sensorimotor and parietal cortex, including corticospinal fibers and the somatosensory radiation.
13. Caudate nucleus (body). The part of the striatum predominantly connected with association cortex.
14. Transverse cerebral fissure. An extension of subarachnoid space, situated above the roof of the third ventricle and containing the internal cerebral veins.
15. Dorsomedial nucleus. Connections with prefrontal association cortex.
16. Anterior nucleus. Afferents from the mammillary body (via the mammillothalamic tract), efferents to the cingulate gyrus.
17. Terminal (thalamostriate) vein, adjacent to the stria terminalis.
18. Mammillothalamic tract. Projection from the mammillary body to the anterior nucleus of the thalamus. Part of the Papez circuit.
19. Lenticular fasciculus (passing through the internal capsule). Part of the projection from the internal segment of the globus pallidus to the thalamus.
20. Claustrum. Reciprocal connections with cerebral cortex, poorly understood function.
21. Ansa lenticularis. Part of the projection from the internal segment of the globus pallidus to the thalamus.
22. Interthalamic adhesion (massa intermedia).
23. Medial zone of the hypothalamus. At this level, includes the ventromedial and dorsomedial nuclei.
24. Lateral hypothalamic nucleus.
25. Location of the basal nucleus (of Meynert). Groups of large cholinergic neurons in the basal forebrain that innervate most forebrain areas.
26. Globus pallidus (internal segment). Afferents from the striatum and subthalamic nucleus, efferents to the thalamus and midbrain reticular formation.
27. Globus pallidus (external segment). Afferents from the striatum, efferents to the subthalamic nucleus and other parts of the basal ganglia.
28. Ventral anterior and ventral lateral (VA/VL) nuclei. Afferents from the cerebellum and basal ganglia, efferents to motor areas of cortex.
29. Reticular nucleus of the thalamus. Afferents from the thalamus and cerebral cortex, GABAergic efferents to the thalamus.
30. Body of the fornix. Efferents from the hippocampus to the septal nuclei, basal forebrain, and mammillary body.

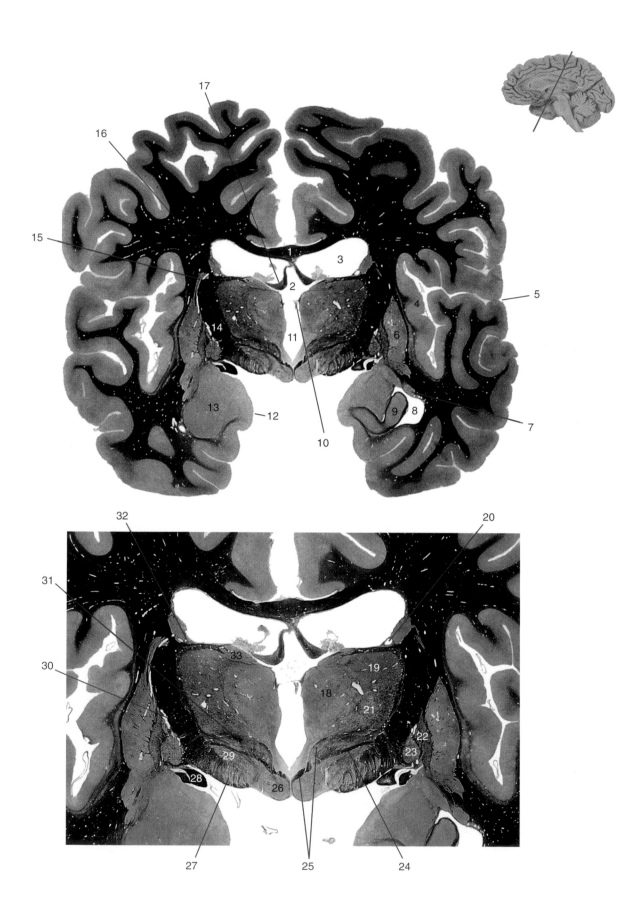

Figure 25-5 Midthalamus; mammillary bodies.

1. Corpus callosum (body). Commissural fibers interconnecting most cortical areas.
2. Transverse cerebral fissure. An extension of subarachnoid space, situated above the roof of the third ventricle and containing the internal cerebral veins.
3. Body of the lateral ventricle.
4. Insula. Includes gustatory and visceral cortex.
5. Lateral sulcus (Sylvian fissure).
6. Putamen. The part of the striatum with predominantly motor connections.
7. Caudate nucleus (tail). The part of the striatum predominantly connected with association cortex.
8. Inferior horn of the lateral ventricle.
9. Anterior end of the hippocampus, the core of one of the two major limbic circuits.
10. Choroid plexus in the roof of the third ventricle.
11. Third ventricle, the slit-shaped cavity of the diencephalon.
12. Uncus. The proximity of the surface of the uncus to the cerebral peduncle can cause clinical problems.
13. Amygdala. A collection of nuclei forming the core of one of the two major limbic circuits.
14. Posterior limb of the internal capsule. Contains projections to and from sensorimotor and parietal cortex, including corticospinal fibers and the somatosensory radiation.
15. Gray bridge between the putamen and caudate nucleus; part of the reason the striatum got its name.
16. Caudate nucleus (body). The part of the striatum predominantly connected with association cortex.
17. Body of the fornix. Efferents from the hippocampus to the septal nuclei, basal forebrain, and mammillary body.
18. Dorsomedial nucleus. Connections with prefrontal association cortex.
19. Ventral lateral (VL) nucleus. Afferents from the cerebellum and basal ganglia (primarily the former), efferents to motor areas of cortex.
20. Terminal (thalamostriate) vein, adjacent to the stria terminalis.
21. Ventral posterolateral (VPL) nucleus. Afferents from the spinal cord (spinothalamic tract) and posterior column nuclei, efferents to somatosensory cortex.
22. Globus pallidus (external segment). Afferents from the striatum, efferents to the subthalamic nucleus and other parts of the basal ganglia.
23. Globus pallidus (internal segment). Afferents from the striatum and subthalamic nucleus, efferents to the thalamus and midbrain reticular formation.
24. Lenticular fasciculus. Part of the projection from the internal segment of the globus pallidus to the thalamus.
25. Mammillothalamic tract. Projection from the mammillary body to the anterior nucleus of the thalamus. Part of the Papez circuit.
26. Mammillary body. Afferents from the hippocampus, efferents to the anterior nucleus of the thalamus. Part of the Papez circuit.
27. Substantia nigra. The reticular part receives inputs from the striatum and projects to the thalamus, midbrain reticular formation, and superior colliculus; the compact part contains pigmented, dopaminergic neurons that project to the striatum and other parts of the basal ganglia.
28. Optic tract. Axons of ganglion cells from half of each retina, on their way to the lateral geniculate nucleus, superior colliculus, and a few other sites.
29. Subthalamic nucleus. Afferents from motor cortex and the external segment of the globus pallidus, excitatory efferents to the internal segment of the globus pallidus and other parts of the basal ganglia.
30. Zona incerta. One more source of direct inputs to the cerebral cortex; function unknown.
31. Thalamic fasciculus. Projections from the cerebellum and basal ganglia to the ventral anterior and ventral lateral nuclei (VA/VL).
32. Stria terminalis. Efferents from the amygdala to the septal nuclei, basal forebrain, and hypothalamus.
33. Lateral dorsal nucleus. Efferents to the cingulate gyrus.

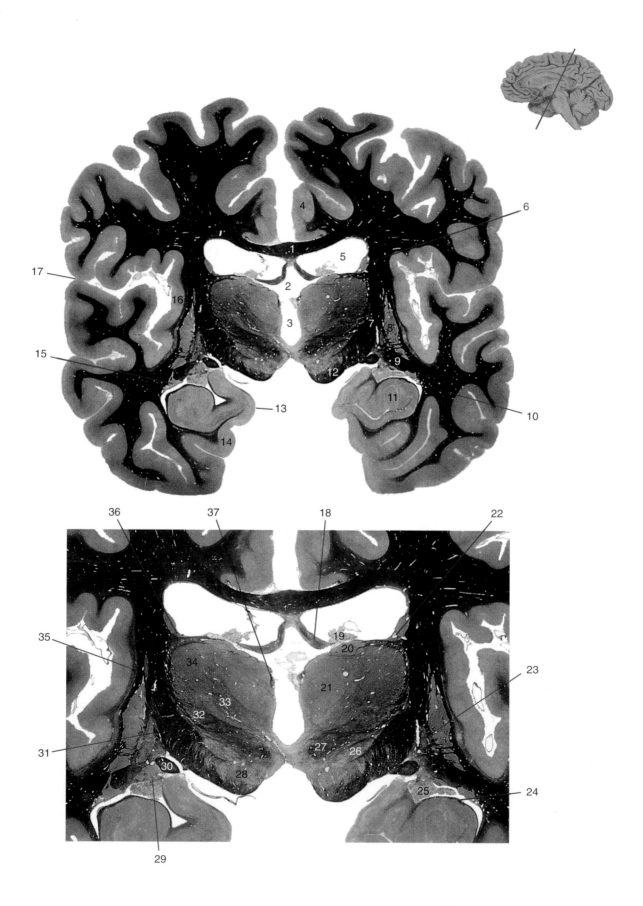

Figure 25-6 Midthalamus.

1. Corpus callosum (body). Commissural fibers interconnecting most cortical areas.
2. Transverse cerebral fissure. An extension of subarachnoid space, situated above the roof of the third ventricle and containing the internal cerebral veins.
3. Third ventricle, the slit-shaped cavity of the diencephalon.
4. Cingulate gyrus. Extensive limbic connections; at posterior levels such as this, mostly in circuits involving the hippocampus.
5. Body of the lateral ventricle.
6. Caudate nucleus (body). The part of the striatum predominantly connected with association cortex.
7. Posterior limb of the internal capsule. Contains projections to and from sensorimotor and parietal cortex, including corticospinal fibers and the somatosensory radiation.
8. Putamen. The part of the striatum with predominantly motor connections.
9. Sublenticular part of the internal capsule. Contains projections to and from temporal and some other cortical areas, including the auditory radiation and part of the optic radiation.
10. Inferior horn of the lateral ventricle.
11. Hippocampus, the core of one of the two major limbic circuits.
12. Cerebral peduncle. Corticospinal, corticobulbar, and corticopontine fibers.
13. Uncus. The proximity of the surface of the uncus to the cerebral peduncle can cause clinical problems.
14. Parahippocampal gyrus. This anterior level is entorhinal cortex, the source of most afferents to the hippocampus.
15. Caudate nucleus (tail). The part of the striatum predominantly connected with association cortex.
16. Insula. Includes gustatory and visceral cortex.
17. Lateral sulcus (Sylvian fissure).
18. Body of the fornix. Efferents from the hippocampus to the septal nuclei, basal forebrain, and mammillary body.
19. Choroid plexus in the body of the lateral ventricle.
20. Lateral dorsal nucleus. Efferents to the cingulate gyrus.
21. Dorsomedial nucleus. Connections with prefrontal association cortex.
22. Terminal (thalamostriate) vein, with adjacent stria terminalis.
23. Globus pallidus (external segment). Afferents from the striatum, efferents to the subthalamic nucleus and other parts of the basal ganglia.
24. Alveus. Hippocampal efferents on the ventricular surface of the hippocampus.
25. Choroid plexus in the inferior horn of the lateral ventricle.
26. Subthalamic nucleus. Afferents from motor cortex and the external segment of the globus pallidus, excitatory efferents to the internal segment of the globus pallidus and other parts of the basal ganglia.
27. Rostral end of the red nucleus, surrounded by cerebellar efferents on their way to the thalamus.
28. Substantia nigra. The reticular part receives inputs from the striatum and projects to the thalamus, midbrain reticular formation, and superior colliculus; the compact part contains pigmented, dopaminergic neurons that project to the striatum and other parts of the basal ganglia.
29. Stria terminalis, which has now emerged from the posterior surface of the amygdala. Efferents from the amygdala to the septal nuclei, basal forebrain, and hypothalamus.
30. Optic tract. Axons of ganglion cells from half of each retina, on their way to the lateral geniculate nucleus, superior colliculus, and a few other sites.
31. Ventral posteromedial nucleus (VPM). Afferents from trigeminal and solitary nuclei, efferents to somatosensory and gustatory cortex.
32. Ventral posterolateral nucleus (VPL). Afferents from the spinal cord (spinothalamic tract) and posterior column nuclei, efferents to somatosensory cortex.
33. Centromedian nucleus, the largest of the intralaminar nuclei. Afferents from the globus pallidus, efferents to the striatum.
34. Ventral lateral nucleus (VL). Afferents from the cerebellum and basal ganglia (primarily the former), efferents to motor areas of cortex.
35. Reticular nucleus of the thalamus. Afferents from the thalamus and cerebral cortex, GABAergic efferents to the thalamus.
36. Stria terminalis. Efferents from the amygdala to the septal nuclei, basal forebrain, and hypothalamus.
37. Stria medullaris of the thalamus. Site of attachment of the roof of the third ventricle, and a route through which septal efferents reach the habenula.

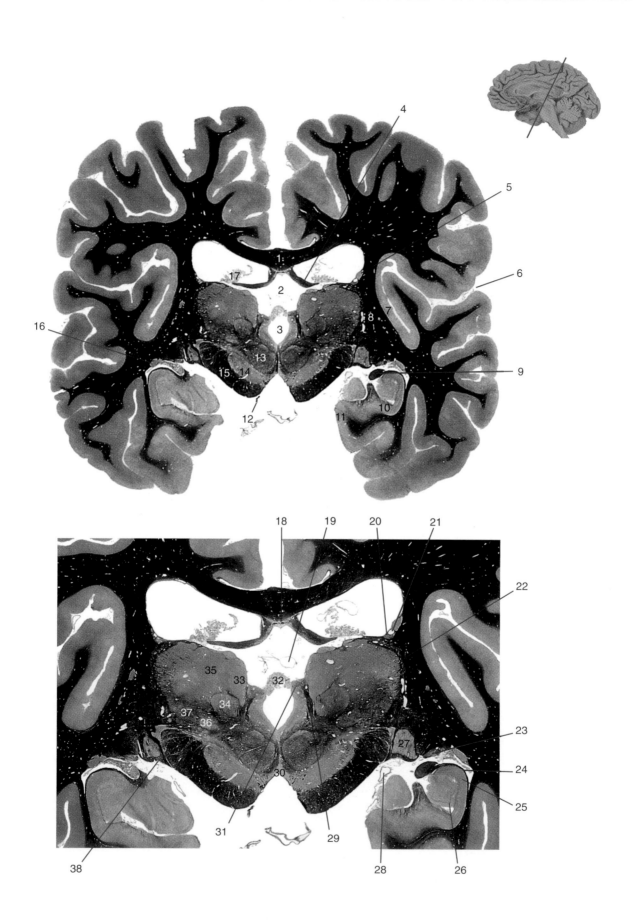

Figure 25-7 Posterior thalamus; habenula.

1. Corpus callosum (body). Commissural fibers interconnecting most cortical areas.
2. Transverse cerebral fissure. An extension of subarachnoid space, situated above the roof of the third ventricle and containing the internal cerebral veins.
3. Third ventricle, near the aqueduct.
4. Body of the fornix. Efferents from the hippocampus to the septal nuclei, basal forebrain, and mammillary body.
5. Caudate nucleus (body). The part of the striatum predominantly connected with association cortex.
6. Lateral sulcus (Sylvian fissure).
7. Insula. Includes gustatory and visceral cortex.
8. Retrolenticular part of the internal capsule. Contains projections to and from the parietal and occipital lobes, including part of the optic radiation.
9. Fimbria of the hippocampus. Hippocampal efferents that have assembled from the alveus, on their way into the fornix.
10. Subiculum, a subdivision of the hippocampus and its principal source of efferents. Afferents from the hippocampus proper.
11. Parahippocampal gyrus. This anterior level is entorhinal cortex, the source of most afferents to the hippocampus.
12. Oculomotor nerve, just emerging from the midbrain.
13. Red nucleus. Afferents from the cerebellum, efferents to the inferior olivary nucleus and a few to the spinal cord.
14. Substantia nigra. The reticular part receives inputs from the striatum and projects to the thalamus, midbrain reticular formation, and superior colliculus; the compact part contains pigmented, dopaminergic neurons that project to the striatum and other parts of the basal ganglia.
15. Cerebral peduncle. Corticospinal, corticobulbar, and corticopontine fibers.
16. Caudate nucleus (tail). The part of the striatum predominantly connected with association cortex.
17. Choroid plexus in the body of the lateral ventricle.
18. Hippocampal commissure. Fibers interconnecting the two hippocampi.
19. Internal cerebral vein, on its way to the great cerebral vein (of Galen).
20. Stria terminalis. Efferents from the amygdala to the septal nuclei, basal forebrain, and hypothalamus.
21. Terminal (thalamostriate) vein, adjacent to the stria terminalis.
22. Reticular nucleus of the thalamus. Afferents from the thalamus and cerebral cortex, GABAergic efferents to the thalamus.
23. Stria terminalis. Efferents from the amygdala to the septal nuclei, basal forebrain, and hypothalamus.
24. Alveus. Hippocampal efferents on the ventricular surface of the hippocampus.
25. Hippocampus proper (cornu ammonis), a subdivision of the hippocampus. Afferents from the dentate gyrus, efferents to the subiculum and septal nuclei.
26. Dentate gyrus, a subdivision of the hippocampus. Afferents from entorhinal cortex, efferents to hippocampal pyramidal cells.
27. Lateral geniculate nucleus. Afferents from the retina, efferents to visual cortex.
28. Posterior cerebral artery, curving around the midbrain on its way to the medial surface of the occipital lobe.
29. Fasciculus retroflexus (the habenulointerpeduncular tract). Conveys limbic output from the habenula to the midbrain reticular formation.
30. Ventral tegmental area. Contains dopaminergic neurons that project to a variety of limbic and neocortical (mostly frontal) areas.
31. Habenula, a relay in caudally directed limbic projections. Afferents from the septal nuclei, efferents to the midbrain reticular formation.
32. Choroid plexus in the roof of the third ventricle.
33. Dorsomedial nucleus. Connections with prefrontal association cortex.
34. Centromedian nucleus, the largest of the intralaminar nuclei. Afferents from the globus pallidus, efferents to the striatum.
35. Lateral posterior nucleus. Connections, similar to those of the pulvinar, with parietal-occipital-temporal association cortex.
36. Ventral posteromedial nucleus (VPM). Afferents from trigeminal and solitary nuclei, efferents to somatosensory and gustatory cortex.
37. Ventral posterolateral nucleus (VPL). Afferents from the spinal cord (spinothalamic tract) and posterior column nuclei, efferents to somatosensory cortex.
38. Optic tract entering the lateral geniculate nucleus.

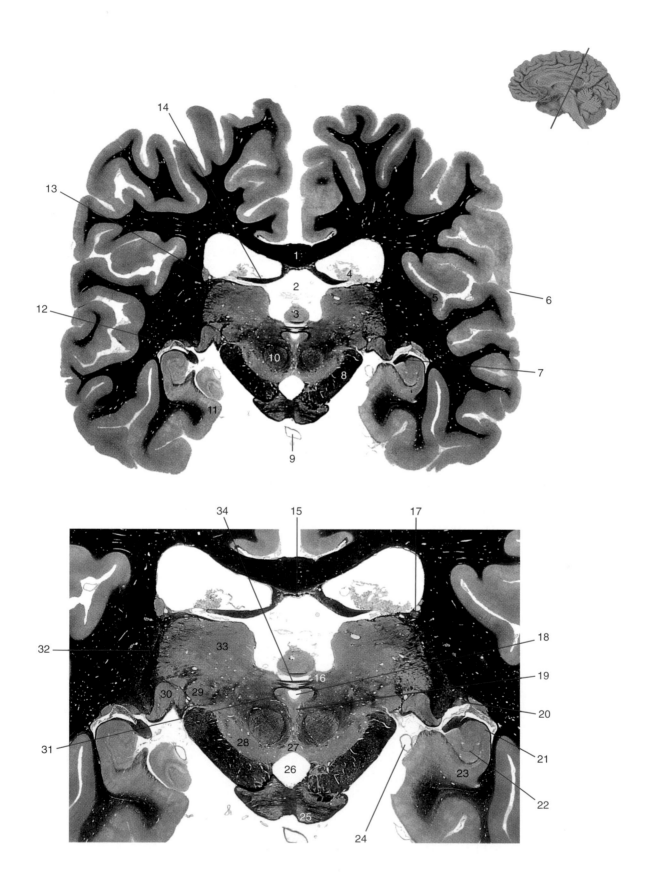

Figure 25-8 Posterior commissure.

1. Corpus callosum (body). Commissural fibers interconnecting most cortical areas.
2. Superior cistern, a subarachnoid cistern continuous anteriorly with the transverse fissure above the roof of the third ventricle.
3. Pineal gland. An endocrine gland important in seasonal cycles and circadian rhythms.
4. Choroid plexus in the body of the lateral ventricle.
5. Insula. Includes gustatory and visceral cortex.
6. Lateral sulcus (Sylvian fissure).
7. Fimbria of the hippocampus. Hippocampal efferents that have assembled from the alveus, on their way into the fornix.
8. Cerebral peduncle. Corticospinal, corticobulbar, and corticopontine fibers.
9. Basilar artery.
10. Red nucleus. Afferents from the cerebellum, efferents to the inferior olivary nucleus and spinal cord.
11. Parahippocampal gyrus. This anterior level is entorhinal cortex, the source of most afferents to the hippocampus.
12. Caudate nucleus (tail). The part of the striatum predominantly connected with association cortex.
13. Caudate nucleus (body). The part of the striatum predominantly connected with association cortex.
14. Body of the fornix. Efferents from the hippocampus to the septal nuclei, basal forebrain, and mammillary body.
15. Hippocampal commissure. Fibers interconnecting the two hippocampi.
16. Pretectal area, part of the pupillary light reflex pathway. Afferents from retinal ganglion cells, efferents to the Edinger-Westphal nucleus.
17. Stria terminalis (adjacent to terminal vein). Efferents from the amygdala to the septal nuclei, basal forebrain, and hypothalamus.
18. Cerebral aqueduct, the connection between the third and fourth ventricles.
19. Oculomotor nucleus. Lower motor neurons for extraocular muscles and the levator palpebrae, preganglionic parasympathetic neurons for the ciliary muscle and pupillary sphincter.
20. Stria terminalis. Efferents from the amygdala to the septal nuclei, basal forebrain, and hypothalamus.
21. Hippocampus proper (cornu ammonis), a subdivision of the hippocampus. Afferents from the dentate gyrus, efferents to the subiculum and septal area.
22. Dentate gyrus, a subdivision of the hippocampus. Afferents from entorhinal cortex, efferents to hippocampal pyramidal cells.
23. Subiculum, a subdivision of the hippocampus and its principal source of efferents. Afferents from the hippocampus proper.
24. Posterior cerebral artery, curving around the midbrain on its way to the medial surface of the occipital lobe.
25. Most rostral pontine nuclei. Afferents from cerebral cortex (via the cerebral peduncle), efferents to contralateral cerebellar cortex (via the middle cerebellar peduncle).
26. Interpeduncular cistern, the subarachnoid cistern between the cerebral peduncles.
27. Ventral tegmental area. Contains dopaminergic neurons that project to a variety of limbic and neocortical (mostly frontal) areas.
28. Substantia nigra. The reticular part receives inputs from the striatum and projects to the thalamus, midbrain reticular formation, and superior colliculus; the compact part contains pigmented, dopaminergic neurons that project to the striatum and other parts of the basal ganglia.
29. Medial geniculate nucleus. Auditory afferents via the inferior brachium, efferents to auditory cortex.
30. Lateral geniculate nucleus. Afferents from the retina, efferents to visual cortex.
31. Periaqueductal gray. Part of a descending pain-control pathway.
32. Reticular nucleus of the thalamus. Afferents from the thalamus and cerebral cortex, GABAergic efferents to the thalamus.
33. Pulvinar. Connections with parietal-occipital-temporal association cortex.
34. Posterior commissure. Crossing fibers dealing with vertical eye movements and the pupillary light reflex.

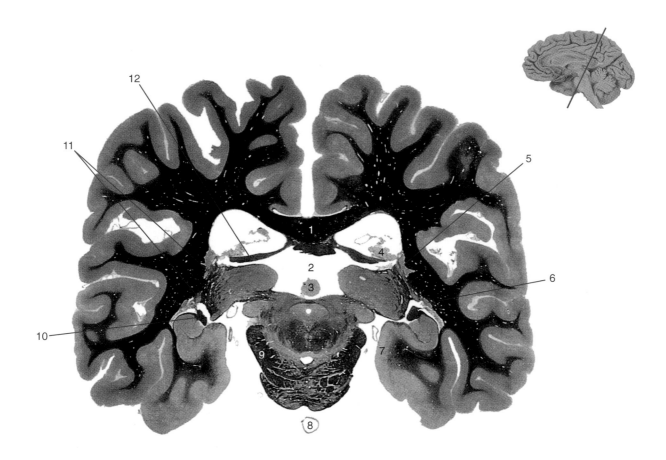

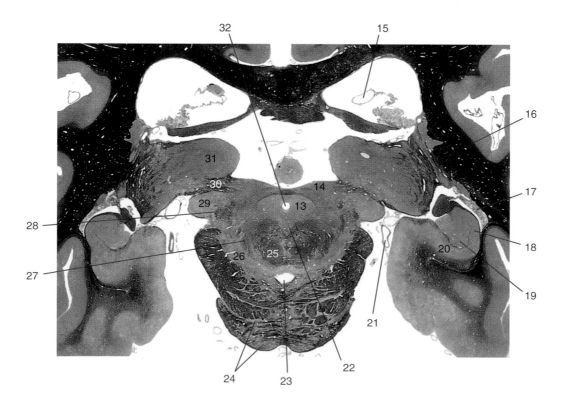

Figure 25-9 Posterior thalamus; midbrain.

1. Corpus callosum (splenium). At this level, commissural fibers interconnecting posterior cortical areas.
2. Superior cistern, a subarachnoid cistern continuous anteriorly with the transverse fissure above the roof of the third ventricle.
3. Pineal gland. An endocrine gland important in seasonal cycles and circadian rhythms.
4. Choroid plexus in the body of the lateral ventricle.
5. Caudate nucleus (body). The part of the striatum predominantly connected with association cortex.
6. Caudate nucleus (tail). The part of the striatum predominantly connected with association cortex.
7. Parahippocampal gyrus, continuous with the cingulate gyrus near the splenium of the corpus callosum.
8. Basilar artery.
9. Cerebral peduncle. Corticospinal, corticobulbar, and corticopontine fibers.
10. Fimbria of the hippocampus. Hippocampal efferents that have assembled from the alveus, on their way into the fornix.
11. Stria terminalis. Efferents from the amygdala to the septal nuclei, basal forebrain, and hypothalamus.
12. Crus of the fornix. Efferents from the hippocampus to the septal nuclei, basal forebrain, and mammillary body.
13. Periaqueductal gray. Part of a descending pain-control pathway.
14. Rostral end of the superior colliculus. Afferents from the retina and visual cortex, efferents to the pulvinar and other structures; functions in visual attention and eye movements.
15. Choroidal vein, draining the choroid plexus of the body of the lateral ventricle.
16. Stria terminalis cut tangentially as it curves around with the lateral ventricle. Efferents from the amygdala to the septal nuclei, basal forebrain, and hypothalamus.
17. Choroid plexus in the inferior horn of the lateral ventricle.
18. Hippocampus proper (cornu ammonis), a subdivision of the hippocampus. Afferents from the dentate gyrus, efferents to the subiculum and septal area.
19. Dentate gyrus, a subdivision of the hippocampus. Afferents from entorhinal cortex, efferents to hippocampal pyramidal cells.
20. Subiculum, a subdivision of the hippocampus and its principal source of efferents. Afferents from the hippocampus proper.
21. Posterior cerebral artery, curving around the midbrain on its way to the medial surface of the occipital lobe.
22. Oculomotor nucleus. Lower motor neurons for extraocular muscles and the levator palpebrae, preganglionic parasympathetic neurons for the ciliary muscle and pupillary sphincter.
23. Interpeduncular cistern, the subarachnoid cistern between the cerebral peduncles.
24. Pontine nuclei. Afferents from cerebral cortex (via the cerebral peduncle), efferents to contralateral cerebellar cortex (via the middle cerebellar peduncle).
25. Crossed superior cerebellar peduncle. Efferents from contralateral deep cerebellar nuclei, on their way to the red nucleus and VL.
26. Substantia nigra. The reticular part receives inputs from the striatum and projects to the thalamus, midbrain reticular formation, and superior colliculus; the compact part contains pigmented, dopaminergic neurons that project to the striatum and other parts of the basal ganglia.
27. Medial lemniscus. Somatosensory afferents from the posterior column nuclei and trigeminal main sensory nucleus, on their way to VPL/VPM.
28. Inferior brachium (brachium of the inferior colliculus). Auditory afferents from the inferior colliculus entering the medial geniculate nucleus.
29. Medial geniculate nucleus. Auditory afferents via the inferior brachium, efferents to auditory cortex.
30. Superior brachium (brachium of the superior colliculus). Contains afferents from the retina and visual cortex to the superior colliculus and pretectal area.
31. Pulvinar. Connections with parietal-occipital-temporal association cortex.
32. Cerebral aqueduct, the connection between the third and fourth ventricles.

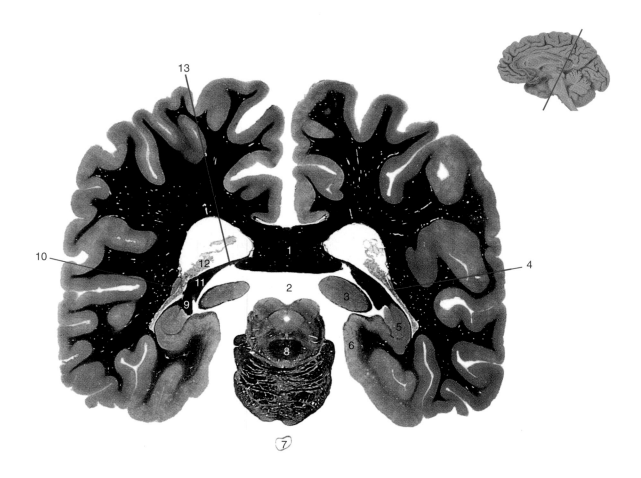

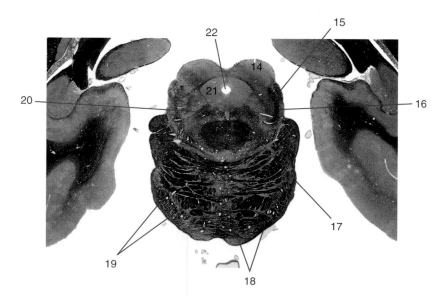

Figure 25-10 Atrium of the lateral ventricle.

1. Corpus callosum (splenium). At this level, commissural fibers interconnecting posterior cortical areas.
2. Superior cistern, a subarachnoid cistern continuous anteriorly with the transverse fissure above the roof of the third ventricle.
3. Pulvinar. Connections with parietal-occipital-temporal association cortex.
4. Choroid plexus, cut tangentially as it curves from the body, through the atrium, and into the inferior horn of the lateral ventricle.
5. Posterior end of the hippocampus, the core of one of the two major limbic circuits.
6. Parahippocampal gyrus, continuous with the cingulate gyrus near the splenium of the corpus callosum.
7. Basilar artery.
8. Decussation of the superior cerebellar peduncles. Efferents from the deep cerebellar nuclei, on their way to the red nucleus and VL.
9. Fimbria of the hippocampus. Hippocampal efferents that have assembled from the alveus, on their way into the fornix.
10. Caudate nucleus, cut tangentially as it curves around with the lateral ventricle.
11. Hippocampal efferent fibers passing from the fimbria of the hippocampus to the crus of the fornix.
12. Glomus, an expanded mass of choroid plexus in the atrium of the lateral ventricle.
13. Crus of the fornix. Efferents from the hippocampus to the septal nuclei, basal forebrain, and mammillary body.
14. Superior colliculus. Afferents from the retina and visual cortex, efferents to the pulvinar and other structures; functions in visual attention and eye movements.
15. Inferior brachium (brachium of the inferior colliculus). Auditory afferents from the inferior colliculus on their way to the medial geniculate nucleus.
16. Medial lemniscus. Somatosensory afferents from the posterior column nuclei and trigeminal main sensory nucleus, on their way to VPL/VPM.
17. Medial longitudinal fasciculus (MLF). Involved in coordinating horizontal eye movements; includes fibers from contralateral abducens interneurons on their way to medial rectus motor neurons.
18. Pontine nuclei. Afferents from cerebral cortex (via the cerebral peduncle), efferents to contralateral cerebellar cortex (via the middle cerebellar peduncle).
19. Corticospinal, corticopontine, and corticobulbar fibers.
20. Central tegmental tract. A complex bundle that contains fibers descending from the red nucleus to the inferior olivary nucleus, ascending gustatory fibers, and ascending and descending fibers of the reticular formation.
21. Periaqueductal gray. Part of a descending pain-control pathway.
22. Cerebral aqueduct, the connection between the third and fourth ventricles.

Glossary

This glossary provides brief descriptions and definitions of the principal neuroscience terms discussed in the preceding chapters. Some editorial judgment was used to keep the length of the glossary reasonable. Terms mentioned tangentially, or those of relatively minor importance, are omitted, as are (for the most part) clinical conditions. Only the meanings most germane to neuroscience are mentioned; for example, of the many meanings of "fovea," only that related to the retina is included. Many items are grouped under more general terms; for example, astrocytes are listed under **glia,** the dentate gyrus is listed under **hippocampus,** and all thalamic nuclei are listed under **thalamus.** Within each entry, terms discussed further in their own entries elsewhere in the glossary are *italicized.*

Many of these definitions were adapted from J.B. Angevine, Jr., *The Human Brain in Photographs and Diagrams,* ed 4, Philadelphia, 2013, Elsevier. Some of these in turn derive, with modifications, from a text by J.B. Angevine, Jr. (with Carl W. Cotman), *Principles of Neuroanatomy,* New York, 1981, Oxford University Press. Thank you to Jay, and also Jeffrey House of Oxford University Press, for permission to draw upon the latter source.

Abducens nerve   The sixth cranial nerve, which emerges anteriorly from the *brainstem* at the junction between the *pons* and *medulla.* It innervates the ipsilateral lateral rectus, causing abduction (hence its name).

Abducens nucleus   The *lower motor neurons* for the ipsilateral lateral rectus, intermingled with interneurons that project through the contralateral *medial longitudinal fasciculus* (MLF) to medial rectus motor neurons; these interneurons provide for conjugate horizontal eye movements. Located near the midline, beneath the floor of the *fourth ventricle* in the caudal *pons.*

Accessory nerve   The eleventh cranial nerve, which originates from the *spinal accessory nucleus* in the *anterior horn* (medulla to C5), emerges laterally from the upper cervical cord, and innervates the sternocleidomastoid and trapezius muscles to mediate turning the head and elevating the shoulder. (The accessory nerve used to be described as having cranial and spinal parts. The spinal part corresponded to the accessory nerve as defined here, and the cranial part corresponded to a series of rootlets that emerge laterally from the caudal *medulla,* join the vagus, and run to the palate, pharynx, and larynx with the *vagus nerve.*)

Accessory oculomotor (Edinger-Westphal) nucleus   A column of small nerve cell bodies near the midline of the *oculomotor nucleus.* Its neurons form the efferent arm of the direct and consensual pupillary light *reflexes*: preganglionic *parasympathetic* neurons effect (via postganglionic neurons in the ciliary ganglion) contraction of the pupillary sphincter to constrict the pupil. Also part of the efferent arm of the near (accommodation) *reflex*: it mediates (again via postganglionic neurons in the ciliary ganglion) ciliary muscle contraction to thicken the lens, and pupillary constriction to increase depth of focus.

Accessory optic nuclei   A series of small nuclei in the rostral *midbrain,* near where the *optic tract* enters the *lateral geniculate nucleus.* They receive inputs from motion-sensitive *ganglion cells* and project to the *vestibular nuclei,* triggering optokinetic movements in response to movement of the visual world across the *retina.* This system is very important for animals without *foveae,* but is poorly developed in humans.

Acetylcholine   A tertiary amine *neurotransmitter* mediating fast excitatory postsynaptic potentials (and end-plate potentials) through nicotinic receptors, and a variety of slower postsynaptic events through muscarinic receptors. Released by *lower motor neurons,* preganglionic *autonomic* neurons, postganglionic *parasympathetic* neurons, and a restricted number of CNS neurons (notably those of the *basal nucleus*). In contrast to most other neurotransmitters, the action of acetylcholine at its synapses is terminated by enzymatic hydrolysis (by acetylcholinesterase).

Action potential   A depolarizing, all-or-nothing electrical signal, typically about a millisecond in duration, that propagates actively and without decrement along *axons* (and sometimes other parts of neurons) to convey information over longer distances than would be possible using *electrotonic* (passive) *spread.*

Adaptation   The progressive decrease in sensitivity shown by most sensory receptors during maintained stimuli. Some receptors adapt rapidly (e.g., *Pacinian corpuscles*), whereas others adapt slowly (e.g., *Golgi tendon organs*). An exception is some *nociceptors,* which become progressively **more** sensitive during a maintained noxious stimulus.

Adenohypophysis   See *pituitary gland.*

Adenosine   A purine derived from ATP, commonly involved in retrograde signaling at synapses. Adenosine binds to *G protein*–coupled receptors (P1 receptors) that are mostly located on presynaptic endings, suppressing transmitter release.

Adequate stimulus   The kind of stimulus energy to which a given sensory receptor is most sensitive (e.g., photons are the adequate stimulus for *photoreceptors*).

Agnosia   Loss of ability to recognize things using a particular sensory system, despite basically normal sensation.

AICA   See *anterior inferior cerebellar artery.*

Alar plate   See *sulcus limitans.*

Allodynia   Pain caused by stimuli that would normally be innocuous, as in wearing clothes over sunburned skin.

Alpha motor neuron   *Lower motor neurons* that innervate the extrafusal fibers of skeletal muscle. They were named for their large axons, which are in the $A\alpha$ range.

Alveus   See *hippocampus.*

Ambient cistern   The combination of the *superior cistern* and sheetlike extensions from it that partially encircle the *midbrain*.

AMPA receptor   A widely distributed type of *ionotropic glutamate* receptor, named for α-amino-3-hydroxyl-5-methyl-4-isoxazole-propionate, a glutamate analog that it binds selectively.

Amygdala   A collection of nuclei in the anteromedial part of the *temporal lobe*, just beneath the *uncus*, forming the core of one of the two major limbic circuits. (The core of the other is the *hippocampus*.)

Angiography   Visualization of blood vessels, traditionally by injecting an x-ray dense substance before an x-ray or *CT* study. Vessels can now also be seen using *MRI* (magnetic resonance angiography, or MRA).

Angular gyrus   That part of the *inferior parietal lobule* formed by the cortex surrounding the upturned end of the superior temporal sulcus; although variable in size and shape, this region is important in language function.

Ansa lenticularis   Part of the projection from the *globus pallidus* to the *thalamus*, with fewer axons than the other part (see *lenticular fasciculus*). It forms a compact, conspicuous cable of myelinated fibers running beneath the *internal capsule* and hooking around its medial edge.

Anterior cerebral artery   The more anterior of the two terminal branches of the *internal carotid artery* (the other is the *middle cerebral*). Anterior cerebral branches (prominently the *pericallosal* and *callosomarginal arteries*) curve around and above the *corpus* callosum to supply *orbital cortex*, the medial surface of the *frontal* and *parietal lobes*, and an adjoining narrow band of cortex along their superior surfaces.

Anterior chamber (of the eye)   The aqueous humor–filled space between the iris and the cornea.

Anterior choroidal artery   A long, thin, branch of the *internal carotid artery* that accompanies the *optic tract* and supplies many structures along the way: the optic tract, *choroid plexus* of the inferior horn of the *lateral ventricle*, part of the *cerebral peduncle*, and deep regions of the *internal capsule, thalamus,* and *hippocampus*.

Anterior commissure   A small, sharply defined bundle of commissural fibers between the rostrum of the *corpus callosum* (to which it is closely related developmentally) and the columns of the *fornix* as they turn down toward the *hypothalamus*; a few inconspicuous anterior fibers interconnect olfactory structures, while its many large posterior fibers link the temporal cortex of the two sides of the brain.

Anterior communicating artery   A short vessel at the anterior end of the *circle of Willis* interconnecting the two *anterior cerebral arteries* just in front of the *optic chiasm*; occasionally it may be very small or, very rarely, absent.

Anterior corticospinal tract   The smaller of the two *corticospinal tracts* (see *lateral corticospinal tract*), consisting of the fibers (about 15%) in each medullary *pyramid* that continue directly into the *anterior funiculus* of the *spinal cord* without decussating; many fibers eventually cross in the anterior white commissure of the cord before terminating, but some end uncrossed. Fibers of the anterior corticospinal tract end (mainly in the cervical and thoracic spinal cord) on spinal motor neurons or nearby interneurons in medial parts of the anterior horn, affecting motor neurons for axial muscles.

Anterior funiculus   One of the three major divisions of the spinal white matter (*funiculus* is Latin for "string" or "cord," as in the old term "funicular" for cable-car), the others being the *lateral* and *posterior funiculi*. The anterior funiculus is located between the anterior median fissure and the exiting *ventral roots*, and contains various tracts (mostly descending), including the *anterior corticospinal tract*.

Anterior horn   One of the three general divisions of the spinal gray matter, the others being the *posterior horn* and the intermediate gray. It contains numerous local-circuit neurons, cell bodies of *alpha (lower) motor neurons*, axons of which enter the *ventral* (anterior) *roots* and end on skeletal muscle, and cell bodies of *gamma motor neurons* that regulate the sensitivity of *muscle spindles*.

Anterior inferior cerebellar artery (AICA)   A long, circumferential branch of the *basilar artery* arising just above the union of the two *vertebrals*. It supplies anterior regions of the inferior cerebellar surface, including the *flocculus*, and parts of the caudal *pons*.

Anterior nucleus   See *thalamus*.

Anterior perforated substance   The inferior surface of the forebrain, roughly between the *orbital gyri* and the *hypothalamus*. So named because numerous *lenticulostriate* and other small *perforating* branches penetrate the brain there.

Anterior root   The anterior, motor root of a *spinal nerve*, coalescing from a variable number of unevenly spaced rootlets that depart the *spinal cord* along its anterolateral sulcus.

Anterior spinal artery   A single midline vessel that originates rostrally as two arteries (one from each *vertebral*) which shortly join and then course within the anterior median fissure along the entire spinal cord. It receives additional blood from the thoracic/abdominal aorta through numerous anastomoses with radicular arteries below the upper cervical region, and gives rise to hundreds of central and circumferential branches that supply the anterior two-thirds of the cord.

Anterolateral system   An umbrella term for the *spinothalamic tract* and closely related ascending fibers, all of which deal with pain, temperature, and to some extent touch, but many of which do not reach the *thalamus*, mostly ending instead in *brainstem* sites such as the *reticular formation*.

Aphasia   Inability to use language (as opposed to a basic motor or sensory deficit that makes it difficult to, for example, articulate or hear). The two broad categories of aphasia are nonfluent aphasias (e.g., Broca's aphasia), in which language production is severely impaired, and fluent aphasias (e.g., Wernicke's aphasia), in which language production is relatively spared but language comprehension may be severely impaired.

Apraxia   Impairment of the ability to perform movements of various types, despite intact strength, coordination, and comprehension.

Aprosodia   Impairment of the ability to either produce or comprehend *prosody* (or both).

Aqueduct (of Sylvius)   The narrow channel through the *midbrain* connecting the *third* and *fourth ventricles*. The aqueduct is a remnant of the lumen of the embryonic *mesencephalon*; it lacks a *choroid plexus* and serves only as a conduit for *CSF* descending through the ventricular system (its stenosis or obstruction is the most common cause of congenital *hydrocephalus*).

Arachnoid The thin meningeal layer that lines and is attached to the *dura mater*, and is interconnected with the *pia mater* by arachnoid trabeculae.

Arachnoid barrier. A layer of arachnoid cells zipped together by tight junctions, preventing diffusion between *subarachnoid space* and the extracellular fluids of the *dura mater*.

Arachnoid granulations. Large collections of arachnoid villi (meaning 1).

Arachnoid trabeculae. Thin strands of collagenous connective tissue that interconnect the arachnoid and *pia*, contributing to the mechanical suspension of the *CNS* within *subarachnoid space*.

Arachnoid villi. 1. Small evaginations of the arachnoid that protrude through the dura mater and into the lumen of a dural sinus of the brain (especially the *superior sagittal sinus*), so that only loosely arranged arachnoid cells and endothelium intervene between *subarachnoid space* and venous blood. Arachnoid granulations are the major (but not exclusive) sites of reabsorption of *cerebrospinal fluid* into the venous system. 2. Small vacation homes for spiders in southern France.*

ARAS See *ascending reticular activating system*.

Archicortex See *cerebral cortex*.

Arcuate fasciculus An association bundle within each *cerebral hemisphere* that curves above the *insula*, interconnecting anterior and posterior parts of the hemisphere. Also called the superior longitudinal fasciculus. Damage to fibers of the arcuate fasciculus passing from *Wernicke's area* to *Broca's area* has traditionally been thought to be the cause of conduction aphasia, although it now appears that cortical damage in the *supramarginal gyrus* is required for the development of this syndrome.

Arcuate nucleus A nucleus in the *periventricular zone* of the tuberal *hypothalamus* containing many of the neurons that produce releasing hormones and inhibiting hormones for control of the *adenohypophysis*, as well as neurons important for the control of feeding behavior.

Area postrema A small region at the caudal end of the fourth ventricle near where the ventricular walls join at the obex. The area postrema is one of several *circumventricular organs* of the brain in which cerebral capillaries are fenestrated and allow free communication between the blood and brain extracellular fluid ("holes" in the blood-brain barrier); it is thought to monitor blood for toxins and to trigger vomiting.

Artery of Adamkiewicz A particularly large radicular artery that joins the *anterior spinal artery* at about spinal cord level T12 in most individuals and supplies most or all of the arterial supply to the cord below that level.

Ascending reticular activating system (ARAS) An umbrella term for the cholinergic, aminergic, and other projections from the *reticular formation* to the *cerebrum* that regulate states of consciousness.

Astrocyte See *glia*.

Ataxia Greek for "lack of order," a term used for incoordinated movements. Although usually taken to indicate cerebellar damage, somatosensory and other deficits can also cause ataxia.

Audiogram A plot of the threshold for hearing pure tones versus the frequencies of those tones. Thresholds are measured in *decibels* relative to the average threshold for normal young ears, and the audiometer compensates for the frequency dependence of our sensitivity to tones. Hence a normal audiogram is a straight line at zero decibels.

Autonomic nervous system The parts of the *PNS* (extending slightly into the *CNS*, to the cell bodies of preganglionic neurons) that control smooth and cardiac muscle and glands. The autonomic system includes *parasympathetic*, *sympathetic*, and *enteric* subdivisions.

Autoregulation The automatic compensatory response of cerebral arterioles to changes in blood pressure. Increases in blood pressure cause the vessels to constrict and decreases cause them to dilate, with the result that cerebral blood flow remains constant over a wide range of pressures.

Axon The single, cylindrical appendage used by most *neurons* to conduct *action potentials* away from the soma and toward axon terminals that make synaptic endings on other neurons.

Axon reflex A "reflex" involving peripheral branches of single *nociceptors*, in which signals initiated in one branch travel not only centrally toward the *CNS*, but also back toward the periphery in other branches. The depolarization traveling peripherally causes the release of *glutamate* and *neuropeptides*, resulting in flare and edema. This is the only known example of a reflex that does not involve at least one synapse in the *CNS*.

Babinski's sign Dorsiflexion of the big toe and fanning of the other toes in response to firm stroking of the lateral part of the sole of the foot. The presence of Babinski's sign, except in infants, indicates *corticospinal tract* damage.

Basal forebrain A loosely used umbrella term for an area at and near the inferior surface of the *telencephalon* between the *hypothalamus* and *orbital cortex*. It includes the *anterior perforated substance* superficially and extends superiorly into the *septal* area and the adjacent, oxymoronically named, *substantia innominata* (see also *basal nucleus*).

Basal ganglia A group of subcortical nuclei, most prominently including the *striatum*, *globus pallidus*, *substantia nigra*, and *subthalamic nucleus*, that collectively modulate the output of frontal cortex. Basal ganglia damage has traditionally been considered to cause disorders characterized by involuntary movements, difficulty initiating movement, and alterations in muscle tone (e.g., Parkinson's disease). However, damage to certain parts of the basal ganglia can cause disturbances of cognition and motivation instead.

Basal nucleus (of Meynert) Groups of large cholinergic neurons in the *substantia innominata* of the *basal forebrain*. Widespread projections of these and nearby *septal* neurons blanket the *neocortex*, *hippocampus*, and *amygdala* with cholinergic endings, suggestive of general regulation of forebrain activity.

Basal plate See *sulcus limitans*.

Basal pons A mass of gray and white matter, oriented transversely and filled with transversely and longitudinally coursing fibers, on the anterior surface of the *pons*. The basal pons looks like a bridge (for which the pons was named) between the two cerebellar hemispheres, but in fact it is a key link between the *cerebrum* and *cerebellum*: *corticopontine* fibers

---

*Thanks to Dr. Tom Finger.

end in its scattered *pontine nuclei*, which in turn project across the midline into the *cerebellum* via the *middle cerebellar peduncle*.

Basal vein (of Rosenthal)   A deep cerebral vein whose tributaries drain the *insula* and some structures near the inferior surface of the forebrain. The basal vein then curves around the *midbrain* and joins the *great cerebral vein*.

Basilar artery   A large vessel formed by union of the two *vertebral arteries*. The basilar artery runs upward along the anterior median surface of the *pons* and gives rise to many *perforating* branches that supply the *pons* and caudal *midbrain*. It also gives rise to the *anterior inferior cerebellar artery* and the *superior cerebellar artery* before bifurcating at the level of the *midbrain* into the two *posterior cerebral arteries*.

Basilar membrane   The portion of the wall of the cochlear duct stretched between the osseous spiral lamina and the spiral ligament, supporting the *organ of Corti*. The basilar membrane is narrow and stiff near the base of the *cochlea*, and becomes progressively wider and floppier toward the apex. Partially as a consequence of the resulting mechanical tuning, the part of the spiral *organ of Corti* near the base of the *cochlea* is most sensitive to high frequencies and the part near the apex to low frequencies.

Blind spot   See *visual field*.

Blood-brain barrier   In a strict sense, the diffusional barrier created by bands of tight junctions joining the endothelial cells of *CNS* capillaries. The term is often used in a broader sense to refer to this barrier in combination with the *arachnoid* barrier and the choroid epithelium, the three of which collectively isolate the extracellular fluids of the CNS from the general extracellular fluids of the body.

Bony labyrinth   See *labyrinth*.

Brachium conjunctivum   See *superior cerebellar peduncle*.

Brachium of the inferior colliculus   Auditory afferents from the *inferior colliculus* on their way to the *medial geniculate nucleus*. Also referred to as the inferior brachium.

Brachium of the superior colliculus   A bundle of fibers that passes over the *medial geniculate nucleus* to reach the *superior colliculus*. Contains afferents from the *retina* that bypass the *lateral geniculate nucleus* and project directly to the *superior colliculus* and *pretectal area*, as well as projections from *cerebral cortex* to the *superior colliculus*. Also referred to as the superior brachium.

Brachium pontis   See *middle cerebellar peduncle*.

Brain   The entire CNS, exclusive of the spinal cord (i.e., the cerebral hemispheres, diencephalon, cerebellum, and brainstem).

Brainstem   In common medical usage, the *midbrain*, *pons*, and *medulla*. (Earlier definitions frequently also included various parts of the *diencephalon* and *telencephalon*, such as the *thalamus* and *basal ganglia*.)

Branchiomeric   Related embryologically to the branchial arches, which play major roles in the development of the face, oral and nasal cavities, larynx, and pharynx.

Broca's area   The *opercular* and *triangular* parts of the *inferior frontal gyrus*, usually on the left. *Broca's area* has traditionally been considered critical for the production of language, but more recent work indicates that other structures such as the *insula* and the head of the *caudate nucleus* may be at least equally important.

Brodmann's areas   A series of 47 areas making up the neocortex, described and numbered by Brodmann based on (sometimes subtle) structural differences. Many of the numbers are still used in reference to cortical areas because specific functions are associated with them.

Brown-Séquard syndrome   Ipsilateral weakness and touch/position deficits combined with contralateral pain/temperature deficits, resulting from damage to one side of the *spinal cord*. A classic example of a crossed syndrome more often associated with *brainstem* damage, in which some symptoms are referred to one side of the body, others to the other.

C fibers   Unmyelinated *PNS* axons. These include the axons of postganglionic *autonomic* neurons, warmth receptors, and many visceral receptors and *nociceptors* (slow pain).

Calcarine sulcus   A prominent, deep cerebral infolding., originating anteriorly in the *temporal lobe* near the splenium of the *corpus callosum* and continuing posteriorly into the *occipital lobe*, where it terminates at the occipital pole. Its upper and lower banks contain the primary visual cortex (*Brodmann's area* 17). Anteriorly along this course the *parietooccipital sulcus* branches off from it.

Callosomarginal artery   A branch of the anterior cerebral artery that follows the cingulate sulcus.

Catecholamine   An amine molecule with a catechol nucleus. The major catecholamine neurotransmitters are *dopamine* and *norepinephrine*; epinephrine is another, but has a more limited role.

Cauda equina   The collection of spinal nerve roots traversing the *lumbar cistern* on their way to the intervertebral foramina through which they leave the vertebral canal.

Caudate nucleus   The more medial part of the *striatum*, bulging into the *lateral ventricle* with its large head in the wall of the anterior horn, tapering body immediately behind, and long slender tail running posteriorly into the atrium and then anteriorly into the inferior horn. It is principally connected with prefrontal and other association areas of cortex, and involved more in cognitive functions and less directly in movement.

Central canal   The narrow, functionless vestige of the lumen of the spinal part of the embryonic *neural tube*, lined by *ependyma* and usually obstructed by epithelial debris. It runs the length of the *spinal cord*, contains traces of *cerebrospinal fluid*, and opens into the *fourth ventricle* at the *obex* of the *medulla*.

Central nervous system (CNS)   The *brain* and *spinal cord*. The formal *CNS/PNS* boundary is near the attachment points of the spinal and cranial nerve roots, where the myelinating glial cells change from *oligodendrocytes* to *Schwann cells*.

Central sulcus (of Rolando)   An anatomically and functionally important infolding of the *cerebral hemisphere*, beginning just medial to the superior border of the hemisphere, proceeding over its superior margin, and descending obliquely forward almost to the *lateral sulcus*. The central sulcus is the boundary between the *frontal* and *parietal lobes*, and the transition zone between primary motor and primary somatosensory cortex.

Central tegmental tract   A complex, heterogeneous tract running centrally through each side of the brainstem *reticular formation* and providing a major highway through which reticular afferents and efferents are distributed. It also contains a major projection from the *red nucleus* to the ipsilateral *inferior olivary nucleus.*

Centromedian nucleus   See *thalamus.*

Centrum semiovale   The white matter of a *cerebral hemisphere* at levels above the *corpus callosum* and *lateral ventricles.* This macroscopically uniform mass consists of interwoven association bundles and fibers on their way to and from the *internal capsule* and *corpus callosum.*

Cephalic flexure   The bend of about 80 degrees between the long axis of the *brainstem* and *spinal cord* and the anterior-posterior axis of the *cerebrum.*

Cerebellar cortex   The three-layered cortex covering the *cerebellum,* comprising a superficial molecular layer (mostly neuronal processes and synapses), a layer of *Purkinje cell* bodies, and a deep layer of vast numbers of granule cell bodies.

Cerebellar peduncles   The three paired fiber bundles connecting the *cerebellum* and *brainstem* and conveying cerebellar afferents and efferents. See *inferior cerebellar peduncle, middle cerebellar peduncle,* and *superior cerebellar peduncle.*

Cerebellomedullary cistern   See *cisterna magna.*

Cerebellopontine angle   The area where the pontomedullary junction adjoins the *cerebellum.* Cranial nerves VII and VIII emerge into this angle.

Cerebellum   A large, convoluted subdivision of the nervous system (*cerebellum* literally means "little brain") that receives inputs from sensory systems, the *cerebral cortex* and other sites and participates in the planning and coordination of movement. Cerebellar outputs arise in a series of deep nuclei, the *fastigial, interposed,* and *dentate nuclei* (listed individually in this glossary).

    Anterior lobe. All of the cerebellum anterior to the primary fissure (partly vermis, partly hemisphere).

    Flocculus. The hemispheral component of the flocculonodular lobe, the part of the cerebellum particularly concerned with the vestibular system and eye movements.

    Hemispheres. The large paired lateral parts, important for motor planning and coordination of the limbs.

    Nodulus. The vermal component of the flocculonodular lobe, the part of the cerebellum particularly concerned with the vestibular system and eye movements.

    Posterior lobe. All of the cerebellum, except for the flocculonodular lobe, posterior to the primary fissure (partly vermis, partly hemisphere).

    Primary fissure. Separates the anterior and posterior lobes of the cerebellum.

    Tonsil. A medial, inferior part of the posterior lobe hemisphere, adjacent to the medulla as it passes through the foramen magnum.

    Vermis. The most medial zone of the cerebellum, straddling the midline. Vermis is Latin for "worm."

Cerebral arterial circle (Circle of Willis)   The anastomotic polygon at the base of the brain, consisting of parts of the *internal carotid, anterior cerebral,* and *posterior cerebral arteries,* interconnected by the *anterior* and *posterior communicating arteries.*

Cerebral cortex   The 1.5- to 4.5-mm thick layer of gray matter that covers the surface of each *cerebral hemisphere.* The cerebral cortex includes olfactory areas (paleocortex) and the hippocampus (archicortex), but most of it is six-layered neocortex. The neocortex is made up of a huge number of columnar functional modules, organized into primary sensory and motor areas, unimodal association areas, multimodal association areas, and limbic areas.

Cerebral hemisphere   The telencephalic derivatives on each side of the CNS, together with a few nontelencephalic but adjoining structures. Includes the *cerebral cortex, striatum, globus pallidus, hippocampus, amygdala,* and the white matter pathways interconnecting them.

Cerebral peduncle   As the term is used in this book, a massive sheaf of tightly packed *corticospinal, corticobulbar,* and *corticopontine* fibers traveling along the base of the *midbrain.* (Others use the term "cerebral peduncle" to refer to all of one side of the midbrain inferior to the aqueduct. In this terminology, the bundle of corticofugal fibers is called the "pes pedunculi," "basis pedunculi," or "crus cerebri.")

Cerebrospinal fluid (CSF)   The clear, colorless fluid that fills the ventricles and the *subarachnoid spaces* surrounding the brain and *spinal cord.* CSF is produced primarily by the *choroid plexus* of the *lateral, third,* and *fourth ventricles,* leaves through the median and lateral apertures of the *fourth ventricle,* and reaches the venous circulation through *arachnoid granulations.*

Cerebrum   The two cerebral hemispheres and the diencephalon.

Choroid (of the eye)   The pigmented, vascular connective tissue layer interposed between the *retina* and the *sclera.* This tissue layer continues anteriorly to form the bulk of the *ciliary body* and *iris.*

Choroid fissure   A C-shaped fissure on the medial surface of each *cerebral hemisphere,* leading into the *choroid plexus* of the *lateral ventricle.*

Choroid plexus   Long, grapevine-like, highly convoluted and vascularized strands in the *lateral, third,* and *fourth ventricles* where most of the *CSF* is produced.

    Choroid epithelium. The cuboidal epithelium covering the ventricular surface of the choroid plexus. Choroid epithelium is continuous with the *ependymal* lining of each ventricle, but is specialized as the secretory epithelium that produces CSF.

    Glomus. An enlarged strand of choroid plexus in the atrium of the *lateral ventricle.* The glomus accumulates calcium deposits with age, and so can often be seen in *CT* images.

Choroidal vein   A tortuous vessel entering the terminal (thalamostriate) vein near the interventricular foramen and draining the choroid plexus of the body of the lateral ventricle.

Chromatolysis   Swelling and apparent loss of *Nissl* substance of a neuronal cell body in response to axonal damage.

Ciliary body   An expanded ring of tissue at the periphery of the iris, containing the ciliary muscle. The ciliary body is covered by the double-layered ciliary epithelium, which produces aqueous humor.

Cingulate gyrus   A broad belt of cortex partially encircling the *corpus callosum.* The cingulate gyrus forms the upper part of the *limbic lobe* (see also *parahippocampal gyrus*) and has extensive limbic connections. Anterior cingulate cortex is closely related to the *amygdala,* posterior cingulate cortex to the *hippocampus.*

Cingulate sulcus A more or less continuous, curved infolding of each *cerebral hemisphere* clearly demarcating the outer margin of the *cingulate gyrus*; posteriorly, a branch (the marginal branch) ascends to the superior margin of the *parietal lobe* immediately behind the upper end of the *central sulcus*.

Cingulum An association bundle located in the white matter underlying the *cingulate gyrus* and interconnecting limbic cortical areas.

Circular sulcus The sulcus outlining the *insula*, demarcating it from the overlying *opercula*.

Circumventricular organs A series of small areas in the ventricular walls near the midline in which the *blood-brain barrier* is lacking, allowing them to monitor various aspects of blood chemistry or to release hormones into the circulation.

Cistern An expanded area of *subarachnoid space*, typically caused by the arachnoid and dura bridging over a substantial indentation in the brain. Major cisterns include the *ambient*, *interpeduncular*, *lumbar*, and *superior cisterns*, *cisterna magna*, and the *transverse fissure*.

Cisterna magna (cerebellomedullary cistern) A large subarachnoid *cistern* between the *medulla* and the inferior *vermis*.

Clasp-knife response The collapse of resistance seen when a *spastic*, hypertonic limb is forcibly flexed or extended.

Claustrum A thin but extensive layer of gray matter beneath the *insula*, separated from it and the underlying *putamen* by the *extreme* and *external capsules*, respectively. The claustrum has reciprocal connections with *cerebral cortex*, but incompletely understood functions.

Climbing fiber A terminal branch of a contralateral *inferior olivary* neuron that wraps around the proximal dendrites of a *Purkinje cell* and forms an extremely powerful distributed synapse. Climbing fibers provide one of the two major excitatory inputs to *cerebellar cortex* (see also *mossy fiber* and *parallel fiber*) and are important in the motor learning functions of the *cerebellum*.

Clonus Rhythmic contractions and relaxations sometimes seen when a *spastic* muscle is stretched.

CNS See *central nervous system*.

Cochlea A cone-shaped, spiral cavity in the temporal bone, containing the cochlear duct (which in turn contains the *basilar membrane* and the *organ of Corti*).

Cochlear nuclei The nuclei in which the primary auditory afferents of the *vestibulocochlear nerve* terminate. The dorsal and ventral cochlear nuclei form a continuous band of gray matter draped over the *inferior cerebellar peduncle* near the pontomedullary junction, and project bilaterally to the *superior olivary nucleus* and into the *lateral lemniscus*.

Collateral sulcus A deep infolding of the inferior surface of the *temporal lobe*, bulging into the wall of the inferior horn of the *lateral ventricle* as the collateral eminence. It separates the *occipitotemporal (fusiform) gyrus* from the *parahippocampal gyrus*.

Coma A pathological state of unconsciousness from which a patient cannot be aroused.

Computed tomography (CT) Computer-aided reconstruction of "slices" in various planes through the head or body. The term is usually used to mean x-ray CT, in which the attenuation of x-ray beams at different angles is used to compute maps of x-ray density.

Conduction velocity The speed at which *action potentials* are propagated along an axon. Small unmyelinated axons conduct at less than 1 m/sec, whereas large myelinated axons conduct at nearly 100 m/sec.

Conductive hearing loss Hearing loss caused by defective function of the outer or middle ear (e.g., middle ear infection), preventing airborne sound vibrations from being conducted to the *cochlea*.

Cone One of the two categories of *retinal* photoreceptors (*rods* are the other kind). Cones are less sensitive than rods but are connected in pathways with relatively little convergence. This allows them to be the receptors for high-acuity vision, particularly in the *fovea* where they are the only receptors present. In addition, there are three different spectral types of cones (long-, middle-, and short-wavelength), allowing cones to subserve color vision.

Confluence of the sinuses The meeting point, near the internal occipital protuberance, where venous blood arrives through the *straight* and *superior sagittal sinuses* and leaves through the *transverse sinuses*.

Conjugate eye movements Movements of both eyes the same amount in the same direction. See also *saccade* and *smooth pursuit*.

Conus medullaris The tapering caudal end of the *spinal cord*, at about vertebral level L1-L2.

Corona radiata Bundles of fibers fanning out above the *internal capsule*, entering or leaving it.

Corpus callosum (Latin for "hard body"), a massive curvilinear bridge of commissural fibers, shaped in sagittal sections like an overturned canoe. The corpus callosum interconnects most cortical areas of the two *cerebral hemispheres* and serves to join them functionally, providing the substrate for a unitary consciousness.

Body. The main arched part of the corpus callosum. Its fibers distribute extensively within each hemisphere.

Genu. The kneelike sharp anterior bend, containing fibers that lead to and from *prefrontal cortex*.

Rostrum. The slender, narrow part beneath the genu, resembling the prow of the (overturned) boat; interconnects *orbital* areas.

Splenium. The thick, rounded posterior bend, containing fibers to and from the *occipital* and *temporal lobes*.

Corticobulbar tract Strictly defined, a large collection of fibers originating in the *cerebral cortex* and descending through the *internal capsule* (immediately anterior to the closely related *corticospinal* fibers) to terminate (via numerous, often intricate routes) in the "bulb" (an old term for the *medulla* or, by extension, for the entire *brainstem*) on neurons of sensory relay nuclei, the *reticular formation*, and motor nuclei of cranial nerves. In common usage, the term refers only to the last fibers of this group. Basically, the equivalent of the *corticospinal tract* for cranial nerve nuclei.

Corticopontine tract A very large collection of fibers originating in *frontal, parietal, occipital*, and *temporal* cortex and descending through the *internal capsule* (both anterior and posterior to the *corticospinal/corticobulbar* projections) to ipsilateral *pontine nuclei*, from which axons pass to the contralateral half of the *cerebellum* through the *middle cerebellar peduncles*.

Corticospinal tract A collection of about a million axons that originate in the *cerebral cortex*, descend through the *internal capsule, cerebral peduncle, basal pons*, and medullary *pyramid*, then reach the *spinal cord*, where they terminate, via the *lateral* and *anterior corticospinal tracts*. Roughly half of them originate in primary *motor cortex*, the rest arising from *premotor* and *supplementary motor areas* and the *parietal lobe* (especially somatosensory cortex). Corticospinal axons end in the spinal cord on cells of the *posterior horn*, intermediate gray, and *anterior horn*, where some synapse directly on *alpha* and *gamma motor neurons*. A single functional role is difficult to specify, but this is the principal pathway for the production of skilled voluntary movements.

Cranial nerves The 12 paired nerves subserving sensory and motor functions for the head and neck. The *olfactory nerve* (CN I) projects directly to the *cerebral hemisphere*, the *optic nerve* (CN II) projects directly to the *diencephalon*, and the *accessory nerve* (CN XI) exits from the upper cervical *spinal cord*; the remaining nine enter or leave the *brainstem*.

Cribriform plate A perforated region of the ethmoid bone in the roof of the nasal cavity. The *olfactory nerve* (CN I)—bundles of axons of olfactory receptor neurons—pass through the perforations to reach the *olfactory bulb*.

CSF See *cerebrospinal fluid*.

CT See *computed tomography*.

Cuneate tubercle A conspicuous swelling on the dorsolateral aspect of the mid-*medulla* overlying the *cuneate nucleus*, which mediates that part of the *posterior column-medial lemniscus pathway* carrying tactile and proprioceptive information from the arm and upper body.

Cuneocerebellar tract Uncrossed fibers from the *lateral cuneate nucleus*, carrying proprioceptive information from the arm to the ipsilateral half of the cerebellar *vermis* and medial *hemisphere* via the *inferior cerebellar peduncle*.

Cuneus The wedge-shaped area of medial *occipital* cortex between the *calcarine* and *parietooccipital sulci*. Includes the upper half of primary visual cortex.

Decibel (dB) A logarithmic measure of sound pressure or sound intensity, relative to some reference level. A tenfold increase in sound pressure level corresponds to a 20 dB change, and the range of normal hearing encompasses about 140 dB.

Declarative memory Memories of facts and events available to consciousness. See also *episodic* and *semantic memory*.

Deep cerebellar nuclei See *fastigial, interposed,* and *dentate nuclei* (listed individually).

Deep tendon reflex The stretch *reflex*—contraction of a skeletal muscle in response to stretch. This is the only monosynaptic reflex, involving muscle spindles and lower motor neurons. So called, even though the responsible receptors are not in tendons, because of the way it is tested clinically.

Deep veins The collection of cerebral veins that eventually drain into the *straight sinus*. Major deep veins include the *basal vein, great cerebral vein, internal cerebral vein,* and *thalamostriate (terminal) vein*.

Delta fibers Thinly myelinated sensory fibers, so called because they conduct in the Aδ range. These include the axons of cold receptors, many touch and visceral receptors, and *nociceptors* (fast pain).

Dendrites Tapering extensions from neuronal cell bodies; the principal but not the only site of synaptic inputs. The dendrites of many neurons have their own extensions, dendritic spines, that may be favored sites for modifying the strength of synapses. See also *neuron*.

Dentate gyrus See *hippocampus*.

Dentate ligament See *denticulate ligament*.

Dentate nucleus The largest and most lateral of the deep cerebellar nuclei, featuring a highly convoluted narrow band of neurons arranged like a bag, with an anteriorly directed opening (hilus) from which efferents emerge to form most of the *superior cerebellar peduncle*. Some dentate outputs reach the *red nucleus* or *inferior olivary nucleus*, but most are bound for the *thalamus*.

Denticulate ligament A thickened, lateral, serrated sheet of *pia mater* on each side of the *spinal cord*, with periodic extensions that attach to the *arachnoid* and *dura*, stabilizing the position of the cord within the dural sac.

Dermatome The area of skin innervated by a single *spinal cord* segment.

Diaphragma sellae A small *dural septum* that covers the *pituitary* fossa.

Diencephalon Literally the "in-between-brain," the caudal subdivision of the embryonic forebrain, giving rise to the *pineal gland, habenula, thalamus, subthalamic nucleus, retina, optic nerve* and *tract, hypothalamus,* and *neurohypophysis*.

Disconnection syndrome A neurological syndrome caused by damage to the white matter interconnecting cortical areas which are themselves undamaged. For example, transection of the axons connecting visual areas to language areas could leave someone able to see but unable to read.

Disinhibition A form of excitation of some part of the *CNS*, caused by inhibiting an inhibitory input. An example is inhibitory inputs to the *globus pallidus* that suppress some part of the tonic inhibition of the *thalamus* by the *globus pallidus*. Suppression of this tonic inhibition allows some thalamic outputs to emerge.

Dopamine A *catecholamine* neurotransmitter used by neurons of the *substantia nigra, ventral tegmental area,* and a few other neuronal types. Nigral dopaminergic neurons project to the *striatum*, whereas those of the nearby *ventral tegmental area* project mostly to *frontal* cortex and *limbic* structures.

Dorsal cochlear nucleus See *cochlear nuclei*.

Dorsal longitudinal fasciculus Ascending and descending fibers traveling through the *periaqueductal* and *periventricular* gray matter, connecting the *hypothalamus* to the *reticular formation* and to preganglionic *autonomic* neurons.

Dorsal motor nucleus of the vagus A prominent *autonomic* efferent nucleus containing most of the preganglionic *parasympathetic* neurons for thoracic and abdominal viscera. Located in the floor of the fourth ventricle in the rostral *medulla*, between the *hypoglossal nucleus* and the *nucleus of the solitary tract*.

Dorsomedial nucleus See *thalamus*.

Dura mater The outermost and most substantial of the three meningeal layers. Intracranial dura mater is firmly attached to the inside of the skull and serves as its periosteum. Spinal dura mater forms a sac, separate from the vertebral periosteum, within which the *spinal cord* is suspended. See also *epidural space, subdural space,* and *venous sinus.*

Dural septa   Inward, sheetlike extensions of dura mater that define intracranial compartments. See also *diaphragma sellae, falx cerebri,* and *tentorium cerebelli.*

Electrotonic conduction or **spread**   The passive spread of a voltage change along a section of neuronal membrane. In contrast to constantly regenerated *action potentials,* the current causing an electrotonic voltage change is progressively lost, either by charging the membrane capacitance or by leaving through ion channels. The resistance and capacitance of the membrane, together with the longitudinal resistances of the neuronal process and the extracellular fluids, determine the length constant for this passive spread and the time constant for reaching a constant voltage. See also *spatial summation* and *temporal summation.*

Emboliform nucleus   See *interposed nucleus.*

Endocannabinoid   Endogenously produced substances, derived from neuronal membranes, that bind to the same *G protein*–coupled receptors that marijuana extracts do. These receptors are most commonly located on presynaptic endings, suppressing transmitter release when activated.

Endolymph   The distinctive high K⁺-low Na⁺ fluid that fills the membranous *labyrinth.*

Endoneurium   Wisps of loose connective tissue that surround the individual nerve fibers within the fascicles of a peripheral nerve.

Enkephalin   Endogenously produced *neuropeptides* that bind to the same *G protein*–coupled receptors that opium extracts do. Prominently involved in pain-control circuitry, but widely distributed in other parts of the *CNS* as well.

Enteric nervous system   The subdivision of the *autonomic nervous system* contained within the walls of the gut. The enteric system includes sensory and motor neurons and interneurons entirely outside the *CNS* and is able to function independently, although normally it is modulated by other *autonomic* elements connected to the *CNS.*

Entorhinal cortex   The cortex covering the anterior part of the *parahippocampal gyrus,* near the *uncus.* Entorhinal cortex receives inputs from the *amygdala,* the *olfactory bulb,* the *limbic lobe* and other cortical association areas, and in turn is the major source of afferents to the *hippocampus.*

Ependyma   Cells forming the lining of the ventricles and the central canal of the *spinal cord.* A specialized ependymal lining (the choroid epithelium) coats the ventricular surface of the *choroid plexus* and secretes *CSF.*

Epidural space   1. In the cranium, the potential space between the periosteal layer of the *dura mater* and the inner surface of the skull. This potential space can become a real space in certain pathological conditions, most commonly as a result of tearing a meningeal artery. 2. In the vertebral canal, the normally present space between the dural sac surrounding the *spinal cord* and the vertebral periosteum.

Epineurium   The outermost and most substantial of the three layers of connective tissue investing peripheral nerves. The epineurium is continuous centrally with the *dura mater.*

Episodic memory   Conscious memory of events, such as the details of a recent party.

Epithalamus   One of the four subdivisions of the *diencephalon;* its most prominent components are the *pineal gland* and the *habenula.*

EPSP (excitatory postsynaptic potential)   See *synapse.*

Equilibrium potential   The potential at which a given ion has no net tendency to move in either direction across a membrane (i.e., the potential at which the ion's concentration gradient is counterbalanced by electrical driving forces). See *Nernst equation.*

External capsule   The sheet of white matter between the *putamen* and *claustrum.* This is the route taken by many cholinergic fibers from the *basal nucleus* on their way to *cerebral cortex,* by some corticostriate fibers, and by some cortical association fibers.

External medullary lamina (of the thalamus)   A thin, curved sheet of myelinated fibers (afferent and efferent), in places fenestrated and in others dense, surrounding the lateral surface of the *thalamus;* enclosed by a thin shell of gray matter, the reticular nucleus (see *thalamus*), which intervenes between it and the *internal capsule.*

Extraocular muscles   The six muscles that together rotate each eye in its orbit: the medial, lateral, superior and inferior rectus muscles, and the superior and inferior obliques.

Extreme capsule   The sheet of white matter between the *insula* and *claustrum.* This is the route taken by fibers interconnecting the *insula* and other cortical areas, and by some cortical association fibers.

Facial colliculus   A swelling in the floor of the *fourth ventricle* in the caudal *pons,* caused by the underlying internal genu of the *facial nerve* looping around the *abducens nucleus.*

Facial nerve   The seventh cranial nerve, which emerges anterolaterally from the *brainstem* along the groove between the *basal pons* and the *medulla.* The facial nerve serves nasopharyngeal, taste, and external ear sensation; controls muscles of facial expression; and regulates secretion by the submandibular, sublingual, and lacrimal glands.

Facial nucleus   A group of lower motor neurons in the caudal *pons* that innervate muscles of the ipsilateral half of the face. Their axons loop over the *abducens nucleus* in the internal genu of the *facial nerve.*

Falx cerebri   The sickle-shaped *dural septum* between the two cerebral hemispheres.

Fasciculus   Latin for "little bundle," a general term used for an anatomically distinct (and usually small) collection of nerve fibers in the *CNS.*

Fasciculus cuneatus   Uncrossed, large, myelinated, primary afferents entering the *posterior column* of the spinal cord rostral to T6 and carrying tactile and proprioceptive information from the arm; many of these fibers ascend to the *medulla* to terminate in *nucleus cuneatus.*

Fasciculus gracilis   Uncrossed, large, myelinated, primary afferents entering the *posterior column* of the spinal cord caudal to T6 and carrying tactile and proprioceptive information from the leg; many of these fibers ascend to the *medulla* to terminate in *nucleus gracilis.*

Fasciculus retroflexus   See *habenulointerpeduncular tract.*

Fastigial nucleus   The most medial of the deep cerebellar nuclei. Its afferents come primarily from the cerebellar *vermis,* and its efferents mainly project bilaterally to the *vestibular nuclei* and *reticular formation.*

Filum terminale   The pial prolongation (literally, the "terminal thread") extending through the *cauda equina,* from the caudal end of the spinal cord (the *conus medullaris*) to the end of the dural sac surrounding the *spinal cord.*

Fimbria   A prominent band of white matter (literally, the "fringe") along the medial edge of the *hippocampus*. The fimbria is an accumulation of myelinated axons (mostly efferent) that first collect on the ventricular surface of the *hippocampus* as the alveus. Near the splenium the fimbria separates from the *hippocampus* as the crus of the *fornix*.

Flocculus   The hemispheral component of the flocculonodular lobe, the part of the *cerebellum* particularly concerned with the vestibular system and eye movements.

FMRI (functional magnetic resonance imaging)   See *magnetic resonance imaging*.

Foliate papillae   See *taste bud*.

Fornix   A prominent paired fiber bundle, mostly containing hippocampal efferents, that interconnects the *hippocampus* of each *cerebral hemisphere* and the ipsilateral *septal area* and *hypothalamus*.

  Body. Upper arched cable formed by the union of the crura beneath the *septa pellucida* in the midline.

  Column. One of the two bundles that diverge from the body, then pass down and back toward the *mammillary bodies*.

  Crus. One of the two origins ("legs") of the body, formed by detachment of the *fimbria* from the *hippocampus*.

  Fimbria. Hippocampal efferents that have assembled from the alveus, on their way into the crus.

  Postcommissural fornix. The continuation of most fornix fibers passing behind the *anterior commissure* and into the *hypothalamus*.

  Precommissural fornix. Fornix fibers that leave the columns just above the *anterior commissure*, bound for the *septal nuclei*, *ventral striatum*, and some nearby cortical areas.

Fourth ventricle   The most caudal of the brain ventricles, shaped like a tent with a peaked roof protruding into the overlying *cerebellum* and a diamond-shaped floor formed by the upper surface of the *pons* and rostral *medulla*; confluent with the *third ventricle* via the *cerebral aqueduct* and open to *subarachnoid space* through three foramina: one median aperture (of Magendie) and two lateral apertures (of Luschka).

Fovea   The central part of the *macula lutea*, containing only *cones* and specialized for color vision of the highest spatial acuity.

Frontal eye field   A *frontal* cortical area prominently involved in voluntary *saccades* to the contralateral side, and in *smooth pursuit* movements as well; located in the posterior part of the *middle frontal gyrus* and in the adjoining walls of the precentral sulcus.

Frontal lobe   The most anterior lobe of each *cerebral hemisphere*. The frontal lobe includes *motor*, *premotor*, and *supplementary motor cortex*, an extensive *prefrontal* region, and a large expanse of *orbital cortex*. The latter two regions have access via long association fibers to all other lobes and also to the limbic system, and are important (in a poorly understood way) in working memory, regulating emotional tone, prioritizing bodily/environmental demands, and stabilizing short- and long-range goal-directed activity.

Fungiform papillae   See *taste bud*.

Funiculus   Latin for "string" or "cord," used in reference to one of the three prominent subdivisions of spinal cord white matter. See *anterior*, *lateral*, and *posterior funiculus*.

Fusiform gyrus   See *occipitotemporal gyrus*.

Fusimotor neuron   See *gamma motor neuron*.

G protein   Shorthand for guanine nucleotide-binding protein. G proteins are signaling molecules that are widely distributed throughout the body. They normally have GDP bound to them, but when activated they exchange this for GTP, dissociate, and trigger some other process (e.g., activation of an enzyme, opening an *ion channel*). In *neurons*, G proteins serve as the link between many *neurotransmitter* receptors and the postsynaptic potentials produced at that *synapse*; for example, muscarinic cholinergic receptors are coupled to G proteins. G proteins are also an integral part of some sensory *transduction* mechanisms, for example those of photoreceptors and olfactory receptors.

GABA (Gamma-aminobutyric acid)   A *glutamate* derivative that is the major *neurotransmitter* for brief, point-to-point inhibitory synaptic events in the *CNS*.

Gamma motor neuron   Small motor neurons that innervate the intrafusal fibers of *muscle spindles*, adjusting the spindles' sensitivity. They were named for their thinly myelinated axons, which are in the Aγ range, and are also known as fusimotor neurons.

Ganglion cell   The neurons of the innermost *retinal* cell layer. Their axons form the *optic nerve*.

Ganglionic arteries   See *perforating arteries*.

Gap junction   An intercellular junction formed by apposed groups of connexons, cylindrical protein assemblies. The connexon channel is large enough to allow the free passage of ions and small molecules between cells, making them the substrate for electrical *synapses* (which are greatly outnumbered by chemical *synapses*).

Generator potential   See *receptor potential*.

Glia   A diverse collection of non-neuronal cell types that perform a wide variety of metabolic, electrical, and mechanical support functions. In the *PNS*, Schwann cells form *myelin*, unsheathe unmyelinated axons, and serve as satellite cells in ganglia. In the *CNS*, oligodendrocytes form *myelin*, astrocytes provide metabolic and mechanical support and help respond to injury, microglia transform into phagocytes in response to injury, and *ependymal* cells line the ventricles.

Globose nucleus   See *interposed nucleus*.

Globus pallidus   A wedge-shaped nucleus medial to the *putamen* that gives rise to most of the efferents from the *basal ganglia*.

  External segment. Afferents from the *striatum* and *subthalamic nucleus*, efferents (via the *subthalamic fasciculus*) to the subthalamic nucleus.

  Internal segment. Afferents from the *striatum* and *subthalamic nucleus*, efferents (via the *ansa lenticularis* and *lenticular fasciculus*) to the thalamus.

Glomus   See *choroid plexus*.

Glossopharyngeal nerve   The ninth cranial nerve. Its rootlets emerge from a shallow groove on the lateral surface of the *medulla* dorsal to the *olive*. This nerve serves naso-oropharyngeal, carotid body/sinus, middle ear, taste, and external ear sensations, assists with swallowing (stylopharyngeus muscle), and regulates salivation (parotid gland).

Glutamate   An amino acid that is the major neurotransmitter for brief, point-to-point excitatory synaptic events in the *CNS*.

Glycine An amino acid that mediates some brief, point-to-point inhibitory synaptic events in the *CNS*, particularly in the *spinal cord*.

Golgi tendon organ A slowly adapting mechanoreceptive ending that monitors muscle tension; found at myotendinous junctions.

Gracile tubercle A conspicuous swelling, just caudal to the *obex*, located dorsomedially on the *medulla* overlying the *nucleus gracilis*, which mediates that part of the *posterior column–medial lemniscus* pathway carrying tactile and proprioceptive information from the leg and lower body.

Great cerebral vein (of Galen) A large, unpaired vessel arising in the *superior cistern* by union of the two *internal cerebral veins*. During its short course it receives the *basal veins* (of Rosenthal), then turns superiorly around the splenium of the *corpus callosum* and joins the inferior sagittal sinus to form the *straight sinus*. The great vein is a key conduit in the deep venous drainage of the brain.

Gyrus rectus A slender, straight convolution ("straight gyrus") that forms the most medial part of *orbital cortex*. Gyrus rectus has extensive limbic connections, particularly in circuits involving the *amygdala*.

Habenula A small mound of neurons on the dorsomedial surface of the caudal *thalamus*, derived from the embryonic *diencephalon*. The habenula receives diverse afferents from the mediobasal forebrain (e.g., *septal nuclei, preoptic area*) that arrive through the superiorly arching *stria medullaris of the thalamus*. Habenular efferents descend to various paramedian midbrain reticular nuclei via the *habenulointerpeduncular tract*. Although it is anatomically evident that the habenula is a relay in caudally directed limbic projections, its exact role is poorly understood.

Habenulointerpeduncular tract A fiber bundle that conveys output from the superiorly coursing *stria medullaris/habenula* route precipitously down again to the paramedian midbrain *reticular formation* (where all other caudally directed limbic projections arrive more expediently by passing inferiorly through the *hypothalamus*). Also called *fasciculus retroflexus*, owing to its lordotic curvature.

Hair cell The characteristic receptor cell type of the auditory and vestibular systems, named for the graduated array of actin-filled microvilli (stereocilia) emerging from its apical surface. Except in the *cochlea*, each hair cell also has a single true cilium (the kinocilium) adjacent to the tallest stereocilia. The graduated array is the basis of a functional polarization of these cells: transduction channels are located near the ends of the stereocilia and deflection of the hair bundle toward or away from the tallest stereocilia causes depolarization or hyperpolarization, respectively, whereas deflection perpendicular to this axis causes no response. Some hair cells are also contractile, allowing outer hair cells of the *organ of Corti* to amplify vibrations of the *basilar membrane*.

Herniation Movement of part of the *CNS* from one compartment to another in response to an expanding mass. Clinically prominent patterns of herniation include herniation of the *cingulate gyrus* under the free edge of the *falx cerebri*, herniation of the *uncus* through the *tentorial* notch, and herniation of the cerebellar *tonsil* through the foramen magnum.

Hippocampus A specialized cortical area rolled into the medial *temporal lobe*. The hippocampus plays a critical role in the consolidation of new *declarative memories*. Anatomi-cally, it has three subdivisions (until recently, usually referred to collectively as the hippocampal formation rather than the *hippocampus*), from within outward as follows:

Dentate gyrus. In cross section, one of two interlocking C-shaped strips of cortex (the hippocampus proper is the other). Afferents from entorhinal cortex, efferents to hippo-campal pyramidal cells.

Hippocampus proper (also called cornu ammonis, or Ammon's horn). Afferents from the dentate gyrus and *septal nuclei*, efferents to the subiculum and *septal nuclei*.

Subiculum. A transitional zone between the hippocampus proper and *entorhinal cortex*, the subiculum receives afferents from the hippocampus proper and is the principal source of efferents from the hippocampus in general. Hippocampal efferents collect on the ventricular surface of the hippocampus proper as a sheet of white matter called the alveus, and from there reach the *fornix* through the *fimbria*.

Histamine A monoamine neurotransmitter derived from histidine, used by neurons of the *tuberomammillary nucleus* of the *hypothalamus*. Like *monoaminergic* neurons in some other nuclei, these have widely branching axons that innervate most of the *CNS*. They participate in the sleep-wake cycle, which presumably explains why antihistamines make people drowsy. In addition, histamine released from mast cells as a result of tissue damage acts on *nociceptors* and is an important mediator of their sensitization.

Homunculus Literally a "little person," the term is used in neuroscience to refer to maps of the body in cortical areas and the cross sections of tracts.

Horner's syndrome The combination of miosis (small pupil), ptosis (drooping eyelid), and enophthalmos (recession of the eyeball; this is more apparent than real). Horner's syndrome can result from damage anywhere along the head/neck *sympathetic* pathway, from *hypothalamic* efferents to preganglionic or postganglionic neurons.

Hydrocephalus Expansion of part or all of the ventricular system. This can occur passively in response to degeneration of some part of the CNS (e.g., expansion of the anterior horns of the *lateral ventricles* in Huntington's disease) or as a result of obstruction in the path of CSF flow. Obstructive hydrocephalus is commonly divided into communicating and noncommunicating types, depending on whether the obstruction is outside or inside the ventricles.

Hyperalgesia Increased sensitivity to stimuli that would normally be only mildly uncomfortable, as in slapping a sunburned back.

Hypocretin See *orexin*.

Hypoglossal nerve The twelfth cranial nerve, whose rootlets emerge from the rostral *medulla* in an anterolateral sulcus between the *pyramid* and the *olive*. It innervates intrinsic and extrinsic skeletal muscles of the tongue.

Hypoglossal nucleus A group of *lower motor neurons* that innervate muscles of the ipsilateral half of the tongue. Located in the floor of the *fourth ventricle* in the rostral *medulla*, near the midline.

Hypoglossal trigone A triangular elevation in the floor of the caudal *fourth ventricle* formed by the underlying *hypoglossal nucleus*.

Hypophysis See *pituitary gland*.

Hypothalamic sulcus A shallow, curved indentation (convex side down) in the wall of the *third ventricle*, extending from the *interventricular foramen* to the opening of the *cerebral aqueduct*. The hypothalamic sulcus is the boundary between the *thalamus* and the *hypothalamus*.

Hypothalamus   The most inferior of the four divisions of the *diencephalon*, the hypothalamus plays a major role in orchestrating visceral and drive-related activities. It has three general zones:

   Anterior region. Includes the *suprachiasmatic, supraoptic,* and *paraventricular nuclei,* projects axons to the *neurohypophysis* and to caudal sites (even including the *spinal cord*).

   Posterior region. Includes the *mammillary* and posterior nuclei and projects to the *thalamus* and *midbrain tegmentum.*

   Tuberal region. Includes the dorsomedial, ventromedial, and *arcuate nuclei.* The latter secretes releasing factors and inhibiting factors into the *pituitary* portal system.

Inferior brachium   See *brachium of the inferior colliculus.*

Inferior cerebellar peduncle   A major input route to the cerebellum, containing crossed olivocerebellar fibers that end as *climbing fibers,* the uncrossed posterior *spinocerebellar* and *cuneocerebellar tracts,* vestibulocerebellar fibers, and other cerebellar afferents. Sometimes referred to as the restiform ("ropelike") body.

Inferior colliculus   A large, rounded mass of gray matter in the roof of the caudal *midbrain.* The inferior colliculus is a major link in the auditory system, receiving the *lateral lemniscus* and giving rise to the *brachium of the inferior colliculus,* which in turn conveys auditory fibers to the medial geniculate nucleus of the *thalamus.*

Inferior frontal gyrus   The most inferior of three longitudinally oriented *frontal* gyri. The *opercular* and *triangular* parts of this gyrus in the dominant hemisphere form *Broca's area,* an area important for the production of spoken and written language.

Inferior olivary nucleus   A large nucleus in the anterolateral *medulla,* shaped like a bag with a convoluted wall of gray matter (like a crumpled, pitted olive). Olivary afferents are diverse (from the *spinal cord, red nucleus,* deep cerebellar nuclei, and other places), but efferents are all olivocerebellar. They pour out of its medially facing mouth (or hilus), cross the midline as *internal arcuate fibers,* join the *inferior cerebellar peduncle,* and blanket the contralateral *cerebellum* as *climbing fibers* that form powerful excitatory synapses on *Purkinje cells* and other neurons.

Inferior parietal lobule   The lower part of the lateral surface of the *parietal lobe,* below the *intraparietal sulcus.* The inferior parietal lobule consists of the *angular* and *supramarginal gyri,* which (in the dominant hemisphere) are functionally related to *Wernicke's area,* and thus are important in the comprehension of language.

Inferior salivary nucleus   Preganglionic *parasympathetic* neurons in the rostral *medulla* whose axons travel through the *glossopharyngeal nerve* to innervate ganglia for the parotid gland.

Inferior temporal gyrus   The most inferior of three longitudinally oriented convolutions visible on the lateral aspect of the *temporal lobe.* The inferior temporal gyrus is part of a large region of visual association cortex occupying most of the *occipital lobe* and much of the *temporal lobe.*

Infundibulum   The hollow, funnel-like stalk of the *pituitary gland,* descending from the *median eminence* of the *hypothalamus* to the posterior lobe of the *pituitary.* The infundibulum arises during embryonic development as a ventral outgrowth of the diencephalic floor, and is later joined by the anterior *pituitary* derived from the roof of the oral cavity.

Inner ear   See *labyrinth.*

Inner hair cell   See *hair cell* and *organ of Corti.*

Insula   The original lateral surface of the embryonic *telencephalic* vesicle overlying an area of fusion with the *diencephalon,* forming in the adult a central lobe of the *cerebral hemisphere,* typically convoluted into about three short gyri (located more anteriorly) and two long gyri. With rapid cerebral expansion during fetal development, the insula is overgrown and by birth concealed by frontal, parietal, and temporal *opercula.* It includes gustatory and autonomic areas, but is less well understood than other cortical areas due to its hidden location.

Intermediate nerve   The smaller, more lateral, sensory subdivision of the *facial nerve,* so named because it is situated between the larger (motor) subdivision and the *vestibulocochlear nerve.*

Intermediolateral cell column   See *lateral horn.*

Internal arcuate fibers   A general term for the large collection of axons that arch across the midline of the *medulla.* Many internal arcuate fibers are axons leaving the *nuclei gracilis* and *cuneatus* to form the contralateral *medial lemniscus;* most others are olivocerebellar fibers on their way to end as *climbing fibers.*

Internal capsule   A compact, curved sheaf of thalamocortical, corticothalamic, and other cortical projection fibers shaped like part of a funnel. The internal capsule is divided into five regions, based on each region's relationship to the *lenticular nucleus:*

   Anterior limb, between the *lenticular nucleus* and the head of the *caudate nucleus.* Connections between the *thalamus* (dorsomedial and anterior nuclei) and *prefrontal* and anterior *cingulate* cortex, plus many frontopontine fibers.

   Genu, at the junction between the anterior and posterior limbs. Connections between the *thalamus* (VA, VL) and *motor/premotor* cortex, plus some frontopontine fibers.

   Posterior limb, between the *lenticular nucleus* and the *thalamus.* Connections between the *thalamus* (VA, VL, VPL/VPM) and *motor,* somatosensory and other parietal cortex, plus *corticobulbar* and *corticospinal* fibers.

   Retrolenticular part, passing posterior to the *lenticular nucleus.* Connections between the *thalamus* (pulvinar, LP) and parietal-occipital-temporal association cortex, plus the upper part of the *optic radiation* (from the lateral geniculate nucleus).

   Sublenticular part, dipping under the posterior part of the *lenticular nucleus.* Projections to and from the *temporal lobe,* including the auditory radiation (from the medial geniculate nucleus) and the lower part of the *optic radiation* (from the lateral geniculate nucleus) before it turns posteriorly through *Meyer's loop* on its way to the *occipital lobe.*

Internal carotid artery   A large distributing artery, originating from the bifurcation of the common carotid artery and running cranially in the neck to enter the base of the skull and eventually the cranial vault. The internal carotid artery branches at the *circle of Willis* into *anterior* and *middle cerebral arteries.* The two internal carotids account for 85% of cerebral blood flow and thus supply most of the blood to the brain.

Internal cerebral vein   The major *deep vein* of each *cerebral hemisphere*, formed at the *interventricular foramen* by the confluence of the smaller *septal* and *terminal (thalamostriate) veins* (the latter receiving the *choroidal vein*, which drains much of the *choroid plexus*). Immediately after its origin the internal cerebral vein bends sharply posteriorly (the bend is called the *venous angle*), proceeds posteriorly in the *transverse fissure*, and fuses with its counterpart in the *superior cistern* to form the unpaired *great vein* (of Galen).

Internal medullary lamina (of the thalamus)   A dense, curved sheet of myelinated fibers within the *thalamus*, demarcating medial and lateral divisions everywhere except posteriorly, where it does not enter the pulvinar, and anteriorly, where it forks into a V-shaped groove for the anterior nucleus. The internal medullary lamina contains several small and two large intralaminar nuclei (the centromedian and parafascicular nuclei).

Interneuron   In the broadest sense of the term, neurons that are located entirely within the *CNS* and interconnect other neurons. However, the term is usually used to refer to small local-circuit neurons, and those with long axons (e.g., *corticospinal* neurons) are called projection neurons.

Internuclear ophthalmoplegia (INO)   Inability to use one medial rectus during attempted lateral gaze, as a result of damage to the ipsilateral *medial longitudinal fasciculus (MLF)*.

Interpeduncular cistern   The subarachnoid *cistern* leading forward from the space between the *cerebral peduncles*, extending under the *diencephalon* and containing the *circle of Willis*.

Interposed nucleus   The deep cerebellar nucleus interposed between the *dentate* and *fastigial nuclei*. The interposed nucleus has two distinct subdivisions, the globose nucleus medially and emboliform nucleus laterally (looks like an embolus in the hilus of the adjoining *dentate nucleus*). Both subdivisions receive input from *cerebellar cortex* of the medial hemisphere, both project (via the *superior cerebellar peduncle*, like the *dentate nucleus*) to the *red nucleus* and ventral lateral nucleus of the *thalamus*.

Interthalamic adhesion (massa intermedia)   A small ovoid area of continuity between the two *thalami* resulting from expansion of the walls of the *third ventricle* during development and their fusion. The interthalamic adhesion is mainly gray matter, containing neurons and axonal and dendritic processes. (This structure is often reduced in size or absent, especially in the brains of elderly persons, but in some mammals, such as rodents, it is massive, reducing the size of the third ventricle but anatomically making the thalamus almost a single unpaired structure.)

Interventricular foramen (of Monro)   The narrow orifice between each *lateral ventricle* and the *third ventricle*.

Intralaminar nuclei   See *thalamus*.

Intraparietal sulcus   A longitudinally oriented sulcus on the lateral aspect of the *parietal lobe*, separating it into a *superior parietal lobule* above and an *inferior parietal lobule* below.

Ion channel   An assembly of protein subunits surrounding a central channel that, at least in some configurations, allows ions to cross the membranes of neurons (and other cells). Some channels switch between closed and open states in response to transmembrane voltage changes, others in response to binding particular ligands (e.g., a particular *neurotransmitter*). Those in sensory receptors may switch states in response to some form of stimulus energy (e.g., heat, mechanical deformation).

Ionotropic receptor   A postsynaptic receptor that is a *neurotransmitter*-gated *ion channel*.

IPSP (inhibitory postsynaptic potential)   See *synapse*.

Iris   The pigmented membrane suspended in front of the lens whose central aperture (the pupil) admits light to the eye. The iris contains two muscles (a sphincter and a dilator) that regulate the size of the pupil.

Juxtarestiform body   Fibers on the medial surface of the inferior cerebellar peduncle that interconnect the cerebellum and the vestibular nuclei.

Labyrinth   The inner ear, consisting of the membranous labyrinth suspended within the bony labyrinth. The bony labyrinth, a *perilymph*-filled channel within the temporal bone, includes the *cochlea*, semicircular canals, and vestibule. The *endolymph*-filled membranous labyrinth includes the cochlear and *semicircular ducts*, the *utricle*, and the *saccule*.

Lamina terminalis   A thin membrane at the anterior end of the *third ventricle*, curving down from the rostrum of the *corpus callosum* to the *optic chiasm* and corresponding (roughly, if not precisely) to the rostral end of the *neural tube*. The lamina terminalis connects the two *telencephalic* vesicles of the embryonic forebrain and provides a route through which commissural fibers that will later comprise the *anterior commissure* and *corpus callosum* begin to grow.

Laminae (of the spinal gray matter)   See *Rexed's laminae*.

Lateral aperture   See *fourth ventricle*.

Lateral corticospinal tract   The larger of the two *corticospinal tracts* (see *anterior corticospinal tract*), comprising the 85% or so of the fibers in each medullary *pyramid* that cross the midline in the *pyramidal decussation* to reach the opposite *lateral funiculus*. The axons of this tract end on spinal *lower motor neurons* or (more often) on smaller *interneurons* that in turn synapse on motor neurons. Its fibers are often said to be arranged somatotopically, with those passing to more caudal cord levels located more laterally, but anatomical evidence does not support this view.

Lateral cuneate nucleus   The equivalent for the arm of *Clarke's nucleus* for the leg. Proprioceptive primary afferents travel through *fasciculus cuneatus* to this nucleus, which then gives rise to uncrossed *cuneocerebellar* fibers that enter the *cerebellum* via the *inferior cerebellar peduncle*.

Lateral dorsal nucleus   See *thalamus*.

Lateral foramina (of Luschka)   See *fourth ventricle*.

Lateral funiculus   One of the three major divisions of the spinal white matter, the others being the *anterior* and *posterior funiculi*. The lateral funiculus contains various ascending and descending tracts, including the *spinocerebellar*, *spinothalamic*, and *lateral corticospinal tracts*.

Lateral geniculate nucleus   See *thalamus*.

Lateral horn   A small, pointed lateral extension of the intermediate spinal gray noted from T1 through L2 or L3. The lateral horn contains the intermediolateral cell column, a long column of preganglionic *sympathetic* neurons serving the entire body. Axons of these preganglionic *sympathetic* neurons leave through the *ventral roots*.

Lateral lemniscus   A flattened ribbon of fibers on the lateral surface of the rostral *pontine tegmentum*, arising from the *cochlear nuclei* and *superior olivary nuclei*. The lateral lemniscus is part of the ascending auditory pathway, conveying information from both ears to the *inferior colliculus*.

Lateral olfactory tract   A small tract (in humans) through which olfactory fibers travel across the surface of the *basal forebrain* to *piriform cortex, entorhinal cortex,* and the *amygdala.*

Lateral posterior nucleus   See *thalamus.*

Lateral sulcus (Sylvian fissure)   A long, deep sulcus on the lateral aspect of each *cerebral hemisphere* resulting from downward and forward expansion of the *temporal lobe* during fetal development. The *insula* lies hidden within the depths of this sulcus, which separates the *temporal lobe* from the *frontal* and *parietal lobes* and provides a route by which the *middle cerebral artery* accesses the lateral convexity.

Lateral ventricle   The large central cavity of each *cerebral hemisphere,* following a C-shaped course throughout the hemisphere and derived from the lumen of the embryonic *telencephalic* vesicle.

>   **Anterior horn.** The frontal horn, in the *frontal lobe* anterior to the *interventricular foramen.*

>   **Atrium (or trigone).** The region near the splenium of the *corpus callosum* where the body and the posterior and inferior horns meet.

>   **Body.** In the *frontal* and *parietal lobes,* extending posteriorly to the region of the splenium of the *corpus callosum.*

>   **Inferior horn.** The temporal horn, curving down and forward into the *temporal lobe.*

>   **Posterior horn.** The occipital horn, projecting backward into the *occipital lobe.*

Lateral vestibulospinal tract   The uncrossed projection from the lateral *vestibular nucleus,* which travels through the ventral part of the *lateral funiculus* to reach the motor neurons for antigravity muscles.

Lemniscus   Greek for "ribbon" and originally used for tracts that are flattened in cross section. Now sometimes used in a more functional sense to refer to tracts that project directly to the thalamus.

Length constant   See *spatial summation.*

Lenticular fasciculus   Part of the projection from the *globus pallidus* to the *thalamus.* It has more axons than the other part (see *ansa lenticularis*) and is more spread out, forming numerous conspicuous bundles of myelinated fibers running medially through the *internal capsule,* like the teeth of a comb. Medial to the *internal capsule* the lenticular fasciculus is joined by the *ansa lenticularis* before both enter the *thalamus.*

Lenticular nucleus   The *putamen* and *globus pallidus* considered as one anatomical structure.

Lenticulostriate (lateral striate) arteries   A collection of about a dozen small branches of the *middle cerebral artery* along its course toward the *lateral sulcus.* They penetrate the overlying brain near their origin and pass upward to supply deep structures (*internal capsule, globus pallidus, putamen*). The lenticulostriate arteries exemplify a large collection of small *perforating* or ganglionic arteries that arise from all arteries around the base of the brain; these narrow, thin-walled vessels are involved frequently in strokes that deprive deep cerebral structures of blood and thus cause neurological deficits out of proportion to their size. Other named groups of *perforating arteries* include the *thalamogeniculate arteries,* arising more posteriorly from the *posterior cerebral artery.* The *anterior choroidal artery* is, in effect, a very large *perforating artery.*

Leptomeninges   The *pia mater* and *arachnoid* considered together.

Limbic lobe   The most medial lobe of the *cerebral hemisphere,* facing the midline and visible grossly only in sagittal section. The limbic lobe consists of a continuous border zone of cortex around the *corpus callosum,* comprising the *cingulate* and *parahippocampal gyri* and their narrow connecting isthmus; this lobe and its many connections, cortical and subcortical, make up and characterize the limbic system.

Limen insulae   Limen is Latin for "threshold," and in this case refers to the transition point from the *anterior perforated substance* to the *insula.* The *circular sulcus,* which surrounds almost the entire *insula,* ends on either side of the limen insulae, allowing access for the *middle cerebral artery.*

Line of Gennari   See *striate cortex.*

Lingual gyrus   The gyrus forming the inferior bank of the *calcarine sulcus.* The lingual gyrus overlaps the posterior portion of the *occipitotemporal gyrus,* separated from it by the *collateral sulcus.*

Locus ceruleus   A column of pigmented, blue-black neurons (locus ceruleus is Latin for "blue spot") near the floor of the *fourth ventricle,* extending through the rostral *pons.* Locus ceruleus neurons provide most of the far-flung noradrenergic innervation of the cerebrum.

Longitudinal fissure   An extensive vertical cleft, oriented sagittally and occupied by the *falx cerebri,* separating the two *cerebral hemispheres* around the margin of the undivided *corpus callosum.*

Long-term depression   A decrease in synaptic efficacy lasting hours or longer. One well-known type involves signaling by *NMDA receptors* that leads to removal of *AMPA receptors,* but there are other mechanisms. Thought to be involved in at least some types of memory.

Long-term potentiation   An increase in synaptic efficacy lasting hours or longer. One well-known type involves signaling by *NMDA receptors* that leads to insertion of additional *AMPA receptors,* but there are other mechanisms. Thought to be involved in at least some types of memory.

Lower motor neuron   The large neurons in the spinal *anterior horn* and in cranial nerve motor nuclei whose axons innervate the extrafusal fibers of skeletal muscle. Also referred to as *alpha motor neurons* and anterior horn cells.

Lumbar cistern   The *CSF*-filled subarachnoid *cistern* extending from the *conus medullaris,* at about vertebral level L1-L2, to the end of the spinal dural sac, at about vertebral level S2. Nerve roots of the *cauda equina* travel through the lumbar cistern.

Macula lutea   A yellowish patch of retina slightly lateral to the *optic disk.* At its center is the *fovea,* a depression in the *retina* containing only elongated *cones* and specialized for vision of the highest acuity.

Magnetic resonance imaging (MRI)   A form of *tomography* based on radiofrequency emissions from particular kinds of atomic nuclei, most commonly hydrogen nuclei. MRI parameters can also be adjusted to produce images of blood vessels (magnetic resonance angiography, or MRA) or to detect increases in blood flow to active areas of the brain (functional magnetic resonance imaging, or fMRI).

Mammillary body A prominent component of the posterior *hypothalamus*. The mammillary body receives afferents from the *hippocampus* (chiefly the subiculum) via the *fornix*, and sends efferents to the anterior nucleus of the *thalamus* via the *mammillothalamic tract*. This is part of a historic neural circuit proposed by James Papez in 1937 as an anatomical substrate for emotion. Although it was derided by some then and viewed as simplistic by others now, the *Papez circuit*—a grand loop from *hippocampus* through *hypothalamus*, *thalamus*, and neocortex back to *hippocampus* again— was unquestionably the impetus for the decades of research that led to the limbic system concept of today.

Mammillothalamic tract The projection from the *mammillary body* to the anterior nucleus of the *thalamus*; part of the *Papez circuit*.

Massa intermedia See *interthalamic adhesion*.

Medial foramen (of Magendie) See *fourth ventricle*.

Medial forebrain bundle A collection of thinly myelinated and unmyelinated fibers running longitudinally through the lateral *hypothalamus* and reaching the *basal forebrain* and the *brainstem tegmentum*. It interconnects the *hypothalamus* with both these areas and also conveys *monoaminergic* fibers on their way from the *brainstem* to widespread cerebral areas.

Medial geniculate nucleus See *thalamus*.

Medial lemniscus Somatosensory afferents originating from the contralateral *posterior column* nuclei and *trigeminal* main sensory nucleus and ascending through the *brainstem* to the *thalamus* (VPL/VPM). The medial lemniscus is the principal ascending pathway for tactile and proprioceptive information.

Medial longitudinal fasciculus (MLF) A longitudinal fiber bundle involved in coordinating eye and head movements. The MLF includes fibers from contralateral *abducens* interneurons to medial rectus motor neurons in the *oculomotor nucleus*. It is also the route of descent for fibers of the medial vestibulospinal tract. See also *internuclear ophthalmoplegia*.

Medial striate artery A large *perforating* branch of the *anterior cerebral artery*, also known as the recurrent artery of Heubner. It supplies the *striatum* in the region of *nucleus accumbens* and also the anterior limb and genu of the *internal capsule*.

Medial vestibulospinal tract Efferents from the medial *vestibular nuclei* of both sides that descend through the *MLF*, then travel through the *anterior funiculus* to reach motor neurons for neck muscles. Important for coordinating eye movements and head movements.

Median aperture See *fourth ventricle*.

Median eminence A swelling at the base of the *hypothalamus* between the *optic chiasm* and the *mammillary bodies* from which the *infundibulum* arises. The median eminence is one of the *circumventricular organs* and is the site at which hypothalamic releasing hormones and inhibiting hormones gain access to the *hypophyseal* portal system.

Medulla (medulla oblongata) The most caudal of the three subdivisions of the *brainstem*, continuous rostrally with the *pons* and caudally with the *spinal cord*. This small structure is important out of proportion to its size: it is crucial to vital functions (respiratory, cardiovascular, visceral activity) and other integrative activities; most sensory and motor tracts of the *CNS* run rostrally and caudally through it.

Meissner corpuscle Rapidly adapting encapsulated mechanoreceptive endings located in the dermal papillae of hairless (glabrous) skin. These endings, together with *Merkel endings*, are largely responsible for the tactile acuity of areas such as fingertips.

Membrane potential The voltage difference between the outside of a cell (defined as zero) and the inside, typically on the order of –65 millivolts (i.e., inside 65 mV negative to outside). All cells have membrane potentials, but neurons specialize in using moment-to-moment changes in this potential as a signaling mechanism. Voltage changes in an inside-positive direction are called depolarizing, and those that make the inside more negative are called hyperpolarizing.

Membranous labyrinth See *labyrinth*.

Merkel ending Slowly adapting disc-shaped mechanoreceptive endings inserted into Merkel cells, which are specialized cells in the basal epidermal layer of both hairy and glabrous skin. These endings, together with *Meissner corpuscles*, are largely responsible for the tactile acuity of areas such as fingertips.

Mesencephalon The second of the three primary embryonic brain vesicles, the only one to remain undivided during subsequent development. See also *midbrain*.

Metabotropic receptor A receptor that produces its postsynaptic effects through intermediate steps, most commonly involving a *G protein*.

Metencephalon The more rostral of the two secondary embryonic brain vesicles derived from the *rhombencephalon*; gives rise to the *pons* and *cerebellum*.

Meyer's loop Geniculocortical fibers representing the contralateral upper visual field that pass through the sublenticular part of the *internal capsule* and loop anteriorly into the *temporal lobe* before turning back toward the *occipital lobe*.

Microfilament A twisted pair of actin filaments, forming the thinnest of the three major types of cytoskeletal elements.

Microglia See *glia*.

Microtubule Cylindrical assembly of 13 strands of tubulin polymers. Microtubules are major cytoskeletal components, and also serve as the "railroad tracks" for fast axonal transport.

Midbrain (mesencephalon) The most rostral of the three subdivisions of the *brainstem*. The midbrain remains tubular in plan but features a great variety of structures: the *superior* and *inferior colliculi* in its roof (tectum), *aqueduct* and *periaqueductal gray*, *oculomotor* and *trochlear nuclei* and *pretectal area*, upper part of the *reticular formation*, *red nuclei*, *substantia nigra*, and *cerebral peduncles*. Like the *medulla*, a small region of enormous importance.

Middle cerebellar peduncle The largest of the cerebellar peduncles, containing fibers from contralateral *pontine nuclei* that end as *mossy fibers* in almost all areas of cerebellar cortex. Sometimes referred to as the brachium pontis (the "arm of the pons").

Middle cerebral artery The more posterior of the two terminal branches of the *internal carotid*. The middle cerebral artery runs laterally beneath the *basal forebrain* to reach the *insula*, where many branches arise and exit from the *lateral sulcus*. It supplies the *insula*, most of the lateral surface of the *cerebral hemisphere*, and the anterior tip of the *temporal lobe*.

Middle ear   The air-filled cavity in the temporal bone through which sound vibrations are transferred by three ossicles (malleus, incus, stapes) from the tympanic membrane to the inner ear.

Middle frontal gyrus   One of three longitudinally oriented *frontal* gyri, situated between the *superior* and *inferior frontal gyri*. It includes part of *premotor cortex*, as well as the *frontal eye field*, which is involved in initiating voluntary eye movements to the contralateral side.

Middle temporal gyrus   One of three longitudinally oriented gyri on the lateral surface of the *temporal lobe* between the *superior* and *inferior temporal gyri*. It contains some visual association cortex, as well as multimodal or heteromodal association cortex.

Miosis   Narrowing of the pupil.

MLF   See *medial longitudinal fasciculus* and *internuclear ophthalmoplegia*.

Monoamine   A molecule containing one amine group. The principal neuroactive monoamines are *dopamine, histamine, norepinephrine*, and *serotonin*.

Mossy fiber   The most abundant form of input to *cerebellar cortex*. Mossy fibers end on granule cells, whose *parallel fibers* in turn innervate *Purkinje cells*. Except for *climbing fibers*, all specific inputs to *cerebellar cortex* (e.g., those from contralateral *pontine nuclei*) terminate as mossy fibers.

Motor cortex   A tapering strip of cortex (*Brodmann's area* 4) in the *precentral gyrus*; the cortical area from which movements are most easily elicited and the source of about half of the corticospinal tract. Also referred to as primary motor cortex.

Motor neuron   See *lower motor neuron* and *upper motor neuron*.

Motor unit   The combination of a single *lower motor neuron* and all the muscle fibers it innervates.

MRA   See *magnetic resonance imaging*.

MRI   See *magnetic resonance imaging*.

Muscle spindle   An encapsulated receptor organ in skeletal muscle containing a few slender intrafusal muscle fibers with sensory endings and the terminals of *gamma motor neurons* applied to them. The sensory endings detect muscle length or its changes, and the gamma endings regulate the sensitivity of the spindle.

Mydriasis   Widening of the pupil.

Myelencephalon   The more caudal of the two secondary embryonic brain vesicles derived from the *rhombencephalon*; gives rise to the *medulla*.

Myelin   Spiral wrappings of Schwann cell (PNS) or oligodendrocyte (CNS) membranes around *axons*, interrupted periodically by *nodes of Ranvier*. Myelin forms a low-capacitance insulating coating around *axons*, greatly increasing their *conduction velocities* by allowing *saltatory conduction*.

Neocortex   See *cerebral cortex*.

Nernst equation   The equation specifying the logarithmic relationship between the concentration gradient of an ion across a semipermeable membrane and its *equilibrium potential*.

Nerve growth factor (NGF)   The first discovered and most famous of the *neurotrophins*. NGF is important for the survival of *sympathetic* ganglion cells and some dorsal root ganglion cells during development.

Neural crest cells   Cells near the crest of each neural fold that are not incorporated into the *neural tube*, but rather migrate widely, form most elements of the *PNS*, and contribute to many other structures.

Neural tube   The tubular epithelial structure formed when the neural groove deepens, closes and detaches from the surface epithelium; the neural tube goes on to form the *CNS*.

Neurofilament   A ropelike assembly of protein polymers; one of three major cytoskeletal components. Neurofilaments aggregate into neurofibrils after some preparation methods, and can be stained and seen microscopically.

Neurohypophysis   See *pituitary gland*.

Neuron   An electrically active cell that forms one of the basic information processing units of the nervous system. Typical neurons are multipolar and have numerous *dendrites* and a single *axon* emerging from an axon hillock, but some are unipolar and others bipolar. Most are wholly contained within the *CNS*, serving as local *interneurons* or projection neurons with long axons, some are partly in the *CNS* and partly in the *PNS* (*lower motor neurons*, preganglionic *autonomic* neurons, many *primary afferent neurons*), and some are entirely in the *PNS* (postganglionic *autonomic* neurons, *enteric* neurons).

Neuropeptide   A short peptide able to function as a *neurotransmitter* (although many neuropeptides do double duty by serving other functions elsewhere in the body). Neuropeptides are derived from larger precursor proteins synthesized in the cell body and shipped by fast axonal transport to synaptic terminals, where they are released from large dense-core vesicles.

Neurotransmitter   A chemical synthesized by neurons and released into synaptic clefts, where it diffuses to other neurons and causes some specific response. Most neurotransmitters are small amine molecules, amino acids, or neuropeptides that are released from vesicles, although some are gases that simply diffuse across neuronal membranes.

Neurotrophins   A small family of neurotrophic factors that includes *nerve growth factor*.

Neurulation   Formation of the *neural tube* by infolding of the neural plate.

Nissl bodies   Clumps of rough endoplasmic reticulum that are prominent in the cell bodies and proximal *dendrites* of *neurons*.

Nitric oxide   A short-lived, gaseous *neurotransmitter* that diffuses across neuronal membranes and stimulates the production of the second messenger cyclic GMP.

NMDA receptor   A special type of *glutamate* receptor that has both transmitter-gated and voltage-gated properties, requiring depolarization in addition to the binding of glutamate to open. Once open it allows Ca^{2+} entry, which in turn sets in motion second-messenger cascades that can alter the properties of the postsynaptic neuron. Thought to be important for the augmentation of synaptic strength underlying some forms of learning and memory.

Nociceptor   A receptor with free nerve endings specifically sensitive to noxious stimuli of one or more types. All have thinly myelinated or unmyelinated axons.

Nodes of Ranvier Periodic gaps in the sheaths of myelinated axons where voltage-gated Na⁺ channels are concentrated and action potentials are regenerated. See also *myelin* and *saltatory conduction*.

Nodulus The *vermal* part of the flocculonodular lobe, involved in postural stability.

Nondeclarative memory Memories not accessible to consciousness, such as sensory and motor skills, learned emotional associations, and conditioned reflexes.

Norepinephrine A *catecholamine* neurotransmitter used by most postganglionic *sympathetic* neurons, and by neurons of the *locus ceruleus* (rostral *pons*) and a few other *brainstem* sites. Locus ceruleus neurons have widely branching axons that innervate most of the *cerebrum* and *cerebellum*.

Nucleus accumbens The most inferior part of the *striatum*, with predominantly limbic connections. Nucleus accumbens was traditionally known as nucleus accumbens septi, reflecting its position immediately lateral to the base of the *septum pellucidum*, as if leaning against it. It is now recognized as the major component of the *ventral striatum*.

Nucleus ambiguus A collection of *lower motor neurons* for laryngeal and pharyngeal muscles, and preganglionic *parasympathetic* neurons for the heart. Located in the *reticular formation* of the rostral *medulla* medial to the *spinothalamic tract*.

Nucleus cuneatus Site of termination of *fasciculus cuneatus* and origin of the arm region of the *medial lemniscus*. Located in the caudal *medulla* (extending a short distance into the rostral *medulla*) lateral to *nucleus gracilis*.

Nucleus dorsalis (of Clarke) A rounded group of large cell bodies in the intermediate spinal gray near the medial edge of the base of the *posterior horn*, from about T1 through L2 or L3. Clarke's nucleus is the origin of the posterior *spinocerebellar tract*, through which stretch receptor and other mechanoreceptive input from the leg reaches the ipsilateral cerebellar *vermis* and medial *hemisphere*.

Nucleus gracilis Site of termination of *fasciculus gracilis* and origin of the leg region of the *medial lemniscus*. Located in the caudal *medulla* medial to *nucleus cuneatus*.

Nucleus of the solitary tract The principal visceral sensory nucleus of the *brainstem*; the site of termination of the visceral *primary afferents* in the *solitary tract*. Located near the floor of the *fourth ventricle* in the rostral *medulla* and caudal *pons*, just lateral to the *sulcus limitans* and surrounding the *solitary tract*.

Nystagmus Rhythmic involuntary eye movements that may be horizontal, vertical, torsional, or some combination of these. The movements may have the same velocity in all directions (pendular nystagmus) or be faster in one direction (jerk nystagmus), in which case it is named for the fast phase. Jerk nystagmus is a normal response at the beginning and end of rotation (rotatory and postrotatory nystagmus), during movement of the visual world across the *retina* (optokinetic nystagmus), or after irrigation of the ear canal with warm or cool water (caloric nystagmus). Nystagmus that is spontaneous or that is triggered or made worse by gaze in some direction is a sign of various kinds of toxicity or pathology.

Obex Apex of the V-shaped caudal fourth ventricle, where the ventricle narrows into the central canal of the caudal *medulla* and *spinal cord*.

Occipital lobe The most posterior lobe of each *cerebral hemisphere*. The occipital lobe includes the primary visual cortex in the banks of the *calcarine sulcus* and adjoining areas of visual association cortex.

Occipitotemporal gyrus (fusiform gyrus) A long gyrus, beginning just lateral to the *uncus* and running posteriorly along the inferior surface of the *temporal lobe* to the *occipital lobe*. Along its course in the *temporal lobe* the occipitotemporal gyrus is bounded laterally by the *inferior temporal gyrus* and medially by the *parahippocampal gyrus*.

Oculomotor nerve The third cranial nerve, emerging into the *interpeduncular cistern* of the *midbrain*. The oculomotor nerve innervates most of the extraocular muscles (see also *oculomotor nucleus*): superior, medial, and inferior recti, inferior oblique, and levator palpebrae superioris. It also conveys preganglionic *parasympathetic* fibers to the ciliary ganglion, where postganglionic fibers arise to innervate the pupillary sphincter and ciliary muscle.

Oculomotor nucleus *Lower motor neurons* for the ipsilateral medial and inferior recti and inferior oblique, the contralateral superior rectus, and the levator palpebrae of both sides. Preganglionic parasympathetic neurons in one of its columns, the *Edinger-Westphal nucleus*, control the ipsilateral pupillary sphincter and ciliary muscle.

Olfactory bulb The knoblike anterior end of the *olfactory tract* on the orbital surface of the *frontal lobe*. The olfactory bulb is the site of central termination of incoming olfactory fibers (CN I) from the *olfactory epithelium* in the nasal cavity. It is large and well laminated in animals depending heavily on the sense of smell, but relatively small and poorly differentiated in the human brain.

Olfactory epithelium A patch of olfactory receptor neurons and supporting cells in the roof and adjoining walls of the nasal cavity. Chemosensitive cilia of the receptor neurons spread out in the mucus layer covering the epithelium and bind odorants.

Olfactory nerve Cranial nerve I, the bundles (olfactory fila) of very thin axons of olfactory receptor neurons that pass vertically through the *cribriform plate* and terminate in the *olfactory bulb*.

Olfactory sulcus A sulcus on the *orbital* surface of the *frontal lobe*, immediately lateral to *gyrus rectus* and harboring the *olfactory bulb* and *tract*.

Olfactory tract Projections from *olfactory bulb* neurons (mitral and tufted cells) to olfactory (*piriform*) cortex and the *amygdala*. The olfactory tract also conveys modulatory efferents traveling from deeper olfactory centers back to the *olfactory bulb*.

Olfactory tubercle A restricted area of the *anterior perforated substance* where some *olfactory tract* fibers terminate. The olfactory tubercle forms a distinct elevation in some animals, but is not very apparent in human brains.

Oligodendrocyte See *glia*.

Olive Protuberance on the lateral aspect of the *medulla*, just dorsolateral to the *pyramid*, caused by the underlying *inferior olivary nucleus*.

Olivocochlear neurons Neurons in the *superior olivary nucleus* that project to the *organ of Corti* and control its sensitivity, either by terminating directly on outer *hair cells* or by terminating on the afferent endings on inner *hair cells*.

Onuf's nucleus   A small cluster of *lower motor neurons* in S2 that innervate the external urethral and anal sphincters.

Opercula (singular, **operculum**)   The parts of the *frontal*, *parietal*, and *temporal lobes* bordering the *lateral sulcus* and overlying the *insula*, hiding it from view.

Opercular part (inferior frontal gyrus)   The most posterior part of the *inferior frontal gyrus*, containing the posterior half of *Broca's area* (see *inferior frontal gyrus*).

Optic chiasm   The site at which *optic nerve* fibers from *ganglion cells* in the nasal half of each *retina* decussate, so that each *optic tract* contains fibers arising in the temporal *retina* of the ipsilateral eye and the nasal *retina* of the opposite eye.

Optic disk   The circular site a few mm medial to the fovea where *optic nerve* fibers turn posteriorly and leave the eye through the lamina cribrosa. There are no photoreceptors in the optic disk, accounting for the blind spot of each eye (see *visual field*).

Optic nerve   The second cranial nerve, containing axons of the various types of retinal *ganglion cells* projecting to the lateral geniculate nucleus of the *thalamus, superior colliculus, pretectal area, suprachiasmatic nucleus* of the *hypothalamus*, and a few other sites.

Optic radiation   A conspicuous, sharply defined, and heavily myelinated bundle of visual fibers originating in the lateral geniculate nucleus, departing the *thalamus* through the retrolenticular and sublenticular parts of the *internal capsule*, curving in a broad fan around the atrium and the posterior and inferior horns of the *lateral ventricle*, and terminating in the primary visual cortex on the upper and lower banks of the *calcarine sulcus*. See also *Meyer's loop*.

Optic tract   Axons of *ganglion cells* from corresponding halves of each *retina* (i.e., temporal half of the ipsilateral *retina* and nasal half of the contralateral *retina*) on their way to the lateral geniculate nucleus, *superior colliculus, pretectal area*, and a few other sites.

Orbital gyri   The variably sulcated (in a pattern often resembling the letter H) group of gyri that comprise the orbital surface of the *frontal lobe*. The orbital gyri are not named individually, in contrast to the *gyrus rectus* immediately medial to them. (The *gyrus rectus* is on the orbital surface, but is usually not included among the orbital gyri.)

Orbital part (inferior frontal gyrus)   The most anterior part of the *inferior frontal gyrus*, so named because it merges with the *orbital gyri*.

Orexin   A wakefulness-promoting *neuropeptide* produced by *hypothalamic* neurons near the *fornix* and distributed to widespread parts of the *CNS*.

Organ of Corti   The receptor organ for hearing. The organ of Corti is a spiral strip of specialized epithelial cells on the surface of the *basilar membrane*, containing a single row of inner hair cells, a row of outer hair cells 3 to 5 cells wide, and an assortment of unique supporting cells. The stereocilia of the outer hair cells are inserted into the overlying tectorial membrane, with the result that vibrations of the *basilar membrane* cause deflections of these stereocilia.

Otoacoustic emission   Faint sounds detectable with a sensitive microphone in the external auditory canal, caused by contractions of outer hair cells. The vibrations of the *basilar membrane* resulting from these contractions propagate backward through the inner ear and middle ear ossicles, vibrating the tympanic membrane.

Otolithic organs   The *utricle* and *saccule*, called this because of the insertion of the stereocilia of their *hair cells* into an overlying otolithic membrane. The otoliths make this membrane more dense than *endolymph*, in turn making the *utricle* and *saccule* sensitive to linear acceleration and gravity.

Outer ear   The auricle and external auditory canal, which together conduct sound vibrations to the tympanic membrane.

Outer hair cell   See *hair cell* and *organ of Corti*.

Pachymeninx   The *dura mater* (pachy is Greek for "thick").

Pacinian corpuscle   A widespread type of mechanoreceptor, consisting of a sensory nerve ending encapsulated by many concentric layers of very thin epithelial cells. Pacinian corpuscles adapt very quickly to maintained touch, but respond well to vibration.

Paleocortex   See *cerebral cortex*.

Papez circuit   The neural loop from *hippocampus* to *mammillary body* to anterior nucleus of the *thalamus* to *cingulate/ parahippocampal* cortex and back to the *hippocampus*. The Papez circuit was originally proposed as the anatomical substrate for emotional experience, but is now known to be more involved in the consolidation of *declarative memories*.

Papilledema   Swelling of the *optic disk*, usually caused by increased intracranial pressure transmitted through the *subarachnoid space* around the *optic nerve*.

Parabrachial nuclei   A collection of nuclei adjacent to the *superior cerebellar peduncle* (brachium conjunctivum) as the latter traverses the rostral *pons*. Various parts of the parabrachial nuclei are involved in transferring visceral sensory information to the *hypothalamus* and *amygdala*.

Paracentral lobule   The extensions of the *precentral* and *postcentral gyri* onto the medial surface of the hemisphere, forming a lobule that surrounds the end of the *central sulcus*.

Parafascicular nucleus   See *thalamus*.

Parahippocampal gyrus   The gyrus immediately adjacent to the *hippocampus*. Its anterior region contains the *entorhinal cortex*, a meeting ground for cortical projections from multiple areas and the source of most afferents to the *hippocampus*.

Parallel fiber   The terminal branches of the T-shaped axon of a cerebellar granule cell. Parallel fibers travel in enormous numbers through the dendritic trees of *Purkinje cells*, conveying *mossy fiber* information to them.

Paramedian pontine reticular formation (PPRF)   A region of the pontine *reticular formation* near the *abducens nucleus*, containing the neurons that generate the timing signals for fast horizontal eye movements (e.g., *saccades*) to the ipsilateral side.

Parasympathetic nervous system   One of the three divisions of the *autonomic nervous system*, also referred to as the craniosacral system because of the location of its preganglionic neurons in the *dorsal motor nucleus of the vagus, nucleus ambiguus*, a few other cranial nerve nuclei, and the sacral *spinal cord* (S2-S4). Preganglionic parasympathetic neurons project to cholinergic postganglionic neurons in ganglia in or near the organs they innervate.

Paraventricular nucleus   A diverse group of neurons in the anterior *hypothalamus*. Some convey oxytocin or vasopressin to the neurohypophysis, others deliver releasing or inhibiting hormones to the *pituitary* portal system, and others project caudally as far as the *spinal cord*.

Parietal lobe A cerebral lobe bounded by the *frontal, temporal,* and *occipital lobes* on the lateral surface of each hemisphere, and by the *frontal, limbic,* and *occipital lobes* on the medial surface. The parietal lobe contains primary somatosensory cortex in the *postcentral gyrus,* areas involved in language comprehension (in the *inferior parietal lobule,* usually on the left), and regions involved in complex aspects of spatial orientation and perception.

Parietooccipital sulcus A deep fissure separating the *parietal* and *occipital lobes* on the medial aspect of the *cerebral hemisphere.* Inferiorly the parietooccipital sulcus joins the *calcarine sulcus,* which continues into the *temporal lobe* as a common stem for both these sulci.

Peduncle A term that literally means "little foot," used to refer a group of fibers that have collected from a fanned-out array into a compact bundle (e.g., the convergence of fibers from the *corona radiata* and *internal capsule* into the *cerebral peduncle*).

Pedunculopontine nucleus A nucleus in the midbrain *reticular formation* adjacent to the decussation of the *superior cerebellar peduncles,* through which *basal ganglia* outputs reach *brainstem* motor programs.

Perforating arteries Small arteries, also referred to as ganglionic arteries, that arise from larger arteries in and near the *circle of Willis* and supply deep cerebral structures such as the *diencephalon* and *basal ganglia.* See also *lenticulostriate arteries* and *thalamogeniculate arteries.*

Periamygdaloid cortex A cortical area covering part of the *amygdala* and merging with it; part of primary olfactory cortex.

Periaqueductal gray An area of gray matter and poorly myelinated fibers surrounding the *aqueduct* in the *midbrain.* The periaqueductal gray is the site of origin of a descending pain-control pathway that relays in nucleus raphe magnus (among other connections).

Pericallosal artery A branch of the *anterior cerebral artery* that travels just above the *corpus callosum.*

Perilymph The high Na^+-low K^+ fluid, continuous with the *CSF* in *subarachnoid space,* that fills the bony *labyrinth* and surrounds the membranous *labyrinth.*

Perineurium A continuation of the *arachnoid,* ensheathing the fascicles of nerve fibers in peripheral nerves. Like the *arachnoid,* the perineurium contains a layer of cells interconnected by bands of tight junctions, forming part of the anatomical basis for the blood-nerve barrier.

Peripheral nervous system (PNS) The total collection of somatic and visceral afferent and efferent fibers that infiltrate virtually the entire body, conveying messages to and from the *CNS.* The formal PNS/CNS boundary is near the attachment points of the spinal and cranial nerve roots, where the myelinating glial cells change from Schwann cells to oligodendrocytes.

Perisylvian language zone Language-related areas bordering the lateral sulcus (Sylvian fissure), usually on the left. Includes Broca's area, Wernicke's area, and the *angular* and *supramarginal gyri.*

Periventricular zone See *hypothalamus.*

PET (positron emission tomography) scan Tomographic images based on the gamma rays emitted from the sites of positron-electron collisions. PET scans following injection of positron-emitting tracers are used to map areas of altered blood flow, glucose uptake, or ligand binding.

Phrenic nucleus A column of lower motor neurons for the diaphragm, located in the anterior horn from about C3 to C5.

Pia mater The innermost and thinnest of the three meninges, attached to the surface of the CNS and connected to the *arachnoid* by arachnoid trabeculae.

PICA See *posterior inferior cerebellar artery.*

Pineal gland A dorsal outgrowth of the *diencephalon,* protruding from the *third ventricle* immediately above and posterior to the paired *habenular* nuclei. The pineal is an endocrine gland important in seasonal cycles of some animals; in humans it secretes melatonin with a circadian rhythm and participates in adjusting the phase of the rhythm.

Piriform cortex A cortical area overlying the *lateral olfactory tract* as it moves toward the *temporal lobe;* part of primary olfactory cortex.

Pituitary gland (hypophysis) The "master gland" through which the *hypothalamus* controls most other endocrine glands. The posterior lobe of the pituitary is an outgrowth of the *diencephalon* and remains connected to the *median eminence* through the infundibular stalk, the posterior lobe and the *infundibulum* together comprising the neurohypophysis; neurons of the hypothalamic *supraoptic* and *paraventricular nuclei* release oxytocin and vasopressin into the bloodstream in the neurohypophysis. The anterior lobe (adenohypophysis), although attached to the posterior lobe and *infundibulum,* is derived embryologically from the roof of the oral cavity. It secretes a variety of hormones that control other endocrine glands, at rates dictated by releasing hormones and inhibiting hormones that reach it from the *hypothalamus* via the hypophyseal portal system.

Planum temporale The superior surface of the *temporal lobe,* posterior to the *transverse temporal gyri.* The planum temporale is usually larger on the left, presumably corresponding to the importance of this and adjoining cortical areas in language functions.

PNS See *peripheral nervous system.*

Pons The second of the three parts of the *brainstem,* continuous rostrally with the *midbrain* and caudally with the *medulla.* The pons is overlain by the *cerebellum* and includes an enlarged basal region (see *basal pons*).

Pontine flexure A flexure in the embryonic *neural tube,* concave side facing dorsally, that results in the walls of the *neural tube* spreading laterally to produce the shape for which the *rhombencephalon* was named.

Pontine micturition center A group of cells in the *reticular formation* of the rostral *pons* that coordinates the various components of normal micturition.

Pontine nuclei A collective term for the many small nuclei in the *basal pons* that receive afferents from *cerebral cortex* (via the *internal capsule* and *cerebral peduncle*) and project to contralateral *cerebellar cortex* (via the *middle cerebellar peduncle*).

Pontocerebellar fibers Projections from *pontine nuclei* to the contralateral *cerebellar cortex,* where they terminate as *mossy fibers* (as do all cerebellar afferents except those from the *inferior olivary nucleus*).

Postcentral gyrus   A vertically oriented convolution of the *parietal lobe* immediately posterior to the *central sulcus*. The postcentral gyrus is the site of primary somatosensory cortex (*Brodmann's areas* 3, 1, and 2).

Posterior cerebral artery   A prominent artery that arises from the bifurcation of the *basilar artery* at the level of the *midbrain*. The posterior cerebral artery forms the posterior part of the *circle of Willis* and supplies the rostral *midbrain*, posterior *thalamus*, medial *occipital lobe*, and inferior and medial surfaces of the *temporal lobe*.

Posterior chamber (of the eye)   The flattened ring of space between the *iris* and the lens, into which aqueous humor is secreted by the ciliary epithelium.

Posterior column   The entire contents of one *posterior funiculus* except for its share of the propriospinal tract (a thin shell of white matter around the gray matter).

Posterior commissure   Crossing fibers interconnecting the two sides of the rostral *midbrain* and *pretectal area*. These crossing fibers are involved in the consensual pupillary light *reflex* and in coordinating vertical eye movements.

Posterior communicating artery   A short vessel connecting the *posterior cerebral artery* to the *internal carotid*, thereby forming one link in the *circle of Willis*. Normally pressures in the *internal carotid* and *posterior cerebral arteries* are balanced so that little or no blood flows around the circle, but if one vessel is occluded the posterior communicating artery may allow anastomotic flow and thus prevent neural damage.

Posterior (dorsal) root   The posterior, sensory root of a *spinal nerve*, which divides into a variable number of regularly spaced rootlets that enter the *spinal cord* along its posterolateral sulcus.

Posterior funiculus   One of the three major divisions of the spinal white matter (see also *anterior* and *lateral funiculus*), principally occupied by ascending collaterals of large myelinated primary afferents carrying impulses from various kinds of mechanoreceptors. This is the first stage of the major pathway to *cerebral cortex* for low-threshold cutaneous, joint, and muscle receptor information.

Posterior horn   One of the three general divisions of the spinal gray matter, the others being the *anterior horn* and the intermediate gray. It contains numerous local-circuit neurons, and cell bodies of projection neurons that will form ascending sensory pathways; capped at all levels by the *substantia gelatinosa*.

Posterior inferior cerebellar artery (PICA)   A long, circumferential branch of the *vertebral artery*, supplying much of the inferior surface of the *cerebellum*; en route it sends shorter branches to the *choroid plexus* of the *fourth ventricle* and to much of the lateral *medulla*.

Posterior perforated substance   The ventral surface of the rostral *midbrain*, between the *cerebral peduncles*. So named because numerous small *perforating* branches of the *posterior cerebral artery* penetrate the brain here, on their way to deep structures such as the *thalamus*.

Posterior spinal artery   A small branch of each *vertebral artery* that travels near the line of attachment of *dorsal roots*, supplying the posterior third of the *spinal cord*. Like the *anterior spinal artery*, it receives additional blood from the thoracic/abdominal aorta through numerous anastomoses with radicular arteries below the upper cervical region.

Posterolateral tract (of Lissauer)   A pale-staining area of white matter between the *substantia gelatinosa* (capping the posterior gray horn of the spinal cord) and the pial surface of the cord. Lissauer's tract stains more lightly than the rest of the spinal white matter because it contains finely myelinated and unmyelinated pain and temperature fibers (derived from the lateral division of each *posterior root* filament) which then distribute into the underlying gelatinosa over several segments.

PPRF   See *paramedian pontine reticular formation*.

Precentral gyrus   A vertically oriented convolution of the *frontal lobe* immediately anterior to the *central sulcus*. The precentral gyrus is the site of primary *motor cortex* (*Brodmann's area* 4).

Precuneus   The part of the *parietal lobe* on the medial surface of the hemisphere, excluding the medial extension of the *postcentral gyrus*.

Prefrontal cortex   The part of the *frontal lobe* anterior to the *premotor* and *supplementary motor areas*. One of the two great areas of multimodal association cortex in human brains, important for working memory, planning, and choosing appropriate responses to social and life situations.

Premotor cortex   A tapering strip of cortex (part of *Brodmann's area* 6) on the lateral surface of the *frontal lobe*, immediately anterior to primary *motor cortex*; important for the planning of voluntary movements.

Preoccipital notch   The midpoint of a shallow, curved indentation along the inferior margin of the lateral aspect of each *cerebral hemisphere*. The preoccipital notch serves as a landmark for synthesizing boundaries for the *parietal, occipital,* and *temporal lobes* on the lateral and medial surfaces of the hemisphere.

Preoptic area   The area in the walls of the *third ventricle* immediately anterior to the *optic chiasm*; traditionally a telencephalic region but structurally and functionally continuous with the *hypothalamus* of the *diencephalon*.

Presynaptic inhibition   Inhibition of transmitter release from a synaptic terminal produced by an axoaxonic synapse on that terminal.

Pretectal area   The region between the *superior colliculus* and caudal *thalamus*. The pretectal area receives afferents from the *retina* and visual association cortex. It projects efferents bilaterally to the *Edinger-Westphal nuclei*, crossing both in the *posterior commissure* and in the ventral *periaqueductal gray*. It is a critical link in the pupillary light *reflex*.

Primary afferent   A neuron with an axon that conveys information from the periphery into the *CNS*. Dorsal root ganglion cells, cranial nerve ganglion cells, and olfactory receptor neurons are prominent examples of primary afferent neurons.

Primary fissure (of the cerebellum)   A deep cleft, particularly noticeable on the medial surface of a hemisected *cerebellum*, that separates most of the *cerebellum* into anterior and posterior lobes.

Proprioception   Perception of the position of parts of the body.

Prosencephalon   The most rostral of the three primary embryonic brain vesicles, giving rise to the *cerebrum*. The prosencephalon (forebrain) subsequently subdivides into the *telencephalon* and *diencephalon*.

Prosody The patterns of emphasis, timing, and pitch that add most of the emotional content and some of the meaning to speech.

Ptosis Drooping of the eyelid, because of either *oculomotor* damage or *sympathetic* damage (e.g., as part of *Horner's syndrome*).

Pulvinar See *thalamus*.

Purkinje cell The distinctive output neurons of *cerebellar cortex*, each with an elaborate, flattened dendritic tree. Purkinje cells receive inputs from *parallel fibers* and *climbing fibers* and project to *deep cerebellar nuclei*.

Putamen The part of the *striatum* involved most prominently in the motor functions of the *basal ganglia*. The putamen receives afferents from *cerebral cortex* (primarily motor and somatosensory areas), and from the *substantia nigra* (compact part) and the centromedian nucleus of the *thalamus*. It projects efferents to the *globus pallidus*, which in turn projects via the *thalamus* (VA/VL) to *premotor* and *supplementary motor areas*. The putamen forms the outer component of the *lenticular nucleus* (the *globus pallidus* is the inner part).

Pyramid *Corticospinal* fibers from the ipsilateral *precentral gyrus* and adjacent areas of *cerebral cortex*, forming a prominent fiber bundle (roughly triangular in cross section, which gave rise to the name) on the ventral surface of the *medulla*.

Pyramidal decussation The site, located at the spinomedullary junction, at which most fibers in each *pyramid* cross the midline to form the contralateral *lateral corticospinal tract*.

Raphe nuclei A series of nuclei extending through the *brainstem* near the midline of the *tegmentum*, collectively providing most of the *serotoninergic* innervation of the *CNS*.

Receptive field The area (e.g., an area of skin or an area of *retina*) in which application of an *adequate stimulus* causes a neuron in a spatially mapped sensory system to change its firing rate.

Receptor potential The electrical response of a sensory receptor to application of its *adequate stimulus*. Depending on the receptor type, receptor potentials may be depolarizing or hyperpolarizing, and may be produced directly by stimulus-gated *ion channels* or indirectly by *G protein*–coupled mechanisms. In vertebrate nervous systems, all receptors with long axons produce only depolarizing receptor potentials, which spread to a trigger zone and generate trains of *action potentials*; hence these receptor potentials are also called generator potentials.

Recurrent artery (of Heubner) See *medial striate artery*.

Red nucleus A two-part nucleus in the rostral *midbrain* involved in *cerebellar* circuitry. In humans the large parvocellular part receives inputs from the contralateral *dentate nucleus* and provides a massive output of uncrossed fibers to the *inferior olivary nucleus*; the small magnocellular part receives inputs from the contralateral *interposed nucleus* and gives rise to a small, crossed *rubrospinal tract*.

Referred pain Pain seeming to originate from some predictable part of the body surface as a result of a damaged internal organ. A common example is angina pectoris, pain in the left side of the chest and the left arm accompanying coronary artery disease.

Reflex An involuntary, stereotyped response to a sensory input. All reflex circuits (other than *axon reflexes*) involve at least a *primary afferent* and a *lower motor neuron* (or a preganglionic and postganglionic *autonomic* neuron). With the exception of the stretch reflex, all reflex arcs also include one or more interneurons.

Corneal (blink) reflex. Blinking of both eyes in response to something touching either cornea; afferent limb CN V, efferent limb CN VII.

Flexor (withdrawal) reflex. Withdrawal of a body part from a noxious stimulus. Typically involves flexion of a limb, but depending on the site of the stimulus extensors may be called into play.

Gag reflex. Gagging caused by something touching the posterior wall of the pharynx; afferent limb CN IX, efferent limb CN X.

Jaw jerk reflex. The stretch reflex of the masseter; afferents in the mesencephalic nucleus of V, efferents in the motor nucleus of V.

Near (accommodation) reflex. Simultaneous bilateral contraction of the medial rectus, ciliary muscle, and pupillary sphincter in response to shifting visual attention to a near object; afferent limb CN II, efferent limb CN III. This is a transcortical reflex, with circuitry involving the lateral geniculate nucleus and visual cortical areas.

Pupillary light reflex. Constriction of the ipsilateral pupil (direct response) and contralateral pupil (consensual response) when light is shone on either retina; afferent limb CN II, efferent limb CN III.

Stapedius (acoustic) reflex. Bilateral contraction of the *stapedius* in response to loud sound in either ear; afferent limb CN VIII, efferent limb CN VII.

Stretch reflex. Contraction of a skeletal muscle in response to stretch. This is the only monosynaptic reflex, involving *muscle spindles* and *lower motor neurons*. Also called a deep tendon reflex (even though the responsible receptors are not in tendons) because of the way it is tested clinically.

Vestibuloocular reflex. Movement of the eyes to compensate for movement of the head, with the result that images stay stable on the *retina*; afferent limb CN VIII, efferent limb CNs III, IV, and VI.

Refractory period The few milliseconds following an *action potential*, during which it is first impossible to elicit another *action potential* (absolute refractory period), then possible only with greater than usual depolarization (relative refractory period). The refractory periods are caused by lack of available voltage-gated Na^+ channels, which were inactivated during the preceding *action potential* and have not yet returned to their "resting" state. Refractory periods ensure that *action potentials* propagate unidirectionally and also limit the maximum firing frequency.

Restiform body See *inferior cerebellar peduncle*.

Reticular activating system See *ascending reticular activating system*.

Reticular formation The central region of the *brainstem*, occupying most of the *tegmentum* of the *midbrain*, *pons*, and *medulla* with a complex netlike fabric of nerve cell bodies and interwoven processes; its myriad multimodal afferents, profusely collateralizing efferents running upward and downward to every level of the *CNS*, and involvement in virtually every activity from visceral functions to consciousness make it a core integrating structure of the brain.

Reticular nucleus   See *thalamus*.

Retina   The innermost tissue layer of the eye, itself double-layered, consisting of the retinal pigment epithelium (adjacent to the choroid) and the neural retina (adjacent to the vitreous). Vertebrate neural retinas are inverted relative to the path of light, with the photosensitive outer segments of *rods* and *cones* interdigitated with processes of pigment epithelial cells, *ganglion cells* that give rise to the *optic nerve* adjacent to the vitreous, and retinal interneurons (horizontal, bipolar, and amacrine cells) in between. The same tissue layer continues anteriorly as the ciliary epithelium and the posterior layers of the *iris*, which contain the pupillary sphincter and dilator.

Rexed's laminae   Terminology for a series of ten layers of neurons described in the spinal cord gray matter. Lamina II, for example, corresponds to the *substantia gelatinosa*, lamina IX to clusters of *lower motor neurons*, and lamina X to the gray matter surrounding the *central canal*.

Rhinal sulcus   A sulcus demarcating the lateral boundary of the *uncus* on the medial aspect of the *temporal lobe*; sometimes continuous with the *collateral sulcus* behind it.

Rhombencephalon   The most caudal of the three primary embryonic brain vesicles. Named for the rhomboid shape of the *fourth ventricle* that develops within it, the rhombencephalon (hindbrain) subsequently subdivides into the *metencephalon* and *myelencephalon*.

Rhombic lips   Thickenings of lateral portions of the alar plate in the rostral part of the embryonic *rhombencephalon* (hindbrain) that will go on to form the *cerebellum*.

Rigidity   Generalized increase in muscle tone, making the limbs inflexible. Rigidity is seen most commonly as a symptom of Parkinson's disease.

RiMLF   See *rostral interstitial nucleus of the MLF*.

Rod   One of the two categories of retinal photoreceptors (*cones* are the other kind). Rods are more sensitive than cones and are able to generate detectable electrical responses to the absorption of single photons. However, they are connected in pathways with a great deal of convergence, are totally absent in the *fovea*, and all contain the same visual pigment (rhodopsin). The net result is that rod vision has low spatial acuity, is effective only in dim light, and cannot be used to discriminate colors.

Romberg's sign   Loss of balance when standing with feet together and eyes closed, indicating defective proprioceptive or vestibular function.

Rostral interstitial nucleus of the MLF (riMLF)   A region of the mesencephalic *reticular formation* near the *oculomotor nucleus*, containing the neurons that generate the timing signals for fast vertical eye movements (e.g., *saccades*).

Rubrospinal tract   Fibers that leave the magnocellular part of the *red nucleus*, cross the midline almost immediately, and project to spinal cord *motor neurons*; important in many mammals, this is apparently a small tract in humans.

Ruffini ending   A widespread, slowly adapting, subcutaneous mechanoreceptor, consisting of sensory endings interwoven with collagen fibers in a thin capsule.

Saccade   Rapid, steplike eye movement used to acquire an image on the *fovea*. Saccades are used for voluntary eye movements in all directions, for reading and other forms of visual scanning, and to look over at something we catch a glimpse of in the periphery; the same neural machinery that generates saccades is used to generate the fast phase of *nystagmus*.

Saccule   One of the dilations of the membranous *labyrinth* within the vestibule, connected to the *cochlea* and the *utricle*. The saccule, like the utricle, is an *otolithic organ* with the stereocilia of its *hair cells* inserted into an otolithic membrane, making it sensitive to linear acceleration and gravity.

Saltatory conduction   Propagation of *action potentials* along a myelinated *axon*, by spreading very rapidly along myelinated segments and then being regenerated at each *node of Ranvier*. See also *myelin* and *nodes of Ranvier*.

Schwann cell   See *glia*.

Sclera   The thick outermost tissue layer of the eye (forming the "white of the eye"), continuous anteriorly with the cornea and posteriorly with the *dural* sheath of the *optic nerve*.

Second messenger   A substance whose concentration changes as a result of binding of a ligand or stimulation of a receptor, and which in turn causes physiological changes in a cell. An example is cyclic GMP, whose concentration in retinal photoreceptors decreases when photons are absorbed, leading to closing of cyclic GMP-gated cation channels.

Secondary neurulation   Extension of the cavity of the *neural tube* into the cell mass at the caudal end of the tube, resulting in formation of the sacral *spinal cord*.

Semantic memory   Conscious memory of facts, such as bits of geography or the meaning of words.

Semicircular ducts   The parts of the membranous *labyrinth* contained within the semicircular canals. Each contains a crista, a transverse ridge covered by *hair cells* and supporting cells. The stereocilia of the hair cells are inserted into a gelatinous diaphragm (the cupula), allowing the duct to detect angular acceleration.

Sensorineural hearing loss   Hearing loss caused by damage to cochlear *hair cells* or the cochlear part of the *vestibulocochlear nerve*, with the result that hearing is equally compromised whether sound is delivered by the normal outer ear-middle ear route or by bone conduction.

Septal nuclei   A component of the medial wall of the *cerebral hemisphere* just beneath the base of the largely glial *septum pellucidum*. The septal nuclei are continuous inferiorly with the *preoptic area* and *hypothalamus*, and are reciprocally connected with the *hippocampus, amygdala, hypothalamus*, and other limbic structures via the *fornix, stria terminalis*, and other tracts. They are also the source of cholinergic input to the *hippocampus*.

Septal vein   A deep cerebral vein that runs posteriorly across the septum pellucidum to join the thalamostriate (terminal) vein and thus form the internal cerebral vein.

Septum pellucidum   A thin, chiefly glial, almost transparent, paired membrane separating the two *lateral ventricles*. (In most brains the two septa pellucida are so closely apposed as to appear as a single structure, and for simplicity they are so labeled in most of the illustrations in this book.)

Serotonin   A *monoamine neurotransmitter* derived from tryptophan, used by neurons of the *raphe nuclei* in the midline of the *brainstem*. Neurons of the raphe nuclei have widely branching axons that innervate most of the *CNS*.

Sigmoid sinus   The continuation of each *transverse sinus* after it leaves the attached edge of the *tentorium cerebelli*. Named for the sinuous course it takes on the way to the internal jugular vein.

Size principle The systematic recruitment of *motor units* in order of increasing size as the force of a muscle contraction increases.

Sleep A reversible state of reduced consciousness and muscle relaxation that we all engage in cyclically for mostly unknown reasons. Periods of sleep include both slow-wave sleep, characterized by synchronized slow waves in EEG recordings, and REM sleep, characterized by rapid eye movements, a desynchronized EEG, and vivid, detailed dreams.

Smooth pursuit Relatively slow eye movements used to keep the image of a moving object on the *fovea*.

Solitary nucleus See *nucleus of the solitary tract*.

Solitary tract *Primary afferents* conveying visceral information from cranial nerves VII, IX, and X to the adjacent *nucleus of the solitary tract* that surrounds it.

Somatotopic Arranged systematically according to parts of the body surface, as in the somatotopic maps in the *precentral* and *postcentral gyri*.

Spasticity A condition of increased muscle tone and increased reflex contraction in response to rapid stretch, usually more pronounced in the flexors of the upper extremity and the extensors of the lower extremity. Spasticity is usually seen accompanied by weakness and *Babinski's sign*, as part of the *upper motor neuron* syndrome.

Spatial summation The adding up of postsynaptic potentials generated at spatially separate sites on a neuron. The degree of spatial summation is directly proportional to the length constant of a neuronal process, the distance over which all but 1/e of a synaptic current leaks out of the process.

Spinal accessory nucleus *Lower motor neurons* for the sternocleidomastoid and trapezius, located in the *anterior horn* from the very caudal *medulla* to about C5.

Spinal cord The most caudal subdivision of the *CNS*, extending from the *pyramidal decussation* to the *conus medullaris* at about vertebral level L1-L2. The human spinal cord has 31 segments and 2 enlargements (cervical, C5-T1, and lumbar, L2-S3).

Spinal nerve The mixed nerve formed by the *dorsal* and *ventral roots* associated with a given *spinal cord* segment. The *dorsal root* contains somatic and visceral sensory fibers with cell bodies in the ganglion of that dorsal root. The *ventral root* contains the axons of *alpha* and *gamma motor neurons* and, from some segments, the axons of preganglionic *autonomic* neurons.

Spinocerebellar tracts

Anterior spinocerebellar tract. Crossed fibers from lumbosacral spinal gray matter, carrying mechanoreceptive and other information related to leg movement. The anterior spinocerebellar tract stays in a lateral position along the *spinal cord* and *brainstem* until the rostral *pons*, and there moves over the *superior cerebellar peduncle* and enters the *cerebellum*, where it largely recrosses.

Posterior spinocerebellar tract. Uncrossed fibers from *Clarke's nucleus*, carrying proprioceptive information from the leg to the ipsilateral half of the cerebellar *vermis* and medial hemisphere via the *inferior cerebellar peduncle*.

Spinocervical tract A small tract of uncertain significance in humans, originating from projection neurons in the ipsilateral *posterior horn* and conveying somatosensory information to the lateral cervical nucleus of C1-C2. The lateral cervical nucleus in turn projects to the contralateral *thalamus* through the *medial lemniscus*.

Spinothalamic tract Crossed fibers from neurons in the *posterior horn* of the *spinal cord* conveying pain and temperature information to the *thalamus* (VPL and other nuclei).

Splenium See *corpus callosum*.

Stapedius A tiny muscle that attaches to the head of the stapes and suppresses vibrations of the middle ear ossicles. The stapedius is innervated by the *facial nerve* and is the effector in the acoustic *reflex*.

Strabismus Misalignment of the eyes, resulting in diplopia.

Straight sinus The final recipient of blood flowing through *deep cerebral veins*. The straight sinus travels in the line of attachment of the *falx cerebri* and *tentorium cerebelli* and empties into the *confluence of the sinuses*.

Stria medullaris (of the thalamus) A horizontal ridge on the medial surface of the *thalamus*, produced by an underlying fiber bundle. The site of attachment of the roof of the *third ventricle* and a route through which *septal* efferents reach the *habenula*.

Stria terminalis A slender, poorly myelinated tract following a long C-shaped course within the thalamostriate groove that separates the *caudate nucleus* from the *thalamus*. The stria terminalis plays a role for the *amygdala* analogous to that played by the *fornix* for the *hippocampus*—it conveys efferents from the *amygdala* to the *septal area* and *hypothalamus*.

Striate cortex Primary visual cortex (*Brodmann's area* 17), located in the banks of the *calcarine sulcus*. Named for the sheet of myelinated fibers (the stripe of Gennari) visible with the naked eye in layer IV.

Striatum An inclusive term for the *caudate nucleus*, *putamen*, and *ventral striatum*. The striatum is the major point of entry into *basal ganglia* circuitry, receiving inputs from most or all cortical areas and projecting inhibitory outputs to the *globus pallidus* and *substantia nigra* (reticular part).

Stripe of Gennari See *striate cortex*.

Strumus (commonly misspelled **strumous**) A primitive *telencephalic* extension that, unlike structures such as the neocortex that have expanded greatly in primates, has remained constant in size and position. It is located rostral to the *lamina terminalis*, medial to *gyrus rectus*, and ventromedial to the *substantia innominata*. Only the anterior and ventral nuclear groups are developed in humans, and these are subdivided cytoarchitectonically into four discrete nuclei: the anteroventral, anterior ventral, and the subdivided anterior and ventral ventral anterior nuclei. The interconnections of the strumus are extensive and complex, but their importance cannot be underestimated. There are four major afferent pathways: a substantial input from a variably present limbic nucleus, the effluvium, traveling through the superior and inferior effluviostrumular tracts; and minor inputs from the trivium and nimbus in the *temporal lobe*. Since the strumus has no known efferent pathways, however, its functional importance has been difficult to justify anatomically. (The frequently mentioned strumulotrivionimboeffluviostrumular loop apparently does not exist.)

The clinical importance of the strumus is based on the disorder subacute combined strumuloma. This is an idiopathic disease of exquisitely rare occurrence and indeterminate symptomatology that forms the basis for the identification of the strumus as the center controlling involuntary higher cortical functions.

Subarachnoid space   The normally present, *CSF*-filled space between the *arachnoid* and the *pia mater*. Subarachnoid space is enlarged in *cisterns*, and is the space through which cerebral and spinal arteries and veins travel over the surface of the *CNS*.

Subcallosal fasciculus   A compact group of lightly staining myelinated fibers in the white matter of each *cerebral hemisphere* (visible mainly in the *frontal lobe*). The subcallosal fasciculus forms a pale arched band subjacent to the *corpus callosum*. It conveys inputs from cortex (chiefly association areas) to the *caudate nucleus*.

Subdural space   Nominally, the potential space between the *dura mater* and the *arachnoid* (although when it occurs it is actually a splitting of the innermost layers of the dura). This potential space can become a real space in certain pathological conditions, most commonly as a result of tearing a cerebral vein at the point where it enters a dural *venous sinus*.

Subgranular zone   The zone near the base of the dentate gyrus, facing the *hippocampus* proper, where new dentate granule cells are produced throughout life.

Subiculum   See *hippocampus*.

Substantia gelatinosa   A distinctive region of gray matter, surmounted by *Lissauer's tract*, that caps the *posterior horn* of the *spinal cord* at all levels. The substantia gelatinosa looks pale in myelin-stained material because its inputs are poorly myelinated or unmyelinated. It deals mostly with pain and temperature sensation, and is an important site for modulating the entry of this information into ascending pathways.

Substantia innominata   A variably used term for parts of the *basal forebrain*, including at least the *basal nucleus* and the *ventral pallidum*.

Substantia nigra   A large nucleus in the *midbrain*, interposed between the *red nucleus* and *cerebral peduncle*. The substantia nigra has two parts: a compact part, containing closely packed, pigmented (with neuromelanin) *dopaminergic* neurons that project to the *striatum*, and a reticular part, containing more loosely arranged neurons, receiving inputs from the *striatum* and projecting to the *thalamus*.

Subthalamic fasciculus   Small bundles of fibers that cross the *internal capsule* like the teeth of a comb. Fibers of the subthalamic fasciculus interconnect the *globus pallidus* and *subthalamic nucleus*, which face each other on either side of the *internal capsule*.

Subthalamic nucleus   A lens-shaped, biconvex mass of gray matter just medial and superior to the junction of the *internal capsule* and *cerebral peduncle*. The subthalamic nucleus is the basis of an indirect route through the *basal ganglia*: striatum → globus pallidus (external segment) → subthalamic nucleus → globus pallidus (internal segment) → thalamus. The *globus pallidus*–subthalamic nucleus connections travel in the *subthalamic fasciculus*.

Subventricular zone   A narrow layer of stem cells underneath the *ependymal* lining of the *lateral ventricles*. Those adjacent to the head of the *caudate nucleus* continually produce newborn neurons that migrate to the *olfactory bulb*.

Sulcus limitans   A longitudinal groove in the embryonic *spinal cord* and *brainstem* that separates the alar plate of gray matter (sensory nuclei) from the basal plate (motor nuclei).

In adult brains it persists as a groove in the floor of the *fourth ventricle* that separates motor nuclei of cranial nerves (now medial to it) from sensory nuclei of cranial nerves.

Superficial veins   The collection of veins on the surface of the *cerebral hemispheres* that avoid the *straight sinus* system (see *deep veins*). Most of them drain into the *superior sagittal sinus*, although some reach the cavernous sinus, the *transverse sinus*, or other sinuses near the outside of the brain.

Superior brachium   See *brachium of the superior colliculus*.

Superior cerebellar artery   A branch of the *basilar artery* that arises just caudal to its bifurcation. Long circumferential branches supply the superior surface of the *cerebellum*, and shorter branches supply much of the rostral *pons* and caudal *midbrain*.

Superior cerebellar peduncle   The major efferent route from the *cerebellum*, containing projections from deep cerebellar nuclei on their way to the contralateral *red nucleus* and *thalamus* (VL/VA). Sometimes referred to as the brachium conjunctivum (a "joined-together arm," named for its course through a decussation with its contralateral counterpart). A descending limb leaves the superior cerebellar peduncle near its decussation and projects to the contralateral *inferior olivary nucleus*.

Superior cistern   The enlarged, *CSF*-filled subarachnoid *cistern* above the *midbrain*, also termed the quadrigeminal cistern and the cistern of the great cerebral vein. The superior cistern is an important radiological landmark, continuous anteriorly and posteriorly with the *transverse fissure* and laterally with thin, curved spaces that partially encircle the midbrain before joining its underlying *interpeduncular cistern*. (The combination of superior cistern and these sheetlike extensions is known as the ambient cistern.)

Superior colliculus   A large, rounded mass of gray matter in the roof of the rostral *midbrain*. The superior colliculus receives afferents from the *retina* and visual cortex, sends efferents to the pulvinar and other structures, and plays a role in directing visual attention and controlling eye movements.

Superior frontal gyrus   The most superior of three longitudinally oriented frontal gyri, continuing onto the medial surface of the hemisphere. The superior frontal gyrus includes *supplementary motor cortex* and part of *premotor cortex*.

Superior longitudinal fasciculus   See *arcuate fasciculus*.

Superior olivary nucleus   A complex of nuclei near the rostral end of the *facial motor nucleus* in the caudal *pons*. The superior olivary nucleus is the first site of convergence of fibers representing the two ears and is the source of many fibers of the *lateral lemniscus*. It is also the origin of both crossed and uncrossed *olivocochlear* bundles, which run centrifugally in the vestibulocochlear nerve and terminate in the *organ of Corti*, modulating cochlear *hair cell* activity.

Superior parietal lobule   The upper part of the lateral surface of the *parietal lobe*, above the *intraparietal sulcus*. The superior parietal lobule contains somatosensory association cortex.

Superior sagittal sinus   A prominent *venous sinus* in the attached edge of the *falx cerebri*. Venous blood traveling posteriorly in this sinus meets up with blood from the *straight sinus* at the *confluence of the sinuses*.

Superior salivary nucleus Preganglionic *parasympathetic* neurons in the caudal *pons* whose axons travel through the *facial nerve* to innervate ganglia for the submandibular and sublingual salivary glands and lacrimal gland.

Superior temporal gyrus The uppermost gyrus of the *temporal lobe*, bordering on the *lateral sulcus*. The superior temporal gyrus includes primary auditory cortex (actually located in the wall of the *lateral sulcus*, in *transverse temporal gyri* crossing the top of the *temporal lobe*), auditory association cortex, and (usually on the left) *Wernicke's area*. This is one example of a region of visibly different size and configuration in the two cerebral hemispheres, typically being more extensive in the left hemisphere.

Supplementary motor area The part of *Brodmann's area* 6 on the medial surface of the hemisphere, in the *superior frontal gyrus* anterior to primary *motor cortex*; important for the planning of complex, self-paced movements.

Suprachiasmatic nucleus A tiny nucleus in the anterior *hypothalamus* that serves as the "master clock" for circadian rhythms. Inputs from retinal *ganglion cells* help keep its oscillations in phase with day-night cycles.

Supramarginal gyrus The part of the *inferior parietal lobule* surrounding the upturned end of the *lateral sulcus*. Although variable in size and shape, the supramarginal gyrus is important in language function.

Supraoptic nucleus A group of *hypothalamic* neurons above the *optic tract* that convey oxytocin or vasopressin to the posterior *pituitary*.

Sylvian fissure See *lateral sulcus*.

Sympathetic nervous system One of the three divisions of the *autonomic nervous system*, also referred to as the thoracolumbar system because of the location of its preganglionic neurons in the *lateral horn* of the T1-L3 spinal cord. Preganglionic sympathetic neurons project to (usually) noradrenergic postganglionic neurons in sympathetic chain ganglia and prevertebral ganglia.

Synapse A point of contact at which one neuron influences another; may be electrical (see *gap junction*), but most are chemical. Typical chemical synapses include a presynaptic element with transmitter-filled synaptic vesicles, a synaptic cleft across which released transmitter diffuses, and a postsynaptic element studded with receptor molecules that bind the transmitter. Depending on the nature of the receptor, a depolarizing EPSP (excitatory postsynaptic potential) or a hyperpolarizing IPSP (inhibitory postsynaptic potential) may result.

Taste bud An ovoid collection of taste receptor cells, supporting cells, and basal cells (which develop into new taste cells). Taste buds are located mainly in small fungiform papillae on the anterior two thirds of the tongue, in foliate papillae on the sides of the posterior tongue, and in the walls of vallate (circumvallate) papillae two thirds of the way back on the dorsal surface of the tongue (although there are also some in the palate and pharynx). Each taste bud has an apical taste pore through which the receptor cells are exposed to substances dissolved in saliva.

Tectorial membrane See *organ of Corti*.

Tectospinal tract A small tract projecting from the *superior colliculus* to the cervical *spinal cord*, probably involved in rotating the head toward objects of interest.

Tectum The *superior* and *inferior colliculi*, the "roof" of the midbrain.

Tegmentum A general anatomical term for the area anterior to the ventricular spaces of the *medulla, pons*, and *midbrain*. "Tegmentum" is a useful umbrella term (Latin for "covering") for all structures covering the basal components of the *brainstem* (*pyramids, basal pons, cerebral peduncles*) and includes the *reticular formation*, nuclei of cranial nerves, most ascending and descending tracts (except the *corticospinal tract*), the *red nuclei*, and *substantia nigra*.

Telencephalon The most rostral of the five secondary embryonic brain vesicles. The paired telencephalic vesicles give rise to the *cerebral hemispheres*.

Temporal lobe The most inferior lobe of each *cerebral hemisphere*, inferior to the *lateral sulcus* and anterior to the *occipital lobe*. The temporal lobe includes auditory sensory and association cortex, part of posterior language cortex, visual and higher-order association cortex, primary and association olfactory cortex, the *amygdala*, and the *hippocampus*. (The *parahippocampal gyrus*, a major part of the *limbic lobe*, is also commonly referred to as part of the medial temporal lobe.)

Temporal summation The adding up of postsynaptic potentials generated in the same neuron at slightly different times. The degree of temporal summation is directly proportional to the time constant of a neuronal process, the time it takes the membrane potential response to a constant current to come within $1/e$ of its final value.

Tentorium cerebelli The *dural septum* between the *cerebellum* and the inferior surfaces of the *occipital* and *temporal* lobes. The *midbrain* passes through a midline notch in the tentorium; this notch provides an aperture through which parts of the medial *temporal lobe* can *herniate* in response to expanding masses.

Terminal vein A *deep cerebral vein* traveling with the *stria terminalis* in the groove between the *thalamus* and the adjacent *caudate nucleus*. It drains much of these two structures. See also *thalamostriate vein*.

Thalamic fasciculus Projections from the cerebellum (via the superior cerebellar peduncle) and basal ganglia (via the ansa lenticularis and lenticular fasciculus), gathered together beneath the thalamus (VA/VL).

Thalamogeniculate arteries *Perforating* branches of the *posterior cerebral artery* lateral to the *circle of Willis* that supply posterior parts of the *thalamus*.

Thalamostriate vein A frequently used alternate name for the *terminal vein*, more useful because it says not only where the vessel is, but also what it does.

Thalamus A collection of nuclei that collectively are the source of most extrinsic afferents to the cerebral cortex. Some thalamic nuclei (relay nuclei) receive distinct input bundles and project to discrete functional areas of the cerebral cortex. Others (association nuclei) are primarily interconnected with association cortex. Still others have diffuse cortical projections, and one has no projections to the cortex at all.

    Anterior nucleus. The thalamic relay for the limbic system. Afferents from the *mammillary body* and other limbic structures, efferents to the *cingulate gyrus*.

    Centromedian nucleus (CM). The largest intralaminar nucleus; afferents from the *globus pallidus*, efferents to the *striatum* (with branches projecting diffusely to widespread cortical areas).

Dorsomedial nucleus (DM). Interconnections with *prefrontal* association cortex and the limbic system.

Intralaminar nuclei. A set of thalamic nuclei, including the centromedian and parafascicular nuclei, so named because they are embedded in the *internal medullary lamina*.

Lateral dorsal nucleus. Efferents to the posterior part of the *cingulate gyrus*; in many ways an extension of the anterior nucleus.

Lateral geniculate nucleus (LGN). The thalamic relay for vision. Afferents from the *retina* via the *optic tract*, efferents to primary visual cortex within, above, and below the *calcarine sulcus*.

Lateral posterior nucleus (LP). Interconnections, similar to those of the pulvinar, with posterior association cortex.

Medial geniculate nucleus (MGN). The thalamic relay for hearing. Afferents from the *inferior colliculus* via the inferior brachium, efferents to auditory cortex in the *transverse temporal gyri*.

Midline nuclei. Nuclei on the medial surface of the thalamus, in the walls of the *third ventricle*, with connections similar to those of the intralaminar nuclei.

Parafascicular nucleus (PF). An intralaminar nucleus with connections similar to those of the centromedian nucleus.

Pulvinar. The largest thalamic nucleus, interconnected with parietal-occipital-temporal association cortex.

Reticular nucleus. An unusual thalamic nucleus with no projections to the cortex. Afferents from the thalamus and *cerebral cortex*, *GABAergic* efferents back to the thalamus.

Ventral anterior nucleus (VA). A thalamic relay for the motor system. Afferents from the *basal ganglia* and *cerebellum*, efferents to motor areas of cortex.

Ventral lateral nucleus (VL). A thalamic relay for the motor system. Afferents from the *cerebellum* and *basal ganglia*, efferents to motor areas of cortex.

Ventral posterolateral nucleus (VPL). The thalamic relay for somatic sensation from the body. Afferents from the *medial lemniscus* and *spinothalamic tract*, efferents to somatosensory cortex in the *postcentral gyrus*.

Ventral posteromedial nucleus (VPM). The thalamic relay for somatic sensation from the head and for taste. Afferents from the *trigeminal* portions of the *medial lemniscus* and *spinothalamic tract* and from the *nucleus of the solitary tract*; efferents to somatosensory cortex in the *postcentral gyrus* and to gustatory cortex in and near the *insula*.

Third ventricle   The single, median, vertically oriented cavity of the *diencephalon*, separating the *thalamus* and *hypothalamus* of the two hemispheres. The third ventricle is confluent anteriorly with both *lateral ventricles* through the *interventricular foramina* and posteriorly with the *fourth ventricle* through the *aqueduct*. It has four small outpocketings:

Infundibular recess. Leads into the hollow *infundibular* stalk.

Optic recess. Small recess just above and anterior to the *optic chiasm*.

Pineal recess. Leads into the stalk of the *pineal gland*.

Suprapineal recess. An outpocketing of the roof of the *third ventricle* just anterior to the *pineal gland*.

Time constant   See *temporal summation*.

Tomography   Literally "making a picture of a slice," *tomography* is a general term for a process that can be implemented in several ways. Tomographic images originally were made using clever photographic tricks, but are now made using computers to map out x-ray density (*CT*), hydrogen nuclei distribution (*MRI*), and changes in blood flow (PET, *fMRI*) in planes.

Tonsil (of the cerebellum)   The lowest lying parts of the cerebellar posterior lobes, adjacent to the foramen magnum.

Transduction   Conversion by a sensory receptor of some form of stimulus energy into a *receptor potential*.

Transverse fissure   An extension of *subarachnoid space*, situated above the roof of the *third ventricle* and containing the *internal cerebral veins*. I use the term in a more extended sense in this book, to refer to the long slit intervening between the *cerebral hemispheres* and structures below them—the cleft normally occupied by the *tentorium cerebelli*, continuing into the *superior cistern*, and from there into the *subarachnoid space* above the roof of the *third ventricle*.

Transverse sinus   The laterally directly sinus on each side in the attached edge of the *tentorium cerebelli*, conveying blood from the *confluence of the sinuses* to the *sigmoid sinus*.

Transverse temporal gyrus (of Heschl)   Gyri (usually two in number) that run transversely across the lower bank of the *lateral sulcus*. The location of primary auditory cortex.

Trapezoid body   Auditory fibers from the *cochlear nuclei* to the *superior olivary nuclei* that cross the midline in a trapezoid-shaped area of the caudal *pontine tegmentum*.

Traveling wave   The wave of mechanical deformation that travels along the *basilar membrane* in response to sound, reaching a maximum at some point determined by the sound frequency.

Triangular part (inferior frontal gyrus)   The middle of the three parts of the *inferior frontal gyrus*, containing the anterior half of *Broca's area* (see *inferior frontal gyrus*).

Trigeminal nerve   The fifth cranial nerve, emerging anterolaterally from the *basal pons*. The trigeminal nerve conveys somatosensory (and some chemosensory) fibers from the ipsilateral half of the head and efferents to ipsilateral muscles of mastication.

Motor root. Small, anterior root containing efferent fibers that distribute through the mandibular division of the nerve.

Sensory root. Massive, posterior root containing afferent fibers that arrive through all three divisions of the nerve.

Trigeminal nuclei

Main sensory. Termination site of large-diameter afferents (the equivalent of a *posterior column* nucleus for the trigeminal system). Most of its efferents project to the contralateral VPM via the *medial lemniscus*; some, however, project to the ipsilateral VPM via the dorsal trigeminal tract.

Mesencephalic. The cell bodies of primary afferents from muscle spindles in muscles of mastication and from other oral mechanoreceptors.

Motor. *Lower motor neurons* for ipsilateral muscles of mastication.

Spinal. The termination site of the spinal *trigeminal tract*. The caudal part of the nucleus (in the caudal *medulla*, merging with the cervical *posterior horn*) looks like the spinal *posterior horn*, has a component similar to the *substantia gelatinosa*, and processes pain and temperature information. Its efferents project to VPM through the *spinothalamic* *tract*. More rostral parts (the interpolar and oral nuclei) transmit trigeminal information to the *cerebellum* and into some trigeminal *reflex* arcs.

Trigeminal tracts

Mesencephalic. Processes of cell bodies in the adjacent mesencephalic *trigeminal nucleus* that send one branch to innervate mechanoreceptors in and around the mouth and others to central termination sites such as the *trigeminal main sensory nucleus*.

Spinal. Central processes of primary afferents from the ipsilateral side of the face, conveying information about pain and temperature (and some tactile information) to the spinal *trigeminal nucleus*.

Trochlear nerve The fourth cranial nerve, emerging as an already-crossed small bundle from the posterior aspect of the *midbrain*, just caudal to the *inferior colliculus*. The trochlear nerve innervates the superior oblique muscle, which helps to intort the eyeball and turn it downward and laterally.

Trochlear nucleus *Lower motor neurons* for the contralateral superior oblique muscle, located in the caudal *midbrain* just caudal to the *oculomotor nucleus*. Trochlear axons exit the paired nuclei, turn caudally in the overlying periaqueductal gray, arch posteriorly to decussate (like the old time ice-tongs used to handle large blocks of ice), and leave the *brainstem* at the *pons-midbrain* junction.

Tuber cinereum A low mound of gray matter on the inferior aspect of the *hypothalamus*, bounded by the *optic chiasm*, *optic tracts*, and anterior edge of the *mammillary bodies*. The tuber cinereum contains the *median eminence* and the beginning of the *infundibular* stalk, and is a region of great importance in hypothalamic hormonal regulation of the anterior *pituitary*.

Tuberomammillary nucleus A relatively small group of neurons in the posterior *hypothalamus*, the source of *histaminergic* fibers that project widely to the *cerebral cortex* and *thalamus*.

Tuberothalamic artery A perforating branch of the posterior communicating artery that supplies the anterior thalamus.

Uncinate fasciculus 1. Fibers of the inferior occipitofrontal fasciculus that curve sharply around the *limen insulae* to interconnect *orbital cortex* and anterior *temporal* structures. 2. *Fastigial* efferents that cross the midline within the *cerebellum* and loop over the *superior cerebellar peduncle* before reaching the *brainstem* through the *juxtarestiform body*.

Uncus A medial protuberance from the anterior end of the *parahippocampal gyrus* caused by the underlying *amygdala*. The proximity of its surface to the adjacent *cerebral peduncle* can cause clinical problems during cerebral edema or as a result of space-occupying masses, because the uncus can *herniate* through the *tentorial* notch and compress the *midbrain*.

Upper motor neuron A neuron whose axon descends from the *cerebral cortex* or *brainstem* to the *spinal cord* (or to a cranial nerve motor nucleus) to affect the activity of *lower motor neurons*; includes *corticospinal*, vestibulospinal, reticulospinal, *tectospinal*, and *rubrospinal* neurons.

Utricle One of the dilations of the membranous labyrinth within the vestibule, connected to the *saccule* and to all three *semicircular ducts*. The utricle, like the saccule, is an *otolithic organ* with the stereocilia of its *hair cells* inserted into an otolithic membrane, making it sensitive to linear acceleration and gravity.

Vagal trigone A small elevation in the floor of the caudal *fourth ventricle* with boundaries forming a triangle just lateral to the *hypoglossal trigone*. Each vagal trigone is a fusiform swelling produced by the underlying *dorsal motor nucleus of the vagus*.

Vagus nerve The tenth cranial nerve, emerging as a series of filaments from a groove dorsal to the *olive*. The vagus has diverse components: efferents to branchial arch muscles arise from *nucleus ambiguus* in the *medulla* and mediate swallowing and phonation; efferents to *parasympathetic* ganglia for thoracic and abdominal viscera arise from the *dorsal motor nucleus of the vagus* and *nucleus ambiguus* in the *medulla*; afferent fibers mediate general visceral sensation, taste from the epiglottis, and cutaneous sensation behind the ear.

Vallate (circumvallate) papillae See *taste bud*.

Venous angle The point at which the newly formed *internal cerebral vein* turns sharply caudally as it leaves the *interventricular foramen*. This is an important radiological landmark indicating the location of the genu of the *internal capsule* and the anterior end of the *thalamus*.

Venous sinus An endothelium-lined channel within the *dura mater*, typically in an attached edge of a *dural septum*. Cerebral veins either merge directly with sinuses (as in the *great vein* entering the *straight sinus*) or, more commonly, penetrate the *arachnoid* and enter a venous sinus through one of its sides.

Ventral amygdalofugal pathway A massive but loosely organized fiber bundle running transversely in the *basal forebrain*. It interconnects the *amygdala* with the *hypothalamus*, *septal area*, *thalamus*, and even the *brainstem*, and is thus an important pathway of the limbic system.

Ventral anterior nucleus See *thalamus*.

Ventral cochlear nucleus See *cochlear nuclei*.

Ventral lateral nucleus See *thalamus*.

Ventral pallidum A limbic extension of the *globus pallidus*, located beneath the *anterior commissure*, with inputs from the *ventral striatum*. The ventral pallidum is part of a *basal ganglia* circuit similar to those involved in motor functions, but that in this case has limbic inputs (*amygdala*, *hippocampus* → *ventral striatum*), and outputs (via the dorsomedial nucleus of the *thalamus*) to *prefrontal* and *orbital cortex*.

Ventral posterolateral nucleus See *thalamus*.

Ventral posteromedial nucleus See *thalamus*.

Ventral striatum The primarily limbic subdivision of the *striatum*, comprising *nucleus accumbens*, adjacent parts of the *caudate nucleus* and *putamen*, and certain nearby parts of the *basal forebrain*.

Ventral tegmental area An unpaired region of the *midbrain* medial to the compact part of the *substantia nigra*, containing *dopaminergic* neurons that project to various limbic and neocortical areas.

Vergence eye movements Nonconjugate eye movements used to get or keep the images of objects at different distances on both foveae, as in the convergence used to look at a near object and the divergence used to switch gaze to a distant object.

Vermis Midline, sinuous zone of the *cerebellum* (vermis is Latin for "worm"), between the two *cerebellar hemispheres*. The vermis includes a representation of the trunk conveyed by the *spinocerebellar tracts*; its outputs, primarily through the *fastigial nucleus*, reach the *vestibular nuclei* and *reticular formation*.

Vertebral artery One of the two major arteries that supply each side of the *CNS* (see also *internal carotid artery*). The vertebral artery originates as the first branch of the subclavian, runs cranially through foramina in cervical vertebrae, enters the base of the skull through the foramen magnum, and ascends along the *medulla*. At the pontomedullary junction it unites with its contralateral counterpart to form the *basilar artery*. The vertebral artery and its *posterior inferior cerebellar* branch (PICA) supply blood to the *medulla* and inferior part of the *cerebellum*, and it supplies the cervical *spinal cord* via the *posterior* and *anterior spinal arteries*.

Vestibular nuclei Four elaborately subdivided secondary sensory nuclei of the vestibular division of the eighth cranial nerve in the floor of the *fourth ventricle*; collectively they project to the nuclei of extraocular muscles (mostly via the *medial longitudinal fasciculus*), the *cerebellum*, the *reticular formation*, the *thalamus*, and the *spinal cord*:
Inferior. Peppered with small bundles of vestibular *primary afferents* that run through it.
Lateral. Origin of the lateral vestibulospinal tract to ipsilateral extensor motor neurons.
Medial. Origin of the medial vestibulospinal tract, projecting bilaterally to cervical motor neurons.
Superior. Ascending and descending connections with nuclei of extraocular muscles (other vestibular nuclei also share in this).

Vestibulocochlear nerve The eighth cranial nerve, emerging anterolaterally from the *brainstem* in the *cerebellopontine angle*. It has vestibular and cochlear divisions innervating *hair cells* in vestibular organs (cristae of the *semicircular ducts* and maculae of the *utricle* and *saccule*) and in the auditory spiral *organ of Corti* in the cochlear duct, respectively.

Visual field The area visible to one eye. By convention and for functional reasons, the *fovea* is at the center of the field, which extends about 90 degrees temporally but is less extensive in other directions. Because the optics of the eye reverse and invert the image on the *retina*, the temporal field is seen by the nasal *retina*, the superior part of the field is seen by the inferior *retina*, and the *blind spot* (corresponding to the *optic disk*) is temporal to the *fovea* in the visual field.

Vomeronasal organ A tubular receptor organ, lined with chemosensitive neurons, in the cartilaginous portion of the nasal septum. Terrestrial vertebrates use the vomeronasal organ to detect pheromones released by other members of their species, but its role in humans appears to be minor at best.

Wallerian degeneration Degeneration and removal of an *axon* and any associated *myelin* distal to a point of transection.

Wernicke's area The posterior part of the *superior temporal gyrus* (*Brodmann's area* 22), usually on the left. Wernicke's area, along with the *angular* and *supramarginal gyri* and parts of the *middle temporal gyrus*, is important for the comprehension of language.

Zona incerta A small sheet of gray matter interposed between the *subthalamic nucleus* and the *thalamus*, enveloped by efferent fibers from the *globus pallidus*. The zona incerta has widespread connections, including direct inputs to *cerebral cortex*, but its function is largely unknown.

Index

Page numbers followed by "f" indicate figures, "t" indicate tables, and "b" indicate boxes.